# Tumors
*of the*
# Soft Tissues

SECOND EDITION

# Tumors
## *of the*
# Soft Tissues

## SECOND EDITION

**Tapas K. Das Gupta, MD, PhD, DSc**
Professor and Head
Department of Surgical Oncology
University of Illinois at Chicago
Chicago, Illinois

**Prabir K. Chaudhuri, MD**
Professor and Chief
Division of Surgical Oncology and
Division of Head and Neck Surgery
Medical College of Ohio
Toledo, Ohio

Appleton & Lange
Stamford, Connecticut

98 99 00 01 02 / 10 9 8 7 6 5 4 3 2 1

Prentice Hall International (UK) Limited, *London*
Prentice Hall of Australia Pty. Limited, *Sydney*
Prentice Hall Canada, Inc., *Toronto*
Prentice Hall Hispanoamericana, S.A., *Mexico*
Prentice Hall of India Private Limited, *New Delhi*
Prentice Hall of Japan, Inc., *Tokyo*
Simon & Schuster Asia Pte. Ltd., *Singapore*
Editora Prentice Hall do Brasil Ltda., *Rio de Janeiro*
Prentice Hall, *Upper Saddle River, New Jersey*

**Library of Congress Cataloging-in-Publication Data**

Das Gupta, Tapas K., 1931–
    Tumors of the soft tissues / Tapas K. Das Gupta, Prabir K.
Chaudhuri.—2nd ed.
        p.    cm.
    Includes bibliographical references and index.
    ISBN 0-8385-9044-6 (case : alk. paper)
    1. Soft tissue tumors.   I. Chaudhuri, Prabir K.   II. Title.
    [DNLM:   1. Soft Tissue Neoplasms.   WD 375 D229t 1998]
    RC280.S66D265    1998
    616.99′2—dc21                                97-40497

Acquisitions Editor: Michael P. Medina
Production Editor: Eileen Pendagast
Designer: Libby Schmitz

ISBN 0-8385-9044-6

PRINTED IN THE UNITED STATES OF AMERICA

# DEDICATION

This book would never have seen the light of day if not for the infinite patience and encouragement of Mrs. Judy Das Gupta. This book is dedicated to her, with our immense thanks.

# CONTENTS

# CONTRIBUTORS

**Robert S. Benjamin, MD**
Internist, Professor of Medicine, and Chairman
Department of Melanoma/Sarcoma Medical Oncology
Medical Director
Multidisciplinary Sarcoma Center
University of Texas, M.D. Anderson Cancer Center
Houston, Texas

**Bina Chaudhuri, MD**
Associate Professor
Department of Pathology
Medical College of Ohio
Toledo, Ohio

**Prabir K. Chaudhuri, MD**
Professor and Chief
Division of Surgical Oncology and
Division of Head and Neck Surgery
Medical College of Ohio
Toledo, Ohio

**Houqi Chen, PhD**
Assistant Professor
Department of Surgical Oncology
University of Illinois at Chicago
Chicago, Illinois

**Robert J. Coombs, MD**
Associate Professor
Department of Radiology
Medical College of Ohio
Toledo, Ohio

**Tapas K. Das Gupta, MD, PhD, DSc**
Professor and Head
Department of Surgical Oncology
University of Illinois at Chicago
Chicago, Illinois

**Tina J. Hieken, MD**
Assistant Professor of Surgery
Rush Medical College
Chicago, Illinois
Attending Surgeon
Rush North Shore Medical Center
Skokie, Illinois

**Norman Jaffe, MD, DSc, Dip. Paed.**
Professor of Pediatrics
Department of Pediatrics
Chief, Long-term Surveillance Clinic
M.D. Anderson Cancer Center
Houston, Texas

**Edward A. Levine, MD**
Associate Professor of Surgery
Chief, Section of Surgical Oncology
Department of Surgery
Louisiana State University School of Medicine
New Orleans, Louisiana

**Mahmood F. Mafee, MD**
Professor of Clinical Radiology
Director, Magnetic Resonance Imaging Facility
Interim Head, Department of Radiology
University of Illinois at Chicago
Chicago, Illinois

**Arno J. Mundt, MD**
Assistant Professor
Department of Radiation and Cellular Oncology
Center for Radiation Therapy
University of Chicago Hospitals
Chicago, Illinois

**Shreyaskumar R. Patel, MD, FACP**
Associate Internist
Associate Professor of Medicine
Department of Melanoma/Sarcoma Medical Oncology
University of Texas, M.D. Anderson Cancer Center
Houston, Texas

**C. Nazenin Shinaver, MD**
Fellow, Neuroradiology
University of Illinois at Chicago
Chicago, Illinois

**Jaroslav J. Stastny, PhD**
Research Assistant Professor
Department of Surgical Oncology
University of Illinois at Chicago
Chicago, Illinois

**Ralph R. Weichselbaum, MD**
Harold Hines, Jr., Professor and Chairman
Department of Radiation and Cellular Oncology
Center for Radiation Therapy
Director, Chicago Tumor Institute
University of Chicago Hospitals
Chicago, Illinois

**Lee S. Woldenberg, MD**
Associate Professor
Department of Radiology
Medical College of Ohio
Toledo, Ohio

# PREFACE

Nothing can be learned unless man proceeds from the known to the unknown. With this thought, we have attempted to synthesize our experience in the diagnosis and treatment of soft tissue tumors with the presently available data on this fascinating group of human neoplasms.

The first section deals with the principles of classification, staging, diagnosis, pathology, and molecular biology. The second section is devoted to the natural history of the benign and malignant tumors arising from each individual tissue type. The third section describes the various models of treatment of soft tissue tumors and the vast strides made in treatment methods. The last section describes the characteristics of childhood sarcomas.

I deeply appreciate all the help and encouragement I have received from my family, colleagues, and friends, and above all, my patients. My gratitude to my co-editor, Dr. Prabir K. Chaudhuri. My thanks to Dr. Bina Chaudhuri for contributing the chapter on Pathology; Drs. Ralph R. Weichselbaum and Arno J. Mundt for the chapter on Radiation Therapy; Drs. Tina J. Hieken and Edward A. Levine for the chapter on Molecular Biology; Dr. Norman Jaffe for the chapter on Childhood Sarcomas; Drs. Mahmood F. Mafee, Lee S. Woldenberg, Robert J. Coombs, and C. Nazenin Shinaver for the chapter on Imaging; Drs. Robert S. Benjamin and Shreyaskumar R. Patel for the chapter on Chemotherapy; and to Drs. Houqi Chen and Jaroslav J. Stastny for the chapter on Immunology and Immunotherapy. My colleagues in the Department of Surgical Oncology, Drs. Henry A. Briele, Arthur W. Boddie, Jr., Michael A. Warso, and Donald K. Wood, made valuable suggestions and corrections. Ms. Anne Skilkaitis is credited for producing the micrographs.

Finally, my limitless thanks to Mr. Kevin Grandfield for editing the entire manuscript.

# INTRODUCTION

Soft somatic tissue (connective tissue) comprises the form and substance of the human body. It accounts for about 40 to 50% of the body weight in adults and 25% in children. Height, weight, and body conformation are largely determined by its distribution. The shapes, such as facial features, are welded in a hereditary pattern by the functional equilibrium of intergrowth of these tissues. The shape, size, and contour of all mature viscera inherently depend on the amount, composition, and geometric configuration of the connective tissue elements.

The mesenchymal constituents of the body mass theoretically have the same risks as the rest of the human body for the development of diseases, tumors, and other morbid conditions. In 1950, Klemperer,[1] in an initial systematized study, offered a nosologic scheme to such apparently diversified pathologic entities of the somatic tissues as rheumatic fever, rheumatoid arthritis, polyarthritis, acute lupus erythematosus, scleroderma, and a host of other diseased conditions. Since then, the subject of diseases of the connective tissue has been well investigated. It appears that, although degenerative diseases, metabolic disorders, and certain muscular afflictions are relatively common, an inverse relationship exists between this large body mass and the development of tumors and tumorlike conditions of the soft somatic tissues. Strangely enough, this curious biologic paradox of a large body mass with a low incidence of tumors did not, for a long time, arouse sufficient interest among clinical scientists to spur a major investigative program.

Of the tumors arising from the primitive mesenchyme, the lymphomas[2] and bone tumors[3,4,5,6] have received most attention. In contrast, soft somatic tissue tumors have been sparsely studied and, until recently, a systematic study of these tumors had not been undertaken.

Stout[7,8] was the first investigator to provide a detailed description of tumors of the soft tissues. Largely on the basis of his original and critical studies, this group of neoplasms was histogenetically classified and their histologic criteria were established. The enormous number of papers by Stout and his colleagues referred to in the body of this text is testimony to his pioneering and enduring work in the field. The fascicle *Tumors of the Soft Tissue* by Stout and Lattes[9] has essentially stood the test of time.

Systemic clinical studies of soft tissue tumors were primarily initiated by Pack and his colleagues.[10] The volume of material published by Pack and his associates is astounding. Even today, most authors reporting on end result studies frequently use the data provided by Pack and his coworkers as the historic reference point. For certain histologic types, Pack's studies are still valid and have been confirmed by more recent publications.

The contributions of Enzinger and his colleagues at the Armed Forces Institute of Pathology have helped to better understand the histology and histogenesis of these tumors. For many of these tumors, they established the histologic criteria for proper diagnosis. The multitude of papers by Enzinger and his co-workers, cited in various chapters of this text, testify to the fundamental nature of his group's contribution to this subject.

In recent years, histopathologists have provided us with elegant morphologic studies, easing histogenetic classification and establishing a sound basis for the management of tumors of the soft tissues.[11] Although a number of excellent clinicopathologic papers, cited elsewhere in this text, have recently been published, in general clinicians have not as yet synthesized and appropriately applied these morphobiologic data to the understanding of the natural history and overall management of these tumors.

With the establishment of the Department of Surgical Oncology at the University of Illinois, we decided that accurate data on all these soft tissue tumors or tumorlike conditions would be maintained on a prospective basis. Along with this sarcoma registry, a sarcoma bank was also established, which has allowed us to pursue molecular, biochemical, immunocytochemical, and receptor studies on these rare tumors. The results of our treatment program have been compared with the burgeoning new clinicopathologic findings, and we have attempted clinicomorphologic correlation of these diverse tumors. The experience derived from the biologic study of these tumors and their benign counterparts constitutes the basis of this book. All patients were evaluated and managed under our supervision.

Since the publication of the first edition, considerable improvements have taken place in the diagnostic radiologic methods. The improvements are of such magnitude that a separate chapter has been dedicated solely to this topic. Experts from both medical centers (the University of Illinois at Chicago and the Medical College of Ohio) have joined together in providing their expertise to produce an excellent addition to this new edition.

The chapter on pathology is written primarily for the clinician and in no way attempts to be a major text reference for histopathology of somatic tissue tumors. However, it has been extensively revised to bring forth the current concepts on the histogenesis and molecular aspects of these unusual tumors. Although the tumors arising from the peripheral nerve tissue are neuroectodermal in origin and are in no way similar in biologic behavior to mesenchymal tumors, because of their similarity in clinical presentation and the concomitant difficulty in management, they are included in this book.

Curiously, in spite of their rarity, malignant mesenchymal tumors have generated considerable interest amongst molecular biologists. A number of molecular markers have been identified as playing a rather significant role in the initiation, growth, and progression of sarcomas. A comprehensive review of all of these is beyond the scope of this book; however, pertinent portions of this knowledge are of clinical relevance and these have been reviewed and synthesized into a separate chapter on the molecular biology of soft tissue sarcomas.

To provide a better perspective for comprehension of the natural history of these diverse mesenchymal and neuroectodermal neoplasms, tumors arising from each tissue type have been individually discussed and the pertinent literature has been summarized. The end results after various types of treatment, as found in the published reports, have been compared with those observed in the patient population treated primarily at the University of Illinois. The operative techniques described in Chapter 16 are those performed by the editors and their group in the Department of Surgical Oncology. However, we do not claim any originality or innovation in the techniques of these often-complex operations.

The field of radiation therapy in the management of sarcomas in general and especially for the treatment of intact primary tumors has grown immensely since the first edition of this book was published. Thus, we asked Drs. Arno Mundt and Ralph Weichselbaum to synthesize the current knowledge on the subject, and, as is evident, the chapter on radiation therapy provides the reader with an excellent overview of current state-of-the-art methods and treatment of soft tissue sarcomas.

The oncologic community has long admired the contributions of Dr. Robert Benjamin and his associates in the chemotherapeutic management of soft tissue sarcomas. We are extremely pleased that he agreed to write the chapter on chemotherapy of malignant mesenchymal tumors. This contribution will certainly enhance the value of this edition of the book. Similarly, we are very grateful that Dr. Norman Jaffe agreed to write the chapter on pediatric sarcomas. His contributions in this field are well known, and his chapter on this topic is an up-to-date summary of the diagnosis and management of these vexing problems in infancy and childhood.

The chapter on immunology and immunotherapy has been entirely revised by Drs. Houqi Chen and Jaroslav J. Stastny, and it essentially summarizes the work performed in the Department of Surgical Oncology as well as other centers. Although clinical immunology for sarcomas is not yet available, it is a burgeoning field, and we believe that within a short time, clinical trials will come into force. Thus, we think that this field is rife with possibilities for further investigations.

It is hoped that our experience with these rare, fascinating tumors, our methods of management, and our data on their natural history and biologic behavior will be useful to all interested in the study of these tumors and tumorlike conditions.

# ■ REFERENCES

1. Klemperer P: The concept of collagen disease. Am J Path 26:505, 1950

2. Gall EA, Mallory TB: Malignant lymphoma: A clinicopathologic survey of 618 cases. Am J Path 18:381, 1942

3. Bloodgood JC: The diagnosis and treatment of benign and malignant tumors of bone. J Radiology 7: 147, 1920

4. Codman EA: Bone Sarcoma. New York, Paul B. Hoeber Inc, 1925

5. Coley BL: Neoplasms of Bone and Related Conditions: Their Etiology, Pathogenesis, Diagnosis, and Treatment. New York, Paul B. Hoeber Inc, 1949

6. Ewing J: Neoplastic Diseases, 4th ed. Philadelphia and London, W. B. Saunders, 1942

7. Stout AP: Panel on Soft-Part Tumors. Proc Nat Cancer Conf, 1949, p 206

8. Stout AP: Tumors of the Soft Tissues. Atlas of Tumor Pathology, Sect 2, Fasc 5. Washington DC, AFIP, 1953

9. Stout AP, Lattes R: Tumors of the Soft Tissues. Atlas of Tumor Pathology, Sect 2, Fasc 1. Washington DC, AFIP, 1967

10. Pack GT, Ariel IM: Tumors of the Soft Somatic Tissues. New York, Paul B. Hoeber Inc, 1958

11. Enzinger FM, Weiss S (eds): Soft Tissue Tumors. Mosby, St. Louis, 1995

# I

# Characteristics of Soft Tissue Sarcomas

# 1

# Epidemiology and Etiology

Although benign tumors of mesenchymal origin are quite common, malignant mesenchymal tumors are relatively rare and comprise less than 1 percent of all malignancies in humans. Malignant soft tissue tumors are highly diverse but have as a common theme of presentation a "mass" and a relatively high incidence of blood-borne metastases and low incidence of lymphatic metastases. Otherwise, the tumors designated as soft tissue tumors have diverse etiology, histogenesis, and histologic appearance. The National Cancer Institute's Surveillance, Epidemiology, and End-Result program (SEER) reports the overall estimated number of soft tissue sarcomas in 1996 as approximately 6,400 new cases per year (3,500 males; 2,900 females) and the number of sarcoma-related deaths as 3,700 (1,800 males and 1,900 females).[1] This shows an increase of approximately 700 new cases of sarcomas and 600 more sarcoma-related deaths compared to what was recorded in 1990. In a study examining cancer trends in the United States comparing a period of mid-1970 to early 1990, DeVesa and colleagues observed no significant increase in the incidence of soft tissue sarcomas.[2] Compared to many other common tumors, such as lung cancer, breast cancer, melanoma, and cancers of the gastrointestinal tract, the number of epidemiologic studies of soft tissue sarcomas conducted is relatively low. Also, an identifiable common etiologic factor in patients with soft tissue sarcoma is lacking in most cases. Chemically and virally induced sarcomas in experimental systems have provided a body of scientific data on their etiologic factors,[3–11] but little of this information applies to human sarcomas. It appears that the incidence of soft tissue sarcoma varies little in different countries. Ryd-

holm and colleagues[12] estimated an annual incidence of 1.4 per 100,000 population. Recently, there has been an increased incidence of soft tissue sarcoma noted in the United States. However, most of this apparent increase can be accounted for by the increased number of Kaposi's sarcomas associated with acquired immunodeficiency syndrome (AIDS). Except for AIDS-related Kaposi's sarcoma, the overall incidence of soft tissue sarcoma in this country appears to have remained relatively stable.

The incidence of soft tissue sarcoma also varies depending on the sex and age of the patient. Soft tissue sarcoma is more common in men; however, this predilection for men over women varies considerably depending on the histologic type of sarcomas. For example, epithelioid sarcoma is more common in male patients, but giant cell tumors of the tendon sheath are more commonly encountered in young women. Also, in adults, the incidence of malignant mesenchymal tumors increases with age; most sarcomas are noted after age 20, and approximately 40 percent affect persons 55 years or older.[13] In a study reported by Rydholm et al.,[12] the incidence of soft tissue sarcoma in patients over age 80 was reported as 8 per 100,000 population, compared to an overall incidence of 1.4 per 100,000 population. Also, racial predilection in soft tissue sarcoma is noted. Sporadic soft tissue sarcomas are rarely found to aggregate in families.[14,15] Genetic factors, environmental exposure, or both, may account for the substantial racial and ethnic differences that appear in the distribution of some types of soft tissue sarcomas. In the spectrum of sarcomas, this is particularly apparent in the incidence of Kaposi's sarcoma, a disease that predominantly affects elderly persons of Eastern European descent. In contrast, Kaposi's sarcoma is a common form of childhood cancer in equatorial Africa. Ewing's sarcoma in children is less common in the black than in the white population. An adequate explanation of these racial and ethnic variances has not been advanced. As noted previously, when all soft tissue sarcomas are considered as a group, there is no definite racial predilection for this type of tumor.

# ■ ETIOLOGY

Although a number of different etiologic factors have been implicated in the genesis of soft tissue sarcoma, determining the exact causative factor of any given tumor is difficult. Well-known etiologic factors of soft tissue sarcoma include genetic predisposition, radiation, chemical carcinogens, viral factor(s), and immunodeficiency state. Occasionally, a soft tissue sarcoma can arise in a preexisting lesion. Sarcomatous transformation of a neurofibroma has been described; however, in most other instances, it is doubtful that soft tissue sarcoma develops from preexisting benign counterparts, such as lipoma converting to liposarcoma or hemangioma developing into angiosarcoma.

# ■ FAMILIAL AND GENETIC FACTORS

## HEREDITARY NEOPLASMS OR SARCOMALIKE CONDITIONS

Only a small proportion of human malignant tumors are inherited in a Mendelian pattern, indicating a single gene transmission that occurs as an inherited trait or as a complication of inherited precursor lesions that are clinically recognizable (Table 1–1). Recognition of this preneoplastic hereditary syndrome would allow for early screening of family members for possible treatment and delineation of biochemical and physiologic mechanisms linking a gene defect to these neoplasms. Familial preneoplastic and neoplastic syndromes related to mesenchymal tumors will be described in detail in various chapters of this book. In this section, they are briefly reviewed to provide a better perspective of the multifactorial influence on the etiology of tumors.

## Gardner's Syndrome

Gardner's syndrome is characterized by the appearance of multiple mesenchymal and skeletal tumors in conjunction with colonic polyposis.[16] The extra-alimentary tumors are usually osteomas, lipomas, or epidermal cysts. The close association of aggressive fibromatosis and low-grade fibrosarcoma in patients with Gardner's

**TABLE 1–1. HEREDITARY NEOPLASTIC SYNDROMES**

Hereditary neoplasms or sarcomalike conditions
  Gardner's syndrome
  Chemodectoma
  Retinoblastoma
  Pheochromocytoma and medullary thyroid carcinoma
Preneoplastic conditions (hamartomatous syndromes)
  Neurofibromatosis
  Tuberous sclerosis
  von Hippel-Lindau syndrome
  Multiple exostoses
  Peutz-Jeghers syndrome

syndrome is well known. This syndrome is described in detail elsewhere (Chapter 8). Gardner's syndrome is inherited as an autosomal dominant trait. The genetic defect appears to be in chromosome 5, locus 21–23. Some of these tumors occur in surgically traumatized sites, which suggests also a possible underlying abnormality in the reparative process.

## Chemodectomas

Chemodectomas are paragangliomas and can arise anywhere in the sympathochromaffin axis (i.e., sympathetic system and interrelated chromaffin organs). The most prominent locations are the carotid bifurcation and the nodose ganglion in the neck. These tumors sometimes produce catecholamines. Familial carotid body tumors are frequently bilateral.[17]

## Retinoblastoma

Inherited retinoblastoma has recently been associated with development of sarcomas, mostly osteosarcomas. Retinoblastoma is an embryonic ocular tumor that occurs in young children, with incidence of about 1 in 20,000; in 5 to 10 percent, the occurrence is familial. Bilateral involvement is more common in familial than in nonfamilial cases. Penetrance is about 80 to 90 percent; therefore, clinically unaffected persons may occasionally transmit the tumors.[18,19] Jensen and Miller[18] suggest that deletion of the D chromosome is a frequent manifestation in retinoblastoma. Associated congenital malformations of varying degrees have been reported.[18–22] Jensen and Miller[18] also found that 53 of the 1,077 evaluated children with retinoblastoma had major congenital malformation. Additionally, 21 were mentally retarded, whereas only 4 to 7 instances would normally be expected. A further finding was that 30 children had a second primary cancer, osteosarcoma being the most common. One case of rhabdomyosarcoma in a child with retinoblastoma has also been reported.[23] Although radiation-induced cancers of the head and neck region are well recognized, the osteosarcomas and fibrosarcomas reviewed by Jensen and Miller[18] were distant from any irradiated area. In our own sarcoma registry, we have two patients who were treated for retinoblastoma in childhood and developed retroperitoneal sarcomas by age 30. One had a grade 1–2 fibrosarcoma, the other a grade 2 leiomyosarcoma.

Recently, retinoblastoma has opened a new dimension in the genesis of soft tissue sarcomas.[24–27] Stratton and associates[28] found that structural alterations of the Rb1 gene were also found in various soft tissue sarcomas. Of the 69 specimens examined, loss of two of the alleles of this gene was detected in leiomyosarcomas. Overall, in 33 percent of the tumors, Stratton and colleagues found a loss of at least one of the alleles. These authors have suggested that the alteration of Rb1 locus plays a role in the pathogenesis of soft tissue sarcomas, particularly in leiomyosarcomas. Similarly, Cance and associates[29] found by both immunocytochemical and Western blot techniques that, when expression of Rb1 gene products is altered, the prognosis of soft tissues sarcomas changes. Apparently, when the expression of Rb1 gene products is substantially lowered in a given sarcomatous tumor, the patient has a considerably poorer prognosis. Although all current data regarding childhood retinoblastoma and development of adult malignant mesenchymal tumors are rather sporadic, the relationship requires further investigation and clarification.

### Pheochromocytoma and Medullary Thyroid Carcinoma

Pheochromocytomas and medullary thyroid carcinomas occur either singly or together.[30–32] The reported penetrance is approximately 85 percent; a higher rate may be found upon careful screening of the patient's family for increased production of catecholamines and calcitonin by otherwise silent tumors. These tumors are usually diagnosed after the second decade of life and tend to arise bilaterally or at multiple foci in the adrenal medulla and the thyroid. The syndrome may also include parathyroid hyperplasia (MEM 2A) and with ganglioneuromas (MEM 2B).

### PRENEOPLASTIC CONDITIONS OR HAMARTOMATOUS SYNDROMES

Structural defects in several organ systems can be identified in this condition. Usually, there are defects in development with incorrect differentiation and random mixing of all the component tissues. One or more of the tissues may proliferate as a localized growth (hamartoma). The hamartomas are classified primarily as malformations as opposed to true benign neoplasms.[33] As with hereditary neoplasms, autosomal dominant inheritance is noted in these syndromes, and there is no evidence that environmental factors contribute to the development.

### Neurofibromatosis

Neurofibromatosis, or von Recklinghausen's neurofibromatosis, occurs in about 1 in 3,000 live births and is characterized by multiple café-au-lait spots and multiple neurofibromas. Frequently, it is associated with lipomas, lymphangiomas, and hemangiomas. A detailed discussion of this syndrome and some of its variants can be found in the chapter discussing nerve sheath tumors (Chapter 10).

Both peripheral neurofibromatosis (neurofibromatosis type-1) and central neurofibromatosis (neurofibromatosis type-2) are associated with malignant soft tissue tumors. Both neurofibromatosis type-1 and type-2 are autosomal dominant diseases. The gene for neurofibromatosis type-1 has been detected in the pericentromeric region of chromosome 17. The gene for neurofibromatosis type-2, characterized by bilateral acoustic neurofibroma, is located in chromosome 22. Young, Eldridge, and Gardner[34] described bilateral acoustic neuromas and concluded that (1) if a patient with unilateral acoustic neuroma is young, or if there is a family history of acoustic neuroma, the possibility of eventual bilateral disease is great; (2) if a diagnosis of bilateral acoustic neuroma is established, the patient should be carefully watched for development of other central nervous system tumor(s) and his or her relatives should be screened for acoustic neuroma; and, (3) tumors that occur both unilaterally and bilaterally, such as acoustic neuroma, neuroblastoma, retinoblastoma, pheochromocytoma, and chemodectoma, are generally sporadic and nonfamilial when unilateral, but when bilateral, are frequently transmitted genetically as an autosomal-dominant trait. Lee and Abbott[35] confirmed the observation of Young and co-workers from the study of their own clinical material.

### Tuberous Sclerosis

Tuberous sclerosis is associated with the clinical triad of adenoma sebaceum, epilepsy, and mental retardation. Characteristic hamartomas occur in the brain, retina, heart, lung, and kidneys. Giant cell astrocytomas of the brain develop in about 1 to 3 percent of these patients.[30]

### von Hippel-Lindau Syndrome

von Hippel-Lindau syndrome features angiomatosis of the retina and cerebellum and often is associated with cysts and angiomas of the viscera and of the cutaneous and subcutaneous tissue. Patients with this syndrome show a predisposition to associated hypernephromas, pheochromocytomas, and ependymomas. Table 1–2

**TABLE 1–2. HEREDITARY NEUROLOGICAL SYNDROMES ASSOCIATED WITH CUTANEOUS AND SUBCUTANEOUS ANGIOMAS**

| Syndrome | Inheritance | Sex | Onset | Skin Lesions | Central Nervous System Findings |
|---|---|---|---|---|---|
| Ataxia, telangiectasia | Autosomal recessive | Equal | Childhood | Telangiectasia increased by sun exposure | Cerebellar ataxia; ocular telangiectasia; nystagmus; mental retardation; dysarthria |
| Fabry's disease | Sex-linked | Males show full syndrome | Childhood | Angiokeratomas in clusters | Cerebrovascular accident; neuronal glycolipid deposition (peripheral neuritis) |
| von Hippel-Lindau syndrome | Autosomal dominant | Equal | Adulthood | Port-wine stain or no lesion; café-au-lait spots | Cerebellar hemangioblastoma and cyst; spinal hemangioblastoma (rarely) |
| Rendu-Osler-Weber disease | Autosomal dominant | Equal | Childhood | Telangiectasia of skin, mucous membrane | Angiomas in brain or spinal cord, with signs of local tumor |
| Sturge-Weber syndrome | Autosomal dominant or not familial | Equal | Birth (in two-thirds of patients) | Port-wine stain in distribution of fifth cranial nerve | Angioma of meninges, intracranial calcifications; mental retardation; epilepsy; hemiparesis; visual impairment |

shows the hereditary neurologic disorders associated with cutaneous and subcutaneous angiomas.

### Multiple Exostosis (Diaphyseal Aclasis)

Multiple exostoses are osteomas occurring at the surface of growing bones. Severe deformities often result, and transformation of chondrosarcoma is reported in approximately 5 to 10 percent of the cases.[30,36]

### Peutz-Jeghers Syndrome

In Peutz-Jeghers syndrome, hamartomatous gastrointestinal polyps are associated with melanin pigmentation of the buccal mucosa and lips. These polyps are usually in the small intestine and rarely become malignant.[30,37]

### ■ CONGENITAL DEFECTS AND SARCOMAS

Certain childhood sarcomas are associated with congenital anomalies.[38–41] Miller[40] found that, among children with Wilms' tumor and neuroblastoma,[41,42] the peak mortality is at about four years of age. A similar mortality pattern was found in patients with primary liver cancer and adrenocortical neoplasia.[43,44] In general, the following congenital defects occur sporadically and may be due to fresh mutation of the genes:[30] sporadic aniridia with Wilms' tumor; congenital hemihypertrophy or visceral cytomegaly with Wilms' tumor; adrenocortical tumor or hepatoblastoma; enchondromatosis or enchondromas and hemangiomas with chondrosarcomas; and gonadal dysgenesis with gonadoblastoma.

### ■ CANCER FAMILIES

The concept of cancer families now includes familial neoplasms of dissimilar types.[30,45] In a study of childhood rhabdomyosarcoma, the tendency for the cancer to aggregate in the siblings was associated with high frequency of various other cancers (especially in the female breast) in parents and other relatives (Li-Fraumeni cancer syndrome).[46] Sarcomas in children are also found in association with adrenocortical carcinoma, brain tumors, and other childhood tumors as second primaries.[47,48] Miller[38] found that siblings of children who died of brain tumors were at excessive risk of sarcomas of the muscles and the bones. Adenomatous polyps of the colon (familial polyposis) may be associated with familial adenocarcinoma[45] and, in familial aggregations, with brain tumors (Turcot syndrome)[39] and various sarcomas.[47]

### ■ TRAUMA

Although the clinician is frequently faced with the patient who historically links sarcoma to an antecedent episode of trauma, there is no evidence to suggest that trauma plays any role in the induction of the human mesenchymal malignant tumors, except for fibromatosis associated with polyposis coli or Gardner's syndrome. In these patients, a sizable number of cases have been reported where the fibromatosis developed in the surgical scar. Also, in rare cases, soft tissue sarcomas have been associated with thermal or acid burns and in the fracture site.[13]

## ■ CHEMICAL FACTORS

Sarcomatous transformation induced by chemical carcinogen in experimental animals has long been described.[11] But, although polycyclic hydrocarbons produced sarcomas in rats, mice, and guinea pigs, chemical carcinogen as an etiologic factor for soft tissue sarcoma is relatively rare.[49–51] In 1979, Hardell reported a case-controlled study evaluating the effect of exposure to phenoxyacetic acid or chlorophenols as a cause for soft tissue sarcoma.[52] The dioxin-containing herbicide 2, 3, 7, 8-tetra-chlorodibenzo-p-dioxin (TCDD) has been implicated in causing various soft tissue sarcomas. Similarly, Agent Orange, a defoliant which contained dioxin, has also been implicated in a higher incidence of soft tissue sarcoma among Vietnam veterans.[53,54] However, none of the studies reported by Collins and co-workers,[55] which examined the mortality rates of workers exposed to dioxin in industrial accidents, found any increased evidence of sarcomas among workers exposed to dioxin alone. Fingerhut et al.[56] and Suruda et al.[57] evaluated prolonged exposure of humans to dioxin and its effect after a long latent period. In their studies, they noted that, among patients with longer than 1 year of exposure and 20 years' latent period, there was a significant increase in risk of mortality from soft tissue sarcoma.[56,57] Polyvinyl chloride exposure has also been implicated in the etiology of angiosarcoma. However, such occurrences are distinctly rare.[58]

## ■ PHYSICAL FACTORS

### ASBESTOS

Asbestos has long been known to be a potent carcinogen. Occurrence of pleural and peritoneal mesothelioma has been strongly linked to asbestos exposure. Asbestos-induced mesothelioma depends on the type of asbestos and intensity and duration of the exposure. Generally, there are two types of asbestos fibers: blue asbestos (crocidolite), which is mined in South Africa and is highly carcinogenic; and white asbestos (chrysolite), which carries a lesser risk to those exposed of developing cancer. Asbestos fibers inhaled in the pulmonary parenchyma and ultimately reaching the pleural surface are associated, after a long latent period, with the development of mesothelioma.[59,60]

### FOREIGN BODY

Sarcoma induction via foreign bodies is much better substantiated. Although the evidence in humans is based on isolated case reports, the fact that such instances are documented should arouse considerable interest among clinical oncologists.

Tumors associated with foreign bodies have been reported intermittently since 1880.[61] Around the 1940s, several investigators[62–64] found that rats may develop sarcoma after a plastic material is implanted in different body sites. These observations were further explored by Oppenheimer and coworkers,[65–67] Nothdurft,[68–71] Zollinger,[72] and Alexander.[73] These elegant studies established the etiologic role of foreign bodies in the induction of sarcomas in experimental animals. By excluding the chemical factors, they concluded that the physical presence and nature of the foreign bodies were singularly responsible for sarcomagenesis. Since artificial implants of various kinds are being used by surgeons for functional and cosmetic reasons, there has been extensive investigation of the biocompatibility of these agents.[64,67,74–79]

Considering the tremendous increase in the frequency of foreign-body implants in humans during the last 30 years, the actual number of sarcomas relative to foreign body reported has been extremely small, compared with the number of foreign-body induced sarcomas in laboratory animals.[65–72] No sarcomas were reported by Ruben and co-workers[80] among 281 patients with facial prostheses, nor by deCholonoky[81] among 1,100 women who underwent augmentation mammoplasty. Similar reports of a lack of sarcoma associated with foreign body have been published by other investigators.[82–85] There have been sporadic studies, however, with reports of sarcomas associated with foreign materials. Burns and associates[86] reported the development of sarcoma 10 years after arterial repair by Teflon-Dacron prostheses. In another instance, a chondrosarcoma developed 18 years after implantation of Lucite spheres in the pleural cavity.[87] In 1970, Ott[61] collected all cases of foreign body-induced sarcomas up to 1966 and found that, in some instances, the latency period was 40 years or more. Foreign materials such as metal implants, steel, plastic, bullets, shrapnel pieces, surgical sponges, and bone wax have all been implicated in sarcomatous development.[88] Human sarcomas associated with implanted plastic material have also been reported by Bischoff.[89] Jennings et al.[90] gathered examples of angiosarcoma associated with foreign material.

Recently, Engle et al.[91] examined the possible effects of breast implants on the development of breast sarcoma in a time-trend analysis based on surveillance, epidemiology, and end-result (SEER) data. They considered a 10-year latency period after breast implantation for the development of sarcoma in the breast.

Compared to the period from 1973 to 1981, there was a tenfold increase in the number of women with breast implant for 10 or more years in 1982 to 1990 (55,000 versus 509,000). However, age-adjusted incidence of breast sarcoma was only 0:13 per 100,000 women for the initial nine-year study period 1973–1981 and 0:12 per 100,000 women for the latter nine-year period. Thus, there appears to be no noticeable increase in the incidence of breast sarcoma secondary to breast implant.[91]

## ■ RADIATION FACTORS

Ionizing radiation in sufficiently high doses acts as a complete carcinogen, serving as both a tumor initiator and promoter. Malignant transformation can be initiated in nearly any tumor or organ of man or experimental animals by the proper choice of radiation dose and exposure schedule. The principal interest in radiation as an environmental carcinogen is not at high dosages. Relatively few patients receive such high dosages, and, in most cases in which they do, the radiation is given as a localized treatment for a malignant tumor.

The induction of bone tumor by radiation was first observed in clock dial painters after accidental ingestion of radium while painting the luminous dials.[92,93] In addition to osteosarcomas, these victims showed an excessive incidence of fibrosarcomas and of carcinomas of the perinasal and mastoid sinuses.[94,95] The latency period for induction of tumors varied inversely with the radium content of the skeleton, being as short as 10 years in persons with 5–6 μCi of radium, and more than 25 years in those with smaller radium burns.[96] The incidence of bone tumors has been interpreted as roughly the square of the terminal concentration of radium in the skeleton, exceeding 20 percent at the level of 5 μCi or more, but with no evidence of tumor induction at levels of less than 0.5 μCi.[97]

The overall incidence of radiation-induced sarcoma after therapeutic radiation appears quite small and probably accounts for less than 0.1 percent of cancer patients treated with radiation. In our experience, radiation-induced sarcoma accounts for less than 2 percent of all sarcoma patients. Arlen et al.[98] outlined the criteria for radiation-induced sarcoma. According to these investigators, for a given sarcoma to be accepted as radiation induced: (1) there must be a latency period of at least three years between completion of the radiation and initiation of the tumor; (2) the tumor must develop in the radiated field; and (3) the region where the radiation-induced sarcoma arises must have been confirmed normal before radiation. Although we have seen radiation-induced angiosarcoma in adolescents, radiation-induced sarcomas are seen mostly in female patients and most frequently in adults. Radiation-induced sarcoma covers a wide spectrum of histologic subtypes; however, malignant fibrous histiocytoma is the most common radiation-induced sarcoma and accounts for approximately 70 percent of all cases. Most radiation-induced sarcomas are high-grade sarcomas and generally have been associated with poor prognosis. Laskin et al.[99] reported a 26 percent survival among 53 patients with radiation-induced soft tissue sarcoma.

## ■ VIRAL FACTORS

Although type C viral particles have been associated in several animal sarcomas,[3,4] there has been no confirmed isolation of infectious type C virus from normal or transformed human tissue. Recently, however, several groups have reported identifying in human tumor tissue nucleic acid sequences or reverse transcriptase from the known well-characterized mammalian type C viruses. Kufe and associates[3] demonstrated that RNA sequence homologous to certain sequences of Rauscher mouse leukemia virus can be detected in human sarcomas. Although these and similar data[4–10] are of interest, direct correlation of a possible association between the type C virus and human neoplasia must await isolation of infectious type C virus from human tissue, or at least the identification of human cell culture that releases human type C virus in high titers. The recent increase in Kaposi's sarcoma in AIDS patients has renewed interest in the role of viruses as etiologic factors for soft tissue sarcoma. However, a disproportionately increased number of Kaposi's sarcoma among male homosexual AIDS patients, as compared to heterosexual AIDS patients and drug abusers, raised the possibility that factors other than the herpes virus type 1 are necessary for oncogenic effect. Several co-factors, including cytomegalic inclusion, have been implicated; however, factors associated with orofecal contamination are apparently important for Kaposi's sarcoma in AIDS patients. Interestingly, Hudson et al.[100] reported angiosarcoma arising at the site of previous herpes zoster-infected areas.

## ■ IMMUNOLOGIC FACTORS

In general, the incidence of malignancy has increased among patients who are immunodeficient or therapeutically immunosuppressed. However, most of these malignant lesions are either lymphomas or are of epithelial origin.[101] Malignancy of mesenchymal origin of different histologic types, although rare, has been described among organ transplant recipients. The exact role of immunodeficiency in Kaposi's sarcoma among AIDS patients is uncertain, but there appear to be other etiologic factors in the increased incidence of Kaposi's sarcoma among AIDS patients. Interestingly, development of lymphangiosarcoma in postmastectomy patients has been proposed to be secondary to regional immunodeficiency associated with loss of immune surveillance secondary to lymphedema.[102] Schenk and Penn[103] compiled a registry of 5,170 transplant recipients consisting of 5,000 with kidney and 170 with heart allograft. In 1 percent, or 52 patients, a neoplasm developed. Twenty-eight were of epithelial origin (skin, cervix, and tongue), 22 were lymphomas, and 2 were leiomyosarcomas. Although these neoplasms are doubtlessly malignant, there is some confusion as to the mechanism of their development in supposedly immunosuppressed patients.[103,104] Therefore, while there may be a risk of soft tissue sarcoma developing in an immunodeficiency state, only rarely does this occur.[105]

## REFERENCES

1. Parker SL, Tong T, Bolden S, et al.: Cancer statistics 1996. CA Cancer J Clin 46(1):5, 1996
2. DeVesa SS, Blot WJ, Stone BJ, et al.: Recent cancer trends in the United States. J Natl Cancer Inst 87(3):175, 1995
3. Kufe D, Hehlmann R, Spiegelman S: Human sarcomas contain RNA related to the RNA of a mouse leukemia virus. Science 175:182, 1972
4. Lieber NM, Todaro GJ: Mammalian type C RNA viruses. In Becker FF (ed): Cancer: A Comprehensive Treatise, vol. 2. New York, Plenum Press, 1975
5. Rauscher FJ, O'Conner TE: Virology. In Holland JF, Frei E III (eds): Cancer Medicine. Philadelphia, Lea & Febiger, 1973, p 15
6. Bernhard W: The detection and study of tumor viruses with the electron microscope. Cancer Res 20:712, 1960
7. Green M: Oncogenic viruses. Ann Rev Biochem 39:735, 1970
8. Ruebner RJ, Todaro GJ: Oncogenesis of RNA viruses as determinants of cancer. Proc Natl Acad Sci 64:1087, 1969
9. Shope RE: Koch's postulates and a viral cause of human cancer. Cancer Res 20:1119, 1960
10. Hanafusa H: Avian RNA tumor viruses. In Becker FF (ed): Cancer: A Comprehensive Treatise, vol. 2. New York, Plenum Press, 1975, p 49
11. Baldwin RW, Price MR: Neoantigen expression in chemical carcinogenesis. In Becker FF (ed): Cancer: A Comprehensive Treatise, vol. 1. New York, Plenum Press, 1975, p 406
12. Rydholm A, Manberg NO, Gullberg B, et al.: Epidemiology of soft tissue sarcoma in the locomotor system: A retrospective population-based study of the inter-relationship between clinical and morphological variables. Acta Pathol Microbiol Immunol Scand 92A:363, 1984
13. Enzinger FM, Weiss SW (eds): Soft Tissue Tumors, 3rd Ed., Chap. 1. St. Louis, Mosby-Yearbook, 1995, p 1
14. Hartley AL, Birch JM, Kelsey AM, et al.: Are germ cell tumors part of the Li-Fraumeni cancer family syndrome? Cancer Genet Cytogenet 42:221, 1989
15. Usui M, Ishii S, Yamawaki S, Hirayama T: The occurrence of soft tissue sarcomas in three siblings with Warner's syndrome. Cancer 54:2580, 1984
16. Gardner EJ, Richards RC: Multiple cutaneous and subcutaneous lesions occurring simultaneously with hereditary polyposis and osteomatosis. Am J Hum Genet 5:139, 1953
17. Wilson H: Carotid body tumors: Familial and bilateral. Ann Surg 171:843, 1970
18. Jensen RD, Miller RW: Retinoblastoma: Epidemiologic characteristics. N Engl J Med 185:307, 1971
19. Falls HF, Neel JV: Genetics of retinoblastoma. Arch Ophthalmol 46:367, 1951
20. Thompson H, Lyons RB: Retinoblastoma and multiple congenital anomalies associated with complex mosaicism with deletion of D chromosome and probably D/C translocation. Hum Chromosome Newsl 15:21, 1965
21. Van Kempen C: A case of retinoblastoma, combined with severe mental retardation and a few other congenital anomalies, associated with complex aberrations of the karyotype. Manndschr Kindergeneeskd 34:92, 1966
22. Pruett RC, Atkins L: Chromosome studies in patients with retinoblastoma. Arch Ophthalmol 82:177, 1969
23. Levene M: Congenital retinoblastoma and sarcoma botryoides of the vagina: Report of a case. Cancer 13:532, 1960
24. Li FP: Hereditary retinoblastoma, lipoma, and second primary cancer. J Natl Cancer Inst 89:83, 1997
25. Fontanesi J, Parham DM, Pratt C, Meyer D: Second malignant neoplasms in children with retinoblastoma: The St. Jude Children's Research Hospital experience. Ophthalmic Genet 16:105, 1995
26. Li W, Fan J, Hochhauser D, et al.: Lack of functional retinoblastoma protein mediates increased resistance to antimetabolites in human sarcoma cell lines. Proc Natl Acad Sci U S A 92:10436, 1995
27. Berner JM, Forus A, Elkahloun A, et al.: Separate amplified regions encompassing CDK4 and MDM2 in human sarcomas. Genes Chromosom Cancer 17:254, 1996
28. Stratton MR, Williams S, Fisher C, et al.: Structural alterations of the Rb1 gene in human soft tissue tumours. Br J Cancer 60:202, 1989
29. Cance WG, Brennan MF, Dudas ME, et al.: Altered expression of the retinoblastoma gene product in human sarcomas. N Engl J Med 323:1457, 1990
30. Fraumeni JF Jr.: Genetic factors. In Holland JF, Frei E III (eds): Cancer Medicine. Philadelphia, Lea & Febiger, 1973, p 7
31. Schimke RN, Hartmann WH, Prout TE, Riomorin DL: Syndrome of bilateral pheochromocytoma, medullary thyroid carcinoma, and multiple neuromas. N Engl J Med 279:1, 1968
32. Wander JV, Das Gupta TK: Neurofibromatosis. In Ravitch MM, Austen WG, Scott HW Jr., et al. (eds): Current

Problems in Surgery, vol. 14. Chicago, Year Book Medical Publishers, 1977

33. Willis RA: Borderland of Embryology and Pathology, 2nd ed. London, Butterworth, 1962, p 341

34. Young DF, Eldridge R, Gardner WJ: Bilateral acoustic neuroma in a large kindred. JAMA 214:347, 1970

35. Lee DK, Abbott ML: Familial central nervous system neoplasia: Case report of a family with von Recklinghausen's neurofibromatosis. Arch Neurol 20:154, 1969

36. Epstein LL, Bixler D, Bennett JE: An incidence of familial cancer including three cases of osteogenic sarcoma. Cancer 25:889, 1970

37. McKusick VA: Genetic factors in intestinal polyposis. JAMA 182:271, 1962

38. Miller RW: Deaths from childhood leukemia and solid tumors among twins and other sibs in the United States, 1960–1970. J Natl Cancer Inst 46:203, 1971

39. Turcot J, Despres JP, St Pierre F: Malignant tumors of the central nervous system associated with familial polyposis of the colon: Report of two cases. Dis Colon Rectum 2:465, 1959

40. Miller RW: Relation between cancer and congenital defects: An epidemiologic evaluation. J Natl Cancer Inst 40:1079, 1968

41. Miller RW, Fraumeni JF Jr., Manning MD: Association of Wilms' tumor with aniridia, hemihypertrophy, and other congenital malformations. N Engl J Med 270:922, 1964

42. Miller RW, Fraumeni JF Jr., Hill JA: Neuroblastoma: Epidemiologic approach to its origin. Am J Dis Child 115:253, 1968

43. Fraumeni JF Jr., Miller RW, Hill JA: Primary carcinoma of the liver in childhood: An epidemiologic study. J Natl Cancer Inst 40:1087, 1968

44. Fraumeni JF Jr., Miller RW: Adrenocortical neoplasms with hemihypertrophy, brain tumors, and other disorders. J Pediatr 70:129, 1967

45. Smith WG: The cancer-family syndrome and heritable solitary colonic polyps. Dis Colon Rectum 13:362, 1970

46. Li FP, Fraumeni JF Jr.: Soft tissue sarcomas, breast cancer, and other neoplasms. A familial syndrome? Ann Intern Med 71:747, 1969

47. Fraumeni JF Jr., Vogel CL, Easton JM: Sarcomas and multiple polyposis in a kindred: A genetic variety of hereditary polyposis. Arch Intern Med 121:57, 1968

48. Li FP, Fraumeni JF Jr.: Rhabdomyosarcoma in children: Epidemiologic study and identification of a familial cancer syndrome. J Natl Cancer Inst 43:1365, 1969

49. Fingerhut MA, Halperin WE, Honchar PA, et al.: An evaluation of reports of dioxin exposure and soft-tissue sarcoma pathology among chemical workers in the United States. Scand J Work Environ Health 10:299, 1984

50. Smith AH, Pearce NE, Fisher DO, et al.: Soft tissue sarcoma and exposure to phenoxyherbicides and chlorophenols in New Zealand. J Natl Cancer Inst 73:1111, 1984

51. Hoar SK, Blair A, Holmes FF, et al.: Agricultural herbicide use and risk of lymphoma and soft-tissue sarcoma. JAMA 256:1141, 1986

52. Hardell L: Case-control study: Soft tissues sarcomas and exposure to phenoxyacetic acids or chlorophenols. Br J Cancer 39:711, 1979

53. Bilar JC: How dangerous is dioxin? N Engl J Med 324:260, 1991

54. Greenwald P, Kovaszany B, Collins DN: Sarcoma of soft tissue after Viet Nam service. J Natl Cancer Inst 73:1107, 1984

55. Collins JJ, Strauss ME, Levinskas JJ, et al.: The mortality of workers exposed to 2, 3, 7, 8-tetra-chlorodibenzo-p-dioxin in a trichlorophenol process accident. Epidemiology 4:7, 1993

56. Fingerhut MA, Halperin WE, Marlow DA: Cancer mortality in workers exposed to 2, 3, 7, 8-tetra-chlorodibenzo-p-dioxin. N Engl J Med 324:212, 1991

57. Suruda AJ, Ward FM, Fingerhut MA: Identification of soft tissue sarcoma death in cohorts exposed to dioxin and to chlorinated naphthalenes. Epidemiology 4:14, 1993

58. Evans DM, Williams WJ, Jung IT: Angiosarcoma and hepatocellular carcinoma in vinyl chloride workers. Histopathology 7:377, 1983

59. Craighead JE: Current pathogenetic concept of diffuse malignant mesothelioma. Hum Pathol 18:544, 1987

60. Craighead JE, Mossman BT: The pathogenesis of asbestos associated disease. N Engl J Med 306:1466, 1982

61. Ott G: Fremdkorpersarkome. Exp Med Pathol Klin 32:1, 1970

62. Alexander P, Homing ES: Observations on the Oppenheimer method of inducing tumors by subcutaneous implantation of plastic films. CIBA Foundation Symposium on Carcinogenesis, 1959, p 24

63. Bischoff F, Bryson G: Carcinogenesis through solid state surfaces. Progr Exp Tumor Res 5:85, 1964

64. Bryson G, Bischoff F: Polymer carcinogenesis. Symposium on Polymer Chemistry, American Chemical Society Western Regional Meeting, 1965

65. Oppenheimer BS, Oppenheimer ET, Danishefsky I, et al.: Further studies of polymers as carcinogenic agents in animals. Cancer Res 15:333, 1955

66. Oppenheimer BS, Oppenheimer ET, Stout AP, et al.: The latent period in carcinogenesis by plastics in rats and its relation to the precancerous stage. Cancer 11:204, 1958

67. Oppenheimer BS, Oppenheimer ET, Stout AP, et al.: Studies of the mechanism of carcinogenesis by plastic films. Acta Unio Int Contra Cancrum 15:659, 1959

68. Nothdurft H: Die experimentelle Erzeugung von Sarkomen bei Ratten und Mausen Durch Implantation von Rundscheiben aus Gold, Silber, Platin Oder Elfenbein. Naturwissenschaften 42:106, 1955

69. Nothdurft H: Uber die Sarkomauslosung durch Fremdkorperimplantationen bei Ratten in abhangigkeit von der Form der Implantate. Naturwissenschaften 42:106, 1955

70. Nothdurft H: Tumorezeugung durch Fremdkorperim-

plantation. Abhandl Deutsch Akad Wiss Derl Klasse Med 3:80, 1960

71. Nothdurft H: Unterschiedliche Ausbeuten an subcutanen Fremdkorpersarkomen der Ratte in Abhangigkeit von der Korpeffegion. Naturwissenschaften 49:18, 1962

72. Zollinger HU: Experimentelle Erzeugung maligner Nierenkapseltumoren bei der Ratte durch Druckreiz Plastic-Kapseln. Schweiz Z Tschr Aflg 15:666, 1952

73. Alexander P: The reactions of carcinogens with macromolecules. Adv Cancer Res 2:1, 1954

74. Milne J: Fifteen cases of pleural mesothelioma associated with occupational exposure to asbestos in Victoria. Med J Austral 2:669, 1969

75. Wagner JC, Berry G: Mesotheliomas in rats following inoculation with asbestos. Br J Cancer 23:567, 1969

76. Brand KG, Buoen LC: Polymer tumorigenesis: Multiple preneoplastic clones in priority order with clonal inhibition. Proc Soc Exp Biol Med 128:1154, 1968

77. Brand KG, Buoen LC, Brand I: Premalignant cells in tumorigenesis induced by plastic film. Nature 213(part 2):810, 1967

78. Brand KG, Buoen LC, Brand I: Carcinogenesis from polymer implants: New aspects from chromosomal and transplantation studies during premalignancy. J Natl Cancer Inst 39:663, 1967

79. Brand KG: Foreign body-associated tumors in man. In Becker FF (ed): Cancer: A Comprehensive Treatise, vol. 1. New York, Plenum Press, 1975, p 486

80. Rubin LR, Bromberg BE, Walden RH: Long-term human reaction to synthetic plastics. Surg Gynecol Obstet 132:603, 1971

81. deCholnoky T: Augmentation mammaplasty: Survey of complications in 10,941 patients by 265 surgeons. Plast Reconstruct Surg 45:573, 1970

82. Calnan JS: Assessment of biological properties of implants before their clinical use. Proc R Soc Med 63:1115, 1970

83. Dukes CE, Mitchley BCV: Polyvinyl sponge implants: Experimental and clinical observations. Br J Plast Surg 15:225, 1962

84. Dutton J: Acrylic investment of intracranial aneurysms. Br Med J 2:597, 1959

85. Spence WT: Form-fitting plastic cranioplasty. J Neurosurg 11:219, 1954

86. Bums WA, Kanhouwand S, Tillman L, et al.: Fibrosarcoma occurring at the site of a plastic vascular graft. Cancer 29:66, 1972

87. Thompson RJ, Entin SD: Primary extraskeletal chondrosarcoma. Cancer 23:936, 1969

88. Benishak O, Carriner H, Brenner B, et al.: Angiosarcoma of the colon developing in a capsule of foreign body. Am J Clin Pathol 97:416, 1992

89. Bischoff F: Organic polymer biocompatibility and toxicology. Clin Chem 18:869, 1972

90. Jennings DA, Peterson L, Axiotis CA, et al.: Angiosarcoma associated with foreign body material: A report of three cases. Cancer 62:2436, 1988

91. Engle A, Lamm SH, Lari SH: Human breast sarcoma and human breast implant: A time trend analysis based on SEER data (1973–1990). J Clin Epidemiol 48(4):539, 1995

92. Martland HS: Occurrence of malignancy in radioactive persons: A general review of data gathered in the study of radium dial painters, with special reference to the occurrence of osteogenic sarcoma and the interrelationship of certain blood diseases. Am J Cancer 15:2435, 1931

93. Looney WB: Effects of radium in man. Science 127:630, 1958

94. Aub JC, Evans RD, Hempelmann LH, Martland HS: The late effects of internally deposited radioactive materials in man. Medicine 31:221, 1952

95. Marinelli LD: Radioactivity and the human skeleton. Am J Roentgenol 80:729, 1958

96. Evans RD: The effect of skeletally deposited alpha-ray emitters in man. Br J Radiol 39:881, 1966

97. National Research Council: The effects on populations of exposure to low levels of ionizing radiation. Report of the Advisory Committee on the Biological Effects of Ionizing Radiation. Washington DC, National Academy of Sciences, 1972

98. Arlen M, Higginbotham NL, Huvos AG, et al.: Radiation-induced sarcoma of bone. Cancer 28:1087, 1971

99. Laskin WB, Silverman TA, Enzinger FM: Post-radiation soft tissue sarcoma: An analysis of 53 cases. Cancer 62:2330, 1988

100. Hudson CP, Hanno R, Callen JP: Cutaneous angiosarcoma in a site of healed herpes zoster. Int J Dermatol 23:404, 1984

101. Melief CJM, Schwartz RS: Immunocompetence and malignancy. In Becker FF (ed) Cancer: A Comprehensive Treatise, vol. 2, New York, Plenum Press, 1975

102. Scheiber H, Barry FM, Russel WC: Stewart-Treves Syndrome: A lethal complication of postmastectomy lymphedema and regional immature deficiency. Arch Surg 114:82, 1979

103. Schenk SA, Penn I: Cerebral neoplasms associated with renal transplantation. Arch Neurol 22:226, 1970

104. Schenk SA, Penn I: De-novo brain tumors in renal transplant recipients. Lancet 1:983, 1971

105. Penn I: The occurrence of cancer in immune deficiencies. Cur Probl Cancer 6(10):1, 1982

# 2

# Classification

Most malignant soft tissue tumors arise de novo. In the benign form, these tumors seldom undergo malignant transformation (i.e., angiomas only rarely convert to malignant angioendotheliomas;[1] synovial sarcomas rarely arise from benign preexisting tumors of the tendon sheath; and lipomas rarely become liposarcomas).[1,2] However, some large lipomas may undergo xanthomatous or myxomatous degeneration, with liposarcoma developing many years later.[3,4] Similarly, certain disease entities appear benign but on long-term follow-up show a rather high incidence of associated malignant tumors, a prime example being type 1 and type 2 neurofibromatosis.[5] Occasionally, a tumor is histologically diagnosed as benign, but its behavior is characterized by local recurrence and distant dissemination. Finally, some tumors are histologically benign, but incomplete excision may result in local recurrence, and multiple recurrences may lead to malignant transformation.[2]

There are myriad different varieties of tumors and tumorlike conditions of the soft somatic tissues. Each is a separate entity and requires a specific plan of treatment. Therefore, even though the morphologic distinction of a given soft tissue tumor might at times be difficult and could be conjectural, every attempt should be made to establish an exact histologic diagnosis. Histologic classification is impeded because most of these tumors are derived from primitive mesenchyme and tend to undergo metaplasia under the stress of neoplasia. Thus, before an attempt is made to develop a practical histogenetic classification of these tumors, it is appropriate to briefly trace the development of tissues from the primitive mesenchyme and to elaborate on the term *metaplasia* in the context of somatic tissue tumors. Neoplasms arising solely from the nervous tissue are, strictly speaking, neither sarcomas nor sarcomatous conditions. However, most are clinically considered sarcomas or variants thereof, and are included in this book.

The term *mesenchyme* embraces all the undifferentiated nonepithelial mesodermal tissue of the embryo or fetus. The derivatives of the mesoderm are (1) epithelium of the gonads; (2) mesothelium, the flat pavement epithelium or endothelium of the celomic cavities; and (3) mesenchyme (Greek, *mesos* = middle; *enchyma* = that which is poured in), the diffusely cellular precursors of the connective, vascular, skeletal, muscular, and hematopoietic tissues. The embryonic mesenchymal cells are fusiform or stellate, and their processes are in intimate contact with those of the adjacent cells, forming a network. In recent years, several authors[6–9] have identified not only some specific mesenchymal factors but also a number of genes that influence both epithelial and mesothelial morphogenesis, thereby creating considerable doubt as to the exact sequence of events that leads to either dedifferentiation or differentiation, resulting in the formation of a given mesenchymal tumor.

During the process of differentiation of primitive mesenchyme into connective tissue, cartilage, and bone, distinct substances (e.g., collagen and elastic fibers, chondroitin or osseomucin, and lime salts) are deposited into it. The mesenchymal cells that line the blood vessels, lymph vessels, and celomic spaces are distinguished as endothelium, and celomic endothelium is called *mesothelium*. The distinction, although descriptively useful, is not absolute and is not of much help in interpreting the biologic behavior of tumors of the primitive mesenchyme. The various kinds of tissues differentiated from mesenchyme are closely allied, as shown not only by their common source in the embryo, but also by their regenerative growth in adult life, when they revert morphologically to the appearance of embryonic mesenchyme and may redifferentiate into other tissues. Thus, proliferating vascular and fibroblastic tissues may form cartilage, bone, smooth muscle, and hematopoietic cells—changes that are called *metaplasia*. The following paragraphs briefly summarize the developmental characteristics of the tissues derived from the primitive mesenchyme and the peripheral nervous tissue.

## ■ CONNECTIVE TISSUE

Fibrous, areolar, mucoid, and adipose tissues differentiate from the cellular mesenchyme. In the human embryo, most of the prospective fibrous tissues are still relatively cellular. The soft intercellular matrix is poor in collagen and rich in mucinous fluid. By the end of the second month of gestation, many of the main tendons, ligaments, fasciae, and other fibrous structures are plainly present as mesenchymal condensations, with appropriately oriented fibroblasts and increasing collagen. Fat cells first appear in the subcutaneous tissue during the fifth fetal month. Mesenchymal cells become plump and rounded. Multiple droplets of fat appear in their cytoplasm, and these enlarge and coalesce to form a single large droplet in each cell. However, Shaw[10] proposed that fat cells arise merely by fat storage in ordinary connective tissue cells, and some support for this concept can be found in adult tissue with metaplasia.

Chondrification in the mesenchyme begins in particular foci of perichondral centers; the cells here become separated by a mucinous intercellular matrix. The prechondral tissue quickly develops into embryonic cartilage with a hyaline basophilic matrix. In the human embryo, chondrification is well advanced by the seventh week (15 to 20 mm), each cartilage and bone being represented by its cartilaginous rudiment.[11]

Bursae and tendon sheaths develop as clefts in the mesenchyme and then undergo synovial differentiations.[12–14] They appear from the third month of gestation onward, although some do not develop until late fetal or postnatal life. The late development of some of these synovial structures indicates the importance of pressure and movement in their formation and prepares us for the metaplastic formation of false bursae over pressure points in adult life.[15]

## ■ VASCULAR OR ANGIOBLASTIC TISSUE

The earliest blood vessels are derived from angioblastic tissue, which differentiates from the mesenchyme in three regions: (1) the surface of the yolk sac; (2) the body of the stalk; and (3) the chorion.[16,17] In the yolk sac and base of the body stalk, small, more or less spherical groups of cells are found early in the third week of gestation. These are termed *blood islands*. Most believe that the peripheral cells of the islands become flattened and form the vascular endothelium, while the central cells convert into primitive red blood cells. Later, these small blood-containing spaces form a continuous network of small vessels.

All blood vessels, even the largest arteries and veins, begin as simple endothelial capillaries. The growth and differentiation of vessels can be observed in the living state in the developing limb buds or tails of tadpoles. A capillary plexus develops in a series of arcades from which new sprouts continuously grow into developing tissues. Certain vessels carrying an inflow of blood enlarge, acquire muscular coats by differentiation of smooth muscle fibers from surrounding mesenchymal cells, and become arteries. Other vessels with a return blood flow enlarge and become veins. By the end of the fourth week of gestation, as the rest of the body grows, the vascular system extends and undergoes increasing elaboration.

## ■ LYMPHATICS

The development of the lymphatics has always been a controversial topic. Sabin[18] and Lewis[19] believed them to be the outgrowths of a developing venous system. Other embryologists have theorized that the lymphatics develop in the local tissues by the confluence of mesenchymal spaces. In the human embryo of two to four months, the lymphatics of the neck, mediastinum, and retroperitoneum are large, easily definable, thin-walled vessels.

## ■ MUSCULAR TISSUE

### SMOOTH MUSCLE

Smooth muscle differentiates in situ from the mesenchyme surrounding the particular organ. This shows condensation and orientation of elongated cells in specific directions, circular or longitudinal with respect to the axis of the viscus or the vessel. As early as the sixth week, this process is evident in the walls of the intestine and many other viscera, but myogenesis from mesenchyme continues throughout the greater part of fetal life.[15]

## SKELETAL MUSCLE

Most of the classic writings on the embryology of the skeletal musculature assert that all somatic muscles, with the exception of certain muscles of the head and neck (which develop from branchial mesenchyme) and the limb muscles (which develop in situ from the mesenchyme of the limb buds), are derived from myotomes. Each myotome divides into dorsal (epaxial) and ventral (hypaxial) regions, the former situated dorsolaterally to the developing vertebral column, and the latter migrating ventrally in the body wall or somatopleure.[20] Willis,[21] however, questioned the validity of this concept.

Using an embryonic myosin heavy chain as a differentiation marker, Schiaffino and colleagues[22] analyzed the histologic characteristics of rhabdomyosarcoma arising at different sites. According to the results of their study, it appears that some of the trunk musculature arises locally from the nonmyotonic mesenchyme. In the differentiation of striated muscle, the primitive muscle cell, the rhabdomyoblast, may arise from either the somatic or nonsomatic primitive mesenchyme. Myoblasts multiply by mitosis; further recruitment from the neighboring mesenchyme also occurs.[20] By the eighth week, however, the pale cytoplasm contains myofibrils, even with cross-striations. From the eighth week onward, rhabdomyoblasts continue to be differentiated and grow until after birth.

## ■ PERIPHERAL NERVOUS SYSTEM

The peripheral nerves and associated ganglia arise by migration of neuroblasts and the outgrowth of nerve fibers from two sources: the neural tube and the neural crest. The main contribution of the neural tube to the nervous system is the outgrowth of motor nerve fibers into the spinal and cranial nerves from neuroblasts in the basal laminae of the cord and the corresponding motor nuclei in the brain stem.

During the fourth week, the neural folds close to form the neural tube, with a longitudinal strip of special ectodermal tissue—the neural crest. The neural crest forms along the dorsal surface of the tube, between this surface and the overlying ectoderm. Its proliferating cells migrate ventrolaterally to form a large mass in each dorsolateral aspect of the neural tube from the midbrain region downward, extending caudally as the neural tube itself elongates. From this mass arise the cranial and sensory nerve ganglia, the spinal posterior root ganglia being particularly promi-

nent during the second month of gestation. Other cells migrate still further ventrally to form neuroblasts of the prevertebral and visceral autonomic ganglia, chromaffin cells of the adrenal medulla, organ of Zuckerkändl, renal and celiac ganglia, the neurilemmomal cells of Schwann, all the peripheral nerves, probably most of the melanoblasts of the skin and of the head and neck region, and possibly the branchial arch skeleton.

## ■ METAPLASIA

Metaplasia signifies transformation of an adult tissue of one kind into a differentiated tissue of another kind in response to abnormal circumstances. It is an acquired condition and must be distinguished from developmental heterotopia or heteroplasia.

Voluminous literature is available on the metaplastic formation of bone or cartilage in scars, hemorrhages, and inflammatory or degenerative lesions, but these topics will not be discussed here. Occasionally, however, such metaplastic changes may create some clinical confusion concerning the diagnosis of a given soft tissue sarcoma. Notable among these are the ossification of scars, especially in the abdominal wall, which must be distinguished from desmoids; and the various types of myositis ossificans from extraskeletal osteosarcoma and chondrosarcoma.[23–30] The capacity of ordinary connective tissue to undergo transformation into adipose tissue has often been disputed. Lipoblasts have frequently been regarded as distinctive cell types.[31] However, some authors[32,33] accept the view that fat cells can form from connective tissue. Under the influence of tumorigenesis, metaplastic changes to adipose cells are sometimes seen. Liposarcomas often contain other kinds of connective tissue; lipomatous, fibromatous, cartilaginous, and myxomatous elements often coexist in the same tumor.[34]

Three distinct questions arise regarding muscular metaplasia: (1) Can new smooth muscle fibers be formed in adult tissue by transformation of nonmuscular cells? (2) Can cross-striated muscle fibers be so formed? (3) Can smooth muscle fibers be transformed into cross-striated fibers? The formation of smooth muscle from nonmuscular tissue in the adult occurs in some cases of endometriosis and in some mixed tumors of the endometrium. Willis[35] documented several instances of metaplastic smooth muscle fibers and striated muscle fibers in neoplastic endometrial stroma. Furthermore, rhabdomyosarcomas are occasionally encountered in adults in organs that normally contain no striated muscle (e.g., breast[36,37] and lung[38–40]). In these cases, it is much more likely that aberrant differentiation has occurred in tumor cells arising from some other mesenchymal tissue than it is that the tumor has arisen from long-dormant, developmentally heterotopic rhabdomyoblasts. However, regarding the question of whether smooth muscle fibers can be transformed into striated fibers, Willis, in 1958,[35] after extensively reviewing the subject, commented, "In spite of the suggestion, based on comparative histology, that two kinds of muscle may be akin and therefore possibly interconvertible, the transformation of smooth to striated muscle remains unproven." Although this statement still holds true, the identification of various mesenchymal growth factors[6-9] and their influence on myogenesis has indicated that, under certain experimental conditions, it will be possible to demonstrate that smooth muscles can be transformed into striated muscles.

Metaplasia occurs only in proliferating cells. It is, in many cases, a form of regeneration accompanied by atypical differentiation. The multiplying cells of a regenerating tissue approach embryonic conditions, and metaplasia is evidence of resumed embryonic activity.

Fig. 2–1 summarizes the ontogenesis of soft tissue sarcomas on the basis of embryologic data of the primitive mesenchyme. Any adult component of the mesenchyme could be the primary site of a sarcoma. This common ancestry of all sarcomas obviously can create

considerable difficulty in actual histogenetic classification. The problem is worse in those instances in which metaplasia is induced in the original adult tissue by neoplastic transformation. The tumor and tumorlike conditions of the peripheral nervous tissue, in contrast, have a different ancestry and can be distinguished from mesenchymal tumors. In a number of instances, however, due to the contribution from the surrounding connective or muscle tissue, these tumors can mimic the histologic appearance of mesenchymal tumors, making the distinction between these tumors difficult. However, with the advances in immunocytochemical techniques and development of sarcoma-specific monoclonal antibodies, it has become considerably easier to classify a given sarcoma. Still, however, occasionally a tumor is encountered which is unclassifiable.

With this background, we have classified the mesenchymal tumors and tumors arising from the peripheral nervous tissue (Table 2–1, pages 17–19), based on Stout's[41,42] original classification, but with modifications in light of recent knowledge. Like most other classifications, this one has its defects, especially since, in some instances, the cell of origin of some tumors is questionable. However, the clinician can use Table 2–1 as a ready reference for the management of these tumors and tumorlike conditions.

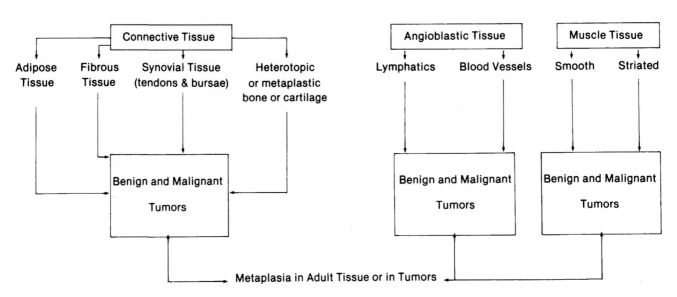

**Figure 2–1.**   Primitive mesenchyme (ontogenesis of mesenchymal sarcoma).

**TABLE 2–1. CLASSIFICATION OF SOFT TISSUE TUMORS**

| Tissue of Origin | Benign Tumors or Tumorlike Conditions | Malignant Tumors |
|---|---|---|
| **Adipose tissue** | Lipoma (cutaneous or deep)<br>Multiple lipomas<br>Angiolipoma<br>Atypical lipoma<br>Lipoblastoma<br>Hibernoma<br>Lipomatoses<br>Idiopathic lipopathies | Liposarcoma<br>Well-differentiated w/various stages of differentiation<br>Dedifferentiated<br>Myxoid<br>Round cell type (poorly differentiated)<br>Pleomorphic type |
| **Fibrous tissue** | Fibroma<br>Fibromatoses (w/all its variants)<br>Juvenile variants<br>Congenital generalized fibromatosis<br>Fibromatous coil<br>Juvenile aponeurotic fibroma<br>Angiofibroma<br>Recurring digital tumors with inclusion bodies<br>Progressive myositis<br>Adult variants<br>Keloid<br>Palmar and plantar fibromatoses<br>Penile fibromatosis<br>Idiopathic retroperitoneal fibrosis<br>Pseudosarcomatous fasciitis<br>Progressive myositis ossificans<br>Paradoxical fibrosarcoma of skin<br>Elastofibroma<br>Aggressive fibromatoses in all locations (w/ or w/o<br>associated paraneoplastic syndromes) | Fibrosarcoma (both adult and congenital or infantile types) |
| **Fibrous histiocytic tumors** | Fibrous histiocytoma (superficial and deep)<br>Juvenile xanthogranuloma<br>Reticulocytoma<br>Xanthoma<br>Intermediate (potential for local recurrence)<br>Atypical fibroxanthoma<br>Dermatofibrosarcoma protuberans<br>Giant cell fibroblastoma<br>Plexiform fibrous histiocytoma<br>Angiomatoid fibrous histiocytoma | Malignant fibrous histiocytoma with the currently<br>identified four variants (e.g., storiform, myxoid,<br>giant cell, and xanthomatous types) |

continued

**TABLE 2–1.  CLASSIFICATION OF SOFT TISSUE TUMORS** continued

| Tissue of Origin | Benign Tumors or Tumorlike Conditions | Malignant Tumors |
|---|---|---|
| **Muscle tissue** | | |
| Smooth muscle | Leiomyoma (cutaneous and deep)<br>Epithelioid leiomyoma<br>Angiomyoma<br>Leiomyomatosis | Leiomyosarcoma<br>Epithelioid leiomyosarcoma |
| Skeletal muscle | Rhabdomyoma (w/all its variants) | Rhabdomyosarcoma (w/all its variants) |
| **Neural tumors** | | |
| Tumors of schwannian origin | Schwannomas (neurilemmomas) and/or neurofibromas, solitary type with multiple phenotypic characteristics and locations<br>Similar tumors in association with generalized neurofibromatosis or other types of neurocutaneous syndromes (paraneoplastic syndromes) | Malignant schwannomas or malignant peripheral nerve sheath tumor (MPNST) (neurofibrosarcomas, solitary type) analogous to the benign counterparts, with malignant phenotypes<br>Malignant transformation in neurofibromatosis or other types of neurocutaneous syndromes<br>Malignant granular cell tumors<br>Clear cell sarcoma of tendon sheath (malignant melanoma of soft parts)<br>Malignant melanocytic schwannoma<br>Neuroepithelioma<br>Possibly extraskeletal Ewing's sarcoma |
| Non-neoplastic traumatic masses | Traumatic neuromas | |
| Tumors of sympathochromaffin axis | Ganglioneuroma (differentiated)<br>Pheochromocytomas | Malignant ganglioneuromas (ganglioneuroblastomas)<br>Neuroblastomas<br>Malignant pheochromocytomas |
| Tumors of the cartoid body and allied structures | Carotid body tumors<br>Paragangliomas | Malignant carotid body tumors<br>Malignant paragangliomas |
| **Synovial tissue** | Synovioma<br>Giant cell tumors of tendon sheath<br>Villonodular synovitis<br>Ganglions | Synovial sarcomas (all histologic types) |
| **Angiomatous tissue** | | |
| Vascular tissue | Hemangiomas (w/all the variants and locations)<br>Angiomatoses | Angiosarcoma (malignant hemangioendothelioma)<br>Kaposi's sarcoma |
| **Perivascular tumors** | Glomus tumor<br>Glomangiomyoma<br>Hemangiopericytoma<br>Lymphangioma<br>Lymphangiomyomata<br>Lymphangiomatosis | Malignant glomus tumor<br>Malignant hemangiopericytoma |
| Lymphatic tissue | | Lymphangiosarcoma |

**TABLE 2–1.** concluded

| Tissue of Origin | Benign Tumors or Tumorlike Conditions | Malignant Tumors |
|---|---|---|
| **Heterotopic bone and cartilage** | Myositis ossificans<br>Extraskeletal chondroma and osteoma | Extraskeletal osteosarcoma<br>Extraskeletal chondrosarcoma (w/all its variants) |
| **Undetermined histogenesis** | Benign mesothelioma<br>Myxoma (w/all its variants)<br>Ossifying fibromyxoid tumors<br>Mesenchymoma<br>Amyxoid tumors | Epithelioid sarcoma<br>Malignant fibrous mesothelioma<br><br>Malignant mesenchymoma<br><br>Alveolar soft part sarcoma<br>Malignant extrarenal<br>rhabdoid tumor<br>Desmoplastic small cell tumor |

## REFERENCES

1. Pack GT, Ariel IM: Tumors of the Soft Somatic Tissues. New York, Hoeber-Harper, 1958, p 44
2. Das Gupta TK, Brasfield RD: Soft tissue tumors: Classification and principles of management. Cancer 18:259, 1968
3. Schiller H: Lipomata in sarcomatous transformation. Surg Gynecol Obstet 27:218, 1918
4. Sternberg SS: Liposarcoma arising within subcutaneous lipoma. Cancer 5:975, 1952
5. Wander JV, Das Gupta TK: Neurofibromatosis. In Ravitch MM, Austin WG, Scott HW Jr., et al. (eds): Current Problems in Surgery, vol 14. Chicago, Year Book Medical Publishers, 1977
6. Bard J: Morphogenesis: The cellular and molecular processes of developmental anatomy. Cambridge, England, Cambridge University Press, 1990
7. Montesano R, Matsumoto K, Nakamura T, Orci L: Identification of a fibroblast-derived epithelial morphogen as hepatocyte growth factor. Cell 67:901, 1991
8. Montesano R, Shaller G, Orci L: Induction of epithelial tubular morphogenesis in vitro by fibroblast-derived soluble factors. Cell 66:697, 1991
9. Gumbiner BM: Epithelial morphogenesis. Cell 69:385, 1992
10. Shaw HB: A contribution to the study of the morphology of adipose tissue. J Anat Physiol 36:1, 1902
11. Keman JD Jr.: The chondrocranium of a 20-mm human embryo. J Morphol 27:605, 1916
12. Black BM: The prenatal incidence, structure, and development of some human synovial bursae. Anat Rec 60:333, 1934
13. Gray DJ, Gardner E: Prenatal development of the human knee and superior tibiofibular joints. Am J Anat 86:235, 1950
14. Gray DJ, Gardner E: Prenatal development of the human elbow joint. Am J Anat 88:429, 1951
15. Willis RA: The Borderland of Embryology and Pathology. London, Butterworth, 1958, p 54
16. Bloom W, Bartelmez GW: Hematopoiesis in young human embryos. Am J Anat 67:21, 1940
17. Hertig AT: Angiogenesis in the early human chorion and in the primary placenta of the macaque monkey. Contr Embryo 25:37, 1935
18. Sabin FR: On the origin of the lymphatic system from the veins and the development of the lymph hearts and thoracic duct of the pig. Am J Anat 1:367, 1902
19. Lewis FT: The development of the lymphatic system in rabbits. Am J Anat 5:95, 1906
20. Warwick R, Williams PL (eds): Gray's Anatomy, 35th ed. London, Longman, 1973, p 124
21. Willis RA: The Borderland of Embryology and Pathology. London, Butterworth, 1958, p 410
22. Schiaffino S, Gorza L, Sartore S, et al.: Embryonic myosin heavy chain as a differentiation marker of developing human skeletal muscle and rhabdomyosarcoma. Exp Cell Res 163:211, 1986
23. Nicholson GW: Heteromorphoses in the human body. Guy's Hosp Rep 71:75, 1922
24. Nicholson GW: Studies on tumour formation: Acquired tissue malformations. Guy's Hosp Rep 72:402, 1922
25. Keith A: Concerning the origin and nature of osteoblasts. Proc R Soc Med 21:1, 1927
26. von Seeman H: Uber die Entstehungsbedingungen metaplastischer Knochenbildungen. Dtsch Z Chir 217:60, 1927
27. Huggins CB: The formation of bone under the influence of epithelium of the urinary tract. Arch Surg 22:377, 1931
28. Huggins CB: The phosphatase activity of transplants of the epithelium of the urinary bladder to the abdominal wall producing heterotopic ossification. Biochem J 25 (pt 1):728, 1931
29. Lloyd-Williams IH: On a case of bony plaques developing in the skin. Br Med J 2:1055, 1929
30. Huggins CB, McCarroll HR, Blocksom BH Jr.: Experiments on the theory of osteogenesis: The influence of local calcium deposits on ossification; the osteogenic stimulus of epithelium. Arch Surg 32:915, 1936
31. Cameron GR, Seneviratne RD: Growth and repair in adipose tissue. J Pathol Bact 59:665, 1947
32. Flemming W: Weitere Mittheilungen zur Physiologie der Fettzelle. Arch Mikv Anat 7:328, 1871
33. Clark ER, Clark EL: Microscopic studies of the new formation of fat in living adult rabbits. Am J Anat 67:255, 1940
34. Enzinger FM, Winslow DJ: Liposarcoma. A study of 103 cases. Virchows Arch Pathol Anat 335:367, 1962
35. Willis RA: Metaplasia. The Borderland of Embryology and Pathology. London, Butterworth, 1958, p 506
36. Sailer S: Sarcoma of the breast. Am J Cancer 31:183, 1937
37. Govan ADT: Two cases of mixed malignant tumour of the breast. J Pathol Bact 57:397, 1945
38. Cumming ARR, Shillitoe AJ: Ball-valve mitral obstruction by a sarcoma of a pulmonary vein. Br Heart J 19:287, 1957
39. McDonald S Jr, Heather JC: Neoplastic invasion of the pulmonary veins and left auricle. J Pathol Bact 48:533, 1939
40. Forbes GB: Rhabdomyosarcoma of bronchus. J Pathol Bact 70:427, 1955
41. Stout AP, Ariel IM: Panel on soft-part tumors. Proc Natl Cancer Conf, 1949, p 206
42. Stout AP: Tumors of the soft tissues. In Atlas of Tumor Pathology. Sect. 2, Fasc 5. Washington DC, AFIP, 1953

# 3

# Principles of Clinical Diagnosis, Staging, and Prognosis

The accuracy of clinical diagnoses of soft tissue sarcomas is always questionable. Although lipomas whose margins apparently slip out of the examining finger are classic, occasionally liposarcomas lurk in these seemingly benign tumors. Thus, a blasé attitude is dangerous to the patient. It is essential to have a systematic approach to diagnosis and therapy of all soft tissue tumors.

The diagnosis of large ulcerating or fungating tumors (Fig. 3–1) is not difficult; problems arise, however, with the small, apparently innocuous variety. Therefore, history-taking is of utmost importance in the diagnosis and treatment of these tumors. Often the clinician is remiss in not obtaining a detailed history of the initial appearance of the tumor and its associated symptoms, which often provides clues to the diagnosis. The case histories appearing below describe classic examples. On the basis of these descriptions, it is possible to develop some general guidelines in the history-taking of soft tissue tumors.

## ■ CASE HISTORIES

**Patient 1**: A 46-year-old woman had noticed a mass in her right thigh about four to six weeks before seeking medical advice. Initially, this tumor was thought to be benign; however, she came to us for a second opinion. The relatively soft tumor in the upper anterior aspect of the thigh was found to be a liposarcoma (Fig. 3–2).

**Patient 2**: A 10-year-old girl was brought to her pediatrician with a small tumor of several weeks' duration in the right temporal region. The pediatric surgeon considered the tumor to be a sebaceous cyst. On excision, it was found to be a rhabdomyosarcoma (Fig. 3–3).

**Patient 3**: A 58-year-old woman was seen with a slowly enlarging tumor in her arm (Fig. 3–4), which had been present for several years without causing any difficulty. The patient previously sought the advice of another physician, but since it was a symptomless mass, no further investigation had been undertaken. Detailed history-taking and clinical examination, however, showed that she had type 1 neurofibromatosis. Because of this association, an incisional biopsy was performed, and the diagnosis of neurofibrosarcoma was established.

**Patient 4**: A 51-year-old man complained that he had had perineal pain radiating to the medial aspect of both thighs for about two years. A careful urologic examination, including cystoscopy, failed to show any abnormalities in the urethra, prostate, or urinary bladder. The patient was diagnosed with pudendal neuralgia. However, after two years, a small tumor in the perineum could be palpated, and an x-ray of the pelvis showed complete destruction of the inferior pubic ramus of the left side (Fig. 3–5). A wedge specimen was taken and microscopic examination established this tumor as a hemangiopericytoma.

**Patient 5**: A 21-year-old man was seen by his physician for a tender swelling of the right buttock. He related that he had sustained a trauma while playing basketball a few weeks prior to his visit. A diagnosis of infected hematoma of the right buttock was made, and the patient was treated with antibiotics. When the mass did not subside, it was incised for adequate drainage. Following this procedure, the tumor fungated out through the wound. An histologic examination established a diagnosis of rhabdomyosarcoma (Fig. 3–6).

**Patient 6**: A skin tumor was noted in the area of the knee joint of a 41-year-old man. The patient was diagnosed with pyogenic granuloma and was treated with antibiotics (Fig. 3–7). When the lesion was found to be

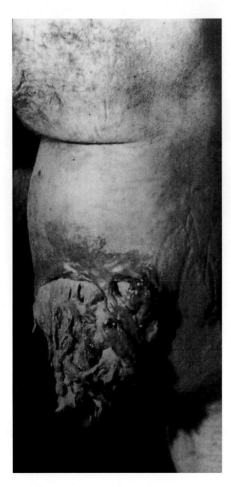

**Figure 3–1.** Fungating tumor in the right posterior thigh of a 55-year-old man. Tumor was subcutaneous for two to three years, then started to grow, but the patient did not seek medical attention until the lesion fungated. Microscopic diagnosis of liposarcoma was established.

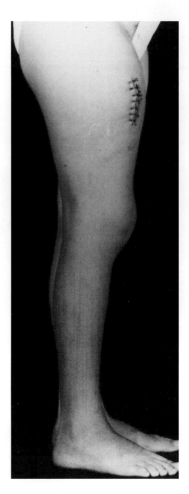

**Figure 3–2.** Tumor in the right thigh of a 46-year-old woman. The mass clinically measured 5 × 8 cm, was relatively soft, and appeared to be a benign lipoma. A wedge biopsy showed it to be a liposarcoma.

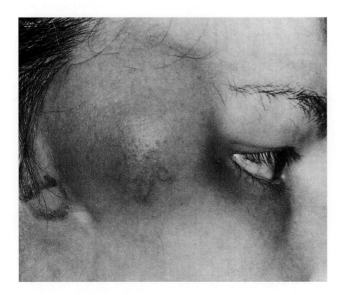

**Figure 3–3.** Close-up view of tumor in right temple of a 10-year-old girl. A glistening of the overlying skin surface can be easily seen. The tumor was found to be a rhabdomyosarcoma.

refractory to conservative treatment, the patient was referred to the University of Illinois Hospital. A wedge biopsy specimen showed the tumor to be a dermatofibrosarcoma protuberans.

**Patient 7**: A four-month-old male infant was found to have a small tumor in the region of the medial malleolus of the right foot. The tumor was excised elsewhere and the patient was diagnosed with fibrosarcoma. On the basis of this diagnosis, a wide excision or an amputation was contemplated. The parents, seeking a second opinion, were referred to the University of Illinois Hospital. They related that the nodule in that area was about 1 cm in diameter when first discovered and had remained mobile for several weeks prior to its relatively rapid increase in size. A clinical diagnosis of fibromatosis was made, which was later confirmed by several pathologists. The child was spared from an extensive operation, since this type of fibromatosis is self-limiting (Fig. 3–8).

These above-mentioned case histories illustrate the basic concept that, as in other disease processes, a thor-

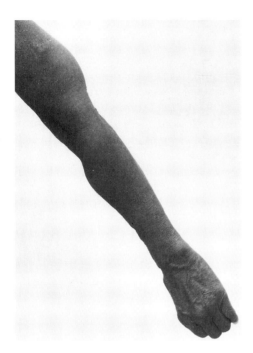

**Figure 3–4.** Tumor of the left arm in a 58-year-old woman. Because of multiple café-au-lait spots on anterior chest wall and posterior trunk, a detailed family history was obtained. Stigmata of type 1 neurofibromatosis were found in patient's siblings and parents. A wedge biopsy of the tumor showed that the tumor was indeed a malignant peripheral nerve sheath tumor (MPNST).

ough clinical history frequently leads to accurate diagnosis. In general, the following guidelines can be used as identifiable clues for the diagnosis of soft tissue sarcomas:

1. A rapid-growing solitary soft tissue tumor in persons who are over forty should be considered with suspicion.
2. A tumor of short duration located in the upper aspect of the thigh, especially in a woman, should be considered malignant until proven otherwise.
3. Although exceptions are occasionally seen, the existence of multiple lipomas in general precludes the possibility of a malignant adipose tissue tumor.
4. Subcutaneous tumors in the head and neck region of a child should be carefully examined to rule out a malignant tumor.
5. All retroperitoneal tumors should be considered sarcomas until proven otherwise.
6. A tumor larger than 10 cm should arouse suspicion of malignancy.
7. An unexplained buttock mass in an adult should be assumed to be a tumor, and injudicious incision and drainage should be avoided even when it resembles an inflammatory mass.

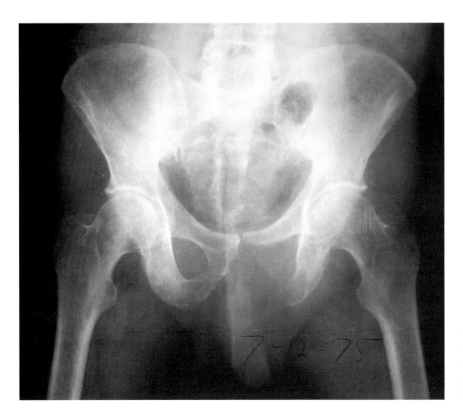

**Figure 3–5.** Roentgenograph of the pelvis of a 51-year-old man showing bony destruction of left inferior ramus of the pubis. This soft tissue mass was revealed on wedge biopsy to be a hemangiopericytoma arising in the perineum.

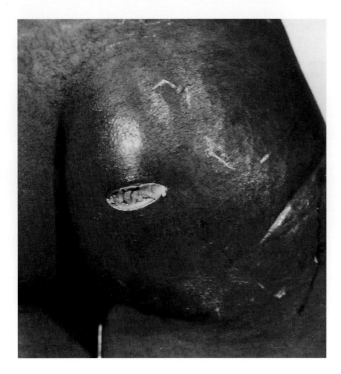

**Figure 3–6.** Large tumor of right buttock of a 21-year-old man, with diagnosis of abscess of the buttock. Two incisions were made. Through one of these incisions, the underlying tumor can be seen to protrude. Because the huge fungating tumor was refractory to radiation therapy, the patient underwent a hemipelvectomy, but died two years later with diffuse metastasis.

8. Soft tissue sarcomas are frequently associated with certain preneoplastic disease states, such as type 1 neurofibromatosis, Gardner's syndrome, and several other varieties of neurocutaneous or mucocutaneous syndromes.

9. In children, small tumors in the distal ends of the extremities are usually benign, and great caution should be taken before any radical therapy is undertaken.

10. Almost all angiomatous tumors in children are benign (Fig. 3–9).

11. The persistence of unexplained pain along the course of one or more major peripheral nerves should be viewed with suspicion, since occasionally pain is caused by a malignant tumor pressing on or infiltrating the fibers of a peripheral nerve or a plexus. Malignant peripheral nerve sheath tumors have frequently been missed because such complaints of pain were not investigated thoroughly. This symptom occurs with all types of cancer and is not produced by soft tissue sarcomas only.

The clinical examination of a patient with a soft tissue tumor likewise must be thorough. A description of systemic examination that is not directly related to the given tumor will not be discussed in this chapter. The focus of this chapter will be on the examination of the primary tumor, the anatomic region in which the tumor is located, and any other associated conditions.

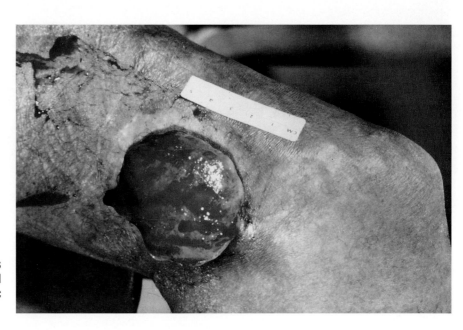

**Figure 3–7.** Dermatofibrosarcoma protuberans in the region of the knee joint of a 41-year-old man. The mass was thought to be a pyogenic granuloma.

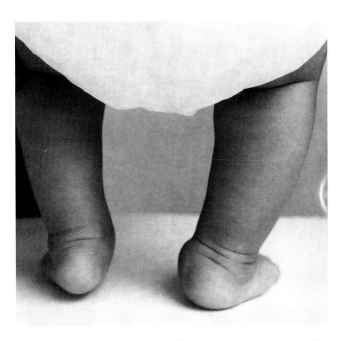

**Figure 3–8.** Posterior view of the ankles of a four-month-old boy. The medial swelling of the right ankle is easily apparent, compared with the left medial aspect. Parents stated that the tumor was discrete at first, then became diffuse.

## ■ CLINICAL EXAMINATION OF THE PRIMARY TUMOR

Examination of the primary tumor, with a clear, concise, and accurate description of the clinical features, is absolutely essential. Failure to do this frequently results in an incorrect assessment. Often, the microscopic description with accurate histologic diagnosis is missed because the clinician failed to examine the primary tumor thoroughly or record the findings meticulously. Clinical examination of the primary tumor can be performed with an cyc toward the following six factors.

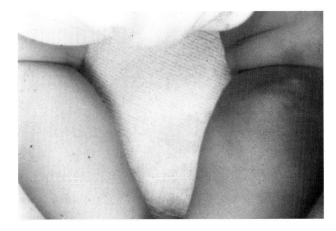

**Figure 3–9.** A localized cavernous hemangioma of the right leg in a six-month-old infant. This type of angioma does not need any treatment unless symptomatic.

## LOCATION

The location of the primary tumor should be ascertained. First, determine the broad anatomic location, that is, whether it is in the head and neck region or the trunk or extremities. Next, determine the specific location in the general anatomic region. A tumor located in the temporal area or in the region of the outer canthus of the eye or along the lateral margin of the nose should arouse suspicion of a rhabdomyosarcoma, especially in a young adult. A lesion located in the upper inner aspect of the thigh has a high possibility of being a sarcoma. Furthermore, especially in the extremities, the prognosis for a patient with a given sarcoma has been linked with whether the tumor is superficial (subcutaneous) or deep (intermuscular or deeper). Generally, the more superficial the tumor, the better the prognosis.[1,2]

## SHAPE

The shape of the primary tumor frequently indicates the type of sarcoma. A malignant tumor of a peripheral nerve usually grows in its long axis and frequently appears as a fusiform mass. A lipoma or a liposarcoma can assume any shape or size (Fig. 3–10) because adipose tissue has more freedom to expand. More commonly a large, round subcutaneous mass is either a lipoma or a liposarcoma. A fibrous tissue tumor usually is ovoid.

## SIZE

Although the size of a given primary tumor usually does not indicate either benignity or malignancy, an accurate documentation of its size is desirable. If the tumor is malignant, then its size helps in the clinicopathologic staging in a given anatomic location. The size of the primary tumor also indicates the most practical type of primary therapy to be instituted. For example, a 2-cm liposarcoma located in the upper outer aspect of the thigh can be adequately treated with wide soft tissue resection; in contrast, a 15-cm liposarcoma in the same location might require a much larger operation, or radiation, or both. Although size alone should not be the determining factor, tumors larger than 10 cm frequently are malignant (Fig. 3–10). Within the same histologic type, malignant tumors measuring less than 5 cm carry a better prognosis for the patient.[2–5]

## CONSISTENCY

The consistency of a primary tumor can frequently lead to a correct clinical assessment. For example, a lipoma is uniformly soft, whereas a liposarcoma can be distinguished by its areas of relatively firm consistency, even though the tumor appears soft on first examination. A uniformly firm or hard soft tissue tumor should be considered malignant, irrespective of its size or location.

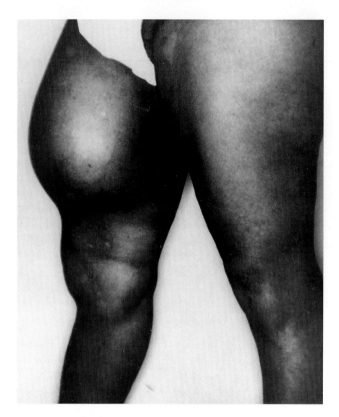

**Figure 3–10.** A large tumor in the anterolateral aspect of the right thigh. The size itself is an indication of possible malignancy (i.e., more than 10 cm). Incision biopsy confirmed diagnosis of liposarcoma. *(Reproduced with permission from Das Gupta TK: Tumors and Tumorlike Conditions of the Adipose Tissue. In Ravitch MM, et al. (eds):* Current Problems in Surgery. *Copyright 1970 by Year Book Medical Publishers, Inc., Chicago.)*

## RELATION TO SURROUNDING TISSUES

It is essential that the clinician evaluate the relationship of a primary tumor to the surrounding adipose tissue, muscles, nerves, major vessels, and bones. This information is not only useful in proper staging but also helps the histologist to arrive at a correct microscopic diagnosis. For example, a tumor consisting of spindle-shaped malignant cells may be designated as spindle cell sarcoma. However, if it is known that the tumor arose from a peripheral nerve or was intimately adherent to the nerve, it is highly likely that this tumor is of neural origin.

Currently, routine use of magnetic resonance (MR) imaging of presumed malignant mesenchymal tumors allows the clinician to reasonably identify the tissue of origin and the extent of the tumor (see Chapter 4 for details). When the detailed morphological findings (i.e., immunocytochemical and/or ultrastructural) of the biopsy specimen are added to the extant data, in most instances, an accurate pretreatment diagnosis can be established. In staging, the relationship of

the surrounding structures is used for T-classification. If a tumor invades the major vessels or the bones, it is classified as $T_3$, indicating a relatively poor prognosis.

## REGIONAL NODES

Soft tissue sarcomas do not metastasize in large numbers to the regional nodes.[6] However, because some do, it is essential that regional nodes be examined in every case of suspected soft tissue sarcoma.

## ■ ASSOCIATED PRENEOPLASTIC OR HAMARTOMATOUS SYNDROMES

Both benign and malignant soft tissue tumors are sometimes associated with preneoplastic or hamartomatous syndromes. For example, a patient with multiple café-au-lait spots presenting with a subcutaneous mass probably has either a benign or malignant neurogenic tumor. An overview of the relationship of these hamartomatous syndromes to soft tissue sarcomas is discussed in the section dealing with epidemiology. The individual syndromes are separately discussed along with those tumors with which they are primarily associated.

## GENERAL EXAMINATION OF THE PATIENT

Following assessment of the primary tumor and any associated conditions, the overall status of the patient should be evaluated, including any preexisting cardiovascular and/or pulmonary problems. Other systemic diseases such as diabetes should also be taken into consideration. Since benign soft tissue tumors far outnumber sarcomas (except in the retroperitoneal region), in most instances, a biopsy should be performed before undertaking an expensive general workup. If the clinicopathologic examination suggests sarcoma, then a complete metastatic workup germane to the histogenetic type of primary tumor should be instituted.

## DIAGNOSTIC AIDS IN SOFT TISSUE TUMORS

Diagnostic aids commonly used to evaluate primary soft tissue tumors can be classified as follows: (1) roentgenologic examinations, (2) radioisotope methods, and (3) biochemical tests. Since the advent of the computed tomography (CT) scan and magnetic resonance imaging (MRI), the radiologic evaluation of soft tissue tumors has undergone revolutionary changes. The art and science of radiological diagnosis of soft tissue sarcomas has advanced so much that a separate chapter is dedicated to this topic (see Chapter 4). Routine plain x-ray of soft tissue tumor has very limited usefulness, but in some cases may resolve some diagnostic riddles (Figs. 3–11 and 3–12).[7,8]

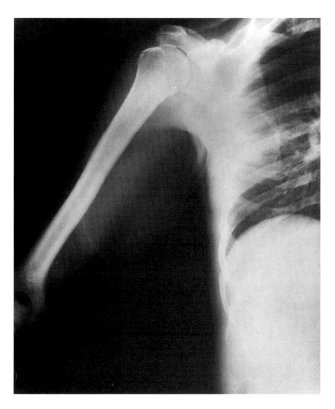

**Figure 3–11.** A large tumor of the medial aspect of the arm of a 60-year-old man. Roentgenogram of this smooth fatty tumor was suggestive of a lipoma, and excision substantiated the diagnosis.

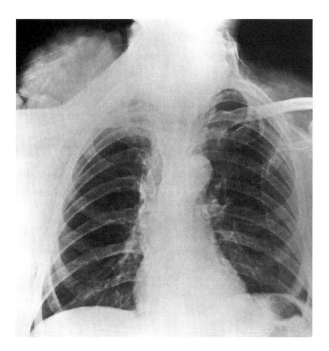

**Figure 3–12.** A multilobulated tumor in the right side of the neck and the shoulder of a 55-year-old man. Roentgenographic examination suggested a malignant fatty tumor (liposarcoma), which was later substantiated by a wedge biopsy.

### Biochemical Tests

Biochemical tests for the diagnosis of soft tissue tumors or sarcomas in general are not specific. In certain sarcomas, prognosis appears to be correlated with local tumor tissue alkaline phosphatase activity. However, at present, these tests have no clinical significance.

Investigations of steroid receptors, fibroblast growth factor, epidermal growth factor, and nerve growth factor in soft tissue tumors are being performed in several laboratories. Similarly, a number of molecular prognostic markers are also being investigated to ascertain whether any of these singly or in combination would help assess either the aggressiveness of the primary sarcoma(s) or the overall influence in survival of patients with soft tissue sarcomas (see Chapter 6 for details).

## ■ MORPHOLOGIC DIAGNOSIS OF SOFT TISSUE TUMORS

The most accurate diagnostic method for establishing the identity and nature of a soft tissue tumor is the microscopic examination of either the entire tumor or a representative portion. Undue haste in establishing a pathologic diagnosis is not only unnecessary but occasionally detrimental to the best interest of the patient. In view of the rarity of soft tissue sarcomas, hasty decisions based on either frozen sections or on an aspiration biopsy are seldom justified, and there is considerable evidence against making such a decision.

The methods used for histologic diagnosis of soft tissue tumors are the following: (1) fine-needle aspiration biopsy, (2) core-needle biopsy, (3) excision biopsy, and (4) incision (wedge) biopsy.

### FINE-NEEDLE ASPIRATION BIOPSY

Fine-needle aspiration biopsy of soft tissue tumors is an accepted diagnostic method in some institutions.[9] In this technique, the clinician infiltrates an appropriate area of skin over the tumor with 1 percent plain Xylocaine. Following achievement of local anesthesia, the tumor is held between the index finger and thumb of one hand, and a long, fine 19g needle attached to a 5-cc syringe, mounted on an aspiration gun, is introduced into the tumor. Constant pressure must be maintained while the gun is manipulated up and down several times so that an adequate number of cells are aspirated. The aspirate is then smeared on glass slides, fixed with preservative, and stained. In larger tumors, the site for obtaining the aspirate depends on the clinician's experience. In general, firm or hard areas should be aspirated. It is essential to recognize that, after placing the needle in the desired area, a constant aspiration pressure must be applied for two to three minutes, with movements in the depth and direction of the needle. The success of fine-needle aspiration biopsy in obtaining sufficient numbers of identifiable cells depends entirely on the aggressiveness and experience of the individual performing the biopsy.

## CORE-NEEDLE BIOPSY

Core-needle biopsy is essentially the same technique as that for aspiration biopsy, the difference being that, instead of a fine needle, a Trucut needle is used to obtain a core of tissue. The area of biopsy is cleaned with an antiseptic, which is followed by infiltration of 1 percent Xylocaine in a small area of overlying skin. Then a 2.0- to 3.0-mm incision is made on the skin at the intended position of introduction of the needle. The needle with overlying sheath is placed just beyond the periphery of the mass, and the central needle is advanced into the mass while the position of the outer sheath is held steady. Following this procedure, the position of the central needle is stabilized, and the outer sheath is advanced over the needle. Then both needles with the sheaths over them are withdrawn simultaneously. This usually gives a 1.5- to 2.0-cm long and 2-mm wide core of tissue. The tissue is then processed for normal histologic examination. Currently, various types of "core-biopsy needles" are available; the clinician should choose the one most suitable for the type of tumor to be biopsied.

This method of needle biopsy, although used in some centers, is not always the most suitable technique for histologic diagnosis of soft tissue tumors. The limitations of this method are the following: (1) only a small piece of tissue is obtained, and it frequently is not a representative area of the tumor; and (2) the relative rarity of these tumors will prevent most pathologists from arriving at a correct diagnosis from this small specimen, even though it may contain the most representative area of a given tumor.

## EXCISION BIOPSY

Excision biopsy is the most commonly used method of morphologic diagnosis. In relatively small soft tissue tumors, it is appropriate to perform an excision of the tumor with local anesthesia. The detailed technical aspects are discussed in Chapter 16. It is essential that the surgeon be careful to observe the location of the tumor and its relation to surrounding structures such as muscle, fibrous tissue, vessels, and nerves. All this information is used in the clinicopathologic staging and prognostication. Although most soft tissue tumors are benign (e.g., lipomas) and frequently can be diagnosed macroscopically, it is still, however, advisable that the final diagnosis be rendered after microscopic examination of the tissues.

## INCISION (WEDGE) BIOPSY

When the tumor is relatively large and there is clinical suspicion that it might be malignant, an incision biopsy is certainly justified. In this method, which is very similar to the method of excision biopsy, an appropriate area of skin overlying the tumor is anesthetized with 1 percent Xylocaine. An incision is made, and a representative wedge of the tumor is excised. It is essential that a large wedge of the tumor be removed from the area most likely to yield the best information. This method has the theoretic disadvantage of cutting into the tumor with resultant spillage of tumor cells; however, if definitive therapy is instituted within one to two weeks of biopsy, no untoward effect has as yet been demonstrated either in terms of longevity, fungation, or local recurrence.

The biopsy material obtained by the aspiration technique, although having the distinct advantage of being the least traumatic and possibly providing an immediate diagnosis, has the major disadvantage of being unreliable. The same criticism is leveled against a core-needle biopsy of soft tissue sarcomas, albeit this method has found renewed use in a variety of other tumors. In centers in which there is a concentration of patients with soft tissue sarcomas, these two methods are routinely being used.

Most patients with soft tissue tumors, therefore, have either an excisional or an incisional biopsy diagnosis. Once the specimen is obtained, it is sometimes possible to immediately freeze a portion and obtain a histologic diagnosis. Simultaneously, definitive therapy can then be recommended. However, in most instances, it is extremely difficult to arrive at an accurate histogenetic diagnosis from examination of the frozen sections. Because of this disadvantage, it is recommended that the specimen thus obtained be divided into three parts. The first part is frozen, and cryostat sections are studied to inform the clinician, if possible, whether the tumor is malignant. If the tumor is obviously benign, then appropriate treatment can be immediately instituted. However, if the tumor is malignant, all attempts to arrive at a definitive diagnosis should be avoided until further study. The second part of the specimen should be processed for conventional light microscopy and immunohistochemistry, and the third part for electron microscopy. Currently, immunocytochemistry has in general replaced the necessity of routine ultrastructural examination of soft tissue sarcomas, but in certain instances, ultrastructural examination is still of immense importance. In most large centers, it is possible to obtain an accurate diagnosis within the first seven days after biopsy. However, if such facilities are not available, it is most appropriate to await consultation with other pathologists and oncologists before any therapeutic decision is undertaken. This delay of a few days does not jeopardize the patient's condition in any way, but instead provides the patient with the maximum therapeutic advantage.

Once a diagnosis of sarcoma is made, the patient must be assessed for metastatic status before definitive therapy for the primary tumor is recommended. Evaluation of the metastatic status depends on the natural history of the specific sarcoma. Most sarcomas have similar patterns of metastatic spread; however, some have specific characteristics. The general workup to determine metastases will be described in the following section; the detailed points regarding specific sarcomas will be discussed in chapters dealing with individual types of tumor.

## ■ GENERAL WORKUP TO DETERMINE METASTASES

The lung is the most common site of metastases from any sarcoma, and the presence of pulmonary metastases must be excluded before any therapy. Small metastatic nodules are often missed in a normal chest x-ray; therefore, a CT scan should be obtained to evaluate for pulmonary and subpleural metastasis. Details on the role of CT scan and MRI are outlined in Chapter 4.

### SCINTIGRAPHY

Investigation with scintigraphy is indicated for evaluation of the liver, brain, and skeletal system. Radionuclide scan of the liver and brain has been largely replaced by CT scan or MRI for greater accuracy. However, it appears that, in the future, imaging with radio-labeled monoclonal antibodies will be of value in detecting occult metastases (see Chapter 20).

Bone remains an infrequent site of metastasis from soft tissue sarcoma. However, certain histologic types such as angiosarcoma may have somewhat higher incidence of bone metastasis; thus, bone scan may be of value in selected cases. Soft somatic tissue tumors, once they are apparent, can be classified as benign or malignant, and the histogenetic type can be properly ascertained in most instances. After the histologic diagnosis is made and the patient adequately evaluated for evidence of metastatic disease, the tumor should be staged.

## ■ STAGING OF SARCOMAS

Soft tissue sarcomas and all the variants thereof should be staged clinicopathologically to adequately assess the mode of treatment and for reporting the end result. Staging methods have varied over the years. The American Joint Committee for Cancer Staging and End-Result Reporting[3] published a minimally acceptable staging method. Although open to considerable criticism, it nevertheless offers a guideline for staging soft tissue sarcomas.

The Soft Tissue Task Force in 1977 proposed the staging system based on the size of tumor and the involvement of the tumor with major vessels, nerves, and bones (T-category); grade of tumor (G-category) in a three-grade system (from cellularity, extent of necrosis, pleomorphism, and mitosis); involvement of lymph nodes (N-category); and presence or absence of metastasis (M-category). This staging system was reviewed, refined, and widely accepted by the International Committee on Soft Tissue Sarcoma Staging.

Among all the parameters for staging the soft tissue tumor, probably the estimation of the grade of the lesion has the most variability. Not only do pathologists differ among the classification of the grade (two-grade, three-grade, or four-grade systems); the parameters considered for determination of grade also vary considerably. These parameters include cellular differentiation, pleomorphism, necrosis, and mitotic count.

In a two-grade system, the tumor is classified as low grade or high grade. This results in a practical problem of classifying a large group of tumors which are neither clearly low grade nor clearly high grade. As such, mostly these tumors are graded either low or high.

In a four-grade system, grade 3 and 4 lesions are considered high grade. By definition, some tumor subtypes are usually considered low grade and others high grade. A third histologic group can be either low or high grade, and, as such, a specific grade in this group must be decided before any therapy is initiated. Table 3–1 shows the usual grades for histologic subtypes.

The international classification for staging of soft tissue sarcoma is based on the TNM classification, adopted from the staging system of soft tissue sarcoma by the Soft Tissue Task Force, and is currently most widely used. The details of this staging system are described below.

### PRIMARY SITE

The exact location of the tumor, its depth from the skin surface, its size, and its relation to the surrounding structures require accurate estimates. This information constitutes the T-classification. This is best accomplished after an MR examination of a given primary tumor whenever possible (see Chapter 4 for details).

### REGIONAL NODES

The lymph node basin relates to the site of origin of the sarcoma and any of the major lymph node compartments that may be at risk (N-classification).

**TABLE 3–1. CORRELATION BETWEEN HISTOLOGIC TYPE AND GRADE OF SOFT TISSUE SARCOMA**

| Mostly Low Grade | Mostly High Grade | May be Either High Grade or Low Grade |
|---|---|---|
| Desmoid | Synovial sarcoma | Fibrosarcoma |
| Dermatofibrosarcoma protuberans | Rhabdomyosarcoma | Leiomyosarcoma |
| Kaposi's sarcoma (non AIDS-related) | Angiosarcoma | Hemangiopericytoma |
| Well-differentiated liposarcoma | Lymphangiosarcoma | |
| Myxoid liposarcoma | Round cell liposarcoma | |
| Alveolar soft part sarcoma | Pleomorphic liposarcoma | |
| | Extraosseous osteosarcoma | |
| | Extraosseous chondrosarcoma | |
| | Extraosseous Ewing's sarcoma | |
| | Malignant fibrous histiocytoma | |
| | Malignant peripheral nerve sheath tumors associated with type 1 neurofibromatosis | |

## METASTATIC SITE

The lung is the most common metastatic site of involvement, but a large variety of other viscera may also be invaded, such as bone, liver, brain, and so forth (M-classification).

## HISTOLOGIC CLASSIFICATION

Determination of the histogenesis of a given tumor (see Table 2–1, Chapter 2) is of primary importance.[3] Once the histologic type is established, the tumor should be graded according to the accepted criteria for malignancy, including cellularity, cellular pleomorphism, and mitotic activity (Figure 3–13A to 3–13D). The tumor grades (G-classification) are expressed as follows:

| | |
|---|---|
| $G_1$ | Well-differentiated |
| $G_2$ | Moderately well-differentiated |
| $G_3$ to $G_4$ | Poorly to very poorly differentiated (undifferentiated) |

Some tumors are highly malignant, regardless of their cellular differentiation, and should be classified as $G_3$; for example, rhabdomyosarcoma in adults, certain types of angiosarcomas, and synovial sarcoma. The currently accepted TNM classification is as follows:

Primary Tumor (T)

| | |
|---|---|
| $T_x$ | Minimum requirements cannot be met |
| $T_0$ | No demonstrable tumor(s) |
| $T_1$ | Less than 5 cm in maximum diameter |
| $T_2$ | Tumor 5 cm or greater in diameter |
| $T_3$ | Tumor showing macroscopic invasion of the surrounding bone, major vessels, or |

major nerves (See Chapter 4 for details regarding the methods of obtaining this information.)

Nodal status (N)

| | |
|---|---|
| $N_x$ | Minimum requirements cannot be met |
| $N_0$ | No histologically verified metastases to regional nodes |
| $N_1$ | Histologically verified regional node metastases |

Distant Metastases (M)

| | |
|---|---|
| $M_x$ | Not assessed |
| $M_0$ | No known distant metastases |
| $M_1$ | Distant metastases present (specific site) |

Specific site according to the following notation:

| | |
|---|---|
| Lung | PUL |
| Osseous | OSS |
| Hepatic | HEP |
| Brain | BRA |
| Lymph nodes | LYM |
| Bone marrow | MAR |
| Pleura | PLE |
| Skin | SKI |
| Eye | EYE |
| Other | OTH |

Following therapeutic excision of the primary tumor, a postsurgical residual tumor reclassification is also indicated.

| | |
|---|---|
| $R_0$ | No residual tumor |
| $R_1$ | Microscopic residual tumor |
| $R_2$ | Macroscopic residual tumor |

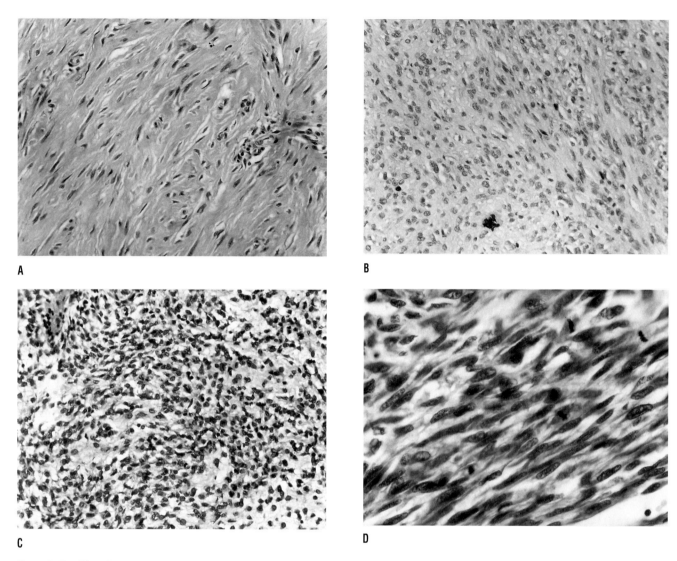

**Figure 3–13. (A)** Well-differentiated fibrosarcoma ($G_1$). (H & E. Original magnification $\times$ 250.) **(B)** Moderately well-differentiated fibrosarcoma ($G_2$). (H & E. Original magnification $\times$ 250.) **(C)** Poorly differentiated or undifferentiated fibrosarcoma ($G_3$ or $G_4$). (H & E. Original magnification $\times$ 250.) **(D)** High-power magnification of a poorly differentiated fibrosarcoma. (H & E. Original magnification $\times$ 250.) The distinction between $G_3$ and $G_4$ is sometimes extremely difficult.

The clinicopathologic information described above helps in staging soft tissue sarcomas. The proposed staging is shown below:

Stage Grouping

Stage I:    $I_A$ $G_1$ $T_1$ $N_0$ $M_0$
Grade 1 tumor, less than 5 cm in diameter with no regional lymph nodal or distant metastases
$I_B$ $G_1$ $T_2$ $N_0$ $M_0$
Grade 1 tumor, 5 cm or greater in diameter with no regional lymph nodal or distant metastases

Stage II:    $II_A$ $G_2$ $T_1$ $N_0$ $M_0$
Grade 2 tumor, less than 5 cm in diameter with no regional lymph nodal or distant metastases

$II_B$ $G_2$ $T_2$ $N_0$ $M_0$
Grade 2 tumor, 5 cm or greater in diameter with no regional lymph nodal or distant metastases

Stage III:    $III_A$ $G_3$ $T_1$ $N_0$ $M_0$
Grade 3 tumor, less than 5 cm in diameter with no regional lymph nodal or distant metastases
$III_B$ $G_3$ $T_2$ $N_0$ $M_0$
Grade 3 tumor, 5 cm or greater in diameter with no regional lymph nodal or distant metastases
$III_C$ Any G $T_{1,2}$ $N_1$ $M_0$
Tumor of any histologic grade or size (no invasion), with regional lymph node metastases but without distant metastases

Stage IV: IV$_A$ Any G T$_3$ Any N M$_0$

Tumor of any histologic grade of malignancy that grossly invades bone, major vessels, or major nerves with or without regional lymph node metastases but without distant metastases

IV$_B$ Any G Any T Any N M$_1$

Tumor with distant metastases

Obviously, the staging system described above is cumbersome. However, it should form the basis for a more practical staging system classifying the primary tumors, local extension, histologic type, grade, and regional and extraregional metastatic status. It appears that, if all patients with soft tissue sarcomas are assessed accordingly, the end-result reporting following one or the other form of treatment program can be properly evaluated among the various groups.

From the experience with soft tissue sarcoma at Memorial Sloan-Kettering Hospital, Hajdu[10] has proposed quite a practical system of staging. Based on size, depth of the lesion, and histologic grade (two-grade system either high or low grade), Hajdu has staged the primary sarcoma from stage 0 (with 3 good prognostic signs) to stage III (with 3 bad prognostic signs). If there is any detectable metastasis, the lesion is classified as stage IV.

Prognostic factors for Hajdu's staging system of soft tissue sarcomas are as follows: Size: less than 5 cm (good prognostic sign), more than 5 cm (bad prognostic sign); Depth: superficial to deep fascia (good prognostic sign), deep to deep fascia (bad prognostic sign); Grade: low grade (good prognostic sign), high grade (bad prognostic sign).

| | |
|---|---|
| Stage 0 | 3 good prognostic signs |
| Stage I | 2 good prognostic signs |
| | 1 bad prognostic sign |
| Stage II | 1 good prognostic sign |
| | 2+ bad prognostic signs |
| Stage III | 3+ bad prognostic signs |
| Stage IV | Patients with evidence of metastases (including regional metastases) |

The attractiveness of this staging system is in its simplicity, and, in the experience of Hajdu, the predictive outcome in such a staging system is accurate. However, the drawback of this staging system is its two-grade system and lack of universal acceptability for comparison of data from different centers.

There has been recent evidence which suggests that local recurrence does not alter the ultimate outcome in patients with soft tissue sarcomas (see section, below, on prognostic parameters); however, a staging system was missing for locally recurrent soft tissue sarcoma to predict its outcome. Recently, Chang et al.[11] outlined a staging system based on growth rate index (GRI) and the presence or absence of necrosis in the tumor.

Growth rate index was calculated from size of the recurrence in centimeters divided by number of months from primary treatment to detection of the recurrence. The presence or absence of necrosis was defined by area of spontaneous necrosis more than 4 mm in size in the microscopic sections of the recurrent tumor. By applying multivariate analysis in locally recurrent sarcoma, as to the significance of the GRI, grade, necrosis, depth, size, vascular invasion, and ploidy, only necrosis and GRI were found to be of any clinical significance. Based on this information, Chang et al.[11] staged the locally recurrent sarcomas in four groups shown below.

| Stage | Factors for Stage | Two Years Metastasis with Survival (percent) |
|---|---|---|
| Stage I | GRI ≤ 0.4 no necrosis | 94 |
| Stage II | GRI < 0.4 no necrosis | 79 |
| Stage III | GRI < 0.4 with necrosis | 61 |
| Stage IV | GRI < 0.4 with necrosis | 6 |

The proposed staging system is based on easily available parameters. This staging system separates a group with excellent outcome from a group with poor outcome. However, the reproducibility of this staging system remains to be substantiated.

## PROGNOSTIC PARAMETERS OF SARCOMAS

In a retrospective review of prognostic factors among 1,005 cases of soft tissue sarcomas, Hashimoto et al.[12] found that, in univariate analysis, cellularity, pleomorphism, differentiation, mitosis, amount of stroma necrosis, and grading were all significant factors. However, in multivariate analysis, the prognostic factors were different for different histologic types.[12] For example, in malignant fibrous histiocytoma and leiomyosarcoma, tumor necrosis and grading were the only two significant factors influencing the overall prognosis. On the other hand, attempts to delineate individual prognostic factors in 60 or so different types of lesions for practical clinical use is also cumbersome. Hence, in this chapter, we will elucidate some of the common clinical, histologic, and molecular factors important to the final outcome in successful management of such lesions.

***Age.*** In general, age is not a consistent prognostic factor in adult soft tissue sarcomas. However, in certain histologic types of lesions such as synovial sarcoma, Pritchard et al.[13] reported that younger patients have better outcomes. With multivariate analysis, these authors also found that older patients with malignant fibrous histiocytoma carry a worse prognosis. Similarly, increasing age was found to be a poor prognostic factor for treatment outcome in multimodal limb salvage procedure using radiation and intra-arterial chemotherapy.[13] However, Chang et al.[11] found that, in 83 extremity liposarcomas, there was no detectable influence of age on patients' outcome. In analysis of soft tissue sarcomas of the extremity and torso, LeVay and co-authors reported that age at diagnosis also influences outcome.[14] From analysis of the existing publications,[11,13,15,16] it appears that, *in most histologic subtypes, age does not exert a strong prognostic influence in adult soft tissue sarcomas.*

### Sex.
Although anecdotal data suggest that women with soft tissue sarcomas carry a better prognosis, when the available data are analyzed, it does not appear that sex plays a significant role in determining the overall prognosis in patients with adult soft tissue sarcomas.[11,13–15,17,18]

### Size.
In most reports, size of the lesion appears to have a significant negative influence on outcome. Larger lesions appear to have poorer prognosis.[11,14,18–20] However, some authors[21–23] reported that size had little influence on the prognosis of soft tissue sarcomas. In our experience, however, the size in general plays an important role: tumors smaller than 5 cm carry a better prognosis than those larger than 5 cm in maximum diameter, and size is a reliable clinical parameter for staging and prognosis.

### Invasion of Surrounding Tissue.
Invasion to major blood vessels, veins, and bones indicates a poorer prognosis. To what extent this appears to contribute to incomplete resection, resulting in recurrence and possible metastases, is unclear. However, many of these lesions are deeply situated, larger in size, and higher in grade, each of which contributes individually to poorer outcome. In the current staging system, involvement of major veins, arteries, or bones makes it a $T_3$ and hence stage 3 lesion. In retroperitoneal sarcomas, however, invasion of surrounding organs only plays a minimal role, if any, provided that the lesion can be completely resected with resection of the involved organ.[15]

### Location of the Tumor.
Anatomic location of a given tumor appears to play a major role in the outcome of sarcoma patients.[24] In general, sarcomas of the extremities and torso have better outcomes than sarcomas of the head and neck area and retroperitoneum. Even within the same histologic type, lesions located deep, rather than superficial, to deep fascia have much worse prognosis.[16,19] Based on this important prognostic factor, Gaynor et al.[19] devised a practical staging system, which appears to have clinical relevance.

### Morphologic and Histologic Prognostic Parameters.
Several morphologic and histologic prognostic parameters have been outlined. Of these, the grade of the tumor is probably the most important. Although occasional small series have failed to show the influence of grade as a significant prognostic parameter,[17,20,25] the evidence to the contrary is overwhelming.[11–13,15,19,21,22,25] The grade of the lesion is determined by taking into consideration a number of different histologic parameters. These parameters may include cellularity, pleomorphism, anaplasia, necrosis, stromal component, and mitosis. Necrosis and mitosis have also been often reported as independent histologic prognostic parameters.[12,15,17,19,21,25,26] None of the grading systems reported to date includes all these parameters in assessing prognosis.

The accuracy and predictive value of these parameters to the biologic behavior of these lesions differs by histologic types. For example, a high mitosis count in infantile fibrosarcoma does not signify a high grade and poor outcome, but high mitotic count in an extremity leiomyosarcoma signifies worse prognosis. Even within the same histologic group, mitosis by itself may not predict the biologic behavior of this tumor. In uterine sarcomas, there may be three to four mitoses/10 high-power fields, and the tumor behaves in a benign manner. In contrast, one to two mitoses/10 high-power fields in extremity leiomyosarcomas will signify aggressive behavior.

Although metastatic lesions in sarcomas usually maintain the grade of the primary tissue, in some cases, a higher grade may be encountered in metastatic lesions. Occasionally, a lower grade or more differentiated lesion is noted in both local recurrence and metastasis. Influence of grade on response to chemotherapy has been evaluated by Van Haelst-Pisani et al.,[27] who suggest that a high-grade tumor responds better and more often to chemotherapy.

## INFLUENCE OF HISTOLOGY ON PROGNOSIS OF SOFT TISSUE SARCOMA

Table 3–1 outlines the usual grading for each histologic classification. Invasion of blood vessels within tumor and lymphatic and lymph node metastasis usually signify much poorer prognosis. However, such invasions are almost always associated with high-grade lesions.

### Margin of Surgical Resection.
Among the clinical parameters, margin of resection is an important prognostic marker. The local failure rate in patients with positive margins is very high, even after adequate radiation therapy. Numerous reports also demonstrate poor outcome in patients with microscopically positive or close margins.[11,13,14,20–22,28–32] LeVay et al.[14] reported correla-

tion between positive margins and local recurrence.[25] Different relapses were also associated with positive margins, and local control of the recurrent disease did not change the incidence of ultimate metastasis. Tanabe and associates[28] showed that microscopically positive margins increased the risk of local recurrence. However, the status of the margins was not an important factor in overall survival. They also suggested that cutting into the tumor during the operation is usually associated with decreased survival. In the analysis of patients with head and neck sarcomas, Kraus and his coauthors[21] found that positivity of the surgical margin is the only predictor for local recurrence, and both margin status and grade of the tumor were predictors for distant failure. Thus, it appears that achieving negative surgical margin is important in improving local control of the disease.

The overall influence of local failure or local recurrence on the ultimate survival of sarcoma patients is a subject of controversy. In the past, it was uniformly believed that local recurrence results in higher incidence of distant failure. However, this basic concept has been recently challenged by several authors. LeVay and coworkers,[14] in review of 389 extremity and soft tissue sarcomas, found that local control indeed was a factor for survival. Patients treated for recurrence in their series had worse survival due to metastasis despite similar local control to primary cases.[25] In a larger series of patients, Gaynor et al.[19] found that local recurrence was not a factor in survival in high-grade lesions. However, for low- and intermediate-grade tumors, local recurrence was associated with higher distant failure. In their experience, they noted local recurrence had more influence in well-differentiated lesions. Similarly, Tomita and co-workers[25] reported that local recurrence of low-grade soft tissue sarcomas significantly reduced the ultimate survival. However, for high-grade sarcoma, local recurrence was not an influencing factor in overall survival. In a review by Stotter et al.[33] of 175 patients with extremity soft tissue sarcomas, the influence of local recurrence on survival was only apparent when considered as a time-dependent variable in multivariate analysis. Rooser and associates[34] have questioned the significance of local recurrence in overall survival. In an analysis of patients with distant metastasis with or without local recurrence, several authors found no difference in time interval or pattern of metastasis.[34–36]

Gustafson et al.[37] observed no difference in survival in 432 patients with extremity and torso sarcomas who were divided into two groups: one with no local recurrence and metastasis; the other with local recurrence but no demonstrable metastasis. However, the group of patients who had both metastases and local recurrence had poorer outcome. In a separate study, Gustafson and associates[38] also cautioned against cor-

relation of local recurrence and metastases. Tanabe et al.,[28] in analysis of extremity soft tissue sarcoma patients undergoing limb salvage procedure, also noted that local failure did not alter the overall survival.

Definitive answers on influence of local recurrence in all types of soft tissue sarcomas are yet undetermined. In a recent report from Memorial Sloan-Kettering Cancer Center, Heslin et al.[39] reviewed the influence of perioperative blood transfusion on recurrence and survival in primary extremity sarcomas. Autologous blood transfusion was found to be a significant prognostic factor in many different carcinomas. However, for adult soft tissue sarcomas, perioperative blood transfusion had no independent influence on local recurrence or metastasis.

The molecular markers that are currently being investigated as prognostic markers are discussed in detail in Chapter 6. Thus, in sum, the parameters summarized in Table 3–2 currently can be used as benchmarks for appropriate prognostication of adult soft tissue sarcomas.

## TABLE 3–2. PROGNOSTIC PARAMETERS IN SOFT TISSUE SARCOMAS

**Clinical Factors**
  Age
  Sex
  Size of the mass
  Location of the mass
  Invasion to surrounding tissue

**Morphologic Factors**
  Histologic type
  Grade of lesion
  Tumor-free margin
  Tumor necrosis
  Blood vessels invasion
  Lymphatics

**Molecular Markers**
  (e.g., chromosomal aberrations, ploidy, proliferative index, and tumor promoter and suppressor genes)

## REFERENCES

1. Soule EH, Geitz M, Henderson ED: Embryonal rhabdomyosarcoma of the limbs and limb girdles. Cancer 23:1336, 1969
2. Pritchard RF, Soule EH, Taylor WF, et al.: Fibrosarcoma: A clinicopathologic and statistical study of 199 tumors of soft tissue of the extremities and trunk. Cancer 33:888, 1976
3. Manual for Staging of Cancer. Chicago, American Joint Committee for Cancer Staging and End-Result Reporting, 1978
4. Suit HD, Russell WD: Soft part tumors. Cancer 39:830, 1977

5. Suit HD, Russell WD, Martin RG: Sarcoma of soft tissue: Clinical and histopathological parameters and response to treatment. Cancer 35:1478, 1975

6. Weingrad DN, Rosenberg SA: Early lymphatic spread of osteogenic and soft tissue sarcoma. Surgery 84:231, 1978

7. Bowden L: The diagnosis and treatment of soft part sarcomas. Virignia Med Monthly 81:463, 1954

8. Jenkins HP, Delaney PA: Benign angiomatous tumors of skeletal muscles. Surg Gynecol Obstet 55:464, 1932

9. Koss LG, Durfee GR: Diagnostic Cytology and its Histopathologic Bases. Philadelphia, J.B. Lippincott, 1961

10. Hajdu SI (ed): History and classification of soft tissue tumors. In Pathology of Soft Tissue Tumors. Philadelphia, Lea & Feibiger, 1979, p 45

11. Chang HR, Gaynor J, Tan C, et al.: Multifactorial analysis of survival in primary extremity liposarcoma. World J Surg 14:610, 1990

12. Hashimoto H, Daimaru Y, Takeshita S, et al.: Prognostic significance of histologic parameters of soft tissue sarcomas. Cancer 70:2816, 1992

13. Pritchard DJ, Reiman HM, Turcotte RE, Ilstrup DM: Malignant fibrous histiocytoma of the soft tissues of the trunk and extremities. Clin Orthop 289:58, 1993

14. LeVay J, O'Sullivan B, Catton C, et al.: Outcome and prognostic factors in soft tissue sarcoma in the adult. Int J Radiat Oncol Biol Phys 27:1091, 1993

15. Catton CN, O'Sullivan B, Kotwall C, et al.: Outcome and prognosis in retroperitoneal soft tissue sarcoma. Int J Radiat Oncol Biol Phys 29:1005, 1994

16. Ravaud A, Bui NB, Coindre JM, et al.: Prognostic variables for the selection of patients with operable soft tissue sarcomas to be considered in adjuvant chemotherapy trials. Br J Cancer 66:961, 1992

17. el-Jabbour JN, Akhtar SS, Kerr GR, et al.: Prognostic factors for survival in soft tissue sarcoma. Br J Cancer 62:857, 1990

18. Frezza G, Barbieri E, Ammendolia I, et al.: Surgery and radiation therapy in the treatment of soft tissue sarcomas of extremities. Ann Oncol 3:S93, 1992

19. Gaynor JJ, Tan CC, Casper ES, et al.: Refinement of clinicopathologic staging for localized soft tissue sarcoma of the extremity: A study of 423 adults. J Clin Oncol 10:1317, 1992

20. Tran LM, Mark R, Meier R, et al.: Sarcomas of the head and neck. Prognostic factors and treatment strategies. Cancer 70:169, 1992

21. Kraus DH, Dubner S, Harrison LB, et al.: Prognostic factors for recurrence and survival in head and neck soft tissue sarcomas. Cancer 74:697, 1994

22. Lucas DR, Nascimento AG, Sim FH: Clear-cell sarcoma of soft tissues. Mayo Clinic experience with 35 cases. Am J Surg Pathol 16:1197, 1992

23. van Unnik JA, Coindre JM, Contesso C, et al.: Grading of soft tissue sarcomas: Experience of the EORTC Soft Tissue and Bone Sarcoma Group. Eur J Cancer 29A:2089, 1993

24. Geer RJ, Woodruff J, Casper ES, Brennan MF: Management of small soft-tissue sarcoma of the extremity in adults. Arch Surg 127:1285, 1992

25. Tomita Y, Kuratsu S, Naka N, et al.: A staging system for soft-tissue sarcoma and its evaluation in relation to treatment. Int J Cancer 58:168, 1994

26. van Geel AN, van Coevorden F, Blankensheijn JD, et al.: Surgical treatment of pulmonary metastases from soft tissue sarcomas: A retrospective study in The Netherlands. J Surg Oncol 56:172, 1994

27. van Haelst-Pisani CM, Buckner JC, Reiman HM, et al.: Does histologic grade in soft tissue sarcoma influence response rate to systemic chemotherapy? Cancer 68:2354, 1991

28. Tanabe KK, Pollock RE, Ellis LM, et al.: Influence of surgical margins on outcome in patients with preoperatively irradiated extremity soft tissue sarcomas. Cancer 73:1652, 1994

29. Frankenthaler R, Ayala AG, Hartwick RW, Goepfert H: Fibrosarcoma of the head and neck. Laryngoscope 100:799, 1990

30. Perry RR, Venzon D, Roth JA, Pass HI: Survival after surgical resection for high-grade chest wall sarcomas. Ann Thorac Surg 49:363, 1990

31. Steinberg BD, Gelberman RH, Mankin HJ, Rosenberg AK: Epithelioid sarcoma in the upper extremity. J Bone Joint Surg Am 74:28, 1992

32. Eeles RA, Risher C, A'Hern RP, et al.: Head and neck sarcomas: Prognostic factors and implications for treatment. Br J Cancer 68:201, 1993

33. Stotter AT, A'Hern RP, Fisher C, et al.: The influence of local recurrence of extremity soft tissue sarcoma on metastasis and survival. Cancer 65:1119, 1990

34. Rooser B, Gustafson P, Rydholm A: Is there no influence of local control on the rate of metastases in high-grade soft tissue sarcoma? Cancer 65:1727, 1990

35. Saddegh MK, Lindholm J, Lungberg A, et al.: Staging of soft-tissue sarcomas. Prognostic analysis of clinical and pathological features. J Bone Joint Surg Br 74:495, 1992

36. Evans RA: Soft tissue sarcoma: The enigma of local recurrence. J Surg Oncol 53:88, 1993

37. Gustafson P, Dreinhofer KE, Rydholm A: Metastasis-free survival after local recurrence of soft-tissue sarcoma. J Bone Joint Surg Br 75:658, 1993

38. Gustafson P: Soft tissue sarcoma. Epidemiology and prognosis in 508 patients. Acta Orthop Scand Suppl 259:1, 1994

39. Heslin MJ, Gaynor JJ, Newman E, et al.: Effect of perioperative blood transfusion on recurrence and survival in 232 primary high-grade extremity sarcoma patients. Ann Surg Oncol 1:189, 1994

# 4

# Imaging of Soft Tissue Sarcomas

Soft tissue sarcomas are relatively uncommon,[1-6] but the role of imaging in the diagnosis and management of soft tissue sarcomas has changed dramatically over the past decade, mostly due to the development of magnetic resonance imaging (MRI). However, x-ray-based imaging in its various forms (plain film, angiography, and computed tomography [CT]) still remains an important part of imaging protocols.

The goals of x-ray-based imaging initially include discovery and description, determination of differential diagnosis, and sometimes assessment of the aggressiveness of certain malignant mesenchymal tumors. In several soft tissues sarcomas, CT still remains a significant tool to help accurately stage a tumor, as well as a guide during fine-needle aspiration biopsy. Angiography may be used to delineate vascular anatomy preoperatively. Finally, CT and MRI are critical in evaluating locoregional extension of the primary tumor and distant sites for recurrence and/or metastasis. Imaging accuracy has taken on even greater significance due to improved survival subsequent to new techniques in limb salvage procedures and advances in adjuvant and neoadjuvant therapies.[7,8] Improved detection (resulting in earlier diagnosis), improved staging, and greater understanding of tumor histology and behavior have led to improved surgical and treatment guidelines.

## ■ PLAIN X-RAY

Plain film radiography, sensitive to the electron density of matter, is limited mainly to evaluation of tumor mineralization or fat content.[8] This ability is most useful when combined with CT. The radiolucency of fat-containing tumors can suggest a well-differentiated liposarcoma or lipoma (see Figs. 3–11 and 3–12),[9] and the density of calcification in chondroid matrix can be seen in soft tissue chondrosarcoma. Phleboliths clustered in the soft tissues indicate underlying hemangioma, quite different from the peripheral pattern of calcification of myositis ossificans or the central pattern more typically seen in osteosarcoma of the soft tissues.[10] Plain x-ray, sometimes using low-Kv techniques to enhance soft tissue detail, can detect underlying bony exostoses, the typical cartilaginous matrix of synovial osteochondromatosis, or the characteristic peripheral calcific pattern of myositis ossificans.[3,8] Similarly, plain x-ray may show bony involvement, cortical erosion, periosteal new bone formation and reaction, destruction of bony matrix, and may even suggest soft tissue extension and invasion in primary bone tumors such as Ewing's sarcoma and osteogenic sarcoma (Fig. 4–1).[10,11]

In the abdomen, an x-ray film can indirectly indicate an underlying mass, as in the case of leiomyosarcoma displacing bowel or an abscess discovered due to the presence of air-fluid level in the soft tissues. Preoperative evaluations have included the intravenous urogram to exclude obstruction and define organ displacement, as well as barium studies to look for mucosal invasion and extrinsic compression. Generally, however, the finding on plain film is nonspecific. While this type of imaging is sometimes useful as an introductory study, computer-derived imaging (based either on the electron density of matter, as in CT, or on proton density as in MRI) has become the imaging modality of choice, depending on the body area of tumor involvement.

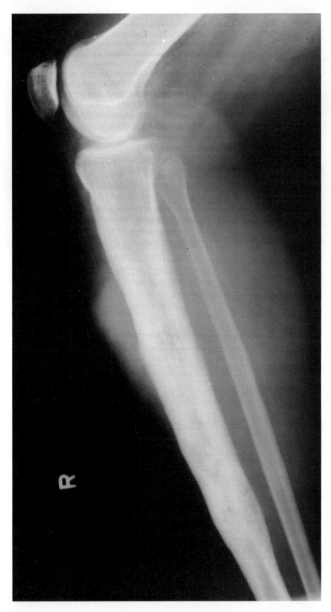

**Figure 4–1.** Soft tissue mass in the right leg of a 24-year-old man. Roentgenogram showed invasion of the periosteum of the tibia. A clinical diagnosis of sarcoma was made, and biopsy examination showed this tumor to be rhabdomyosarcoma.

CT and MRI allow the reconstruction of tissue contrast in true cross-sections (i.e., without being influenced by nearby or distant tissues in the section), with excellent tissue-contrast discrimination (resolution).[12] Both CT and MRI, but particularly MRI, provide the best anatomic cross-sectional imaging technology available to date. The chief advantages of CT in diagnostic radiology are the following: (1) removal of blurred background and superimposed overlying structures commonly seen in standard tomography;[12,13] (2) a true tomographic section is obtained that is almost an exact representation of a tissue attenuation coefficient, which may be used to identify and quantitate particular tissues; and (3) the CT image is stored and displayed digitally so that the image contrast can be manipulated during viewing, giving the most effective diagnostic information.[12,13] Using an intravenous iodinated-contrast medium during CT scanning helps to better differentiate the vascular structures from the adjacent areas. The new generation high-resolution scanner, with a smaller pixel (picture element) and a combination of thin-section (1 to 1.5 mm) and extended bone range (expansion of the Hounsfield unit scale up to 4000 units [i.e., +3000 to −1000]), provides clear definition and differentiation of soft tissue structures, while also providing superior bone detail.

## DYNAMIC COMPUTED TOMOGRAPHY

Conventional CT scanning has the limitation of being a static imaging technique giving essentially an anatomic and morphologic image. The routine iodinated contrast-enhanced CT also provides a static picture of the distribution of the iodinated-contrast material within the various tissues. Development of the high-resolution scanner, which has both short scan time and interscan delay, made it possible to perform rapid-sequence CT imaging (dynamic CT) after the bolus of iodinated-contrast material passes through an organ.[14–16] When contrast material passes through a cross-section, it creates a dynamic image field, exhibiting local density changes during the scan interval.[14] Rapid-sequence CT imaging allows for sequential imaging throughout the arterial, capillary, and venous phases; provides information about vascular anatomy (CT angiography); locates major vessels; and eliminates the possibility of vascular lesions in the differential diagnosis of a head and neck tumor.[14,15] Dynamic CT can also be used to visualize vascular structures via rapid-sequential dynamic CT with automatic table incrementation: "dynamic incrementation scanning."[14,15] This technique allows sequential images throughout the arterial and venous phases, which results in improved delineation of vascular structures and thus resolves a common clinical problem encountered with regular contrast-infusion CT scanning (i.e., whether a rounded image represents a vascular structure, a neoplasm, or both).[14,15] In glomus complex tumors or vascular lesions, dynamic CT scanning clearly visualizes the sequential enhancement of the carotid arteries and jugular veins. The tumor becomes densely opacified for a short time as the intravenously injected bolus of iodinated-contrast material traverses the vascular bed of a particular tissue section.[14–16]

## MAGNETIC RESONANCE IMAGING

One advantage of MRI is its ability to obtain transverse (axial) and direct coronal, sagittal, and oblique images without changing the position of the patient. The contrast relationships of different tissues are different on MRI than on CT scanning. Technical factors of various pulse sequences to obtain an MR image, and the physical and biochemical composition of the sample, play significant roles in tissue contrast in MR images. Water, such as in cerebrospinal fluid (CSF), vitreous chamber, or simple cysts, has long $T_1$ and $T_2$ relaxation times and would appear as a hypointense (dark) image in $T_1$-weighted ($T_1$W) and proton-weighted (PW) (proton-density) scans, and as a hyperintense (bright) image in $T_2$-weighted ($T_2$W) MR scans. The lens has an intermediate signal intensity (gray) in $T_1$W and PW scans and appears as a hypointense image in $T_2$W scans.

Fat has short $T_1$ and intermediate $T_2$ relaxation times, and would therefore appear as a hyperintense image in $T_1$W and PW scans and as a relatively hypointense image in $T_2$W scans. Tissues of intermediate structure (for example, muscles) show an intermediate signal on $T_1$W and PW scans, and a low signal on $T_2$W MR scans. Solid structures, such as cortical bone, enamel, dentin, and fibrous tissues (sclera, tendons, fascia), are hypointense (dark) on $T_1$W, PW, and $T_2$W scans because of their scarcity of mobile hydrogen atoms. The cortical bone would appear black, whereas the medullary cavity would be bright due to signals from fat. Air in paranasal sinuses, because of the lack of hydrogen atoms, appears dark in all MR scans. In most pulse sequences, vascular structures such as carotid arteries and internal jugular veins are readily identified as low-signal intensity (dark) structures. With routine MR pulse sequences, excited spins are carried away from the selected imaging section before a signal (echo) is formed (signal-void phenomenon), creating a dark image with signal intensity similar to that of air, cortical bone, enamel, and dentin.

### Dynamic Magnetic Resonance Imaging

Fast-scan or narrow flip angle MR imaging (dynamic MRI) is performed using the gradient-echo (GRE) pulse sequence such as the "GRASS" imaging technique ("gradient-recalled acquisition in the steady state"). Its prime characteristic is the ability to provide $T_1$, $T_2$, and PW images in a very short time. A striking feature of GRASS images is the high-intensity (bright) appearance of vascular structures, "MR angiography," especially when vessels transect the image slice. All MR scans, except where mentioned, are performed with a superconductive magnet of 1.5 Tesla (Tesla = 10,000 gauss). GRASS images are obtained with TR = 25 to 30 msec, TE = 12 to 15 msec, and a variable flip angle (10 to 30 degrees).

### Tissue Characterization of $T_1$W and $T_2$W Images

Damadian and co-workers[17] showed that malignant tissues, except melanotic tumors, have long $T_1$ and $T_2$ relaxation times. Nonmelanotic tumors, therefore, are often hypointense on $T_1$W scans and would appear as hyperintense images on $T_2$W scans. Melanotic lesions would often appear relatively hyperintense on $T_1$W and PW MR scans and become hypointense on $T_2$W MR scans.[18]

Magnetic resonance imaging is currently superior to CT for imaging soft tissue tumors. No studies have been able to consistently differentiate benign lesions from ones that are malignant. Margins are typically better defined on $T_2$-weighted images; however, benign and malignant cases are not readily distinguished by their margins. Absence of increased signal intensity on $T_2$-weighted images does not indicate benignity.[19]

Disadvantages of MR imaging are as follows: (1) MRI frequently requires 45 to 60 minutes scanning time, during which time any patient motion, including heavy breathing, swallowing, and coughing, results in image degradation; (2) MRI is contraindicated in patients with cardiac pacemakers and cochlear implants and in those harboring ferromagnetic objects in the body; (3) MRI is not readily available, and is, unfortunately, the most expensive of all diagnostic imaging methods.

In the following sections, we will present the strengths and weaknesses of x-ray-based imaging and define the role of each modality in each phase of diagnosis and treatment to ensure the best results and most cost-effective care.

## ■ TUMORS OF THE ADIPOSE TISSUE

### LIPOMATOUS TUMORS

Most benign lipomatous tumors can be categorized into several groups (see Chapter 7).

### Lipoma

Lipomas are well characterized by CT and MRI; on MRI, their signal intensity approximately equals subcutaneous fat, having high-signal intensity on $T_1$-weighted images (Figs. 4–2 and 4–3) and low signal intensity on TW images. These tumors are usually surrounded by a thin capsule and are well circumscribed. There is no enhancement after the administration of intravenous contrast material. Occasionally, they may be septated,

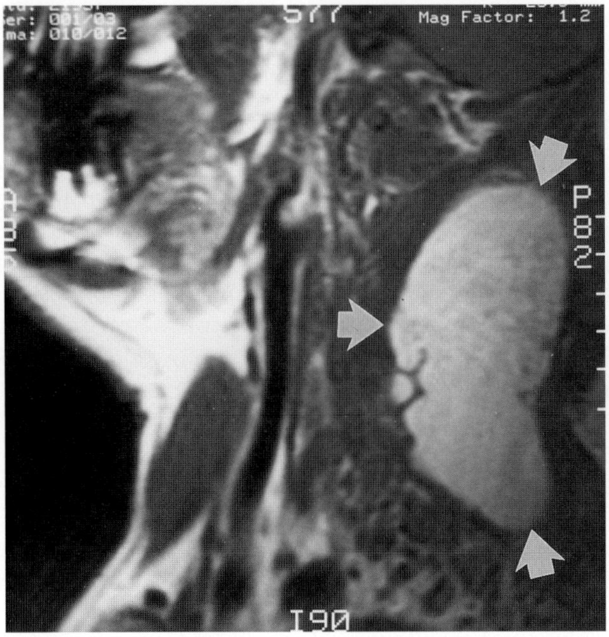

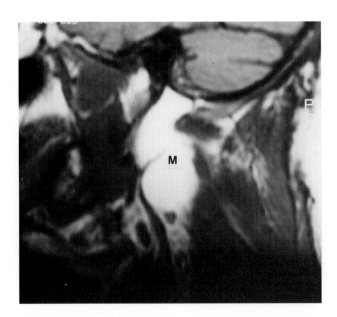

**Figure 4-2.** Lipoma. Sagittal T$_1$W magnetic resonance (MR) scan shows a large high-signal intensity mass *(arrows)* in the posterior aspect of the neck, compatible with a lipoma.

appearing as linear areas of low-signal intensity on both T$_1$- and T$_2$-weighted sequences (Fig. 4-4).[20]

## Angiomyolipoma

Angiomyolipoma (AML) is a specific hamartomatous lesion arising as a solitary or multicentric lesion in one or both kidneys. Multiple and bilateral lesions are less

common. One-third of cases are associated with tuberous sclerosis. Angiomyolipoma occurs more frequently in women, with a median age of 46 years. Two-thirds of cases cause symptoms of abdominal or flank pain, hematuria, or chills and fever. Less commonly, they may be asymptomatic and discovered incidentally. Despite atypical features at times, nearly all AMLs seem to pursue a benign clinical course (see Chapter 7 for clinical details). When enough fatty tissue is present within the tumor, CT and MRI appearances are pathognomonic; attenuations and signal intensities are consistent with fat (Fig. 4-5). However, intratumoral hemorrhage and predominant muscle or vascular components may make the diagnosis difficult.[21]

## Myelolipoma

Myelolipoma is a tumorlike growth of mature fat and bone marrow elements most commonly occurring in the adrenal gland.[22] It can also occur as an isolated soft tissue mass, especially in the pelvic region, in patients without any evidence of hematopoetic disorders.[23,24] Myelolipomas are most commonly encountered in adults 40 years or older. These patients may be asymptomatic or present with abdominal pain, nausea, or

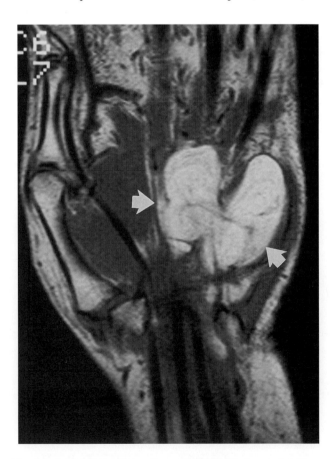

**Figure 4-4.** Hypothenar lipoma. Coronal T$_1$W MR scan shows a hypothenar lipoma *(arrows).*

**Figure 4-3.** Lipoma. Sagittal T$_1$W MR scan shows a large mass (M) extending from the base of the skull into the parapharyngeal space.

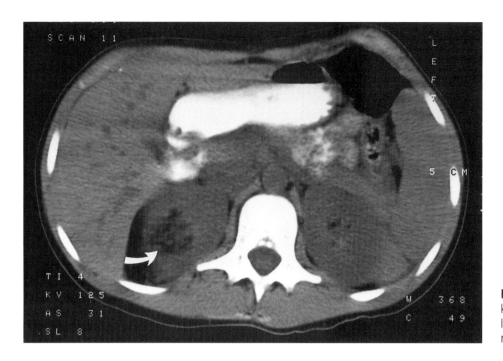

**Figure 4–5.** Angiomyolipoma of right kidney. Axial CT scan shows an irregular low-density mass *(arrow)* involving the right kidney.

constipation.[22] A well-circumscribed nonhomogeneous fat mass with low attenuation and little to no enhancement is usually the finding in a CT examination (Fig. 4–6).[25]

## ■ PELVIC LIPOMATOSIS

Pelvic lipomatosis is essentially a benign condition in which there is abundance of fatty tissue in the peri-rectal and perivesical spaces in the pelvis, giving the impression of a large pelvic tumor (see Figs. 7–7A to 7E in Chapter 7 for further details).

## LIPOSARCOMA

Liposarcomas constitute the second largest group of soft tissue sarcomas, accounting for 17.7 percent.[26] Most patients are in their fourth through seventh dec-

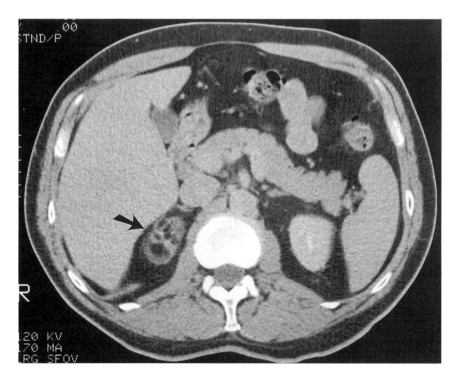

**Figure 4–6.** Myelolipoma of right adrenal gland. Axial CT scan shows a heterogeneous mass *(arrow)* with areas of low density involving the right adrenal gland.

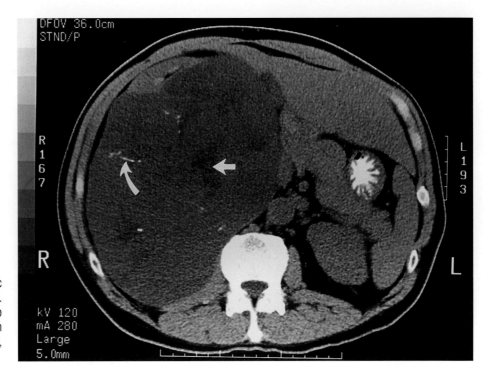

**Figure 4–7.** Retroperitoneal pleomorphic liposarcoma infiltrating liver and muscle. On the original CT, tumor was thought to arise from the kidney. Note low-attenuation areas *(arrows)* consistent with fat density, as well as calcification *(arrowhead)*.

ades, and peak incidence is between 40 and 60 years. Patients with involvement in the retroperitoneum are on average 5 to 10 years older than those with involvement in the extremities. Retroperitoneal liposarcomas cause gradual and diffuse abdominal enlargement (Figs. 4–7 and 4–8). Radiographically, liposarcoma appears as a bulky mass with a pseudocapsule. Margins may be well defined or irregular (Fig. 4–9). The amount of fat varies. Poorly differentiated masses have almost no fat, making histologic diagnosis via radiographic criteria difficult. If any solid or nonfatty component is present in a predominantly fatty tumor, the possibility of sarcomatous changes should be considered.[21]

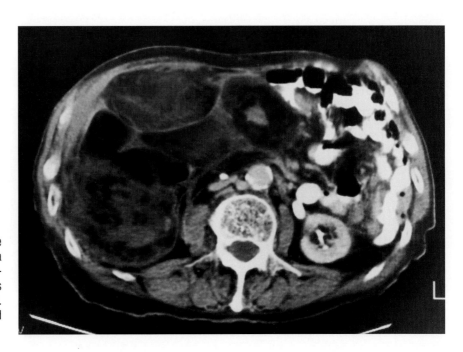

**Figure 4–8.** Liposarcoma in a 62-year-old male with contrasted abdominal CT demonstrating a massive retroperitoneal tumor with both soft tissue and fatty components. This appearance is characteristic of well-differentiated liposarcoma. The right kidney (not seen) has been displaced cephalad and bowel to the left.

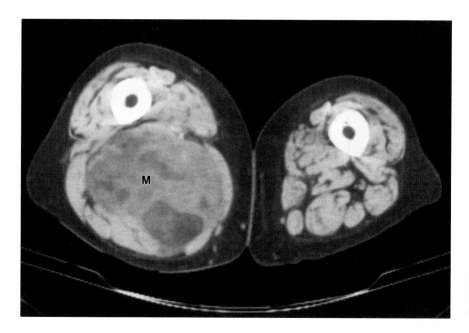

**Figure 4–9.** Liposarcoma of the right thigh. Axial CT scan shows a large heterogeneous mass *(M)* with areas of low density involving the right thigh.

## ■ TUMORS OF THE FIBROUS TISSUE

Fibromatoses are a group of benign fibrous tissue proliferative lesions that can arise in both the superficial and deep regions of the human body. These lesions, by virtue of their proliferative nature, have infiltrative qualities and frequently infiltrate the surrounding structures.[27,28] The superficial variety of fibromatoses is commonly found in the palm or the sole of the foot. Both palmar and plantar fibromatoses have very specific clinical presentation and can be accurately diagnosed by their clinical features. Similarly, superficial fibromatoses located elsewhere can also be diagnosed clinically and seldom require any imaging studies (for further details on fibromatoses, see Chapter 8). In contrast, in spite of the fact that angiofibromas are also benign, imaging studies are essential.

### ANGIOFIBROMA

Angiofibroma is a benign, highly vascular, nonencapsulated neoplasm arising exclusively in adolescents, with intracranial involvement in 20 to 36 percent of patients.[29,30] It is histologically benign but locally aggressive. It almost always arises in the nasopharynx near the pterygopalatine fossa. The tumor spreads into the maxillary sinus, nasal cavity, sphenoid sinus, ethmoid sinus, infratemporal fossa, into the orbit via the inferior orbital fissure, and intracranially.[31]

Radiographic imaging is diagnostic. Angiofibroma demonstrates marked enhancement on CT scans. On dynamic CT scans, it reveals intense enhancement early, characteristic of very vascular lesions. On MR images, this lesion appears as a mass of low-to-intermediate signal intensity on $T_1W$ and PW images and of intermediate-to-high signal intensity on $T_2W$ and GRE images. Multiple flow-void channels may be seen representing the highly vascular nature of this tumor. There is also marked enhancement after gadolinium administration (Fig. 4–10).[31]

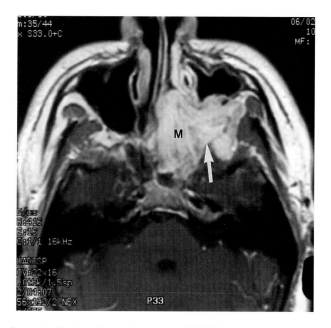

**Figure 4–10.** Angiofibroma. Postcontrast $T_1W$ MR scan shows an enhancing mass *(M)* in the nasopharynx and nasal cavity, with extension in the pterygopalatine fossa *(arrow).*

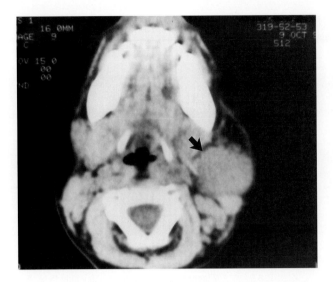

**Figure 4–11.** Aggressive fibromatosis in a 3-year-old patient. Axial CT scan shows a large mass *(arrow)* in the left submandibular space.

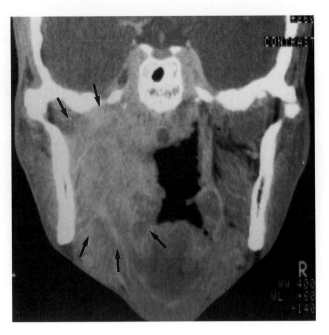

**Figure 4–12.** Aggressive fibromatosis. Postcontrast coronal CT scan shows a large infiltrative mass *(arrows)* involving the left parapharyngeal space. Note infiltration of the lateral and medial pterygoid muscles.

Deep-seated fibromatosis or aggressive fibromatosis was initially described as a separate clinicopathologic entity in 1838 by Müller,[32] who coined the term *desmoid.* Over the years, various terms have been used to describe this interesting, albeit rare, clinicopathologic entity.[33] Currently, however, the term *aggressive fibromatoses* is probably the best descriptive term. Aggressive fibromatoses can occur in every anatomic locale and are characterized by their ability to locally infiltrate the surrounding structures.

Radiologic examination reveals a soft tissue mass with localized periosteal thickening or frank bony destruction.[34] On CT, masses can be both ill defined and well circumscribed. Precontrast scans show variable attenuation relative to muscle. After contrast, they may or may not enhance. Usually, the masses demonstrate higher attenuation than that of skeletal muscle. Magnetic resonance imaging demonstrates a nonhomogeneous mass with low-to-intermediate signal on $T_1$-weighted images relative to muscle. Because its degrees of cellularity vary, attenuation and enhancement on CT also vary, as does signal intensity on MRI (Figs. 4–11 to 4–14). $T_2$-weighted images show variable intensity relative to muscle (Figs. 4–15A and 4–15B).[35] In abdominal wall desmoids, similarly the tumor infiltrates the surrounding structure (Figs. 4–16A and 4–16B).

## MALIGNANT FIBROUS HISTIOCYTOMA

Malignant fibrous histiocytoma (MFH) is the most common adult soft tissue sarcoma of late adult life, comprising greater than one-fourth of all soft tissue sarco-

mas. Most occur in the sixth through eighth decades of life. Rarely do tumors in children have the same histologic features as the adult forms.

Radiologic features demonstrate a nonspecific soft tissue mass. In the extremities, they are usually adjacent

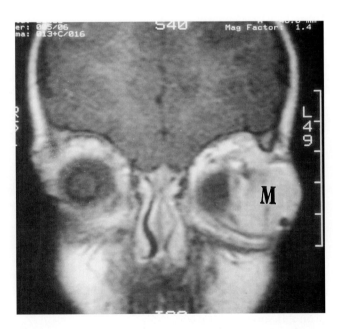

**Figure 4–13.** Aggressive fibromatosis. Postcontrast coronal $T_1$W MR scan shows an enhancing mass, involving the anterolateral aspect of the left orbit in this 2-year-old patient.

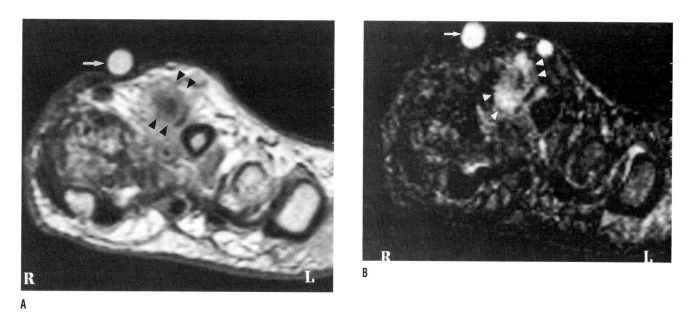

**Figure 4–14.** Aggressive fibromatosis. **(A)** Coronal PW MR scan of the left foot shows a mass with ill-defined margins *(arrowheads)*. White arrow points to a skin marker. **(B)** Coronal T$_2$W MR scan shows the mass *(arrowheads)*.

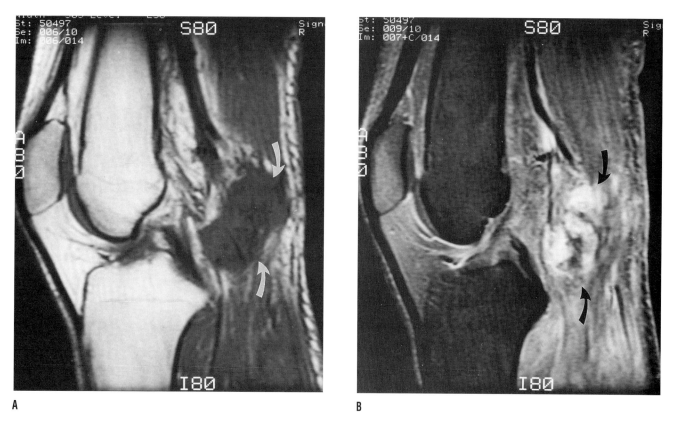

**Figure 4–15.** Desmoid tumor of popliteal fossa. Sagittal T$_1$W **(A)** and T$_2$W **(B)** scans showing a large mass *(arrows)*.

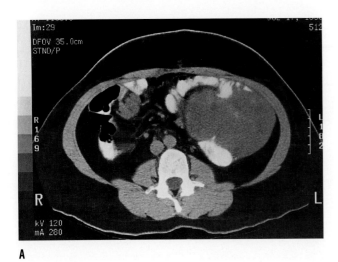
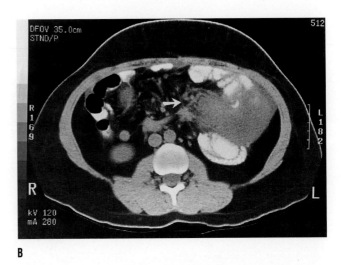

**A**    **B**

**Figure 4–16.** Desmoid tumor of abdomen in a 33-year-old female three years after colon resection. The patient had Gardner's syndrome. While some areas of the mass are well defined **(A)**, there is mesenteric infiltration *(arrow)* **(B)**.

to the diaphyses of long bones. Smooth cortical erosion by direct extension is also possible. In 5 to 20 percent of cases, calcification or ossification has been observed in plain radiographs. CT scan shows a large, lobulated relatively well-defined soft tissue mass that often contains areas of decreased attenuation, centrally corresponding to regions of myxomatous tissue, hemorrhage, or necrosis (Fig. 4–17). After contrast administration, the solid portions of the mass enhance (Figs. 4–18 and 4–19). Computed tomography also helps identify calcifications and cortical erosions in deeply seated masses. The identification of cortical involvement strongly suggests MFH. On MR imaging, MFH demonstrates intermediate signal intensity on $T_1$-weighted images and heterogeneously high signal on $T_2$-weighted images (Fig. 4–20). After gadolinium DTPA contrast material administration, there is enhancement of the solid components.[36]

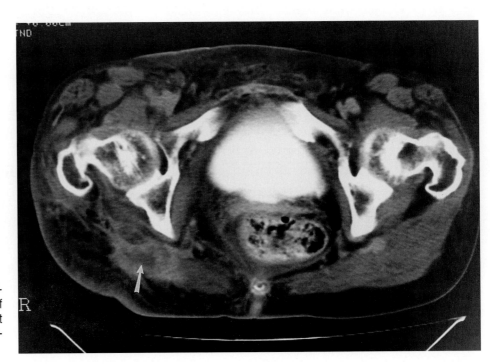

**Figure 4–17.** CT of the pelvis of a 55-year-old female showing recurrence of malignant fibrous histiocytoma in the right gluteal region *(arrow)* nine months following resection.

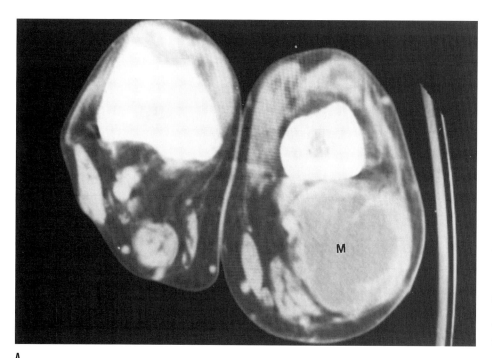

A

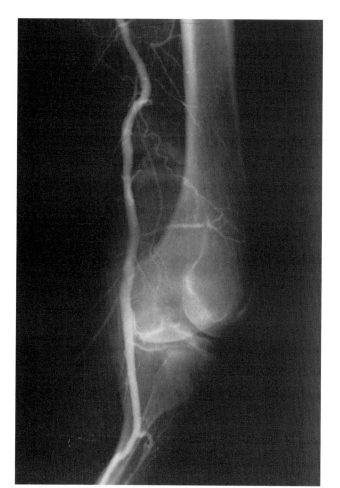

B

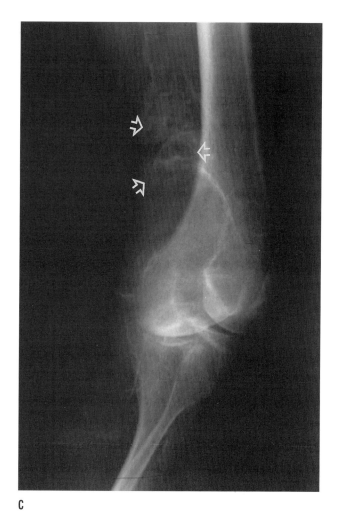

C

**Figure 4–18. (A)** Malignant fibrous histiocytoma. Contrast-enhanced CT scan shows a large mass *(M)* posterior to the lower aspect of femur. The same tumor is visualized by means of an angiogram. **(B)** Early arterial phase angiogram showing normal vasculature, but the tumor can be seen in the background. **(C)** A delayed image shows a faint blush in the region of the mass (note the arrows outlining the tumor).

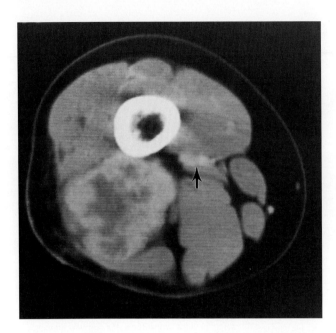

**Figure 4–19.** Contrasted CT of malignant fibrous histiocytoma originating from vastus lateralis in a 26-year-old female. The tumor had well-defined margins, and the adjacent neurovascular bundle *(arrow)* is not involved.

## FIBROSARCOMA

Fibrosarcoma constitutes about 4.1 percent of all soft tissue sarcomas. As with other sarcomas, CT and MR imaging demonstrate nonspecific findings of nonhomogeneous masses varying from well defined (Fig. 4–21) to very invasive.

## ■ TUMORS OF THE MUSCLE TISSUE

### SMOOTH MUSCLE TUMORS

#### Leiomyosarcoma

Leiomyosarcomas are the third most common soft tissue sarcoma, accounting for 10 to 15 percent.[37] These tumors frequently occur in the retroperitoneum (35 percent), mesentery (25 percent), and either the thigh or knee (19 percent).[38] About two-thirds of retroperitoneal leiomyosarcomas occur in women. For tumors arising in the deep soft tissues of the extremities, the gender incidence is equal. Retroperitoneal leiomyosarcomas are highly aggressive and often attain extremely large size before clinical recognition (Fig. 4–22). Computed tomography features show large, sometimes partially calcified, soft tissue mass, often with central necrosis (Fig. 4–23).[21] Five-year survival rates in deep-seated (i.e., intra-abdominal) leiomyosarcoma are poor.[39–41]

#### Rhabdomyosarcoma

Rhabdomyosarcomas comprise 5.4 percent of soft tissue sarcomas. Nearly half of all soft tissue sarcomas occurring in patients younger than 15 are rhabdomyosarcomas. It is the most common soft tissue sarcoma in adolescents and young adults, but it is relatively rare in persons older than 45 years. Adult cases are predominantly male, by a ratio of 1.3:1.[42] The embryonal type (the most common [50 to 60 percent]) usually occurs in the first decade, while the alveolar type (20 percent) occurs in the second and third decades, with a mean

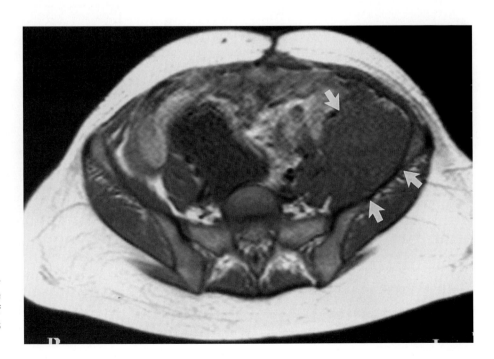

**Figure 4–20.** Malignant fibrous histiocytoma. Axial T$_1$W MR scan shows a large mass *(arrows)* involving the left side of the pelvis, including the illiacus and psoas muscles.

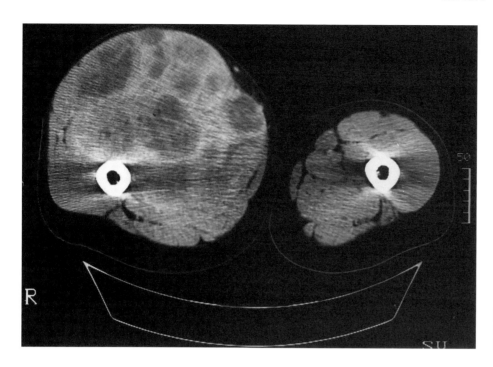

**Figure 4–21.** Fibrosarcoma. Contrast-enhanced axial CT scan shows a heterogeneous mass involving the right leg.

age of 23 years. The head and neck is involved most often, followed by the lower extremities and trunk for embryonal and alveolar types. Botryoid embryonal rhabdomyosarcoma is a variant of embryonal rhabdomyosarcoma and occurs in 5 to 10 percent. It is most often seen in mucosa-lined hollow organs, such as the vagina and urinary bladder. Pleomorphic type accounts

for less than 5 percent of all rhabdomyosarcomas. It may affect patients of any age, but shows peak incidence in patients over 40 years of age and usually affects large muscles such as the thigh.[42]

Computed tomography features include bulky, solid masses with attenuation values similar to muscle tissue (Fig. 4–24).[21] On MRI, the tumor appears hypo-

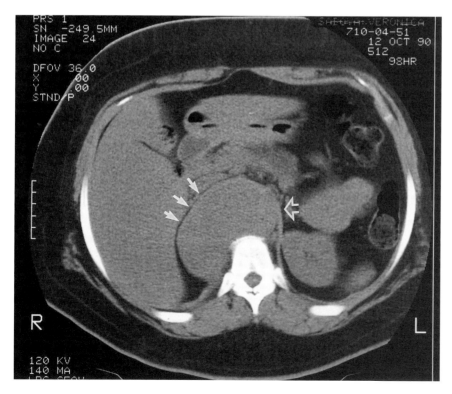

**Figure 4–22.** Retrocrural leiomyosarcoma. Axial CT scan shows a large mass *(arrows)* behind the crura of the diaphragm *(hollow arrow)*.

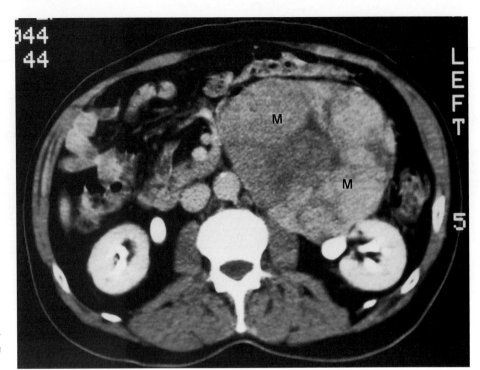

**Figure 4–23.** Leiomyosarcoma of retroperitoneum. Axial CT scan shows a large mass *(M)*.

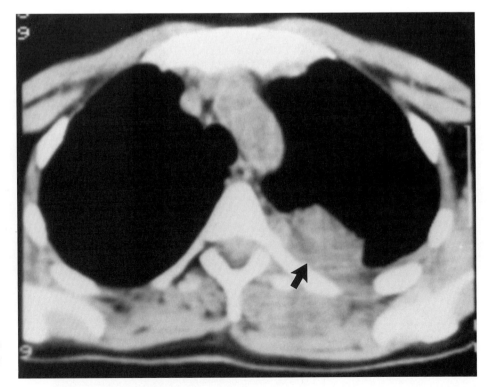

**Figure 4–24.** Rhabdomyosarcoma of the paraspinal muscle. Axial CT scan shows an irregular mass *(arrow)*.

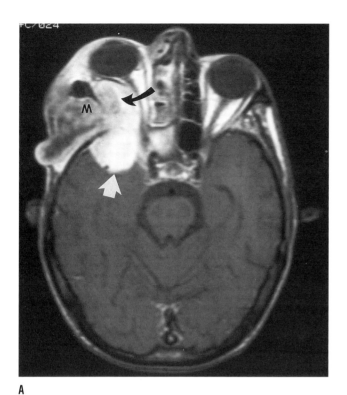
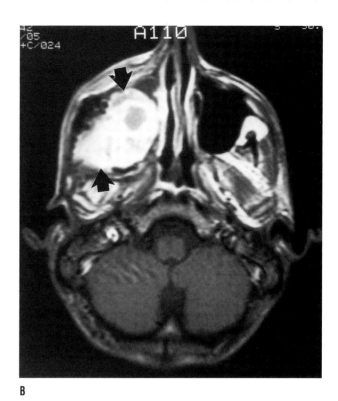

**A**                                      **B**

**Figure 4–25.** Rhabdomyosarcoma. **(A)** Contrast-enhanced T$_1$W MR scan shows a large mass *(M)* in the right temporal fossa, extending into the orbit *(black arrow)* and right middle cranial fossa *(white arrow)*. **(B)** Large tumor in the right temporal fossa *(arrows)*.

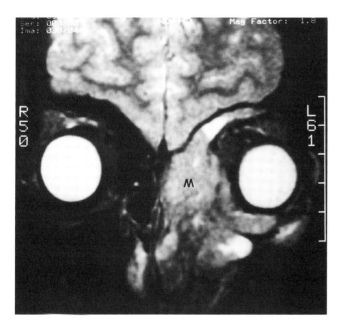

**Figure 4–26.** Rhabdomyosarcoma. Coronal T$_2$W MR scan shows a large tumor *(M)* involving left ethmoid sinus, extending into the left orbit and maxillary sinus.

intense to isointense to muscle tissue on T$_2$-weighted images. Contrast enhancement is moderate to marked (Figs. 4–25 and 4–26)

## ■ TUMORS OF THE PERIPHERAL NERVES

### BENIGN TUMORS OF PERIPHERAL NERVES

#### Neurofibroma/Schwannoma

Neurofibroma is a nerve sheath tumor that can occur as a solitary lesion (versus multiple when in association with neurofibromatosis type-1 [NF-1]). Neurofibromas show low-to-intermediate signal intensity on T$_1$-weighted images, with a slightly higher signal intensity in the central zone than in the peripheral zone. On T$_2$-weighted images, the peripheral zone shows a higher intensity than fat, and the central zone retains intermediate intensity. After contrast, enhancement is seen in the central zone (Fig. 4–27).[43]

Schwannoma or neurilemoma is an encapsulated nerve sheath tumor comprising two components: a highly ordered cellular component (Antoni A) and a

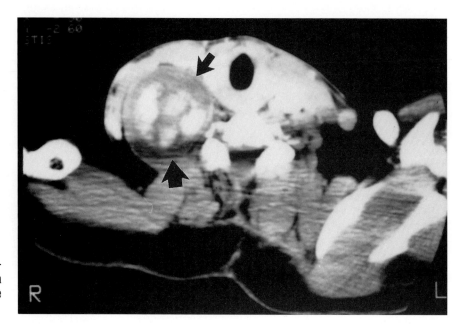

**Figure 4–27.** Neurofibroma with possible malignant transformation. Enhanced CT scan shows a large mass *(arrows)* in the posterior triangle of the right neck.

loose myxoid component (Antoni B) (see Chapter 5 for specific details). There is a predilection for the head and neck, and flexor surfaces of the extremities (Fig. 4–28). Deeply situated masses predominate in the retroperitoneum and posterior mediastinum. They can occur as solitary lesions, but most are multiple (Fig. 4–29) and associated with NF-1.[44] Schwannomas of the vagus, trigeminal, sympathetic chain, and hypoglossal nerves in the parapharyngeal space (Fig. 4–30) present as rounded masses bulging into the nasopharynx.[45,46] The benign nature of the tumor is often predicted by an evaluation of CT and MR scans, which show mass effect but not obliteration or invasion of the fascial planes. Since these tumors are frequently encountered in the head and neck region, even in larger tumors with considerable extension a preoperative assessment of benignity and/or malignancy is highly desirable and in most instances possible (Fig. 4–31).

On MRI, benign schwannomas demonstrate intermediate signal on $T_1$-weighted, and high signal on $T_2$-weighted, sequences with intense enhancement (Figs. 4–32 and 4–33). However, in some cases, heterogeneous enhancement may occur if the mass contains cystic components.

## MALIGNANT PERIPHERAL NERVE SHEATH TUMORS

Computed tomography images demonstrate a bulky soft tissue mass that may have areas of necrosis or calcification (Fig. 4–34). Magnetic resonance imaging may

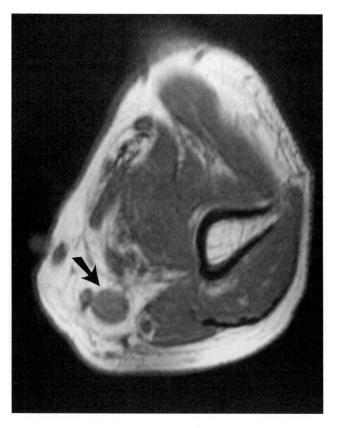

**Figure 4–28.** Neuroma of ulnar nerve. Axial $T_1$W MR scan shows an isointense mass *(arrow)*.

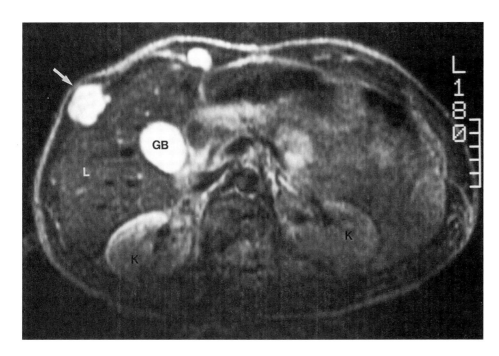

**Figure 4–29.** Schwannoma. Axial T₂W MR scan of abdomen shows a schwannoma *(arrow)* involving the abdominal wall. *GB* = gall bladder; *K* = kidney; *L* = liver.

show variable intensities on both $T_1$- and $T_2$-weighted images, depending on the degree of intratumoral necrosis. The extent and aggressiveness can be evaluated well with MRI.

### Paraganglioma (Glomus tumors)

Paraganglia are specialized neural crest cells that arise in association with the autonomic ganglia throughout the body, including the adrenal medulla, carotid and aortic bodies, vagal body, and small groups associated with the thoracic, intra-abdominal, and retroperitoneal ganglia (see Chapter 10 for detailed discussion). Dynamic CT clearly visualizes the sequential enhancement of the carotid arteries and internal jugular veins, and the tumor becomes densely opacified for a short time as the intravenously injected bolus of contrast material traverses the vascular bed of the tumor (Figs. 4–35 and 4–36). With MRI, paragangliomas can be distinguished from other lesions such as neurofibroma. They are seen as hypointense to brain on $T_1W$ images and become hyperintense on $T_2W$ MR scans.

Glomus complex tumors are highly vascular, which dynamic MR (GRASS) can demonstrate, allowing them to be differentiated from other lesions. They are seen as hypointense to brain on $T_1W$ images and become hyperintense on $T_2W$ MR scans. They usually show signal void (dark) areas due to their increased vascularity (Figs. 4–35 and 4–36). The intracranial extension of a base of the skull lesion is best demonstrated on post-contrast-enhanced CT or MRI scans. For glomus complex tumors, a CT scan reveals the bone destruction and total extent of the disease and gives accurate assessment of the middle ear.

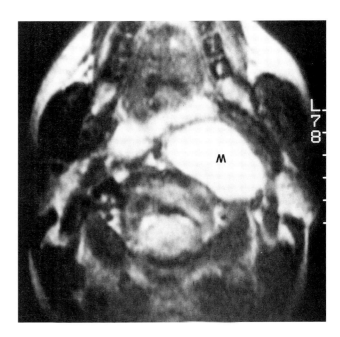

**Figure 4–30.** Schwannoma. Axial T₂W MR scan shows a large mass *(M)* in the left parapharyngeal space.

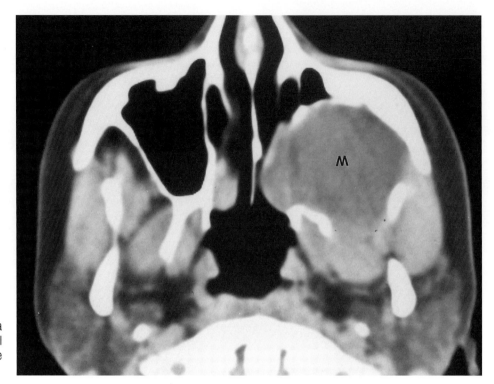

**Figure 4–31.** Axial CT scan shows a large mass *(M)* in the left infratemporal fossa, compatible with a benign nerve sheath tumor.

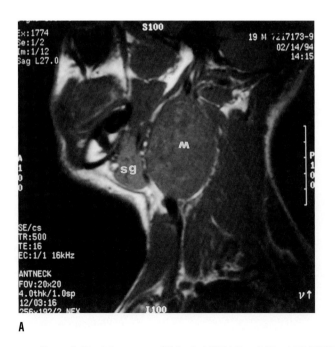

**A**

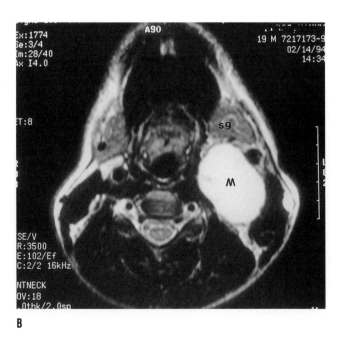

**B**

**Figure 4–32.** Schwannoma. **(A)** Sagittal T₁W MR and **(B)** axial T₂W MR scans showing a large mass *(M)*, behind the left submandibular gland *(sg)*.

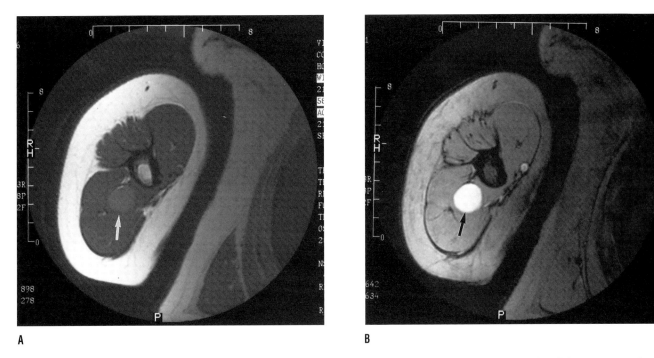

**A**                                                    **B**

**Figure 4–33.** Benign tumor of the radial nerve. Axial T$_1$W MR **(A)** and T$_2$W **(B)** scans showing characteristic signal intensities of a radial nerve neuroma *(arrow)*.

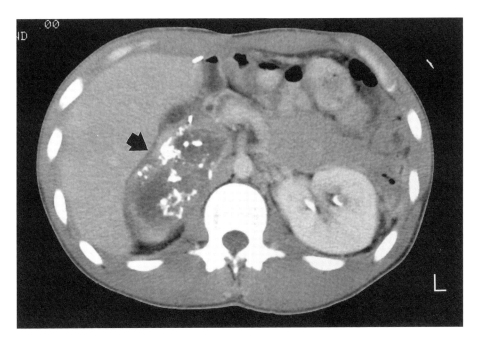

**Figure 4–34.** Malignant schwannoma. Enhanced axial CT scan of the abdomen shows a large heterogeneous mass *(arrow)* with dystrophic calcifications replacing the right kidney.

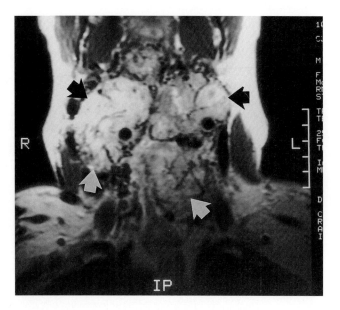

**Figure 4–35.** Bilateral carotid body tumors (chemodectoma). Coronal MR scan shows large masses *(arrows)* with significant vascularity.

## ■ EXTRASKELETAL CARTILAGINOUS AND OSSEOUS TUMORS

Malignant osseous and/or cartilaginous tumors also occur as primary soft tissue neoplasms, but they are much less common than primary osteosarcomas or chondrosarcomas of the bone.[47] A detailed clinico-pathologic description of these interesting, albeit rare, sarcomas will be found elsewhere in the book. From an imaging standpoint, the features are less specific than in some other sarcomas. However, on MRI, most extra-skeletal chondrosarcomas have low-signal intensity on $T_1$-weighted images and increased signal intensity on $T_2$-weighted images (Figs. 4–37A and 4–37B).[48,49] On CT scans, osteogenic sarcomas show as irregular islands of tumor bone formation and marked bone destruction (Figs. 4–38A and 4–38B). Radiologic differentiation between these and osteoblastoma or giant cell tumors is indeed difficult.

Myositis ossificans is a benign ossifying process that is generally solitary and well circumscribed. It is found most commonly in the musculature, but may occur in other tissues, especially tendons and subcutaneous fat.[50] Diagnosis is very difficult, particularly in its early stage, when it is often confused with extraskeletal osteo-sarcoma. Late examples, consisting entirely of mature lamellar bone, are sometimes misdiagnosed as osteo-mas. The initial complaint noted within hours to days after an injury is pain and tenderness followed by dif-fuse soft tissue swelling. Within several weeks, the swelling becomes more circumscribed and indurated, gradually transforming into a hard firm mass. It tends to affect active adolescents and adults, predominantly males. Myositis ossificans is rare in children.[51]

Initial plain radiographs may show an increase in soft tissue density in the affected area. Calcification is rarely seen before the end of the third week after

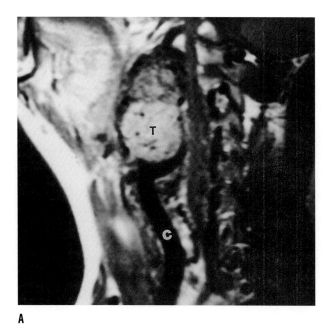

A

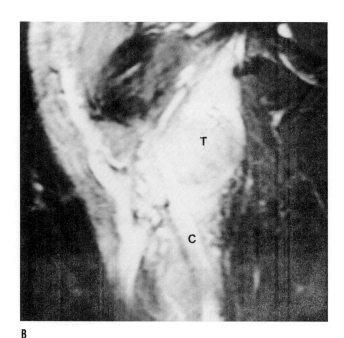

B

**Figure 4–36.** Carotid body tumor. **(A)** Sagittal $T_1$W and **(B)** gradient-echo MR scans show carotid body tumor *(T)* and common carotid arteries *(C)*. Note displacement of internal and external carotid arteries.

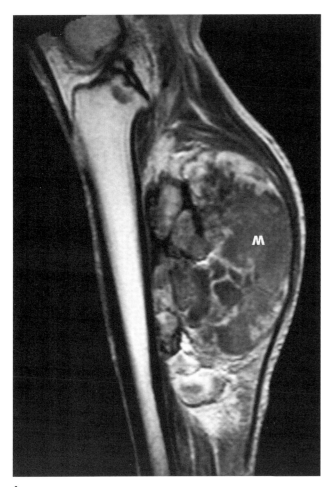

**A**

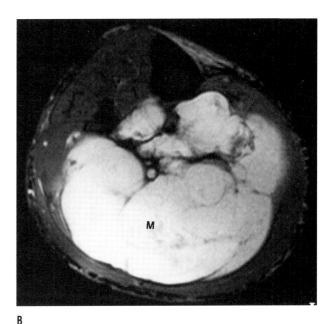

**B**

**Figure 4–37.** **(A)** Sagittal T$_1$W and axial steady states inversion recovery (STIR) of a chondrosarcoma of the right calf. **(B)** MR scans showing a large mass *(M)*, compatible with chondrosarcoma.

injury. When present, it appears as faint, irregular floc-cular radiopacities. As it progresses, it becomes more of a circumscribed soft tissue mass with dense calcifica-tions peripherally.[52] Calcification is seen most clearly four to six weeks after injury. It proceeds from the periphery to the center, which is an important differ-entiating point from osteosarcoma, whose calcifications are more dense in the center and proceed peripherally. A distinct radiolucent cleft separates the mass from the underlying bone, which helps differentiate this from osteochondroma (Figs. 4–39A and 4–39B). Myositis is a self-limiting process with excellent prognosis after local excision.[51] Spontaneous regression has also been ob-served.[53]

Radiologic imagings of various other types of mes-enchymal tumors have been and are being performed. Most of these only show the presence of a deep-seated tumor with no particular characteristic able to provide the clinician with a clue to the morphologic charac-

teristics. Thus, these tumors are not individually cata-logued or illustrated. In effect, MR and CT imaging studies in malignant mesenchymal tumors have revolu-tionized the general principles of staging and manage-ment of soft tissue neoplasms.

Angiographic studies of cavitary tumors, such as retroperitoneal sarcomas, are essential. No patient with a suspected retroperitoneal tumor should be operated on without prior angiographic study. Figs. 4–40 and 4–41 are angiograms of selected patients with retroperi-toneal tumors; the accompanying case histories in the legends show the need for these angiograms.

## VENOGRAPHY

Venography has a limited role in the diagnosis or management of soft tissue tumors. Contrast studies of the inferior vena cava are valuable for the preopera-tive assessment of retroperitoneal soft tissue tumors

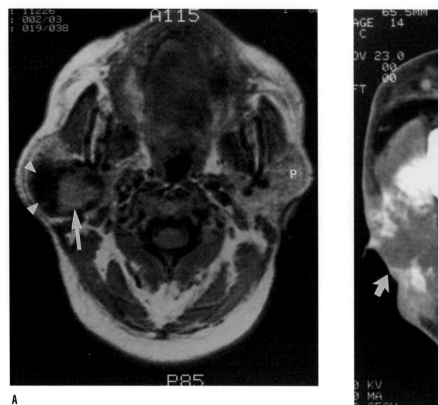

A

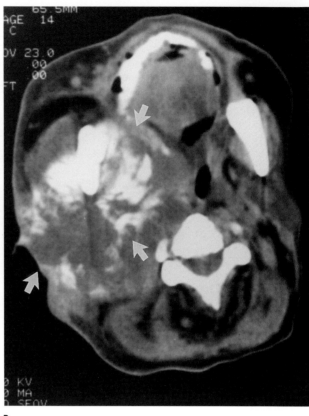

B

**Figure 4–38.** Osteogenic sarcoma in a patient who had a previously resected pleomorphic adenoma. Axial T$_1$W **(A)** MR scan demonstrates a heterogeneous mass involving the right parotid gland. There is a soft tissue component *(arrow)* and a lower intensity bony component *(arrowheads)*. Axial CT scan **(B)** performed on the same patient several months later demonstrates significant enlargement with neoplastic bone formation. *P* = normal parotid gland.

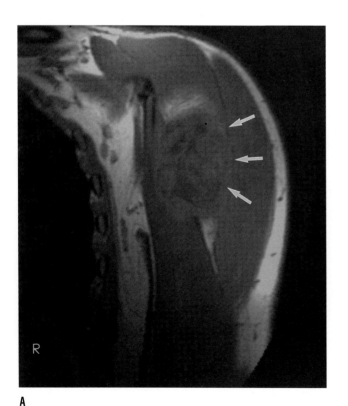

A

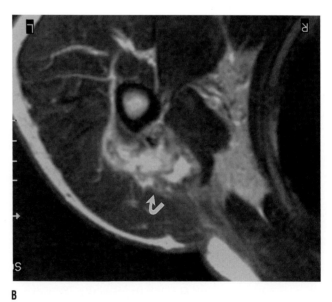

B

**Figure 4–39.** Myositis ossificans. Coronal T$_1$W **(A)** and axial T$_2$W **(B)** MR images of the shoulder demonstrating a heterogeneous mass in the soft tissues separate from the humerus.

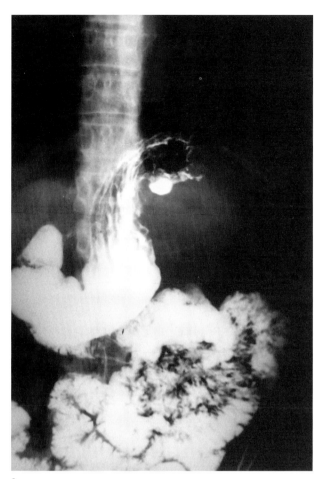

**A**

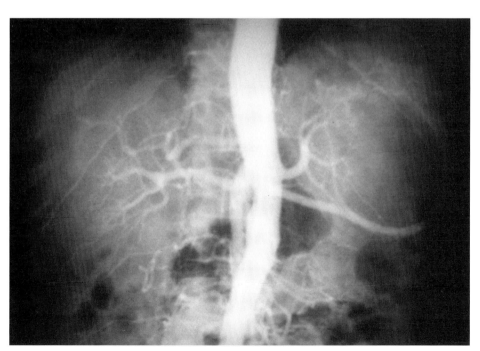

**B**

**Figure 4–40. (A)** Upper gastrointestinal tract series showing the greater curvature of the stomach persistently pushed toward the right, but diagnosis could not be established. Patient was a 45-year-old man with a history of indigestion and vague abdominal discomfort. **(B)** Aortogram showing a tumor of the left retroperitoneum. The neovascularity is suggestive of malignancy.

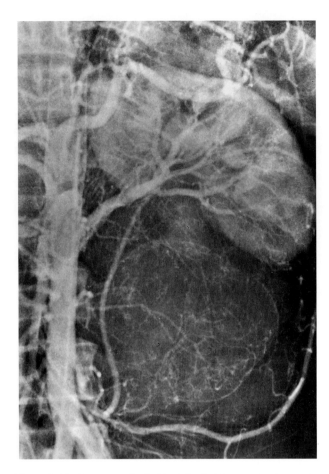

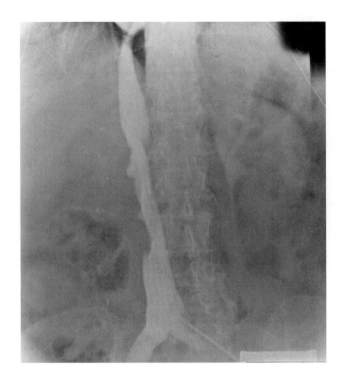

**Figure 4–42.** Inferior venacavogram of a patient with fibrosarcoma of the retroperitoneum. Note involvement of the vena cava.

**Figure 4–41.** Aortogram of palpable abdominal tumors showing a retroperitoneal tumor on the left side. This tumor was found to be a leiomyosarcoma.

(Fig. 4–42). The clinician frequently fails to recognize the extent of a retroperitoneal tumor, even after a flush aortogram is obtained. A large retroperitoneal tumor may press on or adhere to the inferior vena cava, with little systemic manifestation in the patient. Furthermore, the inferior vena cava can occasionally be the site of origin of the retroperitoneal tumor (e.g., retroperitoneal leiomyosarcoma). Although, with dynamic CT, the need for this type of investigation is decreasing, still it must be borne in mind that in certain complex retroperitoneal sarcomas, especially in recurrent tumors, this technique provides additional preoperative information and helps the surgeon avoid some major pitfalls.

## RADIOISOTOPE TECHNIQUES

Using radioisotope scintigraphy to diagnose primary soft tissue sarcoma or determine the extent of meta-

static disease has had limited success. Today, no generally accepted radiopharmaceutical drug is available for the diagnosis of soft tissue sarcomas. The success of imaging of metastatic sarcoma will depend on the availability of sarcoma-specific monoclonal antibodies. In our Department of Surgical Oncology, we are currently investigating the applicability of sarcoma-specific radiolabeled monoclonal antibodies developed in our laboratory for the detection of occult metastatic soft tissue sarcomas. The preliminary results appear to be encouraging and certainly merit further investigation. (See Chapter 20 for further details.)

## REFERENCES

1. Sim FH, Edmonson JH, Wold LE: Soft-tissue sarcomas: Future perspectives. Clin Orthop 289:106, 1993
2. Storm FK, Mahvi DM: Diagnosis and management of retroperitoneal soft-tissue sarcoma. Ann Surg 214(1):2, 1991
3. Arca MJ, Sondak VK, Chang AE: Diagnostic procedures and pretreatment evaluation of soft tissue sarcomas. Semin Surg Oncol 10(5):323, 1994
4. Pino G, Conzi GF, Murolo C, et al.: Sonographic evaluation of local recurrences of soft tissue sarcomas. J Ultrasound Med 12(1):23, 1993

5. Agnarsson BA, Baldeursson G, Benediktsdottir KR, Hrafnkelsson J: Tumors in Iceland. 14. Malignant tumors of soft tissues. Histological classification and epidemiological considerations. Acta Pathol Microbiol Immunol Scand 99:443, 1991

6. Boring CC, Squires TS, Tong T: Cancer statistics CA. Cancer J Clin 41:19, 1991

7. Olson PN, Everson LI, Griffiths HJ: Staging of musculoskeletal tumors. Radiol Clin North Am 32(1):151, 1994

8. Massengill AD, Seeger LL, Eckardt JJ: The role of plain radiography, computed tomography, and magnetic resonance imaging in sarcoma evaluation. Hematol Oncol Clin North Am 9(3):571, 1995

9. Jelinek JS, Kransdorf MJ, Shmookler BM, et al.: Liposarcoma of the extremities: MR and CT findings in the histologic subtypes. Radiol 186(2):455, 1993

10. Kransdorf MJ, Jelinek JS, Moser RP: Imaging of soft tissue tumors. Radiol Clin North Am 31(2):359, 1993

11. Munk PL, Poon PY, Chhem RK, Janzen DL: Imaging of soft-tissue sarcomas. Can Assoc Radiol J 45(6):438, 1994

12. McCullough EC: Basic physics of x-ray computed tomography. In Norman D, Korobkin M, Newton TH (eds): Computed Tomography. St. Louis, CV Mosby, 1977

13. Boyd DP: Physics II computed tomography. In Norman D, Korobkin M, Newton TH (eds): Computed Tomography. St. Louis, CV Mosby, 1977

14. Shugar MA, Mafee MF: Diagnosis of carotid body tumors by dynamic computerized tomography. Head Neck Surg 4:518, 1982

15. Dobben GD, Valvassori GE, Mafee MF, Berninger WH: Evaluation of brain circulation by rapid rotation of computer tomography. Radiol 133:105, 1979

16. Valvassori GE, Mafee MF, Dobben GD: Evaluation of blood circulation of the hindbrain by dynamic computed tomography. Radiol 133:105, 1979

17. Damadian R, Cope FW: NMR in cancer. V. Electronic diagnosis of cancer by potassium (39K) nuclear magnetic resonance: Spin signatures and T1 beat patterns. Physiol Chem Phys 6:309, 1974

18. Mafee MF, Peyman GA, Grisolano JE, et al.: Malignant uveal melanoma and simulating lesions: MR imaging evaluation. Radiology 160:773, 1986

19. Kransdorf MJ, Jelinek JS, Moser RP Jr., et al.: Soft tissue masses: Diagnosis using MR imaging. Am J Roentgenol 153:541, 1989

20. Gelineck J, Keller J, Myhre Jensen O, et al.: Evaluation of lipomatous soft tissue tumors by MR imaging. Acta Radiol 35(4):367, 1994

21. Murphy WA, Totty WG, Destouet JM, et al.: Musculoskeletal system. In Lee JL, Sagel SS, Stanley RJ (eds): Computed Body Tomography with MRI Correlation. 2nd ed. New York, Raven Press, 1989, p 899

22. Enzinger FM, Weiss SW: Benign tumors of the peripheral nerves. In Enzinger FM, Weiss SW (eds): Soft Tissue Tumors. 3rd ed. St. Louis, Mosby-Yearbook, 1995, p 821

23. Benson PA, Janko AB: Pelvic myelolipoma (rare presacral tumor). Am J Obstet Gynecol 92:884, 1965

24. Dodge OG, Evans DMD: Haemopoeisis in a presacral fatty tumor (myelolipoma). J Pathol Bacteriol 72:313, 1956

25. Behan M, Martin EC, Meucke EC, Kazam E: Myelolipoma of the adrenal: Two cases with ultrasound and CT findings. Am J Roentgenol 129:993, 1977

26. Lawrence W Jr, Donegan WL, Natarajan N, et al.: Adult soft tissue sarcomas. A pattern of care survey of the American College of Surgeons. Ann Surg 205:349, 1987

27. Konwaler BJ, Keasbey L, Kaplan L: Subcutaneous pseudosarcomatous fibromatosis fascitis: Report of 8 cases. Am J Clin Pathol 25:241, 1955

28. Stout AP: The fibromatoses. Clin Orthop 19:11, 1961

29. Carter BL: Tumors of the paranasal sinuses and nasal cavity. In Valvassori GE, Buckingham RA, Carter BL, et al. (eds): Head and Neck Imaging. Thieme, Stuttgart, 1988, p 219

30. Norris CM, Goodman ML: Case records of the Massachusetts General Hospital. N Engl J Med 326:1417, 1992

31. Mafee MF. In Valvassori GE, Mafee MF, Carter BL (eds): Imaging of the Head and Neck. Thieme, Stuttgart, 1995, p 303

32. Müller J. Uber den fienern Bau und die Formen der Krankhaften Grechwulste. Berlin, G Reimer, 1838, p 80

33. Enzinger FM, Shiraki M: Musculo-aponeurotic fibromatosis of the shoulder girdle (extra-abdominal desmoid): Analysis of thirty cases followed up for ten or more years. Cancer 20:1131, 1967

34. Enzinger FM, Weiss SW: Fibromatoses. In Enzinger FM, Weiss SW (eds): Soft Tissue Tumors. 3rd ed. St Louis, Mosby-Yearbook, 1995, p 201

35. Casillas J, Sais GJ, Greve JL, et al.: Imaging of intra- and extraabdominal desmoid tumors. Radiographics 11:959, 1991

36. Murphey MD, Gross TM, Rosenthal HG: Musculoskeletal malignant fibrous histiocytoma: Radiologic-pathologic correlation. Radiographics 14:807, 1994

37. Enzinger FM, Weiss SW: Leiomyosarcoma. In Enzinger FM, Weiss SW (eds): Soft Tissue Tumors. 3rd ed., St Louis, Mosby-Yearbook, 1995, p 491

38. Hashimoto H: Incidence of soft tissue sarcomas in adults. Curr Top Pathol 89:1, 1995

39. Wile AG, Evans HL, Romsdahl MM: Leiomyosarcoma of soft tissue: A clinicopathologic study. Cancer 48:1022, 1981

40. Ranchod M, Kempson RL: Smooth muscle tumors of the gastrointestinal tract and retroperitoneum. Cancer 39:255, 1977

41. Shmookler BM, Lauer DH: Retroperitoneal leiomyosarcoma: A clinicopathologic analysis of 36 cases. Am J Surg Pathol 7:269, 1983

42. Enzinger FM, Weiss SW: Rhabdomyosarcoma. In Enzinger FM, Weiss SW (eds): Soft Tissue Tumors. 3rd ed. St Louis, Mosby-Yearbook, 1995, p 539

43. Fumikazu S, Shusuke S, Kunihiro K, et al.: Intrathoracic neurogenic tumors: MR-pathologic correlation. Am J Roentgenol 159:279, 1992

44. Stout AP: The peripheral manifestations of specific nerve sheath tumor (neurilemoma). Am J Cancer 24:751, 1935

45. Hanafee WN: Radiology of the pharynx and larynx—Part IV. In Valvassori GE, Potter GD, Hanafee WN, et al. (eds): Radiology of the Ear, Nose and Throat. Thieme, Stuttgart, 1982

46. Carter BL, Karmody CS: Computed tomography of the face and neck. Semin Roentgenol 3:257, 1978

47. Enzinger FM, Weiss SW: Cartilaginous soft tissue tumors. In Enzinger FM, Weiss SW (eds): Soft Tissue Tumors. 3rd ed. St Louis, Mosby-Yearbook, 1995, p 991

48. Peterson KK, Renfrew DL, Feddersen RM, et al.: Magnetic resonance imaging of myxoid containing tumors. Skeletal Radiol 20:245, 1991

49. Shinaver C, Mafee MF, Chai KH: MRI of mesenchymal chondrosarcoma of the orbit: Case report and review of the literature. Neuroradiology 39:296, 1977

50. Rothberg AS: Tendinitis ossificans traumatica. Am J Surg 58:285, 1942

51. Enzinger FM, Weiss SW: Osseus soft tissue tumors. In Enzinger FM, Weiss SW (eds): Soft Tissue Tumors. 3rd ed. St Louis, Mosby-Yearbook, 1995, p 1013

52. Hutcheson J, Klatte EC, Kremp R: The angiographic appearance of myositis ossificans circumscripta: A case report. Radiology 102:57, 1972

53. Ackerman LV: Extraosseous localized nonneoplastic bone and cartilage formation (so-called myositis ossificans): Clinical and pathological confusion with malignant neoplasms. J Bone Joint Surg 40A:279, 1958

# 5

# Pathology of Soft Tissue Sarcoma

Because of soft tissue sarcoma's relative rarity and the subtle differences in the histologic appearance between benign and malignant tumors arising from mesenchymal tissue, it is difficult for pathologists to always obtain an accurate histologic diagnosis of soft tissue sarcoma. However, with recent improved clinical recognition of these lesions and better-defined histologic criteria for proper pathologic diagnosis, sarcoma is no longer diagnosed only in specialized referral centers, but also in community hospitals. Although routine light microscopic examination of paraffin-embedded sections is still the mainstay of soft tissue sarcoma diagnosis, frequently electron microscopy and immunohistochemistry help establish the proper diagnosis of these lesions. Also, chromosomal abnormality has been studied in some of these soft tissue sarcomas, and specific abnormalities help diagnose some of these tumors. As such, the chromosomal study of soft tissue sarcoma is used with increasing frequency. For example, the chromosomal translocation of synovial cell sarcoma is used as a proof-positive for diagnosis in questionable cases (see Fig. 6–1). Even with all these advancements, still a number of lesions cannot be classified according to their true histogenetic origin, and these lesions are termed *undifferentiated sarcomas*. However, in the last decade, this diagnosis has become less frequent than in the past. We believe that only proper histologic diagnosis and establishment of the histogenetic origin of the tumor, and correlating this information with treatment and outcome, will provide better treatment success, particularly with adjuvant chemotherapy.

The electron microscopic study of tumor tissue is useful in establishing the histogenetic origin in a large number of tumors. Ultrastructural study of normal mesenchymal cells of soft supporting tissue has revealed specific cytoplasmic characteristics and extracellular products indicating specialized forms of cytodifferentiation that enable reasonably certain identification of cell type. Ultrastructural and cellular traits of normal mesenchymal cells appear to be retained in most malignant neoplastic cells to a degree that identifying such characteristics helps establish the proper histogenesis and diagnosis of many soft tissue sarcomas.[1–9] However, electron microscopy has its own limitations: in several instances, overlapping features and variations continue to hamper the accurate histogenetic interpretation. For example, collagen production is not a certain indication that a given sarcoma is a fibrosarcoma or originates from the fibrous tissue. Cells of a neurogenic tumor, presumably derived from Schwann cells, also appear able to form collagen fibrils. Similarly, endothelial cells of an angiosarcoma may not resemble malignant mesenchymal cells; rather, their close intercellular junctions and desmosomes resemble those of other malignant epithelial cells. In such instances, use of immunoperoxidase stains becomes helpful. In the last three decades, immunohistochemical study using both polyclonal and monoclonal antibodies against identifiable specialized protein helped to identify characteristics of many tumors and render proper diagnosis (Fig. 5–1A to 5–1H and Color Plate 2). However, immunoperoxidase stain also has several limitations. In a highly anaplastic sarcoma, it is frequently difficult by immunoperoxidase studies to classify the origin of a given malignant cell. Nevertheless, today ultrastructural confirmation of the tumor and immunoperoxidase

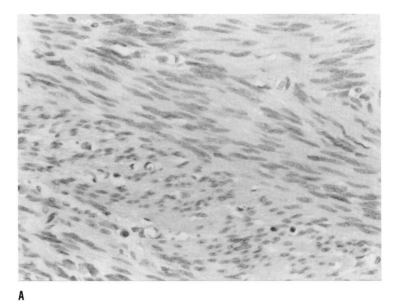

A

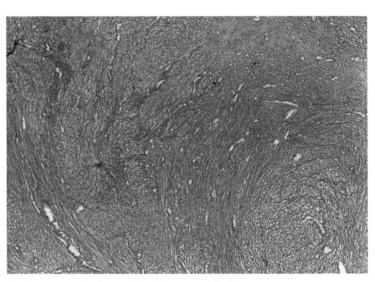

B

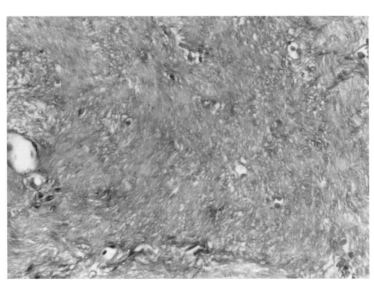

C

**Figure 5–1. (A)** H & E stain of a deep tissue leiomyosarcoma. (Original magnification × 40.) **(B)** Reticulin stain of the same tumor. (Original magnification × 10.) **(C)** Trichrome stain of the same tumor. (Original magnification × 40.) *(Continued.)*

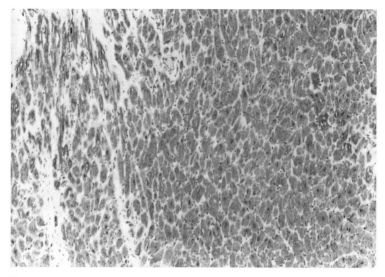

D

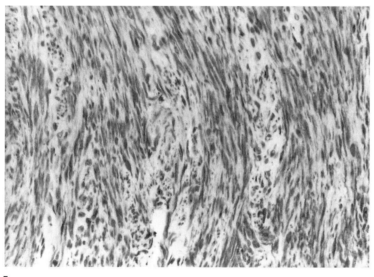

E

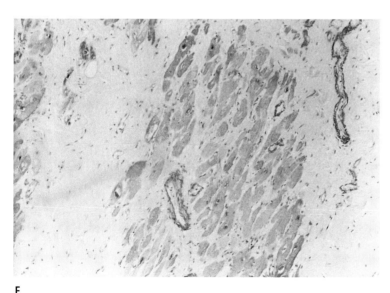

F

**Figure 5–1** *(continued).* **(D)** Desmin control. (Original magnification × 40.) **(E)** Desmin positive for leiomyosarcoma. (Same tumor, original magnification × 40.) **(F)** Actin control. (Original magnification × 10.) *(Continued.)*

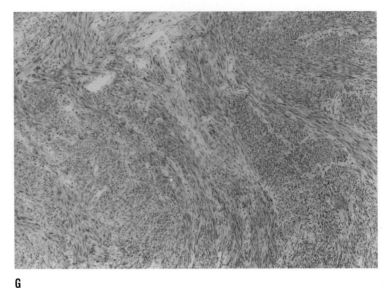

G

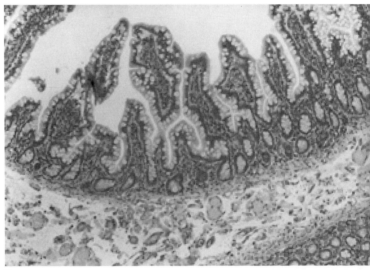

H

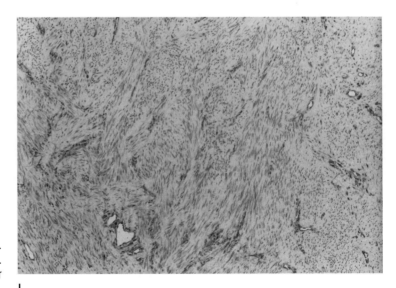

**Figure 5–1** *(continued)*. **(G)** Leiomyosarcoma positive for actin. (Same tumor, original magnification × 10.) **(H)** Vimentin control. (Original magnification × 10.) **(I)** Leiomyosarcoma positive for vimentin. (Same tumor, original magnification × 40.)

I

stains of the paraffin-embedded section help diagnose a given soft tissue sarcoma with greater certainty. Furthermore, in recent years, cytogenetic studies of these mesenchymal tumors have also shed more light on the ontogeny and proper diagnosis of these relatively rare tumors (see Chapter 6).

In this chapter, we will describe and discuss the structure, function, and pathologic aspects of various forms of tumor and tumorlike conditions that arise in soft somatic tissue. The classification of mesenchymal and neural tumors as outlined in Table 2–1, Chapter 2, forms the basis of subsequent discussions. The cytogenetic characteristics of each pertinent tumor type are described below; however, for a better understanding of the proper role of karyotypic studies in relation to molecular biology of soft tissues tumors, the reader is referred to Chapter 6.

## ■ TUMOR AND TUMORLIKE CONDITIONS OF ADIPOSE TISSUE

To better understand tumors and tumorlike conditions of the adipose tissue, it is appropriate to briefly describe the histogenesis and structure of both white and brown adipose tissue. Without such background information, it is difficult to comprehend the complexity of this clinical entity.

Deposition of adipose tissue begins during the fifth month of intrauterine life. Keith[10] stated that certain granular cells of the connective tissue, especially of the subcutaneous layer, secrete fat, which appears first as diffuse droplets. These cells ultimately run together and produce the characteristic outline of the adipose cell. Fat reaches its greatest normal development just before and immediately after birth. At birth, a mass of tissue resembling the interscapular gland of hibernating mammals[11] is frequently found on each posterior triangle of the neck, extending beneath the trapezius muscle. Adipose tissue is then classified into two main types, *white* and *brown*, and tumorlike conditions arising from each type have different characteristics.

## WHITE ADIPOSE TISSUE

White adipose tissue is a white or yellowish-white fatty tissue that is widely distributed throughout the body. The mature adipose cell contains a single large droplet of neutral fat within a thin envelope of cytoplasm (Fig. 5–2). The nucleus is compressed into a crescent shape within the thin rim of cytoplasm. In a well-nourished person, the cells vary in size. In vivo, probably every adipose cell is in contact with a capillary. White adipose tissue appears to be one of the most highly vascularized tissues in the body.

### Histogenesis

The origin of white adipose cells is still unclear. One view, which can be traced back to Flemming,[12] is that both the lobular and the more dispersed adipose tissue are formed by accumulation of fat droplets in unspecialized cells of connective tissue. This view has been widely supported, particularly by Clark and Clark,[13] who observed regular transformation of the fat cells from fibroblasts in transplant chambers built into rabbit ears.

Toldt[14] and Wasserman[15] held that adipose tissue developed from a specialized anlage and that each lobule of adipose tissue develops by enlargement and differentiation of a specific embryonic "primitive" organ composed of mesenchymal cells that are mingled with small blood vessels. Wasserman[15] suggested that, in the human embryo, a thin capsule separates lentiform areas of characteristic structures from the surrounding connective tissue. These lentiform areas consist of a network of capillaries and mesenchymal cells, and these cells are where the fat appears. Both Dabelow[16] and Napolitano[17] provided supporting evidence for the thesis that, even at a very immature stage of development, white adipose cells have specialized structural features

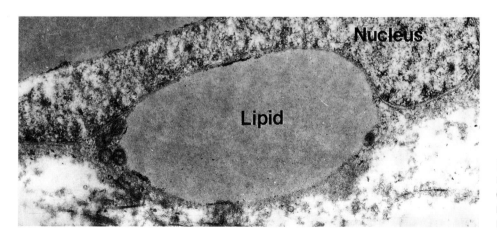

**Figure 5–2.** Electron micrograph of a mature human adipose cell. A single large droplet of lipid fat is compressing the nucleus into a crescent shape. (Original magnification × 31,360.)

and can be distinguished from fibroblasts. Further support of this view stems from the appearance of mature adipose cells in states of extreme nutrition depletion. Such cells lose lipid and assume the form of embryonic adipose cells rather than fibroblasts.[18]

The number of adipose cells apparently increases in mature mammals. Sidman[18] found that, in obese humans, the amount of lipid per cell is elevated, but not sufficiently to account for an increase of 10–30 kg of body fat. The extra lipid, then, must accumulate in the new cells.[19,20]

A number of early reports dealing with tissue culture described the accumulation of fat in cultured connective tissue cells. The relevance of these in vitro reports is uncertain, particularly since it is not yet known whether fatty fibroblasts are true adipose cells. However, transformation of adult fibroblasts into fatty fibroblasts cannot be ruled out. At least for the present, the original concept of Toldt[14] and Wasserman[15] appears valid.

## Structure

A living fat cell in white adipose tissue is a large, brilliant, spherical body. Every mature fat cell contains one large droplet of fat that can be stained with such dyes as osmic acid or Sudan black B (Fig. 5–3). The cytoplasm is reduced to a thin membrane, which surrounds the drop and is taken in the part that contains the flattened nucleus with its central mass of chromatin. The composition of fat in the mature cell can range from simple lipid excess to compound lipids.

The amount of lipid present in fat cells, its chemical composition, and disproportionate volume in comparison to its cytoplasm make it difficult to process the tissue properly for ultrastructure study. Both Sheldon[21] and Napolitano[17] demonstrated that the fine structure of fat cells is essentially the same as that of any other living cell (Fig. 5–4). The intracytoplasmic components are better discerned in fasting animals, owing to depletion of the cytoplasmic lipids.[21] Capillaries are close to the surface of white fat cells. In most instances, they are separated by their respective basement membrane and small bundles of collagen. Neural elements, either myelinated or nonmyelinated, have infrequently been observed in the intercellular region of fat pads.[17]

## BROWN ADIPOSE TISSUE

### Structure

Brown adipose tissue varies from a rich, reddish brown to light tan. The color is mainly contributed by the high concentration of cytochrome pigments in the mitochondria of the adipose cells. Some of its color is due to hemoglobin, which is a highly vascular tissue. The species, distribution, gross anatomy, and histologic structure have been well reviewed by Hammar,[22] Rasmussen,[11] and Johanason and Soderlund.[23] Brown adipose tissue is prominent in most hibernating and many nonhibernating animal species. Although masses of brown fat can be found in the neck, interscapular region, thorax, and axilla, in most species, they are found along the major blood vessels of the thoracic and abdominal cavities, extending to the proximal part of the limbs. Brown fat bodies are usually enclosed in the

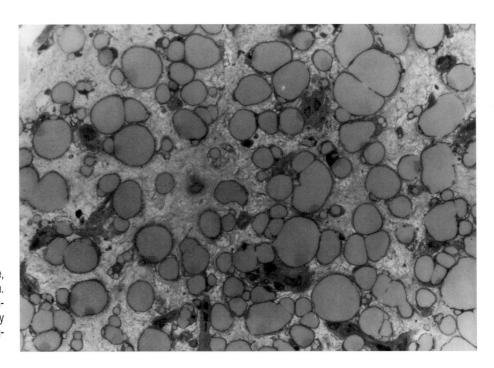

**Figure 5–3.** Mature adipose tissue, Araldite-embedded one-micron section. Osmiophilic lipid droplets are easily discernible. In some cells, the peripherally placed nuclei are also visible. (Original magnification × 310.)

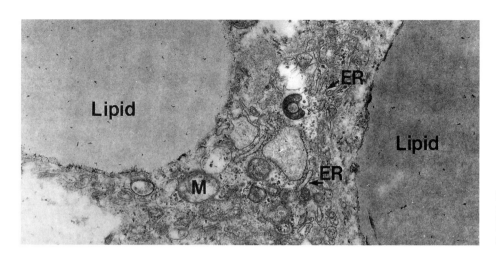

**Figure 5–4.** An adipose cell showing cytoplasmic details. *ER* = endoplasmic reticulum; *M* = mitochondria. (Original magnification × 31,460.)

connective tissue capsule and are sometimes discretely localized.

The fat content of brown adipose cells can increase considerably. This fact raises the question of whether brown and white adipose tissue are separate in origin or represent two stages in the differentiation of one tissue. While there is room for dispute about the source of white adipose cells, it is generally agreed that brown adipose cells arise from a specific anlage at particular body sites at certain times during fetal development and remain concentrated in these body sites; no new areas develop in postnatal life.[24] With advancing age, however, multivacuolar cells of brown adipose tissue are replaced by univacuolar cells, leading to the view that brown adipose tissue is no more than an immature form of white adipose tissue.[24] But when an obese animal is placed on a restricted diet, univacuolar brown adipose tissue cells revert to and keep their multilocular form, whereas true white adipose tissue cells rapidly lose their fat altogether.

The human fetus clearly has brown adipose tissue, and normal adults also have a small amount. In humans, islands of cells of brown fat are best observed in the region of the neck, chest, and periadrenal fatty tissue, which are prominent sites in hibernating rodents.[25] Hibernomas usually occur in these sites. However, none of the studies thus far published has settled the question of whether the two kinds of adipose tissues are distinct from each other.

A normal brown adipose cell, in contradistinction to a white adipose cell, contains a number of small fat droplets. Ultrastructurally, the cell cytoplasm is studded with myriad mitochondria. The brown fat is richly innervated, and nonmyelinated fibers frequently are observed in the connective tissue septa separating the glandlike lobules. Axons may occur in close apposition to brown fat cells. The resulting morphologic relationship is similar to that of the Schwann cell and its C fibers.[26] This observation by Napolitano is consistent with localizations of catecholamine in brown fat.[27,28] Dawkins and co-workers[27] postulated that cytoplasmic localizations of catecholamine, presumably noradrenalin, are clearly appropriate for the activation of lipase in the vicinity of fat droplets and lead to hydrolysis of triglyceride and subsequent oxidation of long-chain fatty acids. Romer[29] demonstrated the presence of corticosteroids and postulated that, under certain conditions, brown fat can take up the functions of the adrenal cortex.

## BENIGN NEOPLASMS OF WHITE ADIPOSE TISSUE

### Lipomas

*Macroscopic Findings.*    The gross appearance of lipomas found in the somatic tissues is essentially that of encapsulated fat. The fatty mass is usually yellow and semifirm and is divided into smaller lobulations by fibrous strands that traverse the tumor. The subcutaneous tumor is generally encapsulated by a thin fibrous layer; however, in the intermuscular variety, the lipomatous tissue frequently extends or infiltrates along the muscle planes, a fact to be considered both from a diagnostic and a therapeutic standpoint—otherwise, an erroneous diagnosis of liposarcoma may be rendered.[30–32] When a comparatively small amount of fibrous tissue is present, the tumor is semi-firm and it is difficult to cut sections. In contrast, in some tumors the fibrous tissue content is high and the tumor firm—these tumors are called *fibrolipomas.* A typical lipoma is thinly encapsulated, presenting a greasy appearance and the yellow coloration of adipose tissue. Occasionally, hemorrhage and xanthomatous or myxoid degeneration may produce patchy discoloration and variegated appearances. Delicate fibrous septa intersect the lipoma and form an irregular supporting structure that carries nutrient blood vessels (Fig. 5–5). At times, the vasculature of the lipoma is extensive, and the term *angiolipoma* is used (Fig. 5–6A and 5–6B). Angiolipomas occur in all sites,

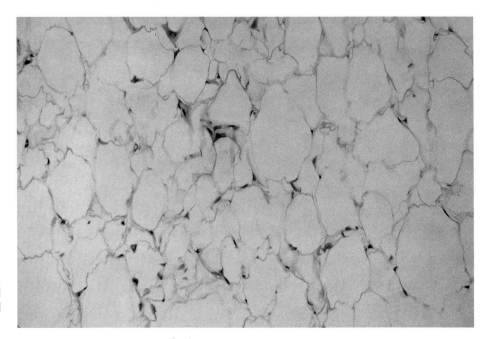

**Figure 5–5.** Solitary subcutaneous lipoma. Delicate fibrous septa and nutrient blood vessels can be easily seen. (H & E. Original magnification × 125.)

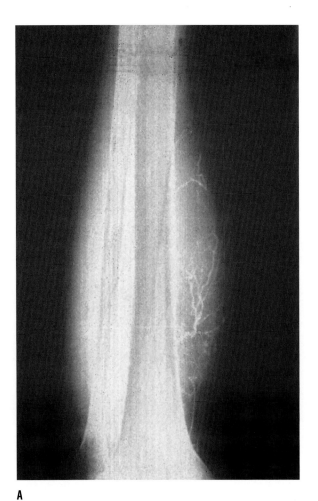

A

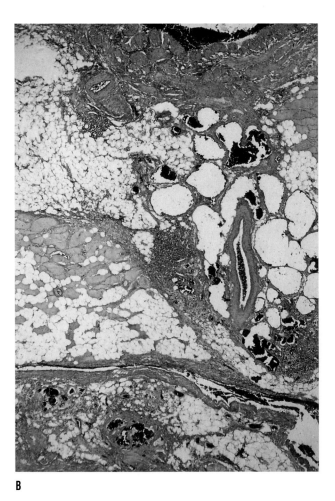

B

**Figure 5–6. (A)** Angiogram of an angiolipoma of the right calf of a 24-year-old man. Clinically this was thought to be a malignant tumor. **(B)** Angiolipoma showing multitude of capillaries with mature fatty tissue. The stroma shows the presence of fibroreticular material around the blood vessels. (H & E. Original magnification × 63). A wide excision of the gross tumor was performed. Although microscopic residual tumor was left behind during the initial operation, patient has remained well for 18 years.

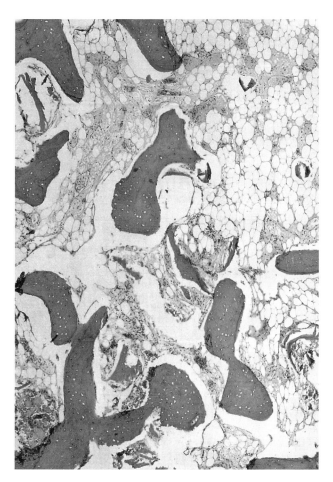

**Figure 5–7.** Osteolipoma in a 65-year-old man with a long-standing history of a subcutaneous tumor in the forearm. Islands of bone are formed within the stroma of a lipoma. (H & E. Original magnification × 63.)

including the viscera. Due to their extensive vascularity, they tend to bleed and clinically may resemble sarcomas. Occasionally, bone formation (ossifying lipoma) and foci of chondrification also occur in lipomas (Fig. 5–7).

**Heterotopic Lipoma.**    Heterotopic lipomas are found in sites other than the adipose tissue. These tumors can be further classified: (1) angiomyolipomas, tumors containing blood vessels and muscle fibers; (2) lipomas of the tendon sheath, tumors connected with collagen tissue; and (3) neurofibrolipomas, tumors containing neural elements. When benign fatty tissue infiltrates surrounding structures and it is difficult to differentiate from well-differentiated liposarcoma, the term *infiltrating* or *diffuse* (neoplastic or non-neoplastic) proliferation of mature fat is used. This group includes diffuse lipomatosis, pelvic lipomatosis (see Fig. 7–17A to 7–17E), symmetrical lipomatosis (Figs. 5–8A to 5–8C), adiposis doloris, and nevus lipomatosis (see Table 2–1) (see Chapter 7 for details).

*Microscopic Findings.*    The tumor cells in common lipomas are usually large, spherical, and distended with fat; some are so laden with fat that the cytoplasm appears to be bound by a barely perceptible membrane surrounding a flattened nucleus (see Fig. 5–5). The cells may also be small, containing less fat, a proportionately greater amount of protoplasm, and a larger, ovoid, centrally placed nucleus. Lipomas have a fairly uniform cytologic appearance and are composed of a mixture of cells of different shapes and sizes, lying close together and sometimes arranged in small groups bound by fibroblasts and collagen. In angiolipomas, the fibrous

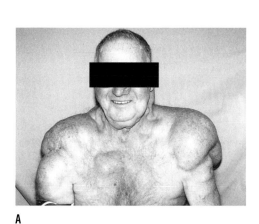
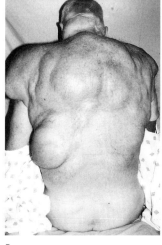
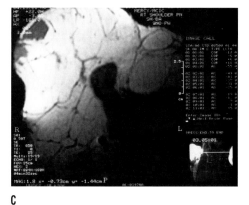

A          B          C

**Figure 5–8. (A)** Anterior view of a 73-year-old man with symmetrical lipomatosis (Madelung's disease). **(B)** Posterior view of the same patient. **(C)** Magnetic resonance imaging of the left shoulder showing numerous septa transversing through lipomas. Microscopically, these are all lipomas with areas of spindled fat cells.

tissue septa contain large numbers of blood vessels (Fig. 5–6B). These capillaries are lined by plump endothelial cells and are surrounded by immature and fusiform fat cells. Rasanen and co-workers[33] calculated the number of vascular channels and concluded that, in angiolipomas, the vascular component ranged from 15 to 40 percent of the fatty tissue.

***Spindle Cell Lipoma.*** Spindle cell lipoma grossly resembles lipoma, with foci of gelatinous areas. Microscopically, it is well circumscribed and composed of mature fat cells and uniform, well-oriented spindle cells associated with bundles of collagen and mucoid material. Occasionally, mast cells and a few thick-walled blood vessels are also seen. Immunostaining of spindles will be positive for S-100 and negative for monocyte/macrophage antigen and laminin.

***Pleomorphic Lipoma.*** Pleomorphic lipoma is usually well circumscribed, and occurs in the subcutaneous tissue of the neck and shoulders of older men. The microscopic features of these tumors are characterized by the presence of floret cells, which are scattered bizarre giant cells with nuclei arranged like a wreath. These lipomas must be separated from adenosing liposarcoma.

*Histochemistry.* A subcutaneous lipoma is intensely stained by Sudan III and oil red 0. Red dyes are selectively absorbed by hydrophobic unsaturated triglycerides, cholesterol esters, and fatty acids. Common subcutaneous lipomas have an extremely low phospholipid content.[34] Gellhorn and Marks[35] reported that the rate of acetate 1-$^{14}$C incorporation into mixed lipids of lipomas and normal subcutaneous adipose tissue from the same subject was faster in tumor than in normal tissue. These authors found that the distribution of radioactivity in lipid components of adipose tissue was about 1 percent of the total activity in free fatty acids, the remainder being in the triglycerides. They concluded that, in lipomas, a disturbance of lipid synthesis is a major factor in fat accumulation. Histochemical staining of enzymes in the common lipomas shows no apparent differences between normal white adipose tissue and lipomas.

*Structure.* A fat cell from a lipoma seldom shows any variations in structure from a normal adult fat cell (see Figs. 5–2 and 5–3).

*Malignant Change.* Malignant change in a lipoma is extremely rare, and most liposarcomas arise as such ab initio. Wright,[36] in 1948, reported a case of liposarcoma arising in a lipoma, and accepted one other from Stout's[37] series. Since then, Sternberg[38] and Sampson et al.[39] have each reported a case of liposarcoma devel-

oping in a subcutaneous lipoma. In none of these cases did the tumor either recur or metastasize after excision. We have seen only one patient in whom a subcutaneous lipoma probably preceded the development of a liposarcoma (Fig. 5–9A and 5–9B).

### Lipoblastoma

Lipoblastoma is a benign tumor of fetal and embryonal adipose tissue, usually found in the extremities of infants and children. Although Jaffe[40] in 1926 coined the term *lipoblastoma* to describe tumors of immature fat cells, the existence of a benign lipoblastic tumor was not widely recognized until 1958, when Vellios and co-workers[41] described it as an entity occurring in the postnatal period. Shear,[42] in 1967, collected seven such cases. In 1975, Chung and Enzinger[43] reviewed 35 cases from the files of the Armed Forces Institute of Pathology and provided the basic morphologic criteria for these tumors. Most of these tumors are lobulated and are found throughout the body, but most commonly in the extremities.[43] We have encountered only one such case, and that was in a 13-year-old girl with a tumor in the left thigh.

The microscopic features are characterized by a lobular arrangement of the tumor cells and a uniform cellular appearance within each tumor lobule (Fig. 5–10). Within each lobule, the fat cells vary in the degree of differentiation. Mature fat cells are interspersed with various types of lipoblasts and spindled or stellate mesenchymal cells. Chung and Enzinger[43] found that histochemical studies of their material did not provide any diagnostic clues. These tumors probably represent a developmental anomaly.[44]

***Atypical Lipoma and Well-differentiated Liposarcoma.*** Kindblom et al.[45] and Evans[46] proposed the term *atypical lipoma* for all tumors formerly classified as well-differentiated liposarcoma, excepting those occurring in the retroperitoneum. Recently, Evans[47] suggested the term *atypical lipomatous tumor* be replaced by *atypical lipoma.* This designation should be restricted to subcutaneous tumors of small size with minimal atypical changes. *Well-differentiated liposarcoma* is a term reserved for deep soft tissue tumors including the musculature of the extremities, the groin, and retroperitoneum. Brooks and Conner[48] have suggested that deep-seated atypical lipomas of the extremities that show areas of dedifferentiation be treated as well-differentiated liposarcoma (i.e., resection with a wider margin).

## MALIGNANT NEOPLASMS OF WHITE ADIPOSE TISSUE

Liposarcomas are relatively common mesenchymal neoplasms of the soft somatic tissue. According to Pack and Ariel,[49] liposarcomas constitute 14.6 percent of all

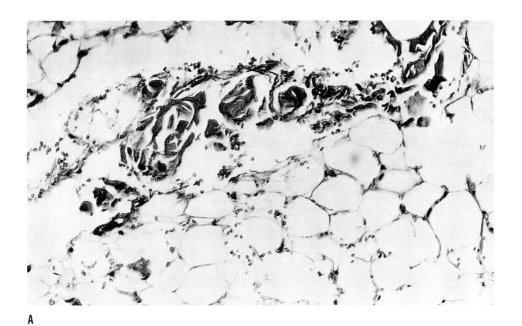

A

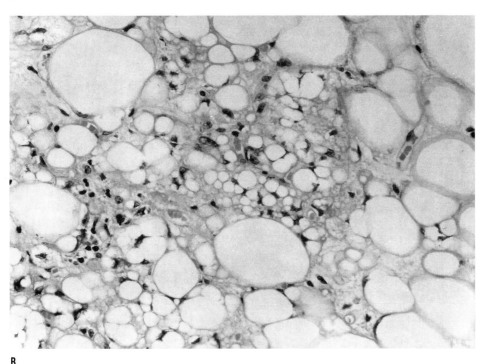

B

**Figure 5–9. (A)** A subcutaneous lipoma located in the gluteal region. The 5-cm tumor was apparently totally excised. (H & E. Original magnification × 100). Ten years later, a 3-cm recurrent tumor was excised from under the scar of the previous tissue. **(B)** This tumor was found to be a well-differentiated liposarcoma. (H & E. Original magnification × 250).

sarcomas of the somatic tissues. Virchow,[50] in 1857, first described a malignant tumor of the fatty tissue in a lower extremity. Following this description, a number of case reports appeared in the contemporary literature emphasizing in particular the large size of these tumors.[49,51] Enzinger and Winslow[52] suggested that, among all mesenchymal sarcomas, liposarcomas are unsurpassed in their wide range of structure and behavior. Stout, in 1944, analyzed 41 cases of liposarcoma,[37]

and subsequently the subject was dealt with in detail by Pack and Pierson,[53] Enzinger and Winslow,[52] Reszel et al.,[54] Enterline et al.,[55] De Weed and Dockery,[51] and Das Gupta.[56]

***Macroscopic Findings.*** Primary liposarcoma is commonly situated deep in the intermuscular or periarticular planes, although subcutaneous locations are not uncommon. They usually range in size from 5 to 10 cm

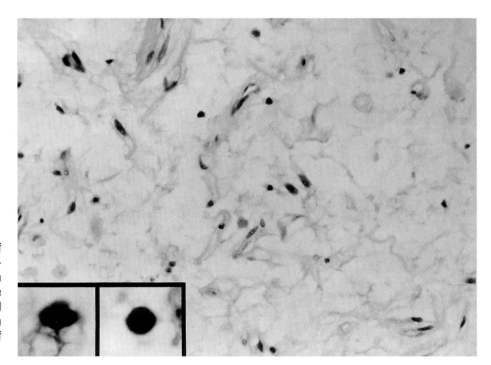

**Figure 5–10.** Lipoblastoma in the thigh of a 13-year-old girl. Note lobular arrangement of the mature fat cells and uniform cellular appearance within each lobule. The stroma is sparsely supplied with blood vessels. (H & E. Original magnification × 125.) Inset shows the different types of lipoblasts. (Original magnification × 600.)

in diameter. However, they may reach enormous size. Delamater,[57] in the Cleveland Medical Gazette, reported probably the largest neoplasm, a liposarcoma weighing 200 pounds at the time of the patient's death. However, reported cases of liposarcomas weighing 50 pounds are not unusual.

Smaller tumors appear to be encapsulated (pseudocapsule). The cut surfaces of these tumors, whether they are large or small, exhibit a variety of col-ors—white, yellow, or red. In large tumors, areas of necrosis, hemorrhage, and cyst formation are often seen (Fig. 5–11). Fibrous septa usually divide the tumor into distinct small lobules. The original primary tumor usually lies between, but does not invade, the muscle belly. In contrast, recurrent liposarcomas invade surrounding bones, muscle, and vessels. In our early series, 115 of 236 patients (48.7 percent) with liposarcomas showed diffuse infiltration of the surrounding tissue.

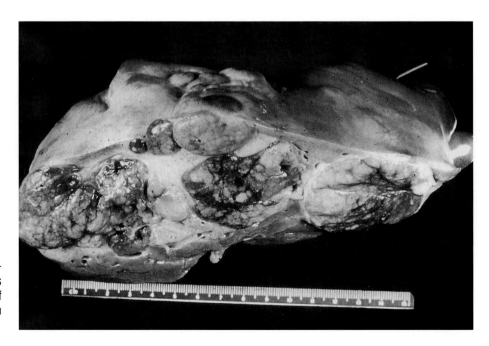

**Figure 5–11.** Cut section of a retroperitoneal liposarcoma. The cut surface shows the characteristic lobulated appearance of mature well-differentiated liposarcoma, with areas of hemorrhage.

Rarely, liposarcomas are of multicentric origin; we have treated 11 such cases.

***Microscopic Findings.***    Opinions differ regarding classification of malignant adipose tissue tumor, but its clinical importance is well appreciated. Careful sampling in each case is important because, in spite of the advent of molecular markers (see Chapter 6), the degree of differentiation and the actual subtype of liposarcoma are still the most reliable parameters in predicting the clinical behavior and in selecting the mode of therapy.

Ewing[58] originally separated liposarcomas into three cell types: adult, myxoid, and granular, relating the last group to brown fat. Stout[37] also classified them into three groups: (1) well-differentiated myxoid, in which the tumor is composed of adult fat cells, embryonal stellate cells, or spindle-shaped lipoblasts with cytoplasmic droplets that stain with Sudan III; (2) poorly differentiated lipoblasts, with various types of nuclei (this tumor carries a poor prognosis); and (3) the round cell type, in which the tumor cells are spherical, with central nucleus and abundant foamy cytoplasm. Frequently, a fourth kind was seen that consisted of mixed cell population. Enzinger and Winslow[52] modified Stout's classification and suggested the following four types: (1) myxoid type; (2) well-differentiated adult; (3) round cell; and (4) pleomorphic.

Currently, liposarcomas are classified as follows: (1) myxoid type, (2) round cell type, (3) well-differentiated with various stages of differentiation, (4) dedifferentiated, and (5) pleomorphic type.

## Myxoid Liposarcoma

According to Enzinger and Winslow,[52] myxoid liposarcoma is the most common type of liposarcoma. These authors found a uniform myxoid pattern, with occasional transition of all other forms of liposarcomas. They aptly pointed out its close similarity to Wasserman's primitive fat organ. As in the primitive fat organ, the tumor is composed of three main elements: proliferating lipoblasts in various stages of differentiation, a plexiform capillary pattern, and a myxoid matrix. Because of the similarity to primitive fat structure, adult cells in certain myxoid liposarcomas are extremely difficult to distinguish from primitive mesenchyme and have sometimes been misinterpreted as mesenchymomas. The abundant capillary network is a hallmark of this type of liposarcoma. The amount of myxoid matrix varies from tumor to tumor (Fig. 5–12). Anastomotic, stellate, and fusiform cells are arranged in a loose intricate network and are accompanied by a variable number of signet cells containing lipids. Mitosis is rarely noted in myxoid liposarcomas. Focal cartilaginous, leiomyomatous, or (very rarely) osseous metaplasia occur in myxoid liposarcoma.

## Round Cell Liposarcoma

Enzinger and Winslow[52] considered that, although round cell tumors are closely related to the myxoid type, they deserve separate consideration because of their aggressive clinical course and frequency of metastases. Microscopically, the tumor is mostly comprised of small round cells of uniform size. The cells usually are

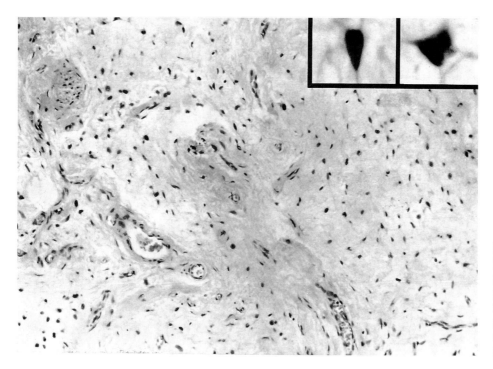

**Figure 5–12.** Myxoid liposarcoma. Vascular network, with the characteristic mucopolysaccharide-rich ground substance, is prominent. Close scrutiny shows anastomosing stellate and fusiform lipoblasts. (H & E. Original magnification × 125.) Inset depicts the morphology of these lipoblasts. (Original magnification × 600.)

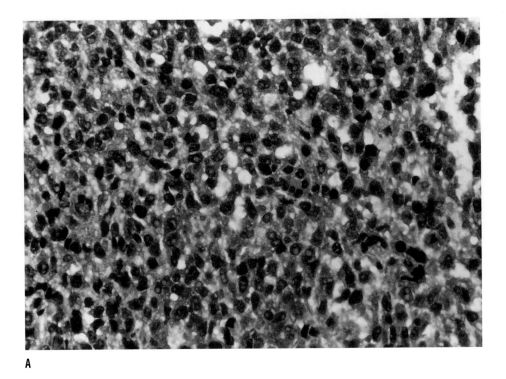

**A**

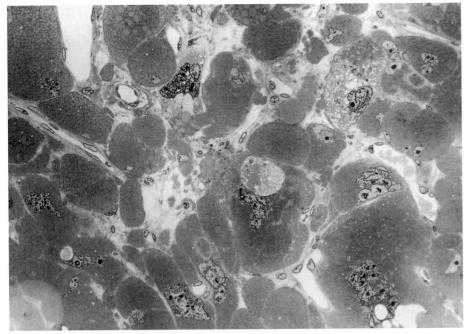

**Figure 5–13.** **(A)** Round cell liposarcoma of the thigh in an 18-year-old girl. The uniform distribution of rounded cells and diminished intercellular material can be seen. Note fat-laden tumor cells and cells in mitosis. (H & E. Original magnification × 250.) **(B)** One-micron section of a round cell liposarcoma. Note the variety of shapes and sizes of multivacuolated lipoblasts, some of which are in direct contact with the capillary lining. (Toluidine blue. Original magnification × 250.)  **B**

not arranged in any particular pattern and may be loosely packed, with occasional areas of increased cellularity (Fig. 5–13). Intracellular lipid formation is scanty. Although there are some areas of myxoid matrix, the capillary vascular prominence characteristic of myxoid liposarcoma is usually not seen. Despite increased cellularity, mitosis is rare.

## Well-differentiated Liposarcoma

The difficulty in distinguishing between a lipoma and well-differentiated liposarcoma has been emphasized by numerous authors.[16,37,52,54,55] These tumors are frequently misdiagnosed as benign deep-seated lipoma (Fig. 5–14). They are usually slow-growing lesions and are not likely to metastasize. Local recurrence is a rule

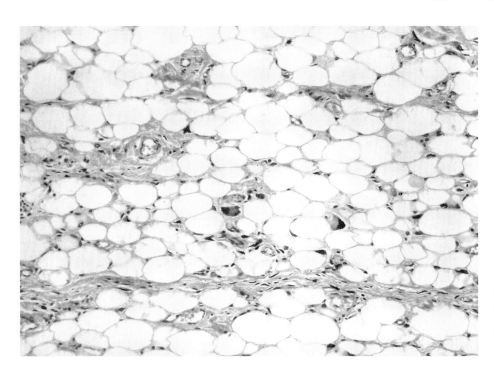

**Figure 5–14.** A well-differentiated liposarcoma of the right iliac fossa in an 80-year-old man. The tumor recurred twice before being treated by us on the third recurrence. (H & E. Original magnification× 125.)

for inadequately excised lesions. Enzinger further classified these lesions into four different varieties: lipoma-like well-differentiated liposarcoma, inflammatory type, sclerosing type, and differentiated type. This classification is more academic than practical.[59]

### Dedifferentiated Liposarcoma

Dedifferentiated liposarcomas occur when two histologic types, such as well-differentiated and poorly differentiated areas, are encountered within the same neoplasm.[60] In cases of recurrence, the tumor may show features of malignant fibrous histiocytoma, rhabdomyosarcoma, or sometimes even leiomyosarcoma. They are most commonly seen in the retroperitoneum, groin, and sometimes in the extremities. This multifaceted morphologic appearance has not been correlated to any known causes (e.g., radiation or other types of carcinogen exposure).

### Pleomorphic Liposarcoma

The distinguishing features of pleomorphic tumors are disorderly growth pattern, extreme degree of cellular pleomorphism, and giant cells (Fig. 5–15A to 5–15D). Some giant cells contain lipid droplets that may either be a single lipid droplet or multiple lipid droplets, giving a scalloped form. In others, the lipoblastic activity is limited, often confined to few cells. The cellular pattern can range from round cells to large giant cells arranged in various configurations, with pyknotic nuclei. Some tumors show polymorphic features, and areas resembling spindle cell fibrosarcoma can be seen. Thus, a pleomorphic liposarcoma can mimic a number

of other types of sarcoma, and the presence of lipoblasts must be demonstrated to establish a prima facie diagnosis of liposarcoma.

The classification proposed by Enzinger and Winslow[52] is theoretically sound and can be used to estimate the biological behavior of liposarcoma. Well-differentiated liposarcoma is commonly infiltrative, and the incidence of local recurrence is higher than for distant metastasis. In contrast, poorly differentiated liposarcomas have a high potential for distant metastasis; from a practical standpoint, however, it is clearly better to estimate the prognosis on the basis of tumor grade, and today this method of prognostication is generally used. In tumors showing areas of varying microscopic features, prognostication must be based on most undifferentiated areas reviewed.

*Histochemistry.* Histochemical studies of liposarcomas have been performed by various investigators,[37,52,61] and, from these studies, it is generally accepted that mucoid material is an integral part of liposarcoma. The mucoid substance is more abundant in the myxoid type than in the pleomorphic or poorly differentiated types and is essentially composed of acid mucopolysaccharide. In some cells, staining demonstrates periodic acid-Schiff-positive material, presumably glycogen. Fat stains show the presence of a large amount of neutral fat (Fig. 5–16). In poorly differentiated tumors, fat is not as well localized as in differentiated types. A fine retrograde network is frequently present (oil red 0 stain of myxoid liposarcoma shows a close association of the cells with the capillaries).

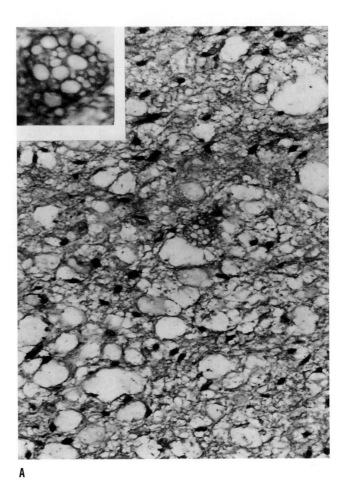

A

**Figure 5–15.** Pleomorphic liposarcoma in the thigh of a 55-year-old man. The disorderly growth pattern in the three areas of the same tumor is a characteristic feature of this type of tumor. **(A)** Area showing rich myxoid stroma with branching capillary network, a multilobulated lipoblast in the center. (H & E. Original magnification × 110.) Inset shows the characteristic features of malignant lipoblasts (Original magnification × 600.) **(B)** Tumor infiltrating the muscle. Lipoblasts and mitosis are visible. (H & E. Original magnification × 250.) *(Continued.)*

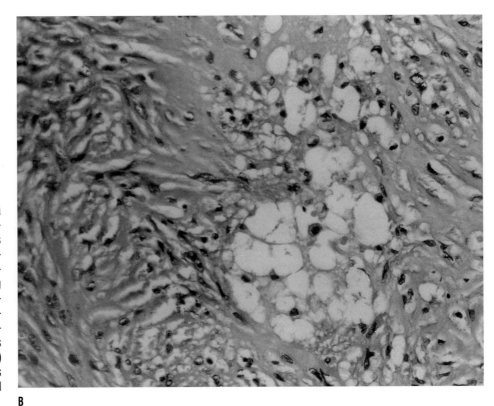

B

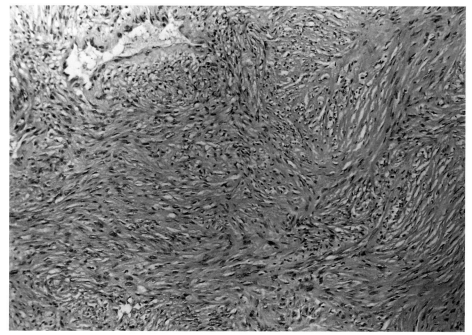

C

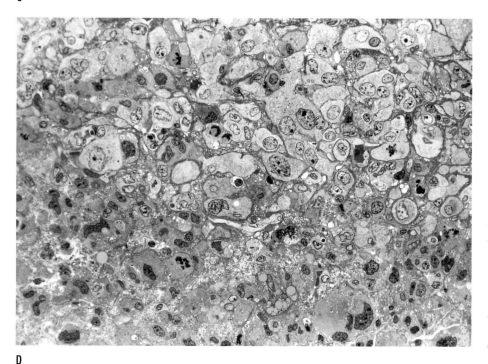

D

**Figure 5–15** *(continued).* **(C)** Area resembling fibrosarcoma. It is composed of uniform spindle cells containing pyknotic solitary nuclei and fibrillary cytoplasm. (H & E. Original magnification × 110.) **(D)** One-micron Araldite-embedded section of a pleomorphic liposarcoma. Multivacuolated lipoblasts, stellate and round mesenchymal cells, and fibroblasts are easily discernible. Several cells show mitotic activity. (Toluidine blue, basic fuchsin stain. Original magnification × 375.)

***Electron Microscopy.***    Ultrastructurally, five types can be identified: multivacuolated tumor cells (liposarcoma cells), stellate mesenchymal cells, round mesenchymal cells, fibroblasts, and normal fat cells (Fig. 5–17A to 5–17C). Large, multivacuolated cells with a peripheral nucleus and abundant cytoplasm contain lipid-laden inclusions and other types of inclusions. Scarpelli and Greider[6] found some of these inclusions did not stain with Sudan black B or oil red 0. Another characteristic feature of cytoplasm is the abundance of microfilament (Fig. 5–17D). In many of these tumors, multiple cytoplasmic inclusions and vacuoles that bear a certain resemblance to one another suggest that they might represent related statuses of similar intercellular processes. Stellate and round mesenchymal cells have a similar appearance and are characterized by hyperchromatic nuclei and basophilic cytoplasm; in some, cytoplasmic processes are abundant, whereas in others,

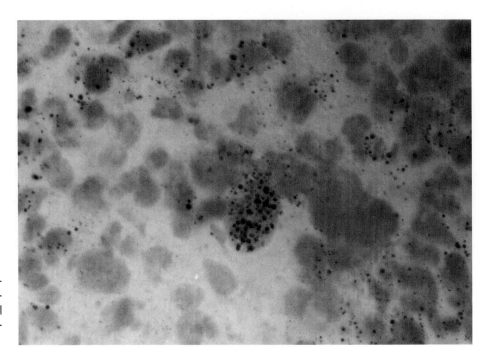

**Figure 5–16.** Oil red O stain of a liposarcoma. Red dye selectively stains hydrophobic unsaturated triglycerides, cholesterol esters, and fatty acids. (Oil immersion. Original magnification × 600.)

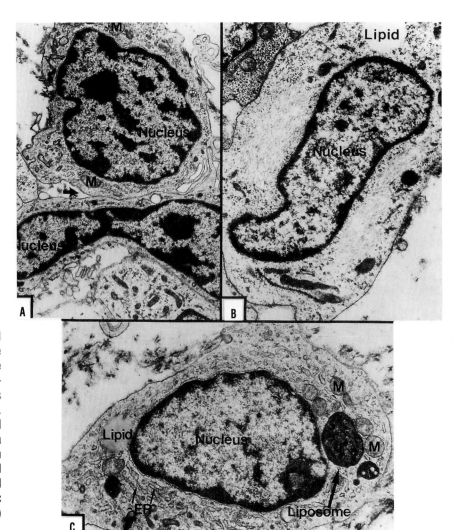

**Figure 5–17.** Electron micrographs of a round cell liposarcoma in the thigh of a 33-year-old male patient. **(A)** Two malignant adipocytes are close without desmosomal contact. Arrow shows the cell-to-cell contact. The upper cell has a round nucleus with scanty cytoplasm and no lipid inclusions. (Original magnification × 11,491.) **(B)** A tumor cell showing one lipid droplet, scanty organelles, and a tenuous filamentous matrix. (Original magnification × 14,833.) **(C)** An immature adipocyte with round nucleus. Scanty cytoplasm containing a defined lipid droplet, mitochondria *(M)*, and endoplasmic reticulum *(ER)*. (Original magnification × 16,758.) *(Continued.)*

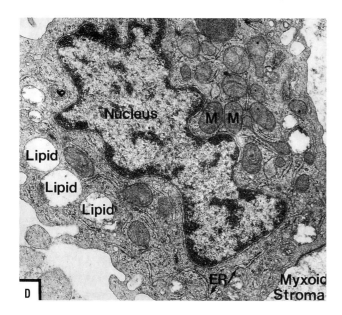

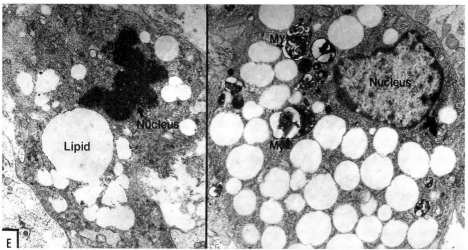

**Figure 5–17** *(continued).* **(D)** Lipoblast from a myxoid liposarcoma with multiple osmiophilic lipid droplets. These are usually composed of neutral lipids. The cytoplasmic processes in this cell are easily discernible. Note the myxoid stroma in the lower right corner of the micrograph. (Original magnification × 31,900.) **(E)** Malignant lipoblast with large coalescing lipid droplets in the cytoplasm from a well-differentiated liposarcoma. Profiles of myelin figures *(My)* are frequently observed. (Original magnification × 14,214.)

the processes are usually absent (Fig. 5–17C and 5–17D). The cytoplasm of these cells is essentially different from that of a multivacuolated cell by the absence of cytoplasmic inclusions (Fig. 5–17E). These cell types are probably all malignant lipoblasts in different stages of evolution. The other two cell types, namely fibroblasts and normal lipoblasts, have the usual characteristics and can be easily identified.

***Immunohistochemical Staining.***   Lipocytes and lipoblasts stain positive with S-100 protein and vimentin, but they vary in intensity in different types of liposarcoma. In some cases, smooth actin may be demonstrated, especially where there are differentiated new muscles.

***Cytogenetic Findings.***   The chromosomal abnormality of liposarcoma depends on the specific type of the lesion. The abnormality usually seen in myxoid liposarcoma

is a balanced translocation of Chromosomes 12 and 16 t(12;16) (q13;p11) and is noted in approximately 80 to 90 percent of the cases.[61–63] The specific abnormality in the chromosomes of myxoid liposarcoma is not seen in any other tumor. In well-differentiated liposarcoma, mostly ring chromosomes involving Chromosome 12 are noted.[65,66] Pleomorphic liposarcoma exhibits a very complex chromosomal aberration and cannot be used for diagnostic purpose. Ring chromosomes have also been demonstrated in typical and atypical lipomas.

Recently, Fletcher and associates[67] have correlated the morphologic features and histologic diagnosis of 178 lipomatous neoplasms with tumor karyotype, using G-banded preparations from short-term cultures. Clonal chromosomal abnormalities were identified in 149 cases (84 percent), and, according to these authors, the karyotype correlated with morphologic diagnosis. Specifically, 26 (96 percent) of 27 myxoid liposarcomas and their poorly differentiated variants showed t(12;16); 29 (78 percent) of 37 atypical lipomas showed ring chromosomes; 74 (80 percent) of 93 subcutaneous and intramuscular lipomas had karyotypic aberrations affecting mainly 12q, 6p, and 13q. Based on these types of findings, these authors concluded that cytogenetic abnormalities are common in lipomatous tumors, correlate reliably with histologic subsets, and can be of diagnostic value in borderline or difficult cases.

***Metastases.*** Liposarcoma, like other soft tissue sarcomas, predominantly metastasizes to the lung. Das Gupta[56] reported an overall incidence of 41 percent in a series of 236 patients, of which 9.3 percent were found on routine postmortem examination. The liver is involved less frequently (only about 10 percent of cases). Metastases are seen to various sites of the body, including the brain, pleura, thyroid, pancreas, and spinal cord. More frequently than any other type of sarcoma, liposarcoma metastasizes to the gastrointestinal tract, usually to the colon (4 percent of cases). Regional lymph node involvement is found in only 3 percent of patients; however, this includes tumors located close to the regional nodes. In the terminal stage or at postmortem, the incidence is much higher, ranging from 10 to 15 percent. Most of the nodal disease probably occurs by direct extension.

## BENIGN NEOPLASMS OF BROWN ADIPOSE TISSUE

### Hibernoma

Benign hibernomas (benign tumors of brown adipose tissue) are lipochrome-rich, tannish-brown, well-encap-sulated solitary tumors. They occur in adults[68–70] and, less commonly, in adolescents[71] and children. The tumors consist of large masses of multiloculated, lipid-rich, closely aggregated, round, oval, or polygonal cells containing sudanophilic granules and centrally placed nuclei (Fig. 5–18). The cells usually are large, in a lobular fashion. These tumors are extensively supplied by capillary blood vessels. The pattern of blood supply is similar to that of organs of hibernating lower mammals.

## MALIGNANT NEOPLASMS OF BROWN ADIPOSE TISSUE

### Hibernoma

Malignant hibernoma or malignant transformation of benign hibernoma has not yet been satisfactorily documented. Symmens[72] in 1944 described a case of a three-month-old boy who died of inanition. On postmortem examination, extensive brown-red nodules were noted throughout the abdominal cavity. Histologic examination suggested that they were brown fat. Pack and Ariel[49] speculated on the possibility of their being malignant hibernomas.

## ■ TUMORS OF THE FIBROUS CONNECTIVE TISSUE

Connective tissue originates from the embryonic primitive mesenchyme. Most prospective fibrous tissue is relatively well formed by the second month of intrauterine life. By the end of the second month, many of the main tendons, ligaments, fascia, and other fibrous structures are present as mesenchymal condensations and are identifiable. Fibrous connective tissue constitutes a major component of the extracellular compartment.

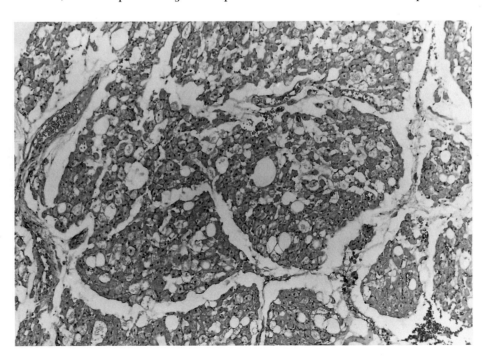

**Figure 5–18.** Hibernoma. Granular, round, or oval fat cells arranged in lobular fashion. (H & E. Original magnification × 65.)

For a better understanding of the diseases and neo-plasms of fibrous connective tissue, adequate back-ground information on the morphology and physiology of the extracellular compartment is necessary.

The discovery of an extracellular compartment influencing the activity of cells has generated many studies providing information trying to explain the morphology and function of this compartment. Today it is generally agreed that the extracellular compart-ment is truly an organ participating actively in many body functions as an autonomous unit. The major area germane to our consideration is that of the connective tissue elements of this compartment.

The components of adult connective tissue can be classified into several groups (Table 5–1). This table takes into consideration the origin of the respective component parts, whether derived locally or from the circulating plasma.[73] The connective tissue consists partly of structural units of local origin forming an enduring organization, and partly of materials in tran-sit between the blood and cells of the region. Morpho-logic division of connective tissue into cells, fibers, and ground substance makes it simple to study the charac-teristics of each group (Fig. 5–19A to 5–19F).

## CELLS

The fibroblast is the characteristic cell in the connec-tive tissue systems, but in specific tissues it appears in the guise of a chondroblast, an osteoblast, an odonto-blast, or a synovioblast. These cells have in common the secretion of collagen, reticulin, elastin, various gly-cosaminoglycans, and glycoproteins.[73,74]

A mature fibroblast has an oval, eccentrically placed nucleus. The cytoplasm is characterized by dilated, rough-surfaced endoplasmic reticulum, a prominent perinuclear Golgi complex, multiple cyto-plasmic granules, and polyribosomes (Fig. 5–19A). Fibroblasts grown in culture show all these characteris-tics, along with the dendritic processes.

Fibroblasts are considered to be the main source of fibrogenesis.[75–78] Extensive studies of the cytoplasmic granules within the fibroblast cytoplasm suggest that these granules are the site of metabolic activity leading to collagen formation.[78–81] Rough endoplasmic reticu-lum is also associated with fibrogenesis.[74,75] However, there is no clear-cut understanding of the role of each cytoplasmic component in fibrogenesis.

Fibrogenesis involves a number of sequential de-velopmental steps. Mechanisms concerned in two of these have received particular attention in tissue cul-ture investigations. One step concerns the determina-tion of the size of the macromolecular particle of the fibrous protein collagen produced by the cell. The other concerns localization of the site or sites where such particles become aggregated into a definitive fi-bril, and, as part of this, the mechanisms involved in enlarging individual collagen fibrils until their charac-teristic size for the particular tissue is attained. The question of the relationship of the fibrous protein and collagen to cells has long been controversial. Undoubt-edly, collagen formation is an active process within the fibroblast cytoplasm (Fig. 5–19F).[82–89]

Collagen is synthesized on polysomes attached to the endoplasmic reticulum, with the nascent chains vec-torially oriented into the cisternae. Residues of colla-gen arise from enzymatic hydroxylation of specific pro-lyl and lysyl residues in peptide linkage in the growing nascent chains. The transcellular movement and se-cretion of procollagen require energy, and the micro-tubular system is required for the translocations of the vacuolar elements. Once secreted from the cell, procollagen is enzymatically converted into collagen. The fibroblast secretes one or more enzymes (procolla-gen peptidase), which separate most of the nonhelical peptides from the ends of the precursor, generating tropocollagen, the triple helical molecule that retains only the abbreviated peptidases. Once generated, tro-pocollagen tends to come out of solution and aggregate in a specific manner to form collagen fibers.[84–88]

## FIBERS

Collagen fibers are the principal structural components of connective tissue. They occur in the body as coarse bundles a few millimeters in diameter and can be seen

## TABLE 5–1. ORGANIZATION AND COMPOSITION OF CONNECTIVE TISSUE

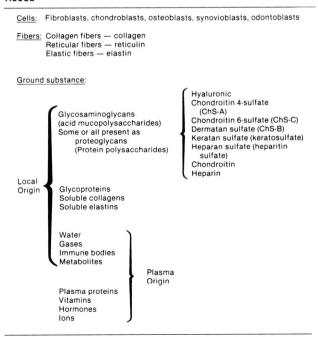

Cells:  Fibroblasts, chondroblasts, osteoblasts, synovioblasts, odontoblasts

Fibers:  Collagen fibers — collagen
Reticular fibers — reticulin
Elastic fibers — elastin

Ground substance:

Local Origin
Glycosaminoglycans (acid mucopolysaccharides) Some or all present as proteoglycans (Protein polysaccharides)
{ Hyaluronic
Chondroitin 4-sulfate (ChS-A)
Chondroitin 6-sulfate (ChS-C)
Dermatan sulfate (ChS-B)
Keratan sulfate (keratosulfate)
Heparan sulfate (heparitin sulfate)
Chondroitin
Heparin }

Glycoproteins
Soluble collagens
Soluble elastins

Water
Gases
Immune bodies
Metabolites

Plasma Origin

Plasma proteins
Vitamins
Hormones
Ions

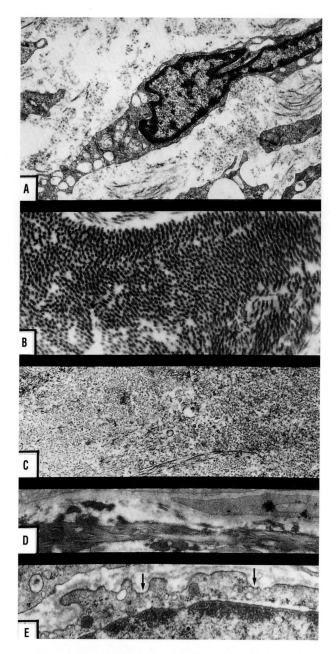

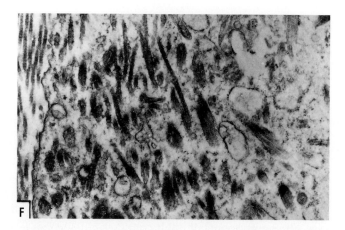

**Figure 5–19** *(continued).* **(F)** Cytoplasm of a fibroblast showing the presence of fibers in different stages of development. (Original magnification × 54,625.)

**Figure 5–19. (A)** A panoramic view of multiple, normal human fibroblasts dispersed in a collagenous matrix. The nuclei are prominent and usually ovoid, but the shape depends on the plane of sectioning. The cytoplasm contains the usual organelles and is crowded with rough endoplasmic reticulum. (Original magnification × 6,500.) **(B)** The mature collagen fibers are seen either in cross section or in different degrees of tangential or longitudinal sections. In the longitudinal section, the characteristic cross-striations can be identified. (Original magnification × 10,200.) **(C)** Reticulin fibers are usually similar to collagen fibers but are generally bunched together and are finer in texture. (Original magnification × 11,450.) **(D)** Elastic lamina of a medium-sized blood vessel. (Original magnification × 45,000.) **(E)** Profile of a basement membrane from an endothelial cell. (Original magnification × 45,000.) *(Continued.)*

under an electron microscope as fine fibrils with a diameter of 600 Å or less, showing a banded structure 640 Å in periodicity. The fundamental chemical unit of collagen that is shared with reticulin is a tropocollagen molecule consisting of three helically wound polypeptide chains.[88] Aggregations of tropocollagen molecules "in phase" lead first to various forms of soluble collagen and finally to relatively insoluble fibrillar collagen. The tropocollagen is a rodlike structure 3,000 Å long and 15 Å wide; hydrogen bonding is responsible for both its internal stability and its capacity to react externally to form bundles (i.e., cross-linking) (Fig. 5–19B). Cross-linkings increase in number with age. Soluble forms of collagen are not seen with the electron microscope and can be classified as ground substance. Other compounds, such as saccharides, may participate in fiber formation. The amount of the carbohydrate-forming part of the intrinsic structure of collagen may be low (0.5 to 1.0 percent in tendon collagen) or quite high (10 percent or more in basement membrane collagen). Collagen has a high content of glycine (about 25 percent) and a low content of aromatic acid. Additionally, it contains two amino acids unique to this class of proteins: hydroxyproline and hydroxylysine.

### Reticulin Fibers

Ultrastructurally, recticulin fibers are similar to collagen fibers but are usually bunched and finer in texture (Fig. 5–19C), with a characteristic distribution in close association with the basement membrane. Reticulin fibers show a strong affinity for silver stains, which has led to the idea that they are formed by the aggregation of tropocollagen molecules in a carbohydrate-rich material that creates these argyrophilic fibers.

## Elastic Fibers

The major component of elastic fibers is the protein elastin, characterized by the presence of two amino acids specific to elastin: desmosine and isodesmosine.[90] These have fine structures that form bridges in a three-dimensional network. The resulting infinitely cross-linked structures are reminiscent of rubberlike polymers, whose behavior they mimic.[90] Elastin is the most important component of large blood vessel walls (Fig. 5–19D).

## Ground Substance

The ground substance of connective tissue is all-inclusive of a larger variety of chemical substances constituting the matrix for the cells to rest on, and is contiguous with the basement membrane.[91] The ground substance is heterogeneous (Table 5–1). It is convenient to divide the components into macromolecules and smaller molecular entities. The macromolecular group includes mucopolysaccharides or glycosaminoglycans, glycoproteins, basement membranes, soluble tropocollagens, elastins not yet polymerized to fibrils, and, finally, serum proteins. In tissue, the acid mucopolysaccharides are complexed with proteins (proteoglycans) to different degrees, and, like fibrin, become relatively water-insoluble. The class of smaller molecular components includes metabolites, vitamins, hormones, gases ($CO_2$, $O_2$, $N_2$), ions, and water.

The ground substance is observed in light microscopic studies (preferably in cryostat vacuum-dried or freeze-dried sections combined with alcohol after fixation) as a homogeneous matrix staining metachromatically with toluidine blue, and pink to red with periodic acid-Schiff (PAS) stain. It is contiguous with the basement membrane of endothelial, epithelial, muscle, fat, and other cells. Because of fixation techniques, ultrastructural studies have been unsatisfactory, and in most instances, only the collagen and reticulin fibers are visible.

## Basement Membrane

Basement membrane characteristically appears as a dense-staining line or sheet interposed between connective tissue and entoderm and highly differentiated mesodermal structures. It stains with PAS and is found contiguous with ground substance. Under the electron microscope, it appears as an electron dense layer and is usually 300 to 500 Å wide, but may reach 3,000 Å or more in a kidney glomerulus (Fig. 5–19E). Most of our knowledge of basement membrane composition is based on glomerular basement membrane. It is commonly thought that the basement membrane arises from the adjoining cells and has antigenic properties characteristic of the cells of probable origin. However, because of the chemical and antigenic complexity of the basement membrane at specific locations, a common origin for all types cannot as yet be proposed.[92,93]

## FUNCTIONS OF CONNECTIVE TISSUE

The function of connective tissue ranges from the minimally extensible joining represented by the collagen-rich tendon, to the elastic recoil of an arterial wall in which elastin is the major connective component. Cartilage is a semi-rigid tissue marked by the presence of the strongly acidic, ion-binding but feebly hydrophilic chondroitin sulfate. The Wharton's jelly of the umbilical cord is composed of a network of collagen fibers embedded in a hydrophilic hyaluronic acid gel and is flexible and rubbery in texture. Skin connective tissue, containing roughly equivalent amounts of hyaluronic acid and chondroitin sulfate, shows considerable water-holding capacity. The limit, in an organized tissue, is reached in the vitreous body, being 99 percent or more water and dissolved substances, 0.1 percent collagen as an extremely fine network, and 0.15 percent hyaluronic acid. The structure is nevertheless self-supporting when physically intact. For the vitreous body, the sine qua non is transparency. The same holds true for the cornea, but here an external protective function is also required. It is composed of highly oriented collagen lamellae in a matrix of keratin and chondroid sulfates. One senses the theme of adaptive evolution in which form and function may have made equal contributions. Other examples of connective tissue functional adaptation are bulk accommodation (uterus), relaxation (symphysis pubis), lubrication (joint interfaces), and the capacity to accumulate and release ions (cartilage, osteoid, and bone).

Changes in connective tissue occur with growth and differentiation. Apart from the manifold phenomena of embryonic induction, the remodeling of tissues as they increase in size implies liability of the extracellular elements.[74] The basement membrane of the skin appears to organize shortly after birth and to become progressively more prominent. Basement membranes tend to disappear after injury and are later regenerated. Striking connective tissue changes occur in the uterus during pregnancy. The process includes an increase in muscle mass, collagen content, and ground substance. Conversely, during involution, all these tissue elements are progressively and rapidly lost. Impairment of this involution process may be the reason for the induction of uterine "fibroids" (leiomyomas).

Hormones may produce increased organ size and vascularity and seem to include, as an integral part of this activity, effects on connective tissue morphology, water content, and ion distribution. Both male and female sex hormones greatly influence the connective tissue. For example, in normal pregnancy, extrauterine fluid accumulates exorbitantly and must be regarded as physiologic edema. Recently, we showed the presence of steroid receptors in several types of human soft somatic tissue sarcomas.[94] The presence of estrogen, androgen, and glucocorticoid receptors in nongynecologic tumors of connective tissue origin, along with other tumors of diverse histogenesis, suggests that hormones probably play a wider role than hitherto suspected in connective tissue physiology and the induction and growth of tumors and tumorlike conditions.

The discovery of the connective tissue enzymes triggered work on the nature of the ground substance. These enzymes are present in testis, many microorganisms, cercariae, snake venom, and leech digestive juices. By 1940, hyaluronic acid and chondroitin sulfates were recognized as the substrates of the spreading factors.[73] The role of these enzymes in the growth and spread of either primary neoplasms of the connective tissue or metastases from elsewhere has been studied. It appears that the spread of these transplantable tumors could in part be influenced by the depolymerizing enzymes (hyaluronidases). The exact role of the connective tissue enzymes in tumor growth and spread is unclear, but they certainly play an important role in the "local factors" that influence the infiltrating ability of a specific tumor type.

In recent years, attention has been focused on "growth factors." Both epidermal growth factor and fibroblast growth factor are being extensively evaluated.[95–103] The influence of these factors in normal organ development and aberrations thereof, as well as the influence on the biologic behavior of human fibrous tissue tumors, are areas of continued interest and research.

Tumors and tumorlike conditions of the connective tissues are not isolated instances of growth of a tumor in a given anatomic site; rather, they probably represent an alteration in one or more local or systemic factors. For example, aggressive fibromatosis occurs frequently among young women, and several types of fibromatoses are associated with various systemic conditions. Although no explanation for these correlations is yet available, these tumors and tumorlike conditions should be reviewed from a new and more critical perspective.

The morphologic characteristics of tumors and tumorlike conditions of the connective tissue are described in Table 2-1. Before describing these individual types, we should comment on three points. The first is to recognize the existence of a specific type of cell "histiocyte" in adult soft tissue tumors. Histiocytes are versatile in behavior and frequently can act either as true fibroblasts or as phagocytes. This versatility makes histologic classification of some of these tumors difficult. Therefore, it is becoming customary to classify them (e.g., dermatofibrosarcoma protuberans and

some giant cell tumors) as fibrous histiocytic tumors. The second point deals with the concept of "facultative fibroblasts." This term, first defined by Stout and Lattes,[104] reminds us that not all fibroblastic cells in tumors or tumorlike conditions originate from preexisting fibroblasts. Under certain circumstances, mesothelial cells, Schwann cells, and lipoblasts can assume the characteristics of fibroblasts and take part in fibrogenesis.[105] The final point is clinicopathologic. Although some tumors are histologically benign, they should not be classified without qualification as benign tumors; clinically, they are aggressive and can be fatal. Therefore, aggressive fibromatosis with all its variants must operationally be assumed to be of low-grade or intermediate malignancy.

## BENIGN FIBROUS TISSUE TUMORS (TUMORLIKE CONDITIONS)

Benign tumors and tumorlike conditions consist of a heterogeneous group of entities, and, since their clinical features, natural history, and presenting features frequently differ, these will be described as distinct clinicopathologic entities. However, it must be recognized that, from a morphologic standpoint, they have a common ontogeny (i.e., fibroblast) and probably can be lumped together.

### Fibroma

True fibrous tissue proliferation leading to the formation of a so-called fibroma is indeed rare. This cutaneous tumor occurs as a pedunculated polypoid structure and usually is excised for cosmetic reasons (see Fig. 8–1). Fibromas rarely occur beneath the skin, despite abundant fibrous tissue. Most fibromas in the somatic tissues are of the mixed variety, for example, myofibroma, angiofibroma, or fibrolipoma, and occasionally osteofibroma or neurofibroma. Cutaneous fibromalike lesions sometimes accompany Gardner's syndrome and tuberous sclerosis. In contrast, the tumor in its pure form can occur in the kidney, liver, or ovary. A fibroma of the ovary is characterized by ascites and pleural effusion (Meigs' syndrome).

***Fibroma of the Tendon Sheath.*** Fibroma of the tendon sheath is a slow-growing dense, fibrous nodule that is attached to the tendon sheath of origin. These tumors are mostly found in adults, usually involve the digits, and sometimes are associated with a history of trauma.[104] Since these tumors are benign, excision is only indicated either for cosmetic reasons or if the tumor is associated with tenderness.

### Fibromatoses with Both Juvenile and Adult Variants

The term *fibromatosis*, as proposed by Stout,[106] comprises a number of broad-based benign fibrous tissue proliferations, which appear benign histologically but biologically occupy an intermediate position between a benign lesion and fibrosarcoma (Table 2–1). They infiltrate the surrounding structures and seldom if ever metastasize (aggressive fibromatoses/desmoids). From a clinical standpoint, these entities can be either superficial or deep.

### Superficial Variant

*Palmar and Plantar Fibromatosis.*    Palmar and plantar fibromatosis are clinical descriptions rather than specific pathologic findings (see Chapter 8 for description).

*Penile Fibromatosis.*    Penile fibromatosis (Peyronie's disease) is a distinctive type of fibromatosis that hardens and deforms the penile shaft. No clear etiologic factor is known.

The superficial variants are primarily of clinical interest and are described in Chapter 8.

### Nodular Fascitis (Pseudosarcomatous Fascitis)

Konwaler, Keasbey, and Kaplan[107] first described nodular fascitis as an entity in 1955. This distinctive fibromatous tumor suddenly proliferates and infiltrates the surrounding tissue (Fig. 5–20). Its periphery is marked by many capillaries and infiltrating inflammatory cells. The fact that it grows rapidly and has high mitotic activity often leads to a mistaken diagnosis of sarcoma.[108,109] A variant of this form in which the tumor infiltrates the periosteum has been described by Hutter and his associates.[110] Proliferative myositis is a variant of pseudosarcomatous fascitis and is characterized by eosinophilic ganglion cells. Adult variants like ossifying fascitis, intervascular fascitis, and cranial fascitis have also been described. Immunohistochemically, nodular fascitis is positive for actin, vimentin, and occasionally desmin staining. Macrophage sometimes stains with CD-68 (KP-1), a marker of lysosomes. This tumor does not stain with S-100.

Juvenile variants of this entity have also been recognized.

1. Juvenile congenital fibromatosis—an extremely rare variant of juvenile fibromatosis. In this condition, the infant is usually born with multiple localized areas of fibromas distributed all over the body; frequently, the infant does not survive long. In a still rarer localized form of the disease, the tumors, usually in the extremities, are known to spontaneously disappear in the course of a few weeks.
2. Fibromatous coli—Another form of highly specialized fibromatosis, fibromatosis coli is usually seen in the neck of newborns. Clinically, it is first recognized as a nodule in the sternomastoid muscle, and the name *torticollis* is applied to these tumorlike conditions.
3. Juvenile aponeurotic fibroma—a highly specialized fibromatosis arising in the hands and feet of children.[111–113] It is prone to calcify and tends to infiltrate locally. Keasbey[112] first drew attention to this tumor; however, Lichtenstein and Goldman[113] have argued that these tumors are cartilaginoid and are also found in adults.

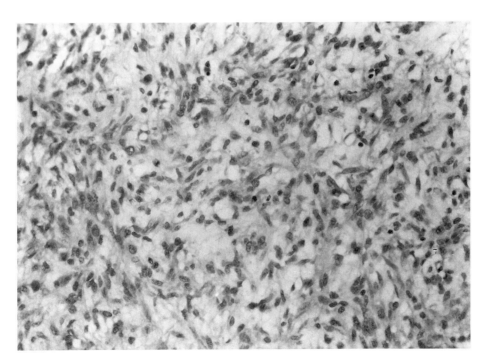

**Figure 5–20.** Pseudosarcomatous fascitis. Note that the lesion consisted of a number of capillaries, fibroblasts, histiocytes, and inflammatory cells scattered on a myxoid matrix. (H & E. Original magnification × 250.)

4. Proliferative fascitis—usually encountered in adults. About two-thirds of the tumors are located in the extremities. They are usually palpable subcutaneous nodules and frequently tender; this tenderness actually draws attention to the presence of these lesions. A deep counterpart of this entity, which usually adheres to the underlying skeletal muscles, is termed *intramuscular myositis*. Similarly, when this is associated with a tendon sheath, it is commonly designated as fibroma of the tendon sheath.

## Progressive Myositis Fibrosa

Progressive myositis fibrosa is a type of fibromatosis in which nodules develop in the muscles and subcutaneous tissue of infants. These nodules likely give rise at a later date to myositis ossificans.

## Nasopharyngeal Angiofibroma

Nasopharyngeal angiofibromas are highly vascular tumors usually seen in the nasopharynx of young adults. Microscopically, they are a highly vascular type of fibrous tissue tumors (Fig. 5–21). The entire tumor is studded with new capillaries and occasional sinusoids. The absence of the elastic lamina is probably the cause of recurrent bleeding episodes, since these vessels do not contract.

## Elastofibroma

In 1969, Jarvi et al.[114] described elastofibroma as an entity characterized by the presence of thick elasticlike fibers coating a reticulin matrix and by conglomeration of elastic material (Fig. 5–22). These lesions usually arise in the scapular region and have not recurred after excision, hence the name *elastofibroma dorsi*.[115] The elastic fibers can frequently be missed, unless a special elastic stain reticulin or trichrome stains are used. These elastic fibers stain positive and sharply outline tangled wavy arrangement of the fibers. The nuclei are either piled up or disbursed in a disarranged fashion between acellular fiber of different length and thickness. Although the exact origin of this type of tumor is controversial, it is probably a degenerative response to some form of trauma.

## Keloid

A keloid is a type of hyperplasia of the fibrous tissue in a scar, usually associated with the swollen appearance of collagen fibers and degenerative changes (Fig. 5–23).

Deep Variants of Aggressive Fibromatosis

1. Abdominal wall fibromatosis (abdominal wall desmoid)
2. Extra-abdominal fibromatosis (extra-abdominal desmoid)

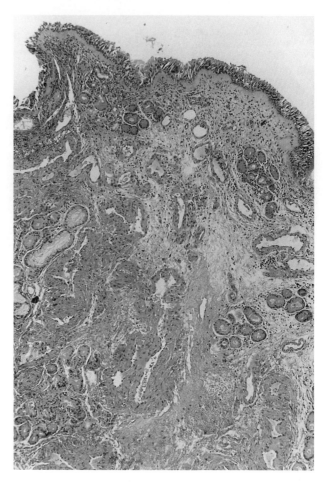

**Figure 5–21.** Juvenile nasopharyngeal angiofibroma. A rich network of thin blood vessels of varying sizes and contours are scattered in a stroma of collagen fibers. The vascular channels are usually lined by a single layer of endothelial cells. (H & E. Original magnification × 65.)

3. Intra-abdominal fibromatosis with or without stigmata of Gardner's syndrome (intra-abdominal desmoid)
4. Intra-abdominal fibrosis (retroperitoneal fibrosis)
5. Desmoplastic fibroma

The phenotypic characteristics of the deep variants are described in this chapter.

## Aggressive Fibromatosis (Desmoids)

Although Bennett gave the first microscopic description of the desmoid in 1849,[116] the term *desmoid tumor* (Greek—*desmos* for "band of tendon") was first coined by Müller in 1838.[117] In 1954, Stout[106,118] used the term *fibromatosis* to describe a broad group of benign fibrous tissue proliferations of similar microscopic appearance that are intermediate in their biological behavior between benign fibrous lesions and fibrosarcomas. Initially, two types were recognized: the abdominal wall desmoid, and the extra-abdominal wall variety. However, another variety is now well recognized: intra-

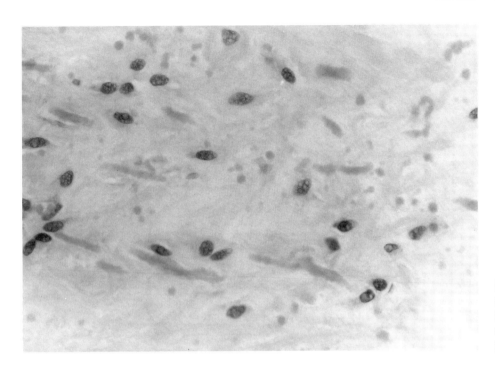

**Figure 5–22.** Elastofibroma dorsi. Microscopically, these tumors are characterized by broad areas of acellular connective tissue bands resembling abnormal fibers (H & E. Original magnification × 375.)

abdominal fibromatosis, which includes pelvic fibromatosis and mesenteric fibromatosis (with or without Gardner's Syndrome.)

***Abdominal Fibromatosis (Abdominal Desmoid).*** Desmoid tumors of the anterior abdominal wall arise from mus-

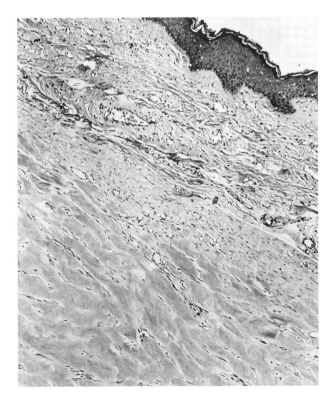

**Figure 5–23.** Keloid is characterized by the replacement of the dermis by scar tissue containing acellular dense collagenous tissue. (H & E. Original magnification × 40.)

cular aponeurotic structures of the abdominal wall, especially the rectus and internal oblique muscles and the fascial covering (Fig. 5–24). They should be considered as low-grade sarcomas with scar-like consistency. These tumors show characteristic features of fibromatosis: poorly cellular, poorly vascularized, and infiltrating tumor engulfing the muscles with no necrosis or degenerations (Fig. 5–25). This tumor usually occurs in young women, and the size ranges from 3.0–10.0 cm. It is locally invasive, and the tumor has a high potential for recurrence if ample margins are not obtained at the time of surgery. It is not known to metastasize.

***Extra-abdominal Aggressive Fibromatosis.*** Although extra-abdominal agressive fibromatosis can occur in any part of the body, the most common location is the shoulder

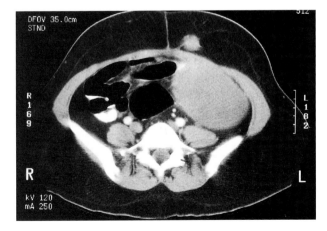

**Figure 5–24.** A computed tomography scan showing a mesenteric and anterior abdominal wall desmoid in a young woman with Gardner's syndrome.

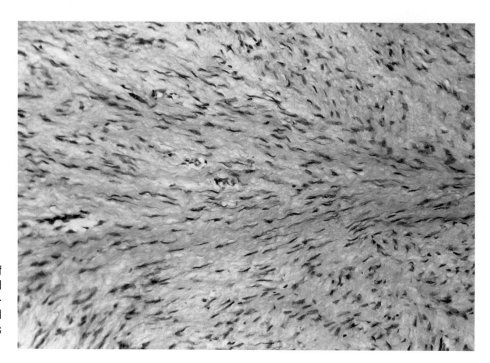

**Figure 5–25.** Aggressive fibromatosis of the abdominal wall desmoid is characterized by hypocellular bands of mature fibrous tissue. Similar histologic features are found in aggressive fibromatosis in all locations (H & E. Original magnification × 125.)

(Fig. 5–26), followed by chest wall and back, and then the thigh and neck. According to Rock et al.,[119] who reviewed 194 patients with fibromatosis, the shoulder, thigh, arms, back, and buttocks are the principle sites of involvement.

Macroscopically, extra-abdominal desmoid tumors are poorly circumscribed and located in the muscular aponeurotic structures, assuming the characteristic of the anatomic region in which they arise. The long axis is usually oriented in the direction of fibers of the muscle bundles. The tumors are firm and rubbery, and on cut section are grayish-white and trabeculated (Fig. 5–26). Aggressive fibromatosis, as the name implies, has a remarkable tendency to infiltrate the surrounding structures, even the periosteum in rare occasions, which leads to erosion of the bones.

The microscopic appearance of aggressive fibromatosis is that of a fibroma or low-grade fibrosarcoma in which the bundles of striated muscles are often found in various stages of atrophy. The tumor consists of moderately hypocellular bands of mature fibrous tissue that infiltrate by extension between individual muscle fibers (Fig. 5–25). Abundant collagenous fibers are arranged in large interwoven and sometimes fascicular bundles. Spindle-shaped fibroblasts with elongated normochromatic nuclei are dispersed between the collagen fibers.

The vascular supply of the desmoid usually appears to be scanty. A capillary network, however, accompanies the proliferative fibrous tissue (Fig. 5–27A). In some lesions, a lymphocytic infiltrate may be found at the advancing periphery. In others, regenerating skeletal

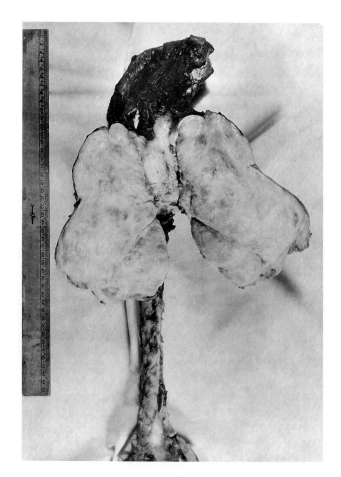

**Figure 5–26.** Aggressive fibromatosis of the extremity. The extensive infiltration of the bone necessitated an amputation.

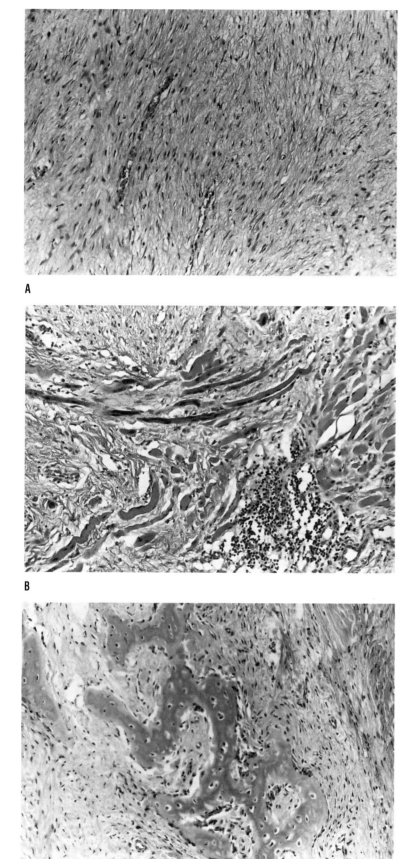

**Figure 5–27. (A)** Capillaries in proliferating fibrous tissue. (H & E. Original magnification × 100.) **(B)** Striated muscle fibers with myxomatous stroma. Note the degenerating muscle fibers with central nuclei and lymphocytic infiltration at the advancing edge. (H & E. Original magnification × 125.) **(C)** Aggressive fibromatosis showing metaplastic bone formation. (H & E. Original magnification × 250.)

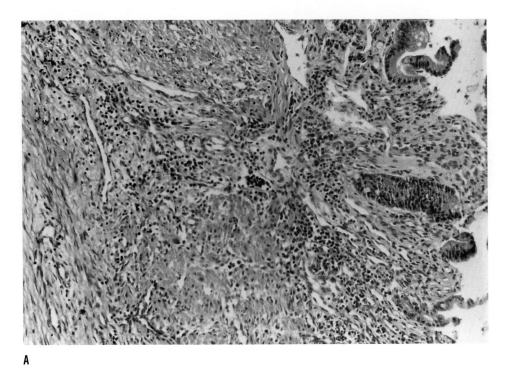

A

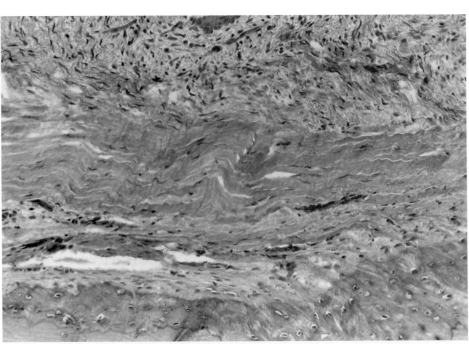

B

**Figure 5–28.** Infiltration of **(A)** wall of small intestine (original magnification × 100), **(B)** periosteum (original magnification × 100). *(Continued.)*

muscle fibers, with centrally placed nuclei, will give a false impression of tumor giant cells (Fig. 5–27B). Foci of myxomatous transformation are found not uncommonly, but metaplastic bone formation is less frequent (Fig. 5–27C). Histologic evidence of infiltration is commonly found (Fig. 5–28A to 5–28D). In certain instances, aggressive fibromatosis might appear moderately cellular with hypertrophic fibroblasts containing hyperchromatic nuclei. However, mitosis is extremely

rare. The general architecture of desmoid is distinctly different from that of well-differentiated fibrosarcoma (Fig. 5–29).

Immunohistochemically, the spindle cells stain with vimentin, alpha smooth muscle actin, muscle actin, and, rarely, polyclonal or monoclonal desmin. Ultrastructural findings of the fibroblastlike cells have nuclei with abundant endoplasmic reticula and mature collagen fibrils in the extracellular space. Some of these

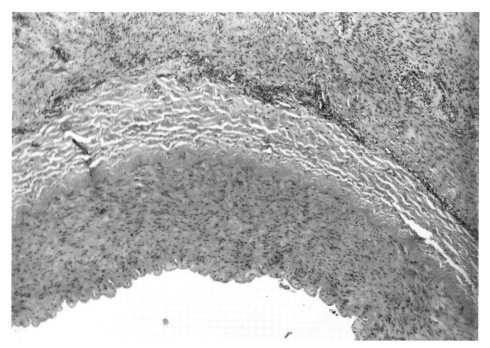

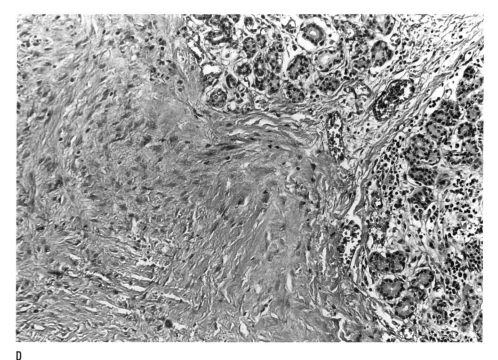

**Figure 5–28.** *(continued).* **(C)** Infiltration of arterial wall (original magnification × 100), **(D)** pancreas (original magnification × 100).

cells have microfilament resembling actin that is 60 nm in diameter. Others have clumped basal lamina along the cell borders. These are all characteristics of myofibroblasts. Typing of the collagen is of little diagnostic value.

***Intra-abdominal Desmoid.***    Intra-abdominal desmoid or fibromatosis is comprised of two main categories, pelvic fibromatosis and mesenteric fibromatosis (Fig. 5–30A

to 5–30C). In aggressive fibromatosis or desmoid tumor associated with Gardner's syndrome, the patient has other clinical characteristics such as polyposis coli, periampullary lesion, osteoma, and multiple sebaceous cysts. Morphologically and histologically, it is similar to intra-abdominal and extra-abdominal fibromatosis.

Pelvic fibromatosis is sometimes mistaken for an ovarian tumor. It is a variant of abdominal fibromatosis. It is asymptomatic and slow-growing, arising in the

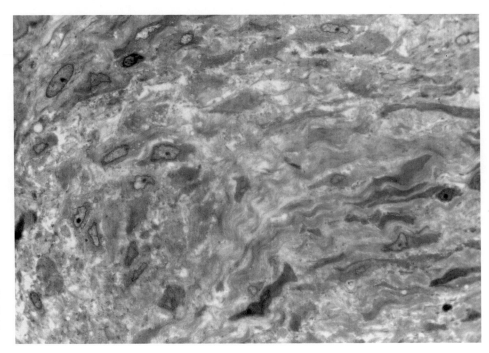

**Figure 5–29.** Cellular desmoid tumor with prominent nuclei, 1-μm Araldite section. (Toluidine blue and basic fuchsin stain. Original magnification × 600.)

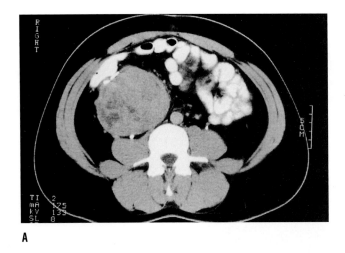

A

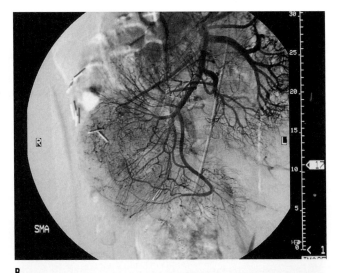

B

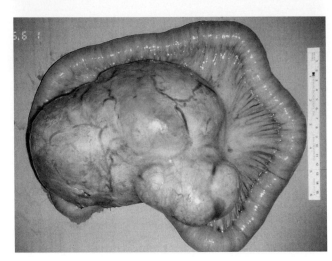

C

**Figure 5–30. (A)** A large mesenteric desmoid in a young man with Gardner's syndrome. **(B)** Angiogram showing the vasculature of the same tumor as in Figure 5–30A. **(C)** Resected specimen with a segment of the jejunum. The tumor measured 20 cm in maximum diameter.

lower portion of the iliac fossa and pelvis. It may be as large as 15 cm in greatest diameter, encircling the urinary bladder, vagina, or rectum, and causing hydronephrosis. Grossly and microscopically, it is like any other abdominal or extra-abdominal fibromatosis, and the therapy is similar.

Mesenteric fibromatosis may also be confused with idiopathic retroperitoneal periuretic fibrosis, which is usually located in deeper tissue.

### Idiopathic Retroperitoneal Fibrosis (Ormond's Disease).

In idiopathic retroperitoneal fibrosis, there is a definite proliferation of the retroperitoneal fibrous tissue accompanied by inflammatory cells and neovascularity.[120] Apparently, the process starts in the pelvis and progresses cephalad. In many instances, an erroneous diagnosis has been made, and underlying sarcoma or lymphoma has been missed.

### Progressive Myositis Ossificans

Progressive myositis ossificans is an unusual disease that is characterized by localized bone formation within the muscle. Occasionally, the entire muscle is replaced by osteoid tissue. As mentioned earlier, probably the initial stage of the disease is represented by progressive myositis fibrosa. Ackerman[121] considered the name of *myositis ossificans* as a misnomer, since this is not an inflammatory lesion, not confined to muscle only, and, in the early stage of the disease, there may not be any appreciable bone formation. This lesion may involve muscle, subcutaneous tissue, and tendon. The exact etiology is uncertain; however, definitive history of trauma at the site of the lesion is not uncommon. Myositis ossificans, although common in young adults, may also be seen in elderly patients. There is a male predominance.

Radiologic appearance of the lesion is important for diagnosis. The characteristic radiologic feature of this lesion is a clear-cut separation of the calcified part of the lesion from underlying bony cortex, and calcification is more predominant in the periphery of lesion, with the central portion of the lesion more or less devoid of calcification.[122,123] Histologically, the periphery of the lesion consists of fibrosis and mature bone formation with occasional areas of cartilage. More centrally, the lesion is devoid of osteoid tissue and consists of proliferative fibroblasts, myofibroblasts with mild to moderate pleomorphism, and mitosis. Inflammatory cells are usually absent, and, when present, they are mostly at the periphery of the lesion.[124]

### MALIGNANT FIBROUS TISSUE TUMORS

### Fibrosarcoma

At one time, the diagnosis of fibrosarcoma was a catchall, and many patients were thought to have fibrosarcoma when in fact the tumor was of a different histo-genesis. Today, after all tumors composed of other cell types that can act as facultative fibroblasts are excluded, the diagnosis of fibrosarcoma is made less often. Sometimes, a microscopic diagnosis is indeed difficult, since the cellularity of a highly cellular fibromatosis frequently resembles that of a fibrosarcoma. Although fibrosarcomas may occur in all parts and organs of the body, they are most common in the extremities.

*Macroscopic Findings.*   These tumors grow in an expansile fashion and usually present as a single gray, firm, round, or lobulated mass that is sharply delineated from the surrounding tissue. There is a pseudocapsule or a compression zone in which tumor invasion is frequently demonstrable (Fig. 5–31A and 5–31B). This tumor can attain enormous size; infrequently, it replaces a whole muscle compartment.

*Microscopic Findings.*   The microscopic features of fibrosarcoma have been conveniently classified into differentiated and undifferentiated types. However, such classification does not imply two distinct clinicopathologic entities, and frequently the histologic features of both types are found in two different areas of the same tumor. The extracellular elements of fibrosarcomas are accompanied by varying amounts of collagen and reticulin. Such fibers and fibrils occur in strands and thick bands that can easily be seen in specially stained sections.

Microscopically (Fig. 5–32A to 5–32C), these tumors are characterized by an interwoven texture of collagen and reticulin fibers, and dispersed between them are the fibrosarcoma cells. In the differentiated areas, intercellular collagen is abundant, and the nuclei of the fibrosarcoma cells are seldom in mitosis. The cytoplasm is scanty, acidophilic, and prolonged into long terminal processes or in spindling fashion. In contrast, the undifferentiated areas are richly cellular, with a few bands of collagen or reticulin displaying mitotic figures. The individual cells show large amounts of cytoplasm with oval nuclei. The presence of giant cells with single or multiple nuclei is not rare.

Fibrosarcomas lend themselves to reliable histologic grading, which in turn influences treatment and prognosis.[125–128] The grading is based on the following criteria: (1) degree of tumor cellularity, (2) degree of cellular anaplasia, (3) production of ground substance, (4) prevalence of mitotic figures, and (5) the presence of giant cells. Grade 1 is the most differentiated, and grades 3 and 4 are the least (Fig. 3–13A). In areas of mixed differentiation, the tumor type should be classified according to the most poorly differentiated area. Based on this grading, a reasonably accurate prognostication is possible; however, to obtain accurate information, at least eight to ten tissue blocks must be sampled.[126]

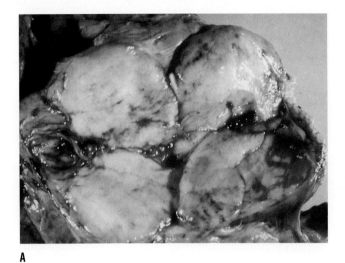

A

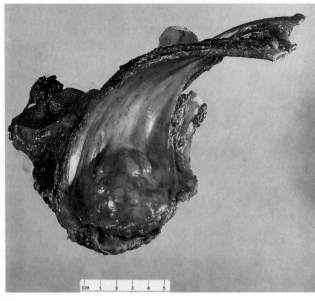

B

**Figure 5–31.** **(A)** A bilobed tumor of the posterior thigh has been bisected. Grayish-tan surface of the tumor is evident; an area of hemorrhage is also discernible. Note the apparent delineation from the surrounding soft tissue. **(B)** An unusual case of a fibrosarcoma of the chest wall viewed from the pleural surface. The extent of this tumor was not comprehensible from clinical examination of the tumor on the chest wall. Note the lobulated appearance of the tumor.

Werf-Messing and van Unnik[129] proposed determining mitotic activity and/or the mitotic index with the degree of fiber formation as a reliable basis for prognostication. They found that, when the mitotic index was 11 or more, distant metastasis was invariably present. Although this technique of determining mitotic index and fiber formation is indeed excellent, in high-grade lesions (grade 4) mitoses might not occur uniformly, and this may lead to an erroneous interpretation. Therefore, scanning a large number of sections and grading of the tumor by an experienced pathologist is probably a more practical way to correlate prognosis.

***Postradiation Fibrosarcoma.*** Postradiation fibrosarcoma is relatively rare, but well recognized. This occurs after a lag period between radiation and tumor formation, varying from 4 to 15 years, and usually requires relatively high-dose radiation (over 4,000 rads). Postradiation fibrosarcoma has been described after radiation therapy for goiter, breast, uterus, seminoma, retinoblastoma, Wilms' tumor, and Hodgkin's disease. The microscopic features show damage such as fat and muscle necrosis with fibrosis, intimal proliferation, atrophy, and presence of atypical fibroblast with scanty cytoplasm, intercellular collagen, and occasional giant cells.

***Fibrosarcoma Arising in Burn Scars.*** After thermal injury or third degree burns, scar tissue may develop into a sarcoma, commonly fibrosarcoma, as reported by Fleming and Rezek and by Pack and Ariel.[130,131] However, chronic burn wounds are more commonly associated with carcinomas than sarcomas. Similar to postradiation fibrosarcomas, these lesions are usually high grade. Desmoplastic or spindle cell carcinoma should be ruled out before the diagnosis of fibrosarcoma is made.

***Congenital and Infantile Fibrosarcoma.*** Congenital or infantile fibrosarcomas are relatively rare. Andersen[132] in 1951, with various tumors of infancy in general, found five fibrosarcomas among a group of 24 soft tissue sarcomas. Stout has also described such lesions. It is different from adult fibrosarcoma in clinical behavior, and it must be distinguished from richly cellular but benign forms of infantile fibromatosis and other types of childhood sarcoma.

*Microscopic Findings.* These lesions are usually similar to other types of fibrosarcoma with prominent reticulin and collagen fibers, but definitely more fasciculated than the adult fibrosarcoma. Infantile fibrosarcomas have abundant collagen. Dahl et al.[133] distinguished between medullary and desmoplastic types of infantile fibrosarcoma based on relative amount of cellularity and collagen tissue in the tumor. As in adult tumor, multinucleated giant cells and mitotic figures are fairly common with scattered chronic inflammatory cells. There are areas of hemorrhage, and these lesions may appear like hemangiopericytoma. However, immuno-

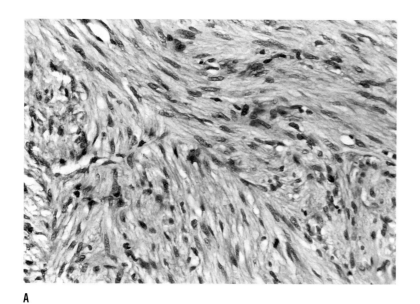

A

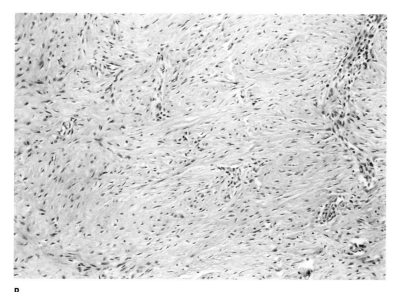

B

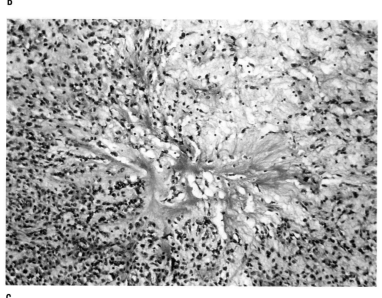

C

**Figure 5–32.** Fibrosarcoma. **(A)** Elongated fibrosarcoma cells are dispersed between a matrix interwoven with collagen and reticulin fibers; occasional mitosis can be seen. (H & E. Original magnification × 110.) **(B)** Well-differentiated fibrosarcoma, showing abundance of collagen with uniform distribution of fibrosarcoma cells. (H & E. Original magnification × 110.) **(C)** Undifferentiated areas of the tumor are richly cellular, and the fibrosarcoma cells are seen with various shapes and configurations; a myxoid matrix in this micrograph is easily discernible. (H & E. Original magnification × 110.)

histochemistry shows they are positive with vimentin but negative for desmin, S-100 protein, and Factor VIII.

Ultrastructural study of the differentiated variety of fibrosarcoma shows malignant myofibroblasts with mature collagen fibers (Fig. 5–33A). The malignant myofibroblastlike cells are basophilic and contain swollen cisternae filled with homogenous substances of moderate electron opacity. Myofilaments are seen in the peripheral part of the cell. The cytoplasm also contains a large number of rough endoplasmic reticula (Fig. 5–33B). In the pleomorphic variety, the spindle-shaped cells have a minimal degree of cell adhesion (Fig. 5–33C). A few collagen fibers are scattered in the intercellular spaces. The cytoplasmic characteristics of these malignant cells are similar to those of fibroblasts, except for the intracytoplasmic myofilaments seen at the periphery of the cytoplasm. Tumors with extreme pleomorphism show very few ultrastructural characteristics leading to a definitive diagnosis.

*Cytogenetic Findings.*   Extra copies of Chromosomes 8, 11, 17, and 20 are characteristic chromosomal changes noted in infantile fibrosarcoma.[134–136] Although most of the time desmoid tumor shows normal cytogenetic appearance, trisomy 8 is seen in approximately 20 percent of the cases.[137,138] Naeem et al.[138] reported the prognostic influence of trisomy 8 in desmoid tumors as a potential marker for high-risk tumor for recurrence. A small number of cases of desmoid tumors in association with Gardner's syndrome have an abnormality of long-arm of Chromosome 5.[139] Similarly, trisomy of Chromosome 8 is occasionally seen in some instances of dermatofibrosarcoma protuberans. However, the most unique characteristic of chromosomal abnormality in dermatofibrosarcoma protuberance is ring chromosome involving Chromosome 17.[137]

*Metastases.*   Metastases from fibrosarcoma occur primarily via the bloodstream, and the most common viscus to be affected is the lung. Distant metastasis is rare in patients with a well-differentiated or grade 1 fibrosarcoma, but the incidence becomes higher as the grade advances, particularly in grade 4. Regional node metastasis is rarely encountered. Metastasis can occasionally be found in viscera other than the lung (e.g., the liver, stomach, pleura, and brain) (Fig. 5–34).

## Fibrous Histiocytic Tumor

Benign fibrous histiocytic tumors have recently been recognized as true clinicopathologic entities, and such diagnoses are being rendered with increasing frequency. Stout and Lattes[104] pointed out that many variants of this process are known to occur, and, as such, several descriptive terms have appeared in the literature.

For descriptive purposes, fibrous histiocytic tumors are divided into two categories: cutaneous and deep. The cutaneous type is usually a solitary, slowly growing tumor and usually appears during early to mid-adult life. It is frequently confused clinically with malignant melanoma, from which it may be distinguished by the presence of central dimpling.[140]

Deeply located benign fibrous histiocytoma is rare. It is usually detected when it is 5 cm or more in size. It occurs between 20 and 40 years of age, and, according to Fletcher,[141] only three cases of fibrous histiocytic tumor involving skeletal muscles were found from 1,000 fibrous histiocytic tumors examined.

Microscopically, cutaneous fibrous histiocytic tumor is a nodular proliferation of tumor cells involving the dermis and is covered by epidermis with acanthosis and hyperplasia (Fig. 5–35). Characteristically, the spindle cells are arranged in storiform pattern. Interspersed in this storiform arrangement are histiocytic cells. They may be mononucleated or multinucleated and often contain lipid and/or hemosiderin granules. Inflammatory cells are also seen. In some cases, they are highly vascularized, giving the appearance of a vascular tumor. Such highly vascular lesions, because of the brown discoloration, are termed *sclerosing hemangioma.* However, Stout and Lattes[104] argued in favor of considering this to be of benign fibrous histiocytic type.

Deep fibrous histiocytic tumors are similar microscopically to those of cutaneous fibrous histiocytoma. The stroma often shows myxoid changes or hyalinization, and, in rare cases, metaplastic osteoid formation is also seen. It can even resemble a giant cell tumor of the soft part. Histochemical, immunohistochemical, and electron microscopic studies are of questionable importance and in fact contribute little to the diagnosis of these tumors.

***Juvenile Xanthogranuloma.***   Juvenile xanthogranuloma is a fibrohistiocytic tumor, usually occurring in infancy and characterized by multiple nodules. These tumors are usually associated with neurofibromatosis and urticaria pigmentosa. It is predominantly seen in the head and neck region and may exhibit features of regression. In rare forms, these cutaneous lesions may be accompanied by lesions in the eyes, lungs, epicardium, oral cavities, and testes. The eye is the most common extracutaneous site and it may be associated with hemorrhage and glaucoma. The prognosis of this disease is usually excellent.

***Reticulohistiocytoma.***   Reticulohistiocytoma is a rare lesion of adult life. Such lesions consist of nodules of eosinophilic histiocytes with multinucleation. These tumors may be associated with destructive arthritis and

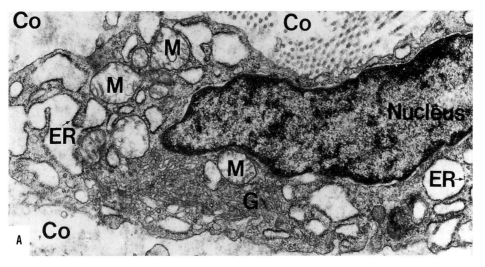

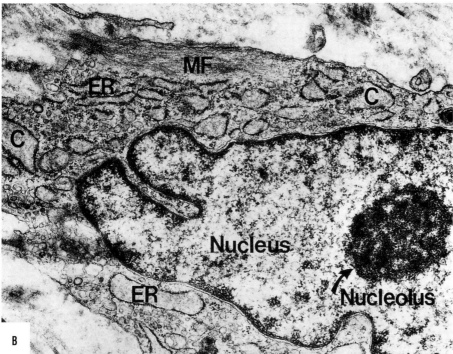

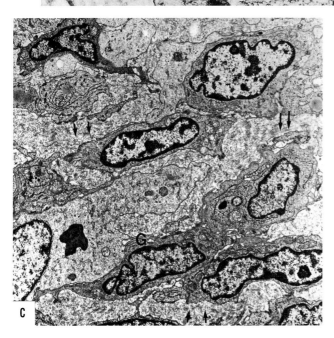

**Figure 5–33.** **(A)** Myofibroblast with mature collagenous stroma. The collagen fibers are seen both in tangential and longitudinal sections. Periodicity of collagen fibers appears to be normal. Cytoplasm shows abundance of rough endoplasm reticulum *(ER)* and mitochondria *(M)*. Myofilament can be seen in the periphery of the cells. (Original magnification × 24,410.) **(B)** High-power view of a myofibroblast. The nucleus has a prominent nucleolus. Cytoplasm is characterized by rough endoplasmic reticulum *(ER)* and swollen cisternae *(C)*. In the peripheral part of the cytoplasm, characteristic bundles of myofilament *(MF)* are easily discernible. (Original magnification × 42,640.) **(C)** Low-power view of pleomorphic (undifferentiated) fibrosarcoma. The spindle-shaped cells are numerous and are scattered all over the stroma, with minimal cell contact. Cytoplasm of most of the myofibroblasts shows peripheral myofilament bundles *(arrows)*. (Original magnification × 42,000.)

99

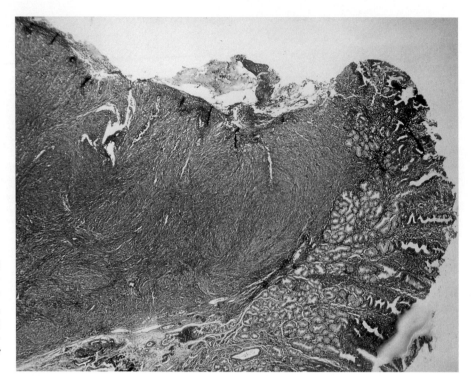

**Figure 5–34.** Fibrosarcoma metastatic to the stomach. Patient presented with upper gastrointestinal bleeding seven years after resection of a grade 3 tumor of the lower extremity. At the time of subtotal gastrectomy, there was no obvious evidence of intra-abdominal extension. (Original magnification × 65.) *(Courtesy of B. Goldsmith, M.D.)*

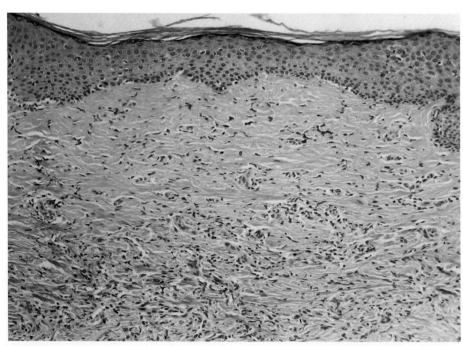

**Figure 5–35.** Sclerosing hemangioma (benign fibrous histiocytoma). The tumor is composed of short spindle or oval cells clustering amid the capillaries. (H & E. Original magnification × 125.) *(Courtesy of Dr. S. G. Ronan, Departments of Pathology and Dermatology, University of Illinois Hospital.)*

constitutional symptoms like multicytic lesions and lipoid dermalarthrosis.

***Xanthoma.*** Xanthoma is a collection of lipid-filled histiocytes. It is thought to be reactive histiocytic proliferation occurring in response to serum lipids. There are five subtypes, and many of them may be associated with primary biliary cirrhosis, diabetes, and occasionally deep soft tissue tumor of tendon or synovium.

## Fibrous Histiocytic Tumors of Intermediate Malignancy

Currently, five types of clinically significant neoplasms fall under the overall category of fibrous histiocytic tumors of intermediate malignancy: (1) atypical fibroxanthoma, (2) dermatofibrosarcoma protuberans; (3) Bednar tumor; (4) angiomatoid fibrous histiocytoma; and (5) plexiform fibrous histiocytic tumors.

***Atypical Fibroxanthoma.*** In 1963, Bourne[142] described an entity that is termed *paradoxical fibrosarcoma of the*

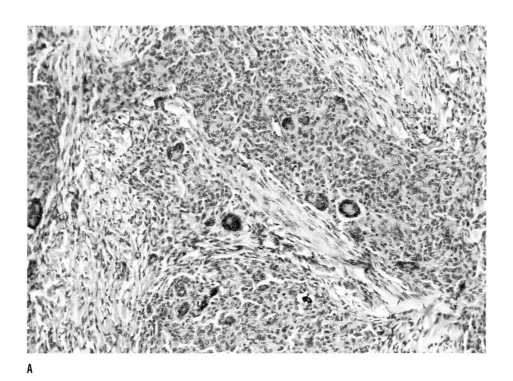

A

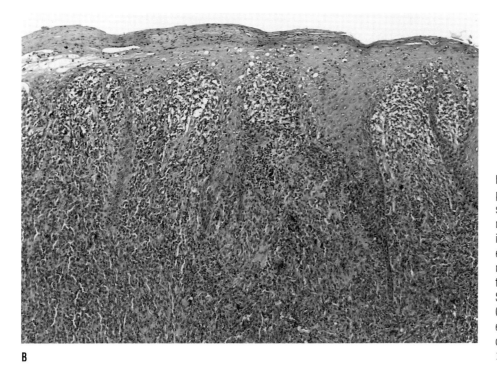

B

**Figure 5–36. (A)** Fibroblastic cells accompanied by reticulin fibers and histiocytes are seen growing in cordlike fashion within the normal structure of the corium. The overlying corium is slightly thickened and is covered by intact epidermis. (H & E. Original magnification × 65.) **(B)** An area showing the fibroblasts, histiocytes, and giant cells. Some of the cells have a foamy cytoplasm. Characteristic examples of multinucleated epulis-type and Touton-type giant cells are obvious. (H & E. Original magnification × 125.)

*skin.* However, Stout and Lattes[104] considered this entity a highly cellular fibromatosis or fibrous histiocytoma. All the data thus far generated[143,144] substantiate the opinion previously expressed by Stout and Lattes.[104] These tumors are predominantly found in the head and neck region.

This tumor is usually covered by epidermis and frequently extends to subcutaneous tissue. It does not have a true capsule, and local extension is seen on occa-

sion. Histologically, fibroblasts, histiocytes, and reticulin fibers are found to grow in cordlike fashion without definitive architecture. Frequently, giant cells are found dispersed among the cordlike arrangements in these lesions (Fig. 5–36A and 5–36B).

***Dermatofibrosarcoma Protuberans.*** The histogenesis of dermatofibrosarcoma protuberans has generated considerable confusion among pathologists. Taylor[145] considered it subcutaneous tumor resembling keloid. Stout[146] considered it a fibrosarcoma of the skin. Taylor and Helwig[147] reviewed 115 cases and concluded this was a fibrous tissue tumor. O'Brien and Stout[148] later included dermatofibrosarcoma protuberans in their group of storiform fibroxanthomas. Today, it is generally agreed that these tumors are a variant of malignant fibrous histiocytoma[104] and that they may occur at all parts of the body.

*Macroscopic Findings.* Grossly, the tumor is firm and fibrous and usually protrudes from the surface of the skin. However, the overlying skin appears normal and seldom shows evidence of ulceration. Sometimes, it is violaceous in color and, on cut section, is often found to be infiltrating the surrounding skin and subcutaneous tissue (Fig. 5–37A and 5–37B).

*Microscopic Findings.* Dermatofibrosarcoma protuberans of the dermis is composed of spindle-shaped cells with the apparent ability to make collagen (Fig. 5–38A). The usual histologic pattern is one of interwoven fibrocellular bands comprised of somewhat uniform spindle-shaped cells and scant collagen. The tumor cells are

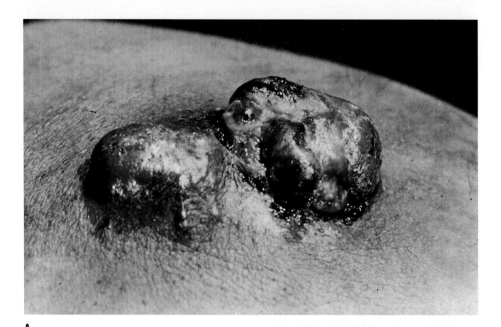

**A**

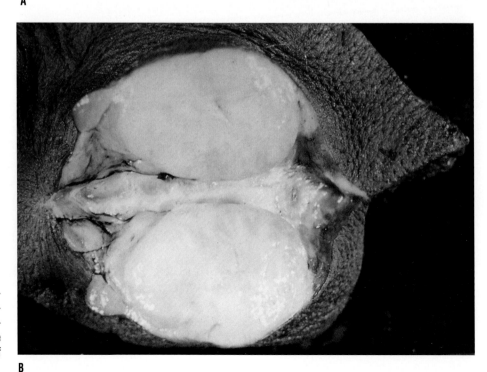

**B**

**Figure 5–37. (A)** A close-up of dermatofibrosarcoma protuberans showing the classical bosselated appearance. **(B)** Cut section of the smaller nodule. Note the glistening white colors and beginning of infiltration in the polar regions.

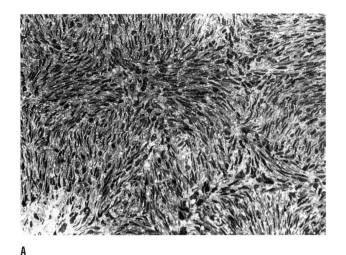

A

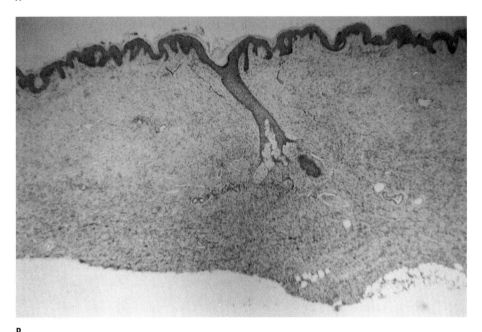

B

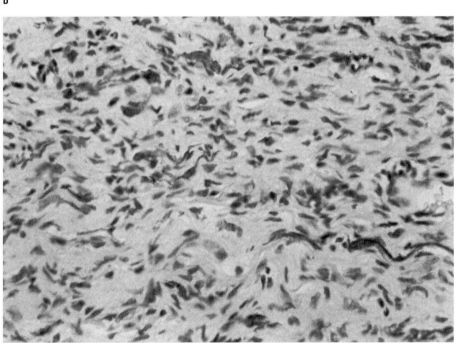

C

**Figure 5–38. (A)** Dermatofibrosarcoma. The classic histologic pattern of interwoven fibrocellular fascicles radiating in a storiform or herringbone fashion is obvious in this 1-μm Araldite-embedded section. (Toluidine blue. Original magnification × 300.) **(B)** Pigmented dermatofibrosarcoma protuberans *(DFP)*. The cells can be seen at the base of the tumors. Note that the entire tumor is below the skin. (H & E. Original magnification × 10.) **(C)** Higher magnification showing melanin-containing cells (H & E. Original magnification × 10.)

mononucleated and spindle-shaped, with nuclei usually arranged in the center of the cytoplasm. At the point of intersection of the bands or fascicle, there may be an acellular collagenous focus from around which these bands are arranged in a storiform pattern. Stout[146] likened this appearance to a spiral nebula and as such, these have been variously designated as storiform, stellate, whorled, cartwheel, twisted strip, or rosettelike. Myxoid areas may be prominent, particularly in recurrent lesion. At times, the intersecting fascicles may simulate a herringbone pattern. The stellate or cartwheel or storiform pattern has been given diagnostic emphasis by Penner[149] and by Taylor and Helwig[147] who encountered it also in differentiated fibrosarcomas arising in the deeper subcutaneous tissue. On the surface of the tumor, there is often a relatively uninvolved zone immediately beneath the atrophic epidermis. However, infiltration of the subcutaneous tissue is a rule. Before a diagnosis of dermatofibrosarcoma protuberans is made, it is perhaps better to consider the total clinical and pathologic presentation than to rely solely on histologic features. In 1967, McPeak and coworkers[150] analyzed 86 patients at Memorial Sloan-Kettering Cancer Center and concluded that the presence of a large number of mitotic figures (eight or more per 10 high-power fields) indicates a metastatic potential of this tumor. However, in nonrecurrent cases, the overall incidence of metastases from dermatofibrosarcoma protuberans is exceedingly rare.

***Bednar Tumor.*** Bednar tumor was originally described by Bednar (Fig. 5–38B and C).[151] In his original description, Bednar presumed this to be a variant of storiform neurofibroma with melanin pigment. However, at present, it is considered to be a variant of dermatofibrosarcoma with melanin pigmentation. However, the ontogenesis of melanin in these mesenchymally derived cells remains unclear.[152]

***Angiomatoid Fibrous Histiocytoma.*** Angiomatoid fibrous histiocytoma was initially termed *angiomatoid malignant fibrous histiocytoma* by Leu and colleagues.[153] Subsequently, Sun et al.[154] described the ultrastructural appearance of angiomatoid fibrous histiocytoma. Enzinger and colleagues[155] refined the diagnostic criteria and described the clinical picture of this lesion in detail. Although it has been described in older age groups, this type of tumor is usually seen in young adults. This tumor is most commonly found in the extremities and presents as a multinodular cyst clinically resembling a hematoma; it carries an excellent prognosis.[156] Twenty percent of the patients can develop local recurrence; however, less than 1 percent exhibit distant metastasis. Complete excision with clear margins is the treatment of choice. Grossly, the tumor is reddish-brown in color with cystic spaces that appear to be filled with old blood. Histologically, Enzinger et al.[155] described the lesion as exhibiting three main features: (1) cystic areas of hemorrhage; (2) solid areas consisting mostly of histiocytelike cells; and (3) infiltration of chronic inflammatory cells. The histiocytic cells are uniform in size and in most cases show very little pleomorphism. Sometimes, these histiocytic cells may have nuclear atypia, and may exhibit hyperchromatic giant cells. Multifocal hemorrhage is almost always present. These blood-filled spaces are lined by tumor cells rather than endothelium. An occasional area of myxoid changes may be seen.

***Plexiform Fibrous Histiocytoma.*** Plexiform fibrous histiocytomas are mostly found in children and young adults, and are common in the upper extremity, followed by the lower extremity. These tumors are usually small, ill-defined lesions involving dermis and subcutaneous tissue. Histologically, the lesion consists of fibroblasts, histiocytes, and multinucleated giant cells. This tumor is arranged in multiple, small nodular areas composed of fibroblastic cells and nests of histiocytic cells with many multinucleated giant cells. These nodular areas are surrounded by fibroblastic cells which form a plexiform growth pattern encompassing these nodules. Pleomorphism and mitosis are relatively uncommon. Histologically, these lesions should be distinguished from granulomatous process by three diagnostic features: histiocytic center without necrosis, absence of surrounding inflammatory cells, and fascicles of fibroblasts encompassing the island of histiocytes and giant cells.

## Malignant Fibrous Histiocytoma

Stout and colleagues should be credited with recognizing and describing this subset of soft tissue sarcomas (Fig. 5–39, A–E). In 1964, O'Brien and Stout[148] reviewed 1,516 cases, of which 979 were fibrous histiocytomas and so-called dermatofibrosarcoma protuberans and 537 were giant cell tumors of the soft somatic tissue, including villonodular synovitis. They observed that, although there had been a few case reports of malignant fibroxanthoma, there was still question as to whether a fibroxanthoma could indeed be termed *malignant.* O'Brien and Stout, however, were convinced that such a malignant tumor did exist, and described 15 cases. Later, Stout and Lattes[104] in 1967 reclassified this tumor and called it malignant fibrous histiocytoma. Since its initial description and subsequent acceptance as a separate entity, controversy has plagued the ontogeny and histogenesis of malignant fibrous histiocytoma, and some authors have questioned the existence of these lesions as a separate entity.[111,157–159] Currently, however, most authors accept their existence as distinct entities and the terminology.[108,111,148,162–166] Malignant fibrous histiocytoma appears to be the most common soft tissue sarcoma encountered in adults.[167] However, this apparent increase may be due to inclusion of a number of other soft tissue tumors with similar features and inclusion of a number of unclassifiable pleomorphic tumors in this entity.[168] Fletcher[168] found that, in a group of 149 tumors purported to be malignant fibrous histiocytoma, when the morphologic features were additionally reviewed by immunohistochemistry, electron microscopy, and more extensive evaluation of samples by light microscopy, only 42 could be accepted as true malignant fibrous histiocytomas. As mentioned previously, the histogenesis of malignant fibrous histiocytoma is also a matter of controversy. Originally, the lesion was thought to be of histiocytic origin.[111,157,164] Some histiocytic markers such as α-1 antichymotripsin are usually positive in malignant fibrous histiocytoma. But these stains are nonspecific as histiocytic markers.

A number of other authors cite immunohistochemical studies suggesting that malignant fibrous histiocytoma is probably of fibroblastic origin rather than histiocytic origin.[150,169,170] Immunocytologic markers such as Leu-3, Leu-M3, T-200, OK-M1, and alphanaphthyl butyrate esterase, which are usually positive in histiocytic cell origin, are almost always negative in malignant fibrous histiocytoma. On the other hand, a fibroblast-associated antigen, which is normally present in fibroblastic tumor, is positive in malignant fibrous histiocytoma and is usually negative in tumors of histiocytic origin. Also, CD-68, a marker for tumors of histiocytic origin, is inconsistently detectable in malignant fibrous histiocytoma.[166]

Although there appears to be a slight male preponderance, the lesion is common in both sexes. In our experience, the most common location of malignant fibrous histiocytoma is the lower limb, but it has been described in almost all anatomic locations and viscera. Grossly, the tumor presents as a mass in the deep soft tissue and is mostly painless and without prior history of trauma. Direct invasion of the adjacent bone is somewhat rare. Grossly, the lesion is solitary and lobulated with grayish-white areas, and, in tumors larger than 5 cm in size, there are areas of necrosis. The cut surface of the tumor may have slightly mucoid appearance; however, this feature is much more prominent in myxoid malignant fibrous histiocytoma.

*Microscopic Findings.*   The main histologic characteristics of malignant fibrous histiocytoma can be summarized as follows: (1) round histiocytes or histiocytelike cells; (2) spindle-shaped or fibroblast type cells; (3) presence of sparse collagenesis; (4) presence of storiform pattern; (5) benign and malignant giant cells; (6) foamy

cells; and (7) lymphocytes (Fig. 5–39A to 5–39E). From histologic appearance, four different subsets of malignant fibrous histiocytoma are described: (1) storiform pattern; (2) a myxoid malignant fibrous histiocytoma; (3) inflammatory type; and (4) giant cell type malignant fibrous histiocytoma. Although the histologic appearance and prognosis of these lesions differ in important ways, the basic pathology is the same. Microscopically, storiform malignant fibrous histiocytoma has a cellular component and a stromal component. The stromal component consists of collagen fibrils around individual cells. This collagen fibril arrangement and the vasculature in the stroma of malignant fibrous histiocytoma can be appreciated better with reticulin stain. The cellular component of malignant fibrous histiocytoma consists of two distinct variations of cellular arrangements of varying proportions. In some areas, the cells are arranged in a storiform pattern around a blood vessel. The cells in the storiform arrangement have a fibroblastic appearance and are usually well-differentiated with very little pleomorphism and moderate to frequent mitosis. In other areas, the tumor appears to be more pleomorphic, with fibroblastic cells exhibiting greater pleomorphism than do storiform areas. Also, in these pleomorphic areas, histiocytic cells and multinucleated hyperchromatic giant cells are rather frequent. Occasionally, a large portion of the tumor may exhibit uniform fascicular growth pattern with scattered giant cells, giving a fibrosarcomatous appearance. However, even in tumors with extensive fascicular pattern, usually small and less defined areas of storiform arrangement can be recognized.

Subsets of malignant fibrous histiocytoma have both diagnostic and prognostic implications. Of the various subsets identified, three (i.e., myxoid malignant fibrous histiocytoma,[162] inflammatory fibrous histiocytoma,[161,171,172] and giant cell type of malignant fibrous histiocytoma) have been found to have prognostic differences.[173] Myxoid malignant fibrous histiocytoma constitutes approximately 25 percent of all malignant fibrous histiocytoma. This variant of malignant fibrous histiocytoma must exhibit at least 50 percent of the tumor as myxoid before being designated myxoid.[162] The myxoid area of this lesion is characterized by myxoid stroma containing cellular areas that are essentially similar to typical malignant fibrous histiocytoma. Within this myxoid background, the cellular areas usually consist of fibroblasts of varying differentiation, some mitotic activity, and occasional giant cells and other inflammatory cells. The blood vessels are usually prominent and are scattered all over the mostly cellular areas, and occasionally are arranged in a plexiform pattern. Other areas of myxoid malignant fibrous histiocytoma exhibit typical features of storiform malignant fibrous histiocytoma described before.

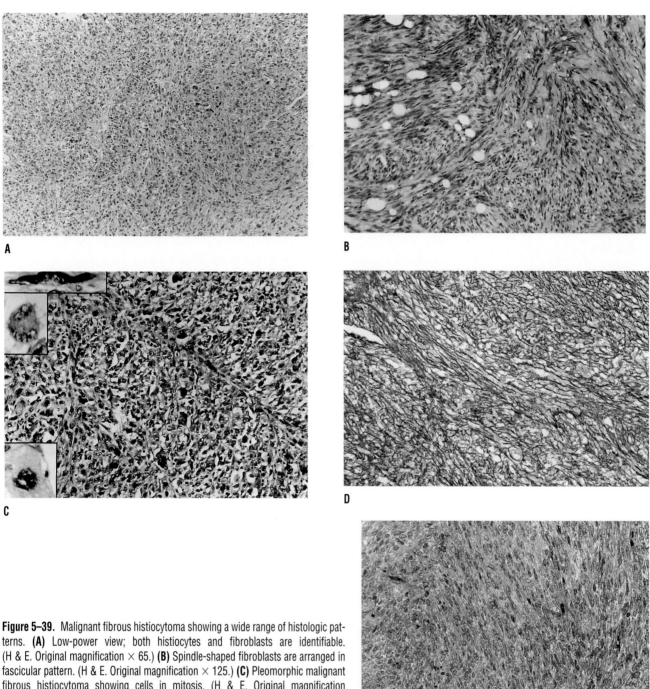

**Figure 5–39.** Malignant fibrous histiocytoma showing a wide range of histologic patterns. **(A)** Low-power view; both histiocytes and fibroblasts are identifiable. (H & E. Original magnification × 65.) **(B)** Spindle-shaped fibroblasts are arranged in fascicular pattern. (H & E. Original magnification × 125.) **(C)** Pleomorphic malignant fibrous histiocytoma showing cells in mitosis. (H & E. Original magnification × 250.) Insert shows the variety of giant cells that are frequently encountered. **(D)** Reticulin stain showing the configuration of reticular fiber distribution. (H & E. Original magnification × 125.) **(E)** One-micron-thick section showing the fibroblasts, histiocytes, giant cells, cells in mitosis, and scanty collagenous stroma. (Toluidine blue. Original magnification × 250.)

Overall, the myxoid malignant fibrous histiocytoma is considered to have a better prognosis. Enzinger and Weiss[166] considered that the majority of myxoid malignant fibrous histiocytomas are grade 2 compared to most storiform malignant fibrous histiocytomas, which are usually grade 3 lesions. This morphologic distinction deserves recognition; however, from a clinical standpoint, these tumors should be managed in a similar manner.

The inflammatory variant of malignant fibrous histiocytoma[165] is characterized by diffuse neutrophilic infiltration unassociated with tissue necrosis. The presence of this acute inflammatory reaction is a unique feature. Kyriakos and Kempson[161] also found interspersed foamy cells, plasma cells, lymphocytes, and Reed-Sternberg type of cells. Inflammatory malignant fibrous histiocytoma is somewhat less common and constitutes less than 10 percent of all malignant fibrous histiocytomas. Although these lesions can be seen in young adults, in our experience they are somewhat more frequent in older patients. Grossly the tumor consists of a homogeneous mass with a striking yellowish coloration due to lipid-laden xanthoma cells constituting most of the tumor. Microscopically, the most characteristic features of these tumors are the acute and chronic inflammatory cells and predominance of xanthoma cells. However, storiform fascicular pattern or growth pattern can usually be recognized. Although both acute and chronic inflammatory cells can be seen, the acute inflammatory cells usually predominate. The histiocytic cells are mostly lipid-laden, giving xanthomatous appearance. In certain areas, the histiocytic cells contain either very little or no lipid and resemble the histiocytic cells seen in storiform malignant fibrous histiocytoma. Hajdu[174] considers the inflammatory variant of malignant fibrous histiocytoma as more aggressive; in contrast, Enzinger and Weiss[166] suggested a somewhat better prognosis in this subset of malignant fibrous histiocytoma.

*Electron Microscopy.*   Fu et al.[165] found that five cell types were clearly identifiable: the fibroblastic cells, the histiocytic cells, the xanthomatous cells, the multinucleated tumor giant cells, and an immature type resembling reticulum cells (Fig. 5–40A to 5–40D). Naturally, the number of cells or their frequency depends on the portion of the tumor section(s) examined, xanthomatous and giant cells being the least common. The cells are attached to each other with several types of intercellular connections. Typical maculae adherents (desmosomes) may be found between fibroblastlike cells, but very rarely between histiocytelike cells. The extracellular space consists mainly of a few well-formed collagen fibers, some immature collagen fibers, and a large number of fibers lacking in periodicity. The small blood vessels in the tumor have a continuous endothelium and are limited by basal lamina. A relatively thick zone, consisting of pericyte process, collagen fibers, and microfibrils, usually surrounds these vessels.

The fibroblasts have large elongated nuclei with one or two nucleoli. The cytoplasm contains multiple cisternae of rough endoplasmic reticulum with well-developed Golgi zones, mitochondria, microfilaments (5–10 nm), and occasional lipid droplets. The histiocytes have oval nuclei with highly developed Golgi zones in the perinuclear area. The cytoplasm is characterized by the presence of an abundance of smooth

endoplasmic reticulum, phagocytic vacuoles, and multivesicular bodies. Frequently, membrane-bound bodies resembling lysosomes can be seen. In addition, the cell membranes are ruffled with numerous pseudopodia. The undifferentiated cells described by Fu et al.[165] are occasionally seen. These cells are small and ovoid with round nuclei and scanty cytoplasm, distinguishable from lymphocytes by their lysosome-like cytoplasmic structure. Xanthomatous cells are characterized by their empty vacuolated cytoplasm or by lipid-filled bodies in the cytoplasm. Fu et al.[165] studied two of these tumors in tissue culture and subsequently processed the cells for light and electron microscopic study. They found that most of the tumor cells maintained similar morphologic characteristics.

*Immunohistochemistry.*   As was mentioned previously, although in earlier studies it was suggested that the malignant fibrous histiocytoma originates from histiocytic cells or is derived from endothelial cells, both hypotheses have been proven erroneous. The presence of $\alpha$-1 antitrypsin and $\alpha$-1 chymotrypsin within the tumor supported the initial thesis of histiocytic origin (Fig. 5–41A to 5–41C and Color Plate 1). However, these enzymes have been demonstrated in other nonhistiocytic sarcomas and carcinomas. More specific histiocytic markers, such as Leu-3, Leu-M3, T-200, OK-M1, and so forth, are absent in malignant fibrous histiocytoma. In contrast, fibroblast-associated antigen stain is positive in most malignant fibrous histiocytomas.

*Cytogenetic Findings.*   Malignant fibrous histiocytoma has a complex clonal and nonclonal aberration resulting in a very complex karyotype.[175–177] However, low-grade lesions such as myxoid malignant fibrous histiocytoma have more consistent chromosomal abnormality. Ring chromosomes are seen in myxoid malignant fibrous histiocytoma in approximately half the cases.[176,178] Nilbert and colleagues[178] correlated the presence of ring chromosomes and MDM2 gene amplification indicating that marker rings of malignant fibrous histiocytoma often harbor material derived from chromosome 12. Rydholm et al.[179] suggested that malignant fibrous histiocytomas with 19 $P^+$ marker chromosome have increased relapse rate and are associated with poor prognosis. However, specific chromosomal abnormality in high-grade malignant fibrous histiocytoma is of very little diagnostic value.

*Metastases.*   Soule and Enriquez[180] found metastases in 13 of 33 patients with malignant fibrous histiocytoma (39 percent). Kempson and Kyriakos[160] reported only three instances in their 30 patients. O'Brien and Stout[148] reported a 75 percent incidence of metastasis. In analysis of 196 patients treated by local excision or

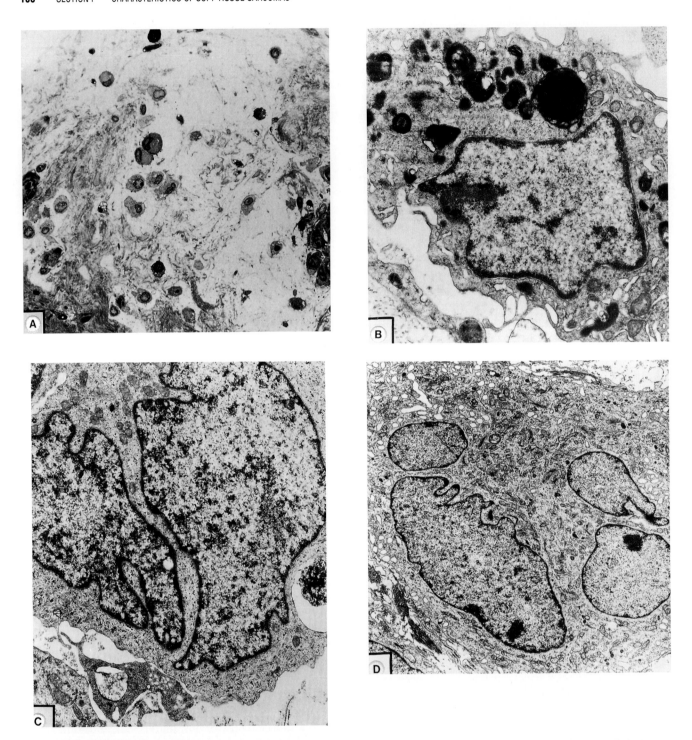

**Figure 5–40.** **(A)** One-micron section of malignant fibrous histiocytoma. Histiocytes are seen in clusters. Several multivacuolated cells and capillaries are scattered in a loose collagenous matrix. (Toluidine blue. Original magnification × 600.) **(B)** One histiocyte from Figure 5–40A. These cells are characterized by an intensely vacuolated outer cytoplasmic fringe that corresponds to the many pseudopodlike processes. The cell body also contains a large variety of inclusion bodies originating from the enzymatic material into secondary lysosomes and residual bodies. (Original magnification × 85,000.) **(C)** A binucleated xanthomatous cell with a lipid inclusion. (Original magnification × 22,000.) **(D)** Portion of a multinucleated giant cell. (Original magnification × 14,500.)

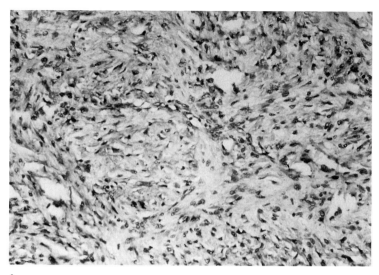

A

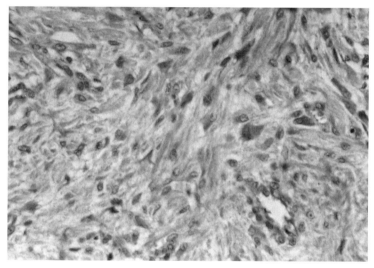

B

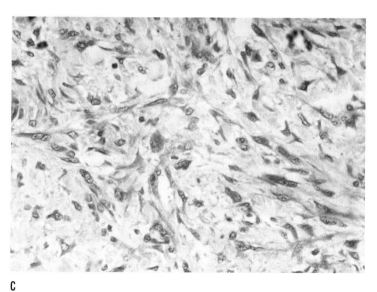

C

**Figure 5–41. (A)** Deep-seated malignant fibrous histiocytoma showing cells in mitosis as well as a number of histiocytes. (H & E. Original magnification × 10.) **(B)** Section from the same tumor showing cells positive for α-antitrypsin. (Original magnification × 20.) **(C)** Similar section positive for α-chymotrypsin. (Original magnification × 20.)

amputation, Weiss and Enzinger[162] reported a 42 percent incidence of distant metastasis. The site of metastases was unknown in 10 patients, but metastasis in the remaining 72 patients was to the lung in 59 patients (82 percent) and lymph nodes in 23 patients (32 percent). Liver, bone, brain, and other body sites were also involved. The incidence of regional node metastasis is difficult to assess in tumors of the extremities. O'Brien and Stout[148] found a 20 percent incidence of lymph node metastasis. Weiss and Enzinger[162] suggested an overall figure of 12 percent. In our own cases, the overall incidence is approximately 20 percent.

Malignant fibrous histiocytoma is aggressive, with a relatively high frequency of metastases: therapeutic planning must take this factor into consideration. Weiss and Enzinger[162] emphasized the association of this tumor with various hematopoietic diseases (e.g., leukemia, Hodgkin's disease, and non-Hodgkin's lymphoma). The relation of hematopoietic disorder to the natural history of malignant fibrous histiocytoma remains to be elucidated.

*Malignant Giant Cell Fibrous Histiocytoma.*  Giant cell type malignant fibrous histiocytoma is synonymous with malignant giant cell tumor of soft parts (Fig. 5–42A and 5–42B). In 1972, Guccion and Enzinger[173] analyzed 32 cases and delineated the clinical and pathologic features of these types of tumors. The patient age is usually between 41 and 80 years. These tumors occur predominantly in males; pain and the presence of a mass are the two most common complaints. The most important laboratory finding is roentgenographic evidence of a soft tissue mass eroding the cortex of the adjacent bone. These tumors are classified into superficial and deep. The superficial tumors are usually less than 5 cm, while the deep ones can grow up to 30 cm. They may be bosselated or oval, with a pseudocapsule. The tumor is tan, with areas of hemorrhage and necrosis. Foci of bone are occasionally noted at the edge.

Histologically, this tumor is characterized by pleomorphic multinucleated giant cells, mononuclear histiocytes, and bizarre to pleomorphic fibroblasts, either arranged around large vascular spaces or clumped in a nodular fashion. The multinucleated giant cells are thought to be neoplastic rather than reactive because of their presence in distant metastasis and blood vessels. They may have formed by fusion or amitotic division, or by phagocytosis of their mononuclear precursor; they contain hemosiderin and osteoid bodies. The osteoid bodies stain best by phosphotungstic acid-hemotoxylin. Chondroblastic and osteoblastic differentiation with formation of cartilage and bone is occasionally observed (Fig. 5–42B).

The formation of bone makes it difficult to differentiate these tumors from the osteocytic variety of osteogenic sarcoma with numerous giant cells.

# ■ TUMORS ARISING IN MUSCLE TISSUE

The muscle tissue constitutes a major element of the body somite and phyllogenetically has been modified into smooth (involuntary), skeletal (voluntary), and cardiac muscle. A brief introductory summary of the embryology, histogenesis, histology, and tissue culture studies would help in understanding the pathologic findings of the tumors and tumorlike conditions of the muscles.

## Smooth Muscle

Myogenesis appears in different organs and regions at different times (e.g., muscularis mucosae develops much later than the main muscular coat in the gastrointestinal tract). In contrast, tracheal muscle is well developed by the eighth intrauterine week. The formation of smooth muscle in the uterus commences in the fourth or fifth month of intrauterine life and continues slowly during infancy and childhood, until just before puberty, when there occurs a great increase of muscle fibers, both in number and in size. Myogenesis in the uterus takes place by continued differentiation of fresh muscle fibers from an undifferentiated subepithelial zone of mesenchyme, the residue of which constitutes the stroma of the adult endometrium, a tissue that retains myogenic power throughout life. Probably this is why endometrial sarcomas develop in women. Little is known of when effective contractility begins in the various muscular organs. However, the degree of differentiation of muscular coats of viscera and arteries suggests that they can function from the second or third month of fetal life.

*Histologic Appearance.*  Smooth muscle, otherwise known as nonstriated or involuntary muscle, differs considerably from the other two types. It is made up of mononuclear spindle-shaped cells varying in length up to 15 μm in the myometrium during pregnancy. In regions where a concentrated contraction in a particular direction occurs, these bundles lie parallel (e.g., separated layers of the external musculature in the intestines). In muscular arteries, nonstriated muscles are present in thick sheets into which capillaries do not penetrate. Within a fasciculus, much of the surface of each cell is coated by a prominent basal lamina, and, between and within the laminae, fine reticulin and collagen fibers form complex networks around each cell, which are separated, except at special points of contact, by a space of 40 to 80 nm.

Individual smooth muscle cells show a centrally placed elongated nucleus, with the cells weakly birefringent, indicating some degree of longitudinal orientation of the cell components. With the electron microscope, the cytoplasm of the cell is seen to consist of closely packed fine filaments lying parallel to the long

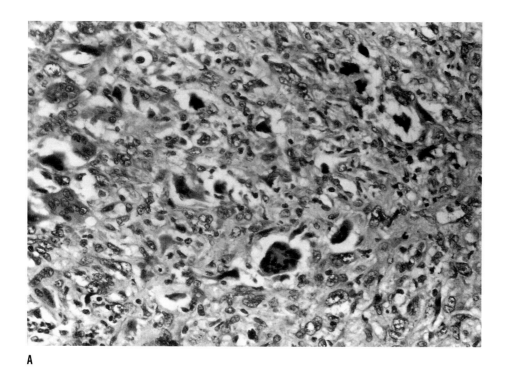

A

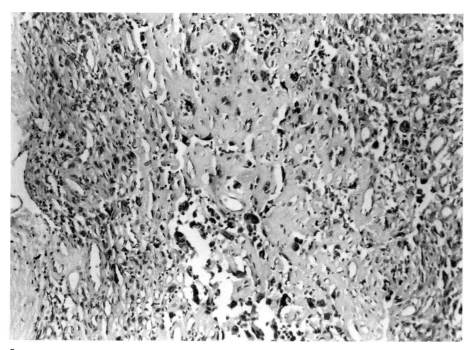

B

**Figure 5–42.** Malignant giant cell tumor. **(A)** The tumor consists of multinucleated giant cells, pleomorphic mononuclear histiocytes, and fibroblasts. (H & E. Original magnification × 250.) **(B)** Low-power view, showing osteoblastic differentiation. (H & E. Original magnification × 125.)

axis of the cell (Fig. 5–43A). Although all the intracytoplasmic constituents are present predominantly in the conical part of the cytoplasm of these cells, most of the cytoplasm contains microfilaments (5 to 8 nm across) that resemble actin filaments of striated muscle. The plasma membrane of the muscle cell contains a number of pinocytotic vesicles, but a system of membranous channels similar to that of skeletal muscle appears to be lacking.

The sarcoplasm, collected in a zone surrounding the nucleus and in the septa between them, contains mitochondria, Golgi materials, and some glycogen. Fusiform densities occur at the sites of confluence of tracts or bundles of myofilaments and at the points where these insert upon the cell membrane. Myofilaments are for the most part organized into parallel bundles oriented along the long axis of the cell. The fibrils are pulled in or pushed out in different directions,

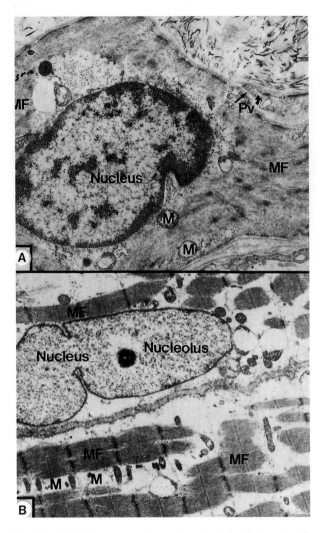

**Figure 5–43.** **(A)** Human normal smooth muscle cell (fallopian tube). The mitochondria and other cytoplasmic organelles occupy a perinuclear position. In the peripheral part of the cytoplasm are the myofilaments *(MF)*, arranged along the longitudinal axis of the cell. These filaments appear to be inserted into the dense bodies. Pinocytotic vesicles *(PV)* are seen along the membrane. There are no transverse striations. (Original magnification × 31,892.) **(B)** Part of a human skeletal muscle cell (sartorius). All the characteristics of a voluntary muscle cell nucleus, with longitudinal arrangement of mitochondria along the contractile elements *(MF)*, are easily discernible. (Original magnification × 14,732.)

crossing one another or fanning out at the periphery of the cell. It is suggested that contractility of smooth muscles is under the control of several internal and external factors.[181] Of interest are the data on hormonal influence[181] and the finding of an association of an acetylcholinelike substance in the activity of the smooth muscle grown in culture.

### Striated or Skeletal or Voluntary Muscle

Although the classic concept that all voluntary muscles develop from paravertebral myotomes or branchial

arches is still accepted by most embryologists and anatomists, the development of rhabdomyosarcomas in unlikely areas, such as the biliary tract,[182] leads one to question the validity of this age-old hypothesis. There appears to be sufficient pathologic[182] and experimental[183] evidence to modify the classic concept, insofar as to add, at least in part, that the somatic musculature is developed from the local nonmyotonic mesenchyme. This point should be borne in mind; otherwise, in some instances a diagnosis of rhabdomyosarcoma might be missed.

In the human embryo of six to seven weeks, the myotomes or other mesenchymal cells destined to become rhabdomyoblasts begin to undergo elongation and form condensed groups with their long axes parallel. They contain either one nucleus or (sometimes) two nuclei and show mitotic proliferation. In most situations, the cytoplasm is devoid of fibrils. In the eight-week-old embryo, some of the rhabdomyoblasts are recognizable, showing the myofibrils with cross-striations. From the eighth week to the fifth month (and possibly still later), new rhabdomyoblasts continue to be differentiated from the mesenchyme. It is believed that, from the fifth month onward, the nuclei take up their surface positions on the fibers, and the fibers acquire distinct sarcolemmal sheaths. Thus, during fetal life, voluntary muscle grows in four ways: (1) differentiation of myoblasts from mesenchyme, (2) mitotic proliferation of the myoblasts that have not yet become fibrillated, (3) longitudinal division of young muscle fibers, and (4) progressive enlargement of fibers, the last becoming relatively more important as the fetus grows. In postnatal life, under normal conditions the growth of muscle is mainly due to the enlargement of the fibers.

Willis[182] reported that, although muscle primordia receive the nerves by the eighth week, the first appearance of motor endplates in muscle is much later (at 20 weeks in the tongue and at 26 to 28 weeks in the limbs). Innervation, though not essential for the development of vertebrate skeletal muscle, is essential for its maintenance. Adult muscles deprived of their nerve supply atrophy and eventually disappear.

***Histologic Appearance.*** Under the light microscope, skeletal muscles appear as closely packed cylinders in longitudinal sections, but with circular, elliptical, or polygonal profiles in cross section. The flattened nuclei of muscle fibers lie peripherally in the zone immediately beneath the cell membrane or sarcolemma; their cytoplasm or sarcoplasm is divided into longitudinal bands or myofibrils each about 1 mm in diameter. In transverse sections, these myofibrils frequently appear aggregated in small groups. In longitudinal sections, the myofibrils are seen to be traversed by striations apparently continuous right across the fiber. Myofibrils vary in their staining characteristics and optical properties, and, on the basis of these characteristics, several bandlike structures can be identified. The significance and behavior of these bands have been described by Huxley and Hanson.[184]

On electron microscopic examination (Fig. 5–43B), each myofibril in longitudinal section is seen to be composed of longitudinally disposed myofilaments. In the resting muscle, these are divided transversely by the Z-bands into serially repeating regions termed *sarcomeres*, each about 2.5 μm long. Two types of myofilaments have been identified: thin (5 nm) and thick (12 nm). These are supposedly actin and myosin, respectively.

The morphology of the rhabdomyoblast has been investigated in skeletal muscles grown in tissue culture, and most of the observations made by electron microscopic examination of fixed tissue specimens have been confirmed. However, the major accomplishment of tissue culture has been a clearer understanding of the histogenesis of rhabdomyoblasts.[185,186] Konigsberg[185] found that skeletal muscle cells in culture pass through a series of morphologic changes resulting in fibrogenesis. Probably a similar mechanism is the underlying reason an anaplastic rhabdomyosarcoma sometimes resembles fibrosarcoma.

## Cardiac Muscle

The development and morphogenesis of cardiac musculature has been investigated extensively, and valuable data have been obtained. However, since tumors of the heart muscle are rare, a detailed discussion is beyond the scope of this treatise.

The foregoing summary of the embryology, histogenesis, histology, and tissue culture studies of smooth and skeletal muscle fibers forms the background for the succeeding description of tumors of myogenic origin.

## TUMORS OF THE SMOOTH MUSCLES

### Leiomyomas

Leiomyoma is a smooth muscle tumor that is considered to be the most common form of primary mesenchymal tumor of the gastrointestinal tract and uterus. In the dermis and subcutaneous tissue, it is rare, and so is a retroperitoneal leiomyoma, which may grow to enormous size (Fig. 5–44).[182,187,188] Occasionally, this tumor may infiltrate the surrounding muscle. This smooth muscle tumor is also found in other locations like kidney,[189] prostate,[189,190] large veins,[191,192] urinary bladder,[193] omentum,[189,194] ureter,[195] spermatic cord,[196] round ligaments,[189] penis,[189] breast,[197] tongue,[197] thyroid,[198] and bone.[199]

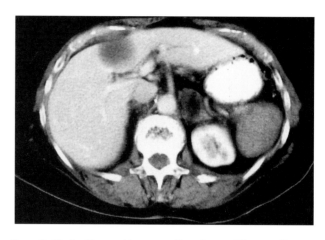

**Figure 5–44.** An 82-year-old woman with an 8-cm solid mass adjacent to the left kidney. Histologically, this was a benign leiomyoma.

***Cutaneous Leiomyoma (Leiomyoma Cutis).*** Cutaneous leiomyoma can essentially be classified into two types: (1) genital leiomyoma, which arises from deep dermis of genital area and (2) extragenital leiomyoma, which is more common and arises from pilar aerector muscle of the skin.[200] The extragenital cutaneous leiomyoma is usually multifocal and often painful. These lesions may be familial and inherited as an autosomal dominant trait.[201–204] Genital leiomyomas are frequently solitary lesions that mostly occur in the scrotum, labia majora, nipple, areola, and penis.

Solitary tumors are round, well-circumscribed, firm nodules that may exceed 2.0 cm in diameter. Solitary lesions may also be found around face, knee joint, and extensor surface of extremities.[104] Microscopically, they are composed of interlacing bands and bundles of spindle cells mixed with little or no fibrous tissue (Fig. 5–45). In cellular leiomyoma, the muscle cells are longer, of greater bulk, and their myofibers are well developed. Lesions in the blood vessels may be quite large; at times, it is difficult to identify the lumen or that a given tumor is of vascular origin. Stout and Lattes[104] stressed that distinguishing between vascular leiomyoma and a venous hemangioma can be difficult. Ultrastructural examination of the leiomyomatous tumors show similar characteristics of a smooth muscle cell. The amount of fibrous matrix depends on the overall cellularity of the tumor.

Stout[205] and Stout and Lattes[104] emphasized the need to recognize a bizarre type of leiomyoma frequently found in the stomach and other parts of the gastrointestinal tract. All these tumors show characteristic macroscopic and microscopic features of a smooth muscle tumor.

***Angiomyoma (Vascular Leiomyoma).*** Angiomyoma is a solitary form of leiomyoma and usually occurs in the

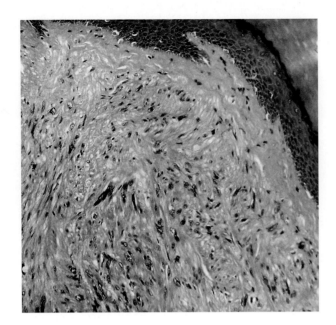

**Figure 5–45.** Cutaneous leiomyoma composed of long, slender, smooth muscle cells arranged in fascicles. Note the long atypical nuclei. (H & E. Original magnification × 125.)

subcutaneous tissue and is composed of numerous thick-walled vessels. In early literature, little attempt was made to separate these tumors from cutaneous leiomyomas, and both were collectively called tuberculum dolorosum because of pain associated with some of these tumors.

***Leiomyoma of Deep Soft Tissue.*** Leiomyomas of the deep soft tissue are sporadic and very uncommon. They may occur at any age and affect both sexes equally. Most are located in the retroperitoneal location or extremity (Fig. 5–44). These tumors produce symptoms depending upon their size and location. Many of them are calcified and a misleading diagnosis of calcifying neurilemoma, synovial sarcoma, or myositis ossificans is made. But grossly and microscopically, they resemble leiomyomas with myxoid or degenerative changes.

***Intravenous Leiomyomatosis.*** Intravenous leiomyomatoses are rare benign neoplasms that usually grow within the blood vessels of the myometrium and occasionally are found at a distance from the body of the uterus. These tumors have also been found in the vena cava and heart.

***Leiomyomatosis Peritonealis Disseminata.*** Leiomyomatosis peritonealis disseminata is a rare condition associated with pregnancy and is more common in African-American women. A history of use of oral contraceptives is usually elicited. These tumors generally regress after pregnancy. The size of the tumors varies from a few mil-

limeters to several centimeters, and the clinical features vary according to the size and location. Microscopically, these tumors resemble smooth muscle nodules.

## Palisade Myofibroblastoma of the Lymph Node (Intranodal Hemorrhagic Spindle Cell Tumor with Amianthoid Fibrils)

Palisade myofibroblastoma of the lymph node is a benign tumor occurring inside a lymph node. This tumor strikingly resembles neurilemomas of the lymph node, as reported by Suster and Rosai.[206] In addition to these spindle cells, there are eosinophilic fibers called *amianthoid fibers* that immunohistochemically can be typed as collagen types I and III. There is a lymphocytic rim at the periphery of the lesion. This is a benign entity and is not to be confused with sarcoma to the nodes.[207]

## Myofibroblastoma of the Breast

Myofibroblastoma of the breast is an uncommon lesion, characterized by spindle cells. Sixteen cases have been reported by Wargotz et al.[208] Most tumors occur in men. It is a well-demarcated mass that does not intermingle with surrounding breast tissue and is composed of spindle cells. At times, it resembles sclerosing lipoma. These tumors rarely have chondroid metaplasia. Mast cells are occasionally encountered. Actin and desmin can be demonstrated by immunohistochemical techniques. Ultrastructural examination shows dense bodies and a basal lamina with pinocytic vesicles. Simple excision is the treatment of choice.

## Angiomyofibroblastoma of the Vulva

Angiomyofibroblastoma of the vulva is described by Fletcher et al.,[209] and it is a distinctly benign tumor of the vulva. The tumor presents with dilated vessels surrounded by smooth muscle, some of which blends with the surrounding muscle cells, and they bleed easily. The tumor has prominent hyaline matrix and can be confused with angiomyxoma. The tumor is less demarcated and is difficult to excise completely. Immunohistochemically, these lesions express desmin and vimentin but not actin.

## Leiomyoblastoma (Epithelioid Smooth Muscle Tumors)

In 1960, Martin and co-workers described an unusual smooth muscle tumor of the stomach, which they termed *myxoid* tumor.[210] In 1962, Stout[205] suggested the term *bizarre leiomyoblastoma.* These tumors cannot be classified as either leiomyomas or leiomyosarcomas, and, though most are benign, some are locally infiltrating or have malignant potential and do metastasize. They have also been designated as epithelioid leiomyomas, clear cell leiomyomas, or plexiform muscle tumors.[205,210,211] According to biologic behavior, these tumors should be classified as either benign or malignant leiomyoblastomas. In some cases, from microscopic appearance, it is difficult to ascertain the malignant potential. Subsequent to the report of Martin and co-workers,[210] these tumors were found in the uterus,[212] retroperitoneum,[213] mesentery,[194] mesocolon,[194,205,214] small intestine,[215] and soft tissue.[214]

***Macroscopic Features.*** Leiomyoblastomas have no special macroscopic features, but tumor size greater than 6 cm must be considered malignant.

***Microscopic Features.*** The tumor cells are polygonal or spindle-shaped, sometimes round, with abundant vacuolated cytoplasm and centrally placed nuclei (Fig. 5–46). In some cases, the existing vacuole may displace the nucleus. Kurman and Norris[211] identified a transition from smooth muscle to clear cell within the tumor. At times, areas containing these clear cells may be mistaken for carcinoma or liposarcoma. The vacuoles are in fact formalin fixation artifacts that are not seen during frozen section or electron microscopy. They are negative for glycogen and fat. In these lesions, multinucleated giant cells are sometimes observed.

In malignant leiomyoblastoma or epithelioid leiomyosarcoma, the cells are pleomorphic with less abundant cytoplasm and are arranged in small clusters of a pseudoalveolar pattern, at times resembling a hemangiopericytoma. They are usually greater than 6.0 cm in size. Mitosis is related to metastatic capability. One mitosis per high-power field indicates a metastatic rate of 2 percent, but more than 10 mitoses per high-power field indicates a metastasis rate of 100 percent.

From a therapeutic standpoint, any lesion containing five or more mitoses per high-power field should be considered malignant.

***Electron Microscopy.*** Electron microscopic examination shows that the overall pattern of the structures does not resemble normal smooth muscles.[216,217] The tumor cells are irregularly shaped and have multiple cytoplasmic processes. The presence of myofibrils provides evidence of smooth muscle origin. In the visceral types, such as leiomyoblastoma of the stomach, micropinocytotic activity is markedly diminished.

Immunocytochemically, muscle-specific actin is present but desmin is absent.[218] According to some, neural markers (neural filaments) may be positive. S-100, neuron-specific enolase, and protein gene product stains may vary.[219–221] The presence of neural elements raises the intriguing possibility that some of these tumors may have a neural origin.

### Leiomyosarcoma

Leiomyosarcoma is a relatively uncommon malignant tumor of the soft somatic tissue. Stout and Hill[222] recorded only 36 cases collected from 19 different institutions. Yannopoulos and Stout[214] added nine others found in children younger than 16 years of age. All leiomyosarcomas are similar in microscopic features. Nonvisceral leiomyosarcomas may be classified in three categories: (1) leiomyosarcoma of the cutaneous and subcutaneous tissue; (2) leiomyosarcoma of the deep tissue, including retroperitoneum and viscera; and (3) leiomyosarcoma of vascular origin.

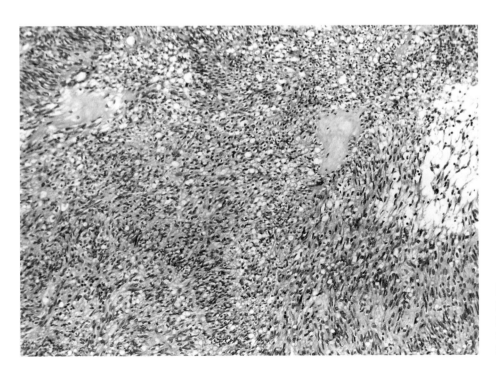

**Figure 5–46.** Leiomyoblastoma. The polygonal epithelioid appearance of the cytoplasm is evident. Vacuolation within these cells can be seen with ease. (H & E. Original magnification × 125.)

***Leiomyosarcoma of the Skin and Subcutaneous Tissue.***
Although the incidence of leiomyosarcoma arising in the smooth muscle of the skin[223,224] is rare, it accounts for about 2 to 3 percent of all superficial soft tissue sarcomas. Soft tissue leiomyosarcoma[222] is most common in women, with a 2:1 or 3:1 ratio over the male rate.[222] According to Stout and Hill,[222] they are found between the fifth and seventh decade of life and are divided into cutaneous and subcutaneous tumors. The cutaneous tumor is less than 2.0 cm in size and has discoloration and umbilication of the overlying surface, while the subcutaneous tumor is more painful and grows larger in size. They are usually solitary in origin.

*Microscopic Findings.*    Most leiomyosarcomas in the superficial soft tissue can be recognized by the elongated cells with centrally located and long nuclei growing in interlacing cords, occasionally suggesting a palisading pattern. Cells of leiomyosarcoma may have anaplastic features, sometimes with bizarre large and occasionally pyknotic nuclei. Stout and Lattes[104] pointed out the difficulty of demonstrating myofibrils in these tumors. Mitotic rate is frequently elevated and provides an excellent guideline for the diagnosis of the leiomyosarcoma. Grading of the tumor is essential for prognosis.

***Leiomyosarcoma of Deep Soft Tissue.***    Leiomyosarcoma of deep soft tissue occurs most commonly in women, and the median age is 60 years. Presenting symptoms depend on location of the tumor (Fig. 5–47) and include nausea, vomiting, weight loss, and other nonspecific symptoms. These lesions can attain huge size,

averaging about 1,600 grams.[225] On cut surface, they are whorled, gray-white masses and may have cyst formation with foci of hemorrhage and necrosis (Fig. 5–48).

*Microscopic Findings.*    Leiomyosarcoma of the deep tissue is characterized by elongated cells with abundant cytoplasm (Fig. 5–49A to 5–49D). The nucleus is classically described as "cigar shaped," occasionally with concave ends. Most tumors are similar to superficial leiomyosarcomas described above. Masson stain and phosphotungstic acid hematoxylin (PTAH) help in diagnosing leiomyosarcoma. Numerous multinucleated giant cells are also seen in this tumor, in addition to cigar-shaped nuclei and interlacing cords and bundles. The delicate network is accentuated by reticulin stain. Glycogen is also present as demonstrated by PAS stain.

At times, the malignant potential of smooth muscle lesions may be difficult to predict from histologic appearance. Also, histologic criteria for malignancy of smooth muscle tumor vary depending on location of the lesion. Traditional parameters, including location, size, pleomorphism, cellularity, necrosis, atypia, and mitosis are all considered in determining the malignant nature of these lesions. However, mitosis remains the most important feature for predicting malignancy of smooth muscle tumors. In retroperitoneal smooth muscle tissue, one or more mitosis per 10 high-power fields is considered malignant. In contrast, uterine lesions with 10 or more mitoses per 10 high-power fields are considered malignant, and lesions with 5 to 9 mitoses per 10 high-power fields are considered borderline. In the gastrointestinal tract, smooth muscle

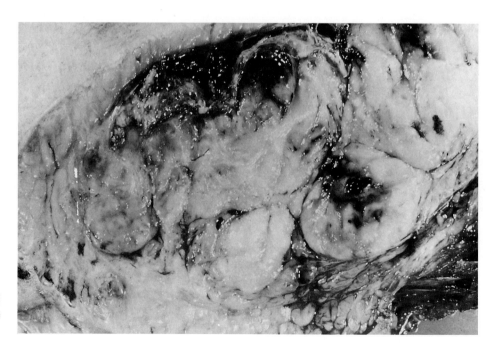

**Figure 5–47.** Cut section of a deep-seated leiomyosarcoma of an extremity. Note peripheral hemorrhagic areas.

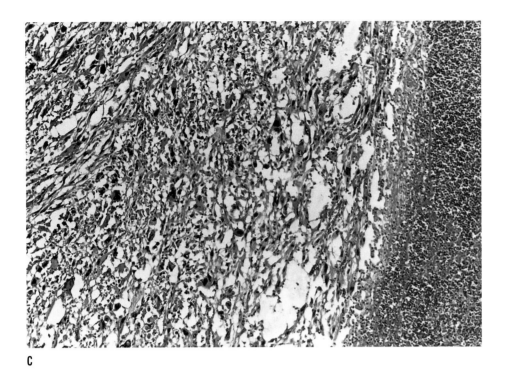

C

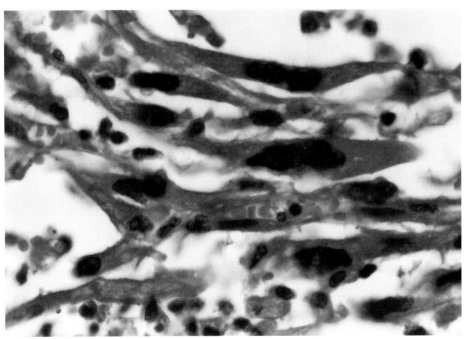

D

**Figure 5–49** *(continued).* **(C)** Another view of a high-grade leiomyosarcoma, of the right arm. Areas of hemorrhage and multiple cells in mitosis, with scanty stroma and tumor giant cells, are seen. (Original magnification × 65.) **(D)** High-power of Figure 5–49C. Smooth muscle cells with longitudinally oriented myofibrils are discernible. (Original magnification × 600.) This patient died within two years of definitive therapy.

reticulum (glycogen tumors). Myofilaments of varying width are found in the periphery of the cytoplasm. Biologically, these are benign tumors and have no relationship to rhabdomyosarcoma. Immunologically, they are immunoreactive to desmin and all of the smooth-muscle antigens. They seem to be less reactive with S-100, vimentin, and Leu-7. Ultrastructurally, existing Z-bands are readily discernible within the I-band. There are also trigonal arrays of actin and myosin filaments which can be seen in cross-striation, and the parallel rows of electron dense particles within the mitochondria.

### Rhabdomyosarcoma
Rhabdomyosarcoma arises in relation to the skeletal muscle in adults and juveniles. However, the tumor is occasionally seen in an anatomic location not known to

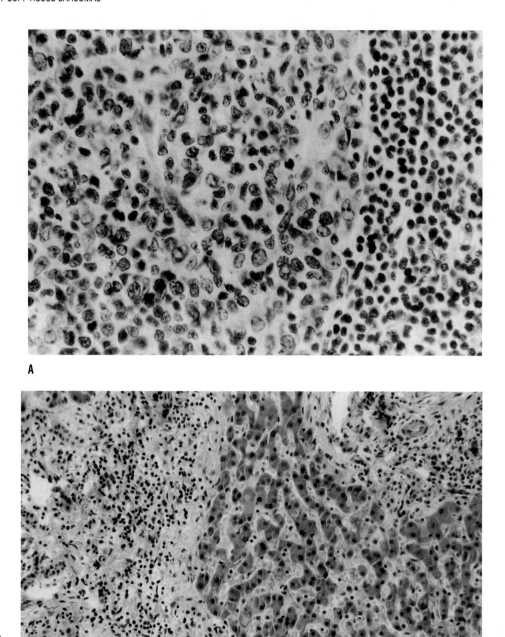

**Figure 5–50. (A)** Leiomyosarcoma metastatic to axillary lymph node. Patient had an axillary node dissection for a leiomyosarcoma of the arm. (H & E. Original magnification × 250.) **(B)** Metastatic leiomyosarcoma to liver. (H & E. Original magnification × 250.)

have an abundance of rhabdomyoblasts, including bladder,[234] urethra,[235] prostate,[189] spermatic cord,[235] vagina,[237,238] uterus,[104,189] round ligament,[189] breast,[189] bronchus,[238] palate,[239–241] tonsils,[239–241] tongue,[239–241] nasopharynx,[239–241] orbit,[49,104,189,241,243] eustachian tube,[243] middle ear,[244] and common bile duct.[245,246]

It is customary to classify rhabdomyosarcoma into three different groups: (1) embryonal, which usually affect children, adolescents, and rarely adults; (2) pleomorphic, which are composed of pleomorphic elements, are usually found in adults and arise in relation to skeletal muscle (only rarely do these occur in children); and (3) alveolar, in which the tumor shows a dis-

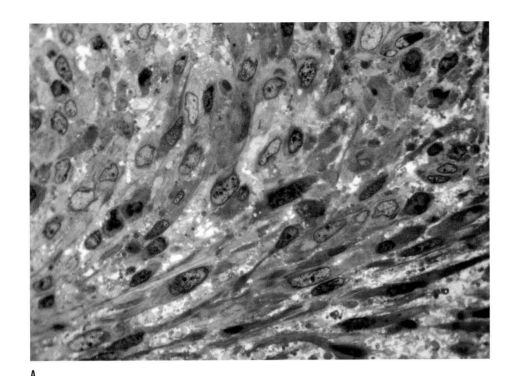

**A**

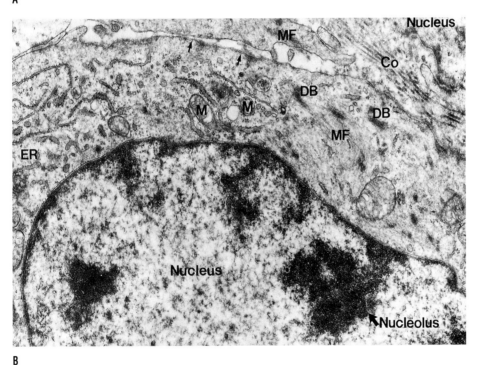

**B**

**Figure 5–51. (A)** One-micron thick Araldite-embedded section of a leiomyosarcoma in the arm of a 55-year-old man. The longitudinal arrangement of the smooth muscle cells is obvious. (Toluidine blue and basic fuchsin stain. Original magnification × 600.) **(B)** Malignant smooth muscle cell from a patient with a retroperitoneal leiomyosarcoma. In this micrograph is seen the major part of one malignant smooth muscle cell, with myofibrils located peripherally within the cytoplasm. The myofibrils *(MF)* appear to be inserted into the dense bodies *(DB)* and the cell membrane *(arrows)*. Cytoplasm contains mitochondria *(M)* and endoplasmic reticulum *(ER)*. In the top of the micrograph, cytoplasm of another muscle cell is identifiable. No desmosomal contacts are present between these two cells. (Original magnification × 35,240.)

tinct alveolar pattern, are found in all age groups but are more common in young adults.

***Embryonal Rhabdomyosarcoma.*** Embryonal rhabdomyosarcoma occurs in children and most commonly in the regions of the head and the neck. Almost 50 to 60 percent of the rhabdomyosarcomas in children are in the head and neck region and most commonly occur below age 15. When it arises near the mucosal surface, it tends to become lobulated and resemble a bunch of grapes, acquiring the descriptive term *botryoid sarcoma.* However, spindle cell rhabdomyosarcoma as a subtype of this embryonal rhabdomyosarcoma is marked by a favorable clinical behavior.

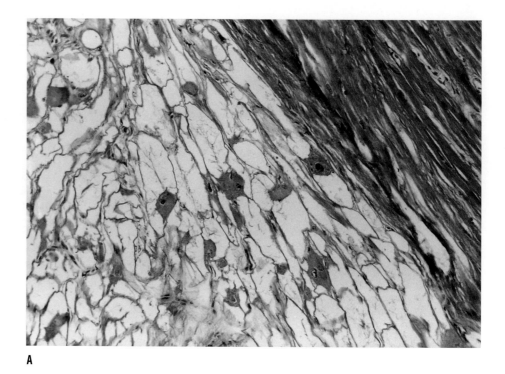

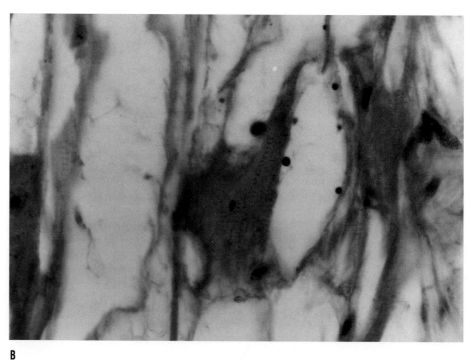

**Figure 5–52. (A)** Rhabdomyoma of the heart. Note arrangement of round cells supported by their stromal trabeculae. (H & E. Original magnification × 125.) **(B)** High-power view with PTAH stain. The cross-striation within the muscle fibers is easily seen. (Original magnification × 375.)

*Macroscopic Findings.* Embryonal rhabdomyosarcoma has no characteristic gross feature by which it can be diagnosed except in locations such as the vagina, anus, nose, palate, or external ear, where the presenting edge truly resembles a cluster of grapes (Fig. 5–53). In all other locations, it resembles any other circumscribed tumor and seldom attains a size of more than 5 cm. Botryoid type accounts for 5 to 10 percent of all rhabdomyosarcomas.

*Microscopic Findings.* Embryonal rhabdomyosarcomas may have a wide spectrum of microscopic appearance

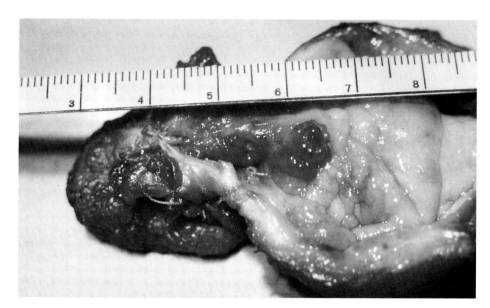

**Figure 5–53.** Specimen of urinary bladder and vagina of four-month-old girl. The primary tumor originated in the urinary bladder and protruded through the urethra to the vagina. The presentation was mistakenly considered a vaginal botryoid sarcoma and inadequately excised. Following recurrence within two months, patient was referred to us (see Table 9–7, Chapter 9 for further clinical details).

resembling various stages of growth of embryonic muscles (Figs. 5–54A to 5–54D). However, most lesions show small round cells with acidophilic cytoplasm or larger elongated cells with cross-striations and acidophilic cytoplasm. Usually, a high rate of mitosis is observed in each high-power field. These cells may be arranged in areas that are tightly packed, intermixed with relatively sparsely populated areas. Some areas may have myxoid background and usually have scanty interstitial collagen. Poorly differentiated lesions show undifferentiated cells, hyperchromatic nuclei with nucleoli, and abundant mitosis. Cytoplasm in these cells is usually scanty or indistinct. Occasional lesions may demonstrate straplike cells, prominent centrally placed nucleus, or racquet-shaped cells with cross-striations.[247] Enzinger and Weiss[247] have also described occasional lesions with foci of immature cartilaginous and osseous tissue. Botryoid sarcomas generally have layers of small round rhabdomyoblasts two to four cell layers thick and have high mitotic activity. These layers of tumor cells in botryoid sarcoma resemble the maximum growth layers of the trunk of a tree and are termed the *cambium layer*.[166]

*Electron Microscopy.*    Nuclei have prominent nucleoli and demonstrate light-staining chromatin and narrow peripheral compact margination (Fig. 5–55A and 5–55B). The immature rhabdomyoblasts manifest a complex cytoplasmic structure within abundant organelles and membranes. The overall morphologic appearance resembles that of an immature rhabdomyoblast grown in tissue cultures.[248] The mitochondria are usually large, with a clear matrix and a parallel array

of cristae. Endoplasmic reticulum varies in quantity and in organization, with numerous small cisternae or smooth endoplasmic reticulum to large cleft lines with rough endoplasmic reticulum. The quantity and type of cytoplasmic fibers are directly proportional to the stage of maturation of the rhabdomyoblasts under study (Fig. 5–55C). In mature rhabdomyoblasts, fully formed intracytoplasmic fibrils are apparent. Most authors[248–252] have not been able to find I- and Z-bands in the myoblasts.

*Metastases.*    Blood-borne metastasis is the major route of systemic spread. However, regional lymph node metastasis in embryonal rhabdomyosarcomas is not uncommon.[239,241,253,254] The lung is the most common site of metastasis.[255] In terminal cases, however, metastasis of embryonal rhabdomyosarcoma may be observed at any anatomic site.

*Pleomorphic Rhabdomyosarcoma.*    Pleomorphic rhabdomyosarcoma is most commonly found in adults and is most common in the extremities.

*Macroscopic Findings.*    The tumor is usually deep-seated within the musculature (Fig. 5–56). It can attain large size and frequently infiltrates the surrounding tissue. The cut sections of the tumor are usually reddish, and often the central part shows hemorrhage or necrosis or both.

*Microscopic Findings.*    The tumor varies so much in pattern and cellularity that, unless convincing evidence of rhabdomyoblast is shown, diagnosis is open to question

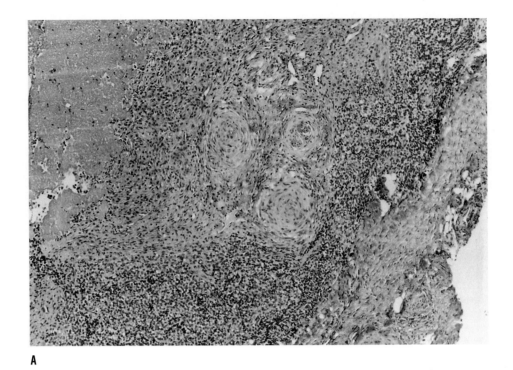

A

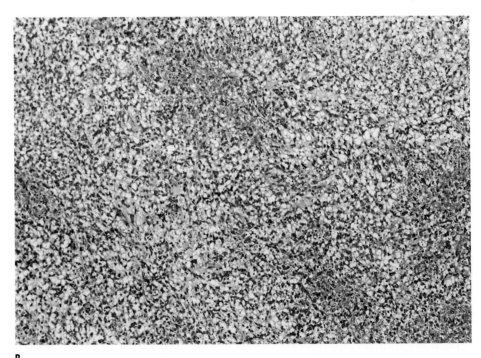

**Figure 5–54. (A)** Embryonal rhabdomyosarcoma. The rhabdomyoblasts are circular. The left-hand corner of the micrograph shows hemorrhage and necrosis; on the right, infiltration of the surrounding muscle bundles can be seen. (Original magnification × 65.) **(B)** Embryonal rhabdomyosarcoma showing a multitude of round cells and areas of myxomatous degeneration. (H & E. Original magnification × 65.) *(Continued.)*

B

(Fig. 5–57A and 5–57B). Rhabdomyoblasts may be rounded or strap-shaped, with more than two nuclear areas in tandem; they may be racquet-shaped with one nucleus; or they may take the shape of a giant cell. Rhabdomyoblast giant cells are usually well-preserved and rarely have pyknotic nuclei. They have large and irregularly shaped vacuoles, peripherally arranged, producing "spider web" cells. The cell cytoplasm tends to be acidophilic, and, in differentiated cells, cross-striations of myofibrils are seen. Under the light microscope, the diagnosis of highly pleomorphic rhabdomyosarcoma is often difficult, and both ultrastructural

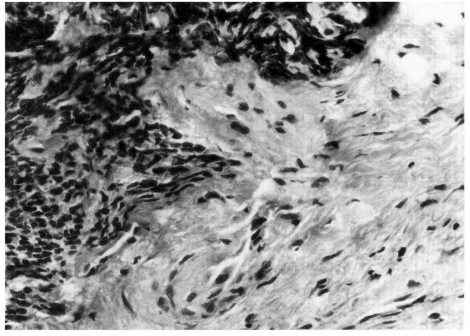

C

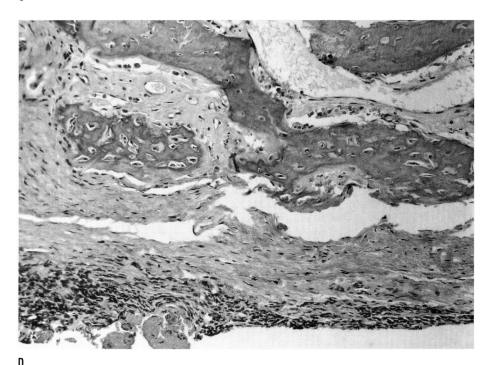

D

**Figure 5–54** *(continued).* **(C)** Infiltration of surrounding muscle in an extremity rhabdomyosarcoma. (H & E. Original magnification × 125.) **(D)** Infiltration of the periosteum in an orbital rhabdomyosarcoma. (H & E. Original magnification × 125.)

and immunohistochemical studies are often required in doubtful cases (see below).

*Immunohistochemistry.*    On immunostaining, these rhabdomyoblasts are positive for myoglobin, muscle-specific

actin, and desmin. These types of muscle-specific cells are not found in malignant fibrous histiocytoma.

*Electron Microscopy.*    Electron microscopic findings of these tumors are similar to those of the embryonal variety just described. The presence of mature rhabdo-

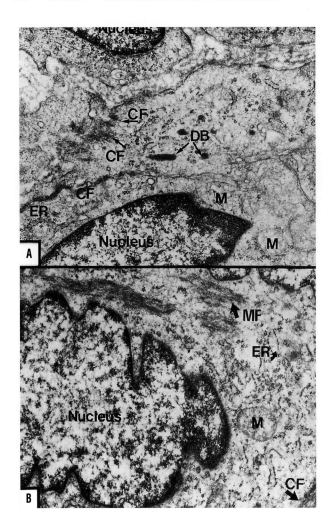

myoblasts with all the cellular characteristics, and of rhabdomyosarcoma giant cells, aids in establishing an accurate diagnosis. In poorly differentiated tumor, a careful search for Z-bands in tumor cells is a valuable step in diagnosis.

*Metastases.*    Pleomorphic rhabdomyosarcoma, like the embryonal variety, metastasizes to the regional nodes and the lungs. The incidence of regional node metastasis, however, is less frequent than in the embryonal variety. In the late stage of the disease, it can metastasize to the pleura, lungs, bones, subcutaneous tissue, kidney, adrenals, pancreas, ovaries, and even the brain.

**Alveolar Rhabdomyosarcoma.**    Alveolar rhabdomyosarcoma usually occurs in children and adolescents, but can be encountered in all age groups. It is found more frequently in the extremities although it can occur in any part of the body. As in the other two types, the tumor infiltrates the surrounding tissue.

*Macroscopic Findings.*    This tumor can attain any size. The transected tissue is firm, grayish-white, and usually shows central necrosis or cystic degeneration.

*Microscopic Findings.*    The cells are round or oval, moderately sized, and apparently unattached to each other. They are contained within spaces lined by the fibrous tissue septum. Frequently, the cells cling to these septa

**Figure 5–55. (A)** Immature malignant rhabdomyoblast, showing various cytoplasmic contents, smooth membrane system, occasional rough endoplasmic reticulum *(ER)*, large mitochondria *(M)*, attempts at cytoplasmic filament formation *(CF)*, and a few dense inclusion bodies *(DB)*. (Original magnification × 34,420.) **(B)** More mature malignant rhabdomyoblasts; formed myofibrillar structures *(MF)* are evident. (Original magnification × 23,520.) **(C)** Cytoplasm of a neoplastic rhabdomyoblast showing an attempt at sarcomere formation. (Original magnification × 46,351.)

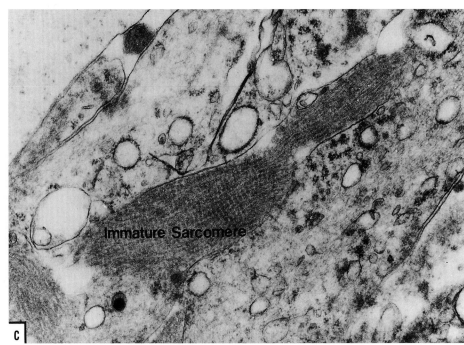

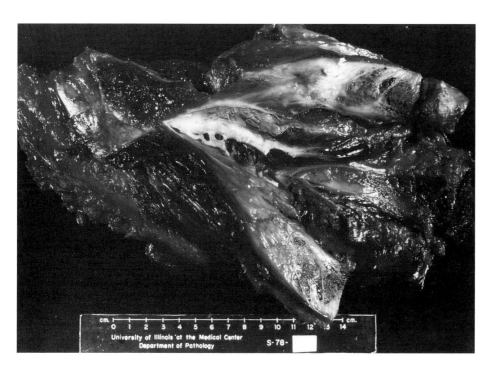

**Figure 5–56.** Cut section of a pleomorphic rhabdomyosarcoma of the lower extremity, with areas of hemorrhage and necrosis.

and may make a pseudoglandular or an alveolar pattern, hence the name (Fig. 5–58A to 5–58C). Occasionally, the cells proliferate, and the alveolar pattern is destroyed. Occasionally, the architecture resembles a neuroblastoma or a malignant lymphoma. The presence of rhabdomyoblasts with all their characteristics, and multinucleated giant cells with peripherally placed wreathlike nuclei determines the nature of the diagnosis.[256]

The incidence of regional node involvement is almost as high as in the embryonal type (Fig. 5–59). Enzinger and Shiraki[257] found 36 of 110 patients (33 percent) to have regional node metastasis. In five of their patients, the diagnosis of primary tumor was made after the biopsy of the palpable regional nodes. In our group of 12 patients, 4 (33 percent) had regional node metastases.

*Cytogenetic Findings.* For rhabdomyosarcoma, cytogenetic study can be used to differentiate the embryonal type from the alveolar variety.[258–262] In alveolar rhabdomyosarcoma, reciprocal translocation of Chromosomes 2 and 13 (t2; 13) (q35;q14) or (t2;13) (q37;q14) is present in approximately 80 percent of the cases. In contrast, in embryonal rhabdomyosarcoma, chromosomes numbering in the hypertriploid range and extensive structural abnormalities along with translocation of 13q to both 1q and 2p were observed.[260] Whereas, in patients with pleomorphic rhabdomyosarcoma, hypo-

diploid tumor with complex translocation involving Chromosomes 5 and 13 and a breakpoint at 13q14 and t(11;12) (q24;q12) can be found. Such abnormality has previously been described in Ewing's sarcoma and related tumors. Embryonal rhabdomyosarcoma usually lacks the specific chromosomal abnormality[259] described above. However, chromosome aberration usually accompanied by loss of gene from short-arm of Chromosome 11 with extra copies of Chromosome 8, 20, and long-arm of Chromosome 2 can occasionally be observed.[139]

## ■ TUMORS DERIVED FROM PERIPHERAL NERVOUS TISSUE

Most nerve fibers are present in muscles and skin by the second month of intrauterine life, but effective functional innervation takes much longer to develop. Appreciation of the structure and function of mammalian nervous tissue began with the pioneering investigations of Ramon y Cajal,[263] von Schwann,[264] del Rio Hortega,[265] His,[266] Sherrington,[267] and Le Gross Clarke[268] in the earlier part of this century, culminating in the description of synapses and synaptosomes by Eccles[269] in the 1960s. Since then, there has been an explosion of knowledge in this area. A description of these elegantly designed studies, the results obtained, and the conclusions drawn, although a fascinating and

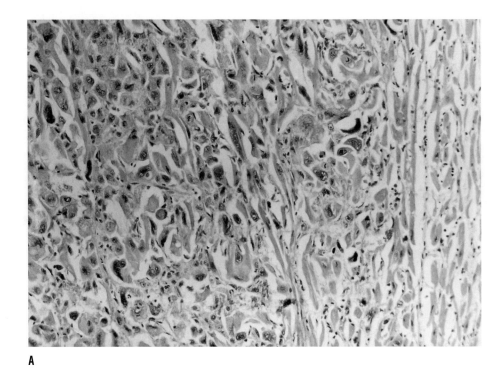

**A**

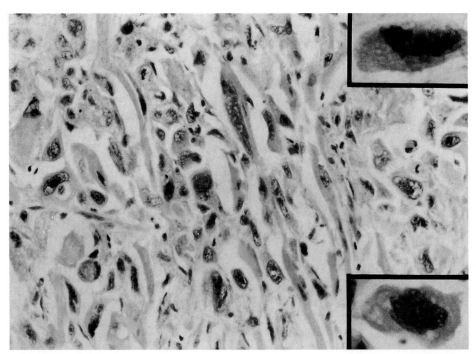

**Figure 5–57. (A)** Pleomorphic rhabdomyosarcoma showing a wide variety of sizes and shapes of the cells. (H & E. Original magnification × 125.) **(B)** High-power view showing the spindle-shaped cells and tumor cells. (H & E. Original magnification × 250.) Inset shows cross-striations in malignant rhabdomyoblast. (Original magnification × 600.)

**B**

romantic study in themselves of the evolution of knowledge in human biology, is not germane to a section on the pathology of neoplasms of the peripheral nerves. However, it is desirable to have a brief summary of the structure and function of normal peripheral nervous

tissue as a point of reference for a better appreciation of the pathologic anatomy of the tumors of the nervous system.

The peripheral nervous system comprises the cerebrospinal and autonomic system of nerves and their associated ganglia-containing nerve cell bodies, together with the cellular and connective tissue elements that ensheathe them.

The structure of the sensory ganglia of the dorsal spinal nerve roots and the corresponding ones on the trunk of the trigeminal, facial, glossopharyngeal, and vagus nerves resemble those of neurons and do not require elaborate description. The autonomic ganglia, in contrast, have a different structure, since their cell bodies are multipolar with dendritic processes that receive synapses from incoming preganglionic visceral motor fibers. Autonomic ganglia are found in the paravertebral sympathetic chains, near the roots of the great visceral arteries in the abdomen, and near or embedded within the walls of various viscera. Autonomic ganglion cells may also be highly modified, as in the case of chromaffin cells of the adrenal medulla, in which the axon is absent.

The nerve trunks and their principal branches are composed of roughly parallel bundles of nerve fibers comprising the efferent and afferent axons, ensheathing Schwann cells, which in some cases produce myelin. These bundles of nerve fibers are surrounded by connective tissue sheaths at different levels of organization. The fibers are grouped together within a trunk in a number of fascicles, each of which may contain from relatively few to many hundreds of nerve fibers. (See Figure 5–60A and 5–60B for details.)

A dense, irregular connective tissue sheath, the epineurium, surrounds the whole trunk, and a similar but less fibrous perineurium encloses each fasciculus. Between these two spaces lies the loose delicate connective tissue network, the endoneurium. These connective tissue planes serve as convenient access for the vasculature of the peripheral nerves that run parallel to the nerve fibers in the endoneurial spaces.

The epineurium is a collagenous adventitial coat with little regular organization; the perineurium, in contrast, has a regular structure of highly flattened laminae of fibroblasts alternating with fine collagenous sheets running in various directions within the sheath (Fig. 5–60A). On the basis of total fiber diameter (i.e., axon and its myelin sheath) and the rate of impulse conduction, the fibers in mixed peripheral nerves have been classified into three major types: A, B, and C. Type A fibers (the largest) consist of various myelinated somatic afferent and efferent fibers; type B, myelinated preganglionic fibers of the autonomic nervous system; and type C, nonmyelinated sensory fibers.

Schwann cells are the chief nonexcitable cells of the peripheral nervous system, enfolding and enwrapping axons over most of their surfaces (Fig. 5–60B). Morphologically, Schwann cells vary with the type of fiber, but generally the nucleus tends to be hetero-

chromatic and ellipsoidal, and the cytoplasm is rich in mitochondria, microtubules, and microfilaments, in addition to prominent lysosomes and well-developed rough endoplasmic reticulum. The basement membrane is found on the external surface, except where it lies adjacent to a nerve cell process. It is a continuous sheath over the abutting Schwann cells at the node of Ranvier, a gap where the axolemma is exposed. Schwann cells have been found not only to provide mechanical support to the nerve cells but also to take part in myriad physicochemical activities.

The larger axons are incorporated in a myelin sheath and are termed *myelinated fibers* (Fig. 5–60A and 5–60B). The fatty composition of the myelin is responsible for the glistening whiteness of the peripheral nerves and white matter centrally. Axons smaller than 0.5 to 1.0 μm generally lack these sheaths and are therefore termed *nonmyelinated fibers*. In routine light microscopic sections, the lipids are removed, and the myelin sheath appears as a vacuolated zone between the axon and the cytoplasm and the nucleus of the Schwann cell. Special stains are required to neutralize myelin; distinguishing these structures by electron microscopy is not difficult.

Schwann cells, autonomic ganglia, chromaffin cells, and other nerve structures can be grown in tissue culture. Schwann cells are known to have myelinating properties even in vitro,[270] and chromaffin cells produce catecholamines.[271] When these cells are fixed and studied under the electron microscope, the ultrastructural characteristics of the cultured cell appear the same as in the fixed tissue specimens.

This brief background on the embryologic and structural aspects allows us to classify the tumors and tumorlike conditions of the peripheral nervous tissue (see Table 2–1, Chapter 2). A purist might take exception to some finer points in this classification, but clinicopathologically such a classification is essential or else the principles of management of these conditions can never be properly defined.

## BENIGN TUMORS

### Solitary Benign Schwannomas, Solitary Neurofibroma, Neurilemmomas, Perineuronal Fibroblastomas, Acoustic Neuromas

A typical neurofibroma of the skin is circumscribed, compressed to the adjacent dermis, and separated from the epidermis with a band of dermis. These characteristics are not found in neurofibroma located in the deep tissues and are indistinguishable from solitary schwannomas. The prominent intracellular component of a neurofibroma is composed of numerous collagen

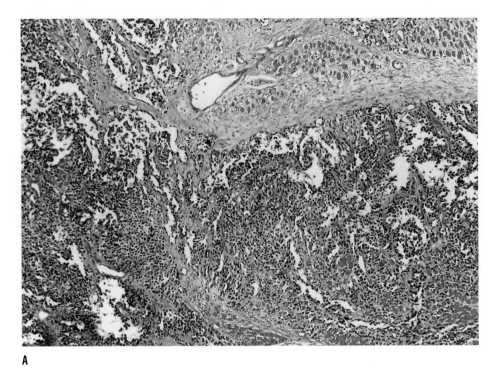

**A**

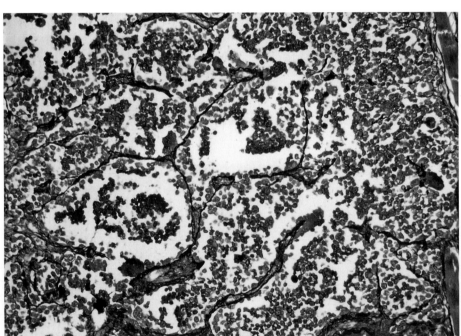

**Figure 5–58. (A)** Alveolar arrangement of an extremity alveolar rhabdomyosarcoma. Infiltration of surrounding structures is apparent. (Original magnification × 65.) **(B)** Reticulin stain outlining the alveolar pattern; unattached rhabdomyoblasts are lying loose within the center of the alveolus. (Original magnification × 125.) *(Continued.)*

**B**

fibers in a nonorganized matrix. The proportion of interstitial collagen in a subcutaneous neurofibroma is higher than in the corresponding solitary schwannoma, and the microscopic distinction between the two can usually be made. Schwann cells are still the principal cells, and the tumor develops because of their proliferation.

*Macroscopic Findings.*   These tumors can vary in size from a few millimeters to more than 20 cm. The small tumors are usually white, fusiform, firm, circumscribed, and encapsulated (Fig. 5–61A), whereas the larger ones are irregularly lobulated, and grayish- or yellowish-white. Cut sections of larger tumors show occasional cystic areas, and some of these cysts contain hemor-

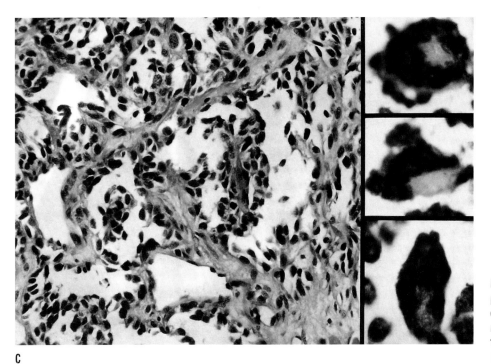

C

**Figure 5–58** *(continued).* **(C)** Under high power, the cellular morphology of the rhabdomyoblasts is apparent. (H & E. Original magnification × 250.) Inset shows the tumor giant cells. (Original magnification × 600.)

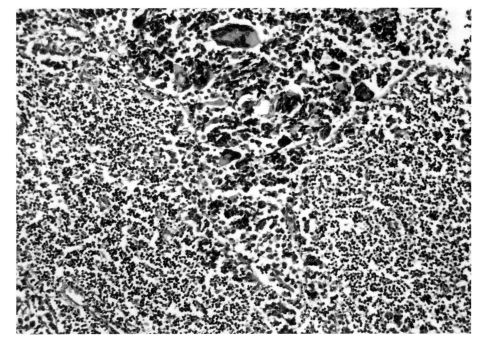

**Figure 5–59.** Axillary lymph node metastases from a primary alveolar rhabdomyosarcoma of the lower end of the arm. (H & E. Original magnification × 125.) Patient is a 28-year-old man, five years postoperative, treated with excision of primary tumor and a simultaneous axillary node dissection. He also received adjuvant chemotherapy.

rhagic fluid. When the nerve of origin is recognized, the tumor usually projects from one side and adheres to the nerve (Fig. 5–61B). Frequently, the nerve of origin is not found.

*Microscopic Findings.*     According to the morphology of the tumor cells and their spatial arrangements, two types of tissues have been described. In type A tissue of

Antoni, the texture is compact and composed of interwoven bundles of long bipolar spindle cells, which in cross-section are seen to be narrow cylinders with tapering ends. The cells have oval or rod-shaped nuclei containing variable amounts of chromatin and inconspicuous nucleoli. In places, the cells form a typical palisading arrangement, with their nuclei in a well-organized pattern. Such foci are termed

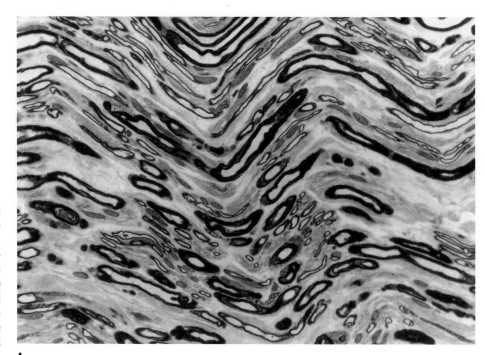

**Figure 5–60. (A)** One-micron-thick section of a normal human sciatic nerve. Myelinated fibers are easily discernible. (Osmium tetroxide stain. Original magnification × 80.) **(B)** Low-power electron micrograph of the same nerve showing the myelinated axons *(Max)* and unmyelinated axons *(Uax)* in different profiles, Schwann cells *(Sch.N)*, with basement membrane *(Bm)*, and the interstitial collagen fibers *(Co)*. (Original magnification × 6,026.) **A**

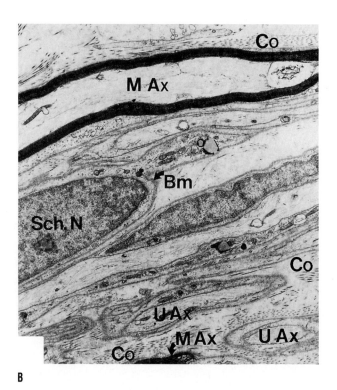

**B**

*Verocay bodies* (Fig. 5–61C). Type B tissue is distinguished by its loose texture and the polymorphism of the tumor cells. Both are highly specific structures of neurilemomas (Fig. 5–61D). Type B distribution is commonly, but not invariably, present in all schwannomas. With hematoxylin-eosin or Alcian blue stains, the matrix stains poorly or not at all. Vessels in schwannomas are usually prominent, with thick, hyalinized walls. Some vessels, particularly large sinusoidal channels, may contain recent or organized thrombi. Lipid-filled foam cells and hemosiderin-laden macrophages, lymphocytes, and mast cells may be found in large numbers, usually around blood vessels.

The electron microscopic appearance of benign schwannomas is characterized by the presence of multiple Schwann cells, with both myelinated and unmyelinated axons interspersed between the interstitial collagen matrix (Fig. 5–61E). Along with Schwann cells, also found within these tumors are a number of fibroblasts, macrophages, lymphocytes, and mast cells.

The presence of mast cells in normal peripheral nerves and in peripheral nerve tumors (Fig. 5–62A and 5–62B) has aroused some interest. Gamble and Goldby[272] found mast cells in the peripheral nerves of a variety of mammals, including man. Ultrastructural study has demonstrated a large number of mast cells in peripheral nerve tumors.[273,274] The function of mast cells in these tumors is not clearly understood, but several possibilities have been suggested. Csaba and asso-

ciates[275] proposed that mast cells inhibit tumor growth by neutralizing tumor polysaccharides. Simpson,[276] in contrast, postulated that epithelial hyperplasia probably causes a local increase in mast cells. The increase in mast cell population may also be related to the increase in endoneurial collagen after nerve degeneration.[277–280] The true significance of these cells, however, still remains unexplained.

Several variants of schwannoma are encountered in any survey of a large series. One variant, cellular schwannoma, requires more clarification, since this type might be misinterpreted as a malignant tumor. Cellular schwannomas are characterized by hypercellularity and nuclear atypism (Fig. 5–63); however, structural characteristics of Antoni types A and B are preserved. Mitoses are occasionally seen, but the prognosis for cellular schwannomas is the same as for all other benign solitary schwannomas.

The totipotential characteristics of the Schwann cell have been emphasized in triton tumors.[281–286] Peripheral nerve tumors can undergo metaplastic changes. The most common benign secondary elements seen in these tumors are cartilage and osteoid, whereas secondary malignant changes include foci of rhabdomyosarcoma, chondrosarcoma, osteogenic sarcoma, and liposarcoma (malignant triton tumors). Woodruff[282] described five nerve sheath tumors containing glands lined with columnar epithelium and mucicarminophilic material. The development of such foci within the substance of nerve sheath tumors is best explained by the multipotential ability of the Schwann cell.

Most investigators believe that encapsulated schwannomas are benign and do not undergo malig-

nant transformation. Only a few documented case reports are found in the literature.[287] We agree with Russell and Rubenstein[288] that documentation of malignant transformation of an apparently benign schwannoma is extremely difficult.

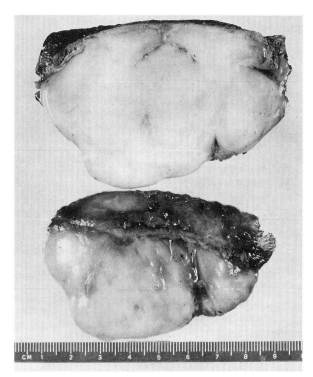

**A**

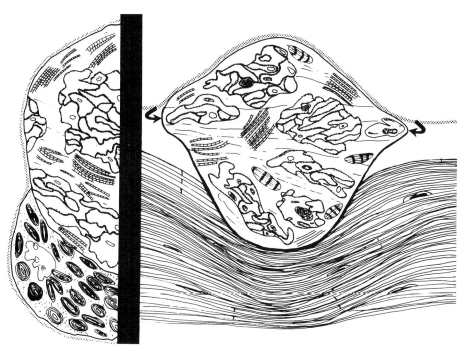

**B**

**Figure 5–61.** **(A)** Cut section of a benign schwannoma showing the glistening white surface. A capsule can easily be seen. *(Fig. 5–61A, 5–61C, and 5–61D Courtesy of Cancer 24:355, 1969)* **(B)** Diagrammatic rendition of a benign schwannoma compressing the adjacent nerve fiber as it increases in size. The tumor is encapsulated, and the main cellular components are neoplastic Schwann cells. The arrows show the plane through which these tumors should be enucleated. *(Modified from Weller and Cervos-Navarro, 1977.) (Continued.)*

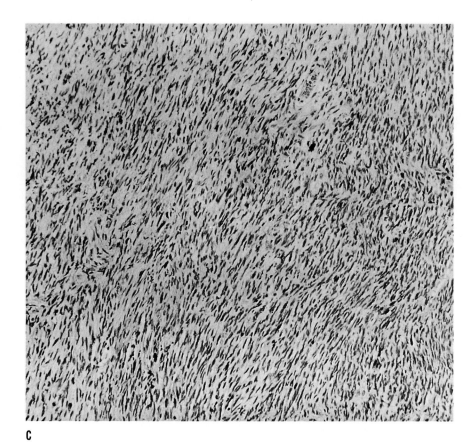

C

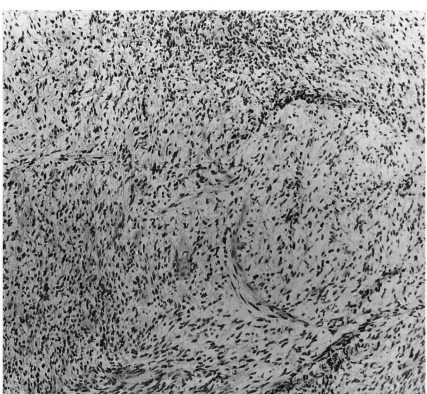

**Figure 5–61** *(continued).* **(C)** Benign schwannoma showing type A tissue of Antoni. Note compact arrangement of interwoven bipolar spindle cells. (H & E. Original magnification × 100.) **(D)** Type B is characterized by loose texture and polymorphism of tumor cells. (H & E. Original magnification × 100.) *(Continued.)*

D

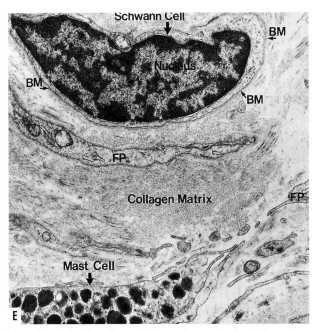

**Figure 5–61.** *(continued).* **(E)** Electron micrograph of a benign schwannoma. Note Schwann cell with its basement membrane *(BM)*, the interstitial collagen matrix, cytoplasmic process of a fibroblast *(FP)*, and a mast cell with its characteristic granules. (Original magnification × 21,300.)

A rare form of benign pigmented schwannian tumor (melanotic schwannoma) is rarely encountered. The tumors are usually laden with melanin pigment and are generally associated with sympathochromaffin axis (e.g., posterior mediastinum).

## Traumatic Neuroma

Traumatic neuroma, or amputation neuroma, is defined as a proliferative non-neoplastic mass found at the site of trauma to a peripheral nerve. It is caused by entrapment of a cluster of Schwann cells, axons, and fibroblasts in a collagenous matrix (Fig. 5–64).

## Type 1 von Recklinghausen's Neurofibromatosis

It is appropriate at this point to describe some salient pathologic features of type 1 von Recklinghausen's neurofibromatosis. Von Recklinghausen's type 1 neurofibromatosis is a hereditary disorder characterized by abnormal cutaneous pigmentations and multiple skin tumors. Frequently, patients with von Recklinghausen's neurofibromatosis have associated neural and epithelial tumors and several syndromes of the neuroendocrine axis. The subject has been extensively dealt with in our previous publications[289,290] and more recently by Friedman and Birch.[291]

Neurofibromatosis is generally considered to be a primary disorder of neural crest derivation, with secondary support from the mesenchymal elements. However, controversy remains as to whether the neural and mesenchymal components of this disease are interrelated or arise independently. Both pigmentary disturbances and neural tumors will be described in this section.

*Café-au-Lait Spots.*   The pigmentation associated with neurofibromatosis is macular and histologically consists of an abnormal deposition of melanin in the basal layers. The characteristic color of this pigmentation has led to the descriptive term of café-au-lait spots, which are essentially equal to large malpighian freckles with melanosis of the basal layers.

The pigmentation in neurofibromatosis is comparable to the pigmented spots in Albright's syndrome.[292]

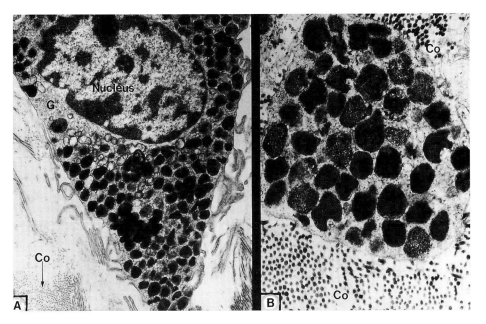

**Figure 5–62. (A)** Mast cell in a benign schwannoma (neurofibroma) from a patient with von Recklinghausen's neurofibromatosis. Cytoplasmic granules are mostly intact. (Original magnification × 14,732.) **(B)** Mast cell cytoplasm from a malignant schwannoma. Note granules in various stages of degranulation. (Original magnification × 46,699.)

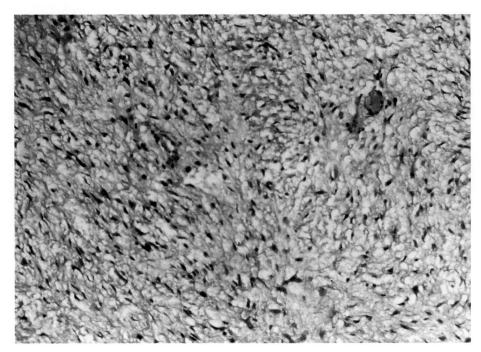

**Figure 5–63.** Cellular schwannoma in a 55-year-old woman. This tumor was initially thought to represent a malignant schwannoma. Careful scrutiny of all areas demonstrated the presence of Antoni A and B types of presentation. (H & E. Original magnification × 100.)

The salient cytologic feature of the pigmentary disturbance in neurofibromatosis is the presence of giant pigment granules in either malpighian cells or melanocytes; such granules are demonstrated in both café-au-lait spots and in normal skin.[275,293] They may vary in size, either filling the whole cell or ranging down to units just at the limit of resolution of the light microscope (0.5 μm). Frequently, they occur in melanocytes and can be seen in preparations not treated

with DOPA. The DOPA reaction, however, enhances their color. In the hyperpigmented lesions of neurofibromatosis, more melanin granules are present in the basal layer than in the surrounding nonpigmented skin. The presence of these giant granules is an important criterion for differentiating between café-au-lait spots occurring in neurofibromatosis, in Albright's syndrome, or in normal subjects.

The question that always perplexes the clinician and the pathologist is the significance of these café-au-lait spots. Although histologically these are hyperpigmented areas and characterize type 1 neurofibromatosis, unlike active junctional nevi, they do not generally change during the individual's lifetime. Giant pigmented nevi and bathing trunk nevi are associated with leptomeningeal melanocytosis in about 20 percent of the cases, and with melanoma in approximately 10 percent.[294] Although most cases of bathing trunk nevi are not associated with von Recklinghausen's neurofibromatosis, giant pigmented nevi do sometimes occur in this disease. Reed and associates[294] recognized the clinical and sometimes microscopic similarity to neurofibroma but considered giant pigmented nevi and neurofibromatosis to be separate and distinct entities. Their opinion is not universally shared.[289,295–298] Histologically, giant pigmented nevi often include several varieties, such as compound nevi, blue nevi, and spindle cell nevi. Brasfield and Das Gupta[289] found histologic characteristics ranging from neurofibroma to plexiform neuroma in the tissues underlying the giant bathing trunk nevi. Additionally, multiple hamartomatous areas of collagen, fat, and neural tissue are also

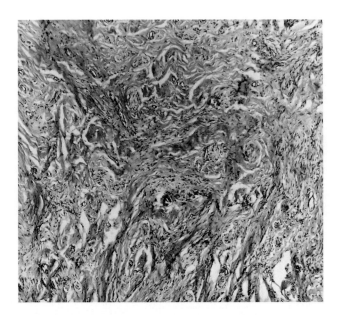

**Figure 5–64.** Micrograph of a traumatic neuroma. Thick axons are seen surrounded by dense fibrous tissue. (H & E. Original magnification × 63.)

one malignant lesion may occur in a patient with type 1 von Recklinghausen's neurofibromatosis.[289]

Involvement of the central nervous system is basic to von Recklinghausen's neurofibromatosis and often has been termed the central form (type 2) of the disease. A variety of neoplasms, including gliomas (glioblastomas, ependymomas, and oligodendrogliomas), meningiomas, and schwannomas can occur in the brain, spinal cord, and meninges.[289,290] Pack and Ariel[49] estimated the incidence of central nervous system involvement to be 5 percent. The two most commonly encountered intracranial anomalies are gliomas of the optic nerve and acoustic neuromas of the auditory nerve. A nerve growth-promoting factor has been isolated in patients with both the central and peripheral forms of the disease.[306,307]

## MALIGNANT TUMORS

### Maligant Peripheral Nerve Sheath Tumors

A malignant schwannoma is a tumor of nerve sheath origin. It infiltrates locally and also metastasizes. As with its benign counterpart, a large number of synonyms are found in the literature: malignant neuroma, malignant neurilemmoma, and neurogenic sarcoma, to name a few. However, there is sufficient justification to consider these tumors as arising from Schwann cells and they are termed either malignant schwannomas or malignant neurilemomas.[288,302,308] In order to avoid these differences in the nomenclature, the World Health Organization has changed the terminology of the lesions to malignant peripheral nerve sheath tumors (MPNST). Malignant peripheral nerve sheath tumors can be found either sporadically or in association with von Recklinghausen's neurofibromatosis.

Harkin and Reed[299] classified MPNSTs into the following four groups: (1) malignant schwannoma, (2) malignant epithelioid schwannoma, (3) nerve sheath fibrosarcoma, and (4) malignant melanocytic schwannoma. According to these authors, group 1 tumors were associated with plexiform neuroma. Groups 2 and 3 were found to be highly malignant. In view of their rarity, little is known about group 4. The histologic features of groups 1 and 3 frequently overlap, and assignment of a given tumor to one or the other category was sometimes arbitrary. Such classifications are of little clinical value. It appears, therefore, that once the histogenetic type of a given tumor has been properly arrived at as being of schwannian origin, a grading according to the degree of anaplasia would be of more clinical significance than such histologic subclassifications. The diagnosis of MPNST is sometimes difficult and elusive because it lacks standardized criteria.

### Solitary Malignant Peripheral Nerve Sheath Tumor or Malignant Schwannoma

Solitary MPNSTs develop in practically every anatomic region. To avoid confusion concerning the histogenesis of primary malignant tumors of the peripheral nerves, D'Agostino and co-workers[309,310] included only tumors that could be shown to arise from major peripheral nerves. This selection was rigorous and excluded a number of patients who might possibly have had malignant schwannomas. Not all MPNSTs arise in large, named, peripheral nerves. A number occur in smaller branches, and the relationship is often overlooked.

*Macroscopic Findings.*    Tumors arising from large peripheral nerves are usually fusiform and appear to be surrounded by a capsule (Fig. 5–67A to 5–67C). Although the nerve appears to enter and traverse the neoplasm, it is impossible to trace it in the tumor. The emergence is obvious in a large peripheral nerve, but, in the mediastinum or in smaller nerves, this feature is not discernible. The cut surface may have a faint-to-marked whorled pattern such as that of a uterine leiomyoma. Areas of cystic degeneration or hemorrhage appear in large tumors. The tumors frequently extend grossly for significant distances within a nerve. We have encountered patients in whom the primary tumor arose in the sciatic nerve in the pelvis and extended through the sciatic notch to the posterior thigh to form a palpable mass (Fig. 5–67A). D'Agostino et al.[310] described one patient in whom the tumor extended all through the median nerve.

*Microscopic Findings.*    Malignant schwannomas are composed of plump spindle cells (Fig. 5–68A to 5–68D). Mitoses are frequently found, and the nuclei are hyperchromatic and vary in size. The pattern of interlacing bundles of tightly packed cells is commonly seen. There is usually a marked uniformity of cell type, producing a monotonous microscopic pattern. Infiltration of the epineurium almost invariably occurs. Infiltration of the perineurium and extension along the fascicles is common enough that the clinician must take this fact into consideration before planning definitive primary therapy.

In addition, other histologic elements may be encountered within MPNSTs. These include squamous differentiation, foci of liposarcomatous areas, and islands of cartilage and bone. Nerve sheath fibrosarcomas are also frequently associated with von Recklinghausen's neurofibromatosis. The tumor cells are thought to be fibroblasts. The matrix may be mucinous, and, on purely morphologic grounds, a diagnosis of fibromyxoid sarcoma can be made. Frequently, such tumors are indistinguishable from common types of

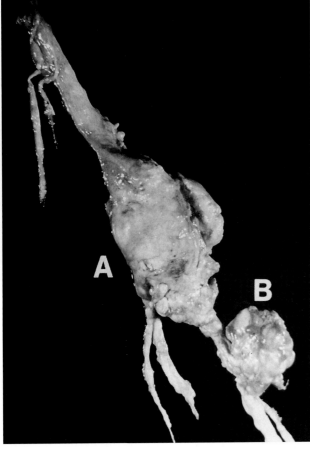

A

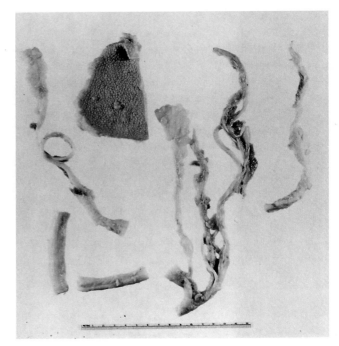

B

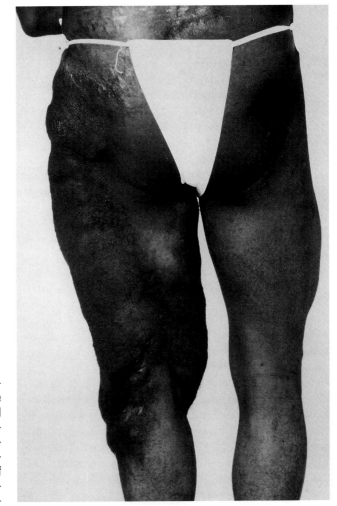

C

**Figure 5–66.** **(A)** Dissected sciatic nerve from a 28-year-old woman with malignant schwannoma arising in the lower part of the nerve, prior to division. The larger mass was malignant. Note smaller pedunculated plexiform neuroma and the beaded appearance of the lower branches. She was treated by a major amputation. *(Dissection of sciatic nerve performed by J. Wander, M.D.)* **(B)** A composite of an elephantoid skin with a small neurofibroma and dissected cutaneous nerves showing the beading characteristic of plexiform neurofibroma of type 1 neurofibromatosis. **(C)** Posterior view of hyperpigmentation and redundancy of skin overlying a plexiform neurofibroma of long duration in a 40-year-old man. *(Continued.)*

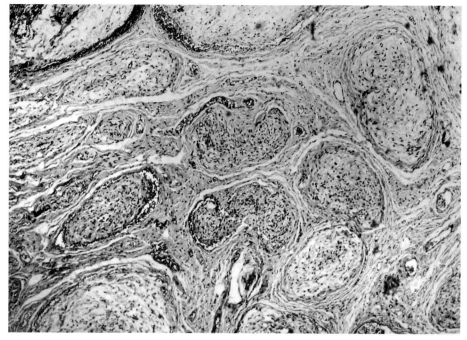

D

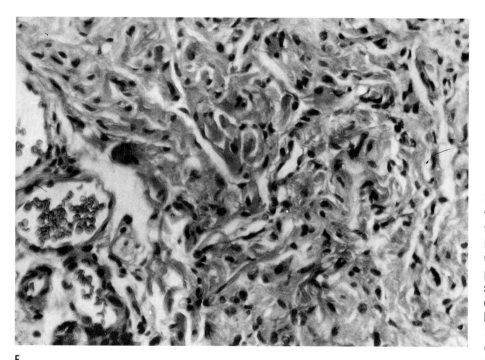

E

**Figure 5–66** *(continued).* **(D)** Low-power view of a plexiform neurofibroma showing the proliferating Schwann cells arranged in bundles separated by fibrous tissue. (H & E. Original magnification × 80.) **(E)** High-power view of sciatic nerve showing preserved myelinated fibers and plump spindle cells embedded in a fibrillary myxomatous background. (H & E. Original magnification × 250.) *(Fig. 5–66A and 5–66D, courtesy of* Current Problems in Surgery, *vol. 14, no. 2, 1977.)*

liposarcoma, even under an electron microscope. Immunohistochemical stains are positive for S-100, Leu-7, and myelin basic protein. Other antibodies against neuron-specific enolase and neurofilament proteins are also present in some cases.

Electron microscopic examination of MPNSTs, like the benign type, shows a large array of Schwann cells, fibroblasts, giant cells, macrophages, and mast cells (see Figs. 5–62A and 5–62B and 5–68D), but a general disorganization is evident. The Schwann cell cytoplasm is frequently in various stages of myelin production. The tumor giant cells and multiple nuclei are common features. Macrophages are seen with a variety of ingested material, probably disintegrated myelin.

The collagen matrix is scanty compared with that in the benign variety.

## Malignant Schwannoma or Malignant Peripheral Nerve Sheath Tumors Associated with von Recklinghausen's Neurofibromatosis

The general morphologic and histologic characteristics of these tumors are similar to those of solitary MPNSTs. The malignant neoplasm that develops along the course of a peripheral nerve is often well demarcated and fusiform. Some are lobulated, and those that extend through an intervertebral foramen assume an hourglass shape. The tumor usually infiltrates the surrounding tissues and the epineurium.

On close microscopic scrutiny, these tumors associated with von Recklinghausen's neurofibromatosis can be distinguished from their solitary counterparts. They consist predominantly of fusiform elements lightly packed in interlacing bundles, closely resembling fibrosarcomas (Fig. 5–69A). Coarse reticulin fibrils may extend in parallel rows among the spindle cells, but adjacent cells may be entwined by delicate fibrils, as in fibrosarcoma. Collagen fibers are usually scanty, and mitoses are common. Frequently, there are foci of pleomorphism, and mononuclear or multinuclear giant cells may be distributed sparingly or plentifully throughout the tumors. In highly anaplastic tumors, bipolar spindle cells and stellate cells are some-

times observed. Electron microscopic examination of these tumors shows that they are more pleomorphic than solitary MPNSTs, with still less interstitial collagen and fewer Schwann cells in varying degrees of maturation (Fig. 5–69B).

Nerve sheath fibrosarcomas are also frequently associated with neurofibromatosis. The tumor cells are

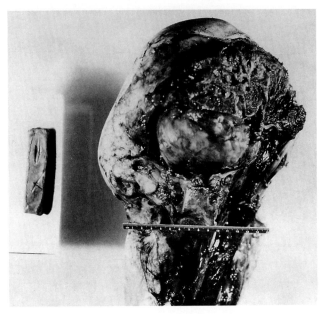

A

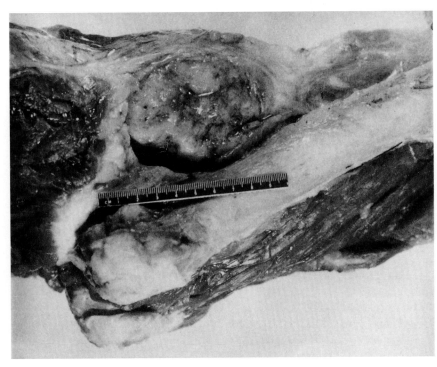

**Figure 5–67. (A)** Malignant schwannoma of the buttock. This tumor was first palpated and visible in the buttock, but actually a part of it was intrapelvic, extending through the sciatic notch and requiring a hemipelvectomy. **(B)** Cut surface of a malignant schwannoma infiltrating the muscle planes. *(Courtesy of Annals of Surgery 175:86, 1972.) (Continued.)*

B

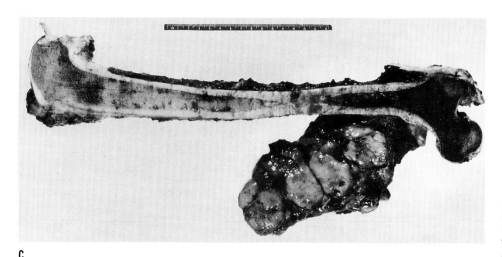

**C**

**Figure 5–67** *(continued).* **(C)** Malignant schwannoma adherent to the femur. The tumor infiltrated the linea aspera, necessitating a hip joint disarticulation.

thought to be fibroblasts. The matrix may be mucinous, and, on purely morphologic grounds, a diagnosis of fibromyxosarcoma can be forwarded. Frequently, such tumors are indistinguishable from common types of fibrosarcoma.

Malignant peripheral nerve sheath tumors can be differentiated into four categories: (1) malignant nerve sheath tumor with rhabdomyoblastic differentiation (malignant triton tumor); (2) malignant peripheral nerve sheath tumor with glandular differentiation; (3) epithelioid malignant peripheral nerve sheath tumor and epithelioid malignant schwannomas; and (4) superficial epithelioid malignant peripheral nerve sheath tumor.

### Malignant Peripheral Nerve Sheath Tumor with Rhabdomyoblastic Differentiation.

As the name implies, it shows both neural and skeletal muscle differentiation and includes neuromuscular hamartoma. This tumor is also called *malignant triton tumor.* These lesions are relatively rare and mostly associated with type 1 neurofibromatosis.[281,311] However, Enzinger and Weiss[312] reported triton lesions unassociated with neurofibromatosis and suggested that the low incidence of sporadic cases is from failure of recognition and diagnosis of such tumors outside the setting of neurofibromatosis. The diagnostic criteria for such lesions are presence of variable number of mature rhabdomyoblasts with eosinophilic cytoplasm in background of typical malignant peripheral nerve sheath tumor.

### Malignant Peripheral Nerve Sheath Tumor with Glandular Differentiation.

In 1892, Garre[313] reported a case of schwannoma with glandular elements. Almost all these patients have type 1 neurofibromatosis. Characteristi-

cally, they have a spindle cell background with muscle, bone, or cartilage in addition to the glands.[314,315] Microscopic appearance of this lesion may closely resemble biphasic synovial sarcoma. Immunohistochemical study helps differentiate because synovial sarcoma is usually keratin-positive with cells in the spindle zone that are rarely S-100-positive, whereas the glandular MPNSTs display focal S-100 protein positivity.

### Epithelioid Malignant Peripheral Nerve Sheath Tumor/Epithelioid Malignant Schwannoma.

In epithelioid MPNSTs, a true rosette is found among large cells with prominent nucleoli. These tumors are often mistaken for melanomas or carcinomas, and the only way to differentiate them is by staining for S-100 and melanin-associated antigens. Eighty percent of these tumors are positive for S-100 but negative for melanoma-associated antigen or keratin. Lodding et al.[316] described metastases to regional lymph nodes in these tumors.

### Superficial Epithelioid Malignant Peripheral Nerve Sheath Tumor.

As the name implies, superficial epithelioid MPNSTs occur in the superficial soft tissue, dermis, and subcutaneous tissue. These lesions are usually encapsulated and well circumscribed. Histologically, they are similar to epithelioid MPNSTs in deep tissues, and the malignant cells stain positive for S-100 protein. These tumors generally are associated with good prognosis.[312]

*Cytogenetic Findings.*   Similar to malignant fibrous histiocytoma, peripheral nerve sheath tumors also show complex chromosomal aberration in high-grade lesion and such chromosomal studies cannot be used for any diagnostic purpose.[317–319]

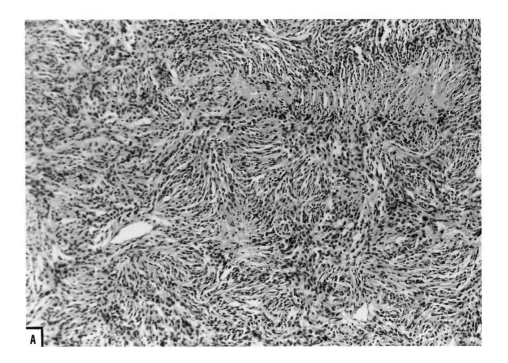

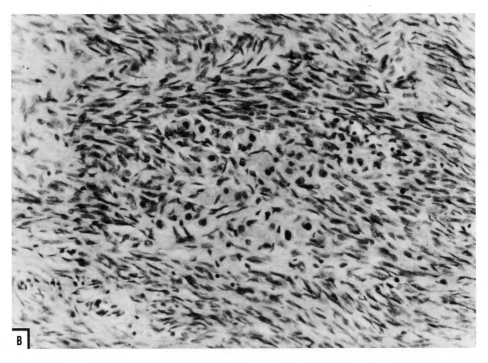

**Figure 5–68. (A)** Malignant schwannoma. The tumor cells are uniform and spindle-shaped, with less collagenous matrix. Multiple blood vessels are also seen. There appears to be a monotony of pattern. Although the tumor is malignant, an Antoni type A presentation still can be seen. (H & E. Original magnification × 63.) **(B)** An undifferentiated malignant schwannoma with multiple ganglionlike cells and a general disorganization. (H & E. Original magnification × 110.) *(Continued.)*

## Clear Cell Sarcoma or Malignant Melanoma of the Soft Parts

Clear cell sarcoma was first described by Enzinger in 1965 (Figs. 5–70A and 5–70B).[320] Its uniform and distinctive clinical and morphologic pattern distinguishes it from other groups of tenosynovial tumors.[163] Clear cell sarcomas are slow-growing and are commonly seen in association with tendons and aponeuroses around the knee and ankle joints.[163,320–326] According to Enzinger,[320] they have a predilection for young women. Because these tumors are intimately adjacent to the sur-

rounding tendons and aponeuroses, simple local excision usually leaves behind a residue of the tumor, with resultant local recurrence and metastasis.

The overall microstructure of these tumors sometimes resembles that of a synovial cell sarcoma (Fig. 5–70A). However, their lack of classic biphasic pattern, the overall rarity of the pseudogangliar cleft, and the presence of intracytoplasmic melanin[321–326] lead one to assume that these tumors are of neural crest origin (Fig. 5–70). The monotony of the microscopic appear-

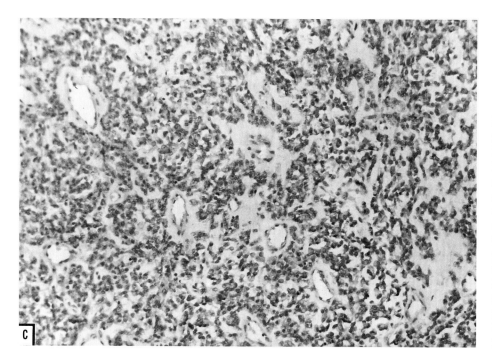

**Figure 5–68** *(continued)*. **(C)** Malignant schwannoma. The cells appear to be epithelioid in nature and are arranged haphazardly. Prominent blood vessels with thick walls are obvious. No area shows the characteristic Antoni A or B configuration. (H & E. Original magnification × 125.) The tumor was excised from the ulnar nerve of a 54-year-old man. **(D)** Electron micrograph from a patient with solitary malignant schwannoma. Profiles of two Schwann cells with basement membrane *(BM)* are easily recognizable. The cells are in a scanty collagenous matrix *(Co)*. A nerve terminal *(NT)* can be easily recognized. (Original magnification × 16,109.)

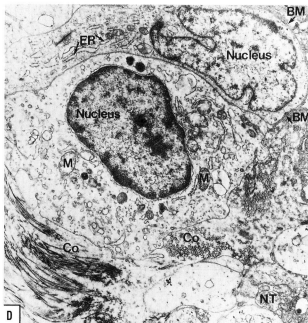

ance associated with the disappearance of PAS-positive material after diastase treatment also separates them from classic synovial sarcoma. Immunohistochemically, these cells are positive for HMB-45 and S-100. Neuron-specific enolase and Leu-7 have also been noted.

## GRANULAR CELL TUMORS

### Benign Tumors

In 1926, Abrikossoff[327] first described a group of tumors arising in the muscles of the tongue, lip, and leg. In view of the presence of granular cells and the close proximity of these tumors to the tongue muscula-

ture and other striated muscles, he assumed these tumors to be of myoblastic origin. With the description of more of these tumors, the proposed myoblastic histogenesis has now come under serious doubt.[189,284,328–331] Because of their frequent intimate relationship with (and occasional presence within) nerve bundles, the granular elements of the myoblastoma cells have been considered to be of neural derivation from Schwann cells or fibroblasts of peripheral nerve sheaths. Pearse,[330] on the basis of histochemical studies, suggested that these tumors are granular cell perineural fibroblastomas, within the cells of which a lipid-containing complex has accumulated. A Schwann cell origin has been suggested by several other authors,[5,329] and this concept has considerable validity. It does not, however, lessen the possibility that these granular cells have histiocytic capacities, since Schwann cells are facultative fibroblasts and can have phagocytic properties. From the available data, it appears prudent to classify granular cell tumors as peripheral nerve tumors.

Granular cell tumors appear as solitary, small nodules with well-defined but not sharply demarcated boundaries. The microstructure of these lesions is characterized by irregularly arranged strands, solid clumps, and nests of large, granular, round or polyhedral, faintly acidophilic cells with vesicular or densely chromatic nuclei (Fig. 5–71). The cluster of cells is surrounded by variable amounts of collagenous tissue or reticulin fibers interspersed with nerve fibers. Frequently, the granular cells are in close apposition to nerve bundles. The histochemistry of these cells may vary considerably from that of muscle cells.

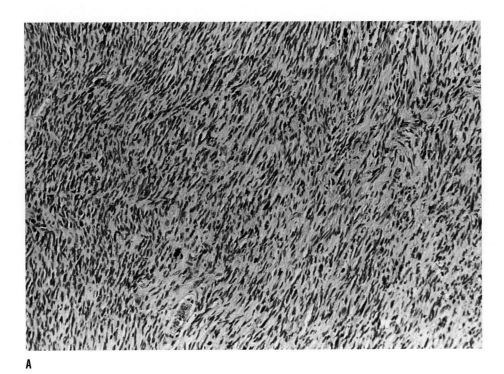

A

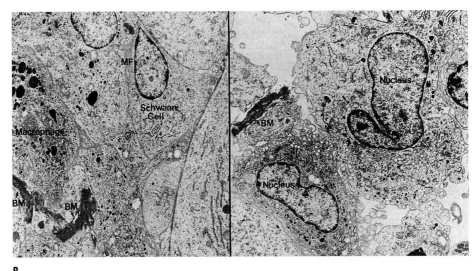

**Figure 5–69. (A)** Malignant schwannoma in type 1 neurofibromatosis. The individual cells and the overall architecture resemble a fibrosarcoma. (H & E. Original magnification × 250.) **(B)** A panoramic view of a malignant schwannoma associated with type 1 neurofibromatosis. Left, one macrophage with various cytoplasmic inclusions and fragmented basal membranes *(BM)* is prominent. However, in the upper right, a Schwann cell is in the process of infolding its membranes *(MF)*, the initial step in the process of myelination. (H & E. Original magnification × 8,185.) Right, various cells in relatively scanty stroma are present. The cell with a kidney-shaped nucleus is identifiable as a neoplastic Schwann cell. (H & E. Original magnification × 6,122.)

B

## Malignant Tumors

The malignant variant of granular cell tumor is rare.[332] The microscopic appearance of the tumor is quite similar to its benign counterpart; however, they are more cellular, and mitotic activity is higher. The final diagnosis is usually rendered based in biologic behavior.

### Tumors of Tissues Secondarily Involving Peripheral Nerves.

Metastases or direct invasion of the perineural spaces is seen in advanced cases of malignancy. In some patients, the direct extension to the adjoining nerve is the only evidence that the presenting tumor is malignant. The mechanism of paralysis in a peripheral nerve was exper-

imentally investigated by Kashef and Das Gupta.[333] These authors found that the primary pathologic change in the sciatic nerves of rats in the presence of Walker 256 carcinosarcoma was segmental demyelination, which appears in most clinical settings to be the initial cause of nerve deficit. However, in long-standing tumors, Wallerian degeneration is often found in the peripheral nerves distal to the tumors (Fig. 5–72A to 5–72C). In the carcinomatous neuromyopathy sometimes seen in patients with terminal cancer, a patchy loss of myelinated fibers has been observed. Croft and co-workers[334] alluded to an immune theory to explain this phenomenon of carcinomatous neuromyopathy in

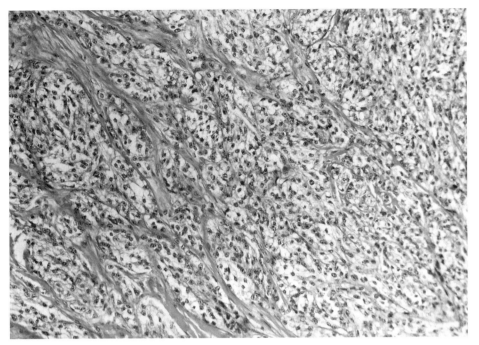

A

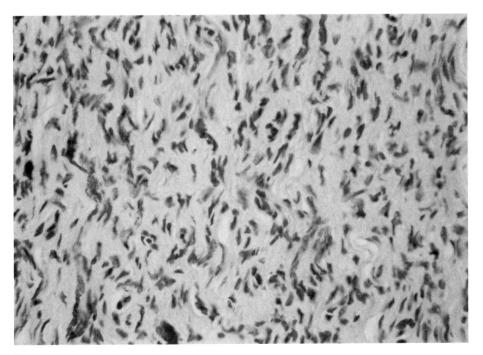

B

**Figure 5–70. (A)** Clear cell sarcoma of tendon sheath. The tumors are composed of clusters of uniform cuboid cells with clear or finely granular cytoplasm and well-delineated cell border. (H & E. Original magnification × 125.) **(B)** The intracytoplasmic melanin as shown in this photomicrograph leads one to conclude that these tumors are of neural crest origin, and the term *melanoma of the soft parts* has become more prevalent.

man. However, the mechanism of this neuromyopathy is still unclear.

*Macroscopic Findings.*   The fully developed lesion is characterized by a fusiform enlargement that bridges the defect in a severed nerve or by a bulbous expansion of the end of an amputated nerve. The nerve fibers disappear in a white, dense, fibrous scar.

*Microscopic Findings.*   In the active phase of growth, the proximal and distal nerve stumps are surrounded by a mucinous matrix that is continuous with the endoneurium and perineurium. In well-formed lesions, Schwann cell cords containing axons thicken, partition, and transform into compact bundles of nerve fascicles (Fig. 5–64). Perineurium condenses around each fascicle, and the adjacent tissue is converted to dense

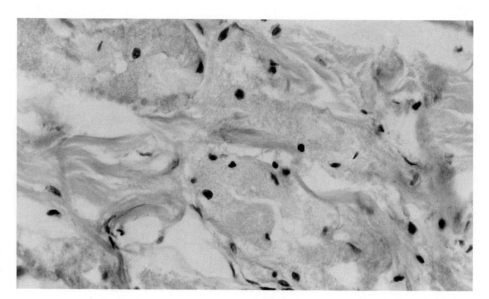

**Figure 5–71.** Granular cell myoblastoma. The cells are uniform, well defined, and granular, with pyknotic nuclei. (H & E. Original magnification × 250.)

fibrous tissue. In the late stage, the whole architecture consists of tangled axons in a dense collagenous matrix, and frequently only Schwann tubes are seen, with no recognizable axons.

## THE SYMPATHOCHROMAFFIN SYSTEM

In the peripheral nervous system, tumors of nerve cell origin occur predominantly in the region of the sympathetic trunk. Sympathogonia are stem cells not only of the sympathoblasts and sympathetic ganglion cells, but also of the chromaffin cells found in the chromaffin tissue dispersed throughout the human body. Thus, two types of tumors occur that correspond to the dichotomy in the development of sympathogonia: (1) sympathetic tumors arising from neuronal cell lines and (2) pheochromocytomas arising from chromaffin cells. Biochemical studies show that sympathetic tumors can synthesize and secrete catecholamines, a well known characteristic of pheochromocytomas. The amount of catecholamines stored in individual tumors, however, varies.[335] It appears that, despite diverse clinicopathologic features, strict sympathetic tumors and classical pheochromocytomas share a common ancestry and can be classified as tumors of the sympathochromaffin system. A brief description of the chromaffin system precedes the description of these tumors.

*Chromaffin system* is an arbitrary but convenient term that brings together various groups of cells which, like those in the adrenal medulla, contain cytoplasmic granules with an affinity for certain salts of chromic acid.[271] Such cells are described as chromaffin elements, or pheochromocytes. There is evidence that these cells are derived, in company with sympathetic neurons, from a common source in the neural crest,

and that the ultimate cell groups so derived preserve considerable topographical relationship with various components of the sympathetic moiety of the autonomic nervous system. Chromaffin cells in the adrenal medulla secrete adrenaline and noradrenaline and are innervated by preganglionic sympathetic fibers, but how far these features are true of chromaffin cells in other situations is not clear. In addition to the medulla of the adrenal gland, the chromaffin tissue includes (1) groups of cells known as paraganglia, (2) para-aortic bodies, and (3) small masses of chromaffin cells scattered irregularly and variably among the ganglia of the paravertebral sympathetic chains, splanchnic nerves, and the great (prevertebral) autonomic plexuses. Coupland[271] described the distribution of the chromaffin tissue in the newborn infant (Fig. 5–73).

The chromaffin cells of the adrenal medulla synthesize and secrete noradrenaline and adrenaline into venous sinusoids, the release being under preganglionic sympathetic control.[271] In several species of mammals, these substances have been identified in two distinct cell types, the noradrenaline-storing cells, which are usually situated more peripherally, and those that store adrenaline, which are centrally located.[336] Chromaffin cells are columnar and arranged in rows one cell thick along the margins of venous sinusoids. The cytoplasm of the chromaffin cell is basophilic and ultrastructurally shows a well-developed granular endoplasmic reticulum, mitochondria, and Golgi complex. Numerous secretory vesicles are also present. In noradrenaline-storing cells, the vesicles are typically rounded or ellipsoidal bodies that, after treatment with aldehyde and osmium, are highly electron-dense. In adrenaline-storing cells, after similar treatment the vesicles have a paler appearance, often with a clear zone

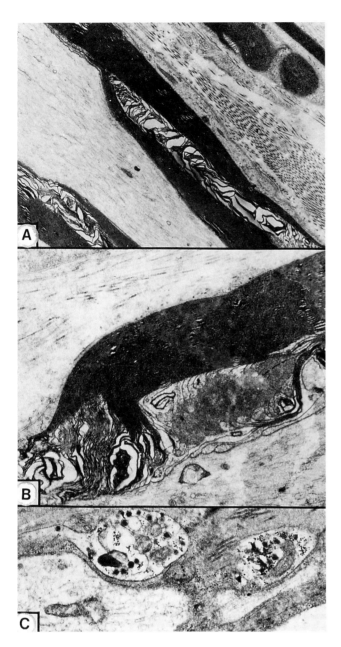

**Figure 5–72.** Sciatic nerve from a patient with a recurrent liposarcoma of the left iliac fossa infiltrating the lateral wall of the pelvis. Patient was treated by a hemipelvectomy. She remained well for 10 years and then moved to another state. Current status is not known. During her first visit to the University of Illinois Hospital, a sciatic nerve deficit was noted. These electron micrographs were taken from the distal sciatic nerve about 5 cm beyond the gross tumor. **(A)** Initiation of segmental changes in the Schmidt-Lanterman incisures at the node of Ranvier. (Original magnification × 19,735.) **(B)** The process of segmental demyelination is apparent. (Original magnification × 34,720.) **(C)** Early phase of Wallerian degeneration can also be seen. (H & E. Original magnification × 34,720.)

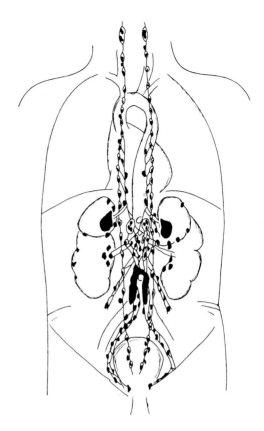

**Figure 5–73.** Diagram of the distribution of chromaffin tissue in the newborn infant. *(Modified from Coupland RE:* The Natural History of the Chromaffin Cell, *1965.)*

between the granular contents and the binding membrane.[336] In human adrenal cells, both types of vesicles have been found, presuming that both may be secreted from the same cell.[337] Chromaffin cells of the adrenal medulla develop and migrate from the neural crests (sympathochromaffin tissue). The chromaffin reaction in the cell is positive in the fifth month of fetal life, but adrenaline is present as early as the third month.[271]

### Paraganglia

Paraganglia are spherical masses of chromaffin cells about 2 mm in diameter, each lying inside or embedded in the capsule of a ganglion of the sympathetic trunk. In the adult, they are generally represented by microscopic remnants only.

### The Para-aortic Bodies (Organs of Zückerkandl)

The para-aortic bodies progressively develop during fetal life and attain their maximum size in the first three years of postnatal life, by which time the largest ones take the form of 1-cm elongated bodies lying on each side of the abdominal aorta in the region of origin of the inferior mesenteric artery. They are usually united across the aorta in the form of an H. The constituent cells undergo dispersal and atrophy and, by age 14, are usually disintegrated.[271] They consist of masses of polygonal chromaffin cells secreting noradrenaline. Other small collections of chromaffin cells are found in fetuses, but these usually regress with age, and only microscopic evidence remains in adults. The function of these chromaffin nests remains unclear.

## Carotid Bodies

The two carotid bodies are reddish-brown ellipsoidal structures situated on each side of the neck in close relation to the carotid sinus. They are about 5 to 7 mm in length and 2.5 to 4 mm in width and vary slightly in position, either posterior to the bifurcation of the common carotid artery or wedged between the commencements of the internal and external carotid arteries. They are attached to, and sometimes partially embedded in, the adventitial layer of these arteries.

The carotid body first appears as a condensation of the mesenchyme around the third pharyngeal arch artery. Its initial nerve supply is mainly from the glossopharyngeal nerve to the third arch. Other similar small bodies are found near the arteries of the fourth and sixth pharyngeal arches; thus, they are close to the arch of the aorta, the ductus arteriosus, and the right subclavian arteries, and are supplied by the superior cervical ganglion and the vagus nerve.

A strong fibrous capsule invests the carotid body, and septa from this capsule pass into the organ and divide it into lobules. Each lobule consists of masses of large polyhedral epithelioid cells (glomus cells or chief cells) and supporting cells, among which are interspersed networks of sinusoidal blood vessels.[338] Each glomus cell contains a large, pale-staining nucleus and a pale, finely granular cytoplasm. The main nerve supply of the carotid body is the carotid branches of the glossopharyngeal nerve, the branches from the superior cervical ganglion, and the vagus nerve. The organ itself is richly innervated by myelinated and nonmyelinated axons. The nonmyelinated nerve endings can form groups. One group terminates in close contact with sinusoid synaptic end bulbs containing 50-nm cholinergic-type clear vesicles associated with the surfaces of glomus cells.[338] Stimulation of the glomus cells alters the chemoreceptor activity in the carotid body.

Electron microscopy of a normal carotid body shows that the glomus cell cytoplasm is characterized by the presence of abundant membrane-limited, osmiophilic granules with generally rounded profiles. These granules range from 100 to 150 nm in outer diameter. Some are separated by a clear zone.

## Tympanic Body (Glomus Jugulare)

The tympanic body is a small ovoid body about 0.5 mm long and 0.25 mm wide located in the adventitia of the upper part of the superior bulb of the internal jugular vein. Its structure is similar to that of the carotid body. It may consist of two or more masses related to the tympanic branch of the glossopharyngeal nerve or the auricular branch of the vagus, as these nerves lie in their canals in the petrous part of the temporal bone.

## Coccygeal Body (Glomus Coccygeum)

The coccygeal body is about 2.5 mm long. It is located anterior or immediately inferior to the apex of the coccyx at the termination of the median sacral vessels that supply afferent and efferent branches to the organ, and is closely related to the ganglion impar of the sympathetic trunk.

## TUMORS OF THE SYMPATHOCHROMAFFIN SYSTEM

The tumors of the sympathochromaffin system can be classified as benign or malignant (see Table 2–1, Chapter 2). The benign tumors are (1) ganglioneuromas, (2) pheochromocytomas, (3) carotid body tumors, and (4) nonchromaffin paragangliomas. The malignant tumors are (1) malignant ganglioneuromas, (2) neuroblastomas, (3) malignant pheochromocytomas, (4) malignant carotid body tumors, and (5) malignant nonchromaffin paragangliomas.

### Benign Tumors

*Ganglioneuroma.*   A comparatively rare benign tumor in which ganglion cells, neurofibrils, and neurilemma cells occur in varying proportions, ganglioneuromas are well known for their ability to mature and become quiescent. In order of decreasing frequency, these tumors are found in the posterior mediastinum, lumbar region, adrenal medulla, and neck.[339–342] Infrequently, they have been found in other locations.[343] Since there is little evidence that mature ganglion cells multiply, it is presumed that during formation a ganglioneuroma is composed of immature neuroblasts. Thus, in a rapidly growing tumor, even if the biopsy specimen suggests a mature ganglioneuroma, a diagnosis of benign tumor should seldom be made.

*Macroscopic Findings.*   A ganglioneuroma is a firm, well-demarcated, usually encapsulated tumor, occasionally of large dimensions. The cut surface is grayish-white and often resembles leiomyosarcoma. Although some of these tumors, notably the mediastinal, attain a large size and extend into the surrounding tissue, infiltrative activity has not been reported.

*Microscopic Findings.*   Mature ganglion cells are characteristic of these tumors. Ganglion cells may occur singly or in clusters and are scattered haphazardly throughout the tumor tissue (Fig. 5–74). Occasionally, a ganglioneuroma structurally resembles a normal ganglion. There is an abundant dense stroma, which may contain stainable neurofibrils and collagen fibers, but the stromal pattern may vary considerably, and arrangements reminiscent of neurofibromas may be seen. In some instances, there is evidence of calcification of individual cells or groups of ganglion cells.

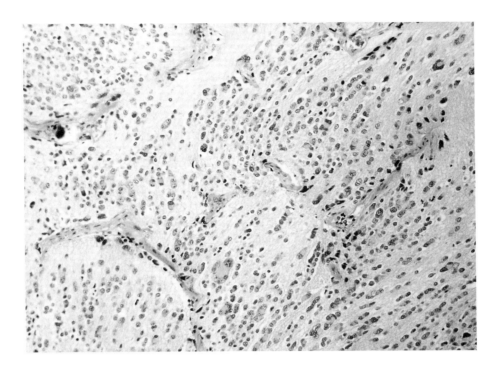

**Figure 5–74.** Ganglioneuroma showing the characteristic fibrillary tissue and ganglion cells. (H & E. Original magnification × 125.)

*Electron Microscopy.* The tumor cells have large nuclei with prominent nucleoli measuring up to 2 μm in diameter. There is abundant cytoplasm, which contains a complex arrangement of various organelles and inclusions. Mitochondria are present in large numbers and are sometimes irregularly shaped. Some are enormous, with short cristae. Both rough and smooth endoplasmic reticula, with a well-developed Golgi complex, is frequently seen.[335]

Numerous granules of different shapes and sizes are present in the cytoplasm. The small membrane-bound granules are uniform in size and shape, are about 100 nm in diameter, and resemble catecholamine granules. They are distributed throughout the perinuclear region and are frequently associated with the Golgi complex. The larger osmiophilic granules are ovoid, with diameters ranging from 250 to several hundred nanometers. Both types of granules are intermingled and frequently coalesce to form larger masses. Multivesicular bodies up to 300 nm are also seen in the cytoplasm of tumor cells.

Much of the space between tumor cells is filled with bundles of cell processes of varying length, some of which are surrounded by Schwann cells. Although multiple myelinated and nonmyelinated axons are seen, typical synapses have not yet been described.[344] Interspersed between these cell processes, collagen fibers and other cells such as fibrocytes or fibroblasts are occasionally observed.

**Pheochromocytoma.** Pheochromocytomas arise in the adrenal glands in approximately 90 percent of patients,

but they can arise wherever sympathochromaffin tissue is found (Fig. 5–73).

*Macroscopic Findings.* Some pheochromocytomas are small, spherical or ovoid masses, usually 1 to 2 cm in diameter but sometimes larger. Size and function, however, are not directly related, since small tumors may be pharmacologically as active as large ones. The larger pheochromocytomas are well demarcated, smooth, and lobulated. The cut surface is brownish-gray, and areas of local hemorrhage are common. In smaller lesions, unless a well-formed capsule separates the tumor, it is difficult to distinguish an area of local hyperplasia of the adrenal medulla from a tumor.

*Microscopic Findings.* The microscopic features of pheochromocytomas correspond well to those of normal adrenal medulla. Frequently, medullary hyperplasia so resembles a pheochromocytoma that distinction between them becomes impossible. Most tumors consist of delicate, richly vascular connective tissue that supports large or small solid alveoli, whorls, cords, or sheets of tumor cells (Fig. 5–75). The cells of a pheochromocytoma are intimately related to thin-walled blood vessels and sinusoids, often lined by tumor cells. The tumor cells are usually larger than normal medullary cells (20 to 30 μm), conspicuously granular, and sometimes vacuolated or foamy. The nucleus is eccentrically placed, hyperchromatic, and often large. This nuclear pleomorphism is a distinguishing feature. These cells stain dark with bichromate salts or chromic acid.

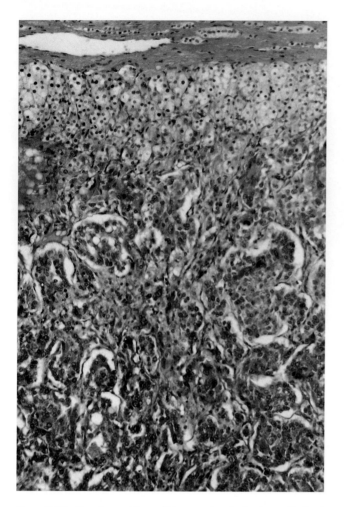

**Figure 5–75.** Pheochromocytoma. This was a functioning tumor. Nests of tumor cells are easily identifiable. (H & E. Original magnification × 125.)

*Electron Microscopy.* The tumor cells resemble adrenal medullary cells. In most areas, the plasma membranes are in close apposition, and the cells are clustered into sheets and nests; however, in some areas, the cells are separated by a rich, collagenous, interstitial tissue. The cytoplasm of the tumor cells contains numerous mitochondria and both smooth and granular endoplasmic reticulum. The characteristic feature, however, is the presence of osmiophilic dense-cored vesicles, which are the site of localization of catecholamines and have been studied extensively.[335]

**Carotid Body Tumors.** Tumors of the carotid body are rare. Most are solitary, usually oval, superficially lobulated, and seldom exceed a few centimeters in diameter. They are resilient and occasionally hard and fibrous, but ordinarily they vary from rubbery to soft; they often adhere firmly to the carotid bifurcation.

*Microscopic Findings.* Essentially, the tumor consists of a complex framework of blood vessels between which

there is a richly cellular, predominantly epithelioid parenchyma. The tumor cells are aggregated in small solid nests, columns, and strands, in close relation to the delicate sinusoids and numerous capillary channels (Fig. 5–76). Frequently, the organoid pattern is repeated and the alveolar pattern is sharply outlined in sections stained for reticulin. The individual tumor cells retain the cytologic features common to normal pheochromocytes.

*Electron Microscopy.* Electron microscopy of carotid body tumors shows that the tumor consists of polygonal cells. The nuclei are generally spherical or oval and occupy either a central or peripheral position. The cytoplasm is rich with mitochondria and both smooth and rough-surfaced endoplasmic reticulum. The cytoplasmic granules usually are of two sizes. The smaller membrane-bound granules are about 0.1 μm and spherical and consist of a central electron-dense core that is separated by a clear zone from the enveloping membrane. The larger variety morphologically is similar to the smaller one, except for the size (0.4 to 0.5 μm). The interstitium of carotid body tumors consists of the usual collagen material, and occasionally some nerve fibers.

**Nonchromaffin Paraganglioma (Glomus Jugulare Tumor).** Nonchromaffin paragangliomas are slow-growing tumors, which are histologically similar to carotid body tumors and usually found either in the glomus jugulare or in the retroperitoneal space. Because of their position behind the tympanic membrane or in the external auditory meatus, glomus jugulare tumors are frequently covered by squamous epithelium. Histologically, these tumors are indistinguishable from carotid body tumors.

**Malignant Tumors**

**Malignant Ganglioneuroma (Ganglioneuroblastoma).** Malignant ganglioneuroma probably represents an intermediate degree of differentiation in the gamut of tumors designated as neuroblastoma, malignant ganglioneuroma, or ganglioneuroblastoma.[345] Some authors have used these terms interchangeably. Operationally, tumors resembling neuroblastoma, with moderate differentiation of the cellular elements located outside the retroperitoneum, may be designated as *malignant ganglioneuromas.* The neck is a common site.[346–348] Malignant ganglioneuroma arising in the vagus nerve has also been described.[349]

These tumors are usually ovoid and fleshy. They are indistinguishable from neuroblastoma on light microscopic examination. The tumor cells, which are small and rounded, show varying degrees of pleomorphism. However, ganglion cells are seen interspersed within a rough collagen matrix. Electron microscopy

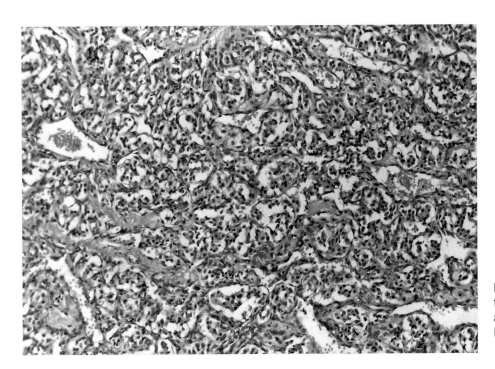

**Figure 5–76.** Carotid body tumor. The tumor cells are arranged in alveolar fashion around vascular channels lined by endothelial cells. (H & E. Original magnification × 125.)

reveals that these tumor cells resemble the cells in pheochromocytoma, with large nuclei and prominent nucleoli. The cytoplasm contains secretory granules containing catecholamines. The interstitium is usually cluttered with unmyelinated axons of varying size and is either partially or completely surrounded by Schwann cell cytoplasm.

**Neuroblastoma.**   Neuroblastoma, although rare, is one of the most common forms of childhood malignancies. This tumor has been observed in fetuses, newborns, and in infants only a few weeks old.[44,350–353] Infrequently, it occurs in adolescents or adults.[345,354] It has also been observed in association with some congenital anomalies[350,355] and von Recklinghausen's neurofibromatosis.[189,356,357]

*Macroscopic Findings.*   Neuroblastomas grow as large, rounded or lobulated, demarcated, soft, vascular, reddish-gray to yellow masses of solid but easily fragmented tissues. Occasionally, they are bilateral and, when they arise near the spine, have a dumbbell appearance. Frequently, there is local infiltration. Necrosis, hemorrhage, and cyst formation within the substance are common.

*Microscopic Findings.*   Neuroblastomas are composed of small, round, or slightly elongated cells with oval hyperchromatic nuclei (Fig. 5–77A and 5–77B). Cellular pleomorphism is a characteristic feature of neuroblastoma. Frequently, areas of totally undifferentiated cells (sympathogonia) and mature ganglion cells are observed in the same tumor. In areas of undifferenti-

ated tumor cells, distinction between a neuroblastoma and an anaplastic lymphosarcoma can be difficult. A distinguishing feature of neuroblastoma, however, is that the lymphocytelike cells are characteristically arranged in a rosette formation. In more differentiated tumors (ganglioblastomas, sympathicoblastomas), the cells have more cytoplasm, and the short processes of the unipolar or bipolar tumor cells can be demonstrated by silver impregnation techniques.

*Immunohistochemistry.*   Immunohistochemically, these tumors do not show glial fibrillary acidic protein, while they do show neuron-specific enolase. The presence of Leu-7, S-100, synaptophysin, neurofilament protein, and chromogranin varies from tumor to tumor, as does the presence of desmin.

*Electron Microscopy.*   There is a remarkable similarity in the fine structure of neuroblastoma and malignant ganglioneuroma.[335,358] Three major ultrastructural types (A, B, and C) can be distinguished in neuroblastoma. In undifferentiated tumors, type A predominates, whereas in most of the common varieties, all three types are encountered in the same tumor.

In type A, the tumor cells are loosely attached to one another, and the cell surfaces are relatively smooth, with fine undulating surfaces devoid of interdigitations; a few desmosomes, however, are apparent. The nuclei are round, elliptical, or polygonal, have a rim of cytoplasm around the nucleus, and contain a few organelles.

In type B areas, the tumor cells are separated by numerous islands of cytoplasm that are actually tangen-

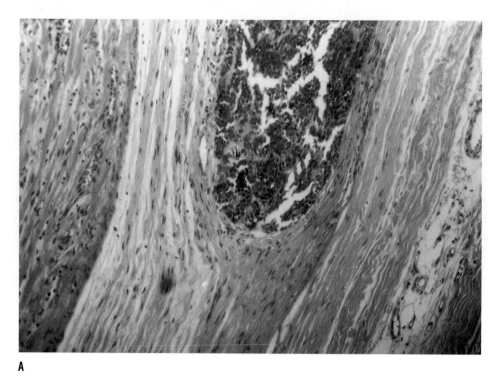

A

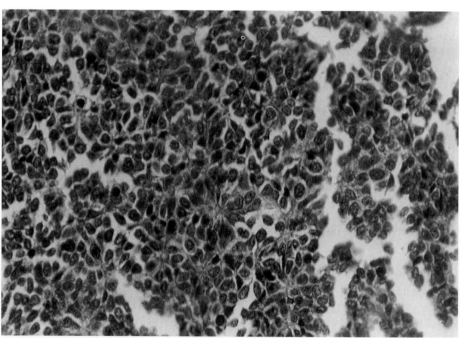

**Figure 5–77. (A)** Neuroblastoma arising in the peroneal nerve of a 25-year-old man. Note the localized area of the tumor along the course of the nerve. (H & E. Original magnification × 65.) **(B)** High-power view of the same tumor showing the classical rosette formation. (H & E. Original magnification × 300.)

B

tial sections of cytoplasmic processes. Occasionally, several cells are arranged in a rosettelike fashion. The nuclei in type B cells are smaller, with a larger cytoplasmic rim containing well-developed endoplasmic reticulum and organelles. In contrast to type A, there are myriad cytoplasmic processes and invagination.

The cells of type C areas have polymorphic nuclei with prominent nucleoli. There is more cytoplasm associated with these cells than with types A and B. The

cytoplasm is characterized by the presence of dense-cored vesicles ranging from 100 to 400 nm in diameter. Numerous unmyelinated axons are also seen in type C areas.

The tumor cells and the cytoplasmic processes in neuroblastoma lack a basement membrane, even where their cell surfaces border a perivascular space. Amorphous homogenous material containing scanty collagen fibers and large numbers of microfibrils fills the intercellular spaces; microfibrillary bundles with characteristic periodic striation are also seen.[335]

Neuroblastoma has the highest rate of spontaneous regression of any solid tumor.[335,339] It is characterized by a spectrum of varying degrees of maturation of the tumor cells. At one end of the spectrum is a highly undifferentiated small cell (type A) and at the other end are ganglioneuromas composed solely of mature cell types. Therefore, the histopathologist is responsible for correlating morphologic features with the biologic behavior of these tumors. In 1968, Beckwith and Martin[360] proposed such a correlation. Their work has since been corroborated by McKinen[361] and by Hughes and co-workers.[362] In contrast, Lauder and Aherne[363] suggested that the prognosis was not related to maturation, but to the degree of lymphocytic infiltration within the tumor.

Histologic grading has been based on the proportional presence of differentiated versus undifferentiated cells. Beckwith and Martin[360] proposed a quantitative classification, whereas McKinen[361] and Hughes and co-workers[362] proposed a simple histologic grading. These methods seem to lead to similar conclusions. The histologic grading proposed by Hughes and co-workers, being more practical, is described in this section.

The tumors can be classified as follows: Grade 1 tumors show a mixed pattern of undifferentiated cells and mature ganglion cells. Grade 2 tumors show a mixed pattern of undifferentiated cells, and some cells show evidence of partial differentiation toward ganglion cells, as indicated by any of the following: (1) vesicular nuclei, (2) the presence of nucleoli, (3) increased cytoplasmic nuclear ratio, (4) formation of the cytoplasmic process. Grade 3 tumors are totally undifferentiated.

Most authors[189,360,361,364,365] have found that the survival rate is excellent with grade 1 and poor with grade 3. Hughes et al.[362] reported only three-year crude survival and found that, of 13 patients with grade 1, 9 (69 percent) survived; of 22 with grade 2, only 2 (9.1 percent) survived; and out of 48 with grade 3, only 3 (6.2 percent) survived. In Beckwith and Martin's[360] series, the patients were classified in finer detail and quantitatively. The five-year survival rate was as follows: with grade 1, 5 out of 5 patients (100 percent); with grade 2, 3 out of 4 (75 percent); with grade 3, 4 of 13 (30 percent); and finally, with grade 4, only 1 of 28 (3 percent).

Most of these tumors in children younger than two years of age are either grade 1 or 2. In older children, the tumors are more undifferentiated and carry an unfavorable prognosis.[363,366,367]

### Malignant Pheochromocytoma.   Malignant pheochromocytomas are so rare that their very existence is ques-

tioned.[368,369] In general, if a pheochromocytoma proves fatal, it is attributable to the action of pressor amines. Although, in some tumors, the microscopic characteristics of hyperchromatic nuclei, giant cells, immature cells, and many mitoses are occasionally seen, there is no evidence that these features indicate a clinically malignant neoplasm. The presence of distant metastases, the tissues of which are chromaffin-positive in locations where chromaffin tissue ordinarily does not occur, is the only proof of a malignant pheochromocytoma.[370]

### Malignant Carotid Body Tumors.   Malignant carotid body tumors are rare.[371] The microscopic criteria generally used to distinguish between a benign and malignant tumor are not reliable. Occasionally, local infiltration might be considered as a sign of low-grade malignancy. If strict criteria for both microscopic and clinical behavior of a malignancy are applied, most reported malignant carotid body tumors will be found to be benign.

### Malignant Nonchromaffin Paraganglioma.   The histogenesis of malignant nonchromaffin paragangliomas is still unclear. Some authors believe that they histologically resemble alveolar soft part sarcoma and should be so classified (see section later in chapter).

Another unusual tumor that is now considered to be a derivative of primitive neuroectodermal tissue is extraskeletal Ewing's sarcoma. From a clinical standpoint, in adults these tumors behave like extraskeletal osteosarcomas or chondrosarcomas. However, because of its ontogeny, this tumor is described in this section.

### Extraskeletal Ewing's Sarcoma.   In 1975, Angervall and Enzinger[372] described the clinicopathologic features of an uncommon extraskeletal neoplasm resembling Ewing's sarcoma of the bone (Fig. 5–78A and 5–78B). These tumors occur mainly in young adults[372,373] and are aggressive. Microscopically, they consist of solidly packed small, round or ovoid, uniform cells arranged in sheets of lobules separated by strands of fibrous connective tissue. The nucleus of the tumor cells contains a finely divided chromatin, a distinct nuclear membrane, and frequently a minute nucleolus. The scanty, ill-defined cytoplasm contains varying amounts of glycogen. Sometimes, the histologic picture is dominated by a "peritheliomatous" pattern, or by large areas of necrosis or hemorrhage. The lungs and the skeleton are the two most common sites of metastases.[372]

## ■ TUMORS AND TUMORLIKE CONDITIONS OF SYNOVIAL TISSUE

Synovial membrane is a derivative of the embryonic mesenchyme lining the nonarticular parts of the syno-

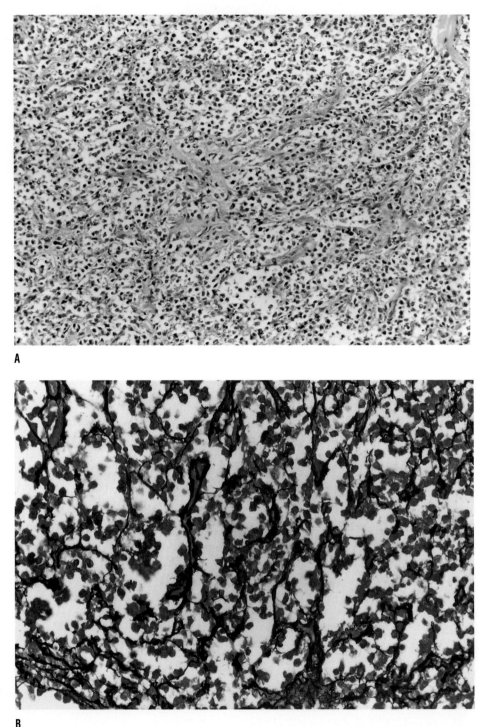

**Figure 5–78. (A)** Monomorphic, predominantly round cells are arranged in sheets in a rich vascular stroma. (H & E. Original magnification × 125.) **(B)** Reticulin stain showing the spatial arrangement of the tumor cells. (Original magnification × 125.)

vial joints, the synovial bursae, and the synovial tendon sheaths.[182,374]

In the human embryo at five weeks, the skeletal blastema of each limb is a continuous unsegmented core of condensed mesenchyme. In this core, the prechondral and, later, cartilaginous centers of individual bones differentiate and extend. As they approach each other, parts of the undifferentiated blastema are left between them. These are the interchondral discs, the rudiments of the future joints. From these discs develop all the joint tissues, including the synovial membrane. Where the synovial and cartilaginous tissues are continuous, distinction is indefinite between the two, and between them and the neighboring tissues. The close histogenetic kinship of fibrous, osseous, cartilaginous, and synovial tissue is nowhere better displayed than in these junctional tissues of joints. Here, the normal histologic features might show many metaplastic changes of mesenchymal tissues.

In postnatal life, the synovial tissue is a pink, smooth, moist, shiny membrane, lining the nonarticular parts of the synovial joints, bursae, and tendon sheaths. Although the free surfaces are formed by cells, they are not aligned in a continuous layer. Rather, they are intermittently arranged and embedded in surrounding collagenous tissue. This provides the nidus for synovial cells away from the actual joint cavity.[182,374] The inner surface of the synovial membrane is occasionally lined with synovial villi; elsewhere, the membrane is thrown into numerous folds projecting into the joint cavity. An accumulation of adipose tissue is characteristic of synovial membrane.

Structurally, synovial membrane varies considerably in different regions, but essentially it consists of a cellular intima resting upon a vascular connective tissue, the subintima (subsynovial tissue). The subintima is loose and areolar but often contains organized laminae of collagen and elastin fibers running parallel to the membrane surface, between which are scattered fibroblasts, macrophages, lipoblasts, and mast cells, frequently contributing to confusion in the diagnosis of these tumors. The subintimal adipose cells that accumulate as fat pads are arranged in compact lobules surrounded by fibroelastic interlobular septa. In contrast, where the synovial membrane lines intrinsic ligaments or intercapsular tendons, the subintima is difficult to distinguish as a separate zone, since it is formed of fibrous tissue that merges with that of the adjacent capsule or tendon.

A synovioblast is the stem cell for all types of synovial cells. Ultrastructurally, two cells types, A and B, have been recognized,[375] but cells with intermediate characteristics are common, and perhaps the differences described merely reflect stages of functional activity rather than distinct cell lineages (Fig. 5–79).

Type A synovial cells predominate and are characterized by surface filopodia, plasma membrane invaginations, and associated micropinocytotic vesicles. Their cytoplasm contains numerous mitochondria, varieties of lysosomes, a system of cytoplasmic filaments, a particularly prominent Golgi apparatus, and associated smooth-walled vesicles, but profiles of endoplasmic reticulum are scanty. Neighboring cells are separated by distinct gaps, but where they approach closely, their surfaces may be complex and interdigitated. Synovial type A cells are the sites of hyaluronate synthesis.[374] In type B synovial cells, most of the above characteristics are poorly developed; however, they contain a wealth of rough endoplasmic reticulum, varying from small, round or oval profiles to a large, flattened, intercommunicating cisternae, together with scattered free cytoplasmic ribosomes. Both cell types contain glycogen deposits, but lipid inclusions are rare, as are perinuclear centrioles.

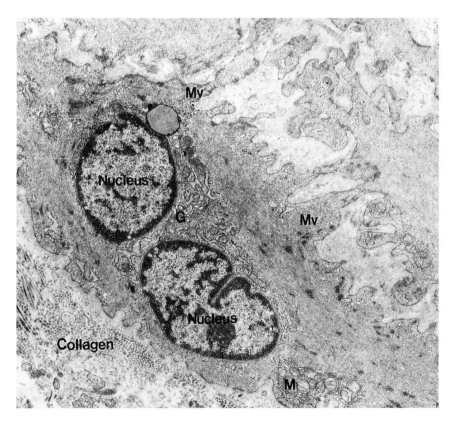

**Figure 5–79.** Electron micrograph of a human synovial membrane showing the predominant cell types. Type A cytoplasm contains occasional inclusion bodies, mitochondria *(M)*. The cytoplasm is uniquely devoid of rough-surfaced endoplasmic reticulum. Type B cell cytoplasm is characterized by relative abundance of rough-surfaced endoplasmic reticulum. In this micrograph, subsynovial tissue is not seen. *Mv*, microvilli; *G*, Golgi zone. (Original magnification × 22,800.)

The tumors and tumorlike conditions are distinctive growths that reproduce many of the histologic and cytologic features of normal synovial tissue. These features include the coexistence of pleomorphic synovial cells and fibroblastic tissue, indications of the persistence of developmental clefts and crypts, the formation of spaces and papillary processes lined by synovial cells, and the presence of mucopolysaccharides and extracellular mucin. However, a number of authors[163,376–379] believe that the term implies only that neoplastic mesenchymal cells have reached a characteristic pattern of differentiation resembling the morphology of synovial membrane.

Although most benign growths of the synovial tissue are structurally characteristic and simple in form, the existence of a truly benign neoplasm of the synovial tissue has been questioned. Jaffe[380] preferred to regard these growths as hyperplastic inflammatory responses rather than true neoplasms. Arthritic overgrowths of the synovial tissue around a knee joint are often difficult to distinguish from true neoplasms. Frequently, these lesions have a villous configuration and contain giant cells, lipid-laden phagocytes, and hemosiderin. For these lesions, the term *pigmented villonodular synovitis* was introduced.[380] But whether true neoplasms arise in these florid hyperplastic villous reactions of synovial tissue, or how many of the so-called benign synoviomas are only tumorlike conditions, is still a matter of controversy. Although this histologic question is intriguing, the clinical significance of such a discussion is important only insofar as determining whether these lesions require any treatment, whether after excision there is a tendency for recurrence, and finally, whether there is

any evidence that some or any of these tumors, at any stage of their evolution, become malignant.

Frequently, these tumefactions are seen as a single solid tumor in and around a joint and tendon sheath, and excision becomes necessary to rule out the possibility of a malignant tumor. The anatomic relationship of the growth to the surrounding tendon sheaths and joints determines the completeness of its removal, thereby influencing the likelihood of recurrence. Tumors that recur almost invariably have a high degree of cellularity, and there are infrequent reports of malignancy developing in the recurrence of previously histologically benign lesions.[189] However, malignant transformation of a villonodular synovitis is highly unlikely.

From this morass of cytologic detail, it is probably appropriate to seek a clinically acceptable classification of tumor and tumorlike conditions relating to synovial tissue. A simplified classification is given below:

A.  Benign tumorlike conditions
    1.  Synovioma
    2.  Villonodular synovitis
    3.  Giant cell tumor of the tendon sheath
    4.  Ganglion
B.  Malignant Tumors
    1.  Synovial sarcoma (malignant synovioma)

## BENIGN TUMORLIKE CONDITIONS

### Synovioma

Infrequently, a localized swelling around the knee joint is encountered in synoviomas (Fig. 5–80). Morphologically, these tumors consist of fibrous stroma in which

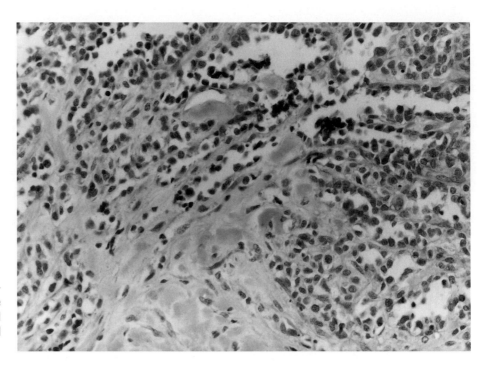

**Figure 5–80.** Benign synovioma. Photomicrograph of a well-delineated tumor of the joint showing slitlike spaces lined by cuboid cells with bland nuclei. (H & E. Original magnification × 250.)

mature synovial cells are interspersed. The clefts are reminiscent of the synovial spaces in the joint capsule, and the overall histologic appearance is somewhat similar to that of synovial sarcoma. There is some controversy as to whether this entity should be separately classified or is indeed a form of villonodular synovitis.

### Villonodular Synovitis
Villonodular synovitis is a relatively common entity frequently seen in conjunction with the flexor tendons of the fingers, wrist, toes, and ankles, but seldom around a large, weight-bearing joint. These lesions can be single or multiple and frequently take the shape of the tendon with which they are associated or to which they are attached. Depending on the local extension, the incidence of recurrence can be high. Although the general histologic appearance resembles that of localized benign synoviomas, these lesions exhibit a preponderance of inflammatory cells (Fig. 5–81A and 5–81B). Hemosiderosis is almost a constant accompaniment.

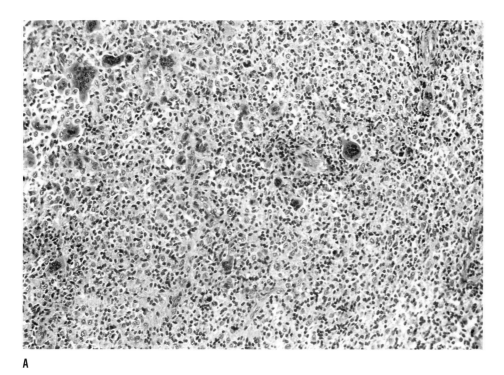

A

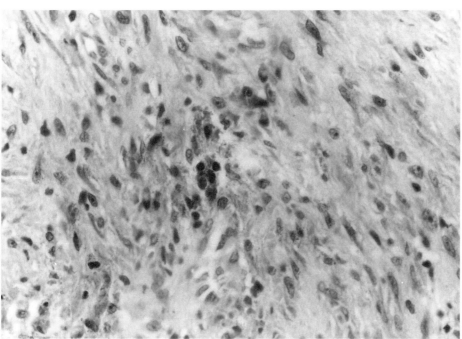

B

**Figure 5–81. (A)** Villonodular synovitis. Note the blending of histiocyte foam cells, stromal cells, and inflammatory cells. A few giant cells are scattered throughout the field. (H & E. Original magnification × 125.) **(B)** High-power view showing the fibrous stroma with loose scattering of histiocytes and hemosiderin granules. (H & E. Original magnification × 375.)

The presence of iron lends the characteristic color to these tumors.

### Giant Cell Tumor of the Tendon Sheath

Giant cell tumors of the tendon sheath are fibrous growths that vary in appearance, depending upon the number of fibroblasts and multinucleated giant cells of the foreign body type (Fig. 5–82).

### Ganglion

Ganglions are cystic swellings of the tendon sheaths of the joint capsules, especially of the tendons of the hands and the feet. Mainly, they are of myxoid tissue. Sometimes the high content of mucopolysaccharides leads to the development of multilocular cysts obliterating the peripheral cells.

## MALIGNANT TUMORS

### Synovial Sarcoma (Malignant Synovioma)

Synovial sarcomas usually arise from the soft tissues of the extremities of young adults.[376–378,381] Frequently, they are found around joints, tendons, and bursae, but some are relatively remote from a specific joint (e.g., those in the neck,[382–384] chest, or abdominal wall,[376,385] or even larynx[386]). Common sites for synovial sarcoma include the wrist, ankle, hands and feet, shoulder region, and hip and knee.[189,376–378,381,387] Seldom do these tumors arise from the lining of a joint cavity, and if the synovial membrane is involved, it is usually due to direct extension.[189,248]

*Macroscopic Findings.* The appearance of these tumors depends on the site of origin, duration, and rate of growth (Fig. 5–83A and 5–83B). In general, they are limited by a pseudocapsule of compressed and attenuated adjacent tissue. They develop as a firm, lobulated, gray or light brown mass of varying size that grows chiefly by expansion, and they can be predominantly vascular. In bulky tumors, areas of necrosis or cystic spaces containing a jellylike amorphous material are common.

*Microscopic Findings.* Synovial cell sarcoma consists of two distinct histologic components: epithelial cell and spindle cell (Fig. 5–84A to 5–84C). Depending on the relative extent of these two components, synovial cell sarcoma can be classified as (1) biphasic, where both components are easily distinguishable and present; (2) monophasic, where either epithelial or spindle cell type predominates; and (3) poorly differentiated. The light microscopic appearance of synovial sarcoma has been well described by several authors. The diagnosis of monophasic synovial sarcoma can be a problem, particularly where the second component is extremely sparse. Differentiating the diagnosis of monophasic spindle cell synovial cell sarcoma from fibrosarcoma can also be difficult. However, with immunoperoxidase stain and chromosomal study, the diagnosis is now somewhat easier.

*Microscopic Appearance of Biphasic Synovial Sarcoma.* Biphasic type is the predominant variety of synovial sarcoma.

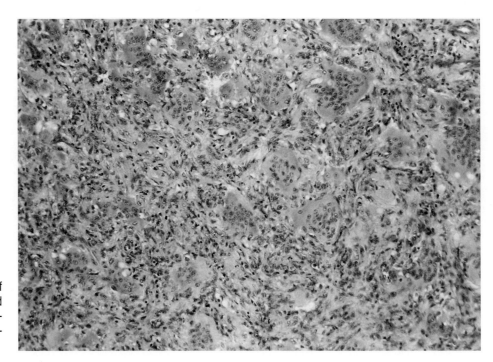

**Figure 5–82.** Benign giant cell tumor of the tendon sheath. Note the uniform round or oval histiocytes and numerous multinucleated giant cells. (H & E. Original magnification × 125.)

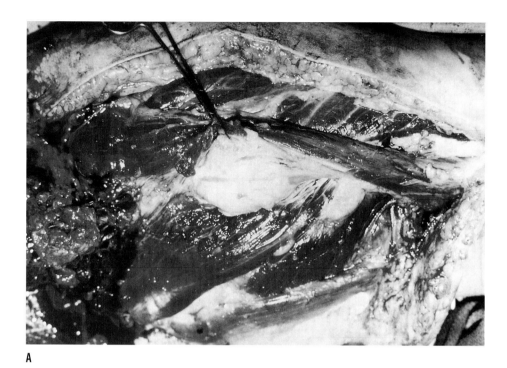

A

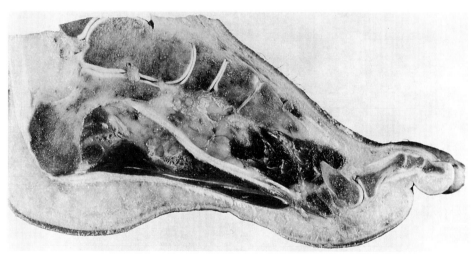

B

**Figure 5–83. (A)** Recurrent synovial sarcoma of the medial thigh in a 31-year-old woman. The lesion was locally excised six months previously. A hip joint disarticulation with groin dissection and adjuvant chemotherapy was the treatment. Note tumor infiltrating the adductor group of muscles. Proximally, the tumor extended up to the base of the femoral triangle. Patient has lived free of disease for 18 years. **(B)** Sagittal view of the bisected specimen of synovial sarcoma of the left foot. The tumor has extended to several compartments. *(Fig. 5–83B, courtesy of Drs. R.M. Barone and S. Saltzstein of San Diego, CA.)*

This is composed of fibroblastlike spindle cells and a cuboid to tall columnar epithelial component. In biphasic type, the spindle cells or fibrous component are the most prominent feature. These spindle cells are plump, with uniform appearance, and usually possess scant cytoplasm. They are commonly arranged in a herringbone pattern, with long sweeping bundles and sometimes irregular nodular arrangements. However, most of the time, mitosis is scanty. Type III collagen surrounding these spindle cells is also identifiable.

The epithelial component of biphasic synovial sarcoma usually consists of cells that are large, round to oval in shape, and have abundant pale-staining cyto- plasm. These cells may be arranged in a different fashion of nests or cords, and they border irregular cleftlike or seroglandular areas. These cleftlike areas should be distinguished from cleftlike blood vessels of hemangiopericytoma and from tissue artifact. These cleftlike areas are bordered by epithelial cells resembling normal synovial tissue. Infrequently, a papillary structure covered with cuboid or flattened epithelial cells may be seen. Also, in rare cases, squamous metaplasia or outright formation of squamous pearls may be observed. Inflammatory cells and multinucleated giant cells are very rarely seen in synovial sarcoma. However, the presence of mast cells in predominantly spindle cell areas of

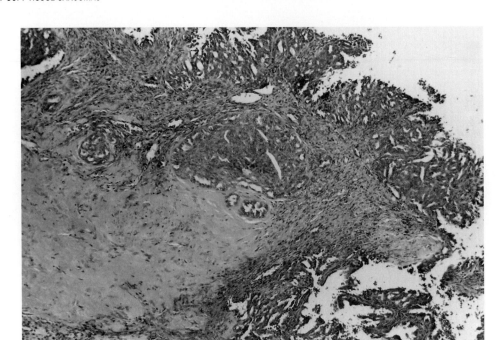

A

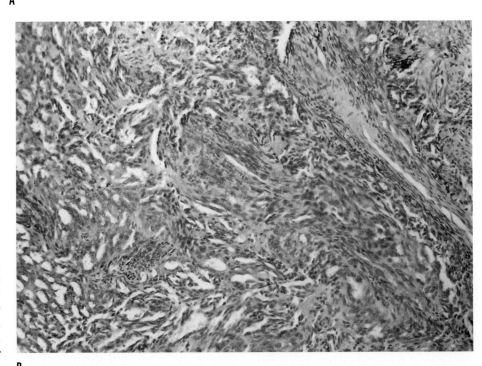

**Figure 5–84.** Synovial cell sarcoma. **(A)** The papillary nature of the tumor is apparent. (Original magnification × 65.) **(B)** Two types of cells can be seen: cuboid cells forming or trying to form glands, which are engulfed by spindle-shaped cells. (H & E. Original magnification × 250.) *(Continued.)*

B

the neoplasm is a typical finding in the biphasic variety of synovial cell sarcoma. Mitotic figures are sparse, and scattered areas of calcification can be found in 30 to 35 percent of the tumors.

*Microscopic Appearance of Monophasic Synovial Sarcoma.* As mentioned previously, monophasic synovial sarcoma can be spindle cell type, fibrosarcomatous type, or epithelial type, depending on the presence of the predominant cell type. Spindle cell monophasic synovial sarcoma is far more common than the epithelial type. In the spindle cell type of monophasic synovial sarcoma, the spindle cells predominate, with only rare foci of epithelial differentiation. Such lesions also possess other characteristics of synovial sarcoma, such as sparse giant cells, presence of mast cells, rare mitoses, absence

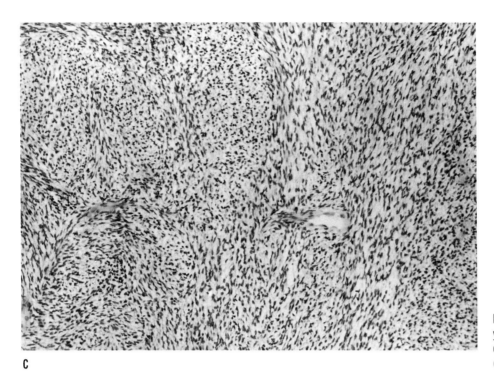

**C**

**Figure 5–84** *(continued).* **(C)** After five years, the tumor recurred and only the spindle cells were noted, making it monophasic. (Original magnification × 125)

of inflammatory cells, and cleftlike areas. By taking into account the patient's age, location of tumor, PAS-positive material within the cell, and sparse Type III collagen, the diagnosis can be established. However, in the absence of minute glandular areas or foci of glandular areas, a diagnosis of monophasic synovial sarcoma can be difficult.

In the past, diagnosis of monophasic synovial sarcoma in the absence of minute foci of epithelial differentiation has been difficult. However, recent studies have shown that a balanced translocation of Chromosome 18 and X Chromosome is a unique feature of synovial sarcoma and is present in approximately 75 percent of the cases. Such chromosomal study helps establish diagnosis in difficult cases (see Chapter 6). The epithelial variant, like its fibrous or spindle cell counterparts, consists almost entirely of glandular tissue with rare spindle cells. The differential diagnosis includes metastatic carcinoma, carcinosarcoma, malignant schwannoma, and melanoma. This is indeed a difficult diagnostic challenge, especially in the absence of any spindle cell areas. Similar to the fibrous or spindle cell counterparts, these lesions also have occasional calcification, PAS-positive material, and mast cells. Inflammatory cells and giant cells are rare or absent.

*Microscopic Appearance of Poorly Differentiated Synovial Cell Sarcoma.* Poorly differentiated synovial cell sarcoma is aggressive and presents a diagnostic problem for the pathologist. The overall incidence of this type of tumor is probably less than 20 percent. This tumor is usually composed of small spindle cells or oval cells, with very little tendency for differentiation. A reticulin stain helps to differentiate a biphasic pattern of epithelial type from a spindle cell type of the lesion. Also, thin-walled, slitlike vascular spaces are seen scattered throughout the section(s). Mitotic figures are more common in poorly differentiated synovial sarcoma than in either the biphasic or monophasic types and may exhibit more than two mitotic figures per high-power field.

*Electron Microscopy.* Examination of ultrathin sections usually reveals a distinct biphasic cell population: the columnar epitheliumlike cells forming the pseudoglandular structures, and the stromal cells resembling fibroblasts (Fig. 5–85A to 5–85D). In a low-power view, the epithelial stroma junction is differentiated by a discrete basement membrane of varying thickness. Roth and associates[383] calculated that the thickness varies from 1,500 to 5,500 Å. In undifferentiated tumors, the basement membrane is frequently disrupted, with resultant continuity of stromal and epithelial type cells.[388]

The epithelial type cells are usually of different cytoplasmic density and, according to the degree of osmiophilia, can be classified into light and dark cells (types A and B); frequently, an intermediate variety is encountered.

The light cells (type A) contain oval nuclei with evenly dispersed chromatin. The cytoplasm of these cells has abundant smooth-surfaced endoplasmic retic-

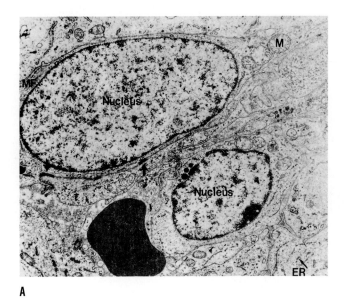

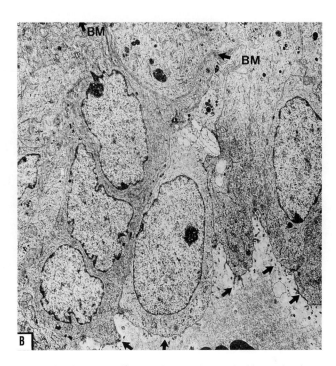

**Figure 5–85.** **(A)** Monophasic synovial cell sarcoma. In this micrograph, profiles of two type A cells are seen. The cytoplasm is characterized by an abundance of microfilaments *(MF)* and smooth membrane system. Also note the quality of fine granules in the rough endoplasmic reticulum *(ER)*. A number of inclusion bodies resembling lysosomes are apparent. The two cells are connected by means of multiple desmosomes shown by arrows. Profiles of cytoplasmic processes are apparent. (Original magnification × 31,900.) **(B)** Panoramic view of a biphasic synovial cell sarcoma. Both type A and type B cells are apparent. The basal lamina (basement membrane) is discrete and can be seen in the upper part *(BM)* of the micrograph. The lower part of the micrograph shows that several epithelioid cells containing microvilli *(arrows)* are bordering the cleftlike lumen. The lumen is filled with amorphous material. (Original magnification × 22,000.) *(Continued.)*

ulum. Fine granular material is commonly observed within the dilated spaces of rough endoplasmic reticulum. Microfilaments, which frequently accompany the epithelial type cells, are usually found in abundance in the light cells.

The dark cells (type B) contain irregularly shaped nuclei with coarse chromatin clumping. The general cytoplasmic morphology of these cells is similar to that of their counterparts, but there is less osmiophilia. However, few differences are noted on close scrutiny. In the cytoplasm of the dark cells, there is lower concentration of endoplasmic reticulum, resulting in lower concentration of fine granular material within the dilated spaces. These cells also generally have fewer microfilaments and microtubules. Desmosomes and interdigitating cytoplasmic processes are frequently seen.

Synovial cell sarcomas involve regional nodes, albeit less frequently than has been reported.[389] However, these data reflect the incidence during the entire natural history of the disease. Therefore, as a general guideline, it can be assumed that the incidence of regional metastases is higher in locally advanced cases and in highly pleomorphic tumors. Unlike other sarcomas, synovial sarcoma in some instances metastasizes to the pancreas (Fig. 5–86).

***Cytogenetic Findings.*** Chromosomal study of synovial sarcoma can be of immense diagnostic value, especially in monophasic spindle cell synovial sarcoma, where it is difficult to differentiate from fibrosarcoma in the absence of occasional glandular area or epithelial element. A number of authors have reported a high degree of consistent chromosomal abnormality in synovial sarcoma, ranging from 75 to 90 percent of the time.[175,390–392] Both biphasic and monophasic synovial cell sarcoma exhibit balanced translocation of Chromosome 18 and X Chromosome at short-arm p11 and long-arm q11, and it is termed as t(X;18) (p11; q11). There are several other variations that have been reported in a number of synovial sarcomas. Although this helps in establishing the diagnosis, such chromosomal abnormality has not been correlated to the prognosis.

## ■ TUMORS AND TUMORLIKE CONDITIONS OF THE VASOFORMATIVE AND PERIVASCULAR TISSUES

Primitive angioblastic tissue differentiates from the mesenchyme in the chorionic end of the body stalk and in the mesoderm lining the chorion. The cells of the

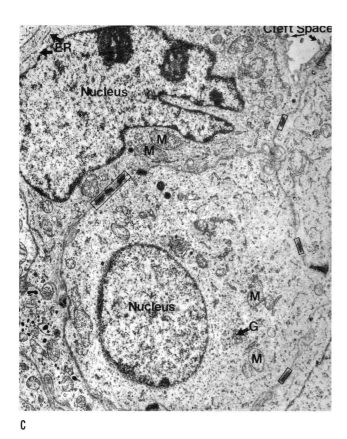

C

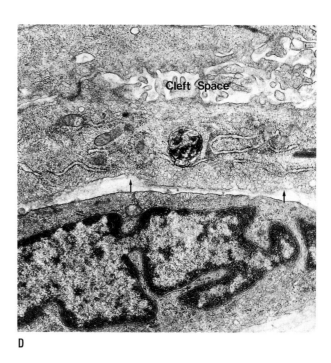

D

**Figure 5–85** *(continued).* **(C)** High-power view. Note the multiple desmosomal contacts (marked by boxes) that type A cells have with surrounding cell processes and one type B cell above. Prominent Golgi zone *(G)* in the type A cells is easily seen. Upper right-hand corner shows the microvilli *(arrows)* lining a cleft space. (H & E. Original magnification × 30,800.) **(D)** High-power view showing the protruding microvilli in the cleftlike space of a biphasic synovial cell sarcoma. (Original magnification × 46,460.)

mesoderm give rise to solid strands of angioblasts, each of which coalesces and eventually becomes a blood vessel. The earliest blood vessels, therefore, develop at several separate sites. From the walls of these vessels, buds grow outward, become canalized, and anastomose with

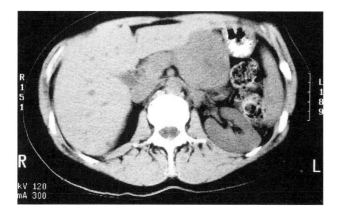

**Figure 5–86.** Computed axial tomography scan of the abdomen with synovial sarcoma metastases to head and body of pancreas. Although rare, the pancreas can be the initial site of metastases in synovial sarcomas.

neighboring vessels, forming a rich vascular network. By the end of the fourth week, the human embryo has a well-developed vascular system with a beating heart.[182] Willis[182] found that, in the healing of granulation tissue, embryonic methods of new vessel formation come into operation. A similar phenomenon probably can explain the histogenesis of some of the benign and malignant vascular angiomas.

There are two divergent views as to the initial stages of development of the lymphatic system.[182] In the early part of this century, it was thought that lymphatic spaces commence as clefts in the mesenchyme and that their living cells take on the characteristics of the endothelium. These spaces coalesce and form a network from which the lymph sacs (e.g., cisternae chyli) develop. In 1969, Kampmeier[393] concluded that the balance of argument favors their developing independently of the venous system. In the human embryo of two to four months, the lymphatics of the neck, mediastinum, and retroperitoneum are relatively large, easily identifiable, thin-walled vessels. In hamartomas of the lymphatic system, these spaces are unusually enlarged and become clinically important.

## VASCULAR TUMORS

Vascular tissue can be the site of several types of benign and malignant neoplasms. They can be classified as follows.

A. Benign tumors
   1. Hemangioma
   2. Angiomatosis
B. Malignant tumors
   1. Angiosarcoma (malignant hemangioendothelioma)
   2. Kaposi's sarcoma

### Benign Tumors

*Hemangioma.* The exact definition of hemangiomas has been a matter of debate over the years. They appear to be hamartomatous disorders. The term *hamartoma* signifies a tumorlike, but primarily non-neoplastic, malformation or inborn error of tissue development characterized by an abnormal mixture of tissues indigenous to the part, with an excess of one or more of the component structures constituting the tissue. Although the excessive tissue in hamartomas is essentially malformational and not neoplastic, it sometimes gives rise to a true neoplasm.[182] That hemangiomas are not true tumors is shown by the following observations: (1) Most are congenital or appear soon after birth (e.g., birthmarks). Visceral angiomas, however, are usually discovered later in life, although a number of these tumors, along with systemic angiomatosis, are diagnosed in children (see Fig. 12–11, Chapter 12). (2) No sharp line of demarcation can be drawn between "angiomas" and acknowledged vascular malformations (e.g., cirsoid aneurysms). (3) Common angiomas do not grow disproportionately and indefinitely as true neoplasms do. Most grow along with the tissues of the part and do not involve a greater territory than the original part affected. Indeed, some, such as strawberry nevi, spontaneously regress after an initial burst of growth.[394] Accidental complications, such as traumatic hemorrhage, inflammation, thrombosis, or cystic changes, might cause an angioma to suddenly change in size and apparently suggest malignant transformation of a preexisting benign tumor. For the sake of convenience and clarity, in this treatise hemangiomas are discussed as benign tumors.

The histopathologic findings of these lesions are difficult to describe without a review of the normal histologic appearance of the blood vessels.[395–397] The capillaries are composed of a lining of endothelial cells, a supporting sheath of reticulin and fibroblasts, and pericytes scattered over the outer surface of the sheath (Fig. 5–87). The capillaries consist of a tube lined by a single layer of polygonal endothelial cells that show

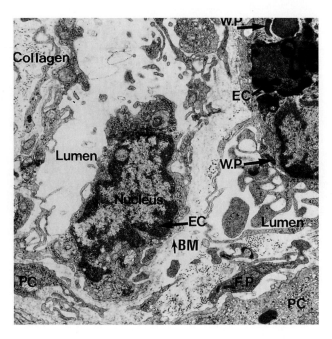

**Figure 5–87.** Electron micrograph of a human capillary from the skin showing the continuous endothelial lining, the endothelial cell *(EC)*, pericyte *(PC)*, and the basal lamina *(BM)*. The endothelial cell contains Weibel-Palade bodies *(WP)*. Several cytoplasmic processes of fibroblasts *(FP)* are also seen. (Original magnification × 15,000.)

variations in their fine structure and intercellular junctions, and a capillary may be continuous or fenestrated.[398] Surrounding the endothelial tube is usually a typical glycoprotein basal lamina, which, at isolated points over the capillary, splits to enclose flattened or branching perivascular cells (pericytes). The basal lamina usually merges into an adventitial layer of fine reticular tissue, with occasional fibroblasts or mast cells, which borders the perivascular spaces. Variations in all these features form the basis of a variety of classifications, but broadly, a capillary may be considered as either continuous or fenestrated.

Angiomas have been classified according to their composition (Fig. 5–88A and 5–88B). A hemangioma comprised of capillaries alone is termed a *capillary hemangioma*. In this variety, the capillaries are arranged haphazardly, and, if they are widely dilated, the resulting tumor is called a *cavernous hemangioma*. Sometimes, capillary angiomas in infants and children show proliferation of the endothelial layer. Stout and Lattes[104] coined the term *benign hemangioendothelioma* for these lesions. However, this distinction is not of great significance except for interpreting a true hemangioendothelioma.[399]

*Immunohistochemistry.* These lesions express a variety of antigens and can be stained immunohistochemically for Factor VIII, EN-4, PAL-E, OKM-5, Anti E-92, throm-

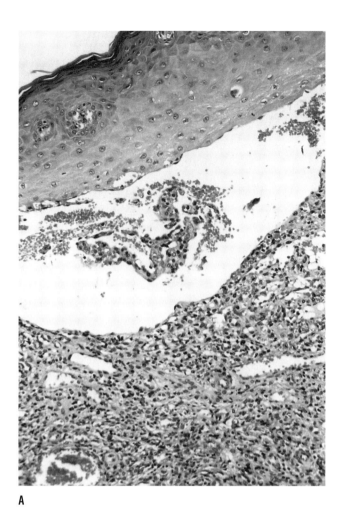

A

bomodulin, alkaline phosphatase, B-721, CD-34 (human hemopoietic progenitor cell antigen), and CD-31 (platelet-endothelial cell adhesion molecule).

*Electron Microscopy.* These lesions show basal lamina confined to endothelial cells containing Weibel-Palade bodies.

***Angiomatosis.*** Infrequently, angiomas arise in a multitude of tissues. They are observed as a large dilation of vascular spaces both in the somatic tissues and in the viscera. This widespread distribution suggests a common developmental error. A description of these entities will be found in the section dealing with the clinical features of angiomas (Chapter 12).

## Malignant Tumors

***Angiosarcomas.*** A wide spectrum of morphologic appearance of malignant lesions arising from the blood vessels resulted in the use of various nomenclature in the literature for these tumors, including angiosarcoma, hemangioendothelioma, hemangioblastoma, lymphangioendothelioma, lymphangiosarcoma, and so forth. Perhaps the designation of angiosarcoma would be more appropriate for all malignant tumors of the endothelium. Morphologically and histologically, the malignant tumors arising from the endothelium of lym-

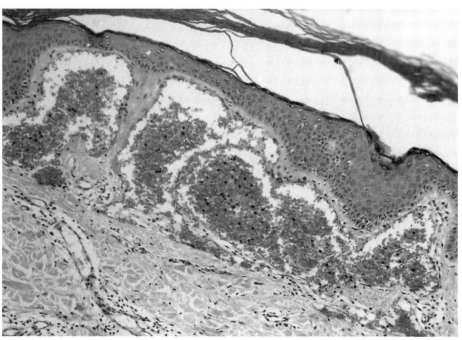

B

**Figure 5–88. (A)** Capillary hemangioma of the skin. All the capillaries are well developed and full of red blood cells. Note the compression of dermal structures. (H & E. Original magnification × 125.) **(B)** Cavernous hemangioma; large blood spaces are lined by a single layer of endothelium. (H & E. Original magnification × 125.)

phatics, so-called lymphangiosarcoma, are very difficult to differentiate from angiosarcoma. Clinically, however, a malignant vascular tumor arising from a lymphedematous area can be very easily recognized and termed *lymphangiosarcoma.* Enzinger and colleagues[398] suggested using the term *hemangioendothelioma* for a tumor of vascular origin of intermediate malignancy. The presentation and, to some extent, the clinical behavior of malignant tumors arising from endothelial cells vary according to the location of the tumor. However, the histologic appearance varies only minimally, depending on the type of angiosarcoma. For the purpose of clinical description, angiosarcomas can be divided into the following categories: (1) cutaneous angiosarcoma; (2) cutaneous angiosarcoma associated with either acquired or congenital lymphedema, or so-called lymphangiosarcoma; (3) radiation-induced angiosarcoma; (4) angiosarcoma of the soft tissue; and, (5) visceral angiosarcoma.

*Macroscopic Findings.* Angiosarcomas, irrespective of the site of origin, are very vascular and have a cystic or spongy appearance. The tumors are usually poorly demarcated, and the infiltrative margin of the lesions extends far beyond the gross appearance of the tumors.

*Microscopic Findings.* The microscopic variations of these lesions are striking (Fig. 5–89A and 5–89B). These tumors are generally composed of anastomosing capillary channels lined by an aggregation of the atypical endothelial lining cells. Sometimes the lining consists of one layer of polygonal or more rounded cells, which are usually larger than normal endothelial cells and more hyperchromatic. In a well-differentiated tumor, the mitosis is usually scanty. At times, the

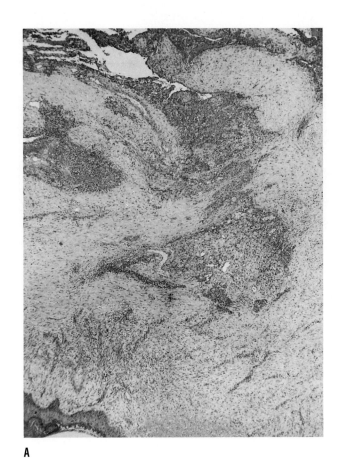

A

**Figure 5–89. (A)** Angiosarcoma of the soft tissues. Part of the skin can be seen in the lower left-hand corner. (H & E. Original magnification × 25.) **(B)** Close-up of the area seen in the upper left-hand corner of Figure 5–89A: Plump cuboid tumor cells are seen projecting into the lumen in a papillary fashion. (H & E. Original magnification × 250.) *(Continued.)*

B

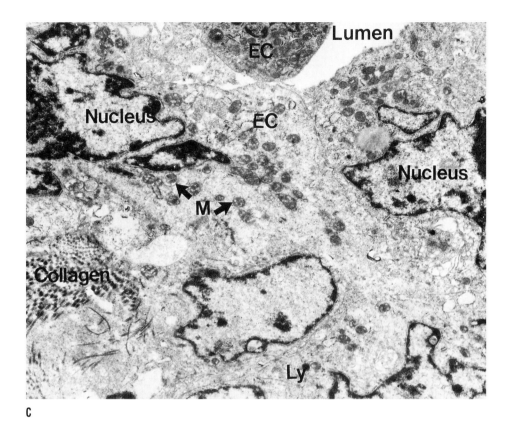

C

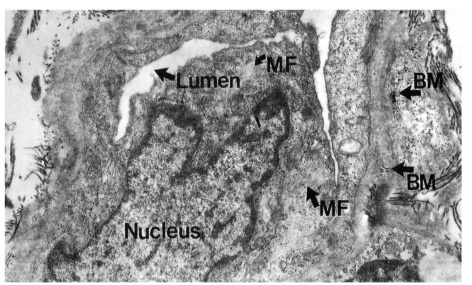

D

**Figure 5–89** *(continued).* **(C)** Micrograph of an angiosarcoma of the extremities. The neoplastic endothelial cells *(EC)* are protruding into the lumen, almost obliterating it. Proliferating endothelial cells are haphazardly scattered throughout, with the usual cytoplasmic components. (Original magnification × 17,140.) **(D)** High-power view of a malignant endothelial cell protruding into the lumen. Note the cytoplasmic microfilaments *(MF)*. Also note the intact basal lamina *(BM)* in this micrograph. (Original magnification × 20,540.)

endothelial cells are in several layers and tend to form areas of heaped-up cells, giving the appearance of a papillary pattern. Extension into the surrounding tissue by the coalescent capillarylike anastomosis is common. At times, there may be areas of more solid structures; however, these areas are usually much more cellular and the tumor cells are less differentiated and have frequent mitosis. Occasionally, a reticulin stain may be necessary to demonstrate that these tumor cells are located within the vascular channel. In so-called spindle hemangioendothelioma, multinucleated giant cells are frequently seen, giving this tumor an appearance like choriocarcinoma.

*Electron Microscopy.*    Ultrastructural examination of the tumor shows the following characteristics (Fig. 5–89C and 5–89D).

1. *Vasculature.* There is an overgrowth of the endothelial cells manifested by an overall increase in the vasculature without conspicuous change in the endothelial lining. The numerical increase in the endothelial cells is evident

when these cells almost clog the lumen by bridging across it.

2. *Tumor cells.* These cells lie between the vascular channels throughout the tumor and vary considerably in morphology. These cells are scattered randomly, and intracellular attachments are seldom seen. Cytoplasmic microfilaments are frequently observed, although inclusions of any type are rare.

3. *Interstitial matrix.* The interstitial matrix is composed of fine fibrillar or flocculent material.

*Immunohistochemistry.*   Although angiosarcomas are expected to maintain some of the antigenicity of endothelial cells, the presence of Factor VIII antigen is relatively uncommon in angiosarcoma (Fig. 5–90A to 5–90C and Color Plate 3). Furthermore, the presence of Factor VIII antigen in tumors, such as epithelioid sarcoma, synovial cell sarcoma, and even some carcinomas, complicates the interpretation of a specific Factor VIII antigen-positive tumor. Similar problems have been associated with various other antibodies normally used for diagnosis of tissue of endothelial origin, for example thrombomodulin, human hemopoietic progenitor cell antigen. Staining of the tumor cells for platelet endothelial cell adhesion molecule cell antigen (CD-31) appears to be more accurate than any other immunohistochemical staining for angiosarcoma. However, the positivity of this immunocytochemical stain does not allow differentiation between a benign and a borderline malignant tumor of endothelial cell origin.

***Kaposi's Sarcoma.***   Kaposi's sarcoma was first described in 1872.[400] Since then, voluminous information has been obtained on this disease. Recent increase in the incidence of this type of sarcoma is largely related to the increased incidence of Kaposi's sarcoma in AIDS patients. Although the exact origin of Kaposi's sarcoma is debated, most malignant cells in Kaposi's sarcoma resemble endothelial cells.[401,402] Current evidence suggests that Kaposi's sarcoma may be virally associated. Good response of Kaposi's sarcoma to various alkylating agents also lends credence to the hypothesis that Kaposi's sarcoma may be similar in origin to Burkitt's lymphoma.[403] The typical Kaposi's sarcoma that used to be seen in elderly male patients of Eastern European descent usually consisted of multiple purple, usually vascular nodules that initially appeared in the dermis of the distal parts of the extremities. Later, smaller lesions coalesced to form a bigger nodular lesion in the skin. However, in this variation of the disease, involvement of the surrounding soft tissue, regional node, bone, and viscera was frequently seen. The gross appearance of the Kaposi's sarcoma in AIDS patients is quite different. The early stage of the lesion presents as a cutaneous patch consisting of proliferation of small vessels surrounded by larger, more dilated vessels. At this stage, this lesion has very little, if any, induration and infiltration to the deeper structure. The more advanced stage is characterized by a plaquelike area with elevation of the skin, which involves most of the dermis and may extend into the deeper tissue. Microscopically, this lesion, composed of capillaries showing free anastomosis and the space between the blood vessels, is filled with red blood cells and lined with spindle-shaped cells and reticulin fibers (Fig. 5–91A to 5–91C). In a well-differentiated lesion, the spindle cell component is displayed around the proliferating vascular channels. In a more advanced lesion, the spindle cells intersect with each other, forming an arclike area.[404] Various areas of the tumor may show the presence of pigment deposits and various types of inflammatory cells. Occasionally, areas of intracellular and extracellular hyalinized globules may be observed.[404] A more aggressive-appearing Kaposi's sarcoma is usually observed in AIDS-related Kaposi's sarcoma patients. These lesions have tumor cells that are much more pleomorphic and have frequent mitosis and occasionally will be very difficult to differentiate from an aggressive angiosarcoma. Even histochemical stain for Kaposi's sarcoma can be very inconsistent. Only a few of these lesions stain positive for Factor VIII antigen. EN-4, which is a monoclonal antibody directed against endothelium, and PAL-E, an antibody against vascular endothelium, are positive in Kaposi's sarcoma. Immunostaining with OKM-5, anti-E92, and HCL, which react with capillary endothelium but not lymphatic endothelium may also stain positive in Kaposi's sarcoma. The presence of mRNA for alpha-smooth muscle actin in Kaposi's sarcoma suggests that the tumor may be of vascular smooth muscle cell origin.[405]

*Electron Microscopy.*   The electron microscopic examination of Kaposi's sarcoma shows that the tumor is composed mainly of two types of cells: hypertrophic endothelial cells and a fibrocytic fibroblast. The endothelial cells show a small number of lysosomes with sparsely distributed ferritin. The remaining characteristics of the endothelial cells are well preserved. The fibroblasts, in contrast, resemble macrophages with numerous cytoplasmic phagosomes and ferritin-containing organelles. The interstitial area, as in other types of vascular tumor, is clear with scanty collagen. Even histochemical study shows moderate localization of alkaline phosphatase, acid phosphatase, nonspecific esterase, and intense reaction to amino peptides activity. No phosphorized activity is seen.[406]

## PERIVASCULAR TUMORS

Recent classification of soft tissue tumors adopted by the World Health Organization[407] included such

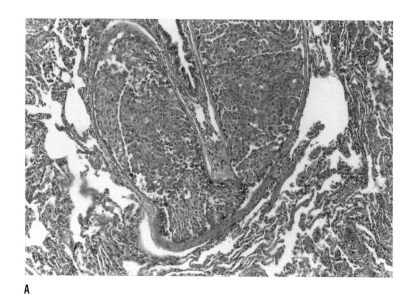

A

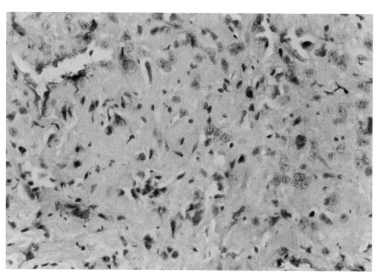

B

C

**Figure 5–90.** **(A)** A thrombus of angiosarcoma blocking the capillary. (PAS stain. Original magnification × 100.) **(B)** PAS stain showing focally positive angiosarcoma. (Original magnification × 40.) **(C)** Factor VIII-positive metastatic angiosarcoma to lung. (Original magnification × 40.)

tumors as glomus tumors and hemangiopericytomas arising from cells that support blood vessels (i.e., pericytes and glomus cells rather than cells which feature endothelial differentiation). Conceptually, it appears to be more logical; thus, these tumors are included in this chapter under the subheading of perivascular tumors.

## Glomus Tumor (Glomangioma)

Glomus tumors are commonly seen as painful nodules in the subungual region. It was first accurately described by Masson.[408] Glomus tumors seldom are larger than a few centimeters and are sporadically found elsewhere in the body.[409–411] Of the viscera, glomus tumors have been described in the stomach,[412–414] heart,[189] and uterus.[415] Interosseous variants are occasionally seen in the terminal phalanges.[416]

The lesion is usually circumscribed and often limited by a well-defined fibrous capsule. Most glomus tumors are characterized by a collection of thick-walled vessels, between which there are interspersed innumerable unmyelinated axons. Different degrees of glomus cell proliferation and varying ratios of cellular vascular elements are exhibited by these tumors (Fig. 5–92A and 5–92B). The morphologic characteristics of these cells are similar to those of pericytes. Based on in vitro studies, Murray and Stout[417] concluded that these cells probably are pericytes. However, in recent years, the actual histogenesis of the glomus tumor has been reassessed.[418–426] Ultrastructural studies by Venkatacha-

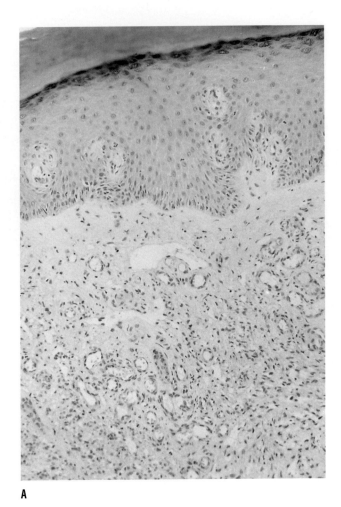

**A**

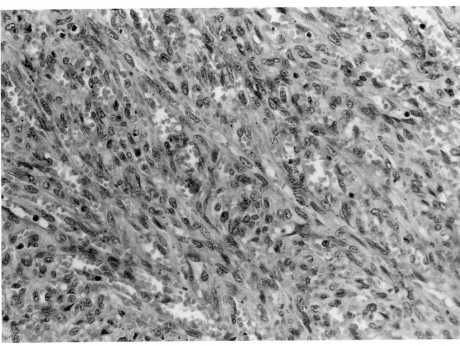

**Figure 5–91. (A)** Cutaneous nodule of Kaposi's sarcoma. In the dermis, multiple capillaries with intervening spindle-shaped cells can be seen. (H & E. Original magnification × 125.) *(Courtesy of Dr. S.G. Ronan, Departments of Pathology and Dermatology, University of Illinois.)* **(B)** The dermis showing the capillaries with malignant spindle-shaped cells. These are filled with red blood cells. (H & E. Original magnification × 375.) *(Continued.)*

**B**

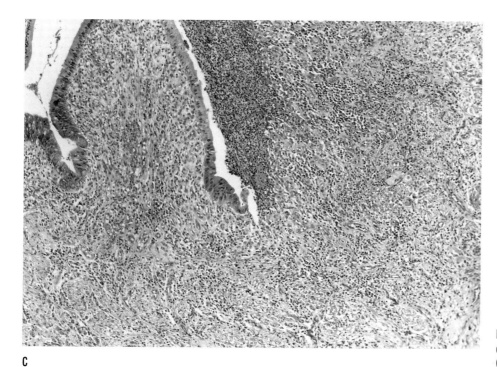

C

Figure 5–91 *(continued).* **(C)** Kaposi's sarcoma involving the small intestine. (H & E. Original magnification × 65.)

lam and Greally,[9] Murad and coworkers,[418] Toker,[424] and Tarnowski and Hashimoto[427] all tend to show that glomus cells morphologically resemble smooth muscle cells. All these authors have concluded that, although glomus tumors frequently show phenotypic characteristics of a smooth muscle origin, they still should be grouped with tumors arising form the perivascular tissue. Glomangiomyomas are a variant of the glomus tumor in which a gradual transition from glomus cells to elongated smooth muscle cells can be traced. These transitions are not obvious in large vessels. The natural history and treatment of this tumor are similar to conventional glomus tumors.

### Benign Hemangiopericytoma

Pericytes referred to above can proliferate as rounded or elongated cells just outside the reticulin sheath of the capillary and develop into a hemangiopericytoma. The tumor has been observed in many parts of the body and may involve a number of viscera, including brain, lung, ovary, bone, and parotid glands.

Due to lack of specific light microscopic and electron microscopic features, the diagnosis of hemangiopericytoma is based on architectural pattern and exclusion of diagnosis of other lesions with similar histologic appearance. Another major problem in the diagnosis of hemangiopericytoma is differentiation between benign and malignant, particularly in borderline or intermediate cases.

The tumor is usually comprised of lightly packed cells with round or oval nuclei arranged surrounding thin-walled blood vessels of varying sizes. The tissue or blood vessel is surrounded by a single layer of endothelium. At times, spindle cells may be arranged in a palisading pattern mimicking neural tumor. In benign lesions, the tumor cells show very little pleomorphism. To render a diagnosis of benign hemangiopericytoma, the mitosis count should be less than two per 10 high-power fields. However, it must be understood that, although the low mitotic count signifies benign nature in most lesions, it does not eliminate the biologic possibility of an aggressive behavior.

### Papillary Endothelial Hyperplasia (Intervascular Hemangioendothelioma, or Intervascular Hemangiomatosis)

Although papillary endothelial hyperplasia was long considered to be a neoplasm, Henschen[428] convincingly argued in 1932 in favor of a reactive response of the endothelial cells to an inflammatory response. These lesions occur in a preexisting vascular lesions, usually hemangioma or pyogenic granuloma. They are small and confined by a pseudocapsule, and can be confused with angiosarcomas, from which they differ by their well-circumscribed nature and lack of necrosis, degeneration, or pleomorphism. Mitosis is rare, and prognosis is excellent. These tumors occur in adults of both genders but may be associated with oral contraceptive use. They present as a well-defined, deep-seated, painful red nodule. Microscopically, they are well defined and show vacuolated cells arranged in a cordlike fashion, sometimes resembling cartilaginous tissue because of its myxoid matrix. The intracytoplas-

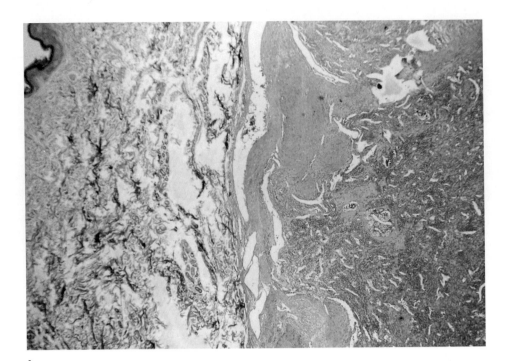

A

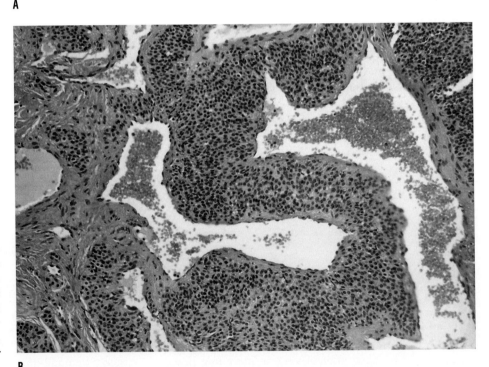

B

**Figure 5–92. (A)** Small foci of a subcutaneous glomus tumor. The glomus cells are arranged in cords along the blood spaces. (H & E. Original magnification × 25.) **(B)** Glomus cells arranged in layers lying in a hyaline matrix. (H & E. Original magnification × 125.) *(Courtesy of Dr. S.G. Ronan, Departments of Pathology and Dermatology, University of Illinois Hospital.)*

mic globule is mucin-negative. Reticulin stain may help to delineate small nests of cells. They usually do not have any mitosis, but have atypia.

***Immunohistochemistry.*** Immunohistochemically, these lesions share the same properties as hemangioma described in the earlier part of this chapter.

***Electron Microscopy.*** Ultrastructurally, these lesions have characteristics of endothelial cells with Weibel-

Palade body. The behavior of this lesion may be unpredictable. Although an occasional case tends to metastasize, the overall prognosis following adequate excision is excellent.

### Malignant Hemangiopericytoma

Malignant hemangiopericytoma is a rare tumor of soft tissues that is formed by proliferation of the pericytes around the blood vessels. It is usually well-encapsulated with a highly vascularized pseudocapsule. It can be found in all parts of the body, including mediastinal, meningeal, nasal, and paranasal locations. However, the most common site in our experience is the thigh. Hemangiopericytomas as a group (both malignant and benign) constitute approximately 3 percent of all soft tissue sarcomas. As mentioned in the section on benign hemangiopericytoma, it is difficult to accurately predict clinical behavior of these lesions solely from histologic appearance.

***Macroscopic Findings.*** The gross appearance has no specific characteristics. Occasionally, the cut surface of the large tumor may show variable extent of necrosis, cyst formation, and hemorrhage (Fig. 5–93A and 5–93B). Sometimes the x-ray finding, particularly angiogram, suggests a vascular tumor with both the venous and arterial phases with increased vascularity and features of arteriovenous shunt.

***Microscopic Findings.*** This lesion arises from pericytes and lacks any typical characteristic features that can readily suggest the diagnosis. Although histologic appearance is subject to considerable variation, all hemangiopericytomas have three essential characteristics: (1) numerous thin-walled vessels lined by a single layer of endothelial cells separated from tumors by a layer of collagen tissue; (2) proliferating parenchymal cells with ill-defined cytoplasm and small oval or round nucleus, occasional areas of spindle cells sometimes arranged in palisading fashion; and (3) a distinct reticulin pattern (Fig. 5–93C and 5–93D).

The diagnosis of hemangiopericytoma is based more on an architectural pattern than on morphology of tumor cells. At times, it is difficult to make a definitive diagnosis on light microscopy (Fig. 5–94A to 5–94C). Under light microscopy, this tumor may be difficult to differentiate from fibrosarcoma or monophasic synovial cell sarcoma. Occasionally, interstitial mucinous substance may also give the lesion a myxoid liposarcomatous appearance. Lack of spindle cells arranged in long bundles or fascicles, absence of lipoblast and plexiform capillaries, and presence of thin-walled vascular channels with single layer endothelium separated by layer of collagen from tumor cells should help establish the diagnosis. At times, it is nearly impossible to make the diagnosis without electron microscopy.

***Electron Microscopy.*** Electron microscopic appearance confirms the pericytic origin of tumor, and the tumor cells are separated from endothelial cells by basal laminae. The tumor cells have elongated cytoplasmic process, round or oval nucleus, sparse organelles, and almost constant presence of pinocytotic vesicles.

The malignant nature of this lesion is difficult to predict from histologic appearance. Although pleomor-

phism of tumor cells is somewhat more pronounced in malignant hemangiopericytoma than its benign counterpart, mitotic activity is the most important feature in predicting the malignant nature of these lesions. The presence of three or more mitoses per ten high-power fields indicates increased malignant potential.

***Immunohistochemistry.*** Vimentin is positive in hemangiopericytoma, together with Factor XIII-A and HLA-DR antigen. CD-34 is occasionally positive. The tumor, however, is negative for Factor VIII, epithelial membrane antigen (EMA), cytokeratin, desmin, and myoglobin. Occasionally, S-100 and Leu-7 will be positive, as will myelin-associated glycoprotein as described by Dictor et al.[429]

***Cytogenetic Findings.*** Chromosomal abnormality is seen frequently in hemangiopericytoma involving the long-arm of Chromosome 12.[430,431] However, such rearrangement of Chromosome 12 has also been described in other spindle cell tumors; hence, it cannot be used as a diagnostic criteria for hemangiopericytoma. No specific chromosomal abnormalities, used for either diagnostic or prognostic purposes, have been noted in tumors of the vascular origin.

# ■ TUMORS OR TUMORLIKE CONDITIONS OF THE LYMPHATIC SYSTEM

These tumors or tumorlike conditions can be classified as follows.

A. Benign Tumors
  1. Lymphangiomas
    a. Papillary
    b. Cavernous
    c. Cystic hygroma
  2. Lymphangiectasis
    a. Local
    b. Regional
  3. Lymphangiomyoma and Lymphangiomyomatosis
B. Malignant Tumors
  1. Lymphangiosarcoma
    a. Postmastectomy (Stewart-Treves syndrome)
    b. Not associated with mastectomy (e.g., arising from congenital edema of extremity)

## BENIGN TUMORS

### Lymphangioma
A lymphangioma, like its vascular counterpart, the angioma, is not a true neoplasm but a hamartomatous malformation. However, for the sake of clarity, it will be discussed here. Proliferation of lymphatic vessels is less

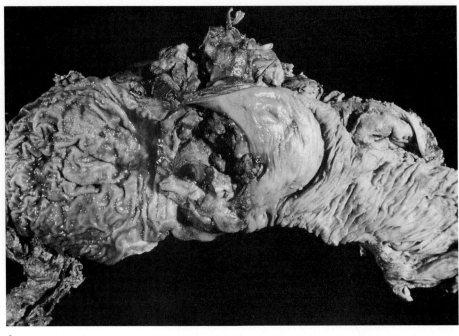

**A**

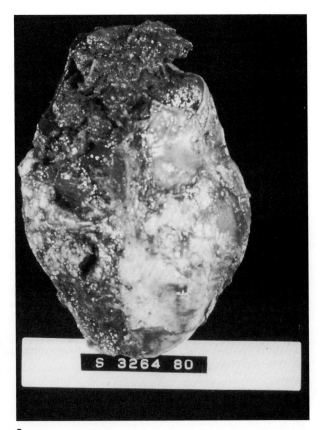

**Figure 5–93.** This recurrent hemangiopericytoma of the anterior abdominal wall was removed from a 26-year-old man. He required excision of the anterior wall, part of the right lobe of the liver, the head of the pancreas, duodenum, and 60 percent of the stomach and transverse colon. **(A)** Specimen of resected anterior abdominal wall with tumor invading first part of the duodenum. This was the cause of preoperative upper gastrointestinal bleeding. After a disease-free interval of four years, he had intra-abdominal recurrence. **(B)** Tumor is invading the spleen. *(Continued.)*

**B**

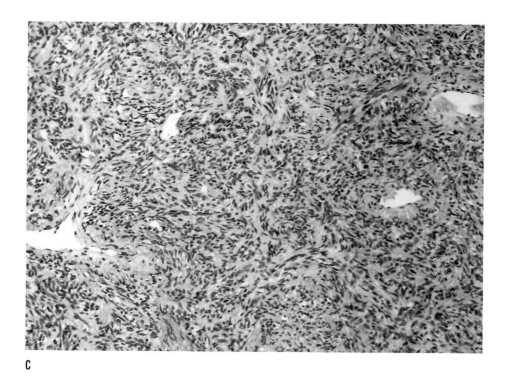

C

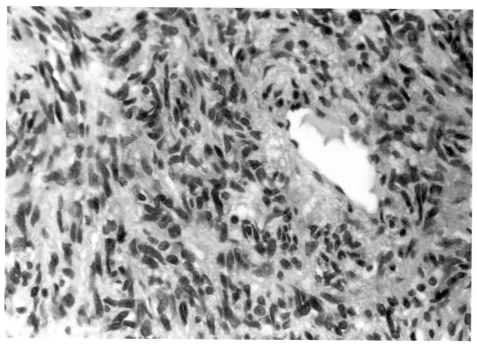

D

**Figure 5–93** *(continued).* **(C)** Hemangiopericytoma, showing many vascular channels. The crowding of the neoplastic cells is outside the walls of the vascular spaces. (H & E. Original magnification × 125.) **(D)** High-power view, showing the predominantly oval and spindle-shaped pericytes. Apparently, normal endothelium is separated from the malignant cells by an amorphous collagenous matrix. (H & E. Original magnification × 375.)

common than in the blood vessels. Generally, lymphangiomas are present at birth as diffuse proliferations that ultimately give the associated structures a grotesque appearance (e.g., gigantism of an extremity). In another form, cystic dilations of enormous size are found, especially in the neck, giving rise to the term *cystic hygroma.* Infrequently, this type of cyst is found in the omentum and mesentery. Microscopically, the lesion is seen to consist of a honeycomb formed of large and small thin-walled cysts separated by bands of fibrous tissue (Fig. 5–95).

## Lymphangiomyomatosis

Lymphangiomyomatosis is a rare condition[432,433] characterized by proliferation of the smooth muscle fibers that participate in the formation of lymphatic channels

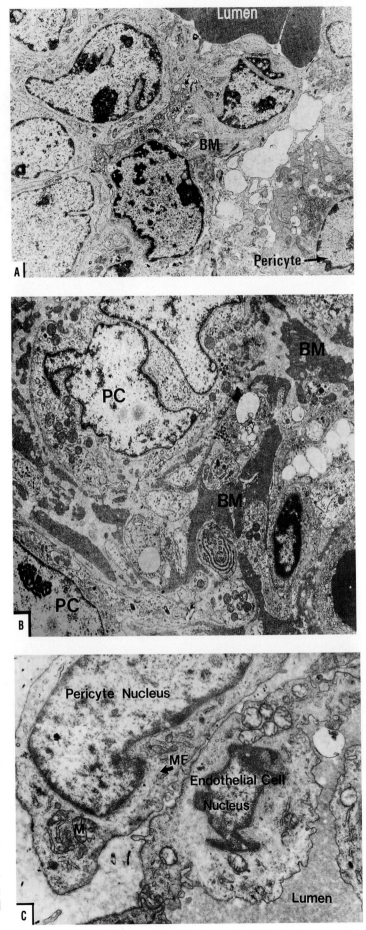

**Figure 5–94. (A)** Low-power view of a hemangiopericytoma. A capillary filled with two attenuated red blood cells is surrounded by neoplastic pericytes. Note the thin discontinuous basal lamina surrounding the neoplastic pericytes. Cytologic details of pericytes are obvious. (Original magnification × 10,470.) **(B)** Another low-power view from a patient with recurrent pelvic hemangiopericytoma. Note the haphazard distribution of basal lamina. (Original magnification × 7,013.) **(C)** High-power view of a neoplastic pericyte. Note the relation of the pericyte with the endothelial cell. This is from a 20-year-old woman with an atypical hemangiopericytoma of the groin.

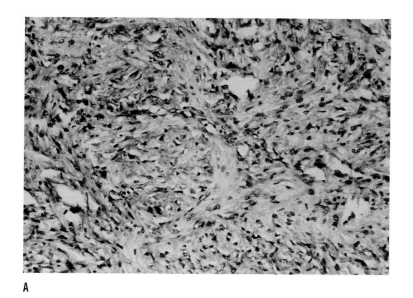

A

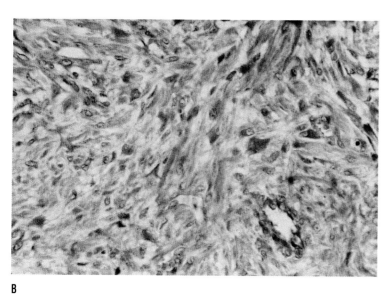

B

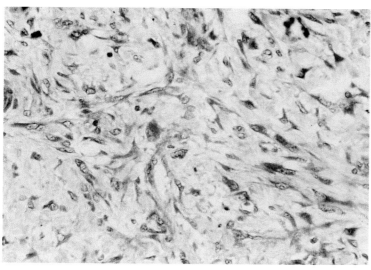

C

**Color Plate 1. (A)** Deep-seated malignant fibrous histiocytoma showing cells in mitosis as well as a number of histiocytes. (H & E. Original magnification × 10.) **(B)** Section from the same tumor showing cells positive for α-antitrypsin. (Original magnification × 20.) **(C)** Similar section positive for α-chymotrypsin. (Original magnification × 20.)

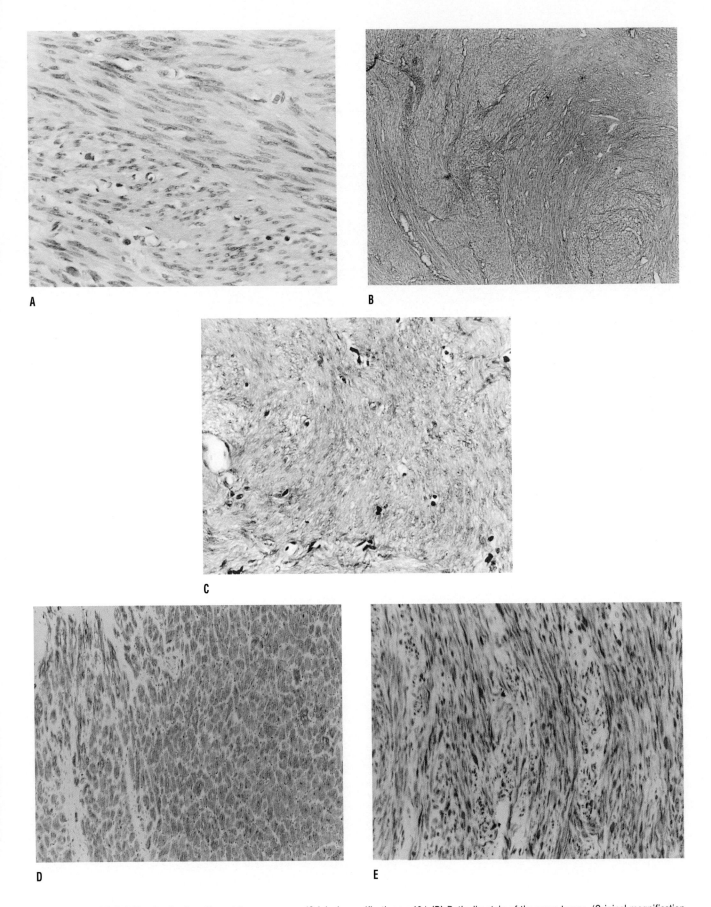

**Color Plate 2.** **(A)** H & E stain of a deep tissue leiomyosarcoma. (Original magnification × 40.) **(B)** Reticulin stain of the same tumor. (Original magnification × 10.) **(C)** Trichrome stain of the same tumor. (Original magnification × 40.) **(D)** Desmin control. (Original magnification × 40.) **(E)** Desmin positive for leiomyo-sarcoma. (Same tumor, original magnification × 40.) *(Continued.)*

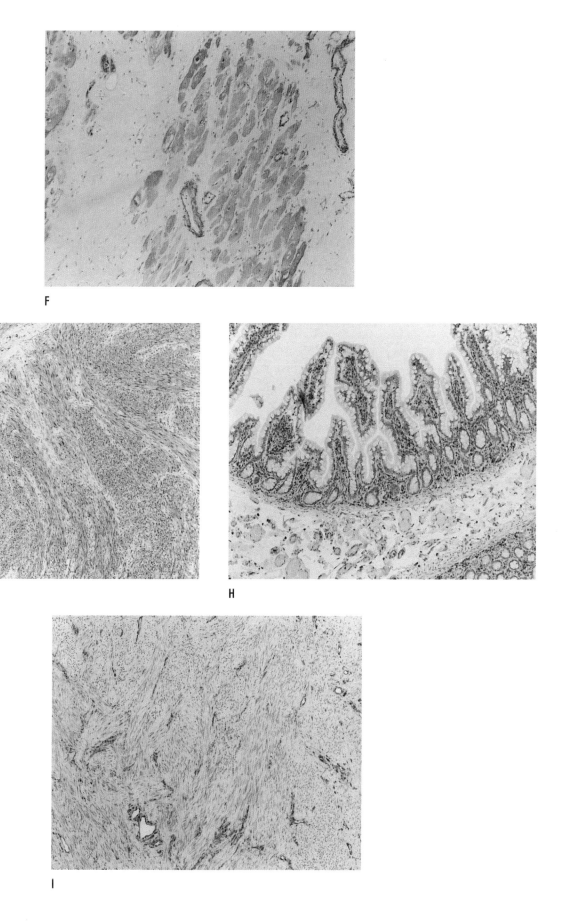

**Color Plate 2** *(continued).* **(F)** Actin control. (Original magnification × 10.) **(G)** Leiomyosarcoma positive for actin. (Same tumor, original magnification × 10.)
**(H)** Vimentin control. (Original magnification × 10.) **(I)** Leiomyosarcoma positive for vimentin. (Same tumor, original magnification × 40.)

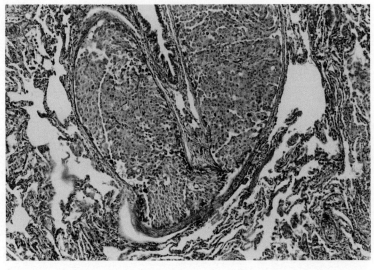

A

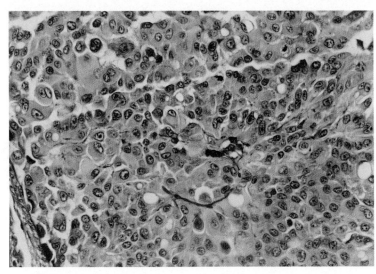

B

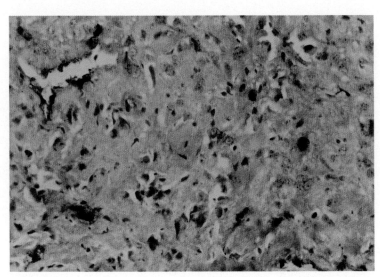

C

**Color Plate 3. (A)** A thrombus of angiosarcoma blocking the capillary. (PAS stain. Original magnification × 100.) **(B)** PAS stain showing focally positive angiosarcoma. (Original magnification × 40.) **(C)** Factor VIII-positive metastatic angiosarcoma to lung. (Original magnification × 40.)

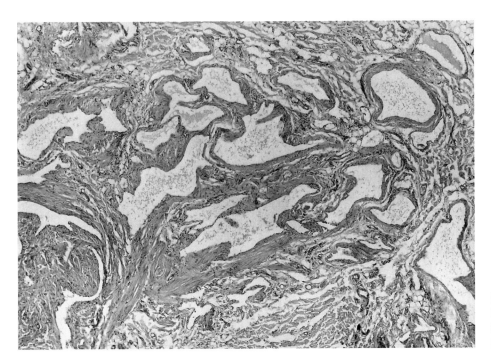

**Figure 5–95.** Lymphangioma showing the honeycomb appearance of thin-walled cystic spaces filled with amorphous material. (H & E. Original magnification × 40.)

throughout the body. Clinically, however, it usually presents with chylothorax, dyspnea, and pneumothorax.[434] Extrapulmonary symptoms include chylous ascites and edema of the extremities (for details, see Chapter 13).

## MALIGNANT TUMORS

### Lymphangiosarcoma

In 1948, Stewart and Treves[435] first recognized the syndrome of postmastectomy lymphangiosarcoma. This is usually associated with lymphedema after radical mastectomy and is often associated with radiation as an adjuvant to radical mastectomy. However, postmastectomy lymphangiosarcoma has also been described in nonlymphedematous postmastectomy patients and in various other congenital and acquired lymphedematous areas.

Lymphangiosarcoma is recognized by its characteristic bluish-red or purplish well-defined macular or papular cutaneous lesions in a lymphedematous extremity or lymphedematous area.

***Microscopic Findings.*** Histologically, this lesion is very difficult to differentiate from an angiosarcoma (Fig. 5–96A and 5–96B). However, the presence of this malignant lesion with histologic appearance of angiosarcoma located in a lymphedematous area helps establish the diagnosis of lymphangiosarcoma. The lesion is usually composed of small capillary channels lined by malignant endothelial cells, has a similar appearance to angiosarcoma, and usually infiltrates the skin, subcutaneous, and deeper tissue. At times, the presence of red blood cells within the capillaries further confuses the diagnosis with angiosarcoma.

***Cytogenetic Findings.*** Although some malignant tumors of endothelial origin exhibit nonclonal deletion and translocation, they lack any characteristic cytogenetic finding.

## ■ TUMOR AND TUMORLIKE CONDITIONS ARISING IN HETEROTOPIC BONE AND CARTILAGE

The histogenesis of either extraskeletal osteogenic sarcoma or chondrosarcoma is still unclear. Most of this is probably related to osseous or cartilaginous metaplasia of soft tissues. Metaplastic ossification occurs in voluntary muscles[182] and other locations.[182] Huggins[436] stressed the concept of metaplasia of connective tissue into bone as a result of unknown influences. In 1940, Binkley and Stewart[432] made an extensive study of the morphogenesis of extraskeletal osteogenic sarcoma and pseudo-osteosarcoma. They proposed that the most important underlying causes of the development of the tumors were localized vascular stasis and concomitant tissue anoxia. Brookes,[438] in 1966, produced experimental osteogenesis by elevation of carbon dioxide tension and red cell count. It appears, therefore, that histologic[436] and experimental[438] evidence is available to support the concept of metaplasia of connective tissue cells into bone. Willis[182] found that new bone or cartilage formation has been described in all tissues of the body.

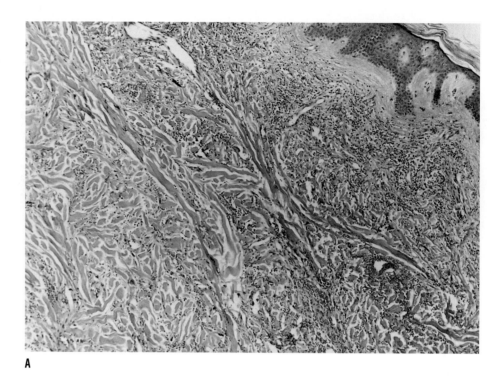

A

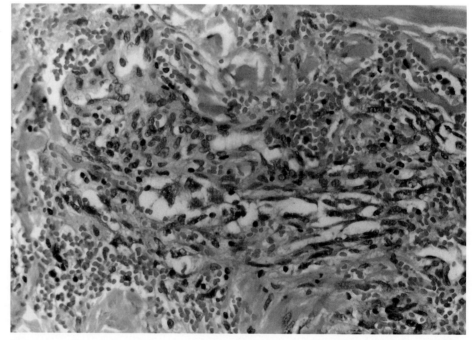

B

**Figure 5–96. (A)** Postmastectomy lymphangiosarcoma. A focus of disorderly growth of vascular channels lined by atypical spindle-shaped cells is seen invading the skin. (H & E. Original magnification × 65.) **(B)** Lymphatic channels of various sizes are lined by pleomorphic endothelial cells. (H & E. Original magnification × 250.)

The bony metaplasia in voluntary muscles, or myositis ossificans, is not, strictly speaking, a tumor; however, because of an occasional clinical presentation of what resembles a tumor, this entity is briefly described. Metaplastic ossification occurs in skeletal muscles in two forms: localized myositis ossificans and a progressive generalized form of unknown cause. The localized form is usually the result of chronic trauma. The most celebrated form of this entity is so-called rider's bone, which is seldom seen nowadays. Microscopically, the histologic picture of new bone extending into inflamed fibrosing muscle is diagnostic. Care must be taken not to confuse this benign self-limiting entity with osteosarcoma. A rare progressive form of this disease is described in Chapter 14.

Benign extraskeletal chondromas of the soft parts are rare. The predominant site is the finger, where over 80 percent of these tumors have been encountered.

## EXTRASKELETAL OSTEOGENIC SARCOMA

Extraosseous osteogenic sarcoma is indeed rare. Since the original description by Boneti[439] in the year 1700, only a handful of documented cases have been reported.[113,437,440–444]

### Macroscopic Findings

These tumors are usually surrounded by a tough connective tissue capsule that intimately adheres to surrounding structures, making dissection extremely difficult (Fig. 5–97). The overlying skin is occasionally ulcerated. The size of the tumor varies. The color of the cut surfaces of the tumors ranges from red to grayish-white to yellowish-white; often, several combinations can be seen in different areas of the same tumor. Areas of hemorrhage and necrosis are common. The central part is usually cystic, whereas the periphery is firm. Rarely, specks of calcification or bone formation can be seen. The remarkable ability of this tumor to infiltrate the surrounding muscles, tendons, and adipose tissue should be borne in mind during gross examination of the tumor. In rare instances, the lesion is in contact with the periosteum of the underlying long bone.

### Microscopic Findings

A striking histologic feature is the nodular arrangement of the tumor (Fig. 5–98A to 5–98C). The nodules are quite cellular and contain both spindle and giant cells, frequently arranged in cords similar to those in fibrosarcoma. The nuclei in the spindle cells vary in shape, size, and staining quality, and frequently are hyperchromatic. Although the degree of cellular pleomorphism and the number of giant cells vary from field to field, there is uniform cellular morphology throughout the tumor. Tumor giant cells with multiple nuclei are most commonly seen in the fibrous part of the tumor. In some instances, 25 or more nuclei are present in a single giant cell. Mitoses are occasionally observed.

Bone formation can be seen in all parts of the tumor, and often a transformation zone from fibrous stroma can be demonstrated. Calcification of osteoid and fibrous tissue can also be observed at various sites in the lesion. Vascularity is not a marked feature, and frequently blood vessels are not seen in several sections. Malignant cells may invade and penetrate the capsule, extending into the surrounding tissue. However, invasion of blood vessels by tumor cells does not commonly occur.

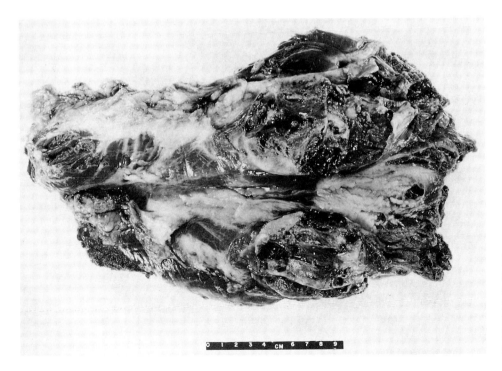

**Figure 5–97.** Cut section of extraskeletal osteosarcoma. The primary tumor was excised from the posterior thigh. Note the infiltrating quality of this tumor. Multiple muscle bundles have been infiltrated on the right. An area of hemorrhage is clearly visible on the upper right.

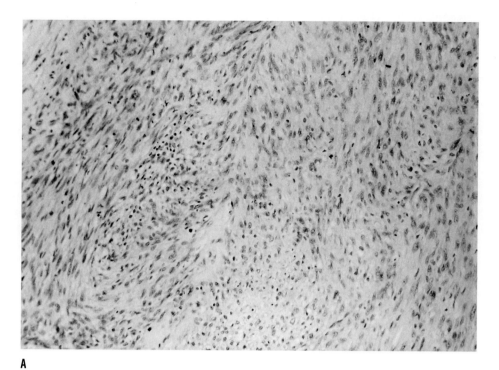

A

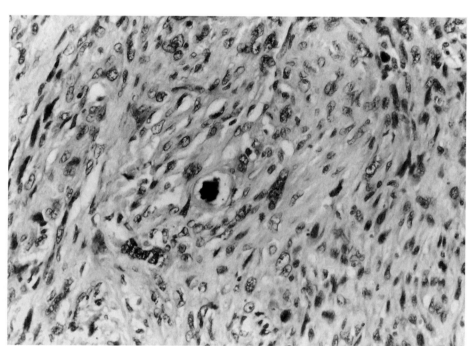

B

**Figure 5–98. (A)** Extraskeletal osteosarcoma. The tumor is highly cellular with scanty stroma, but arrangement resembles that of a fibrosarcoma. (H & E. Original magnification × 125.) **(B)** The nuclei of spindle cells are hyperchromatic, with giant cells and immature osteoid formation. (H & E. Original magnification × 125.) *(Continued.)*

## EXTRASKELETAL CHONDROSARCOMA

Malignant cartilaginous tumors not connected with bone are exceedingly rare (Fig. 5–99A to 5–99C). Stout and Verner[445] described seven cases. These tumors resemble chondrosarcomas of the bone, except that they frequently exhibit conspicuous areas of stellate and round cells set in a poorly differentiated myxomatous matrix, with relatively few foci of hyaline cartilage.[445–448] Enzinger and Shiraki[446] reviewed a series of 34 patients and, on the basis of their light microscopic findings, described the tumors as multinodular, consisting of small, uniform, rounded or elongated cells with a narrow eosinophilic cytoplasm. The cells are

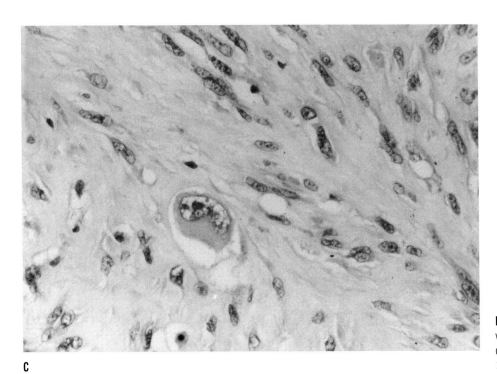

C

**Figure 5–98** *(continued)*. **(C)** High-power view, showing the profile of a malignant osteoblast. (H & E. Original magnification × 375.)

arranged in cords, strands, nests, or clusters. The myxoid ground substance stains deep red with mucicarmine, blue with alcian blue, and deep purple with aldehyde-fuchsin. These staining reactions are not altered by pretreatment with hyaluronidase.[446]

These tumors sometimes resemble myxoid liposarcomas, and careful histologic criteria must be used for a correct diagnosis.[446] Currently, these tumors are morphologically classified as extraskeletal myxoid chondrosarcoma and extraskeletal mesenchymal chondrosarcoma. It is generally agreed that the myxoid variety carries a better prognosis than the mesenchymal counterpart.

# ■ TUMORS AND TUMORLIKE CONDITIONS OF UNDETERMINED HISTOGENESIS

Although more variants of soft tissue tumors are being classified, several still have undefined histogenesis. In benign tumors or tumorlike conditions, the need for such classification is not acute, but in the malignant variety, further investigation is essential. For the present, all these tumors are classified into benign and malignant types as follows:

A. Benign Tumors
   1. Myxoma with all its variants
   2. Ossifying fibromyxoid tumors of the soft tissues
   3. Mesenchymoma
   4. Amyxoid tumors
B. Malignant Tumors
   1. Alveolar soft part sarcoma
   2. Malignant mesenchymoma
   3. Epithelioid sarcoma
   4. Malignant fibrous mesothelioma

## BENIGN TUMORS

### Myxoma

Myxomas are usually diagnosed by their gross appearance. The tumors are spheroidal in shape and, on cut section, show a glistening white matrix filled with abundant gelatinous mucoid material. The microscopic appearance is quite benign as well, with a few cells and a filigree of reticulin fibers.

***Intramuscular Myxomas.*** Intramuscular myxomas occur in all parts of the body, including the heart. These tumors vary from small subcutaneous tumors to large intermuscular types.[49,104] These tumors are composed of cells with elongated pyknotic nuclei and long graceful cytoplasmic processes (Fig. 5–100). The ground substance stains with alcian blue or mucicarmine stains, and the myxoid material can be digested by prior treatment with hyaluronidase.

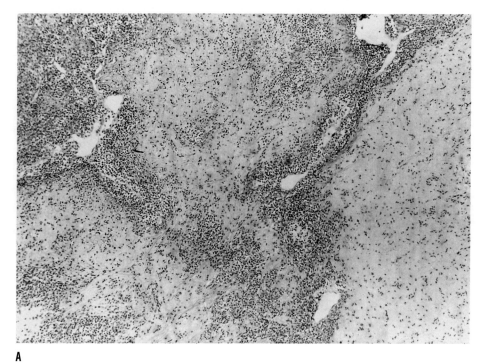

A

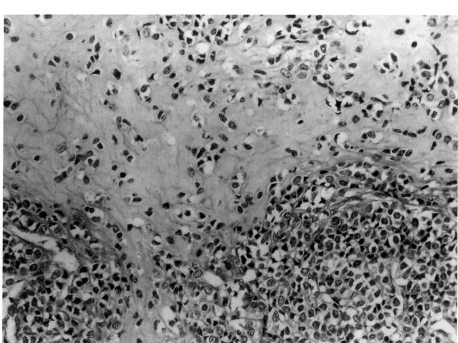

B

**Figure 5–99. (A)** Uniform distribution of homogenous undifferentiated mesenchymal cells and chondrocytes. (H & E. Original magnification × 65.) **(B)** Most malignant mesenchymal cells are either oval or spindle-shaped, intimately interspersed with pleomorphic clumped chondrocytes. (H & E. Original magnification × 250. *(Continued.)*

## Benign Mesenchymoma

Benign mesenchymomas are circumscribed rare tumors usually encountered in the region of the kidney and perirenal tissue,[104] although they can occur elsewhere in the body.[104] These tumors are composed of a mixture of mesenchymal tissues and fibrous tissue.

They are recognizable by the haphazard distribution of adipose tissue, smooth muscle cells, and blood vessels (Fig. 5–101). They tend to locally infiltrate, thereby giving a false impression of malignancy.

There are other benign tumors (e.g., ossifying fibromyxoid tumors, amyxoid tumors of the soft tis-

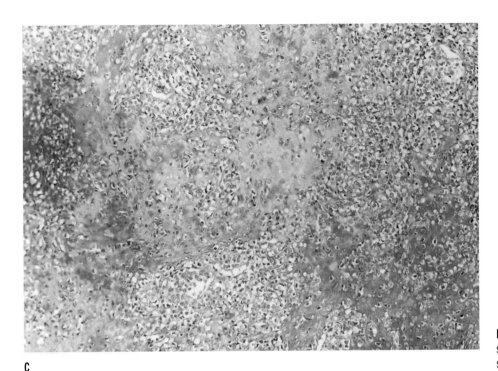

C

**Figure 5–99** *(continued).* **(C)** Alcian blue stain showing the myxoid ground substance. (Original magnification × 125.)

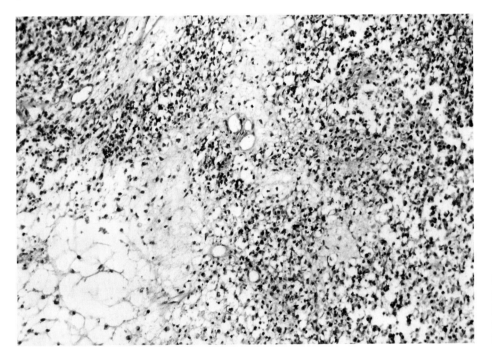

**Figure 5–100.** Intramuscular myxoma; note the fibrillar stellate cells with long fibrillar processes in a mucopolysaccharide-rich stroma. (H & E. Original magnification × 65.)

sues). These are invariably benign and for all practical purposes are variants of benign mesenchymoma and should be treated as such.

## MALIGNANT TUMORS

### Alveolar Soft Part Sarcoma

One group of sarcomas of undetermined histogenesis is the alveolar soft tissue sarcoma, first described by

Christopherson, Foote, and Stewart in 1952.[449] Characteristically, these slow-growing but definitely malignant tumors are found in young adults, more often in women. In 1951, Smetana and Scott[450] described a group of 14 similar cases with a distinctive organized pattern resembling that of a carotid body neoplasm. They considered this tumor to be homologous to bronchial chemodectomas and called them *malignant nonchromaffin paragangliomas.* Since then, lesions of

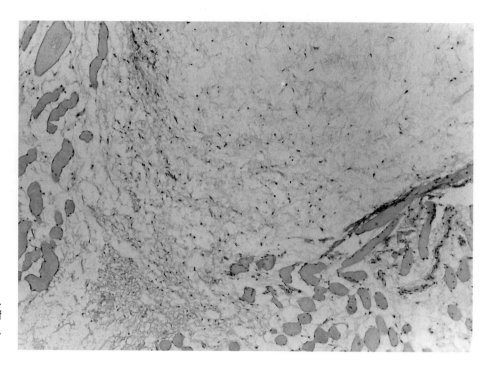

**Figure 5–101.** Benign mesenchymoma. Haphazard distribution of various types of mesenchymal cells can be easily recognized. (H & E. Original magnification × 125.)

identical appearance with organized structures have been reported by other authors.[451,452] Although there is disagreement concerning the histogenesis and consequently the taxonomy and terminology, there is no doubt that these tumors have a distinctive histologic appearance and constitute a rare group of malignant tumors.

***Light Microscopy.***    The organized endocrinelike pattern is striking and uniform. The tumor cells are arranged in round or cordlike discrete groups bound by collagen fibers (Fig. 5–102A and 5–102B). The individual cells are rounded and contain distinctive granules in the cytoplasm. These granules are always diastasis-resistant and PAS-positive.

***Electron Microscopy.***    Shipkey and associates[453] showed unique cytoplasmic crystals in cellular components by electron microscopy examination. These crystals in osmium tetroxide fixed tissue show a lattice pattern.[454,455]

Ultrastructurally, the nuclei exhibit a moderate amount of chromatin and usually contain a solitary nucleolus. The mitochondria tend to be arranged in clusters, frequently separated from one another by strands of close endoplasmic reticulum. The Golgi structures are well developed. All tumor cells contain a varying number of intracytoplasmic crystalline inclusion exhibiting a variety of geometric configuration. These are, for the most part, bound by a solitary limiting membrane. This structure is comprised of parallel laminary filamentous material measuring 36 to 90 Å in thickness and arranged in the periodicity of 58–100 Å. In some cross-grade arrangements, square filamentous arrays are evident (Fig. 5–102C).

Fischer and Reidbord[454] compared the ultrastructural features of the alveolar soft part sarcoma with those of granular cells of myoblastoma, melanoma, carotid body tumor, and alveolar rhabdomyosarcoma. They found sufficient cytomorphologic evidence at the ultrastructural level to consider this tumor a unique type of rhabdomyosarcoma. Obviously, until this histogenetic controversy is resolved, these tumors will remain histogenetically unclassified. Welsh and coauthors[455] in 1972 argued that, while the alveolar soft part sarcoma and nonchromaffin paraganglioma shared a close homology and thus are of related histogenesis, they are different entities. They further argued that malignant granular cell myoblastoma exhibits structural difference to such extent that it is completely unrelated. Unni and Soule[456] have confirmed the observation of Welsh and his associates.

***Immunohistochemistry.***    Alveolar soft part sarcomas do not stain with antibodies against cytokeratin, EMA,

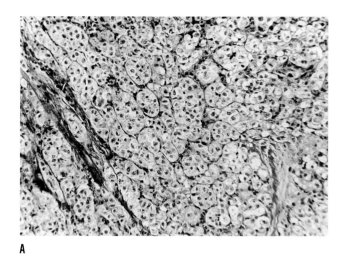

A

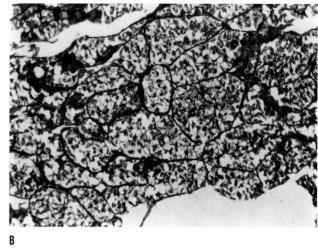

B

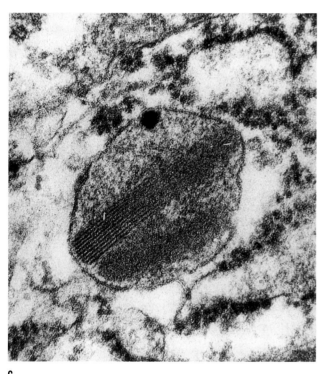

C

**Figure 5–102. (A)** Alveolar soft part sarcoma. The discrete rounded arrangement (organoid) is obvious. (H & E. Original magnification × 125.) **(B)** Reticulin stain clearly showing the organoid pattern. (Original magnification × 125.) **(C)** The classical intracytoplasmic, crystalline, membrane-bound inclusion. Note the parallel laminary filament. (Original magnification × 45,600.)

GFAB, neurofilament serotonin, and neuron-specific enolase.[457,458] However, most can be stained with vimentin, muscle-specific actin, desmin, and, rarely, S-100.

## Epithelioid Sarcoma

Epithelioid sarcoma is an unusual tumor that is often confused histologically with several other neoplasms, including malignant melanoma, granuloma-tous lesions, and, occasionally, metastatic adenocarcinoma.[112,459–464] In 1970, Enzinger[461] analyzed 62 cases and named this entity *epithelioid sarcoma.* This descriptive term is now generally accepted.

Epithelioid sarcoma is commonly seen as a subfascial or subcutaneous lesion, usually originating in the extremities. Infrequently, it occurs in the trunk and scalp, and two cases have been reported arising in the penile shaft.[465]

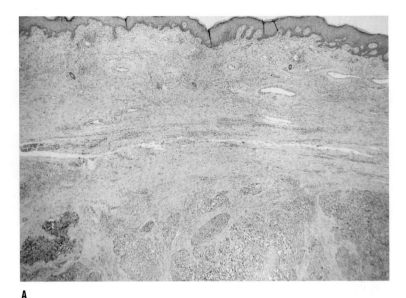

A

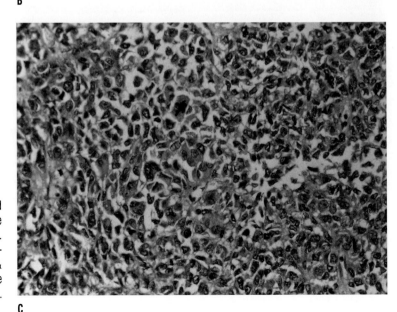

B

C

**Figure 5–103.** Epithelioid sarcoma. **(A)** The tumor is located close to the skin. (H & E. Original magnification × 25.) **(B)** The microscopic architecture is clear in a relatively high-power view. The tumor is composed of clusters of clear oval cells with central necrosis. The necrosis is obvious in the cluster at left. (H & E. Original magnification × 40.) **(C)** High-power view, same area, showing pleomorphic nuclei and abnormal mitosis. (H & E. Original magnification × 250.)

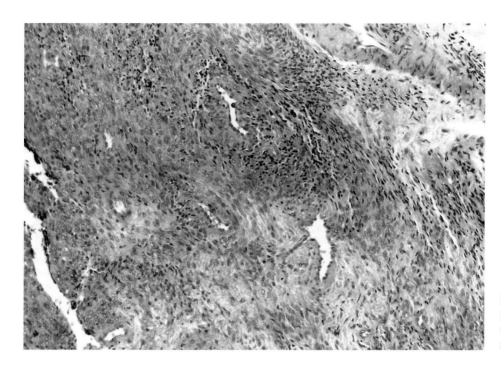

**Figure 5–104.** A malignant mesenchymoma showing the characteristics of a number of cell types. (H & E. Original magnification × 125.)

***Macroscopic Findings.*** The appearance of these tumors varies according to their location. When they occur in the vicinity of a tendon near a joint, multiple nodular tumors along the course of the tendon sheath are observed. When located deep in the subcutaneous tissue, there is no characteristic feature other than a relatively diffuse tumor.

***Light Microscopy.*** The microscopic appearance of these lesions has been well described by Enzinger,[461] Santiago et al.,[466] Gabbiani et al.,[467] and Pratt et al.[459] (Fig. 5–103A to 5–103C). In general, the histologic appearance of epithelioid sarcomas can be divided into the following five types: (1) granulomatous, (2) pseudocarcinomatous, (3) melanomalike, (4) angiosarcomatous, and (5) undifferentiated sarcomatous pattern. Either all or most of these features can be seen in different areas of a given tumor. Santiago and associates[466] suggested that the angiosarcomatous pattern probably represents a fixation artifact. Cytologically, the tumor cells are large, round, or polygonal, with abundant eosinophilic cytoplasm and round or oval nuclei with prominent nucleoli. Poorly differentiated spindle cells with collagenous ground substance are interspersed throughout the tumor.

***Electron Microscopy.*** Ultrastructural studies of these tumors have been published by Enzinger,[461] Gabbiani et al.,[467] Frable et al.,[468] and by Bloustein and associates.[469] These tumors consist of epithelial-like cells similar to those found in normal synovial membrane,[375] synovial sarcoma,[383,388] and clear cell sarcomas of the tendon sheaths and aponeurosis.[325]

## Malignant Mesenchymoma

*Malignant mesenchymoma* is a descriptive term applied to those soft tissue sarcomas in which there are two or more unrelated malignant elements (Fig. 5–104). In the past, the term was frequently used for tumors with extreme pleomorphism. Today, this diagnosis is seldom rendered.

## Malignant Fibrous Mesothelioma

Several acceptable cases have been recorded, primarily in the pleura[104,189,470] and the peritoneum.[190,471] In recent years, the association of asbestos exposure and pleural mesotheliomas has generated considerable interest in these tumors, but, because of their rarity and their anatomic location, they are seldom treated as malignant fibrous tissue tumors.

Tumors arising in relation to serous surfaces show either a predominantly spindle cell or epithelial cell appearance. The two cell types can be found together (as in synovial cell sarcoma) or can be distributed in separate areas of a given tumor. Thus, some areas resemble spindle cell fibrosarcoma and some show other mesenchymal characteristics. The cytoplasm of the epithelial cells is basophilic, and mitosis is seldom encountered.

## REFERENCES

1. Lazarus SS, Med S, Trombetta LD: Ultrastructural identification of a benign perineurial cell tumor. Cancer 41: 1823, 1978
2. Feiner H, Kaye GI: Ultrastructural evidence of myofibroblasts in circumscribed fibromatosis. Arch Pathol 100:265, 1976
3. Napolitano LM: Observations on the fine structure of adipose cells. Ann N Y Acad Sci 137:34, 1965
4. Zimmerman LE, Font RL, Ts'o MOM, Fine BS: Application of electron microscopy to histopathologic diagnosis. Trans Am Acad Ophthalmol Otolaryngol 76:101, 1972
5. Fisher ER, Wechsler H: Granular cell myoblastoma—A misnomer: Electron microscopic and histochemical evidence concerning its Schwann cell derivation and nature (granular cell schwannoma). Cancer 13:936, 1962
6. Scarpelli DG, Greider MH: A correlative cytochemical and electron microscopic study of a liposarcoma. Cancer 15:776, 1962
7. Nystrom SHM: Electron microscopical structure of the wall of small blood vessels in human multiforme glioblastoma. Nature 184:65, 1959
8. DeRobertis E, Setelo JR: Electron microscope study of cultured nervous tissue. Exp Cell Res 3(suppl 2):433, 1952
9. Venkatachalam MA, Greally JG: Fine structure of glomus tumor: Similarity of glomus cells to smooth muscle. Cancer 23:1176, 1969
10. Keith A: Human Embryology and Morphology, 6th ed. London, Edward Arnold and Company, 1948
11. Rasmussen AT: The so-called hibernating gland. J Morphol 38:147, 1923
12. Flemming W: Weitere Mittheilungen zur Physiologie der Fettzelle. Arch Mikr Anat 7:328, 1871
13. Clark ER, Clark EL: Microscopic studies of the new formation of fat in living adult rabbits. Am J Anat 67:255, 1940
14. Toldt C: Lehubuch der Gewebelehre mit voraugsweiser Berucksichtingung des menschlichen Korpers, 3rd ed. Stuttgart, F Enke, 1888, p 724
15. Wasserman E: The concept of the "fat organ." In Rodahl K, Issekutz B (eds): Fat As a Tissue, Symposium Monograph. New York, McGraw-Hill, 1962, p 22
16. Dabelow A: Anat Anz, Erg Heft Band 104, Verh Anat Ge, 54 Vers, Frieburg I Br 1957, p 83
17. Napolitano LM: The differentiation of white adipose cells. An electron microscope study. Cell Biol 18:663, 1963
18. Sidman RL: Adipose tissue. In Willmer EN (ed): Cells and Tissues in Culture, Methods, Biology and Physiology, vol. 2. New York and London, Academic Press, 1965
19. Thomas LW: The chemical composition of adipose tissue of man and mice. Quart J Exp Physiol 47:179, 1962
20. Hellman B, Hellerstrom C: Cell renewal in the white and brown fat tissue of the rat. Acta Pathol Microbiol Scand 51:347, 1961
21. Sheldon H: The fine structure of the fat cell. In Rodahl K, Issekutz B (eds): Fat As a Tissue, Symposium Monograph. New York, McGraw-Hill, 1962
22. Hammar JA: Zur Kenntniss de Fettgewebes. Arch Mikr Anat 45:512, 1902
23. Johanason L, Soderlund S: Intrathoracic lipoma. Acta Chir Scand 126:558, 1963
24. Sidman RL: Adipose tissue. In Willmer EN (ed): Cells and Tissues in Culture, Methods, Biology and Physiology, vol 2. New York and London, Academic Press, 1965
25. Toldt C: Lehubuch der Gewebelehre mit voraugsweiser Berucksichtingung des menschlichen Korpers, 3rd ed. Stuttgart, F Enke, 1888, p 724
26. Napolitano LM: Observations on the fine structure of adipose cells. Ann N Y Acad Sci 137:34 1965
27. Dawkins MJR, Duckett S, Pearse AGE: Localization of catecholamines in brown fat. Nature 209:1144, 1966
28. Wirsen C, Hamberger B: Catecholamines in brown fat. Nature 214:625, 1967
29. Romer TE: Corticosteroids in brown fat by a histochemical method. J Histochem 12:646, 1964
30. Dionne GP, Seemayer TA: Infiltrating lipomas and angiolipomas revisited. Cancer 33:732, 1974
31. Enzinger FM, Harvey DA: Spindle cell lipoma. Cancer 36:1852, 1975
32. Kindblom L-G, Angervall L, Stener B, Wickbom I: Intermuscular and intramuscular lipomas and hibernomas. Cancer 33:754, 1974
33. Rasanen O, Nohteri H, Dammert K: Angiolipoma and lipoma. Acta Chir Scand 133:461, 1967
34. Weller RO, Baylis OB, Abdulla YH, Adams CWM: The electron histochemical demonstration of phosphoglyceride. J Histochem Cytochem 13:690, 1965
35. Gellhorn A, Marks PA: The composition and biosynthesis of lipids in human adipose tissues. J Clin Invest 40: 925, 1961
36. Wright CJE: Liposarcoma arising in a single lipoma. J Pathol Bacteriol 60:483, 1948
37. Stout AP: Liposarcoma—Malignant tumor of lipoblasts. Ann Surg 119:86, 1944
38. Sternberg SS: Liposarcoma arising within a subcutaneous lipoma. Cancer 5:975, 1952
39. Sampson CC, Saunders EH, Gree WE, Larey JR: Liposarcoma developing in a lipoma. Arch Pathol 69:506, 1968
40. Jaffe RH: Recurrent lipomatous tumor of the groin. Arch Pathol 1:381, 1926
41. Vellios F, Baez JM, Shumacker HB: Lipoblastomatosis: A tumor of fetal fat different from hibernoma. Report of a case, with observations of the embryogenesis of human adipose tissue. Am J Pathol 54:1149, 1958
42. Shear M: Lipoblastomatosis of the cheek. Br J Oral Surg 5:173, 1967
43. Chung EB, Enzinger FM: Benign lipoblastomatosis: An analysis of 35 cases. Cancer 32:482, 1975
44. Willis RA: The Pathology of the Tumours of Children. Pathological Monographs II. Edinburgh, Oliver and Boyd, 1962, p 100
45. Kindblom LG, Angervall L, Fassina AS: Atypical liposarcoma. Acta Pathol Microbiol Scand 90A:27, 1982
46. Evans HL: Liposarcomas and atypical lipomatous tu-

mors: A study of 66 cases followed for a minimum of 10 years. Surg Pathol 1:41, 1988

47. Evans HL: Liposarcoma: A study of 55 cases with a reassessment of its classification. Am J Surg Pathol 3:507, 1979

48. Brooks JJ, Conner AM: Atypical lipoma of the extremities and peripheral soft tissues with dedifferentiation: Implications for management. Surg Pathol 3:169, 1990

49. Pack GT, Ariel IA: Tumors of the Soft Somatic Tissue: A Clinical Treatise. NY, Hoeber-Harper, 1958

50. Virchow R: Edin fall von bosartigen: Zum Thiel in der Form des neurons auftretende Fettgeschwulsten. Virchows Arch Pathol Anat 11:281, 1857

51. De Weed JH, Dockery MD: Lipomatous retroperitoneal tumors. Am J Surg 84:397, 1952

52. Enzinger FM, Winslow DJ: Liposarcoma: A study of 103 cases. Virchows Arch Pathol Anat 335:367, 1962

53. Pack GT, Pierson JC: Liposarcoma: A study of 105 cases. Surgery 36:687, 1954

54. Reszel PA, Soule EH, Coventry MB: Liposarcoma of the extremities and limb girdles. J Bone Joint Surg 48A:229, 1966

55. Enterline HT, Culberson JD, Rochlin DB, Brady LW: Liposarcoma: A clinical and pathological study of 53 cases. Cancer 13:932, 1960

56. Das Gupta TK: Tumors and Tumorlike Conditions of the Adipose Tissue. Current Problems in Surgery. Chicago, Year Book, March, 1970

57. Delamater J: Mammoth tumor. Cleveland Gaz 1:31, 1859

58. Ewing J: Neoplastic Diseases, 4th ed. Philadelphia, Saunders, 1940

59. Enzinger FM, Weiss SW, eds.: Soft Tissue Tumors, Chap. 10, St. Louis, CV Mosby, 1983, p 250

60. Elgar F, Goldblum JR: Well-differentiated liposarcoma of the retroperitoneum: A clinicopathologic analysis of 20 cases, with particular attention to the extent of low-grade dedifferentiation. Mod Pathol 10:113, 1997

61. Kauffman SL, Stout AP: Lipoblastic tumors of children. Cancer 12:912, 1959

62. Eneroth M, Mandahl N, Heim S, et al.: Localization of the chromosomal breakpoints of the t(12;16) in liposarcoma to subbands 12q13.3 and 16p11.2 Cancer Genet Cytogenet 48:101, 1990

63. Sreekantaiah C, Karakousis CP, Leong SPL, et al.: Cytogenetic findings in liposarcoma correlate with histopathologic subtypes. Cancer 69:2484, 1992

64. Turc-Carel C, Limon J, Dal Cin P, et al.: Cytogenetic studies of adipose tissue tumors. II. Recurrent reciprocal translocation t(12;16)(q13;p11) in myxoid liposarcomas. Cancer Genet Cytogenet 23:291, 1986

65. Karakousis CP, Dal Cin P, Turc-Carel C, et al.: Chromosomal changes in soft-tissue tumors. Arch Surg 122:1257, 1987

66. Dal Cin P, Kools P, Sciot R, et al.: Cytogenetic and fluorescent in situ hybridization investigation of ring chromosomes characterizing a specific pathologic subgroup of adipose tissue tumors. Cancer Genet Cytogenet 58:85, 1993

67. Fletcher CD, Akerman M, Dal Cin P, et al.: Correlations between clinicopathological features and karyotype in lipomatous tumors: A report of 178 cases from the chromosomes and morphology (CHAMP) collaborative study group. Am J Pathol 148:623, 1996

68. Jennings RC, Behr G: Hibernoma (granular cell lipoma). J Clin Pathol 8:4310, 1955

69. Mesara BW, Batsakis JG: Hibernoma of the neck. Arch Otolaryngol 85:95, 1967

70. Alvine G, Rosenthal H, Murphey M, Huntrakoon M: Hibernoma. Skeletal Radiol 25:493, 1996

71. Brines OA, Johnson MH: Hibernoma: A special fatty tumor. Am J Pathol 25:467, 1949

72. Symmens D: Spindle and giant cell sarcoma arising from unidentified precordial bodies. Arch Pathol 37:180, 1944

73. Catchpole HR: Connective tissue: Capillary permeability. In Zweifach BW, Grant L, McCluskey RT (eds): The Inflammatory Process, vol. 2, 2nd ed. New York, Academic Press, 1973

74. Movat HZ, Fernando NVP: The fine structure of connective tissue. 1. The fibroblast. Exp Mol Pathol 1:509, 1962

75. Kulonen E, Pikkarainen J (eds): Biology of Fibroblast. New York, Academic Press, 1973

76. Daniel MR, Glauert AM, Dingle JT, Lucy JA: The action of vitamin A (retinol) on the fine structure of rat dermal fibroblasts in culture. Strangeways Res Lab Rep, 1965, p 13

77. Davis R, James DW: Electron microscopic appearance of close relationships between adult guinea-pig fibroblasts in tissue culture. Nature 194:695, 1962

78. Fitton Jackson S: Connective tissue cells. In Urachet J, Mirsky AE (eds): The Cell, vol. 6. New York, Academic Press, 1964

79. Ramachandran GN (ed): Treatise on Collagen, vol. 1, Chemistry of Collagen. New York, Academic Press, 1967

80. Gross J: Collagen biology, structure, degradation and disease. Harvey Lect 68:351, 1974

81. Gallop PM, Paz MA: Post-translational protein modifications, with special attention to collagen and elastin. Physiol Rev 55:418, 1975

82. Cameron DA: The fine structure of osteoblasts in the metaphysis of the tibia of the young rat. J Biophys Biochem Cytol 9:883, 1961

83. Bornstein P, Piez KA: Collagen: Structural studies based on the cleavage of methionyl bonds. Science 143:1353, 1965

84. Bornstein P: The biosynthesis of collagen. Ann Rev Biochem 143:567, 1974

85. Goldberg B, Sherr CJ: Secretion and extracellular processing of procollagen by cultured human fibroblasts. Proc Natl Acad Sci 70:361, 1973

86. Gross J: The behavior of collagen units as model in morphogenesis. J Biophys Biochem Cytol 2(suppl):261, 1956

87. Doyle BB, Hukins DWL, Hulmes DJS, et al.: Collagen polymorphism: Its origins in the amino acid sequence. J Mol Biol 91:79, 1975

88. Veis A, Brownell AG: Collagen biosynthesis. Crit Rev Biochem 2:417, 1975

89. Nakajima Y, Miyazono K, Kato M, et al.: Extracellular fibrillar structure of latent TGF beta binding protein-1: Role in TGF beta-dependent endothelial mesenchymal transformation during endocardial cushion tissue formation in mouse embryonic heart. J Cell Biol 136:193, 1997

90. Ross R, Bornstein P: Elastic fibers in the body. Sci Am 224:44, 1971

91. Balazs EA (ed): Chemistry and Molecular Biology of the Intercellular Matrix, vol. 2: Glycosaminoglycans and Proteoglycans; vol. 3: Structural Organization and Function of the Matrix. New York, Academic Press, 1970

92. Kefalides NA: Comparative biochemistry of mammalian basement membranes. In Balazs EA (ed): Chemistry and Molecular Biology of the Intercellular Matrix, vol. 1. New York, Academic Press, 1970, p 553

93. Wallon UM, Overall CM: The hemopexin-like domain (C domain) of human gelatinase A (Matrix metalloproteinase-2) requires Ca2+ for fibronectin and heparin binding. Binding properties of recombinant gelatinase A C domain to extracellular matrix and basement membrane components. J Biol Chem 272:7473, 1997

94. Chaudhuri PK, Walker MJ, Beattie CW, Das Gupta TK: Presence of steroid receptors in human soft-tissue sarcomas of diverse histological origin. Cancer Res 40:861, 1980

95. Dodson JW, Hay ED: Secretion of collagen by corneal epithelium. II. Effect of the underlying substratum on secretion and polymerization of epithelial cell products. J Exp Zool 189:51, 1974

96. Gospodarowicz D, Greenburg G, Birdwell CR: Determination of cellular shape by the extracellular matrix and its correlation with control of cellular growth. Cancer Res 38:4155, 1978

97. Cohen M, Tayler JM: Epidermal growth factor chemical and biological characterization. Recent Prog Horm Res 30:533, 1974

98. Pandit SD, O'Hare T, Donis-Keller H, Pike LJ: Functional characterization of an epidermal growth factor receptor/RET chimera. J Biol Chem 272:2199, 1997

99. Coffey RJ, Hawkey CJ, Damstrup L, et al.: Epidermal growth factor receptor activation induces nuclear targeting of cyclooxygenase-2, basolateral release of prostaglandins, and mitogenesis in polarizing colon cancer cells. Proc Natl Acad Sci U S A 94:657, 1997

100. Zheng JL, Helbig C, Gao WQ: Induction of cell proliferation by fibroblasts and insulin-like growth factors in pure rat inner ear epithelial cell cultures. J Neurosci 17:216, 1997

101. Hernandez-Sanchez C, Werner H, Roberts CT Jr.: Differential regulation of insulin-like growth factor-I (IGF-I) receptor gene expression by IGF-I and basic fibroblastic growth factor. J Biol Chem 272:4663, 1997

102. Zhou Z, Zuber ME, Burrus LW, Olwin BB: Identification and characterization of a fibroblast growth factor (FGF) binding domain in the cysteine-rich FGF receptor. J Biol Chem 272:5167, 1997

103. Agocha A, Sigel AV, Eghbali-Webb M: Characterization of adult human heart fibroblasts in culture: A comparative study of growth proliferation and collagen production in human and rabbit cardiac fibroblasts and their response to transforming growth factor-beta1. Cell Tissue Res 288:87, 1997

104. Stout AP, Lattes R: Tumors of the Soft Tissues. In Firminger HI (ed): Atlas of Tumor Pathology. Sect. 2, Fasc 2. Washington D.C., AFIP, 1967

105. Pulitzer DR, Martin PC, Reed RJ: Fibroma of tendon sheath: A clinicopathologic study of 33 cases. Am J Surg Pathol 13:472, 1989

106. Stout AP: The fibromatoses. Clin Orthop 19:11, 1961

107. Konwaler BE, Keasbey L, Kaplan L: Subcutaneous pseudosarcomatous fibromatosis (fascitis). Am J Clin Pathol 25:241, 1955

108. Chung EB, Enzinger FM: Proliferative fascitis. Cancer 36:1450, 1975

109. Culbertson JD, Enterline HT: Pseudosarcomatous fascitis: A clinicopathological entity. Report of three cases. Ann Surg 151:235, 1960

110. Hutter RVP, Stewart FW, Foote FW: Fascitis: A report of 70 cases with follow-up proving benignity of the lesion. Cancer 15:992, 1962

111. Kauffman SL, Stout AP: Histiocytic tumors (fibrous xanthoma and histiocytoma) in children. Cancer 14:469, 1961

112. Keasbey LE: Juvenile aponeurotic fibroma (calcifying fibroma). A distinctive tumor arising in the palms and soles of young children. Cancer 6:338, 1953

113. Lichtenstein L, Goldman RL: Cartilage tumors in soft tissues, particularly in the hand and foot. Cancer 17:1203, 1964

114. Jarvi OH, Saxen AK, Hopsu-Havu VK, et al.: Elastofibroma—A degenerative pseudotumor. Cancer 23:42, 1969

115. Naylor MF, Nascimento AG, Sherrick AD, McLeod RA: Elastofibroma dorsi: Radiologic findings in 12 patients. Am J Roentgenol 167:683, 1996

116. Bennet JH: On cancerous and cancroid growths. Edinburgh, Southerland & Knox, 1849, p 176

117. Müller J: Uber den feinern Bau und die Formen der Krankhaften Greschwiilste. Berlin, Reimer, 1838, p 80

118. Stout AP: Fibrosarcoma, well-differentiated (aggressive fibromatosis). Cancer 7:953, 1954

119. Rock MG, Pritchard DJ, Reiman HM et al.: Extra-abdominal desmoid tumors. J Bone Joint Surg 66A:1369, 1984

120. Mitchison MJ: The pathology of idiopathic retroperitoneal fibrosis. J Clin Pathol 23:681, 1970

121. Ackerman LV: Extraosseus localized non-neoplasm bone and cartilage formation (so-called myositis ossificans): Clinical and pathological confusion with malignant neoplasms. J Bone Joint Surg 40A:279, 1958

122. Norman A, Dorfman HD: Juxtacortical circumscribed myositis ossificans: Evaluation and radiographic features. Radiology 96:301, 1970

123. Kramsdorf MJ, Meis JM, Jelinek JS: Myositis ossificans MR appearance with radiologic pathologic correlation. Am J Roentgenol 157:1243, 1991

124. Enzinger FM, Weiss SW (eds): Soft Tissue Tumors, 3rd ed., Chap. 35, St. Louis, Mosby-Yearbook, 1995, p 1013

125. Manual for Staging of Cancer. Chicago, American Joint

Committee for Cancer Staging and End Result Reporting, 1978

126. Pritchard DJ, Soule EH, Taylor WF, Ivins JC: Fibrosarcoma: A clinicopathological and statistical study of 199 tumors of the soft tissue and trunk. Cancer 33:888, 1974

127. Soule EH, Geitz M, Henderson ED: Embryonal rhabdomyosarcoma of the limbs and limb girdles. Cancer 23:1336, 1969

128. Suit HD, Russell WD, Martin RG: Sarcoma of soft tissue: Clinical and histopathological parameters and response to treatment. Cancer 35:1978, 1975

129. Werf-Messing BV, Van Unnik JAM: Fibrosarcoma of the soft parts. Cancer 18:1113, 1965

130. Fleming RM, Rezek PR: Sarcoma developing in old burn scar. Am J Surg 54:457, 1941

131. Pack GT, Ariel IM: Fibrosarcoma of the soft somatic tissue: A clinical and pathological study. Surgery 31:443, 1952

132. Andersen DH: Tumors of infancy and childhood: A survey of those seen in the pathology laboratory of the Babies Hospital during the years 1935–1950. Cancer 4:890, 1951

133. Dahl I, Angervall L, Save-Suderbergh J: Atypical fibroblastic tumors in early infancy. Acta Pathol Microbiol Scand 81A:224, 1973

134. Adam LR, Davison EV, Malcolm AJ, et al.: Cytogenetic analysis of a congenital fibrosarcoma. Cancer Genet Cytogenet 52:37, 1991

135. Dal Cin P, Brock P, Casteels-Van Daele M, et al.: Cytogenetic characterization of congenital or infantile fibrosarcoma. Eur J Pediatr 150:579, 1991

136. Schofield DE, Fletcher JA, Grier HE, et al.: Fibrosarcoma in infants and children: Application of new techniques. Am J Surg Pathol 18:14, 1994

137. Dal Cin P, Sciot R, Aly MS, et al.: Some desmoid tumors are characterized by trisomy 8. Genes Chromosom Cancer 10:131, 1994

138. Naeem R, Fletcher JA: Trisomy 8 is a potential marker of high risk in desmoid tumors. Am J Hum Genet 51:A279, 1992

139. Scrable J, Witte D, Shimada H, et al.: Molecular differential pathology of rhabdomyosarcoma. Genes Chromosom Cancer 1:23, 1989

140. Fitzpatrick TB, Gilchrest BA: Dimple sign to differentiate benign from malignant cutaneous lesion. N Engl J Med 296:1518, 1977

141. Fletcher CD: Benign fibrous histiocytoma of subcutaneous tissue and deep soft tissue: A clinicopathological analysis of 21 cases. Am J Surg Pathol 14:801, 1990

142. Bourne RG: Paradoxical fibrosarcoma of the skin (pseudosarcoma): A review of 13 cases. Med J Aust 50(1):504, 1963

143. Finlay-Jones LR, Nicol P, Ten Seldam REJ: Pseudosarcoma of the skin. Pathology 3:215, 1971

144. Woyke S, Domagala W, Olszewski W, Korabiec M: Pseudosarcoma of the skin. An electron microscopic study and comparison with the fine structure of the spindle-cell variant of squamous carcinoma. Cancer 33:970, 1974

145. Taylor RW: Sarcomatous tumors resembling in some respects keloid. J Cutan Genitourin Dis 8:384, 1890

146. Stout AP: Fibrosarcoma: The malignant tumors of fibroblasts. Cancer 1:30, 1948

147. Taylor HH, Helwig EB: Dermatofibrosarcoma protuberans. Cancer 15:717, 1962

148. O'Brien JE, Stout AP: Malignant fibrous xanthomas. Cancer 17:1445, 1964

149. Penner DW: Metastasizing dermatofibrosarcoma protuberans. Cancer 4:1083, 1951

150. McPeak CJ, Cruz T, Nicastri AD: Dermatofibrosarcoma protuberans: An analysis of 86 cases—Five with metastasis. Ann Surg 166:805, 1967

151. Bednar B: Storiform neurofibroma in core of a naevocellular nevi. J Pathol 101:199, 1970

152. Dupree WB, Langless JM, Weiss SW: Pigmented dermatofibrosarcoma protuberans (Bednar tumor): A pathologic, ultrastructural and immunohistochemical study. Am J Pathol 9:630, 1985

153. Leu HJK, Malik M: Angiomatoid malignant fibrous histiocytoma. Arch Pathol Lab Med 110:2010, 1997

154. Sun CC, Toker C, Brietniker R: An ultrastructural study of angiomatoid fibrous histiocytoma. Cancer 40:2013, 1982

155. Enzinger FM, Weiss SW (eds): Soft Tissue Tumors, 3rd ed., Chap. 14, St. Louis, Mosby-Yearbook, 1995, p 325

156. Costa MJ, Weiss SW: Angiomatoid malignant fibrous histiocytoma: A follow-up study of 108 cases with evaluation of possible histologic predictors of outcome. Am J Surg Pathol 14:1126, 1990

157. Ozzello L, Stout AP, Murray MR: Cultural characteristics of malignant histiocytomas and fibrous xanthomas. Cancer 16:331, 1963

158. Dehner LP: Malignant fibrous histiocytoma: Non-specific morphologic pattern, specific pathologic entity, or both? (editorial) Arch Pathol Lab Med 112:236, 1988

159. Wood GS, Beckstead JH, Turner RR, et al.: Malignant fibrous histiocytoma tumor cells resemble fibroblasts. Am J Surg Pathol 10:323, 1986

160. Kempson RL, Kyriakos M: Fibroxanthosarcoma of the soft tissues: A type of malignant fibrous histiocytoma. Cancer 29:961, 1972

161. Kyriakos M, Kempson RL: Inflammatory fibrous histiocytoma: An aggressive and lethal lesion. Cancer 37:1584, 1976

162. Weiss SW, Enzinger FM: Myxoid variant of malignant fibrous histiocytoma. Cancer 39:1672, 1977

163. Hajdu SI, Shiu MH, Fortner JG: Tenosynovial sarcoma: A clinicopathological study of 136 cases. Cancer 39:1201, 1977

164. Weiss SW, Enzinger FM: Malignant fibrous histiocytoma: An analysis of 200 cases. Cancer 41:2250, 1978

165. Fu YS, Gabbiani G, Kaye GI, Lattes R: Malignant soft tissue tumors of probable histiocyte origin (malignant fibrous histiocytomas): General considerations and electron microscopic and tissue culture studies. Cancer 35:176, 1975

166. Enzinger FM, Weiss SW (eds): Soft Tissue Tumor, 3rd ed., Chap. 15. St. Louis, Mosby-Yearbook, 1995, p 351

167. Weiss SW, Enzinger FM: Malignant fibrous histiocytoma. An analysis of 200 cases. Cancer 41:2250, 1978

168. Fletcher CD: Pleomorphic malignant fibrous histiocy-

toma: Fact or fiction? A critical re-appraisal based on 159 tumors diagnosed as pleomorphic sarcoma. Am J Surg Pathol 16:213, 1992

169. Roholl PJ, Prinsen I, Rademakers LP, et al.: Two lines with epithelial cell-like characteristic established from malignant fibrous histiocytomas. Cancer 68:1963, 1991

170. Binder SW, Said JW, Shintaku IP, et al.: A histiocyte-specific marker in the diagnosis of malignant fibrous histiocytoma: Use of monoclonal antibody KP-1 (CD-68). Am J Clin Pathol 97:759, 1992

171. Kahn LB: Retroperitoneal xanthogranuloma and xanthosarcoma (malignant fibrous xanthoma). Cancer 31:411, 1973

172. Rosas-Uribe A, Ring AM, Rappaport H: Metastasizing retroperitoneal fibroxanthoma (malignant fibroxanthoma). Cancer 26:827, 1970

173. Guccion JG, Enzinger FM: Malignant giant cell tumor of soft parts: An analysis of 32 cases. Cancer 29: 1518, 1972

174. Hajdu SI (ed): Pathology of Soft Tissue Tumors: Tumors of Fibrous Tissue. Chap. 2. Philadelphia, Lea & Febiger, 1979, p 57

175. Fletcher JA, Kozakewich HP, Hoffer FA, et al.: Diagnostic relevance of clonal chromosome aberrations in malignant soft-tissue tumors. N Engl J Med 324:436, 1991

176. Mandahl N, Heim S, Arheden K, et al.: Rings, dicentrics and telometric association in histiocytoma. Cancer Genet Cytogenet 30:23, 1988

177. Mandahl N, Heim S, Willen H, et al.: Characteristic karyotypic anomalies identify subtypes of malignant fibrous histiocytoma. Genes Chromosom Cancer 1:9, 1989

178. Nilbert M, Rydholm A, Willen H, et al.: MDM$_2$ gene amplification correlates with ring chromosome in soft tissue tumors. Genes Chromosomes Cancer 9:261, 1994

179. Rydholm A, Mahdahl N, Heim S, et al.: Malignant fibrous histiocytomas with a 19p+ marker chromosome have increased relapse rate. Genes Chromosom Cancer 2:296, 1990

180. Soule EH, Enriquez P: Atypical fibrous histiocytoma, malignant fibrous histiocytoma, malignant histiocytoma and epithelioid sarcoma: A comparative study of 65 tumors. Cancer 30:128, 1972

181. Murray MR: Muscle. In Willmer EN (ed): Cells and Tissues in Culture, Methods, Biology and Physiology, vol. 2, Chap. 8. New York, Academic Press, 1965, p 311

182. Willis RA: The Borderland of Embryology and Pathology. London, Butterworth, 1958, p 411

183. Murray MR: Skeletal muscle tissue in culture. In Bourne GH (ed): Structure and Function of Muscle. New York, Academic Press, 1960, p 111

184. Huxley HE, Hanson J: Changes in the cross-striation of muscle during contraction and stretch and their structural interpretation. Nature 173:973, 1954

185. Konigsberg I: Clonal analysis of myogenesis. Science 140:1273, 1963

186. Reporter MC, Konigsberg IR, Strehler BL: Kinetics of accumulation of creatine phosphokinase activity in developing embryonic skeletal muscle in vivo and in monolayer culture. Exp Cell Res 30:410, 1963

187. Golden T, Stout AP: Smooth muscle tumors of the gastrointestinal tract and retroperitoneal tissue. Surg Gynecol Obstet 73:784, 1941

188. Melicow PJ: Primary tumors of the retroperitoneum: A clinicopathologic analysis of 162 cases. Review of the literature and tables of classification. J Int Col Surg 19:401, 1953

189. Ashley DJB: Evans' Histological Appearance of Tumors, vol. 1, 3rd ed. Edinburgh, Churchill Livingstone, 1978, p 30

190. Smith BH, Dehner LP: Sarcoma of the prostate gland. Am J Clin Pathol 58:43, 1962

191. Light HG, Peskin GW, Ravdin IS: Primary tumors of the venous system. Cancer 13:818, 1960

192. Thijs LG, Kroon TAJ, Vanheeuwen TM: Leiomyosarcoma of the pulmonary trunk associated with pericardial effusion. Thorax 29:490, 1974

193. Silbar JD, Silbar SJ: Leiomyosarcoma of the bladder: Three case reports and review of the literature. J Urol 73:103, 1955

194. Yannopoulos K, Stout AP: Primary solid tumors of the mesentery. Cancer 16:914, 1963

195. Werner JR, Klingensmith W, Denko JV: Leiomyosarcoma of the ureters: Case report and review of literature. J Urol 82:68, 1959

196. Jenkin DG, Subbuswany SG: Leiomyosarcoma of the spermatic cord. Br J Surg 59:408, 1972

197. Craig JM: Leiomyoma of female breast. Arch Pathol 44:314, 1947

198. Hendrick JW: Leiomyoma of thyroid gland: Report of a case. Surgery 42:597, 1957

199. Evans DMD, Sanerkin NG: Primary leiomyosarcoma of bone. J Pathol Bact 90:348, 1965

200. Enzinger FM, Weiss SW (eds): Soft Tissue Tumors, Chap. 11, St. Louis, CV Mosby, 1983, p 282

201. Archer CB, Whittaker S, Greaves MW: Pharmacological modulation of cold-induced pain in cutaneous leiomyomata. Br J Dermatol 118:255, 1988

202. Engelke H, Christophers E: Leiomyomatosis cutis et uteri. Acta Derm Venereol 59(suppl 85):51, 1979

203. Jansen LH, Driessen FML: Leiomyoma cutis. Br J Dermatol 70:446, 1958

204. Prabhakar BR, Davessar K, Chitkara NL, et al.: Leiomyoma of the areolar region of the breast. Ind J Cancer 6:260, 1969

205. Stout AP: Bizarre smooth muscle tumors of the stomach. Cancer 15:400, 1962

206. Suster S, Rosai J: Intranodal hemorrhagic spindle-cell tumor with "amianthoid" fibers: Report of six cases of a distinctive mesenchymal neoplasm of the inguinal region that simulates Kaposi's sarcoma. Am J Surg Pathol 13:347, 1989

207. Eyden BP, Harris M, Greywoode GI, et al.: Intranodal myofibroblastoma: Report of a case. Ultrastruct Pathol 20:79, 1996

208. Wargotz ES, Weiss SW, Norris HJ: Myofibroblastoma of the breast: Sixteen cases of a distinctive benign mesenchymal tumor. Am J Surg Pathol 11:493, 1987

209. Fletcher CD, Tsang WY, Fisher C, et al.: Angiomyofibroblastoma of the vulva: A benign neoplasm distinct from aggressive angiomyxoma. Am J Surg Pathol 16:373, 1992

210. Martin JF, Bazin F, Feroldi J, Cabanne F: Tumours myoides intramurales de l'estomac: Consideration

microscipiques a propos de 6 cast. Ann Anat Path (Paris) 5:484, 1960

211. Kurman RJ, Norris HJ: Mesenchymal tumors of the uterus. VI. Epitheloid smooth muscle tumors including leiomyoblastoma and clear cell leiomyoma. Cancer 37:1853, 1976

212. Rywlin AM, Reecher L, Benson J: Clear cell leiomyoma of the uterus. Cancer 17:100, 1964

213. Lavin P, Hajdu SI, Foote FW: Gastric and extragastric leiomyoblastomas. Cancer 29:305, 1972

214. Yannopoulos K, Stout AP: Smooth muscle tumors in children. Cancer 15:958, 1962

215. Gerszten E, Kay S: Light and electron microscopic study of a leiomyoblastoma of the duodenum. Am J Dig Dis 14:350, 1969

216. Salazar H, Totten RS: Leiomyoblastoma of the stomach. An ultrastructural study. Cancer 25:176, 1970

217. Cornog JL: Gastric leiomyoblastoma: A clinical and ultrastructural study. Cancer 34:711, 1974

218. Ma CK, Amin MB, Kintanar E, et al.: Immunohistochemical characterization of gastrointestinal stromal tumors: A study of 82 cases compared with 11 cases of leiomyomas. Mod Pathol 6:139, 1993

219. Fujimoro T, Hirayana D, Gotoh A, et al.: Different origin of leiomyoblastoma by immunohistochemical study. Gastroenterol Jpn 27:187, 1992

220. Wang XJ, Tang WH, Yu PL: Histological and immunohistochemical study and AgNOR analysis of smooth muscle tumors of the digestive tract. Chung Hua Chung Liu Tsa Chih 16:128, 1994

221. Swanson PE, Stanley MW, Scheithauer BW, et al.: Primary cutaneous leiomyosarcoma: A histologic and immunohistochemical study of 9 cases with ultrastructural correlations. J Cutan Pathol 15:129, 1988

222. Stout AP, Hill WT: Leiomyosarcoma of the superficial soft tissues. Cancer 11:844, 1958

223. Stout AP: Solitary cutaneous and subcutaneous leiomyoma. Am J Cancer 29:435, 1937

224. Johnson S, Rundell M, Platt W: Leiomyosarcoma of the scrotum: A case report with electron microscopy. Cancer 41:1830, 1978

225. Schmookler BM, Lauer DH: Retroperitoneal leiomyosarcoma: A clinicopathologic analysis of 36 cases. Am J Surg Pathol 7:269, 1983

226. Aaro LA, Symmonds RE, Dockerty MB: Sarcoma of the uterus: A clinical-pathological study of 177 cases. Am J Obstet Gynecol 94:101, 1966

227. Pritchett PS, Fu YS, Kay S: Unusual ultrastructural features of a leiomyosarcoma of the lung. Am J Clin Pathol 63:901, 1975

228. Kevorkian J, Cento JP: Leiomyosarcomas of the large arteries and veins. Surgery 73:39, 1973

229. Hedinger E: Ueber intima sarkomatose von venen und arterien in sarkomatoesen strumen. Virchows Arch [A] 383:207, 1979

230. Boghosian L, Dal Cin P, Turc-Carel C, et al.: Three possible cytogenetic subgroups of leiomyosarcoma. Cancer Genet Cytogenet 43:39, 1989

231. Sreekantaiah C, Davis JR, Sandberg AA: Chromosomal abnormalities in leiomyosarcomas. Am J Pathol 142:293, 1993

232. Fletcher JA, Morton CC, Pavelka K, et al.: Chromosome aberration in uterine smooth muscle tumors: Potential diagnostic relevance of cytogenetic instability. Cancer Res 50:4092, 1990

233. Moran JJ, Enterline HT: Benign rhabdomyoma of the pharynx. A case report and review of the literature and comparison with cardiac rhabdomyoma. Am J Clin Pathol 42:174, 1964

234. Mostofi RK, Morse WH: Polypoid rhabdomyosarcoma (sarcoma botryoides) of bladder in children. J Urol 67:681, 1952

235. Tanimura H, Furuta M: Rhabdomyosarcoma of the spermatic cord. Cancer 22:1215, 1968

236. Salm R: Botryoid sarcoma of the vagina. Br J Cancer 15:220, 1961

237. Hilgers RD, Malkasian GD, Soule EH: Embryonal rhabdomyosarcoma (botryoid type) of the vagina: A clinicopathologic review. Am J Obstet Gynecol 107:484, 1970

238. Forbes GG: Rhabdomyosarcoma of bronchus. J Pathol Bacteriol 70:427, 1955

239. Masson JK, Soule EH: Embryonal rhabdomyosarcoma of the head and neck. Report on eighty-eight cases. Am J Surg 110:585, 1965

240. Dito WR, Batsakis JG: Intraoral pharyngeal and nasopharyngeal rhabdomyosarcoma. Otolaryngology 77:123, 1963

241. Donaldson SS, Castro JR, Wilbur JR, Jesse RH: Rhabdomyosarcoma of head and neck in children. Combination treatment by surgery, irradiation, and chemotherapy. Cancer 31:26, 1973

242. Jones IS, Reese AB, Draut J: Orbital rhabdomyosarcoma: An analysis of 62 cases. Am J Ophthalmol 61:721, 1966

243. Horn RC, Enterline HT: Rhabdomyosarcoma: A clinicopathological study and classification of 39 cases. Cancer 11:181, 1958

244. Deutsch M, Leen R, Mercado R: Rhabdomyosarcoma of the middle cranial fossa. Cancer 31:1193, 1973

245. Farinacci RJ, Fairchild JP, Sulak MH, Gilpatrick CW: Sarcoma botryoides (form of embryonal rhabdomyosarcoma) of common bile duct: Report of two cases. Cancer 9:408, 1956

246. Horn RC, Yakovac WC, Kaye R, Koop CE: Rhabdomyosarcoma (sarcoma botryoides) of the common bile duct. Report of a case. Cancer 8:468, 1955

247. Enzinger FM, Weiss S, (eds): Soft Tissue Tumors, 3rd ed., Chap. 22. St. Louis, Mosby-Yearbook, 1995, p 523

248. Corbeil LB: Differentiation of rhabdomyosarcoma and neonatal muscle cells in vitro. Cancer 20:572, 1967

249. Morales AR, Fine G, Horn RC Jr.: Rhabdomyosarcoma: An ultrastructural appraisal. Pathol Ann 7:81, 1972

250. Toker C: Embryonal rhabdomyosarcoma: An ultrastructural study. Cancer 21:11964, 1968

251. Horvat BL, Caines M, Fisher ER: The ultra structure of rhabdomyosarcoma. J Clin Pathol 53:555, 1970

252. McAllister RM, Nelson Rees WA, Johnson KY, et al.: Disseminated rhabdomyosarcomas formed in kittens by cultured human rhabdomyosarcoma cells. J Natl Cancer Inst 47:603, 1971

253. Pack GT, Eberhart WF: Rhabdomyosarcoma of skeletal muscle. Report of 100 cases. Surgery 32:1023, 1952

254. Stout AP: Rhabdomyosarcoma of skeletal muscle. Ann Surg 123:447, 1946

255. Hajdu SI, Koss LG: Cytologic diagnosis of metastatic myosarcomas. Acta Cytol 13:545, 1969

256. Chung A, Ringus J: Ultrastructural observations on the histogenesis of alveolar rhabdomyosarcoma. Cancer 41:1355, 1978

257. Enzinger FM, Shiraki M: Alveolar rhabdomyosarcoma: An analysis of 110 cases. Cancer 24:18, 1969

258. Douglass EC, Shapiro DN, Valentine M, et al.: Alveolar rhabdomyosarcoma with the t(2;13) cytogenetic findings and clinicopathologic correlations. Med Pediatr Oncol 21:83, 1993

259. Sheng W-W, Soukup S, Ballard E, et al.: Chromosomal analysis of sixteen rhabdomyosarcomas. Cancer Res 48:983, 1988

260. Whang-Peng J, Knutsen T, Theil K, et al.: Rhabdomyosarcoma. Genes Chromosom Cancer 5(4):299, 1992

261. Shapiro DN, Parham DM, Douglass EC, et al.: Relationship of tumor cell ploidy to histologic subtype and treatment outcome in children and adolescents with unresectable rhabdomyosarcoma. J Clin Oncol 9:159, 1991

262. Barr FG, Holick J, Nycum L, et al.: Localization of the t(2;13) breakpoint of alveolar rhabdomyosarcoma on a physical map of chromosome 2. Genomics 13:1150, 1992

263. Ramon y Cajal S: Histologie du Systeme Nerveux de L'Homme et des vertebres 2 vols (1909–1911). London, Oxford University Press, 1928

264. von Schwann TH: Microscopical Researches into the Structure and Growth of Animals and Plants. Translated by Henry Smith. London, Sydenham Society, 1847

265. del Rio Hortega P: Le nevroglie et le troisieme element des centres nerveuc. Bull Soc Sci Med Biol Montpellier Vol. 5, 1924

266. His W: Zur Geschichte des Menslichen Ruckenmarks und der Nerven wurzlen. Abh Gesch Math 13:477, 1887

267. Sherrington CS: The Integrative Action of the Nervous System. New Haven, Yale University Press, 1947

268. Le Gross Clark WE: The Anatomical Patterns on the Essential Basis of Sensory Discrimination. Oxford, Clarendon Press, 1947

269. Eccles JC: The Physiology of Synapses. Berlin, Springer-Verlag, 1964

270. Murray ME: Nervous tissue in vitro, Chap 9. In Willmar EN (ed): Cells and Tissues in Culture, Methods, Biology and Physiology, vol. 2. New York, Academic Press, 1965, p 373

271. Coupland RE: The Natural History of the Chromaffin Cell. London, Longmans, 1965

272. Gamble HJ, Goldby S: Mast cells in peripheral nerve trunk. Nature 189:766, 1961

273. Pineda A: Mast cells: Their presence and ultrastructural characteristics in peripheral nerve tumors. Arch Neurol 13:372, 1965

274. Isaacson P: Mast cells in benign nerve sheath tumors. J Pathol 119:193, 1976

275. Csaba G, Acs T, Horvath C, Mold K: Genesis and function of mast cells: Mast cells and plasmacyte reaction to induced homologous and heterologous tumors. Br J Cancer 15:327, 1961

276. Simpson WL: Distribution of mast cells as a function of age and exposure to carcinogenic agents. Ann NY Acad Sci 103:4, 1963

277. Gambel HF, Eames RA: An electron microscopic study of the connective tissues of human peripheral nerves. J Anat 98:665, 1964

278. Nathaniel EJH, Pease DC: Degenerative changes in rat dorsal roots during Wallerian degeneration. J Ultrastruct Res 9:511, 1963

279. Nathaniel EJH, Pease DC: Collagen and basement membrane formation by Schwann cells during nerve regeneration. J Ultrastruct Res 9:550, 1963

280. Ramon y Cajal S: Degeneration and Regeneration of the Nervous System, 2nd ed. New York, Hafner, 1959

281. Woodruff JM, Chernick NL, Smith M, et al.: Peripheral nerve tumors with rhabdomyosarcomatous differentiation (malignant "triton" tumors). Cancer 32:426, 1973

282. Woodruff JM: Peripheral nerve tumors showing glandular differentiation (glandular schwannoma). Cancer 37:2399, 1976

283. Bricklin AS, Ruston HW: Angiosarcoma of venous origin arising in radial nerve. Cancer 39:1556, 1977

284. Usui M, Ishii S, Yamawaki S, et al.: Malignant granular cell tumor of the radial nerve: An autopsy observation with electron microscopic and tissue culture studies. Cancer 39:1547, 1977

285. Kuo TT: Observation of nervous tissue in a Wilm's tumor: Its histogenetic significance. Cancer 39:1105, 1977

286. Krumerman MS, Stingle W: Synchronous malignant glandular schwannomas in congenital neurofibromatosis. Cancer 41:2444, 1978

287. Das Gupta TK, Brasfield RD, Strong EW, Hajdu RI: Benign solitary schwannomas (neurilemomas). Cancer 24:355, 1969

288. Russell DS, Rubenstein LJ: Pathology of Tumors of the Nervous System, 3rd ed. Baltimore, Williams & Wilkins, 1971, p 311

289. Brasfield RD, Das Gupta TK: Von Recklinghausen's disease: A clinical pathologic study. Ann Surg 175:86, 1972

290. Wander JV, Das Gupta TK: Neurofibromatosis. Current Problems in Surgery, vol. 14, no. 2. Chicago, Year Book Medical Publishers, 1977

291. Friedman JM, Birch PH: Type 1 neurofibromatosis: A descriptive analysis of the disorder in 1,728 patients. Am J Med Genet 70:138, 1997

292. Albright F, Butler AM, Hampton AO, Smith P: Syndrome characterized by osteitis fibrosa disseminata, areas of pigmentation and endocrine dysfunction, with precocious puberty in females: Report of 5 cases. N Engl J Med 226:727, 1937

293. Jimbow K, Szabo G, Fitzpatrick TB: Ultrastructure of giant pigment granules (macromelanosomes) in the cutaneous pigmented macules of neurofibromatosis. J Invest Dermat 61:300, 1973

294. Reed WB, Becker SW Sr., Becker SW Jr., Nicke WR: Giant pigmented nevi, melanoma and leptomeningeal melanocytosis: A clinical and histopathological study. Arch Dermat 91:100, 1965

295. Conway H: Bathing trunk nevus. Surgery 6:585, 1939
296. Crowe FW, Schull WJ, Neel JV: A Clinical, Pathological, and Genetic Study of Multiple Neurofibromatosis. Springfield, Ill., Thomas, 1956
297. Pack GT, Davis J: Nevus giganticus pigmentosus with malignant transformation. Surgery 49:347, 1961
298. Rook A, Wilkinson DS, Ebling FJG: Textbook of Dermatology. Oxford, Blackwell, 1972, p 164
299. Harkin JC, Reed RJ: Tumors of the peripheral nervous system. In Atlas of Tumor Pathology, Sect. 2, Fasc 3. Washington, DC, AFIP, 1969
300. Feigin I, Popoff N: Regeneration of myelin in multiple sclerosis. The role of mesenchymal cells in such regeneration and in myelin formation in the peripheral nervous system. Neurology 16:364, 1966
301. Feigin I: The nerve sheath tumor, solitary and in von Recklinghausen's disease: A unitary mesenchymal concept. Acta Neuropathol (Berlin) 17:188, 1971
302. Rubinstein LJ: Tumors of the Central Nervous System, Fasc. 6, Washington DC, AFIP, 1972
303. Hirata K, Kitahara K, Momosaka Y, et al.: Diffuse ganglioneuromatosis with plexiform neurofibromas limited to the gastrointestinal tract involving a large segment of small intestine. J Gastroenterol 31:263, 1996
304. Gordon MD, Weilert M, Ireland K: Plexiform neurofibromatosis involving the uterine cervix, endometrium, myometrium, and ovary. Obstet Gynecol 88(4 pt 2):699, 1996
305. Hosoi K: Multiple neurofibromatosis (von Recklinghausen's disease) with special reference to malignant transformation. Arch Surg 22:258, 1931
306. Schenkein I, Bucker ED, Helson L, et al.: Increased nerve-growth stimulating activity in disseminated neurofibromatosis. N Engl J Med 290:613, 1974
307. Siggers DC, Boyer SH, Eldrige R: Letter-Nerve growth factor in disseminated neurofibromatosis. N Engl J Med 292(21):1134, 1975
308. Das Gupta TK, Brasfield RD: Solitary malignant schwannomas. Ann Surg 171:419, 1970
309. D'Agostino AN, Soule EH, Miller RH: Primary malignant neoplasms of nerves (malignant neurilemomas in patients without manifestations of multiple neurofibromatosis [von Recklinghausen's disease]). Cancer 16:1003 1963
310. D'Agostino AN, Soule EH, Miller RH: Sarcomas of the peripheral nerves and somatic soft tissues associated with multiple neurofibromatosis (von Recklinghausen's disease). Cancer 16:1015, 1963
311. Brooks JS, Freiman M, Enterline HT: Malignant "Triton" tumor: Natural history and immunohistochemistry of nine new cases with literature review. Cancer 39:1556, 1977
312. Enzinger FM, Weiss SW (eds): Soft Tissue Tumors, 3rd ed., Chap. 32. St. Louis, Mosby-Yearbook, 1995, p 889
313. Garre C: Uber sekundare Maligne Neurome. Beitr Z Chir Z 9:465, 1892
314. Brooks JJ, Draffen RM: Benign glandular schwannoma. Arch Pathol Lab Med 116:192, 1992
315. Bigorgne C, Thomine E, Hemet J, Lauret P: Benign glandular schwannoma and Recklinghausen disease. Ann Pathol 12:114, 1992
316. Lodding P, Kindblom LG, Angervall L: Epithelioid malignant schwannoma: A study of 14 cases. Virchow Arch [A] 409:433, 1986
317. Bello MJ, de Campos JM, Kusak E, et al.: Clonal chromosome aberrations in neurinomas. Genes Chromosom Cancer 6:206, 199
318. Fletcher JA, Lipinski KK, Corson JM, et al.: Cytogenetics of peripheral nerve sheath tumors. Cancer Genet Cytogenet 41:224A, 1989
319. Becker R, Wake N, Gibas Z, et al.: Chromosome changes in soft tissue sarcomas. J Natl Can Inst 72(4):823, 1984
320. Enzinger FM: Clear cell sarcoma of tendons and aponeuroses—An analysis of 21 cases. Cancer 18:1163, 1965
321. Budreaux D, Waisman J: Clear cell sarcoma with melanogenesis. Cancer 41:1387, 1978
322. Bearman RM, Noe J, Kempson RL: Clear cell sarcoma with melanin pigment. Cancer 36:977 1975
323. Hoffman GJ, Carter D: Clear cell sarcoma of tendons and aponeuroses with melanin. Arch Pathol 95:22, 1973
324. Kubo T: Clear cell sarcoma of patellar tendon studied by electron microscopy. Cancer 24:948, 1969
325. Mackenzie DH: Clear cell sarcoma of tendon and aponeuroses with melanin production. J Pathol 114:231, 1974
326. Toe TK, Saw D: Clear cell sarcoma with melanin—Report of two cases. Cancer 41:235, 1978
327. Abrikossoff A: Uber Myome Ausgehend von der quergestreiften Wilkurlichen Muskulatus. Virchows Arch [A] 260:215, 1926
328. Aparicio SR, Lumsdeu CE: Light and electron microscopic studies on the granular cell myoblastoma of the tongue. J Pathol 97:339, 1969
329. Solbel HJ, Schwarz R, Marquet E: Light and electron microscopic study of the origin of granular cell myoblastoma. J Pathol 109:101, 1973
330. Pearse AGE: The histogenesis of granular cell myoblastoma. Am J Clin Pathol 19:522, 1949
331. Garancis JC, Komorowski RA, Kuzma JF: Granular cell myoblastoma. Cancer 25:542, 1970
332. Hunter DT Jr., Dewar JP: Malignant granular cell myoblastoma: Report of a case and review of the literature. Am Surg 26:554, 1960
333. Kashef R, Das Gupta TK: Segmental demyelination of peripheral nerves in the presence of malignant tumours. Br J Cancer 21:411, 1967
334. Croft PB, Henson RA, Urich H, Wilkinson PC: Sensory neuropathy with bronchial carcinoma: A study of four cases showing serological abnormalities. Brain 88:501, 1965
335. Weller RO, Cervos-Navarro J: Pathology of Peripheral Nerves. London, Butterworth, 1977, p 188
336. Coupland RE, Pyper AS, Hopwood DA: Method for differentiating between noradrenaline- and adrenaline-storing cells in the light and electron microscope. Nature 201:1240, 1964
337. Brown WJ, Barjas L, Latte H: The ultrastructure of human medulla with comparative studies of white rats. Anat Rec 169:173, 1970
338. Biscoe TJ: Carotid body: Structure and function. Physiol Rev 51:437, 1971

339. Olson JL, Salyer WR: Mediastinal paragangliomas (aortic body tumor): A report of four cases and a review of the literature. Cancer 41:2405, 1978

340. Kay S, Montague JW, Dodd RW: Non-chromaffin paraganglioma (chemodectoma) of thyroid region. Cancer 36:582, 1975

341. Olsen JR, Abell MR: Nonfunctional, nonchromaffin paragangliomas of the retroperitoneum. Cancer 23:1358, 1969

342. Stout AP: Ganglioneuromata of the sympathetic nervous system. Surg Gynecol Obstet 84:101, 1947

343. Dahl WV, Waugh JM, Dahlin DE: Gastrointestinal ganglioneuromas: Brief review with report of duodenal ganglioneuroma. Am J Pathol 33:953, 1957

344. Yokoyama M, Okad K, Takayasa H, Yamada R: Ultrastructural and biochemical study of benign ganglioneuroma. Virchows Arch [A] 361:195, 1973

345. Franks LM, Bollen A, Seeger RC, et al: Neuroblastoma in adults and adolescents: An indolent course with poor survival. Cancer 79:2028, 1997

346. deLorimer AA, Bragg KV, Linden G: Neuroblastoma in childhood. Am J Dis Child 188:441

347. Young LW, Rubin P, Hanson RE: The extra-adrenal neuroblastoma: High radiocurability and diagnostic accuracy. Am J Roentgenol Rad Ther Nucl Med 108:75, 1970

348. Dawson DA: Nerve cell tumors of the neck and their secretory activity. J Laryngol Otol 84:203, 1970

349. Pack GT, Ariel IM, Miller TRA: Malignant ganglioneuroma of the ganglion nodosum of the vagus nerve. Arch Surg 67:545, 1953

350. Koyoumdjian AO, McDonald JJ: Association of congenital renal neuroblastoma with multiple anomalies including unusual oropharyngeal cavity (imperfect buccopharyngeal membrane). Cancer 4:784, 1951

351. Horn RC, Koop CE, Kisen Wetter WB: Neuroblastoma in childhood. J Lab Invest 5:016, 1956

352. Birrier WF: Neuroblastoma as a cause of antenatal death. Am J Obst Gynecol 82:1388, 1961

353. Encinas A, Matute JA, Gomez A, et al.: Primary neuroblastoma presenting as a paratesticular tumor. J Pediatr Surg 32:624, 1997

354. Marsden HG, Steward JK: Tumors in children. Recent Results in Cancer Research, vol. 13. Berlin, Springer-Verlag, 1968

355. Sy WM, Edmandson JH: The developmental defects associated with neuroblastoma—Etiologic implications. Cancer 22:234, 1968

356. Knudson AG, Amromin GD: Neuroblastoma and ganglioneuroma in a child with multiple neurofibromatosis. Cancer 19:1022, 1966

357. Bolande RP, Towler WF: A possible relationship of neuroblastoma to von Recklinghausen's disease. Cancer 26:162, 1970

358. Greenberg R, Rosenthal I, Fall GS: Electron microscopy of human tumors secreting catecholamines: Correlation with biochemical data. J Neuropathol Exp Neurol 179:475, 1969

359. Everson TC, Cole WH: Spontaneous Regression of Cancer. Philadelphia, WB Saunders, 1966

360. Beckwith JB, Martin RB: Observations on the histopathology of neuroblastomas. J Pediatr Surg 3:106, 1968

361. Mckinen J: Microscopic patterns as a guide to prognosis of neuroblastoma in childhood. Cancer 29:1637, 1972

362. Hughes M, Marsden HB, Palmer MK: Histologic patterns of neuroblastoma related to prognosis and clinical staging. Cancer 34:1706, 1974

363. Lauder I, Aherne W: The significance of lymphocytic infiltration in neuroblastoma. Br J Cancer 26:321, 1972

364. Hoehner JC, Gestblom C, Hedborg F, et al.: A developmental model of neuroblastoma: Differentiating stroma–poor tumors' progress along an extra-adrenal chromaffin lineage. Lab Invest 75:659, 1996

365. Halperin EC: Long-term results of therapy for stage C neuroblastoma. J Surg Oncol 63:172, 1996

366. Iwafuchi M, Utsumi J, Tsuchida Y, et al.: Evaluation of patients with advanced neuroblastoma surviving more than 5 years after initiation of an intensive Japanese protocol: A report from the Study Group for Japan for Treatment of Advanced Neuroblastoma. Med Pediatr Oncol 27:515, 1996

367. Leavey PJ, Odom LF, Poole M, et al.: Intra-operative radiation therapy in pediatric neuroblastoma. Med Pediatr Oncol 28:424, 1997

368. Plouin PF, Chatellier G, Fofol I, Corvol P: Tumor recurrence and hypertension persistence after successful pheochromocytoma operation. Hypertension 29:1133, 1997

369. Tato A, Orte L, Diz P, et al.: Malignant pheochromocytoma, still a therapeutic challenge. Am J Hypertens 10:479, 1997

370. Barnes HM, Richardson PJ: Benign metastasizing fibroleiomyoma. J Obstet Gynecol Br Commonw 80:569, 1973

371. Brown JW, Burton RC, Dahlin DC: Chemodectoma with skeletal metastases. Report of two cases. Mayo Clinic Proc 42:551, 1967

372. Angervall L, Enzinger FM: Extraskeletal neoplasm resembling Ewing's sarcoma. Cancer 36:240, 1975

373. Soule EH, Newton W, Moon TE, Tefft M: Extraskeletal Ewing's sarcoma. Cancer 42:259, 1979

374. Ghadially FN, Roy S: Ultrastructure of Synovial Joints in Health and Disease. London, Butterworth, 1969

375. Garland P, Novikoff AB, Hamerman D: Electron microscopy of the human synovial membrane. J Cell Biol 14:207, 1962

376. Cadman NL, Soule EH, Kelly PJ: Synovial sarcoma. An analysis of 134 tumors. Cancer 18:613, 1965

377. Mackenzie DH: Synovial sarcoma: A review of 58 cases. Cancer 19:169, 1966

378. Ariel IM, Pack GT: Synovial sarcoma: Review of 25 cases. N Engl J Med 268:1272, 1963

379. Ichinose H, Powell L, Hoerner HE, et al.: The potential histogenetic relationship of the peripheral nerve to synovioma. Cancer Res 39:4270, 1979

380. Jaffe HL: Tumors and Tumorous Conditions of the Bones and Joints. London, Kimpton, 1958, p 584

381. Van Andel JG: Synovial sarcoma: A review and analysis of treated cases. Radiol Clin Biol 41:145, 1972

382. Krugman ME, Rosin HD, Toker C: Synovial sarcoma of the head and neck. Arch Otolaryngol 98:53, 1973

383. Roth JA, Enzinger FM, Tannenbaum M: Synovial sarcoma of the neck: A follow-up study of 24 cases. Cancer 35:1243, 1975

384. Attie JN, Steckler RM, Platt N: Cervical synovial sarcoma. Cancer 25:785, 1970

385. Hale JE, Calder ILM: Synovial sarcoma of the abdominal wall. Br J Cancer 24:471, 1970

386. Miller LH, Sanatella-Latimer L, Milly T: Synovial sarcoma of the larynx. Trans Am Acad Ophthalmol Otolaryngol 80:488, 1975

387. Haagensen CD, Stout AP: Synovial sarcoma. Ann Surg 120:826, 1944

388. Gabbiani G, Kaye GI, Lattes R, Jajoni G: Synovial sarcoma: Electron microscopic study of a typical case. Cancer 29:1031, 1971

389. Weingrad DN, Rosenberg SA: Early lymphatic spread of osteogenic and soft tissue sarcomas. Surgery 84:231, 1978

390. Dal Cin P, Rao U, Jani-Sait S, et al.: Chromosomes in the diagnosis of soft tissue tumors. I. Synovial sarcoma. Mod Pathol 5:357, 1992

391. Limon J, Mrozek K, Mandahl N, et al.: Cytogenetics of synovial sarcoma: Presentation of ten new cases and review of the literature. Genes Chromosom Cancer 3:338, 1991

392. Turc-Carel C, Dal Cin P, Limon J, et al.: Involvement of chromosome X in primary cytogenetic change in human neoplasia: Nonrandom translocation in synovial sarcoma. Proc Natl Acad Sci U S A 84:1981, 1987

393. Kampmeier OF: Evolution and comparative morphology of the lymphatic system. Springfield, Ill., Thomas, 1969

394. Walsh TS, Tompkins VN: Some observations on the strawberry nevus of infancy. Cancer 9:869, 1956

395. Rhodin JAC: Ultrastructure of mammalian venous capillaries, venules, and small collecting veins. J Ultrastruct Res 25:452, 1968

396. Karnofsky MJ: The ultrastructural basis of capillary permeability studied with peroxidase as a tracer. J Cell Biol 35:213, 1967

397. Simionescu N, Simionescu M: The cardiovascular system. In Weiss L, Greep RO (eds): Histology, 4th ed. New York, McGraw-Hill, 1977

398. Harano A, Dembitzer HM, Zimmerman HM: Fenestrated blood vessels in neurilemoma. Lab Invest 27:305, 1972

399. Enzinger FM, Weiss SW (eds): Soft Tissue Tumors, 3rd. ed., Chap. 25 St. Louis. Mosby-Yearbook, 1995, p 641

400. Kaposi M: Idopathisches multiples pigment sarkom der Haut. Arch Dermatol Syph 4:265, 1872

401. Ramos CV, Taylor HB, Hernandez BA, Tucker EF: Primary Kaposi's sarcoma of lymph nodes. Am J Clin Pathol 66:948, 1976

402. Taylor JF, Iverson OH, Bjerknes R: Growth kinetics of Kaposi's sarcoma. Br J Cancer 35:470, 1977

403. Reynolds WA, Winkleman RK, Soule EH: Kaposi's Sarcoma: A clinicopathologic study with particular reference to its relationship to the reticuloendothelial system. Medicine 44:419, 1965

404. Enzinger FM, Weiss SW (eds): Soft Tissue Tumors, 3rd ed., Chap. 26. St. Louis, Mosby-Yearbook, 1995, p 658–669

405. Weich HA, Salahuddin SZ, Gill P, et al.: AIDS-associated Kaposi's sarcoma-derived cells in long-term culture expresses and synthesizes smooth muscle alpha actin. Am J Pathol 139:1251, 1991

406. Hashimoto K, Lever WF: Kaposi's sarcoma: Histochemical and electron microscopic studies. J Invest Derm 43:539, 1964

407. Weiss SW, Sobin LH: WHO Classification of Soft Tissue Tumors. Berlin, Springer-Verlag, 1994

408. Masson F: Les glomus cutanes de l'homme. Bull Soc Fran Dermatol Syphil 42:1174, 1935

409. Banner EA, Winkelman RK: Glomus tumour of the vagina. Report of a case. Obstet Gynecol 9:326, 1957

410. Hrubam Z, Evans W, Humphreys E: An unusual form of a neurovascular hamartoma. Arch Pathol 69:672, 1960

411. Bindley GV: Glomus tumor of the mediastinum. J Thorac Surg 18:417, 1949

412. Appelman HD, Helwig EB: Glomus tumors of the stomach. Cancer 24:230, 1969

413. Allen RA, Dahlin DC: Glomus tumor of the stomach: Report of two cases. Mayo Clin Proc 29:429, 1954

414. Kay S, Calahan WP, Murray MR, et al.: Glomus tumors of the stomach. Cancer 4:726, 1951

415. Borghard-Erdle AM, Hirsch EF: Glomus tumors of the uterus. Arch Pathol 65:244, 1958

416. Mackenzie DH: Intraosseous glomus tumors: Report of two cases. J Bone Joint Surg 44B:648, 1962

417. Murray MR, Stout AP: The glomus tumor: Investigation of its distribution and the identity of its "epithelioid" cell. Am J Pathol 18:183, 1942

418. Murad TM, von Haam E, Murphy MSN: Ultrastructure of a hemangiopericytoma and a glomus tumor. Cancer 22:1239, 1968

419. Battifra H: Hemangiopericytoma. Ultrastructural study of five cases. Cancer 31:1418, 1973

420. Hahn MJ, Dawson R, Esterly JA, Joseph DJ: Hemangiopericytoma: An ultrastructural study. Cancer 31:255, 1973

421. Harris M: Ultrastructure of a glomus tumor. J Clin Pathol 25:520, 1971

422. Popoff NA, Malinin TI, Rosomoff HL: Fine structure of intracranial hemangiopericytoma and angiomatous meningioma. Cancer 34:1187, 1974

423. Ramsey HJ: Fine structure of haemangiopericytoma and haemangioendothelioma. Cancer 19:1005, 1966

424. Toker C: Glomangioma: An ultrastructural study. Cancer 23:487, 1969

425. van den Oord JJ, De Wolf-Peeters C: Perivascular spaces in endocrine spiradenoma: A clue to its histological diagnosis. Am J Dermatopathol 17:266, 1995

426. Calonje E, Fletcher CD: Cutaneous intraneural glomus tumor. Am J Dermatopathol 17:395, 1995

427. Tarnowski WM, Hashimoto K: Multiple glomus tumors: An ultrastructural study. J Invest Dermatol 52:474, 1969

428. Henschen F: L'endovasculite proliferente thrombopoietigne dans la lesion vasculaire locale. Ann Anat Pathol (Paris) 9:113, 1932

429. Dictor M, Elnar A, Anderson T: Myofibromatosis-like hemangiopericytoma metastasizing as a differentiated vascular smooth muscle and myosarcoma: Myopericytes as a subset of myofibroblast. Am J Surg Pathol 16:1239, 1992

430. Mandahl N, Orndal C, Heim S, et al.: Aberrations of chromosome segment 12q13-15 characterize a subgroup of hemangiopericytomas. Cancer 71:3009, 1993

431. Perez-Atayde AR, Kozakewich HP, McGill T, et al.: Hemangiopericytoma of the tongue in a 10-year-old child: Ultrastructural and cytogenetic observations. Hum Pathol 25:425, 1994

432. Enterline HT, Roberts B: Lymphangiopericytoma. Cancer 8:582, 1955

433. Cornog JL Jr, Enterline HT: Lymphangiomyoma—A benign lesion of chyliferous lymphatics synonymous with lymphangiopericytoma. Cancer 19:1909, 1966

434. Corrin D, Liebow AA, Friedman PJ: Pulmonary lymphangiomyomitosis. Am J Pathol 79:347, 1975

435. Stewart FW, Treves N: Lymphangiosarcoma in postmastectomy lymphedema: A report of six cases in elephantiasis chirugica. Cancer 1:64, 1948

436. Huggins CB: The formation of bone under influence of epithelium of the urinary tract. Arch Surg 22:377, 1931

437. Binkley JS, Stewart FW: Morphogenesis of extraskeletal osteogenic sarcoma and pseudo-osteosarcoma. Arch Pathol 29:42, 1940

438. Brookes M: The vascular factors in osteoarthritis. Surg Gynecol Obstet 123:1255, 1966

439. Boneti T: De ventris tumors. In: Sepulchretum, sive anatomic practice excadaveribus morbo denatis, vol. 3, sect. 21, ObsGeneva, Cramer et Parachon, 1700, p 522

440. Fine G, Stout AP: Osteogenic sarcoma of the extraskeletal soft tissue. Cancer 9:1027, 1956

441. Das Gupta TK, Hajdu SI, Foote FW Jr.: Extraosseous osteogenic sarcoma. Ann Surg 168:1011, 1968

442. Dahm LJ, Schaefer SD, Carder HM, Vellios F: Osteosarcoma of the soft tissue of the larynx. Report of a case with light and electron microscopic studies. Cancer 42:2343, 1978

443. Rao U, Cheng A, Didolkar S: Extraosseous osteogenic sarcoma: Clinicopathological study of eight cases and review of literature. Cancer 41:1488, 1978

444. Huvos AG: Osteogenic sarcoma of bones and soft tissues in older persons: A clinicopathologic analysis of 117 patients older than 60 years. Cancer 57:1442, 1986

445. Stout AP, Verner EW: Chondrosarcoma of the extrakeletal soft tissue. Cancer 6:581, 1953

446. Enzinger FM, Shiraki M: Extraskeletal myxoid chondrosarcoma: An analysis of 34 cases. Human Pathol 3:421, 1972

447. Goldenberg RR, Chen P, Steinlauf P: Chondrosarcoma of the extraskeletal soft tissues. J Bone Joint Surg 49A:1487, 1967

448. Chung EB, Enzinger FM: Chondroma of soft parts. Cancer 41:1414, 1978

449. Christopherson WM, Foote FW, Stewart FW: Alveolar soft part sarcomas: Structurally characteristic tumors of uncertain histogenesis. Cancer 5:100, 1952

450. Smetana GF, Scott WF Jr.: Malignant tumors of the nonchromaffin paraganglia. Milit Surg 109:330, 1951

451. Udekwu FA, Pulvertaft RJV: Studies of an alveolar soft tissue sarcoma. Br J Cancer 19:744 1966

452. Karnauchow PN, Magner D: The histogenesis of alveolar soft part sarcoma. J Pathol Bacteriol 86:169, 1963

453. Shipkey FH, Lieberman PH, Foote FW, Stewart FW: Ultrastructure of alveolar soft part sarcoma. Cancer 17:821, 1964

454. Fisher ER, Reidbord H: Electron microscopic evidence suggesting the myogenous derivation of the so-called alveolar soft part sarcoma. Cancer 27:150, 1971

455. Welsh RA, Bray DM, Shipkey FH, Meyer AT: Histogenesis of alveolar soft part sarcoma. Cancer 29:191, 1972

456. Unni KK, Soule EH: Alveolar rhabdomyosarcoma. An electron microscopic study. Mayo Clin Proc 50:59, 1975

457. Auerbach HE, Brooks JJ: Alveolar soft part sarcoma: A clinicopathologic and immunohistochemical study. Cancer 60:66, 1987

458. Ordóñez NG, Ro JY, Mackay B: Alveolar soft part sarcoma: An ultrastructural and immunocytochemical investigation of its histogenesis. Cancer 63:1721, 1989

459. Pratt J, Woodruff JM, Marcove RC: Epithelioid sarcoma: An analysis of 22 cases indicating the prognostic significance of vascular invasion and regional lymph node metastasis. Cancer 41:1472 1978

460. Bryan RS, Soule EH, Dobyns JH, et al.: Primary epithelioid sarcoma of the hand and forearm: A review of thirteen cases. J Bone Joint Surg 56A:458, 1974

461. Enzinger FM: Epithelioid sarcoma: A sarcoma simulating a granuloma or a carcinoma. Cancer 26:1029, 1970

462. Males JL, Lain KC: Epithelioid sarcoma in XO/XX Turner's syndrome. Arch Pathol 94:214, 1972

463. Rao BN, Pappo A, Bowman L, et al.: Epithelioid sarcoma in children. J Pediatr Surg 31:1663, 1996

464. Evans HL, Baer SC: Epithelioid sarcoma: A clinicopathologic and prognostic study of 26 cases. Semin Diagn Pathol 10:286, 1993

465. Moore SW, Wheeler TE, Hefter LG: Epithelioid sarcoma masquerading as Peyronie's disease. Cancer 35:1706, 1976

466. Santiago H, Feinerman LK, Lattes R: Epithelioid sarcoma. Hum Pathol 3:133, 1972

467. Gabbiani G, Fu YS, Kaye GI, et al.: Epithelioid sarcoma: A light and electron microscopic study suggesting a synovial origin. Cancer 30:486, 1972

468. Frable WJ, Kay S, Lawrence W, Schatzki PF: Epithelioid sarcoma: An electron microscopic study. Arch Pathol 95:8, 1973

469. Bloustein PA, Silverberg SG, Waddell WR: Epithelioid sarcoma: Case report with ultrastructural review, histogenetic discussion, and chemotherapeutic data. Cancer 38:2390, 1976

470. Hernandez FJ, Fernandez BB: Localized fibrous tumors of pleura: A light and electron microscopic study. Cancer 34:1667, 1974

471. Chan PSF, Balfour TW, Bourke JB, Smith PG: Peritoneal mesothelioma. Br J Surg 62:576, 1975

# 6

# Molecular Biology of Soft Tissue Tumors

The past decade has witnessed important advances in our understanding of the molecular biology of soft tissue tumors. Tremendous technical advances in the field of tumor genetics have led to the discovery and characterization of molecular events underlying cytogenetic abnormalities in soft tissue tumors. Genes associated with an inherited predisposition to the development of soft tissue tumors have been identified and cloned for further study. The complex interactions among oncogenes, tumor suppressor genes, transcription factors, and their regulators are under investigation. Some of these developments have already shown clinical applicability as diagnostic aids and prognostic markers for soft tissue tumors. Pilot studies in the treatment of other solid tumors imply that biologic and gene-based treatments for soft tissue tumors are not far off. This chapter summarizes some of these advances in cytogenetics, molecular genetics, and molecular biology, with special emphasis on the existing or potential translational value of these observations.

## ■ CYTOGENETICS AND GENETICS

Recent discoveries have greatly increased our awareness and understanding of the numerous molecular genetic events underlying the development, progression, and metastasis of soft tissue tumors. This section briefly reviews specific chromosomal abnormalities seen in various soft tissue tumors, as well as some recent discoveries resulting from the application of new methods.

A number of specific, consistent clonal abnormalities have been described in soft tissue tumors subjected to cytogenetic analysis. More information has accumulated as molecular genetic methods such as fluorescence in situ hybridization (FISH) and comparative genomic hybridization (CGH) have supplanted analysis of metaphase preparations.[1–4]

Balanced reciprocal chromosome translocations are frequently seen in soft tissue tumors, and some are unique to particular tumor types. The resultant fusion genes and their protein products are now being identified by both candidate gene searches and positional cloning methods. These techniques are expanding our knowledge of the ontogeny of these tumors. In addition, several of these translocations have practical value in the diagnosis and classification of soft tissue tumors. These characteristic translocations are summarized in Table 6–1 and are discussed below.

## TUMORS OF THE ADIPOSE TISSUE

Myxoid liposarcomas are characterized by a translocation t(12;16)(q13.3;p11.2), often as the sole cytogenetic abnormality.[4–10] This results in the fusion of the CHOP and TLS/FUS genes and their subsequent transcriptional dysregulation.[11–14] Normally, CHOP encodes a dominant negative-acting transcription factor involved in adipocyte differentiation.[15] The translocation t(12;16)(q13,p11) has also been observed in some round cell liposarcomas,[16] although complex karyotypes not involving t(12;16) have also been reported in round cell liposarcomas.[7,10] Well-differentiated liposarcomas may contain large marker chromosomes and

**TABLE 6–1. CHARACTERISTIC CHROMOSOME TRANSLOCATIONS IN SOFT TISSUE SARCOMAS**

| Histologic Type of Tumor | Translocation | Molecular Alteration | Frequency (percent) |
|---|---|---|---|
| Myxoid liposarcoma | t(12;16)(q13.3;p11.2) | CHOP-TLS (FUS) | 80 |
| Alveolar rhabdomyosarcoma | t(2;13)(q35;q14) | PAX3-FKHR | 70 |
| | t(1;13)(p36;q14) | PAX7-FKHR | 20 |
| Ewing's sarcoma and peripheral neuroectodermal tumors | t(11;22)(q24;q12) | EWS-FLI1 | Together, |
| | t(21;22)(q22;q12) | EWS-ERG | 95 |
| Clear cell sarcoma | t(12;22)(q13;q12) | EWS-ATF1 | 50–90 |
| Synovial cell sarcoma | t(X;18)(p11.2;q11.2) | SYT-SSX | 95 |
| Extraskeletal myxoid chondrosarcoma | t(9;22)(q22–31;q12) | EWS-? | 50–70 |

ring chromosomes.[9,17] Ring chromosomes have been reported to correlate with MDM2 gene amplification in liposarcomas.[18,19] A recent study employing CGH demonstrated amplification of another chromosome region, 1q21–22, in six of eight well-differentiated liposarcomas.[20] Pleomorphic liposarcomas usually have various complex karyotypes.[4,9]

About two-thirds of benign lipomas are characterized by translocations involving chromosome 12q13–15.[9,21] The lipoma breakpoint does not appear to involve the CHOP or GLI genes.[11,22] A few lipomas have also been found to have ring chromosomes, in some cases associated with MDM2 amplification.[19] The chromosome region 12q13–15 contains a number of genes that have been reported to be amplified or otherwise altered in various soft tissue tumors, including ATF-1, CHOP, CDK4, GLI, MDM2, and the newly described gene OS-9,[23–26] implying that this region is important in mesenchyme differentiation and malignant transformation.

## TUMORS OF THE FIBROUS TISSUE

Malignant fibrous histiocytoma frequently has a complex karyotype, and these types of tumors are quite heterogeneous cytogenetically.[3,7,27,28] Pathognomonic clonal abnormalities have not yet been identified, although rearrangements involving 1q11–12 have been observed in about 40 percent of tumors studied, and ring chromosomes occur in about 20 percent of cases.[19,28]

A supernumerary ring chromosome was observed in each of the few cases of dermatofibrosarcoma protuberans analyzed.[4] Desmoid tumors (aggressive fibromatosis) frequently show karyotypic abnormalities including rearrangements of 5q.[29] Recently, a FISH-based analysis of 20 desmoids revealed trisomy 8 in four tumors, whereas only one had this abnormality detected by conventional banding analysis.[30] Another study has linked trisomy 8 to the recurrence potential of these types of tumors.[31]

## TUMORS OF THE MUSCLE TISSUE

Alveolar rhabdomyosarcoma is characterized by a translocation t(2;13)(q35;q14) in most cases.[32–35] This results in fusion of the DNA-binding domain of the PAX-3 gene (a transcription factor involved in myoblast differentiation) with the 5′ end of the FKHR gene, a newly identified member of the forkhead family of transcription factors.[36–38] A small subset of alveolar rhabdomyosarcomas display a variant translocation t(1;13) (p36;q14) that produces the PAX7-FKHR fusion gene.[39,40] These tumor-specific derivative chromosomes may be visualized by FISH.[41]

Embryonal rhabdomyosarcomas most often have complex structural chromosome rearrangements, frequently including loss of chromosomal region 11p15.5.[42] This is the locus for Beckwith-Wiedemann syndrome, a hereditary disorder characterized by growth dysregulation, exomphalos, macroglossia, and partial gigantism, as well as an increased frequency of adrenal tumors, Wilms' tumors, and embryonal rhabdomyosarcoma.[43] Imprinting—differential activation or deactivation of a gene depending upon the parental origin of the allele—appears to be involved in this hereditary disorder.[44,45] Evidence from subchromosomal DNA-transfer experiments supports the presence of a candidate tumor suppressor gene between the β-globin and insulin genes at this locus.[46]

Although no chromosome abnormality specific for leiomyosarcoma has been identified, and most of these tumors show complex abnormalities, 25 percent show rearrangements of 1q32 by conventional banding techniques.[3,28] By CGH, which detects DNA sequence copy number alterations without the need for specific probes, amplification of 1q21–22 was seen in all three leiomyosarcomas so analyzed.[20]

## TUMORS OF THE PERIPHERAL NERVES

Ewing's sarcoma, which may occur in soft tissue or bone, is a small round cell tumor that has been reclassified, based on both immunohistochemical and ultrastructural features, as a derivative of neuroectodermal tissue. Furthermore, on the basis of two characteristic translocations, t(11;22)(q24;q12) and t(21;22)(q22;q12), it appears that extraskeletal Ewing's tumors share the same ancestory as other primitive neuroectodermal tumors (PNET) as well as some other tumors of neuroectodermal origin.[47–51] Suitable probes now permit detection of these translocations by FISH on short-term cultures of fresh tissue, touch preparations, frozen sections, or paraffin-embedded sections, greatly expanding their clinical usefulness as diagnostic markers. These translocations result in the fusion of the EWS gene on chromosome 11q22 to either the FLI1 gene from chromosome 11q24[52–55] or ERG on 21q22.[56,57] Some small round cell tumors of this class also contain similar chimeric genes, including EWS-WT1[58,59] and EWS-E1A-F.[60] These genes are transcriptional activators or repressors. E1A-F is known to be a transcriptional activator of matrix metalloproteinases and thus may be important in tumor invasion and may prove to be a marker of metastatic potential.

Another soft tissue tumor of neuroectodermal origin, clear cell sarcoma (malignant melanoma of soft parts), is characterized by a translocation t(12;22)(q13;q12) resulting in the formation of a fusion protein EWS-ATF-1, a chimera of the EWS protein and the transcription factor ATF-1.[61–66] The fusion protein appears to function as a constitutive transcriptional activator and deregulates gene expression.[66] The presence of this characteristic translocation in clear cell sarcoma, but not in cutaneous malignant melanoma, supports a biologic distinction between these two entities. Detection of this translocation may aid in distinguishing clear cell sarcoma from morphologically similar tumors such as epithelioid sarcoma.

## SYNOVIAL CELL SARCOMA

Synovial cell sarcomas are characterized by the translocation t(X;18)(p11.2;q11.2)[67–71] (Fig. 6–1). This translocation is found in nearly all cases of synovial cell sarcoma analyzed by banding or FISH and can be determined using paraffin-embedded tissue sections.[72] Recently, two distinct translocation breakpoints for monophasic (Xp11.21/SSX2 locus) and biphasic (Xp11.23/SSX1 locus) synovial cell sarcomas have been demonstrated,[73,74] although two additional studies failed to confirm this relationship with histologic subtype.[75,76] These translocations result in fusion of the SYT gene to the SSX1 or SSX2 gene, and these fusion transcripts can be detected by reverse transcription polymerase chain reaction (RT-PCR) on paraffin-embedded tissue sections from synovial cell sarcomas.[76] This technique may help differentiate monophasic synovial cell sarcoma from other types of soft tissue sarcomas.

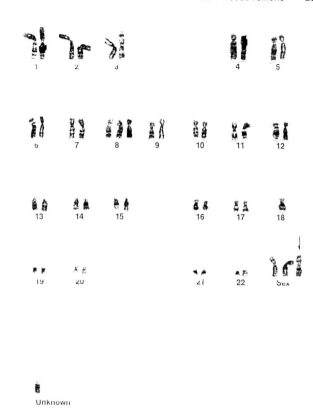

**Figure 6–1.** Karyotype of our synovial cell sarcoma cell line UISO SYN-1 exhibiting the characteristic translocation t(X;18)(p11;q11). *(Courtesy of Mr. Albert Green.)*

## TUMORS OF THE PERIVASCULAR TISSUE

Hemangiopericytomas are another type of soft tissue sarcoma that can exhibit rearrangements of chromosome 12q13–15, a region implicated in mesenchymal differentiation.[3,4,25] To date, no diagnostic cytogenetic abnormalities have been reported in Kaposi's sarcoma.[4]

## TUMORS OF THE HETEROTOPIC BONE AND CARTILAGE

Extraskeletal myxoid chondrosarcoma exhibits a characteristic translocation t(9;22)(q22–31;q12).[77–80] Recent analysis by molecular cloning has shown that the translocation breakpoint on 22q12 involves the EWS gene, suggesting that EWS is important in the development of extraskeletal myxoid chondrosarcoma, as well as neuroectodermal tumors.[80]

## TUMORS OF UNDETERMINED HISTOGENESIS

Alveolar soft part sarcoma is an unusual soft tissue neoplasm of uncertain origin. To date, four of six reported cases have demonstrated abnormalities of the long arm of Chromosome 17.[81–83] Further investigation of the specific nature of these genetic changes is underway and may help elucidate the histogenesis of this tumor.

## ■ FAMILIAL SYNDROMES

Several hereditary syndromes that predispose individuals to the development of benign and/or malignant mesenchymal tumors have been described. Also, familial clustering of soft tissue sarcomas has been observed. These neoplastic and preneoplastic syndromes are summarized in Tables 6–2 and 6–3. As with the study of other familial tumors, genetic alterations in hereditary cases of soft tissue tumors have lead to insight into the molecular events underlying the genesis of the more commonly occurring sporadic soft tissue tumors. This section will review some of these hereditary syndromes, highlighting recent advances in molecular genetics.

### RETINOBLASTOMA

A milestone in understanding hereditary predisposition to bone and soft tissue tumors came from studies of retinoblastoma and the discovery of the RB-1 gene. Retinoblastoma is an uncommon embryonal tumor of the retina seen in young children. Although a family history of the disorder is present in only 10 percent of cases, it is now known that the hereditary form accounts for 30 to 40 percent of cases, three-quarters of which result in bilateral retinoblastomas.[84,85] After successful treatment of retinoblastoma, 30 to 50 percent of patients with the hereditary form of the disease will develop a second nonocular cancer, mostly osteosarcomas and soft tissue sarcomas.[86–90]

In the 1970s, Knudson and others[91,92] proposed that retinoblastoma developed after two mutations rendered both alleles of a "tumor suppressor gene" inactive. Subsequently, the prototype tumor suppressor gene, RB-1, on chromosome 13q14, was identified and characterized.[93–95] The RB-1 protein is variably phosphorylated throughout the cell cycle and normally functions as a negative regulator of cell division.[96,97]

The absence of RB-1 RNA and/or protein in 70 to 100 percent of retinoblastomas studied[95,98] and in many of the secondary bone and soft tissue sarcomas[86,99] confirms the role of RB-1 in the etiology of these tumors. RB-1 expression in sporadic soft tissue sarcomas will be discussed later in this chapter, in the section on tumor suppressor genes.

### NEUROFIBROMATOSIS

Neurofibromatosis (NF), or von Recklinghausen's neurofibromatosis, is actually two distinct heritable disorders of neuroectoderm characterized by neurofibromas and central nervous system tumors. NF-1, the more common form, is an autosomal dominant disorder, affecting 1 in 5,000 people.[100,101] It is characterized by café-au-lait spots, axillary freckling, Lisch nodules of the iris, optic nerve gliomas, and cutaneous, subcutaneous, and visceral plexiform neurofibromas.[101–103] The NF-1 gene, located on chromosome 17q11.2, was identified in 1990 by positional cloning.[104,105] It encodes a protein, neurofibromin, that is important in neuroectodermal differentiation and cardiac development.[106] NF-1 appears to be a tumor suppressor gene, and its loss or functional inactivation may activate the Ras signaling pathway.[107] Children with NF-1 have an increased risk of developing tumors of the central nervous system, Wilms' tumor, and lymphoma, and 10 to 30 percent will develop malignant schwannomas.[103,108] NF-1-associated malignant peripheral nerve sheath tumors may be multiple and tend to occur at a younger age than their sporadic counterparts.[103,108] There is also an increased incidence of other soft tissue sarcomas, especially rhabdomyosarcoma, among these patients.[108–113]

NF-2, affecting 1 in 50,000 people, is also inherited in an autosomal dominant fashion and is distinguished by bilateral eighth cranial nerve tumors, meningiomas,

**TABLE 6–2. HEREDITARY NEOPLASTIC SYNDROMES ASSOCIATED WITH SOFT TISSUE TUMORS**

| Syndrome | Molecular Defect | Manifestations |
|---|---|---|
| Hereditary retinoblastoma | RB-1 gene deletion or rearrangement | Retinoblastoma, bilateral 70%<br>Osteosarcoma, other soft tissue sarcoma in 30–50% |
| Li-Fraumeni cancer syndrome | Germline mutation of p53 | Breast cancer<br>Soft tissue sarcoma<br>Other neoplasms |
| Hereditary multiple exostoses | Constitutional mutation of EXT1, also abnormalities at the EXT2 and EXT3 loci | Multiple osteochondromas of long bones<br>Chondrosarcomas in 5–25%<br>Other soft tissue sarcomas |
| Gardner's syndrome | Germline mutation of APC | Multiple adenomatous polyps<br>Colon cancer<br>Abdominal and mesenteric desmoid tumors in 8–20% |
| Chemodectoma | Unknown | Chemodectomas, often bilateral<br>Pheochromocytoma, occasionally |

**TABLE 6–3. HEREDITARY PRENEOPLASTIC SYNDROMES ASSOCIATED WITH SOFT TISSUE TUMORS**

| Syndrome | Molecular Defect | Manifestations |
|---|---|---|
| Neurofibromatosis type-1 | NF1 | Multiple plexiform neurofibromas<br>CNS tumors<br>Café-au-lait spots<br>Associated malignancies: malignant schwannomas (PNST), other soft tissue sarcomas, malignant CNS tumors, Wilms' tumor, lymphoma |
| Neurofibromatosis type-2 | NF2 | Multiple plexiform neurofibromas<br>Bilateral vestibular schwannomas (PNST)<br>Associated malignancies: malignant schwannomas (PNST), malignant CNS tumors |
| Peutz-Jeghers syndrome | Unknown | Multiple gastrointestinal hamartomatous polyps<br>Associated malignancies: GI tract, ovarian, testicular or other cancers in 50% |
| Hereditary multiple exostoses | Constitutional mutation of EXT1, also abnormalities at the EXT2 and EXT3 loci | Multiple osteochondromas of long bones<br>Associated malignancies: chondrosarcomas in 5–25%, other soft tissue sarcomas |
| von Hippel-Lindau syndrome | VHL | Multiple angiomas<br>Associated malignancies: renal cell carcinoma (25–40%), pheochromocytoma |
| Tuberous sclerosis | TS1 locus chromosome 9<br>TS2 | Multiple CNS hamartomas<br>Renal angiomyolipomas<br>Adenoma sebaceum<br>Associated malignancies: giant cell astrocytoma (2%), renal cell carcinoma |

*Abbreviations: CNS, central nervous system; GI, gastrointestinal; PNST, peripheral nerve sheath tumors.*

and the dermal, subcutaneous, and plexiform neurofibromas seen in NF-1. Mutation of the NF-2 gene on 22q usually results in the formation of a truncated protein, although rare missense mutations have been implicated in a milder, later-onset form of NF-2.[114] Somatic NF-2 mutations have also been reported in nonfamilial vestibular schwannomas and meningiomas.[115] The clinical manifestations and treatment of neurofibromatoses are discussed in Chapter 10.

## LI-FRAUMENI CANCER SYNDROME

Li-Fraumeni cancer syndrome, a syndrome of multiple cancers, including osteosarcoma, soft tissue sarcoma, brain tumors, breast cancer, and other neoplasms,[116,117] results from a germline mutation of the p53 gene.[118–120] The p53 gene, located on human chromosome 17p13, is a tumor suppressor gene involved in transcriptional regulation, DNA repair, cell cycle control, cell differentiation, and apoptosis.[121–129] It is the most frequently mutated gene in (sporadic) human solid tumors.[129,130] Mutation or functional inactivation of the p53 gene occurs in many types of soft tissue sarcomas and will be discussed in detail later in this chapter.

## GARDNER'S SYNDROME

Gardner's syndrome encompasses the classic triad of colonic polyps, bone tumors (especially osteomas of the

skull), and soft tissue tumors.[131,132] After linkage studies implicated a locus on chromosome 5q21,[133,134] it was discovered that germline mutations of the APC gene are responsible for this syndrome.[135–137] The soft tissue tumors associated with Gardner's syndrome include desmoid tumors (aggressive fibromatosis), which occur in 8 to 20 percent of afflicted persons, and fibrosarcoma. The desmoid tumors of Gardner's syndrome frequently involve the abdominal wall and extend into the intestinal mesentery, contributing to the death of up to 20 percent of these patients.[138–142] Study of desmoids occurring in patients with Gardner's syndrome has shown somatic mutations of the APC gene, suggesting that inactivation or deletion of both alleles of the APC gene is an important step in their development.[143] This entity is discussed in greater detail in Chapter 8.

## HEREDITARY MULTIPLE OSTEOCARTILAGINOUS EXOSTOSES (DIAPHYSEAL ACLASIS)

Hereditary multiple osteocartilaginous exostoses is the most common major skeletal genetic disorder and is transmitted in an autosomal dominant fashion with a high degree of penetrance.[144,145] The exostoses are osteochondromas of the metaphysis of growing bone, and, although these lesions appear to become quiescent after growth is completed, malignant transformation (to chondrosarcoma or other sarcomas) will occur in 5 to 25 percent of afflicted children.[146,147] Thus far, three genetic loci involved in this disorder have been identified. The genetic defect on chromosome 8q24.1 involves the recently cloned gene EXT1, which appears to function as a tumor suppressor gene.[148] The EXT2 locus is pericentromeric on chromosome 11, and EXT3 is located on chromosome 19p.[149,150]

## BECKWITH-WIEDEMANN SYNDROME

Beckwith-Wiedemann syndrome is a rare disorder (1 out of 13,700 live births) characterized by growth dysregulation, macroglossia, and partial gigantism, associated with an increased frequency of subsequent adrenal tumors, Wilms' tumors, hepatoblastomas, and embryonal rhabdomyosarcoma.[43,151] Experimental evidence suggests that inactivation of a tumor suppressor gene at 11p15.5 contributes to the development of this syndrome.[44–46,152] Other genes at this locus, including IGF2 (insulin-like growth factor II) and H19 may also be involved.[153]

## PEUTZ-JEGHERS SYNDROME

Peutz-Jeghers syndrome is included here for the sake of completeness, as it frequently leads to sarcomatous changes in the polyps of the small intestine. Peutz-Jeghers syndrome includes the constellation of mucocutaneous pigmentation and gastrointestinal polyposis, inherited in an autosomal dominant fashion. The polyps are hamartomas and may occur anywhere in the gastrointestinal tract. They may manifest with intestinal bleeding, intussusception, or obstruction as they increase in size. There is an increased frequency of cancers in these patients, nearly 50 percent by age 50,[154] most often adenocarcinoma of the gastrointestinal tract, Sertoli cell tumors of the ovary or testicle, breast cancer, and biliary tree adenocarcinoma.[155–158] It remains to be shown whether the hamartomas themselves undergo malignant transformation or whether cancers develop from coexistent adenomatous foci.

## CHEMODECTOMA

Chemodectomas are paragangliomas that most commonly occur at the carotid bifurcation, but they may occur in the paraganglia throughout the body. These tumors may be functional, producing catecholamines and other peptides.[159] Familial carotid body tumors, about 10 percent of cases, are often bilateral and follow an autosomal dominant mode of transmission.[160–163] Malignant chemodectomas are extremely rare. These tumors are discussed in detail in Chapter 10.

## TUBEROUS SCLEROSIS

Tuberous sclerosis is an autosomal dominant condition characterized by multiple hamartomas of the central nervous system and other organs, especially angiomyolipomas of the kidneys (80 percent), along with acneiform skin lesions, cardiac rhabdomyoma, and variable degrees of mental deficiency.[164,165] An association with the TSC1 locus on chromosome 9q34 and/or the TSC2 gene on chromosome 16p13.3 is evident in these patients.[165,166] The latter encodes a putative tumor suppressor protein that may function as a GTPase-activating protein for Rap1 and, not unexpectedly, plays a role in neural development and differentiation.[167,168] The brain abnormalities in tuberous sclerosis predispose to epilepsy as well as various glial tumors, and 2 percent of patients will develop giant cell astrocytomas. Patients with tuberous sclerosis are also at risk of developing renal cell carcinoma.[169]

## VON HIPPEL-LINDAU SYNDROME

von Hippel-Lindau syndrome is another inherited disorder of mesenchyme transmitted in an autosomal dominant fashion with variable expression. It is characterized by angiomatosis of the retina and cerebellum, along with visceral, subcutaneous, and cutaneous angiomas and cysts. In this preneoplastic disorder, patients are prone to develop pheochromocytoma or ependymoma, and 25 to 40 percent eventually develop renal cell carcinoma.[170–172] The gene for von Hippel-Lindau syndrome, VHL, has recently been identified.[173] Mutations of VHL occur not only in the germline of affected family members, but also in some sporadic renal cell carcinomas, hemangioblastomas, and pheochromocytomas.[174–176]

## ■ PLOIDY/CELL CYCLE KINETICS

Prognostication for adults with primary soft tissue sarcoma is currently based on tumor size, histologic grade, depth, location, histologic subtype, and the presence or absence of distant metastases.[177–181] However, recent studies suggest that proliferation markers may improve the prognostic value of standard clinicopathologic markers.[182–200] Some studies have shown that tumor cell proliferative activity and/or DNA content are related to the outcome of patients with soft tissue sarcoma. Several methods have been used to assess cell proliferation, including enumeration of mitotic figures, thymidine labeling indices, DNA-flow cytometric analysis, and immunohistochemical analysis of proteins associated with proliferation.

Clearly, the simplest assessment of proliferative activity of soft tissue sarcoma can be accomplished by counting the mitoses on routine histologic preparations. While interobserver variability compromises this approach,[177,190] assessment of the number of mitotic figures remains an integral part of histologic grading of soft tissue sarcoma.[191] Another method of measuring rates of proliferation is the method of thymidine labeling indices.

Analysis of DNA content has been suggested to be a prognostic indicator for soft tissue sarcoma.[182,183,185,186,188,189,192–195] Studies have found that nondiploid tumors have a poorer prognosis and are more likely to metastasize,[188] but not all investigations have confirmed this relationship.[195,196]

We recently analyzed DNA content in the soft tissue sarcomas of 50 patients and correlated the results with outcome.[197] Our results support the association of DNA content with prognosis, in contrast to findings in two studies of pediatric soft tissue sarcoma.[194,198] In our study of adults, when compared to patients with aneuploid tumors, those individuals with diploid tumors showed more than twofold greater five-year, disease-free, and overall survival rates (Fig. 6–2). Further, multivariate analysis revealed that DNA content was an independent prognostic indicator in our study. The widespread availability of DNA analysis by flow cytometry and image analysis, as well as the magnitude of the difference in predicted survival, suggest that DNA analysis may be useful clinically, for example in selecting candidates for adjuvant systemic therapy. However, such determinations will require further study.

Some studies have shown that S-phase fraction, either alone or in combination with ploidy determinations, has prognostic value for soft tissue sarcoma patients.[199,200] In addition, one study suggested that S-phase fraction predicted the early response of soft tissue sarcomas to chemotherapy.[201] However, the relationship of DNA content and/or S-phase fraction to histologic grading and clinical staging is not well defined. Thus, the use of either of these parameters as a clinical indicator of prognosis remains controversial.

The Ki-67 antigen was described in 1983 as a human nuclear antigen associated with cellular proliferation.[202] Furthermore, study of this antigen has shown that it is normally expressed during late G1, S, G2, and M phases of the cell cycle.[184,187] Immunohistochemical staining for the Ki-67 antigen correlates with the growth fraction of tumors.[203] Previous studies in soft tissue sarcoma and in other tumors have suggested that increased Ki-67 expression is associated with adverse clinical outcome.[184,204–209] Ki-67 expression has been found to be related to other proliferation markers and to p53 mutations.[205,207,209] However, Ki-67 expression may be related to histologic grade of a given soft tissue sarcoma; thus, its value as a prognostic indicator remains uncertain.

We recently evaluated Ki-67 and its relationship to outcome in 49 adult soft tissue sarcoma cases.[197] To date, the threshold value of immunohistochemical staining for Ki-67 expression that defines a high-risk lesion for Ki-67 expression is unclear. We chose 40 percent as a "positive" level of expression. The findings in our study of these 49 patients revealed significantly better survival in patients with low-level versus high-level expression (Fig. 6–3). Although our findings confirm the findings reported by other authors,[187] it appears that a prospective long-range observation in a larger number of patients incorporating all histologic subsets will be required to establish the clinical impact of these markers.

## ■ ONCOGENES

Rapid advances in molecular techniques have made possible definition of specific genetic alterations associated with the malignant phenotype. These "oncogenes" may be classified as dominant or recessive (tumor suppressor genes) depending on if their increased or decreased (respectively) function is associated with malignancy. Soft tissue sarcomas are associated primarily with tumor suppressor genes, but a role for dominant oncogenes has also been reported.

### Ras

The ras gene family consists of three genes: N-, H-, and K-ras, respectively located on chromosomes 1, 11, and 12.[210] Each gene consists of four exons which code for similar 21-kilodalton (kd) proteins. The proteins are related via complex interactions to membrane GTPase activity and intracellular pathways.[211]

Although ras genes have been the subject of many articles and are commonly expressed in adenocarcinomas, their role in soft tissue sarcoma has not been extensively explored. Occasional reports of isolated cases of ras activation in soft tissue sarcoma have been published.[212–214] Several small series of soft tissue sarcomas have shown low incidence of ras mutations—in the range of 3 to 35 percent.[215–217] We recently analyzed 54 leiomyosarcomas for K-ras mutations and found 9 out of 54 (17 percent) to contain mutations. The clinical ramifications of K-ras mutations remain obscure. High rates of K-ras expression have been reported in angiosarcomas with codon 13 mutations.[218] Although ras mutations are demonstrable in some types of soft tissue sarcomas, it is doubtful that this represents the original stimulation for malignant transformation.

### c-erbB2

c-erbB2, or Her-2/neu, is located on human chromosome 17 and encodes a 185-kd transmembrane protein (p185) which has remarkable homology with the epidermal growth factor receptor (EGFR).[219] This oncogene has been most extensively studied in breast cancer, and, in general, amplification of c-erbB2 and/or

Disease Free Survival DNA

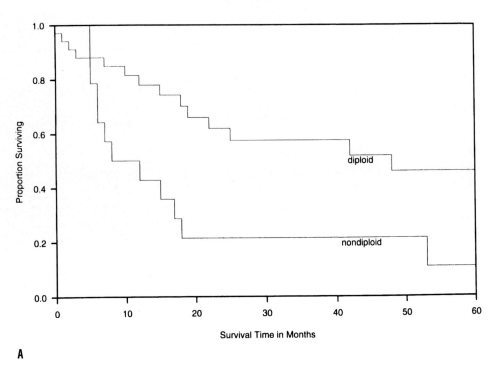

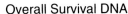

A

Overall Survival DNA

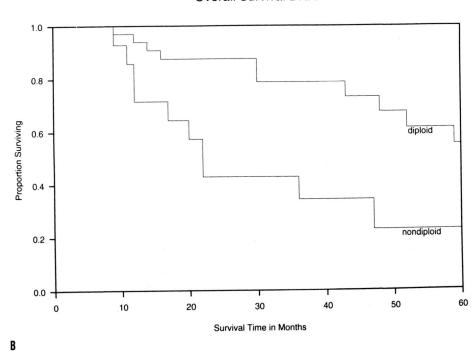

**Figure 6–2. (A)** Disease-free survival by DNA content. Sixty-month survival was 42 percent for diploid tumors versus 16 percent for aneuploid, $p = .010$. **(B)** Overall survival by DNA content. Sixty-month survival was 56 percent for diploid tumors versus 26 percent for aneuploid, $p = .015$.

B

overexpression of p185 is associated with a poor prognosis, especially for patients with lymph node involvement.[220–227] Recent clinical trials suggest that anti-p185 monoclonal antibody has some efficacy in the treatment of metastatic breast cancers overexpressing this oncoprotein.[228]

A few reports have analyzed c-erbB2 amplification or overexpression in soft tissue sarcoma.[229,230] Amplification in soft tissue sarcoma seems to be unusual, occurring in only six of 105 cases in one report.[230] However, p185 overexpression has been found in up to 37 percent of sarcomas.[229,230] One report found

### Disease Free Survival Ki-67

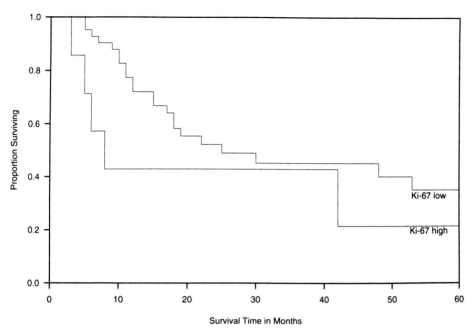

**A**

### Overall Survival Ki-67

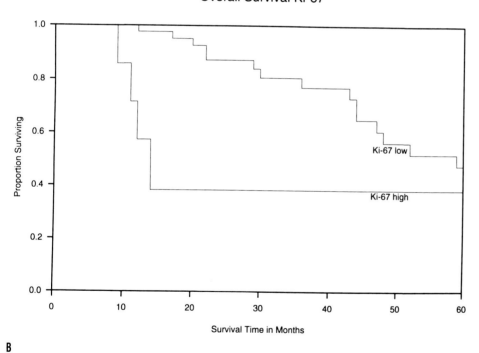

**B**

**Figure 6–3. (A)** Disease-free survival by level of Ki-67 expression. Sixty-month survival was 35 percent for low levels of expression versus 21 percent for high level, $p$ = NS. **(B)** Overall survival by level of Ki-67 expression. Sixty-month survival was 47 percent for low level of expression versus 35 percent for high level, $p$ = .0019.

c-erbB2 expression detected by immunohistochemistry in 78 percent of chondrosarcomas.[231] No studies have attached clinical significance to c-erbB2 amplification and/or overexpression. Furthermore, the low rates of c-erbB2 alterations do not suggest a role in the initiation or progression of soft tissue sarcomas.

### myc

The myc oncogene codes for a 65-kd nuclear phosphoprotein, which binds to DNA and can transform cells both in vitro and in vivo.[232] This gene is normally a single copy on chromosome 2. Amplification of myc has been shown to be a poor prognostic indicator for children with neuroblastoma.[233]

Several reports have been published of myc expression in soft tissue sarcoma.[234–239] In one report, amplification was found in a metastatic lesion but not in the primary tumor.[237] Another report in a study of rhabdomyosarcomas suggested that myc amplification is limited to the alveolar subtype.[236] A study of 23 soft tissue sarcoma cases found myc amplification in 30 percent and suggested it was correlated with higher grade and poorer survival.[234] Although the data for myc expression/amplification suggest a putative relationship between myc with progression and survival, confirmatory studies are needed before determination of myc can be suggested in routine clinical practice.

## MDM2

The MDM2 (murine double minute 2) gene was cloned in 1992.[240] This gene encodes a nuclear phosphoprotein that interacts with both the wild-type and mutant forms of the p53 protein.[241–244] MDM2, a zinc-finger protein, can bind to the amino-terminus of p53 protein to functionally inactivate both wild-type and mutant forms of p53.[244] Since earlier papers describing p53 mutations and MDM2 amplification as mutually exclusive events,[245] it has been shown that p53 mutations and/or MDM2 amplification or overexpression occur in a substantial proportion of soft tissue sarcomas.[246–250] Amplification of this gene, alone or in conjunction with expression of mutant p53 protein, has been shown to correlate with adverse outcome in a variety of soft tissue sarcoma patients.[246,247,251]

## ■ TUMOR SUPPRESSOR GENES

As discussed above, some familial syndromes associated with soft tissue tumors are attributable to germline mutations in tumor suppressor genes. Data from studies of the heritable soft tissue tumors that occur in these patients imply an etiologic role for tumor suppressor gene inactivation. Investigations have documented that (somatic) mutations of these tumor suppressor genes occur in a significant proportion of cases of the sporadic, more commonly occurring forms of soft tissue sarcoma.[115,235,245,246,252–259] Thus, the isolation and functional characterization of familial cancer syndrome genes has emerged as a major strategy for understanding tumorigenesis in general. This section will summarize the role of tumor suppressor genes in soft tissue sarcoma, including some work from our laboratory.

## p53

The p53 gene, located on human chromosome 17p13, encodes a nuclear phosphoprotein involved in transcriptional regulation, translational control, DNA repair, cell-cycle control, cell differentiation, and apoptosis.[121–123,127–129,260,261] Most p53 mutations are missense mutations that produce an altered protein.[129,262] Mutant p53 protein not only lacks the beneficial, tumor suppressive effect of the wild-type protein, but appears to act as an oncogene.[121] Because of its role in apoptosis and DNA repair, p53 may also be involved in mechanisms of drug resistance.[129,263]

The p53 gene is the most commonly mutated gene in human solid tumors[130,264,265] and has been studied extensively in soft tissue sarcomas. Mutation or functional inactivation of the p53 gene has been reported to occur in many types of soft tissue sarcomas.[245,246,248,252–257,266–268] In addition, a few immunohistochemical studies indicate that nuclear accumulation of p53 protein in some types of soft tissue sarcomas is associated with disease recurrence and diminished survival.[207,255,268–270] These studies have suggested a causal relationship between poor prognosis and the presence of mutant p53 protein in soft tissue sarcoma.

Some of our work on mutant p53 expression in soft tissue sarcomas has been an attempt to correlate quantitative analysis of the amount of mutant p53 protein expressed by soft tissue tumors with long-term survival. Our focus has been on how these observations might be used clinically. We previously reported our findings on the significance of mutant p53 protein expression as a prognostic marker in well-differentiated soft tissue sarcomas.[271] In that study, we used an enzyme-linked immunosorbent assay (ELISA) employing mutant p53 Ab240 as the capture antibody to quantitate mutant p53 protein expression in 47 grade 1 soft tissue sarcomas. The p53 Ab240 recognizes an epitope (amino acids 212–217) revealed by a common conformational change or an extensive unfolding of the core domain, and occurring in most mutant p53 proteins.[262,272]

Of the 47 tumors analyzed, we found detectable mutant p53 protein ($> 0.25$ ng of mutant p53 protein/mg total protein) in 16 tumors (34 percent). After a mean follow-up of 112 months, 63 percent of patients with mutant p53-positive tumors, but only 16 percent of patients with mutant p53-negative tumors, had died of disease ($p < 0.001$). Mutant p53 expression of greater than or equal to 4.5 ng/mg total protein predicted even greater reduction in survival, with the mean overall survival dropping from 110 months for patients with mutant p53-negative tumors, to 82 months for patients whose tumors expressed from 0.25 to 4.5 ng of mutant p53, to 32 months for those whose tumors expressed greater than 4.5 ng of mutant p53 protein. These data demonstrate the prognostic significance of quantitative determination of mutant p53 protein expression in low-grade sarcomas.

We have now studied mutant p53 expression by ELISA in 213 soft tissue sarcomas, and we have found detectable levels of mutant p53 protein in 130 (61 percent) of these tumors.[273] Mutant p53 expression was associated with younger patient age and higher tumor grade, as shown in Tables 6-4 and 6-5. Both the proportion of tumors exhibiting mutant p53 expression and the prognostic significance of these observations varied among the histologic types of sarcoma, shown in Table 6-6. For the group as a whole, mutant p53 expression correlated significantly with both disease-free and overall survival, as shown in Fig. 6-4A and 6-4B. In addition, the highest levels of mutant p53 expression ($>10$ ng/mg total protein) were associated with the shortest survival times. Whereas 45 of 83 patients (54 percent) with mutant p53-negative tumors relapsed and 25 of 83 (30 percent) died of disease, 69 of 95 (73 percent) patients with tumors expressing 0.25 to 10 ng of mutant p53 protein/mg total protein relapsed and 54 of 94 (57 percent) died of disease; 28 of 35 patients (80 percent) whose tumors expressed greater than 10 ng of mutant p53 protein relapsed and 23 out of 35 (66 percent) died of disease ($p = 0.0063$ for recurrence and $p = 0.0001$ for death from disease). Mutant p53 expression appears to be better at predicting which patients with low-grade tumors have poor prognoses than which patients with high-grade tumors have relatively good prognoses. This may be because p53 mutations are a relatively early or intermediate event in the progression of these tumors, or because a greater number of null mutations or deletions, which are not detected by this methodology, occur in higher grade tumors. Also, other factors which functionally inactivate p53 protein (e.g., MDM2 overexpression) may have relatively greater importance in these tumors.

We have also studied mutant p53 expression in lung metastases from soft tissue sarcoma patients. In our study of 30 patients, the median survival for the few patients (n=12) with mutant p53-negative lung metastases was $39 \pm 9$ months versus $17 \pm 3$ months for those patients (n=18) with mutant p53-positive lung metastases.[274] Most of these patients received chemotherapy in addition to resection of their metastatic disease, suggesting that mutant p53 may permit the growth of chemoresistant micrometastatic tumor cells.

There are several mechanisms by which altered p53 protein expression may facilitate tumor progression. Tumor-derived p53 mutants often lose sequence-specific DNA binding ability and lack the ability to activate gene transcription. One manifestation of this is the loss of p53-mediated cell cycle checkpoint control, permitting propagation of cells with damaged DNA.[122,125,127,128,262,275,276] The p53 gene also regulates transcription of the GADD45 gene (growth-arrested and DNA damage-inducible gene) which can form a complex with proliferating cell nuclear antigen

### TABLE 6-4. RELATIONSHIP OF MUTANT p53 EXPRESSION IN 213 SOFT TISSUE SARCOMAS TO DEMOGRAPHIC PARAMETERS

| Parameter | Mutant p53+, proportion (%) | p Value |
|---|---|---|
| Gender | | |
| Female | 64/108 (59%) | 0.59 |
| Male | 66/105 (63%) | |
| Age | | |
| Younger than 50 | 73/107 (68%) | 0.03 |
| 50 years or older | 57/106 (54%) | |

### TABLE 6-5. RELATIONSHIP OF MUTANT p53 EXPRESSION IN 213 SOFT TISSUE SARCOMAS TO TUMOR CHARACTERISTICS

| Parameter | Mutant p53+, proportion (%) | p Value |
|---|---|---|
| Grade | | |
| 1 | 20/52 (38%) | 0.0001 |
| 2-3 | 110/161 (68%) | |
| Size | | |
| Less than or equal to 5 cm | 30/46 (65%) | 0.79 |
| Larger than 5 cm | 100/167 (60%) | |
| Location | | |
| Superficial | 71/114 (62%) | 0.69 |
| Deep | 59/99 (60%) | |

### TABLE 6-6. MUTANT p53 EXPRESSION IN VARIOUS HISTOLOGIC TYPES OF SOFT TISSUE SARCOMA

| Tumor Type | Mutant p53+, proportion (%) | Prognostic Value: mutant p53+ vs. mutant p53- |
|---|---|---|
| Liposarcoma | 23/51 (45%) | yes ($p = 0.0001$) |
| Malignant fibrous histiocytoma | 26/46 (57%) | no ($p = 0.11$) |
| Leiomyosarcoma | 27/34 (79%) | no ($p = 0.26$) |
| Malignant schwannoma | 20/26 (77%) | no ($p = 0.98$) |
| Synovial cell sarcoma | 12/18 (67%) | no ($p = 0.53$) |
| Rhabdomyosarcoma | 10/15 (67%) | yes ($p = 0.04$) |
| Fibrosarcoma | 6/10 (60%) | yes ($p = 0.03$) |
| Extraskeletal myxoid chondrosarcoma | 5/9 (56%) | no ($p = 0.07$) |
| Hemangiopericytoma | 0/2 (0%) | — |
| Clear cell sarcoma | 1/1 (100%) | — |
| Undifferentiated | 0/1 (0%) | — |

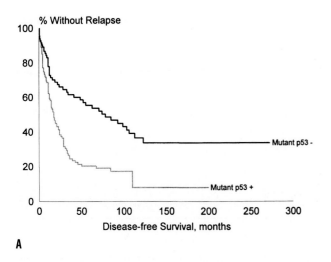

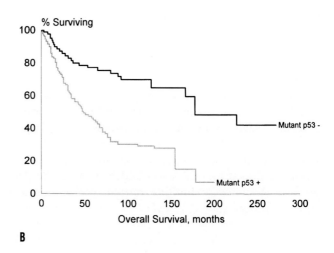

**Figure 6–4. (A)** Disease-free survival curves for soft tissue sarcoma patients with mutant p53+ (n = 130) and mutant p53− (n = 83) tumors. The difference in recurrence-free survival was statistically significant with a *p* value of < 0.0001. **(B)** Overall survival curves for soft tissue sarcoma patients with mutant p53+ (n = 130) and mutant p53− (n = 83) tumors. The difference in recurrence-free survival was statistically significant with a *p* value of < 0.0001.

(PCNA), a DNA-damage-inducible gene, to regulate DNA excision repair.[277,278] The PCNA promoter can also be transcriptionally activated by p53.[279] In addition, therapeutic modalities that act through p53-dependent apoptotic pathways (including doxorubicin and ionizing radiation) are disabled by expression of mutant p53 protein.[280–283] Recent studies also have demonstrated that p53 mutations facilitate angiogenesis either by down-regulating the expression of angiogenesis inhibitors[284] and/or by inducing protein kinase C stimulation of vascular growth factors.[285] p53 can also interact with other tumor suppressor genes known to be involved in the development and/or progression of soft tissue tumors, including RB1.

### RB1

The human retinoblastoma gene, RB1, located on chromosome 13, is another tumor suppressor gene involved in the genesis of soft tissue tumors. As discussed earlier in this chapter, germline mutations of RB1 result in the hereditary form of retinoblastoma. In addition, somatic mutations of this gene and/or absent p110$^{RB}$ protein expression have been observed in various human tumors and tumor cell lines.[97,286–292] Alterations in RB1[235,252,258,259] or p110$^{RB}$ protein expression[288,293–295] have been observed in up to 70 percent of soft tissue tumors studied, but do not appear to consistently have clinical prognostic value.[294] In addition, RB1 is not ubiquitously involved in all types of sarcoma in one study; no p110$^{RB}$ alterations have been reported in pediatric rhabdomyosarcomas studied.[296] The RB1 gene product, depending on its phosphorylation state,

appears to regulate cell growth by modulating transcription factor activity.[96,97,297,298] Loss of p110$^{RB}$ function has been implicated in the development of resistance to certain chemotherapeutic agents.[299] Evidence from murine models of tumorigenesis suggest that RB1 interacts with p53 pathways.[300,301] Indirect support for this interaction in human tumors comes from studies at both the DNA and protein levels.[252,297]

### MTS1

The multiple tumor suppressor 1 gene, MTS1 or p16/CDKN2, was recently identified on Chromosome 9 by linkage studies focusing on familial malignant melanoma.[302,303] This gene encodes an inhibitor of the cyclin-dependent kinase cdk4. Little is known about this gene in either familial or sporadic forms of soft tissue sarcoma. One recent study found MTS1/CDKN2 deletions in two of eight malignant schwannomas and two of five rhabdomyosarcomas studied.[304] The clinical significance of either germline or somatic mutations of this gene in soft tissue sarcoma patients remains to be elucidated.

### ■ DRUG-RESISTANT GENES

Resistance to chemotherapy, a common clinical problem in many neoplastic diseases, is also encountered in patients with soft tissue sarcomas. This resistance may be present at the initiation of chemotherapy or may be acquired by the tumor during the course of therapy. Only within the last decade have the specific mechanisms of biochemical resistance to cytotoxic chemotherapy begun to be understood. Such mechanisms can confer resistance to a single drug; however, clinical drug resistance is frequently characterized by resistance to a number of different drugs, possibly via several mechanisms.

The term *multidrug resistance* (MDR) describes a phenomenon by which a neoplasm becomes resistant to many drugs simultaneously.[305–307] The best known MDR phenotype is mediated via the MDR-1 gene, which is a single-copy gene located on the long arm of Chromosome 7.[307,308] This gene is over 100 kilobases in length and is composed of 27 introns with 28 exons.[305,308–310] MDR-1 codes for a 1,280 amino-acid transmembrane glycosylated protein of 170 kd, p-glycoprotein (P-gp).[308] P-gp functions as an energy-dependent efflux pump for lipophilic drugs. Several commonly used antineoplastic drugs are lipophilic substrates for P-gp; therefore, expression of P-gp results in decreased intracellular accumulation of these drugs.[305–307] The ability of P-gp to keep such drugs from reaching their intracellular targets has resulted in clinical drug resistance.[206,311–315] Substrates of P-gp include vinca alkaloids, epipodophyllotoxins, mitomycin-C, taxol, and anthracyclines such as doxorubicin—the latter being the most active single agent in the treatment of soft tissue sarcomas.[307,310,316,317]

Expression of P-gp has been shown to be related to clinical drug resistance[311,318–322] and poor prognosis[312,313,321] in several types of malignant tumors. Previous studies, predominantly in pediatric soft tissue sarcoma,[313,314,323] evaluated MDR-1/P-gp in soft tissue sarcoma using a variety of methods and showed expression ranging from 0 to 83 percent.[311,318,319,323–325] Further, few studies evaluating P-gp expression in soft tissue sarcoma have correlated findings with clinical course or outcomes.[311,312,314,323,325]

Several techniques have been used to study the MDR-1/P-gp system.[307] The expression of MDR-1 mRNA can be measured using slot-blot,[318,319] northern analysis, or polymerase chain reaction (PCR)-based methods.[206,321,322,326] While the PCR technique seems to be the most sensitive, all are bulk tissue assays and therefore limited by potential sampling error. We analyzed 65 snap-frozen soft tissue sarcoma specimens for the MDR-1 gene using an RT-PCR technique.[197,327] MDR-1 expression was found in 51 percent of the cases. Expression was quantitated using the KB cell lines (with known rates of MDR-1 expression). Low-level expression was found in 42 percent and high-level in 9 percent. No patient with high-level expression survived more than three years. When the results were stratified into three levels of expression (none, low, and high), patients showed significantly different overall and disease-free survival ($p = .016$ and $p = .0035$, respectively), as shown in Fig. 6–5A and 6–5B.

Immunohistochemistry-based techniques employing several antibodies have been used to detect P-gp.[312,313,315,325] Unfortunately, previously used antibodies have suffered from nonspecific binding, which has limited their use.[328] While immunohistochemical methods may not be as sensitive as PCR techniques for detecting very low levels of P-gp expression, the former have the advantage of specificity because each cell can be evaluated microscopically to confirm its malignant character. We believe that the monoclonal antibody, UIC-2 (developed by Igor Roninson, Ph.D., Department of Molecular Biology and Genetics, UIC), represents an improvement in specificity over previously available antibodies.

In a recent study, we used UIC-2 directed against an external epitope of P-gp, which has been shown to be highly specific with low levels of background staining.[328,329] We studied 50 soft tissue sarcoma specimens and correlated the results to outcomes.[197,327] Our results show that expression of P-gp is a marker of a poor prognosis, as determined by the disease-free survival in stages II and III soft tissue sarcoma (see Fig. 6–6A and 6–6B). There was no significant difference in overall survival, stratified by P-gp staining, in this study for stages II and III. However, since the number of patients in this group was relatively small, it is quite possible that this lack of statistical significance in overall survival represents a type I error. Our findings are consistent with previous studies in patients with pediatric soft tissue sarcomas[312] and Ewing's sarcoma.[323]

The use of MDR-1/P-gp assays to predict the sensitivity of a specific tumor to various antineoplastic therapies remains a very active area of investigation.[305–309] Several retrospective studies have yielded data supporting the use of MDR-1/P-gp analysis in this regard for pediatric soft tissue sarcoma,[312] neuroblastoma,[313] leukemia,[330] and other solid tumors.[331,332] Clearly, this aspect of P-gp demands further research, which may best be done prospectively.

Our data imply that soft tissue sarcomas with MDR-1/P-gp expression have a poorer prognosis, independent of response to chemotherapy. Similar findings have been reported in patients with osteosarcoma.[333,334] One explanation for this finding could be increased expression of MDR-1/P-gp stimulated by other genes that are also poor prognostic indicators. Recent studies have shown increased MDR-1/P-gp expression with activation of protein kinase C,[335] oncogenes HER-2/neu,[331] myc,[336] ras,[336,337] and inactivation of the p53 tumor suppressor gene.[337] Further, MDR-1/P-gp expression has been shown to relate to other drug resistance factors, such as glutathione

### Overall Survival MDR-1 Expression

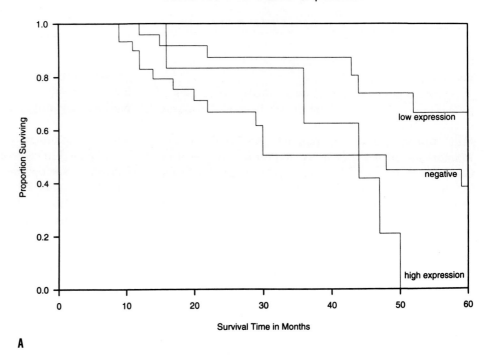

**A**

### Disease Free Survival MDR-1 Expression

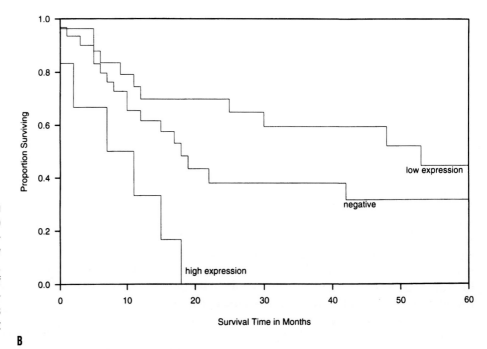

**Figure 6–5. (A)** Overall survival found in cases of high (n = 6), low (n = 27), and no expression (n = 32) of MDR-1 mRNA. Differences between groups were significantly different by univariate analysis, $p$ = 0.016. **(B)** Disease-free survival found in cases of high (n = 6), low (n = 27), and no expression (n = 32) of MDR-1 mRNA. Differences between groups were significantly different by univariate analysis, $p$ = 0.0035.

**B**

S-transferase, and topoisomerase II.[332] Such associations with MDR-1/P-gp expression are likely critical to our understanding of clinical drug resistance.[338–340]

In addition to the MDR-1/P-gp system, other genes have been associated with clinical multidrug resistance. Non-MDR-1-mediated multidrug resistance has also been shown for MRP (multidrug resistance-associated protein).[341,342] However, MRP did confer multidrug resistance to a fibrosarcoma cell line.[343] To date, there has been scant clinical information regarding MRP expression in soft tissue sarcoma. A recent study of MRP expression using an immunohistochemical assay

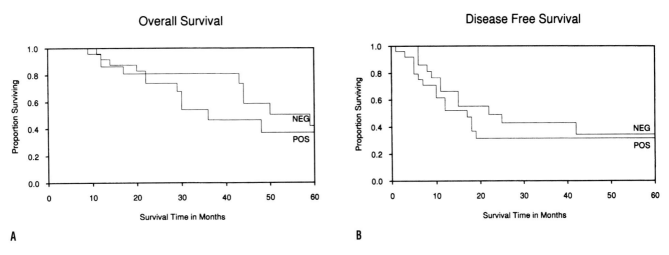

**Figure 6–6. (A)** Overall survival for high-grade tumors without metastases, stages II and III[197,328] (n = 26). The 5-year survival for P-gp negative (NEG) is 54 percent versus 14 percent for P-gp-positive (POS) (*p* = 0.071). **(B)** Disease-free survival for high-grade tumors without metastases, stages II and III,[178] (n = 26). The five-year disease-free survival for P-gp-negative (NEG) is 25 percent versus 19 percent for P-gp-positive (POS) (*p* = .039).

found 0 out of 14 soft tissue sarcomas expressing MRP, with low levels found in all 14 specimens using RT-PCR.[344] The clinical relevance of MRP and other markers of drug resistance is not yet established.[345]

### ■ CONCLUSIONS

Great strides have been made over the past decade in our understanding of the molecular events responsible for soft tissue sarcoma development and progression. However, we are still at the beginning of the journey in our understanding of these molecular phenomena. By analyzing soft tissue sarcomas with increasingly powerful molecular and cytogenetic techniques, we have begun to lift the etiologic shroud that has hung over these unusual tumors.

The genetic changes found in familial forms of sarcoma are also present in some sporadically occurring forms of these tumors. Most have proven to be mutations in tumor suppressor genes, such as the p53 gene. To date, there appears to be little role for dominant-acting oncogenes in the development and/or progression of soft tissue sarcoma. Investigation of the relevance of drug-resistance markers, proliferation markers and DNA analysis in soft tissue sarcomas suggests that prospective studies are warranted for a variety of potential prognostic markers in sarcomas. Such information may help us to select appropriate candidates for adjuvant therapy and even to design appropriate biologic treatment.

Currently, the constantly expanding molecular database in soft tissue sarcoma has only found clinical use by providing diagnostic aids and prognostic markers. Although molecular markers may eventually determine optimal therapeutic measures, they have only recently found use in current clinical trials. Other areas that merit future investigation in soft tissue sarcomas include the role of adhesion molecules, matrix proteins, immunobiology, and other factors that may govern both the site and likelihood of metastasis.

The tremendous developments in our understanding of sarcoma biology of the past few years encourage us to believe that continued investigation will be fruitful from the standpoint of both scientific inquiry and therapeutic value. As our ability to manipulate genetic material improves, we may eventually be able to repair the molecular derangements responsible for soft tissue sarcoma.

### REFERENCES

1. Sandberg AA, Turc-Carel C, Gemmill RM: Chromosomes in solid tumours and beyond. Cancer Res 48: 1049, 1988
2. Kallioniemi A, Kallioniemi O-P, Sudar D, et al.: Comparative genomic hybridization for molecular cytogenetic analysis of solid tumors. Science 258:818, 1992
3. Mitelman F: Catalog of Chromosome Aberrations in Cancer, 5th ed. Wiley-Liss, New York, 1994
4. Heim S, Mitelman F: Cancer Cytogenetics, 2nd ed. Wiley-Liss, New York, 1995
5. Turc-Carel C, Limon J, Da Cin P, et al.: Cytogenetic studies of adipose tissue tumors. II. Recurrent reciprocal translocation of t(12;16)(q13;p11) in myxoid liposarcomas. Cancer Genet Cytogenet 23:291, 1986
6. Mertens F, Johansson B, Mandahl N, et al.: Clonal chro-

mosome abnormalities in two liposarcomas. Cancer Genet Cytogenet 28:137, 1987

7. Molenaar WM, DeJong B, Buist J, et al.: Chromosomal analysis and the classification of soft tissue sarcomas. Lab Invest 60:266, 1989

8. Eneroth M, Mandahl N, Heim S, et al.: Localization of the chromosomal breakpoints of the t(12;16) in liposarcoma to sub-bands 12q13.3 and 16p11.2. Cancer Genet Cytogenet 48:101, 1990

9. Sreekantaiah C, Karakousis CP, Leong SPL, Sandberg AA: Cytogenetic findings in liposarcoma correlate with histopathologic subtypes. Cancer 69:2484, 1992

10. Ohjimi Y, Iwasaki H, Kaneko Y, et al.: Chromosome abnormalities in liposarcomas. Cancer Genet Cytogenet 64:111, 1992

11. Aman P, Ron D, Mandahl N, et al.: Rearrangement of the transcription factor gene CHOP in myxoid liposarcomas with t(12;16)(q13;p11). Genes Chromosom Cancer 5:278, 1992

12. Crozat A, Aman P, Mandahl N, Ron D: Fusion of CHOP to a novel RNA-binding protein in human myxoid liposarcoma. Nature 363:640, 1993

13. Rabbitts TH, Forster A, Larson R, Nathan P: Fusion of the dominant negative transcription regulator CHOP with a novel gene FUS by translocation t(12;16) in malignant liposarcoma. Nature Genet 4:175, 1993

14. Panagopoulos I, Mandahl N, Ron D, et al.: Characterization of the CHOP breakpoints and fusion transcripts in myxoid liposarcomas with the 12;16 translocation. Cancer Res 54:6500, 1994

15. Ron D, Habener JF: CHOP, a novel developmentally regulated nuclear protein that dimerizes with transcription factor C/EBP and LAP and functions as a dominant negative inhibitor of gene transcription. Genes Dev 6:439, 1992

16. Knight JC, Renwick PJ, Dal Cin P, et al.: Translocation t(12;16)(q13;p11) in myxoid liposarcoma and round cell liposarcoma: Molecular and cytogenetic analysis. Cancer Res 55:24, 1995

17. Heim S, Mandahl N, Kristoffersson U, et al.: Marker ring chromosome—A new cytogenetic abnormality characterizing lipogenic tumors? Cancer Genet Cytogenet 24:319, 1987

18. Pedeutour F, Suijkerbuijk RF, Forus A, et al.: Complex composition and co-amplification of SAS and MDM2 in ring and giant rod marker chromosomes in well-differentiated liposarcoma. Genes Chromosom Cancer 10:85, 1994

19. Nilbert M, Rydholm A, Willen H, et al.: MDM2 gene amplification correlates with ring chromosomes in soft tissue tumors. Genes Chrom Cancer 9:261, 1994

20. Forus A, Weghuis DO, Smeets D, et al.: Comparative genomic hybridization analysis of human sarcomas: I. Occurrence of genomic imbalances and identification of a novel major amplicon at 1q21–q22 in soft tissue sarcomas. Genes Chromosom Cancer 14:8, 1995

21. Sreekantaiah C, Leong SPL, Karakous C, et al.: Cytogenetic profiles of 109 lipomas. Cancer Res 51:422, 1991

22. Paulien S, Sandberg AA, Herz J, Gemmill RM: Putative apolipoprotein receptor gene (LRP, A2MR) is not rearranged in either myxoid liposarcoma or lipomas with translocations in 12q13–14. Cancer Genet Cytogenet 60:125, 1992

23. Khatib ZA, Matsushime H, Valentine M, et al.: Coamplification of the CDK4 gene with MDM2 and GLI in human sarcomas. Cancer Res 55:5535, 1993

24. Su YA, Hutter CM, Trent JM, Meltzer PS: Complete sequence analysis of a gene (OS-9) ubiquitously expressed in human tissues and amplified in sarcomas. Mol Carcinog 15:270, 1996

25. Mandahl N, Örndal C, Heim S, et al.: Aberrations of chromosome segment 12q13-15 characterize a subgroup of hemangiopericytomas. Cancer 71:3009, 1993

26. Forus A, Flørenes VA, Maelandsmo, et al.: The protooncogene CHOP/GADD153, involved in growth arrest and DNA damage response, is amplified in a subset of human sarcomas. Cancer Genet Cytogenet 78:165, 1994

27. Mandahl N, Heim S, Willén H, et al.: Characteristic karyotypic anomalies identify subtypes of malignant fibrous histiocytoma. Genes Chrom Cancer 1:9, 1989

28. Örndal C, Rydholm A, Willén H, et al.: Cytogenetic intratumor heterogeneity in soft tissue tumors. Cancer Genet Cytogenet 78:127, 1994

29. Bridge JA, Sreekantaiah C, Mouron B, et al.: Clonal chromosomal abnormalities in desmoid tumors. Implications for histopathogenesis. Cancer 69:430, 1992.

30. Dal Cin P, Sciot R, Aly MS, et al.: Some desmoid tumors are characterized by trisomy 8. Genes Chrom Cancer 10:131, 1994

31. Fletcher JA, Naem R, Xiao S, Corson JM: Chromosome aberrations in desmoid tumors. Trisomy 8 may be a predictor of recurrence. Cancer Genet Cytogenet 79:139, 1995

32. Turc-Carrel C, Lizard-Nacol S, Justrabo E, et al.: Consistent chromosomal translocations in alveolar rhabdomyosarcoma. Cancer Genet Cytogenet 19:361, 1986

33. Douglass EC, Valentine M, Etcubanas E, et al.: A specific chromosomal abnormality in rhabdomyosarcoma. Cytogenet Cell Genet 45:148, 1987

34. Wang-Wuu S, Soukup S, Ballard E, et al.: Chromosomal analysis of sixteen human rhabdomyosarcomas. Cancer Res 48:983, 1988

35. Whang-Peng J, Knutsen T, Theil K, et al.: Cytogenetic studies in subgroups of rhabdomyosarcoma genes. Chromosome Cancer 5:299, 1992

36. Barr FG, Galili N, Holick J, et al.: Rearrangement of the PAX3 paired box gene in the paediatric solid tumour alveolar rhabdomyosarcoma. Nat Genet 3:113, 1993

37. Galili N, Davis RJ, Fredericks WJ, et al.: Fusion of a fork head domain gene to PAX3 in the solid tumour alveolar rhabdomyosarcoma. Nat Genet 5:230, 1993

38. Shapiro DN, Sublett JE, Li B, et al.: Fusion of PAX3 to a member of the forkhead family of transcription factors in human alveolar rhabdomyosarcoma. Cancer Res 53:5108, 1993

39. Douglass EC, Rowe ST, Valentine M, et al.: Variant translocations of chromosome 13 in alveolar rhabdomyosarcoma. Genes Chromosom Cancer 3:480, 1991

40. Davis RJ, D'Cruz CM, Lovell MA, et al.: Fusion of PAX7

to FKHR by the variant t(1;13)(p6;q14) translocation in alveolar rhabdomyosarcoma. Cancer Res 54:2869, 1994

41. Biegel JA, Nycum LM, Valentine V, et al.: Detection of the t(2;13)(p35;q14) chromosomal translocation of PAX3-FKHR fusion in alveolar rhabdomyosarcoma by fluorescence in situ hybridization. Genes Chromosom Cancer 12:186, 1995

42. Scrable HJ, Witte DP, Lampkin BC, et al.: Chromosomal localization of the human rhabdomyosarcoma locus by mitotic recombination mapping. Nature 329:645, 1987

43. Wiedemann HR: Tumours and hemihypertrophy associated with Wiedemann-Beckwith syndrome. Eur J Pediatr 141:129, 1983

44. Scrable H, Cavenee W, Ghavimi F, et al.: A model for embryonal rhabdomyosarcoma tumorigenesis that involves genome imprinting. Proc Natl Acad Sci U S A 86: 7480, 1989

45. Zhan S, Shapiro DN, Helman LJ: Activation of an imprinted allele of the insulin-like growth factor II gene implicated in rhabdomyosarcoma. J Clin Invest 94:445, 1994

46. Koi M, Johnson LA, Kalikin LM, et al.: Tumor cell growth arrest caused by subchromosomal transferable DNA fragments from chromosome 11. Science 260:361, 1993

47. Whang-Peng J, Triche TJ, Knutsen T, et al.: Chromosomal translocation in peripheral neuroepithelioma. N Engl J Med 311:584, 1984

48. Whang-Peng J, Triche TJ, Knutsen T, et al.: Cytogenetic characterization of selected small round cell tumors of childhood. Cancer Genet Cytogenet 21:185, 1986

49. Turc-Carel C, Auria A, Mugneret F, et al.: Chromosomes in Ewing's sarcoma. 1. An evaluation of 85 cases and remarkable consistency of t(11;22)(q24;q12). Cancer Genet Cytogenet 32:229, 1988

50. Donner LR: Cytogenetics and molecular biology of small round cell tumors and related neoplasms. Current status. Cancer Genet Cytogenet 54:1, 1991

51. McManus AP, Gusterson BA, Pinkerton CR, Shipley JM: Diagnosis of Ewing's sarcoma and related tumours by detection of chromosome 22q12 translocations using fluorescence in situ hybridization on tumour touch imprints. J Pathol 176:137, 1995

52. Delattre O, Zucman J, Plougastel B, et al.: Gene fusion with an ETS DNA-binding domain caused by chromosomal translocation in human tumors. Nature 359:162, 1992

53. May WA, Gishizky ML, Lessnick SL, et al.: Ewing sarcoma 11;22 translocation produces a chimeric transcription factor that requires the DNA-binding domain encoded by FLI1 for transformation. Proc Natl Acad Sci U S A 90:5752, 1993

54. Sorensen PHB, Shimada H, Liu XF, et al.: Biphenotypic sarcomas with myogenic and neural differentiation expression Ewing's sarcoma EWS/FLI1 fusion gene. Cancer Res 55:1385, 1995

55. Zucman J, Delattre O, Desmaze C, et al.: Cloning and characterization of the Ewing's sarcoma and peripheral neuroepithelioma t(11;22) translocation breakpoints. Genes Chromosom Cancer 5:271, 1992

56. Sorensen PHB, Lessnick SL, Lopez-Terrada D, et al.: A second Ewing's sarcoma translocation, t(21;22), fuses the EWS gene to another ETS-family transcription factor, ERG. Nat Genet 6:145, 1994

57. Giovannini M, Biegel JA, Serra M, et al.: EWS-erg and EWS-FLI1 fusion transcripts in Ewing's sarcoma and primitive neuroectodermal tumors with variant translocations. J Clin Invest 94:489, 1994

58. Ladanyi M, William G: Fusion of the EWS and WT1 genes in the desmoplastic small round cell tumor. Cancer Res 54:2837, 1994

59. Argatoff LH, O'Connell JX, Mathers JA, et al.: Detection of the EWS-WT1 gene fusion by reverse transcriptase-polymerase chain reaction in the diagnosis of intra-abdominal desmoplastic small round cell tumor. Am J Surg Pathol 20:406, 1996

60. Urano F, Umezawa A, Hong W, et al.: A novel chimera gene between EWS and E1A-F, encoding the adenovirus E1A enhancer-binding protein, in extraosseous Ewing's sarcoma. Biochem Biophys Res Commun 219:608, 1996

61. Bridge JA, Sreekantaiah C, Neff JR, et al.: Cytogenetic findings in clear cell sarcoma of tendons and aponeuroses: Implication for histogenesis. Cancer Genet Cytogenet 52:101, 1991

62. Stenman G, Kindblom LG, Angervall L: Reciprocal translocation t(12;22)(q13;q13) in clear cell sarcoma of tendons and aponeuroses. Genes Chromosom Cancer 4:122, 1992

63. Mrozek K, Karakousis CP, Perez-Mesa C, Bloomfield CD: Translocation 5(12;22)(q13;q12.2–12.3) in a clear cell sarcoma of tendons and aponeuroses. Genes Chromosomes Cancer 6:249, 1993

64. Zucman J, Delattre O, Desmaze C, et al.: EWS and ATF-1 gene fusion induced by t(12;22) translocation in malignant melanoma of soft parts. Nat Genet 4:341, 1993

65. Limon J, Debiec-Rychter M, Nedoszytko B, et al.: Aberrations of chromosome 22 and polysomy of chromosome 8 as non-random changes in clear cell sarcoma. Cancer Genet Cytogenet 72:141, 1994

66. Fujimura Y, Ohno T, Siddique H, et al.: The EWS-ATF-1 gene involved in malignant melanoma of soft parts with t(12;22) chromosome translocation, encodes a constitutive transcriptional activator. Oncogene 12:159, 1996

67. Limon J, Dal Cin P, Sandberg AA: Translocations involving the X chromosome in solid tumors: Presentation of two sarcomas with t(X;18)(q13;p11). Cancer Genet Cytogenet 23:87, 1986

68. Turc-Carel C, Dal Cin P, Limon J, et al.: Involvement of chromosome X in primary cytogenetic change in human neoplasia: Nonrandom translocation in synovial sarcoma. Proc Natl Acad Sci U S A 84:1981, 1987

69. Limon J, Mrozek K, Mandahl N, et al.: Cytogenetics of synovial sarcoma: Presentation of ten new cases and review of the literature. Genes Chrom Cancer 3:338, 1991

70. Dal Cin P, Rao U, Jani-Sait S, et al.: Chromosomes in the diagnosis of soft tissue tumors. I. Synovial sarcoma. Mod Pathol 5:357, 1992

71. Knight JC, Reeves BR, Smith S, et al.: Cytogenetic and

molecular analysis of synovial sarcoma. Int J Oncol 1: 747, 1992

72. Nagao K, Ito H, Yoshida H: Chromosomal translocation t(X;18) in human synovial sarcomas analyzed by fluorescence in situ hybridization using paraffin-embedded tissue. Am J Pathol 148:601, 1996

73. de Leeuw B, Suikerbuijk RF, Olde Weghuis D, et al.: Distinct Xp11.2 breakpoint regions in synovial sarcoma revealed by metaphase and interphase FISH: Relationship to histologic subtypes. Cancer Genet Cytogenet 73:89, 1994

74. Renwick PJ, Reeves BR, Dal Cin P, et al.: Two categories of synovial sarcoma defined by divergent chromosome translocation breakpoints in Xp11.2, with implications for the histologic sub-classification of synovial sarcoma. Cytogenet Cell Genet 70:58, 1995

75. Crew AJ, Clark J, Fisher C, et al.: Fusion of two genes, SSX1 and SSX2, encoding proteins with homology to the Kruppel-associated box in human synovial sarcoma. EMBO J 14:2333, 1995

76. Shipley J, Crew J, Birdsall S, et al.: Interphase fluorescence in situ hybridization and reverse transcription polymerase chain reaction as a diagnostic aid for synovial sarcoma. Am J Pathol 148:559, 1996

77. Hinrichs SH, Jaramillo MA, Gumerlock PH, et al.: Myxoid chondrosarcoma with a translocation involving chromosome 9 and 22. Cancer Genet Cytogenet 14:219, 1985

78. Turc-Carel C, Dal Cin P, Rao U, et al.: Recurrent breakpoints at 9p31 and 22q12.2 in extraskeletal myxoid chondrosarcoma. Cancer Genet Cytogenet 30:145, 1988

79. Hirabayashi Y, Ishida T, Yoshida MA, et al.: Translocation (9;22)(q22;q12): A recurrent chromosome abnormality in extraskeletal myxoid chondrosarcoma. Cancer Genet Cytogenet 81:33, 1995

80. Stenman G, Andersson H, Mandahl N, et al.: Translocation t(9;22)(q22;q12) is a primary cytogenetic abnormality in extraskeletal myxoid chondrosarcoma. Int J Cancer 62:398, 1995

81. Sreekantaiah CS, Li FP, Weidner N, Sandberg AA: Multiple and complex abnormalities in a case of alveolar soft part sarcoma. Cancer Genet Cytogenet 55:167, 1991

82. Cullinane C, Thorner PS, Greenberg ML, et al.: Molecular genetic, cytogenetic, and immunohistochemical characterization of alveolar soft-part sarcoma: Implications for cell of origin. Cancer 70:2444, 1992

83. Van Echten J, Van den Berg E, Van Baarlen J, et al.: An important role for chromosome 17, band q25, in the histogenesis of alveolar soft part sarcoma. Cancer Genet Cytogenet 82:57, 1995

84. Kitchen FD, Ellsworth RM: Pleiotropic effects of the gene for retinoblastoma. J Med Genet 11:244, 1974

85. Abramson DH, Ellsworth RM, Kitchin D, Tung G: Second nonocular tumors in retinoblastoma survivors: Are they radiation induced? Ophthalmology 91:1351, 1984

86. Hansen MF, Koufos A, Gallie BL, et al.: Osteosarcoma and retinoblastoma: A shared chromosomal mechanism revealing recessive predisposition. Proc Natl Acad Sci U S A 82:6216, 1985

87. Draper GJ, Sanders BM, Kingston JE: Second primary neoplasms in patients with retinoblastoma. Br J Cancer 53:661, 1986

88. Roarty JD, McLean IW, Zimmerman LE: Incidence of second neoplasms in patients with bilateral retinoblastoma. Ophthalmology 11:1583, 1988

89. Helton KJ, Fletcher BD, Kun LE, et al.: Bone tumors other than osteosarcoma after retinoblastoma. Cancer 71:2847, 1993

90. Fontanesi J, Parham DM, Pratt C, Meyer D: Second malignant neoplasms in children with retinoblastoma: The St. Jude Children's Hospital experience. Ophthalmic Genet 16:105, 1995

91. Knudson AG: Mutation and cancer: Statistical study of retinoblastoma. Proc Natl Acad Sci U S A 68:820, 1971

92. Comings DE: A general theory of carcinogenesis. Proc Natl Acad Sci U S A 70:3324, 1973

93. Friend SH, Bernards R, Robeli S, et al.: A human DNA segment with properties of the gene that predisposes to retinoblastoma and osteosarcoma. Nature 323:643, 1986

94. Lee WH, Bookstein R, Hong F, et al.: Human retinoblastoma susceptibility gene: Cloning, identification and sequence. Science 235:1394, 1987

95. Fung YKT, Murphree AL, T'Ang A, et al.: Structural evidence for the authenticity of the human retinoblastoma gene. Science 236:1657, 1987

96. Buchkovich K, Duffy LA, Harlow E: The retinoblastoma protein is phosphorylated during specific phases of the cell cycle. Cell 58:1097, 1989

97. Xu H, Xu S, Cagle PT, et al.: Absence of retinoblastoma protein expression in primary non-small cell lung carcinomas. Cancer Res 51:2735, 1991

98. Friend SH, Horowitz JM, Gerber MR, et al.: Deletions of a DNA sequence in retinoblastomas and mesenchymal tumors: Organization of the sequence and its encoded proteins. Proc Natl Acad Sci U S A 84:9059, 1987

99. Toguchida J, Ishizaki K, Saski MS, et al.: Chromosomal reorganization for the expression of recessive mutation of retinoblastoma susceptibility gene in the development of osteosarcoma. Cancer Res 48:3939, 1988

100. National Institutes of Health Consensus Development Conference: Neurofibromatosis: Conference Statement. Arch Neurol 45:575, 1988

101. Riccardi VM: Neurofibromatosis: Past, present and future. N Engl J Med 324:1283, 1991

102. Brasfield RD, Das Gupta TK: von Recklinghausen's disease: A clinicopathological study. Ann Surg 175:86, 1972

103. Das Gupta TK: Tumors of the peripheral nerves. Clin Neurosurg 25:574, 1978

104. Viskochil D, Buchberg AM, Xu RM, et al.: Deletions and a translocation interrupt a cloned gene at the neurofibromatosis type 1 locus. Cell 62:187, 1990

105. Wallace MR, Marchuk DA, Andersen LB, et al.: Type 1 neurofibromatosis gene: Identification of a large transcript disrupted in three NF1 patients. Science 249:181, 1990

106. Brannan CI, Perkins AS, Vogel KS, et al.: Targeted disruption of the neurofibromatosis type-1 gene leads to developmental abnormalities in heart and various neural crest-derived tissues. Genes Dev 8:1019, 1994

107. Bollag G, Clapp DW, Shih S, et al.: Loss of NF1 results in activation of the Ras signaling pathway and leads to aberrant growth in haematopoietic cells. Nat Genet 12:144, 1996

108. Matsui I, Tanimura M, Kobayashi N, et al.: Neurofibromatosis type 1 and childhood cancer. Cancer 72:2746, 1993

109. McKeen EA, Bodurtha J, Meadows AT, et al.: Rhabdomyosarcoma complicating multiple neurofibromatosis. J Pediatr 93:992, 1978

110. Hartley AL, Birch JM, Kelsey AM, et al.: Sarcomas in three generations of a family with neurofibromatosis. Cancer Genet Cytogenet 45:245, 1990

111. Bader JL: Neurofibromatosis and cancer. Ann N Y Acad Sci 486:56, 1986

112. Chan GC, Nicholls JM, Lee AC, et al.: Malignant peripheral neuroectodermal tumor in an infant with neurofibromatosis type II. Med Pediatr Oncol 26:215, 1996

113. Yang P, Grufferman S, Khoury MJ, et al.: Association of childhood rhabdomyosarcoma with neurofibromatosis type 1 and birth defects. Genet Epidemiol 12:467, 1995

114. Kluwe L, Mautner VF: A missense mutation in the NF2 gene results in moderate and mild clinical phenotypes of neurofibromatosis type 2. Hum Genet 97:224, 1996

115. Kley N, Whaley J, Seizinger BR: Neurofibromatosis type 2 and von Hippel-Lindau disease: From gene cloning to function. Glia 15:297, 1995

116. Li FP, Fraumeni JF Jr.: Soft-tissue sarcomas, breast cancer, and other neoplasms: A new familial syndrome? Ann Intern Med 71:747, 1969

117. Li FP, Fraumeni JR Jr., Mulvihill JJ, et al.: A cancer family syndrome in twenty-four kindreds. Cancer Res 48:5358, 1988

118. Malkin D, Li FP, Strong LC, et al.: Germ line p53 mutations in a familial syndrome of breast cancer, sarcomas and other neoplasms. Science 25:1233, 1990

119. Srivastava S, Zou Z, Pirollo K, et al.: Germ-line transmission of a mutated p53 gene in a cancer-prone family with Li-Fraumeni syndrome. Nature 348:747, 1990

120. Malkin D, Jolly KW, Barbier N, et al.: Germline mutations of the p53 tumor-suppressor gene in children and young adults with second malignant neoplasms. N Engl J Med 326:1309, 1992

121. Levine AJ: The p53 tumor-suppressor gene (editorial). New Engl J Med 326(20):1350, 1992

122. Farmer G, Bargonetti J, Zhu H, et al.: Wild-type p53 activates transcription in vivo. Nature 358:83, 1992

123. Seto E, Usheva A, Zambetti GP, et al.: Wild-type p53 binds to the TATA-binding protein and represses transcription. Proc Natl Acad Sci U S A 89:12028, 1992

124. Culotta E, Koshland DE: p53 sweeps through cancer research. Science 262:1958, 1993

125. Harper JW, Adami GR, Wei N, et al.: The p21 Cdk-interacting protein Cip1 is a potent inhibitor of G1 cyclin-dependent kinases. Cell 75:805, 1993

126. Harris CC: p53: At the crossroads of molecular carcinogenesis and risk-assessment. Science 262:1980, 1993

127. El-Deiry WS, Tokino T, Velculescu VE, et al.: WAF1, a potential mediator of p53 tumor suppression. Cell 75:817, 1993

128. El-Deiry WS, Harper JW, O'Connor PM, et al.: WAF1/Cip1 is induced in p53-mediated G1 arrest and apoptosis. Cancer Res 54:1169, 1994

129. Greenblatt MS, Bennett WP, Hollstein M, Harris CC: Mutations in the p53 tumor suppressor gene: Clues to cancer etiology and molecular pathogenesis. Cancer Res 54:4855, 1994

130. Hollstein M, Sidransky D, Vogelstein B, Harris CC: p53 mutations in human cancers. Science 253:49, 1991

131. Gardner EJ, Stephens FE: Cancer of the lower digestive tract in one family group. Am J Hum Genet 2:41, 1950

132. Halling F, Merten HA, Lepsien G, Honig JF: Clinical and radiological findings in Gardner's syndrome. Dentomaxillofac Radiol 21:93, 1992

133. Bodmer WF, Baily C, Bodmer J, et al.: Localization of the gene for familial adenomatous polyposis on chromosome 5. Nature 328:614, 1987

134. Leppert M, Dobbs M, Scambler P, et al.: The gene for familial polyposis coli maps to the long arm of chromosome 5. Science 238:1411, 1987

135. Kinzler KW, Nilbert MC, Su LK, et al.: Identification of FAP locus genes from chromosome 5q21. Science 253:661, 1991

136. Groden J, Thliveris A, Samowitz W, et al.: Identification and characterization of the familial adenomatous polyposis coli gene. Cell 66:589, 1991

137. Joslyn G, Carlson M, Thliveris A, et al.: Identification of deletion mutations and three new genes at the familial polyposis locus. Cell 66:601, 1991

138. Lofti AM, Dozois RR, Gordon H, et al.: Mesenteric fibromatosis complicating familial adenomatous polyposis: Predisposing factors and results of treatment. Int J Colorectal Dis 4:30, 1989

139. Berk T, Cohen Z, McLeod RS, et al.: Management of mesenteric desmoid tumors in familial adenomatous polyposis. Can J Surg 35:393, 1992

140. Tsukada K, Church JM, Jagelman DG, et al.: Systemic cytotoxic chemotherapy and radiation therapy in familial adenomatous polyposis. Dis Colon Rectum 35:29, 1992

141. Bertario L, Presciuttini S, Sala P, et al.: Causes of death and postsurgical survival in familial adenomatous polyposis: Results from the Italian registry. Semin Surg Oncol 10:225, 1994

142. Anthony T, Rodriguez-Bigas MA, Weber TK, Petrelli NJ: Desmoid tumors. J Am Coll Surg 182:369, 1996

143. Miyaki M, Konishi M, Kikuchi-Yanoshita R, et al.: Coexistence of somatic and germ-line mutations of the APC gene in desmoid tumors from patients with familial adenomatous polyposis. Cancer Res 53:5079, 1993

144. Solomon L: Hereditary multiple exostoses. J Bone Joint Surg Br 45B:292, 1963

145. Epstein LL, Bixler D, Bennett JE: An incidence of familial cancer including three cases of osteogenic sarcoma. Cancer 25:889, 1970

146. Unni KK, Dahlin DC: Premalignant tumors and conditions of bone. Am J Surg Pathol 3:47, 1979

147. Wicklund CL, Pauli RM, Johnston D, Hecht JT: Natural history study of hereditary multiple exostoses. Am J Med Genet 55:43, 1995

148. Ahn J, Ludecke HJ, Lindow S, et al.: Cloning of the putative tumour suppressor gene for hereditary multiple exostoses (EXT1). Nat Genet 11:137, 1995

149. Raskind WH, Conrad EU, Chamsky H, Matsushita M: Loss of heterozygosity in chondrosarcomas for markers linked to hereditary multiple exostoses loci on chromosomes 8 and 11. Am J Hum Genet 56:1132, 1995

150. Wuyts W, Ramlakhan S, Van Hul W, et al.: Refinement of the multiple exostoses locus (EXT2) to a 3-cM interval on chromosome 11. Am J Hum Genet 57:82, 1995

151. Vaughan WG, Sanders DW, Grosfeld JL, et al.: Favorable outcome in children with Beckwith-Wiedemann syndrome. J Pediatr Surg 30:1042, 1995

152. Matsuoka S, Thompson JS, Edwards MC, et al.: Imprinting of the gene encoding a human cyclin-dependent kinase inhibitor, p57KIP2, on chromosome 11p15. Proc Natl Acad Sci U S A 93:3026, 1996

153. Morison IM, Becroft DM, Taniguchi T, et al.: Somatic overgrowth associated with overexpression of insulin-like growth factor II. Nat Med 2:311, 1996

154. Giardiello FM, Offerhaus JG: Phenotype and cancer risk of various polyposis syndromes. Eur J Cancer 31A:1085, 1995

155. Scully RE: Sex cord tumor with annular lobules: A distinctive ovarian tumor of the Peutz-Jeghers syndrome. Cancer 25:1107, 1970

156. Ferry JA, Young RH, Engel G, Scully RE: Oxyphilic Sertoli cell tumor of the ovary: A report of three cases, two in patients with the Peutz-Jeghers syndrome. Int J Gynecol Pathol 13:259, 1994

157. Spigelman AD, Arese P, Phillips RK: Polyposis: The Peutz-Jeghers syndrome. Br J Cancer 82:1311, 1995

158. Giardiello FM, Welsh SB, Hamilton SR, et al.: Increased risk of cancer in the Peutz-Jeghers syndrome. N Engl J Med 316:1511, 1987

159. Le Bodic MF, Fiche M, Aillet G, et al.: Immunohistochemical study of 6 multiple familial cervical paragangliomas with lymph node metastasis in one case. Ann Pathol 11:176, 1991

160. Wilson H: Carotid body tumors: Familial and bilateral. Ann Surg 171:843, 1970

161. Sobol SM, Dailey JC: Familial multiple cervical paragangliomas: Report of a kindred and review of the literature. Otolaryngol Head Neck Surg 102:382, 1990

162. Ridge BA, Brewster DC, Darling RC, et al.: Familial carotid body tumors: Incidence and implications. Ann Vasc Surg 7:190, 1993

163. Netterville JL, Reilly KM, Robertson D, et al.: Carotid body tumors: A review of 30 patients with 46 tumors. Laryngoscope 105:115, 1995

164. Monteforte WJ, Kohnen PW: Angiomyolipomas in a case of lymphangiomyomatosis syndrome: Relationship to tuberous sclerosis. Cancer 34:317, 1974

165. Taylor RS, Joseph DB, Kohaut EC, et al.: Renal angiomyolipoma associated with lymph node involvement and renal cell carcinoma in patients with tuberous sclerosis. J Urol 141:930, 1989

166. Henske EP, Kwiatkowski DJ: A 5.4-Mb continuous pulsed-field gel electrophoresis map of human 9q34.1 between ABL and D92114, including the tuberous sclerosis (TSC1) region. Genomics 28:105, 1995

167. Wienecke R, Konig A, DeClue JE: Identification of tuberin, the tuberous sclerosis-2 product. J Biol Chem 270:16409, 1995

168. Geist RT, Gutmann DH: The tuberous sclerosis 2 gene is expressed at high levels in the cerebellum and developing spinal cord. Cell Growth Differ 6:1477, 1995

169. Washecka R, Hanna M: Malignant renal tumors in tuberous sclerosis. Urology 37:340, 1991

170. Horton WA, Wong V, Eldridge R: von Hippel-Lindau disease: Clinical and pathological manifestations in nine families with 50 affected members. Arch Intern Med 136:769, 1976

171. Loughlin KR, Grittes RF: Urological management of patients with von Hippel-Lindau's disease. J Urol 136:789, 1986

172. Neumann HPH, Berger DP, Sigmund G, et al.: Pheochromocytomas, multiple endocrine neoplasia type 2 and von Hippel-Lindau disease. New Engl J Med 329:1531, 1993

173. Latif F, Tory K, Gnarra J, et al.: Identification of the von Hippel-Lindau disease tumor suppressor gene. Science 260:1317, 1993

174. Whaley JM, Gablich J, Glabert L, et al.: Germ-line mutations in the von Hippel-Lindau tumor suppressor gene are similar to somatic von Hippel-Lindau aberrations in sporadic renal cell carcinoma. Am J Hum Genet 55:1092, 1994

175. Gnarra JR, Tory K, Weng Y, et al.: Mutations of the VHL tumor suppressor gene in renal carcinoma. Nat Genet 7:85, 1994

176. Shuin T, Kondo K, Torigoe S, et al.: Frequent somatic mutations and loss of heterozygosity of the von Hippel-Lindau tumor suppressor gene in primary human renal cell carcinomas. Cancer Res 54:2852, 1994

177. Shiu MH, Brennan MF: Surgical Management of Soft Tissue Sarcoma. Philadelphia, Lea & Febiger, 1989

178. American Joint Committee on Cancer: Manual for Staging of Cancer, 4th ed. Philadelphia, J. B. Lippincott, 1992

179. Gaynor JJ, Tan CC, Casper ES, et al.: Refinement of clinicopathologic staging for localized soft tissue sarcoma of the extremity: A study of 423 adults. J Clin Oncol 10:1317, 1992

180. Hajdu SI, D'Ambrosio FG: Histopathologic classification of limb sarcomas in relation to prognosis. Surg Oncol Clin N Amer 2:509, 1993

181. Singer S, Corson JM, Demetri GD, et al.: Prognostic factors predictive of survival for truncal and retroperitoneal soft-tissue sarcoma. Ann Surg 221:185, 1995

182. Kreicbergs A, Tribukait B, Willems J, et al.: DNA flow analysis of soft tissue tumors. Cancer 59:128, 1987

183. Matsuno T, Gebhardt MC, Schiller AL, et al.: The use of flow cytometry as a diagnostic aid in the management of soft-tissue tumors. J Bone Joint Surg 70:751, 1988

184. Ueda T, Aozasa K, Tsujimoto M, et al.: Prognostic significance of Ki-67 reactivity in soft tissue sarcomas. Cancer 63:1607, 1989

185. Alvegard TA, Berg NO, Baldetorp B, et al.: Cellular DNA

content and prognosis of high-grade soft tissue sarcoma: The Scandinavian Sarcoma Group Experience. J Clin Oncol 8:538, 1990

186. Ferno M, Baldetorp B, Akerman M: Flow cytometric DNA analysis of soft tissue sarcomas: A comparative study of fine needle aspirates and postoperative fresh tissues and archival material. Anal Quant Cytol Histol 12:251, 1990

187. Zehr RJ, Bauer TW, Marks KE, Weltevreden A: Ki-67 and grading of malignant fibrous histiocytomas. Cancer 66:1984, 1990

188. Bauer HCF, Kreicbergs A, Tribukait B: DNA content prognostic in soft tissue sarcoma: 102 patients followed for 1–10 years. Acta Orthop Scand 62(3):187, 1991

189. Zapulski MM, Maclorowski Z, Ryan JR, et al.: DNA content parameters of paraffin-embedded soft tissue sarcomas: Optimization of retrieval technique and comparison to fresh tissue. Cytometry 14:327, 1993

190. Baak JPA: Mitosis counting in tumors. Hum Pathol 21:683, 1990

191. Van Unnik JAM, Coindre JM, Contesso C, et al.: Grading of soft tissue sarcomas: Experience of the EORTC soft tissue and bone sarcoma group. Eur J Cancer 29A:2089, 1993

192. Michie BA, Black C, Reid RP, Hamblen DL: Image analysis derived ploidy and proliferation indices in soft tissue sarcomas: Comparison with clinical outcome. J Clin Pathol 47:443, 1994

193. Chengyu L: DNA content and morphological parameters in synovial sarcoma and synovioma. Chin Med J 108:692, 1995

194. Pappo AS, Crist WM, Kuttesch J, et al.: Tumor-cell DNA content predicts outcome in children and adolescents with clinical group III embryonal rhabdomyosarcoma. J Clin Oncol 11:1901, 1993

195. Kuratsu S, Tomita Y, Myoui A, et al.: DNA ploidy pattern and cell cycle stage of tumor cells in soft-tissue sarcomas: Clinical implications. Oncology 52:363, 1995

196. Huuhtanen RL, Blomqvist CP, Wiklund RA, et al.: S-phase fraction of 155 soft tissue sarcomas: Correlation with clinical outcome. Cancer 77:1815, 1996

197. Levine EA, Roninson IB, Kim DK, et al.: MDR-1 expression in soft tissue sarcoma. Surg Forum 45:503, 1994

198. Kilpatrick SE, Teot LA, Geisinger KR, et al.: Relationship of DNA ploidy to histology and prognosis in rhabdomyosarcoma. Comparison of flow cytometry and image analysis. Cancer 74:3227, 1994

199. el-Naggar AK, Garcia GM: Epithelioid sarcoma: Flow cytometric study of DNA content and regional DNA heterogeneity. Cancer 69:1721, 1992

200. Barrios C, Castresana JS, Falkmer UG, et al.: c-myc oncogene amplification and cytometric DNA ploidy pattern as prognostic factors in musculoskeltal neoplasms. Int J Cancer 58:781, 1994

201. Schmidt RA, Conrad EU, Collins C, et al.: Measurement and prediction of the short-term response of soft tissue sarcomas to chemotherapy. Cancer 72:2593, 1993

202. Gerdes J, Schwab U, Lemke H, et al.: Production of a mouse monoclonal antibody reactive with a human nuclear antigen associated with cell proliferation. Int J Cancer 31:13, 1983

203. Kroese MC, Rutgers DH, Wils IS, et al.: The relevance of the DNA index and proliferation rate in the grading of benign and malignant soft tissue tumors. Cancer 65:1782, 1990

204. Hall PA, Richards MA, Gregory WM, et al.: The prognostic value of Ki-67 immunostaining in non-Hodgkin's lymphoma. J Pathol 154:223, 1988

205. Swanson SA, Brooks JJ: Proliferation markers Ki-67 and p105 in soft-tissue lesions. Am J Pathol 137:1491, 1990

206. De Riese WT, Crabtree WN, Allhoff EP, et al.: Prognostic significance of Ki-67 immunostaining in nonmetastatic renal cell carcinoma. J Clin Oncol 11:1804, 1993

207. Drobnjak M, Latres E, Pollack D, et al.: Prognostic implications of p53 overexpression and high proliferation index of Ki-67 in adult soft-tissue sarcomas. J Natl Cancer Inst 86:549, 1994

208. Scotlandi K, Serra M, Manara C, et al.: Clinical relevance of Ki-67 expression in bone tumors. Cancer 75:806, 1995

209. Yang P, Hirose T, Hasegawa T, et al.: Prognostic implication of the p53 protein and Ki-67 antigen immunohistochemistry in malignant fibrous histiocytoma. Cancer 76:618, 1995

210. Bos JL: The ras gene family and human carcinogenesis. Mutat Res 195:255, 1988

211. Hall A: The cellular functions of small GTP binding proteins. Science 346:696, 1990

212. Pulciani S, Santos E, Lauver AV, et al.: Oncogenes in solid tumors. Nature 299:171, 1982

213. Kusakabe H, Yonobayashi K, Sakatani S, et al.: Metastatic epithelial sarcomas with an N-ras oncogene mutation. Am J Dermatopathol 16:294, 1994

214. Gill S, Stratton MR, Patterson H, et al.: Detection of transforming genes by transfection of DNA from primary soft-tissue tumours. Oncogene 6:1491, 1991

215. Cooper CS, Stratton MR: Soft tissue tumours: The genetic basis of development. Carcinogenesis 12:155, 1991

216. Wilke W, Maillet M, Robinson R: H-ras-1 point mutations in soft tissue sarcomas. Mod Pathol 6:129, 1993

217. Stratton MR, Fisher C, Gusterson BA, Cooper CS: Detection of point mutations in n-ras and k-ras genes of human embryonal rhabdomyosarcomas using oligonucleotide probes and the polymerase chain reaction. Cancer Res 49:6324, 1989

218. Marion MJ, Froment O, Trepo C: Activation of k-ras gene by point mutation in human liver angiosarcoma associated with vinyl chloride exposure. Mol Carcinog 4:450, 1991

219. Coussens L, Yang-Fen TL, Liao YC: Tyrosinase receptor with extensive homology to the EGF receptor shares chromosomal location with the neu oncogene. Science 230:1132, 1985

220. Berns EMJJ, Klijn JGM, Van Staveren IL, et al.: Prevalence of amplification of the oncogenes c-myc, HER2/neu, and int-2 in one thousand human breast tumours: Correlation with steroid receptors. Eur J Cancer 28:697, 1992

221. Slamon DJ, Clark GM, Wong SG, et al.: Human breast cancer: Correlation of relapse and survival with amplification of the HER-2/neu oncogene. Science 235:177, 1987

222. Clark GM, McGuire WL: Follow-up study of HER-2/neu amplification in primary breast cancer. Cancer Res 51: 944, 1991

223. Hartmann LC, Ingle JN, Wold LE, et al.: Prognostic value of c-erbB2 overexpression in axillary lymph node positive breast cancer: Results from a randomized adjuvant treatment protocol. Cancer 74:2956, 1994

224. Seshadri R, Firgaira FA, Horsfall DJ, et al.: Clinical significance of HER-2/neu oncogene amplification in primary breast cancer. J Clin Oncol 11:1936, 1993

225. Perren TJ: c-erbB-2 oncogene as a prognostic marker in breast cancer. Br J Cancer 63:328, 1991

226. Lönn U, Lönn S, Nilsson B, Stenkvist B: Prognostic value of erb-B2 and myc amplification in breast cancer imprints. Cancer 75:2681, 1995

227. Tetu B, Brisson J: Prognostic significance of Her-2/neu oncoprotein expression in node-positive breast cancer. Cancer 73:2359, 1994

228. Baselga J, Tripothy D, Mendelsohn J, et al.: Phase II study of weekly intravenous recombinant humanized anti-p185 Her2 monoclonal antibody in patients with Her-2/neu-overexpressing metastatic breast cancer. J Clin Oncol 14:737, 1996

229. Wang D, Barros D'Sa AAB, Johnston CF, Buchanan KD: Oncogene expression in carotid body tumors. Cancer 77:2581, 1996

230. Duda RB, Cundiff D, August CZ, et al.: Growth factor receptor and related oncogene determination in mesenchymal tumors. Cancer 71:3526, 1993

231. Wrba F, Gullick WJ, Fertl H, et al.: Immunohistochemical detection of the c-erbB-2 proto-oncogene product in normal, benign and malignant cartilage tissues. Histopathology 15:71, 1989

232. Persson H, Leder P: Nuclear localization and DNA binding properties of a protein expressed by human c-myc oncogene. Science 225:718, 1984

233. Brodeur GM, Seeger RC, Schwab M, et al.: Amplification of n-myc in untreated human neuroblastoma correlates with advanced disease stage. Science 224:1121, 1984

234. Barrios C, Castresana JS, Kriecbergs A: Clinicopathologic correlations and short-term prognosis in musculoskeletal sarcoma with c-myc oncogene amplification. Am J Clin Oncol 17:273, 1994

235. Ozaki T, Ikeda S, Kawai A, et al.: Alterations of retinoblastoma susceptible gene accompanied by c-myc amplification in human bone and soft tissue sarcomas. Cell Mol Biol (Noisy-le-grand) 39:235, 1993

236. Dias P, Kumar P, Marsden HB, et al.: N-myc gene is amplified in alveolar rhabdomyosarcoma (RMS) but not in embryonal RMS. Int J Cancer 45:593, 1990

237. Garson JA, Clayton J, McIntyre P, et al.: N-myc oncogene amplification in rhabdomyosarcoma at release. Lancet 1:1496, 1986

238. Mitani K, Kurosawa H, Suzuki A, et al.: Amplification of n-myc in a rhabdomyosarcoma. Jpn J Cancer Res 77: 1062, 1986

239. Tsuda H, Shimasato Y, Upton MP, et al.: Retrospective study of amplification of n-myc and c-myc genes in paediatric solid tumors and its association with prognosis and tumor differentiation. Lab Invest 59:321, 1988

240. Oliner J, Kinzler K, Meltzer P, et al.: Amplification of a gene encoding a p53-associated protein in human sarcomas. Nature 358:80, 1992

241. Oliner J, Pietenpol J, Thiagalingam S, et al.: Oncoprotein MDM2 conceals the activation domain of tumour suppressor p53. Nature 263:857, 1993

242. Chen J, Marechal V, Levine AJ: Mapping of the p53 and mdm-2 interaction domains. Mol Cell Biol 13:4107, 1993

243. Barak Y, Gottlieb E, Juven-Gershon T, Oren M: Regulation of mdm2 expression by p53: Alternative promoters produce transcripts with nonidentical translation potential. Genes Dev 8:1739, 1994

244. Chen J, Lin J, Levine AJ: Regulation of transcription functions of the p53 tumor suppressor by the mdm2 oncogene. Mol Med 1(2):142, 1995

245. Leach F, Tokino T, Meltzer P, et al.: p53 Mutation and MDM2 amplification in human soft tissue sarcomas. Cancer Res 53:2231, 1993

246. Cordon-Cardo C, Latres E, Drobnjak M, et al.: Molecular abnormalities of MDM2 and p53 genes in adult soft tissue sarcomas. Cancer Res 54:794, 1994

247. Nakayma T, Toguchida J, Wadayama B, et al.: Mdm2 gene amplification in bone and soft tissue tumors: Association with tumor progression in differentiated adipose-tissue tumors. Int J Cancer 64:342, 1995

248. Flørenes VA, Maelandsmo GM, Forus A, et al.: MDM2 gene amplification and transcript levels in human sarcomas: Relationship to TP53 gene status. J Natl Cancer Inst 86:1297, 1994

249. Bueso-Ramos CE, Yang Y, Manshouri T, et al.: Molecular abnormalities of MDM-2 in human sarcomas. Int J Oncol 7:1043, 1995

250. Kindblom LG, Ahlden M, Meis-Kindblom JM, Stenman G: Immunohistochemical and molecular analysis of p53, mdm2, proliferating cell nuclear antigen and Ki67 in benign and malignant peripheral nerve sheath tumours. Virchows Arch 427:19, 1995

251. Hieken TJ, Das Gupta TK: Co-expression of mutant p53 and MDM2 proteins in liposarcoma. Surg Forum 47:500, 1996

252. Stratton MR, Moss J, Warren W, et al.: Mutation of the p53 gene in human soft tissue sarcomas: Association with abnormalities of the RB1 gene. Oncogene 5:1297, 1990

253. Toguchida J, Yamaguchi T, Ritchie B, et al.: Mutation spectrum of the p53 gene in bone and soft tissue sarcomas. Cancer Res 52:6194, 1992

254. Andreassen Å, Øyjord T, Hovig E, et al.: p53 abnormalities in different subtypes of human sarcomas. Cancer Res 53:468, 1993

255. Wadayama B, Toguchida J, Yamaguchi T, et al.: p53 expression and its relationship to DNA alterations in bone and soft tissue sarcomas. Br J Cancer 68:1134, 1993

256. Latres E, Drobnjak M, Pollack D, et al.: Chromosome 17 abnormalities and TP53 mutations in adult soft tissue sarcomas. Am J Pathol 145:345, 1994

257. Castresana JS, Rubio MP, Gomez L, et al.: Detection of TP53 gene mutations in human sarcomas. Eur J Cancer 31A:735, 1995

258. Weichselbaum RR, Beckett M, Diamond A: Some retinoblastomas, osteosarcomas, and soft tissue sarcomas may share a common etiology. Proc Natl Acad Sci U S A 85:2106, 1988

259. Wunder JS, Czitrom AA, Kandel R, Andrulis IL: Analysis of alterations in the retinoblastoma gene and tumor grade in bone and soft tissue sarcomas. J Natl Cancer Inst 83:194, 1991

260. Vogelstein B, Kinzler KW: p53 function and dysfunction. Cell 70:523, 1992

261. Ewen ME, Miller SJ: p53 and translational control. Biochim Biophys Acta 1242:181, 1996

262. Cho Y, Gorina S, Jeffrey PD, Pavletich NP: Crystal structure of a p53 tumor suppressor-DNA complex: Understanding tumorigenic mutations. Science 265:346, 1994

263. Lee JM, Bernstein A: Apoptosis, cancer, and the p53 tumour suppressor gene. Cancer Metastasis Rev 14:149, 1995

264. Nigro JM, Baker SJ, Preisinger AC, et al.: Mutations in the p53 gene occur in diverse human tumour types. Nature 342:705, 1989

265. Bartek J, Bartkova J, Vojtesek B, et al.: Aberrant expression of the p53 oncoprotein is a common feature of a wide spectrum of human malignancies. Oncogene 6:1699, 1991

266. Mulligan LM, Matlashewski GJ, Scrable HJ, Cavenee WK: Mechanisms of p53 loss in human sarcomas. Proc Natl Acad Sci U S A, 87:5863, 1990

267. Brachman DG, Hallahan DE, Beckett MA, et al.: p53 gene mutations and abnormal retinoblastoma protein in radiation-induced human sarcomas. Cancer Res 41:6393, 1991

268. Taubert H, Würl P, Meye A, et al.: Molecular and immunohistochemical p53 status in liposarcoma and malignant fibrous histiocytoma: Identification of seven new mutations for soft tissue sarcomas. Cancer 76:1187, 1995

269. Kawai A, Noguchi M, Beppu Y, et al.: Nuclear immunoreaction of p53 protein in soft tissue sarcomas: A possible prognostic factor. Cancer 73:2499, 1994

270. Toffoli G, Doglioni C, Cernigoi C, et al.: p53 overexpression in human soft tissue sarcomas: Relation to biologic aggressiveness. Ann Oncol 5:167, 1994

271. Hieken TJ, Das Gupta TK: Mutant p53 expression: A marker of diminished survival in well-differentiated soft tissue sarcoma. Clin Cancer Res 2:1391, 1996

272. Gannon J, Greves R, Iggo R, Lane DP: Activating mutations in p53 produce a common conformation effect. A monoclonal antibody specific for the mutant form. EMBO J 9:1595, 1990

273. Hieken TJ, Das Gupta TK: Quantitation of mutant p53 expression: A marker of the biologic behavior of soft tissue sarcoma (forthcoming).

274. Hieken TJ, Mcnini P, Kim D, Das Gupta TK: Mutant p53 expression in resected soft tissue sarcoma lung metastases predicts treatment outcome. Proc Amer Assoc Cancer Res (abstr) 37:574, 1996

275. Cross SM, Sanchez CA, Morgan CA, et al.: A p53-dependent mouse spindle checkpoint. Science 267:1353, 1995

276. Leveillard T, Andera L, Bissonnette N, et al.: Functional interactions between p53 and the TFIIH complex. EMBO J 15:1615, 1996

277. Smith ML, Chen I, Zhan Q, et al.: Interaction of the p53-regulated protein Gadd45 with proliferating cell nuclear antigen. Science 266:1376, 1994

278. Kastan MB, Zhan Q, El-Deiry WS, et al.: A mammalian cell cycle checkpoint pathway utilizing p53 and GADD45 is defective in ataxia-telangiectasia. Cell 71:587, 1992

279. Morris GF, Bischoff JR, Matthews MB: Transcriptional activation of the human proliferating-cell nuclear antigen promoter by p53. Proc Natl Acad Sci U S A 93:895, 1996

280. Lowe SW, Rule HE, Jacks T, Housman DE: p53-dependent apoptosis modulates the cytotoxicity of anticancer agents. Cell 74:957, 1993

281. Lowe SW, Bodis S, McClatchey A, et al.: p53 status and the efficacy of cancer therapy in vivo. Science 266:807, 1994

282. Fujiwara T, Grimm EA, Mukhopadhyay T, et al.: Induction of chemosensitivity in human lung cancer cells in vivo by adenovirus-mediated transfer of the wild-type p53 gene. Cancer Res 54:2287, 1994

283. Aas T, Borresen AL, Geister S, et al.: Specific p53 mutations are associated with de novo resistance to doxorubicin in breast cancer. Nat Med 2:811, 1996

284. Dameron KM, Volpert OV, Tainsky MA, Bouck N: Control of angiogenesis in fibroblasts by p53 regulation of thrombospondin-1. Science 65:1582, 1994

285. Kieser A, Weich HA, Brandner G, et al.: Mutant p53 potentiates protein kinase C induction of vascular endothelial growth factor expression. Oncogene 9:963, 1994

286. Lee EYP, To H, Shew J, et al.: Inactivation of the retinoblastoma susceptibility gene in human breast cancer. Science 241:218, 1988

287. Varley JM, Armour J, Swallow JE, et al.: The retinoblastoma gene is frequently altered leading to loss of expression in primary breast tumors. Oncogene 4:725, 1989

288. Cance WG, Brennan MF, Dudas ME, et al.: Altered expression of the retinoblastoma gene product in human sarcomas. N Engl J Med 323:1457, 1990

289. Venter DJ, Bevan KL, Ludwig RL, et al.: Retinoblastoma gene deletions in human glioblastomas. Oncogene 7:445, 1991

290. Kornblau SM, Chen N, del Giglio A, et al.: Retinoblastoma protein expression is frequently altered in chronic lymphocytic leukemia. Cancer Res 54:242, 1994

291. Phillips SM, Barton CM, Lee SJ, et al.: Loss of the retinoblastoma susceptibility gene (RB1) is a frequent and early event in prostatic tumorigenesis. Br J Cancer 70:1252, 1994

292. Hamann U, Herbold C, Costa S, et al.: Allelic imbalance on chromosome 13q: Evidence for the involvement of BRCA2 and RB1 in sporadic breast cancer. Cancer Res 56:1988, 1996

293. Shew J-Y, Ling N, Yang X, et al.: Antibodies detecting abnormalities of the retinoblastoma susceptibility gene product (pp110RB) in osteosarcomas and synovial sarcomas. Oncogene Res 1:205, 1989

294. Karpeh MS, Brennan MF, Cance WG, et al.: Altered pat-

terns of retinoblastoma gene product expression in adult soft-tissue sarcomas. Br J Cancer 72:986, 1995

295. Wang J, Coltrera MD, Gown AM: Abnormalities of p53 and p110RB tumor suppressor gene expression in human soft tissue tumors: Correlations with cell proliferation and tumor grade. Mod Pathol 8:837, 1995

296. De Chiara A, T'Ang A, Triche TJ: Expression of the retinoblastoma susceptibility gene in childhood rhabdomyosarcoma. J Natl Cancer Inst 85:152, 1993

297. Weintraub SJ, Prater CA, Dean DC: Retinoblastoma protein switches the E2F site from positive to negative element. Nature 358:259, 1992

298. Zacksenhaus E, Bremner R, Phillips RA, Gallie BL: A bipartite nuclear localization signal in the retinoblastoma gene product and its importance for biological activity. Mol Cell Biol 13:4588, 1993

299. Li W, Fan J, Hochhauser D, et al.: Lack of functional retinoblastoma protein mediates increased resistance to antimetabolites in human sarcoma cell lines. Proc Natl Acad Sci U S A 92:10436, 1995

300. Howes KA, Ransom N, Papermaster DS, et al.: Apoptosis or retinoblastoma: Alternative fates of photoreceptors expressing the HPV-16 E7 gene in the presence or absence of p53. Genes Dev 8:1285, 1994

301. Morgenbesser SD, Williams BO, Jacks T, DePinho RA: p53-dependent apoptosis produced by Rb-deficiency in the developing mouse lens. Nature 371:72, 1994

302. Kamb A, Shattuckeidens D, Eeles R, et al.: Analysis of the p16 gene (cdkn2) as a candidate for the chromosome 9p melanoma susceptibility locus. Nat Genet 8:22, 1994

303. Nobori T, Miura K, Wu DJ, et al.: Deletions of the cyclin-dependent kinase-4 inhibitor gene in multiple human cancers. Nature 368:753, 1994

304. Maelandsmo GM, Berner JM, Florenes VA, et al.: Homozygous deletion frequency and expression levels of the CDKN2 gene in human sarcomas: Relationship to amplification and mRNA levels of CDK4 and CCND1. Br J Cancer 72:393, 1995

305. Pastan I, Gottesman M: Multiple-drug resistance in human cancer. N Engl J Med 316:1388, 1987

306. Gerlach JH, Kartner N, Bell DR, et al.: Multidrug resistance. Cancer Surv 5:25, 1986

307. Gottesman MM, Pastan I: Biochemistry of multidrug resistance mediated by the multidrug transporter. Ann Rev Biochem 62:385, 1993

308. Roninson IB (ed): Molecular and cellular biology of multidrug resistance in tumor cells. New York, Plenum Press, 1991, p 189

309. Chen C-J, Clark D, Ueda K, et al.: Genomic organization of the human multidrug resistance (MDR-1) gene and origin of P-glycoproteins. J Biol Chem 265: 506, 1990

310. Ford JM, Hait WN: Pharmacology of drugs that alter multidrug resistance in cancer. Pharmacol Rev 42:155, 1990

311. Tawa A, Inoue M, Ishihara S, et al.: Increased expression of the multidrug-resistance gene in undifferentiated sarcoma. Cancer 66:1980, 1990

312. Chan HSL, Thorner PS, Haddad G, Ling V: Immunohistochemical detection of P-glycoprotein: Prognostic correlation of soft tissue sarcoma of childhood. J Clin Oncol 8:689, 1990

313. Chan HSL, Haddad G, Thorner PS, et al.: P-glycoprotein expression as a predictor of the outcome or therapy for neuroblastoma. N Engl J Med 325:1608, 1991

314. Gerlach JH, Bell DR, Karakousis C, et al.: P-glycoprotein in human sarcoma: Evidence for multidrug resistance. J Clin Oncol 5:1452, 1987

315. Itsubo M, Ishikawa T, Toda G, Tanaka M: Immunohistochemical study of expression and cellular localization of the multidrug resistance gene product P-glycoprotein in primary liver carcinoma. Cancer 73:298, 1994

316. Antman K, Crowley J, Balcerzak SP, et al.: An Intergroup Phase III randomized study of doxorubicin and dacarbazine with or without ifosfamide and mesna in advanced soft tissue and bone sarcomas. J Clin Oncol 11: 1276, 1993

317. Blum RH: An overview of studies in adriamycin in the United States. Cancer Chemother Rep 6:247, 1975

318. Fojo AT, Ueda K, Slamon DJ, et al.: Expression of a multidrug-resistance gene in human tumor and tissues. Proc Natl Acad Sci U S A 84:265, 1987

319. Goldstein LJ, Galski H, Fojo A, et al.: Expression of a multidrug resistance gene in human cancers. J Natl Cancer Inst 81:116, 1989

320. Robey-Cafferty SS, Rutledge ML, Bruner JM: Expression of a multidrug resistance gene in esophageal adenocarcinoma. Am J Clin Pathol 93:1, 1990

321. Wunder JS, Bell RS, Wold L, Andrulis IL: Expression of the multidrug resistance gene in osteosarcoma: A pilot study. J Orthop Res 11:396, 1993

322. Holzmayer TA, Hilsenbeck S, Von Hoff DD, et al.: Clinical correlates of MDR-1 (P-glycoprotein) gene expression in ovarian and small cell lung carcinomas. J Natl Cancer Inst 84:1486, 1992

323. Roessner A, Ueda Y, Bockhorn-Dworniczak B, et al.: Prognostic implication of immunodetection of P-glycoprotein in Ewing's sarcoma. J Cancer Res Clin Oncol 119:185, 1993

324. Noonan KE, Beck C, Holzmayer TA, et al.: Quantitative analysis of MDR1 (multidrug resistance) gene expression in human tumors by polymerase chain reaction. Proc Natl Acad Sci U S A 87:7160, 1990

325. Cordon-Cardo C, O'Brien JP, Boccia J, et al.: Expression of the multidrug resistance gene product (P-glycoprotein) in human normal and tumor tissues. J Histochem Cytochem 38:1277, 1990

326. Levine EA, Holzmayer TA, Roninson IB, Das Gupta TK: MDR-1 expression in metastatic malignant melanoma. J Surg Res 54:621, 1993

327. Levine EA, Holzmayer J, Bacus S, et al.: Evaluation of newer prognostic markers for adult soft tissue sarcoma. J. Clin Onc 15:3249, 1997

328. Schinkel AH, Arceci RJ, Smit JJM, et al.: Binding properties of monoclonal antibodies recognizing external epitopes of the human MDR1 P-glycoprotein. Int J Cancer 55:478, 1993

329. Mechenter EB, Roninson IB: Efficient inhibition of P-glycoprotein-mediated multidrug resistance with a monoclonal antibody. Proc Natl Acad Sci U S A 89: 5824, 1992

330. Campos L, Guyotat D, Archimbaud E, et al.: Clinical significance of multidrug resistance P-glycoprotein expres-

sion on acute non-lymphoblastic leukemia cells at diagnosis. Blood 79:473, 1992

331. Schneider J, Rubio M-P, Barbazan M-J, et al.: P-glycoprotein, HER-2/neu, and mutant p53 expression in human gynecologic tumors. J Natl Cancer Inst 86:850, 1994

332. Volm M, Kastel M, Mattern J, Efferth T: Expression of resistance factors (P-glycoprotein, glutathione transferase p, and topoisomerase II) and their interrelationship to proto-oncogene products in renal cell carcinomas. Cancer 71:3981, 1993

333. Baldini N, Scotlandi K, Barbanti-Brodano G, et al.: Expression of P-glycoprotein in high-grade osteosarcomas in relation to clinical outcome. N Engl J Med 333:1380, 1995

334. Pinedo HM, Giuseppe G: P-glycoprotein—A marker of cancer-cell behavior. N Engl J Med 333:1417, 1995

335. Chaudhary PM, Roninson IB: Induction of multidrug resistance in human cells by transient exposure to different chemotherapeutic drugs. J Natl Cancer Inst 85:632, 1993

336. Niimi S, Nakagawa K, Yokata J, et al.: Resistance to anticancer drugs in NIH 3T3 cells transfected with c-myc and/or c-H-ras genes. Br J Cancer 63:237, 1991

337. Chin K-V, Ueda K, Pastan I, Gottesman KM: Modulation of activity of the promoter of the human MDR-1 gene by ras and p53. Science 255:459, 1992

338. Benchimol S, Ling V: P-glycoprotein and tumor progression. J Natl Cancer Inst 86:814, 1994

339. Sikic BI: Modulation of multidrug resistance: At the threshold. J Clin Oncol 9:1629, 1993

340. Raderer M, Scheithauer W: Clinical trials of agents that reverse multidrug resistance. Cancer 72:3553, 1993

341. Cole SP, Bhardway G, Gerlach JH, et al.: Overexpression of a transporter gene in a multidrug-resistant human lung cancer cell line. Science 258:1650, 1992

342. Barrand MA, Heppell-Parton AC, Wright KA, et al.: A 190 kilodalton protein overexpressed in non-P-glycoprotein-containing multidrug-resistant cells and its relationship to the MRP gene. J Natl Cancer Inst 86:110, 1994

343. Brueninger LM, Paul S, Gaughan K, et al.: Expression of multidrug resistance-associated protein in NIH/3T3 cells confers multidrug resistance associated with increased drug efflux and altered intracellular drug distribution. Cancer Res 55:5342, 1995

344. Nooter K, Westerman AM, Flens MJ: Expression of the multidrug resistance-associated protein (MRP) gene in human cancers. Clin Cancer Res 1:1301, 1995

345. Armstrong DK, Gordon GB, Hilton J, et al.: Hepsulfam sensitivity in human breast cancer cell lines: The role of glutathione and glutathione S-transferase in resistance. Cancer Res 52:1416, 1992

# Natural History of Individual Tumors

# 7

# Tumors of the Adipose Tissue

## ■ PHYSIOLOGY

The concept of adipose tissue as a dynamic organ able to participate in metabolic processes is now generally accepted. Body fat can be viewed as a reservoir of stored calories in the form of triglycerides, with high calorie density. However, this reservoir is composed of living cells with different functions.

The number of calories converted to fat derives from two variables: energy intake and energy expenditure. The body of a young adult man in caloric balance may contain an average of 14 percent pure fat. The relative amount of body fat, however, increases with age; for example, at age 55 it is approximately 25 percent of body weight.[1] In obese persons, the amount of body fat may reach more than 40 percent of body weight. The lipids extracted from normal human adipose tissue comprise more than 98 percent triglycerides, 1.3 percent total cholesterol, and 0.1 percent phospholipids.[2]

Twenty-two different fatty acids have been identified in the adipose tissue triglycerides. Six of these—palmitic, myristic, palmitoleic, steric, oleic, and linoleic—account for 95 percent of the fatty acid composition in man. Dietary effects on the fatty acid composition occur slowly. Two separate metabolic compartments exist in the white adipose tissue. The larger compartment may serve as a relatively inert storage site, exchanging only slowly with dietary fat. The smaller pool, turning over more rapidly, is in equilibrium with dietary, serum, and liver lipids, and may also be the major site of active synthesis from carbohydrates. Lipomas apparently constitute a relatively inert storage site and exchange slowly with dietary fat. This has probably given rise to the erroneous conclusion that adipose tissue metabolism has no influence on subcutaneous lipomas.

Adipose tissues contain the whole series of mammalian enzymes for carbohydrate and lipid metabolism.[3] A review of the dynamic aspects of adipose tissue metabolism suggests that metabolic regulation of this tissue has a recognizable and reproducible pattern.

Lipid deposition in the body is a result of two processes: incorporation of preformed lipid from the circulation, and de novo synthesis of lipid from carbohydrate directly in the adipose cell itself. Preformed lipid may be derived from the diet or from lipid synthesized in the liver. After absorption by the intestine, dietary lipids (as long-chain fatty acids and monoglycerides) enter the circulation via the thoracic duct as protein-lipid aggregates. The particles may be removed directly by adipose tissue, or they may be removed by the liver and returned to the circulation with modification of the lipid or protein content. They may be hydrolyzed to free fatty acid and reesterified to triglyceride in the liver, then returned to the circulation for eventual incorporation into adipose tissue.

The triglyceride-protein aggregate, no matter what route it has taken, is hydrolyzed on or within the wall of the adipose tissue, and the glycerol and protein are returned to the circulation. The enzyme catalyzing this hydrolysis, lipoprotein lipase, is located at or near the capillary endothelium, and its activity is increased by carbohydrate feeding and probably by insulin or heparin. This type of hydrolysis provides control over the adipose pool by regulating the inflow of fatty acids from circulating triglycerides. The fatty acids, once released from circulating triglycerides by lipoprotein lipase, are reesterified into triglyceride inside the adipose cell, then incorporated into the central droplet. Glycerol in its free form cannot be used for triglyceride synthesis, since adipose tissue lacks the enzyme needed to activate glycerol to glycerol phosphate. Glycerol phosphate must therefore be derived from glucose metabolism. Thus, there is a second controlling mechanism, since the entry of glucose into the adipose tissue is regulated by insulin.[4] Insulin activity controls another extremely important mechanism in the regulation of the body's lipid content: namely, lipogenesis from glucose. Adipose tissue stores little glycogen, and most of the glucose is converted into fatty acids and stored as such. Under the influence of insulin, these fatty acids are esterified with glycerol phosphate and end up in the central droplet of triglyceride. This probably explains why zinc insulin injected subcutaneously over a prolonged period produces fatty tumors phenotypically similar to lipomas.

Mobilization of adipose tissue triglyceride may be in a steady state with the concentration of free fatty acids inside the cell if there is adequate glycerol phosphate. If the supply of glycerol phosphate is inadequate, free fatty acids are released because of inadequate reesterification. Likewise, if lipolysis is accelerated, free fatty acids may accumulate more rapidly than they can be reesterified and, as a result, be released into the circulation. In other words, the release of free fatty acids depends on the relative rates of lipolysis and reesterification.

Adipose tissue may perform functions other than simply serving as an energy storage site. It provides mechanical protection (interarticular pads, buccal cheek pouch), and its role as an insulating agent in subcutaneous sites is well known. The continuous synthesis and breakdown of triglyceride, a heat-producing process, may play a role in thermogenesis. There is evidence that this is indeed true for brown adipose tissue, and a similar role has been suggested for white adipose tissue.

Tumors or tumorlike conditions arising in fat present with protean clinical findings because of the universal distribution of fat. Certain endocrinopathies, idiopathic lipopathies, and true neoplasms are clinically similar and often phenotypically indistinguishable, posing a difficult problem in the management of affected patients. The main diseases of white adipose tissue can be classified as follows: (1) lipopathies, (2) lipodystrophies, (3) primary hyperlipidemia or hypolipidemia producing a tumorlike condition, (4) endocrinopathic disorders, and (5) benign and malignant neoplasms. Only hibernomas (neoplasms) are found to arise in brown adipose tissue.

A detailed discussion of all these disease entities is beyond the scope of this book. They are briefly alluded to and discussed when germane to a presentation on tumors or tumorlike conditions of the adipose tissue.

## ■ DISEASES OF WHITE ADIPOSE TISSUE

### LIPOPATHIES

The term *lipopathies* refers to a group of unrelated diseases of fatty tissue, particularly subcutaneous fat. Lipomas have often been included in this category, but, in this presentation, lipomas will be classified and described in the section on tumors. It is recognized, however, that lipomas may histologically resemble any of the other lipopathies. The following clinical conditions are considered lipopathies: (1) adiposis dolorosa, (2) relapsing febrile nodular nonsuppurative panniculitis, (3) foreign body granuloma, (4) fat necrosis, (5) systemic multicentric lipoblastosis, and (6) steatopygia.

#### Adiposis Dolorosa (Dercum's Disease)

Dercum,[5] in 1892, described a rare disease characterized by adiposity, asthenia, pain, and psychic disturbances. Adiposis dolorosa occurs largely in women during the menopause. It manifests itself either as nodules or, commonly, as a more or less extensive accumulation of subcutaneous fat. Usually, lumpy encapsulated masses are found on the thighs, abdomen, or in the axillary region (Fig. 7–1A and 7–1B). Intra-abdominally, most often, the disease is encountered in the greater omentum, where multiple tumors arranged like "beads" in a chain are the usual finding. Often, these patients are operated on for intractable pain without a correct diagnosis or a diagnosis of pain related to pancreatic biliary disorders. On the abdomen, these masses hang like an apron, and, in other sites, they look like hanging sacs. Subjective symptoms vary from patient to patient, ranging from mere tenderness to spontaneous severe attacks of pain. The cause of this pain is unknown, but even superficial pressure against fatty masses may elicit it. The tenderness and pain cannot be explained on a morphologic basis, since the fatty lesions resemble ordinary lipomas.

Various theories have been proposed to explain the nature of this entity, the most popular being related endocrine disturbance, particularly of the pituitary. A hereditary relationship has also been proposed.[6] Although the exact etiologic factor is unknown, the concept of a combined endocrine deficiency seems logical.[7] Pain is the only distinguishing feature by which Dercum's disease can be differentiated from multiple lipomatosis. Because of its extreme rarity, there is no

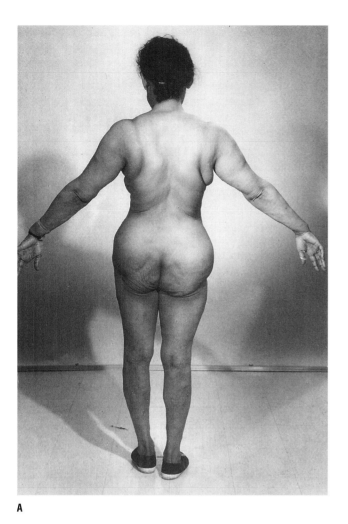

**A**

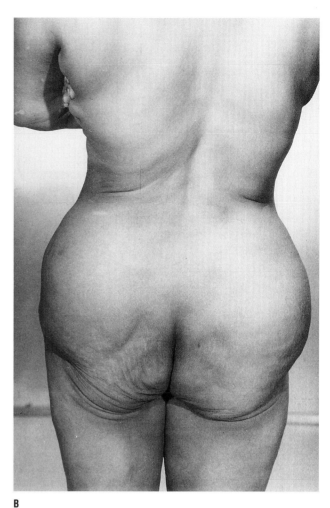

**B**

**Figure 7–1.** (**A**) Bilateral axillary fat pad swelling in a 55-year-old woman who complained of incapacitating pain. Relief of symptoms was achieved after excision. (**B**) Same patient, showing accumulation of gluteal fat. This was less tender than the axillary swellings and was not touched.

accepted definitive therapy. In some extremely tender areas, the excess fat resembling lipomas can be excised, resulting in temporary symptomatic relief.

### Relapsing Febrile Nodular Nonsuppurative Panniculitis (Weber-Christian Disease)

Pfeifer,[8] in 1892, was the first to describe nodular non-suppurative panniculitis as an entity. In 1916, Gilchrist and Ketron[9] reported the second case. However, Weber[10] actually coined the term *relapsing nodular non-suppurative panniculitis* and Christian,[11] in 1928, added the adjective *febrile*. Since then, the entity has been called *Weber-Christian disease*. Lever[12] reviewed the literature and found occasional fatalities. Usually, it is self-limiting and characterized by the intermittent appearance of subcutaneous nodules and plaques caused by degeneration of fatty tissue, with subsequent inflammation.

Recurrent subcutaneous nodules located in the lower extremities constitute the characteristic clinical feature of this entity. The overlying skin is usually erythematous (Fig. 7–2). Lever[13] stated that, occasionally, the skin breaks down and liquid fat drains through the open wound. Clinically, the asymptomatic lesions resemble lipomas. Malaise and slight-to-moderate pyrexia often accompany the appearance of new nodules. Infrequently, this entity develops in the mesentery of obese persons, and they may have acute abdominal symptoms. Clinical distinction from acute appendicitis is often impossible, since in both diseases the patients have fever, leukocytosis, and tenderness in the abdomen. An exploratory celiotomy shows mesenteric panniculitis in Weber-Christian disease (Fig. 7–3). The histologic changes can be divided into three stages. In the first stage, there is focal degeneration of adipose cells, accompanied by an acute inflammatory infiltrate. In

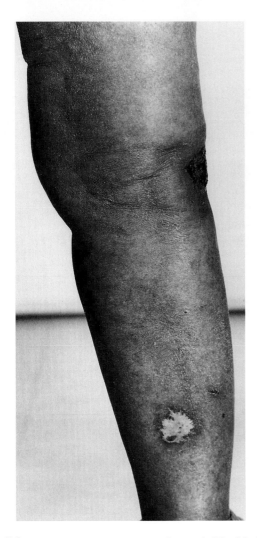

**Figure 7–2.** Example of relapsing nonsuppurative panniculitis of the left lateral aspect of the knee joint. The overlying skin has broken down, with resultant ulcerating lesions. Liquid fat drained for eight weeks before the wound spontaneously healed. Lower tibial area shows healing.

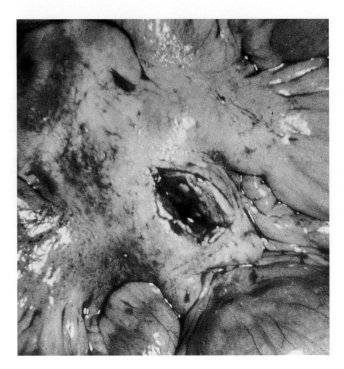

**Figure 7–3.** Mesentery in a case of Weber-Christian disease. Patient was a 39-year-old woman with a 48-hour history of pain in the abdomen similar to acute appendicitis. On exploration, inflamed mesentery was found. Histologic examination of a wedge of tissue showed inflammatory reaction, with a number of macrophages characteristic of this disease *(Reproduced with permission from Das Gupta TK: Tumors and Tumor-Like Conditions of the Adipose Tissue. In Ravitch MM, et al. (eds): Current Problems in Surgery. Copyright March 1970 by Year Book Medical Publishers, Inc., Chicago.)*

the second stage, a number of macrophages with foamy cytoplasm and a varying number of lymphocytes, plasma cells, and histiocytes are seen. In the third stage, fibrosis supervenes. No effective treatment exists for Weber-Christian disease. Steroids will curtail the period of acute manifestation in fulminating cases. Because the entity is self-limiting, only conservative management, to alleviate symptoms, is recommended.

### Foreign Body Granulomas

Many foreign substances, when injected or accidentally implanted in the subcutaneous tissue, produce a foreign body reaction, and often a localized mass develops. These masses can be misdiagnosed as lipomas, especially in the region of the buttocks, unless history of an injection is elicited. Granulomas that follow injection of an oily substance (called lipid granulomas) occur as irregular, hard, nodular subcutaneous swell-

ings. Although clinically they can be mistaken for adipose tissue tumors, the histologic feature is so characteristic that an error in tissue diagnosis is not likely.

### Fat Necrosis

In 1882, Balzer[14] first described fat necrosis as an entity, and ascribed it to acute hemorrhagic pancreatitis. The mechanism of subcutaneous fat necrosis is not clearly understood. An increase in lipase is thought to be the initiating factor, but the cause of the increased tissue lipase content in a specific area of the human body is unknown. Subcutaneous fat necrosis is seen in both adults and children.

Idiopathic fat necrosis sometimes occurs in women with pendulous breasts, presenting as a breast tumor. Adair and Munzer[15] reported its incidence to be 2.76 percent in patients considered to have primary operable carcinoma of the breast. Early fat necrosis is confined to several well-defined fat droplets. Clinically, the firm lesions of fat necrosis resemble carcinoma more than any other benign lesion of the breast. Fat necrosis in the subcutaneous tissue of the buttock or abdomen of obese persons is also well recognized. These lesions closely resemble fatty tumors, and diagnosis usually is made following excision.

Subcutaneous fat necrosis is commonly seen in the newborn and should be differentiated from scleroderma neonatorum, edema neonatorum, and scleroderma occurring in infancy. Lesions of fat necrosis usually appear near the end of the first week after birth, although the time of onset may range from 1 to 42 days.[16] The lesions are deep-seated, indurated masses that may vary in size from several centimeters to large plaques. The distribution often is symmetrical, and the sites of predilection are the back, cheeks, arms, thighs, and buttocks. The smaller lesions freely move over the underlying structures, and the borders of the lesions ordinarily are sharply defined. In the newborn, the usual form of subcutaneous fat necrosis is self-limiting, and no active therapy is required, since most lesions resolve in three to four months. In some unusual instances, subcutaneous fat necrosis in the newborn is associated with hypercalcemia and serious systemic symptoms. Treatment always poses a problem, and fortunately these patients are rare. The exact mechanism of fat necrosis in the newborn is not understood.[16]

### Systemic Multicentric Lipoblastosis

In rare instances, multiple fatty tissue growths are present in subcutaneous as well as visceral fat. Systemic multicentric lipoblastoses tend to recur after excision. These lesions differ from lipomas in that mesenchymal cells and primitive fat cells are frequently found in microscopic sections. Although they present a primitive appearance, no case of malignant degeneration or metastasis has been recorded.

### Steatopygia

Steatopygia (excessive fatness of the buttocks) is normal in some women. Pack and Ariel[17] commented on a female Bushman who was exhibited as an example of callipygia at the Paris exhibition in 1815, and whom Cuvier[17] described as a "Hottentot Venus." There is no need for therapy, and this condition is mentioned merely for the sake of descriptive completeness.

### Lipodystrophy

Lipodystrophy is a rare disease characterized by localized or progressive loss of subcutaneous fat, without subjective symptoms. The cause of progressive lipodystrophy is thought to be a disturbance of autonomic trophic regulation. No therapy exists.

### Primary Hyperlipidemia or Hypolipidemia

Primary hyperlipidemia and hypolipidemia constitute one of the most fascinating problems in the realm of metabolic disorders, but a detailed classification or discussion is beyond the scope of this book. Occasionally, in cases of essential hypercholesterolemia, xanthomatous tumors develop in the extremities. These tumors

have the clinical features of soft tissue tumors and should be distinguished from common lipomas. Usually, they are intradermal, whereas lipomas are subcutaneous.

### Endocrinopathic Disorders

Certain fatty accumulations, the result of metabolic derangements such as Fröhlich's syndrome (which is caused by pituitary or adrenal disturbances), exophthalmos, abnormal accumulation of fat within the orbit secondary to thyroid disturbances, and so forth, are not dealt with in this book, because none of these conditions can be confused with tumors of the adipose tissue.

## ■ NEOPLASMS OF WHITE ADIPOSE TISSUE

A neoplasm of the white adipose tissue can be benign (lipoma) or malignant (liposarcoma).

### LIPOMAS

The etiologic factors of lipomas are unknown. In 1935, Ewing[18] postulated that the major causes for initiation and development of lipomas were the following: (1) heredity (as evidenced by multiple symmetrical lipomas), (2) lipogenesis of tissues, and (3) congenital predisposition toward disturbances in the development of fat. Considerable doubt exists as to the validity of these postulates, but, to date, there are no alternative plausible hypotheses for the development of lipomas, the most common of mesenchymal tumors.

Clinically, lipomas can be classified as (1) solitary, (2) multiple, or (3) congenital diffuse lipomatosis.

### Solitary Lipomas

Solitary lipomas are the most common types of fatty tumor. Pack and Ariel[17] reported the ratio of lipomas to liposarcomas as 120:1, and Stout[19] saw only 21 (1.4 percent) cases of liposarcoma in a series of 1,454 fatty tumors. Solitary lipomas can arise in any part of the human body. They are subclassified according to the site of origin as (1) subcutaneous (most frequent site), (2) intermuscular and intramuscular, (3) intrathoracic, (4) intraperitoneal or retroperitoneal, (5) intraoral, (6) arising in various organs, (7) arising in the central or peripheral nervous systems, and (8) synovial and bone lipomas.

***Subcutaneous Solitary Lipomas.***   In our experience, lipomas occurred in all parts of the human body. Pack and Pierson[20] studied the distribution of 352 lipomas in 134 patients and observed no predilection for any particular site.

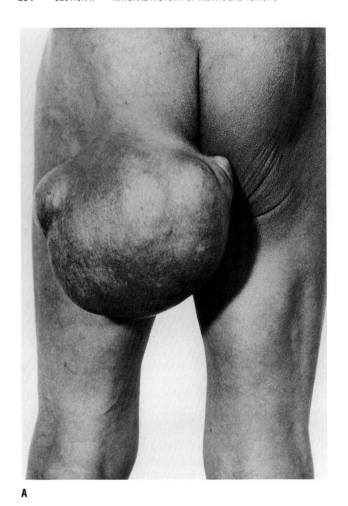

**A**

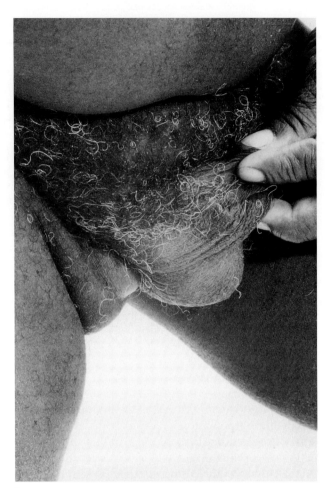

**B**

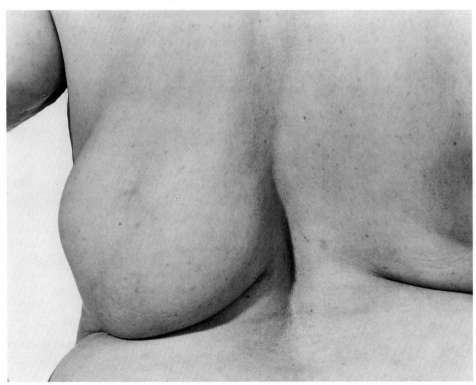

**C**

**Figure 7–4.** (**A**) Lipoma of the left buttock, which was neglected for a long period of time, resulting in saclike appearance.(**B**) Lipoma of the perineum molding to the fold. (**C**) Lipoma of the dorsilumbar region molding to the location.

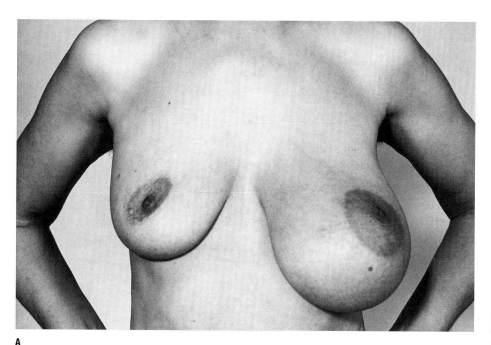

**A**

**Figure 7–5.** (**A**) A 39-year-old woman with a large lipoma of the left breast. (**B**) Xeroradiograph of the same breast.

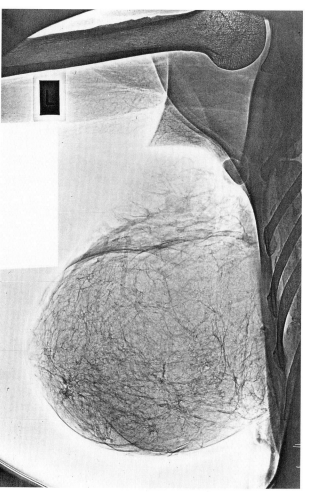

**B**

Generally, lipomas can be diagnosed clinically by a long history of a subcutaneous tumor. The tumors are palpable and can be of any size. In smaller lipomas, the margins of the tumor can easily be palpated. The shape and size of subcutaneous lipomas are frequently molded according to the location (Fig. 7–4A and 7–4C). Those that arise from the subcutaneous tissue of the perineum, the vulva, or the neck become sacculated and hang like fat bags (Fig. 7–4B). Subcutaneous lipomas that arise in the axilla are often attached to the skin and are difficult to diagnose. Occasionally, lipomas of the breast are confused with carcinoma of the breast or fibrocystic disease. Since breast lipomas are rare, the diagnosis should always be made on the basis of histologic examination. Occasionally, a large lipoma of the breast is seen (Fig. 7–5A and 7–5B); however, care should be taken to exclude the possibility of a liposarcoma.

Booher[21] discussed the clinical manifestation of lipomas of the hands and feet, stressing their relative rarity in these sites. He reviewed the literature up to 1965 and found only 65 cases of palmar lipomas, 19 being in his own patients. In our series of 170 lipomas of the upper extremities, 15 were in the hand (Fig. 7–6). Booher[21] described 32 lipomas of the dorsum and wrist, including five cases of his own. We have encountered only four such cases. Table 7–1 shows the incidence of lipomas in the hand in five large series.[21–23] Lipomas of the feet are rarer still. Booher[21] had only three such cases, and we have had six. Clinical diagnosis of lipomas in these areas is difficult.

The lipomas that arise in the head and neck region require special consideration for management. We

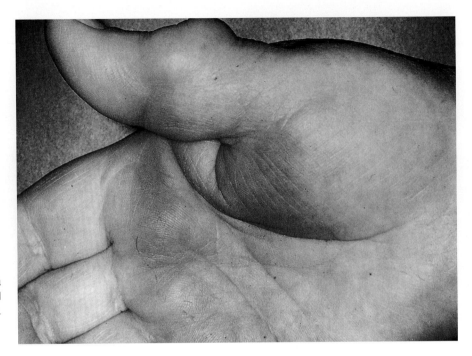

**Figure 7–6.** Lipoma in the thenar eminence of a 55-year-old man. Of interest, he sought medical opinion because of the ganglion in this thumb. Both lesions were excised without difficulty.

have had several patients with lipoma of the parotid region. Although a fine-needle aspiration biopsy might provide a definitive diagnosis, in general these tumors are better managed by resorting to superficial parotidectomy. Lipomas of the forehead, scalp, and neck require care in excision; otherwise, the cosmetic deformity following excision could be far worse than the innocuous small tumor.

## Angiolipoma

Angiolipoma (Fig. 7–7) is a variant of subcutaneous lipoma. The borderline between common solitary lipomas and angiolipomas is still not defined. Clinically, angiolipomas are somewhat tender to the touch, and occasionally there is a history of trauma. Howard and Helwig,[24] in a review of the files of the Armed Forces Institute of Pathology (AFIP), described the distribution of 262 angiolipomas and noted that the tumors arose predominantly in the extremities and trunk, including the retroperitoneum. The management of these tumors is similar to that of common lipomas.

However, there is a distinct group of angiolipomas that infiltrate the surrounding tissue (infiltrating angiolipoma). A curative excision of this variety may at times be extremely difficult. Since these are benign tumors, radical excision, amputation, or radiation therapy in which vital tissues are sacrificed is not in order (Fig. 7–8A and 7–8B).

Infiltrating angiolipomas are rare. We have treated 12 such cases. When the first edition of this book was written, including our then series of four patients, only 27 cases were reported.[25–32] Since 1981, we have treated an additional eight patients. The clinical features of these patients are usually quite similar to subcutaneous lipomas; in spite of their infiltrating character, these tumors are essentially benign (Table 7–2). Occasionally, retroperitoneal angiolipomas may bleed, leading to an abdominal emergency. In rare instances, one or more abdominal viscera require excision. In young women, occasionally the kidney is involved and can rupture during pregnancy, and emergency nephrectomy is required for hemostasis. After excision, local recurrence is rare.

**TABLE 7–1. LIPOMAS OF THE HAND: FIVE SERIES**

| Authors | Date of Publication | No. Cases | Accompanying Symptoms | Comments |
|---|---|---|---|---|
| Booher[21] | 1965 | 31 | Mass and occasional pain | Excised, one recurrence, no nerve pain |
| Phalen et al.[22] | 1971 | 15 | Mass and pain | Six caused nerve compression; all excised |
| Paarlberg et al.[23] | 1972 | 59 | Mass and occasional pain | Excised |
| Das Gupta[32] | 1983 | 15 | Mass and occasional pain | No nerve deficit, all excised; no local recurrence |
| Current series | 1996 | 23[a] | Mass and occasional pain | No nerve deficit, all excised; no local recurrence |

[a]Includes the 15 cases reported in 1983.

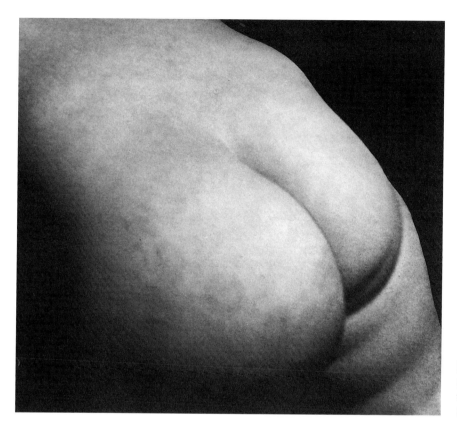

**Figure 7-7.** Angiolipoma of the left buttock in a child. Note spiderweb distribution of subcutaneous venous plexus. *(Courtesy of* Current Problems in Surgery, *1970.)*

## Intermuscular and Intramuscular Lipomas

Intermuscular lipomas have been recognized for many years. In 1913, Kuttner and Landors[33] reviewed 27 cases from the literature, and, since then, several other series have been reported.[34–36] Congenital intermuscular lipomas have also been described. These tumors have been reported to arise within the inner surface of the cheek, just inside the masseter muscle. Probably, most of these represent normal sucking pads of infants.[37]

The exact location of a lipoma arising in the depths of the soft tissue is always confusing. These tumors can be either intermuscular, submuscular, or intramuscular. The intermuscular type grows between the large muscle bundles, probably arising from the intramuscular fascial septa. These lesions form a large central tumor that secondarily infiltrates adjacent muscles. The intramuscular type, on the other hand, originates between the muscle fibers and infiltrates the adjacent muscles by passing through intermuscular septa.

Often, however, it is difficult to establish the exact site of origin, as some of these tumors may develop within the muscle but extend into the intermuscular spaces (Fig. 7–9). Therefore, these tumors should all be considered intermuscular lipomas and managed in a uniform manner.

We have treated 64 cases of intermuscular and/or intramuscular lipomas: 19 in the upper extremities, 37

in the lower extremities, and 8 in the trunk. Kindbloom and co-workers[35] found a similar anatomic distribution in their 43 patients.

The intermuscular lipomas usually are deeply situated but can often be identified by soft tissue roentgenography (Fig. 7–10). They appear as translucent encapsulated masses. Radiolucency is usually characteristic of these tumors, and they are seldom mistaken for cysts or other types of tumors. In the extremities, the deep lipomas may feel soft and flat when the muscles are relaxed, and hard and spherical when the muscles are contracted. The diagnosis must be made after histologic examination of the tissue.

These tumors tend to recur if inadequately excised. Usually, they grow expansively and are not well encapsulated, and fatty off-shoots are frequently left behind, leading to recurrence. It must be emphasized that, although every effort should be made to avoid a recurrence, a major amputation and/or debilitating muscle group excision must not be performed in order to obtain an adequate margin of normal tissue.

## Intrathoracic Lipomas

In 1781, Fothergill[38] reported the first case of intrathoracic lipoma. Krause and Ross[39] reviewed the literature in 1962 and, including their own three patients, compiled a series of 80 patients with intrathoracic lipomas.

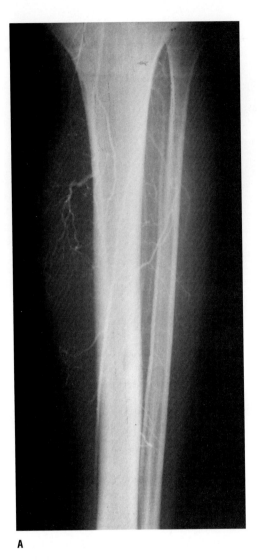

**A**

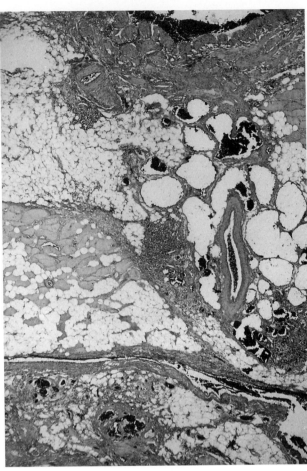

**B**

**Figure 7–8.** (**A**) Angiogram of an angiolipoma of the right calf of a 24-year-old man. Clinically, this was thought to be a malignant tumor. (**B**) Angiolipoma showing multitude of capillaries with mature fatty tissue. The stroma shows the presence of fibroreticular material around the blood vessels. (H & E. Original magnification × 63.) A wide excision of the gross tumor, including gastrocnemius muscle, was performed. Although microscopic residual tumor was left behind during initial operation, the patient has remained well 20 years.

Although solitary lipomas can occur in any site within the thorax, the most common site is the mediastinum,[40] where they can grow to enormous size. The literature is replete with case reports of excision of massive mediastinal lipomas.

Intrathoracic lipoma can be entirely within the thorax or have an hourglass shape, with extension to the neck or through the chest wall into an intercostal space. The presenting feature of an intrathoracic lipoma depends on the size and location of the tumor. In general, the diagnosis is made by a chest roentgenogram that shows a mediastinal mass. Staub et al.[41] found that approximately 50 percent of patients with mediastinal lipomas are symptomatic, the common symptoms being a nonproductive cough, dyspnea, and a feeling of pressure in the chest. Correct diagnosis usually is achieved after an exploratory thoracotomy and excision of the tumor. Complete excision is almost always possible.

### Intraperitoneal or Retroperitoneal Lipomas

Benign fatty tumors are occasionally encountered in the peritoneal cavity or in the retroperitoneum. Within the peritoneal cavity, the most likely place would seem to be the omentum, because of the presence there of a large quantity of fatty tissue. In truth, however, omental lipomas are extremely rare. Elfving and Hastbacka[42] found only one tumor that could remotely be consid-

**TABLE 7–2. SUMMARY OF 12 INFILTRATING ANGIOLIPOMAS**

| Case No. | Age/Sex | Site of Lesion | Comments |
|---|---|---|---|
| 1 | 22/M | Right calf | Tumor of right calf, infiltrating the medial head of the gastrocnemius muscle. Gross tumor excised, leaving tumor behind. No recurrence in three years. |
| 2 | 69/F | Retroperitoneum | Left retroperitoneal area, 15 × 10 × 12 cm mass infiltrating the paravertebral muscles and surrounding structures. Excised, with no recurrence in two years. |
| 3 | 34/F | Retroperitoneum | Diagnosed during pregnancy, created major abdominal catastrophe due to retroperitoneal hemorrhage. Required left nephrectomy and cesarean hysterectomy. Both mother and child doing well one year later. Patient was treated elsewhere and was seen by the author on consultation. |
| 4 | 59/M | Thigh | Large infiltrating mass in right medial thigh infiltrating adductor muscles. Excision of tumor with margin of the muscles has resulted in apparent cure for 2.5 years. |
| 5 | 30/M | Left scapular region | Ovoid tumor causing erosion of scapula and pain. No recurrence after 10 years. |
| 6 | 32/F | Calf muscle | Infiltrating gastrocnemius with pain operated on twice elsewhere, once a wide excision. |
| 7 | 24/F | Lumbar region | Soft mass 20 cm in diameter, destruction of transverse processes, required a major excision but margins were not clear; has remained well for twelve years. |
| 8 | 27/M | Right heel | 5 × 5 × 3 cm mass treated by resection with 1-cm margin, no recurrence. |
| 9 | 51/F | Lateral side of thigh | Painful mass (4 × 3 × 2 cm); wide excision, no recurrence. |
| 10 | 53/M | Shoulder | Mass infiltrated trapezius muscle; lesion excised with a small margin of the muscle. |
| 11 | 55/F | Posterior neck | 5 × 4 × 3 cm mass; excised with portion of muscle. |
| 12 | 44/M | Right upper arm | 12 × 15 × 10 cm mass invading deltoid muscle, excised with 1-cm muscle margin, no recurrence. |

ered a lipoma of the omentum. We have never encountered such a case.

Lipomatous tumors occur more frequently in the retroperitoneal space than in the intraperitoneal region. The retroperitoneal tumors are more often malignant than benign, whereas in other locations the reverse is true. Pack and Ariel[17] reported that, out of a series of 19 retroperitoneal fatty tumors, only 2 were benign. Brasfield and Das Gupta[43] found that 35 of a series of 39 retroperitoneal fatty tumors were malignant. In our current experience, we have encountered only two additional cases where the retroperitoneal tumors were microscopically diagnosed as lipomas. It is our opinion that, when a diagnosis of retroperitoneal lipoma is rendered, repeated efforts should be made to systematically assess the resected specimen so that a low-grade liposarcoma is not misdiagnosed.

The fatty tumors in this location are clinically quiescent during their early period of development, and, because of the nature of the anatomic site, they grow unhampered and attain huge size. Delamater,[44] in 1859, reported a classic case of a 179-pound retroperitoneal tumor in a 36-year-old woman whose original weight was 90 pounds. Symptoms usually are ill defined.

DeWeerd and Dockerty[45] reported the female-to-male ratio in retroperitoneal fatty tumors to be 1.3:1.0; however, in Pack and Ariel's[17] series, the female-to-male ratio was 3:1. Our own experience suggests that it is more common in women. The age range commonly is 40 to 50 years. The ideal method of treatment is excision, but both operative mortality and morbidity are associated with operations for large retroperitoneal tumors.

### Intraoral Lipomas

Submucous lipomas in the oral cavity are extremely rare. Seldin and co-workers[46] reported 26 cases, the lesions being distributed as follows: cheek, 11; buccal fold in the region of mental foramen, 2; lower buccal fold, 2; lip, 3; palate, 2; floor of the mouth, 2; and gingiva, 4. Hatziotis[47] reviewed the published material and described 145 cases over a 22-year period ending in

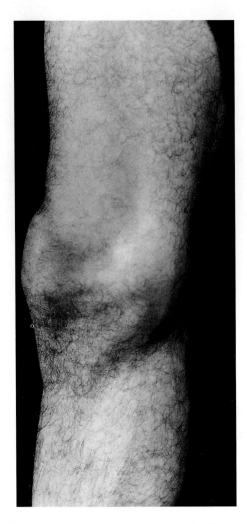

**Figure 7–9.** Intermuscular lipoma attached to the semitendinosus muscle in a 53-year-old man—an uncommon location. *(Courtesy of* Current Problems in Surgery, *1970.)*

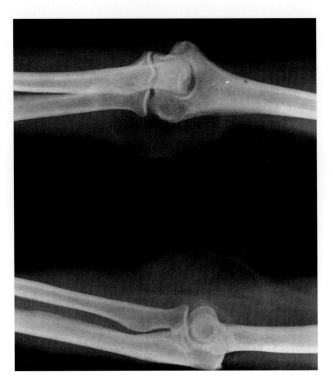

**Figure 7–10.** Roentgenogram of an intermuscular lipoma located in the antecubital fossa. The tumor was within the muscle bundles and was firm on palpation.

1967. Seven new cases were added by Burzynski et al.[48] in 1971. Greer and Richardson[49] analyzed 16 cases seen at the Boston University School of Dentistry and outlined the criteria for accepting intraoral tumors as lipomas. The management of these lesions is excision.

### Lipomas Arising in the Organs

***Lipomas of the Gastrointestinal Tract.*** Lipomas of the gastrointestinal tract, though benign and relatively uncommon, require consideration because they mimic several other types of benign and malignant tumors of the alimentary tract. In 1963, Mayo and associates[50] collected all the lipomas of the alimentary tract in the Mayo Clinic file and found only 186 cases over a period of 27 years (Table 7–3). They further studied the relationship of gastrointestinal lipomas to other gastrointestinal neoplasms, both benign and malignant. The incidence and type were as follows: gastric carcinoma, 1; colon carcinoma, 47; adenomatous polyps, 35; multiple poly-

posis, 8; cavernous hemangioma (sigmoid), 2; and villous adenoma (rectum), 1. These investigators also found various other gastrointestinal diseases in this series, for example, duodenal ulcer, ulcerative colitis, and anal fissures. Feldman[51] studied the relationship of associated conditions in autopsied patients with lipoma of the gastrointestinal tract. Of the 78 cases in his series, 20 were multiple (25.6 percent), growing in widely separated segments of the digestive tract. Frequently, these lipomas were associated with other benign tumors of the gastrointestinal tract: 18 percent with leiomyomas and 23 percent with polyps.

***Esophageal Lipomas.*** Esophageal lipomas are extremely rare. In the series of cases reported by Mayo et al.,[50] only 3 of the 186 cases were located in the esophagus. Diagnosis was based on histologic examination of the material. We have encountered only one such patient, in whom a lipoma (2 cm in diameter) was removed from the lower third of the esophagus.

***Lipomas of the Stomach.*** In 1925, Eliason and Wright[52] compiled a list from the literature of 610 benign stomach tumors and found that lipomas comprised 4.8 percent. These same authors found only one gastric lipoma in 8,000 autopsies. A review of the literature from 1835 to 1940 by Rumold[53] produced 33 cases of submucous gastric lipoma, 17 of which were found at

**TABLE 7–3. LIPOMAS OF THE GASTROINTESTINAL TRACT (MAYO CLINIC): DISTRIBUTION BY ANATOMIC SITE, SEX OF PATIENT, AND PATHOLOGIC NATURE OF LESION**

| Anatomic Site | Sex | | Pathologic Diagnosis | | | | Total |
|---|---|---|---|---|---|---|---|
| | *Male* | *Female* | *Lipomas* | *Fibrolipomas* | *Lipomatosis* | *Lipid Granulomas* | |
| Esophagus | 2 | 1 | 1 | 2 | — | — | 3 |
| Stomach | 4 | 2 | 6 | — | — | — | 6 |
| Small intestine | 21 | 37 | — | — | — | — | 58 |
| Duodenum | 5 | 2 | 6 | 1 | — | — | (7) |
| Jejunum | 2 | — | 2 | — | — | — | (2) |
| Ileum | 7 | 8 | 14 | 1 | — | — | (15) |
| Ileocecal valve | 7 | 27 | 16 | — | 18 | — | (34) |
| Large intestine | 57 | 62 | — | — | — | — | 119 |
| Cecum | 7 | 24 | 27 | — | — | 4 | (31) |
| Ascending colon | 6 | 11 | 16 | 1 | — | — | (17) |
| Transverse colon | 12 | 12 | 21 | 3 | — | — | (24) |
| Descending colon | 12 | 6 | 18 | — | — | — | (18) |
| Sigmoid colon | 10 | 5 | 14 | 1 | — | — | (15) |
| Rectosigmoid | 2 | 1 | 3 | — | — | — | (3) |
| Rectum | 8 | 3 | 8 | 1 | — | 2 | (11) |
| Total | 84 | 102 | 152 | 10 | 18 | 6 | 186 |

*Courtesy of* Surgery *53:598, 1963.*

necropsy and 16 at operation. In 1946, Scott and Brunschwig[54] collected five additional cases from the literature that occurred after 1941 and added one case of their own. In 1948, Alvarez, Lastra, and Leon[55] collected four more cases from the literature, following the report of Scott and Brunschwig,[54] and described a case of their own, bringing the total to 44. In 1958, Pack and Ariel[17] commented on 58 cases of gastric lipomas. Since then, occasional case reports have appeared in the literature. Thompson and Oyster[56] calculated the incidence of gastric lipomas to be 1.1 percent of all benign gastric tumors. Notably, no single clinician has a large personal experience to draw from.

These tumors usually are seen in older individuals and are about equally distributed between the sexes. Structurally, lipomas of the stomach are no different from subcutaneous lipomas. They may range in size from a few millimeters to 9 or 10 centimeters in diameter. They can be sessile or penduncular, single or multiple. When they are submucous, they protrude into the lumen of the stomach and may cause erosions and ulcerations of the mucosa, with bleeding.[57] Submucosal and pedunculated lipomas can produce pyloric obstruction or intussusception.[58]

The gastric lipomas are juxtaposed to the pylorus or antrum in about 60 percent of cases. Although they can arise anywhere in the stomach wall, about 96 percent are submucosal. Pain is the usual symptom; occasionally, ulceration of a polypoid tumor may produce hematemesis and melena. Roentgenologic examina-

tion of a symptomatic patient might point to the presence of a benign tumor. Although the diagnosis can frequently be made by endoscopy and biopsy, assessment of a gastric lipoma can be made only at the operating table. Removal by polypectomy, enucleation, or partial gastrectomy is curative.

***Lipomas of the Small Intestine.*** Lipomas of the small intestine (Fig. 7–11A and 7–11B) are rare and are seldom solitary. Furste and co-workers[57] described a series of 19 cases of gastrointestinal lipomas, of which 11 were in the small intestine. Mayo et al.[50] had 21 such cases in their series of 186. The two most common symptoms in lipomas of the small intestine, as in all other small intestinal tumors, are bleeding and intussusception. Symptomatic patients should be treated by exploratory laparotomy and appropriate resection. Ling and co-workers[59] reported one case of intestinal lipomatosis diagnosed preoperatively. In this case, the patient had resection of the segment containing the ileocecal intussusception, with part of the distal ileum. The specimen was 195 cm long and contained 107 submucosal lipomas.

***Lipomas of the Ileocecal Region and Colon.*** Although a lipoma of the colon is relatively rare, it is generally agreed that this tumor is one of the most common forms of benign mesenchymal tumors of the colon.[50,60] D'Jarid[60] reviewed the cases published between 1844

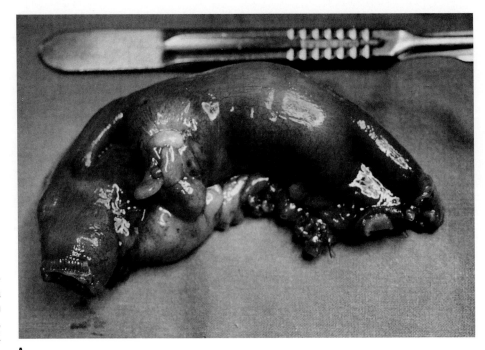

**Figure 7–11.** **(A)** Segment of ileum; the intramural tumor is obvious. Overlying serosa smooth and not infiltrated. **(B)** The lumen opened along the antemesenteric border, showing the lipoma in situ. *(Courtesy of H. Abcarian, M.D.)* **A**

and 1958 and found 278. Analysis showed that these tumors occurred about equally in both sexes and that the age at onset was usually in the sixth decade. A high proportion of lipomas involved the ileocecal junction and the colon. In the series reported by Mayo and his colleagues,[50] 110 of 186 were in the large intestine. These tumors are commonly single (Fig. 7–12A and 7.12B). Intermittent intussusception is the characteristic symptom of colonic lipomas, almost all of which are submucosal in location.

A correct preoperative diagnosis of asymptomatic colonic lipoma can be made by colonoscopy. In cases of obscure intermittent abdominal pain with periods of complete freedom, a diagnosis of intussusception due to a benign tumor should be considered. The possibility of these tumors being adenomas is greater than the likelihood of their being lipomas. In the past, radiographic studies showing either a polypoid tumor or the characteristic filling defect of a colonic intussusception were the only way to diagnose a colonic lipoma preoperatively. However, currently, most of these lipomas are diagnosed by a colonoscopy.

***Lipomas of the Genitourinary Tract.*** Lipomas of the kidney, ureter, and bladder have all been described. In the kidney, angiolipomas are the most common type.[61] It has been suggested that lipomas develop in atrophic kidneys.[62]

***Renal Angiolipoma.*** Renal angiolipomas constitute the most controversial of the benign tumors of the kidney. They are often encountered in the kidneys of patients

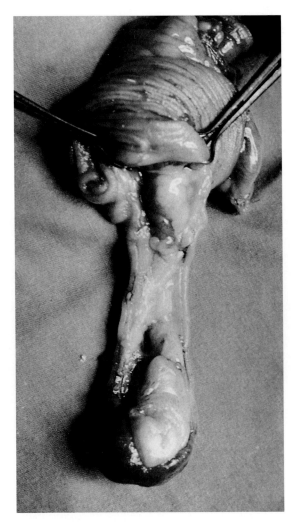

**B**

with the tuberous sclerosis complex and are usually asymptomatic. In patients in whom the renal neoplasm is not associated with tuberous sclerosis, the tumors can become quite large and symptomatic, necessitating resection. Price and Mostofi[61] found 30 cases in the files of the Kidney Tumor Registry of the Armed Forces Institute of Pathology. This lesion occurs more frequently in women than in men. We have only three cases of renal angiolipoma in our files.

The clinical picture ranges from an acute abdominal emergency to that of renal colic. In one of our patients, the abdominal symptoms were misconstrued as tubal pregnancy. Computed tomography scan of the kidney and retroperitoneum may be of considerable help in diagnosis. These tumors are usually large, and the characteristic feature is the associated hemorrhage within the renal parenchyma. Adequate treatment usually entails a nephrectomy. No instance of recurrence after nephrectomy has been reported.

Although rare, lipomas of the female genital tract are a well-accepted clinical entity and may occur at any location.[62,63] Lipomas of the female external genitalia are somewhat more common than those of the genitourinary tract, and a number of such cases are encountered in any busy gynecologic practice. Although lipomas of the spermatic cord are encountered not infrequently, lipomas of the scrotum and testes are indeed rare. There is some controversy concerning the classification of scrotal lipomas because of uncertainty in the determination of the exact primary site. Thus the term paratesticular (covering all structures) has been advocated[64] and is in general use.

### Lipomas of the Respiratory Tract.

Lipoma of the upper respiratory tract is rare. In the past, a number of cases have been mistakenly classified as lipomas. Zakrewski,[65] in 1965, found 68 reported cases of lipomas of the larynx, of which 54 were in the extrinsic and 14 in the intrinsic larynx. He also reported one case of a subglottic lipoma. These tumors behave like all other submucosal lipomas, and the symptoms of obstruction and irritation are relieved by excision. Pulmonary or endobronchial lipomas are extremely rare[66] and are seldom diagnosed before death.

### Lipomas of the Heart.

Lipoma of the heart is a rare entity that is usually diagnosed postmortem. Although these tumors are most commonly incidental necropsy findings, Estevez and associates[67] found a total of 37 cases of cardiac lipoma, including 2 of their own, in which the patients were symptomatic and eventually died.

### Lipomas of the Spleen.

Easler and Dowlin[68] reported one case of primary lipoma of the spleen and found only one other case in the literature. We have no case in our files.

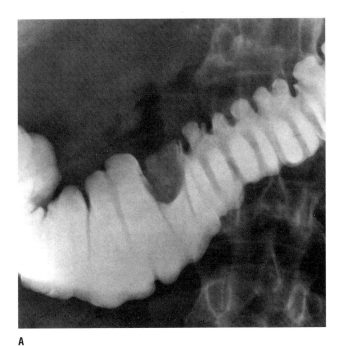
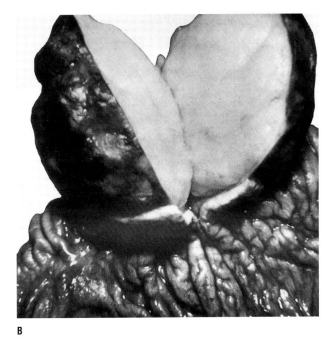

A

B

**Figure 7–12.** (**A**) Roentgenogram of a lipoma of the colon. The smooth contour suggests a benign tumor, but such a preoperative diagnosis should be made with extreme caution. (**B**) A large solitary lipoma of the transverse colon in a 47-year-old man. Patient presented with symptoms of bowel obstruction. An intussusception was found, which could be reduced. The segment containing the lipoma was excised. *(Courtesy of* Current Problems in Surgery, *1970.)*

## ■ LIPOMAS OF THE CENTRAL AND PERIPHERAL NERVOUS SYSTEM

Rokitansky,[69] in 1856, accidentally found the first case of a lipoma of the corpus callosum. Intracranial lipomas are extremely rare, and about 50 percent occur in the corpus callosum. Ewing[70] collected six patients with intracranial lipoma of the pia. The exact number of reported brain lipomas is hard to establish. Manganiello and co-authors[71] reported a total of 69 lipomas of the corpus callosum. These tumors often produce symptoms of obstructive hydrocephalus. Preoperative diagnosis of intracranial lipoma is impossible, and most of these tumors are diagnosed after craniotomy for a presumed brain tumor.

Intraspinal lipomas, which constitute a small percentage of all primary intraspinal tumors, can be either intradural or extradural. The intradural lipomas are of greater interest because they occur in a region supposedly devoid of fat cells. Ehni and Love[72] collected only 29 cases of intradural lipomas. Usually, they are congenital and there is commonly a long history of symptoms. Collins and Henderson[73] stated that symptoms usually appear at one of three age periods: before the third year, in adolescence, and at about the age of 40 years. They often are present for many years before producing serious disability.

The extradural lipomas, on the other hand, are not congenital, occur at all ages, and usually have a short history. There is no characteristic segmental distribution, and they often are associated with the multiple lipomas of obesity. In 1973, Thomas and Miller[74] published their experience of 60 intraspinal lipomas from the Mayo Clinic. They suggested that a history of discomfort of long duration, a midline soft tissue mass, roentgenologic evidence of bony anomaly, and myelographic demonstration of a large dural sac and low-lying conus medullaris are all suggestive of an intraspinal lipoma. Today, however, a magnetic resonance imaging (MRI) study will not only provide the diagnosis but also will clearly delineate the extent of the tumor. Thomas and Miller[74] recommended excision, and a 10-year follow-up showed the results to be favorable. However, when excision was not feasible, a decompressing laminectomy was recommended.

Lipomas of the peripheral nerves are extremely rare. Only recently have these tumors been described.[75–79] However, the diagnosis has been confused with fatty infiltration of the nerves by many authors.[80–82] Lipofibromatous hamartoma infrequently can give rise to macrodactyly. Stout's[83] admonition that such a diagnosis should be accepted with skepticism still holds true.

## ■ SYNOVIAL AND BONE LIPOMAS

Synovial lipomas are not infrequently present within the joint capsule, the popliteal space being one of the common sites.[83] These lipomas can arise within the joint either by penetrating the synovial membrane or as a result of overgrowth of fat within the intra-articular synovial tissue. Extra-articular lipomas are occasionally seen around the hip and knee joints. Intra-articular lipomas are also known as *lipoma arborescens.* They produce a characteristic treelike growth within the synovial membrane. Pack and Ariel[17] emphasized the need for distinguishing this type of lipoma from villous synovitis, an inflammatory overgrowth of the synovia. Lipoma arborescens can simulate pigmented villonodular synovitis, rheumatoid arthritis, and synovial hemangioma. Arthrography and arthroscopy have been used to make a preoperative diagnosis of lipoma arborescens.

Lipomas of the bone are seldom encountered. Bartlett[84] reported two patients in whom the lipomas arose from the periosteum and extended into the contiguous soft tissues. Dahlin,[85] in 1978, described five cases of lipomas of bones, including the roentgenographic findings. Association of a translucent mass in intimate contact with the diaphysis of a long bone and a hyperostotic reaction penetrating the tumor are classic findings. After excision, the patient's progress is good. Occasionally, lipomas occur in the sacroiliac joint, producing symptoms of low back pain.[86] These tumors probably represent benign variants of periosteal fibrous tissue. Lipomas arising in bone should not be confused with ossifying lipomas. In such cases, areas of bone formation are infrequently encountered in the center of a long-standing subcutaneous lipoma (Fig. 7–13).

## ■ MULTIPLE LIPOMAS

Multiple lipomas are unquestionably inherited, and the mode of inheritance is a simple dominant gene.[87] The number varies from 2 or 3 to as many as 500 in one person. Although usually small and subcutaneous, they become large and confluent, producing a knobby contour of the extremities or the trunk that may be disfiguring. Pack and Ariel[17] described one patient with about 400 such lipomas. Several patients with hundreds of lipomas have been treated in our center.

In patients with von Recklinghausen's neurofibromatosis, a large number of lipomas are encountered along with cutaneous neurofibromas, and often clinical distinction between the two types is impossible without histologic examination. Adair et al.[88] suggested that

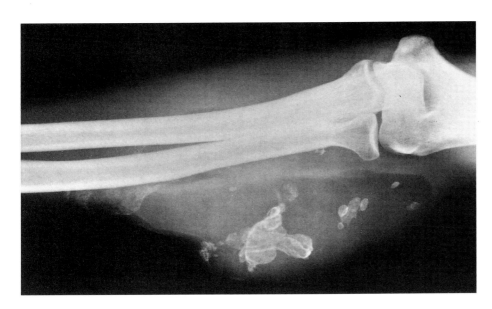

**Figure 7–13.** Areas of ossification in a long-standing solitary lipoma of the forearm. (See also Figure 5–7, Chapter 5.)

multiple lipomas are connected with peripheral nerves and are essentially neurolipomas of neurogenic origin. These authors were impressed by the symmetrical arrangement of multiple lipomas, often corresponding to the course of a peripheral nerve; by their appearance in situations in which fat is usually absent; by their occurrence in young adults; and by a familial tendency to both multiple lipomas and neurofibromatosis, with pigmented cutaneous lesions present in both conditions. However, there is no evidence to support a thesis that multiple lipomas or lipomas in general have any relation to peripheral nerves. Multiple lipomas may be associated with angiomas and, less frequently, with diaphyseal aclasis; or they may be associated with multiple endocrine abnormalities.[89] Pain may suddenly develop in one of the lipomas and gradually extend to involve more and more discrete lipomas. This is not related to adiposis dolorosa.

The treatment of multiple lipomas is a perplexing problem. It is often technically impossible to remove all the hundreds of lipomas, even though total excision might be desirable from a cosmetic viewpoint. The inevitable question is, Do these tumors ultimately become malignant? Fortunately, they rarely do. We have come across only a few such instances. A description of one such patient follows:

*Case Report.*
A 43-year-old man was referred to us for consultation regarding the management of two separate primary liposarcomas. He gave a family history of multiple lipomas. He had had his painful lipomas excised at regular intervals over the past 10 to 15 years. Recently, however, two tumors, one in the neck and the other in the anterior abdominal wall, had rapidly increased in size. His surgeon excised these two lesions and found them to be liposarcomas. A review of the slides confirmed the histologic diagnosis. Examination of the patient showed multiple small lipomas and several large ones. Excision of these tumors was recommended, along with wider excision of the already diagnosed liposarcomas. The patient underwent the suggested therapy. Examination of all the resected lesions showed that he had nine independent primary liposarcomas. He is still doing well 15 years later.

It is not possible to define guidelines for the management of multiple lipomas. Generally, in view of the rarity of malignant degeneration, the reason for excision should be either pain relief or cosmesis. However, if any individual lipoma suddenly enlarges in size, then excision of that lipoma is indicated.

## ■ CONGENITAL LIPOMATOSIS

Congenital lipomatosis is a malformation of the adipose tissue in which the lipoblasts not only form discrete tumors, but also infiltrate the surrounding structures. For clarity of description, the patients are grouped according to the anatomic locations in which lipomatosis is most commonly seen. These are as follows:

1. Congenital diffuse lipomatosis of the extremities
2. Congenital lipomatosis of the trunk
3. Pelvic lipomatosis

*Congenital Diffuse Lipomatosis of the Extremities.* Congenital diffuse lipomatosis of the extremities is usually confined to one or two limbs and commonly is associated

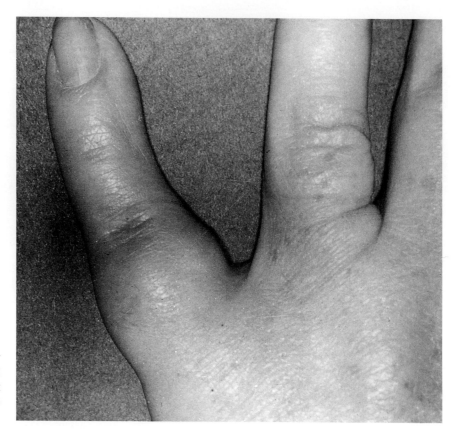

**Figure 7–14.** Lipoma of the palm and index finger in a patient with multiple lipomatosis. The local gigantism of the index finger is evident and was not altered even after excision of the lipoma at the base of the finger.

with corresponding gigantism (Fig. 7–14). Frequently, it is found with a cavernous hemangioma. The condition becomes apparent soon after birth, and usually there is progressive enlargement. The lipomatous tumors commonly infiltrate the surrounding musculature and have an unusual propensity for recurrence, even after relatively wide excision. We have encountered one patient[90] who required a forequarter amputation (Fig. 7–15).

Lipomatosis of discrete parts of the skeletal muscle has been described in Maffucci's syndrome. Cameron and McMillan[91] described a patient with the symptoms of Maffucci's syndrome who had a tumorlike adipose infiltration of the semitendinosus muscle and short head of the biceps femoris.

From a clinician's standpoint, the differential diagnosis is between intermuscular lipomas (page 237) and lipomatosis. Caution is advised, since lipomatosis does not require any therapeutic intervention, whereas intermuscular lipomas need excision.

### Congenital Lipomatosis of the Trunk

The underlying pathologic findings of congenital lipomatosis of the trunk are similar to those of the extremities. In most patients, these tumors are found in the lumbodorsal and scapular regions. Nixon and Scobie[92] reported three cases, all in the lumbodorsal region.

Another type of lipomatosis that may occur at any age is Madelung's disease (Fig. 7–16; Also see Fig. 5–8, A–C), in which the neck and axillae are symmetrically enlarged. The disease has also been called adenolipomatosis, since it occurs in the neck, axillary, and antecubital regions, although it has no relation to lymph nodes.

### Pelvic Lipomatosis

Pelvic lipomatosis (Fig. 7–17A to 7–17E) as a distinct clinical entity has been recognized only since Fogg and Smyth[93] first described it in 1968. However, Engels[94] was the first to recognize the entity on a radiologic basis. It is essentially a benign condition in which there is an abundance of fatty tissue in the perirectal and perivesical spaces in the pelvis.

The cause of this disorder is unknown. Although four patients in the series reported by Engels underwent laparotomy and had large amounts of fatty tissue in the pelvis, they also had extensive pelvic adhesions. Engels concluded that these adhesions were the underlying cause of the distortion of the bladder and sigmoid colon. Rosenberg et al.[95] reported a case of sciatica in a 50-year-old man in whom they had made a diagnosis of Dercum's disease. The patient had painful tender masses on the arms, legs, and right side of the rectum. A barium enema and urographic studies were sugges-

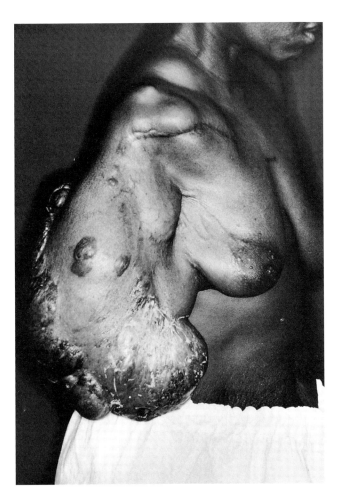

**Figure 7–15.** A 42-year-old woman who had gigantism of the right upper extremity since infancy. She had had multiple operations, and lipomatous tissue was sequentially excised. At age 8, she had an above-elbow amputation. She was first seen with massive enlargement 34 years after above-elbow amputation. The remainder of the upper arm was heavy and painful. She complained of pain, tenderness, and loss of balance. Because of the extreme discomfort, a forequarter amputation was recommended. *(Courtesy of* Current Problems in Surgery, *1970.)*

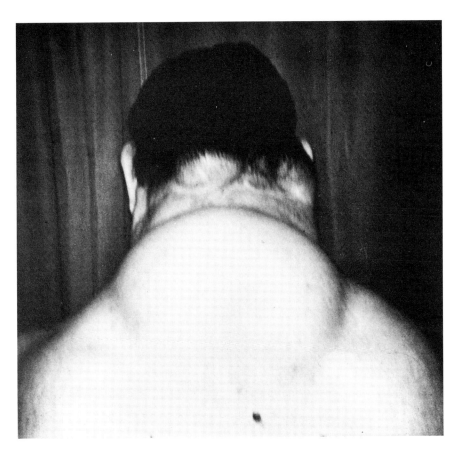

**Figure 7–16.** Typical case of Madelung's deformity. Note the Buffalo hump on the back. *(Courtesy of* Current Problems in Surgery, *1970.)*

247

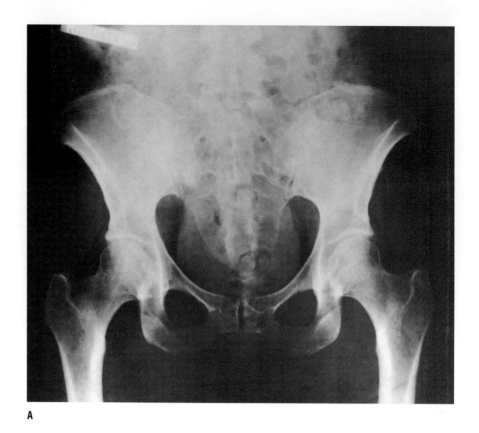

A

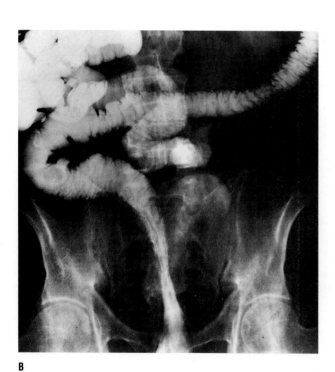

B

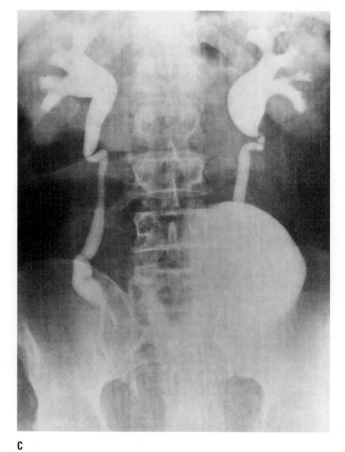

C

**Figure 7–17.** (**A**) Anteroposterior roentgenogram of the pelvis in pelvic lipomatosis. Note the ground glass shadow of the pelvic fatty tissue, the outline of which is smooth. (**B**) Barium enema in a man with pelvic lipomatosis. The vertical straightening and foreshortening of the rectosigmoid is obvious and frequently is diagnostic. (**C**) Displacement of right ureter. *(Continued.)*

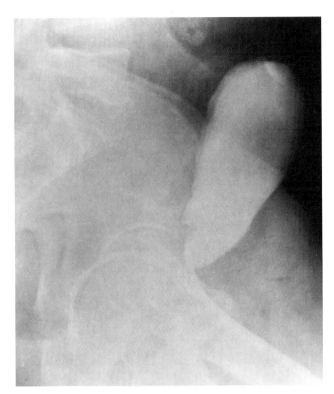

D

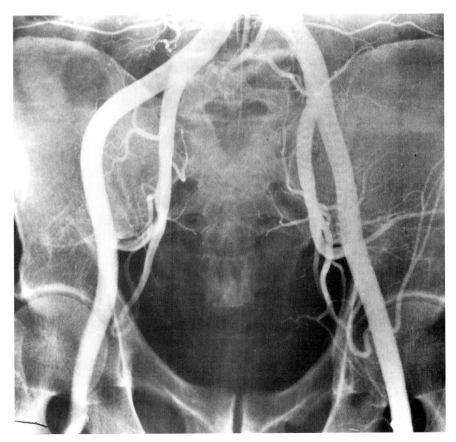

E

**Figure 7–17** *(continued).* (**D**) Dye-filled urinary bladder in pelvic lipomatosis. The bladder appears vertically elongated. (**E**) Aortogram in pelvic lipomatosis, showing the displacement of the iliac vessels. Displacement of the right iliac is most marked.

tive of pelvic lipomatosis. Fogg and Smyth[93] suggested that pelvic lipomatosis is comparable to Weber-Christian disease and sclerosing lipogranulomatosis. It is apparent that different authors have applied various fanciful theories regarding the cause of this unusual clinical entity. However, in reality, no known systemic or local factor or factors can be shown to have a cause-and-effect relationship. Certainly these tumors are not pelvic lipomas, although in one of our patients it was tempting to consider this as a variant of infiltrating angiolipoma.

The term *pelvic lipomatosis* aptly describes the anatomic and pathologic essence of this entity, which consists of an excessive proliferation of fibroadipose tissue in the pelvis. Cook et al.[96] reviewed 29 published cases, 27 in men and 2 in women. At the University of Illinois, we have seen 17 such cases, 11 in men and 6 in women. Clinical correlation varies, with symptoms of lower urinary tract obstruction, vague pelvic pain, constipation, and even hypertension. However, in a large number of these patients, the diagnosis of pelvic lipomatosis is considered only after roentgenograms are obtained for evaluation of these nonspecific complaints.

Physical findings are not consistent, but an ill-defined mass in the suprapubic region has been found most frequently. Prostatic enlargement has been mentioned by some authors.[95–99] Elongation of the membranous and bulbous portions of the urethra has also been observed.[100]

Several authors have mentioned the difficulty of performing cystoscopy because of the elongated bladder or the distorted trigone, or both.[94,96–99] Cystoscopic findings ranged from normal to marked bullous edema.[96] Most authors report that examination of the colon shows tubular narrowing and vertical straightening, with upper displacement of the rectum and the sigmoid colon. Sigmoidoscopy, when performed, reveals no intrinsic lesion, but merely a straightening of that part of the colon.

Plane films of the abdomen demonstrate increased radiolucency in the pelvis; the lucency indicates increased fatty tissue. The bladder appears vertically elongated as a result of fatty infiltration of the pelvis. Hydronephrosis and hydroureters are found when the fat impinges upon the pelvic structures. In our patients, marked hydronephrosis or hydroureters have not been a major problem.

Cook and co-workers,[96] in their review of the various forms of treatment used for these patients, found that 20 patients were operated on and showed masses of fat in the pelvis. In one patient, we found the pelvis totally occupied by globulated fatty tissue without any specific macroscopic or microscopic characteristics. Although reports are found in which urinary diversion has been necessary because of lower urinary tract

obstruction, none of our patients required such diversion.

In our judgment, pelvic lipomatosis is a relatively innocuous entity, and aggressive therapy is unnecessary. Possibly, most of these cases can be diagnosed by x-rays, and an operation can be avoided. There is no place for either radical operation or radical radiation therapy. Furthermore, neither urinary nor fecal diversion should be performed unless the patient is symptomatic in either of these areas.

## ■ TREATMENT OF LIPOMAS

The management of these lesions is operative. The solitary subcutaneous lipomas should be locally excised. Although enucleation via a small incision is usually adequate, care should be taken to avoid leaving fragments of lipomatous tissue behind.

Intermuscular lipomas should be excised, along with a portion of the muscle; however, no major nerve or blood vessel should be sacrificed. Gastrointestinal lipomas should be locally excised via gastrotomy or enterotomy, unless obstruction requires bowel resection.

Multiple lipomas should be excised if they are larger than 5 cm, or if they grow rapidly and produce symptoms. Excision for cosmetic reasons should be an individual decision for each patient. Congenital lipomatosis may require no treatment; however, functional or cosmetic disability may require partial removal, or digital or extremity amputation. Associated orthopedic procedures to stop overgrowth of bone may also be required.

### LIPOBLASTOMA AND LIPOBLASTOMATOSIS

Lipoblastoma and lipoblastomatosis are uncommon benign neoplasms of the adipose tissue that usually occur in children. Coffin and Dehner[101] reported 190 cases of soft tissue tumors in the first year of life; of these, 3 percent were lipoblastomas. We have experience with only six children with lipoblastoma. The oldest was a nine-year-old girl, and the remainder were between three and six years of age. Vellios and his colleagues[102] first coined the term *lipoblastoma* and established this rare form of neoplasm as a distinct clinical entity in the pantheon of pediatric neoplasms. Although these tumors may show karyotypic changes and differ from lipomas by their cellular immaturity and close resemblance to myxoid type of low-grade liposarcomas,[103] these are benign self-limiting entities. After a review of a number of case reports[104–109] and our own material, we conclude that limited excision is

**TABLE 7–4. ANATOMIC DISTRIBUTION OF LIPOSARCOMA (UNIVERSITY OF ILLINOIS SERIES)**

| Anatomic Site | No. Patients[a] | Percent |
|---|---|---|
| Head and neck | 6 | 2.3 |
| Trunk | 32 | 12.2 |
| Retroperitoneal region | 19 | 7.0 |
| Upper extremities | 52 | 20.0 |
| Lower extremities | 154 | 58.5 |
| Total | 263 | 100.0 |

[a]Four patients had multiple primary liposarcomas.

**TABLE 7–5. DISTRIBUTION OF LIPOSARCOMAS IN THE LOWER EXTREMITIES**

| Anatomic Site | No. Patients | Percent |
|---|---|---|
| Buttocks | 18 | 12.0 |
| Thigh | 101 | 65.5 |
| Groin | 12 | 8.0 |
| Leg | 19 | 12.0 |
| Foot | 4 | 2.5 |
| Total | 154 | 100.0 |

the therapy of choice. Any attempt of a radical operation and/or radiation therapy is not indicated.

## LIPOSARCOMAS

### Anatomic Distribution

Liposarcomas seem to have a predilection for the deeper soft tissues, unlike benign solitary lipomas, which more commonly arise in the subcutaneous tissues. In our series of 263 patients, the distribution of the liposarcomas consisted of 154 (58.5 percent) in the lower extremities and 52 (20 percent) in the upper extremities (Table 7–4). In most series,[43,90,100,110–113] the highest incidence of liposarcomas has been found in the lower extremities, upper extremities, retroperitoneum, and trunk, in that order. The sites of occurrence of the 263 liposarcomas in our series at the University of Illinois are shown in Table 7–4. The distribution of these tumors in the various anatomic sites corresponds with the distribution pattern reported in other series.[43,90] In the lower extremities (Table 7–5), the thigh and the buttock are the most common sites. In the upper extremities, there is no apparent predilection for any specific anatomic site.

An uncommon site for liposarcoma is the head and neck region. In 1979, Saunders and co-workers[114] reviewed the literature and found 25 such cases, to which they added 4 of their own, making a total of 29. We have treated six patients with liposarcoma of the head and neck region. One of these patients was a 36-year-old man with a primary tumor located in the scalp. Two years after excision of the primary tumor, he developed a solitary metastasis to the right lobe of the liver, necessitating an extended right lobe lobectomy. He remained well for about 18 months and died of diffuse metastases.

### Clinical Features

In our series of 263 patients, 55 percent were women. In women in their fifth decade, a rapid-growing mass in the upper inner aspect of the thigh is most apt to be a liposarcoma. The age at onset may be as early as six months, with a peak incidence of 55 percent occurring between the ages of 40 and 60 years.[90] The tumor is seen in all races and nationalities, and no predisposing epidemiologic factor is known.

A liposarcoma usually starts as an inconspicuous swelling of the soft tissues and continues to grow steadily (Fig. 7–18A to 7–18E). The patient's usual complaint is the gradual enlargement of a perceptible tumor. Pressure symptoms are felt only when the tumor reaches a certain size. It is almost impossible to arrive at a correct diagnosis by physical examination alone. However, liposarcomas are firmer, more deeply situated, and are more widely attached to the surrounding tissues than are common solitary subcutaneous lipomas. The accuracy of preoperative diagnosis of liposarcoma has increased considerably with the advent of MR imaging. Lipoma is one of the few benign tumors that does not show any signal in MRI on $T_1$-weighted images after administration of Gd-DTPA. This is in contrast to liposarcoma, in which signal density is increased in the nonlipomatous areas of the tumor (see Chapter 4 for details).

### Treatment

***Surgical.*** The fundamental principle in primary management is radical excision, based on anatomic location, size, and local extension of the tumor. In the extremities, the choice of an appropriate type of operation depends on numerous factors, such as regional location, degree or grade of malignancy, fixity to the surrounding tissue (or mobility), the stage of the primary tumor, and the presence or absence of regional metastases.

The dissection should be performed with meticulous, gentle care, and retraction should always be away from, rather than toward, the tumor. The soft tissues encompassing the liposarcoma must never be handled roughly. Most primary liposarcomas can be well treated by means of wide soft tissue resection. Although amputation of an extremity for a liposarcoma is a mutilating procedure and should be performed only when ab-

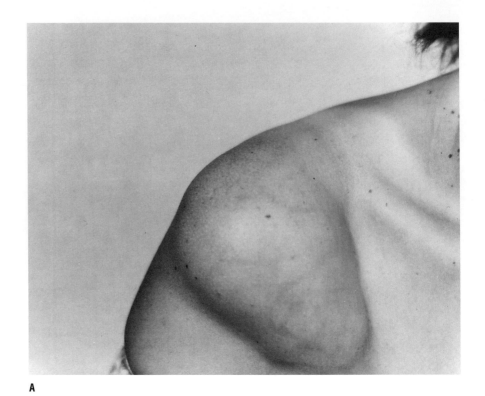

A

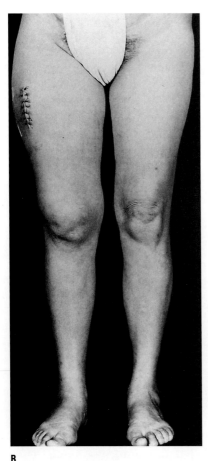

B

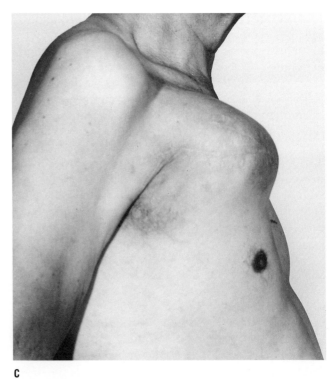

C

**Figure 7–18.** (**A**) The tumor started as an insidious soft subcutaneous swelling. After it attained the present size, it was excised and a well-differentiated liposarcoma was found. (**B**) Liposarcoma of the right thigh in a 48-year-old woman. The primary tumor was 8 cm in maximum diameter before a wedge biopsy was performed. (**C**) Liposarcoma of the chest wall in a 54-year-old man. Medical attention was sought when the mass rubbed against the arm and was a source of irritation. *(Continued.)*

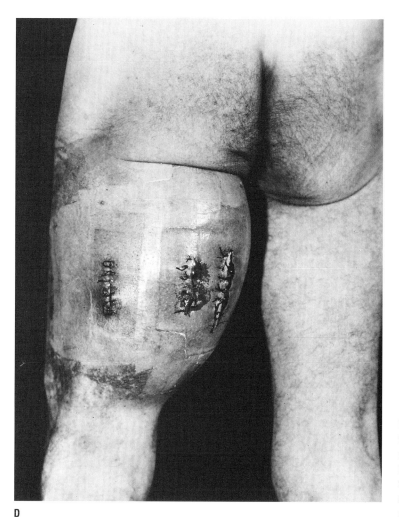

D

**Figure 7–18** *(continued).* (**D**) Liposarcoma of the right posterior thigh. Patient had multiple biopsies before being referred. (**E**) A neglected case of liposarcoma in a 52-year-old man. He had 18 local excisions prior to his visit to the University of Illinois Hospital. A palliative hip joint disarticulation was performed. Following amputation he remained symptom-free for 9 months and died of metastatic liposarcoma 14 months after amputation.

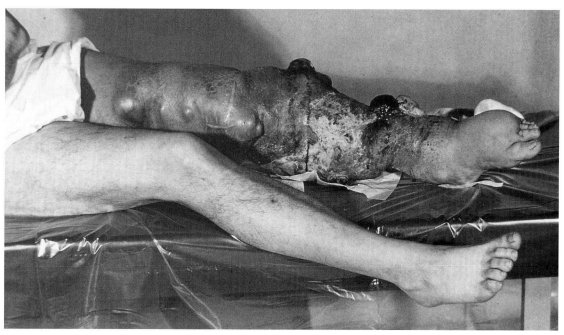

E

solutely indicated, if and when required, the operation should not be denied to the patient. Frequently, an initial inadequate operation results in local recurrence and lowers the overall salvage rate of patients with this type of tumor (Fig. 7–18E).

The technical considerations for wide excision and its variants for major amputations are described elsewhere. Unless all indications and contraindications for each of the types of operations are taken into consideration, the results of treatment will be less than optimal.

***Radiation Therapy.*** In general, the most important role of radiation therapy in the management of primary liposarcoma is in an adjuvant setting. Edland[115] considered radiation therapy more useful as an adjunct to surgery than as a primary form of treatment. Pack and Ariel[17] suggested that the radiosensitivity of liposarcoma is greater than the radiocurability. In their series of 12 patients treated entirely by radiation therapy, only 2 had complete regression of the tumor; 1 had a cure of 10 years or more. Sixteen percent of their patients had complete clinical regression, and 60 percent had partial regression of their primary tumor when preoperative radiation therapy was used. However, microscopic examination of the resected specimens showed residual tumor in most of the patients. McNeer and associates[116] concluded that radiation therapy has an adjuvant role in the treatment of liposarcomas. Preoperative irradiation sometimes converts an otherwise unresectable tumor into a resectable one, as in the case of this bulky retroperitoneal tumor (Fig. 7–19). However, the instances in which such a stratagem will be useful are rather rare, and, in most instances, the best results are obtained when radiation therapy is used after all gross tumor(s) have been resected. The role of postoperative radiation therapy was evaluated by Lindberg and associates.[117] Although the details of the current application of postoperative adjuvant radiation therapy are described in detail in Chapter 17, it is important to mention here that, with advancing technology and improved techniques, the combination of surgery and radiation therapy has considerably reduced the need for major amputations of the extremities.

***Chemotherapy.*** In general, primary liposarcomas do not respond well to any form of conventional systemic chemotherapy. Local infusion or perfusion with any specific agent has not yet shown any specific advantage, especially in well-differentiated or even moderately differentiated liposarcomas. The only exception is highly pleomorphic and/or round cell liposarcomas, in which systemic modern chemotherapeutic regimens might show some instances of reduction in size of a given pri-

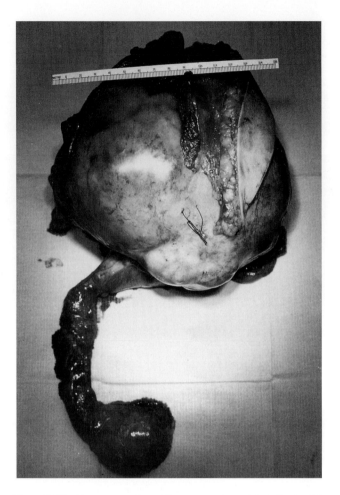

**Figure 7–19.** A huge retroperitoneal liposarcoma that originated in the right spermatic cord. The patient was 58 years old when first seen with a mass extending from the root of the penis to the right subcostal margin. Clinically, the tumor appeared unresectable. A course of preoperative radiation therapy was given. The tumor shrank considerably and three weeks later was resected. Patient remained well for 19 years and died of unrelated causes.

mary liposarcoma. This subject is discussed in detail in Chapter 18 and Chapter 19.

## End Results

The clinical behavior of liposarcomas can be prognosticated by the anatomic site of location and the type and grade of the tumors. Histologic classification of liposarcomas, as proposed by several authors,[100,110–113,118–121] has tended to show that, in well-differentiated tumors, the five-year survival rate is highest and the recurrence rate lowest. Currently, liposarcomas are histologically classified as (1) well-differentiated, (2) myxoid, (3) round cell type, (4) dedifferentiated, and (5) pleomorphic.

During the last decade, reassessment of the histologic subtypes of liposarcoma has resulted in more refined classification of this entity: for example, the well-differentiated variety has been further subclassified into atypical lipoma (lipomalike), inflammatory and sclerosing types, along with the well-established types of myxoid, round cell, and pleomorphic varieties. A relatively newer form (i.e., dedifferentiated) has been added to the histologic classification of liposarcomas.

The term *dedifferentiated liposarcoma* to denote a histologic entity was first coined by Evans[121] in 1979, in an analogy to dedifferentiated chondrosarcoma. This tumor is usually characterized by the coexistence of well-differentiated and poorly differentiated nonlipogenic areas in the same tumor. The dedifferentiated areas show appearances variably resembling pleomorphic malignant fibrous histiocytoma, fibrosarcoma, and the like (see pages 76–80, Chapter 5 for further details). Although no anatomic site and/or size is immune from the development of these tumors, most are larger than 10 cm in diameter and occur in deep-seated sites like the retroperitoneum.[119] McCormick et al.[122] recently analyzed a series of 32 cases and found that 28 (88 percent) of the primary tumors were greater than 10 cm in diameter and that 16 (50 percent) occurred in the retroperitoneum and pelvis. Weiss and Rao,[123] in a review of 92 well-differentiated liposarcomas, observed that 11 (12 percent) had areas of dedifferentiation. Of these 11, 73 percent arose in the retroperitoneum and groin. These authors[123] concluded that the average interval between first diagnosis and dedifferentiation of recurrent tumors is 7.9 years. Several authors[122–125] have proposed a number of theories as to the cause of these areas of dedifferentiation and whether they are encountered ab initio or appear during the course of subsequent recurrence. However, from a therapeutic standpoint, it appears that any large (larger than 10 cm) and/or deep-seated liposarcoma should be considered dedifferentiated even if at first glance it appears to be a well-differentiated liposarcoma.

However, it appears that, as long as the truly well-differentiated variety is correctly separated from the remaining four types, the management program of therapy need not be changed. Therefore, even today, the well-differentiated variety with all of its subtypes can be adequately treated with wide excision maintaining an adequate normal tissues margin. Furthermore, if most retroperitoneal or deep-seated large (larger than 10 cm) liposarcomas are assumed to be dedifferentiated and treated accordingly, the incidence of locoregional recurrence and/or metastases will be reduced. Finally, all the other types, depending on the circumstances and location, will probably be best treated with multimodal therapy.

Enzinger and Winslow,[111] in 1962, reported that, in patients with myxoid liposarcomas, the local recurrence rate was 53 percent and the five-year survival was 77 percent. With the round cell type, the local recurrence rate was 85 percent and the five-year survival rate 18 percent. For the well-differentiated type, the local recurrence rate was 53 percent and the five-year survival rate 85 percent. In the pleomorphic type, the tumor recurred locally in 73 percent of cases, and the five-year salvage rate was only 21 percent. Similarly, the data from the Mayo Clinic published in 1966 showed that the survival rate and rate of local recurrence were similar and likewise dependent on histologic type.

Analysis of our own series of 95 patients in 1981 showed that, in the well-differentiated variety, the local recurrence rate was 0 percent and five-year survival was 83 percent; in the myxoid type, local recurrence was 11 percent and five-year survival was 80 percent. In contrast, the results were more dismal in round cell and pleomorphic types, in which local recurrence rates were 10 percent and 9 percent respectively and five-year survival was 25 percent and 43 percent respectively.

In the current series of 263 patients with liposarcoma, 221 were eligible for five-year survival analysis. In 189 of these patients, the primary tumor could be staged according to the system proposed by the American Joint Committee for Cancer Staging and End-Results Reporting (SEER).[126] Of the 189 patients studied, 109 were treated by surgery alone, and 80 were treated by supplemental radiation therapy. Eighty-eight (81 percent) have remained free of disease for five years, and, of the remaining 80 patients that were treated with supplemental radiation therapy, 52 (65 percent) remained disease-free at the end of 5 years (Table 7–6).

Over the years, the accent in the management of primary liposarcoma has been on operative treatment. In all major reported series, the authors[19,43,90,100,110–113,127,128] in general agreed with the

**TABLE 7–6. FIVE-YEAR RESULTS IN 189 PATIENTS WITH LIPOSARCOMA ACCORDING TO STAGE AND GRADE (UNIVERSITY OF ILLINOIS SERIES)[126]**

| Stage | No. Patients | No. Surviving Free of Disease |
|---|---|---|
| $T_1G_1N_0M_0$ | 28 | 27 (96%) |
| $T_2G_1N_0M_0$ | 38 | 34 (89%) |
| $T_1G_2N_0M_0$ | 25 | 13 (52%) |
| $T_2G_2N_0M_0$* | 28 | 21 (75%) |
| $T_1G_3N_0M_0$[†] | 28 | 12 (43%) |
| $T_2G_3N_0M_0$[†] | 23 | 17 (74%) |
| $T_3G_3N_0M_0$[†] | 19 | 11 (58%) |
| Total | 189 | 141 (75%) |

*Ten of 28 patients received radiation therapy.
[†]All patients received additional radiation therapy, and some received adjuvant chemotherapy as well.

**TABLE 7–7. TYPES OF CURATIVE OPERATION AND END RESULTS IN 189 PATIENTS ELIGIBLE FOR FIVE-YEAR SURVIVAL ANALYSIS**

| Type of Operation | No. Patients | Five-Year NED |
|---|---|---|
| Wide soft tissue excision | 37 | 32 (86%) |
| Muscle group resection | 43 | 37 (86%) |
| Wide excision with node dissection | 14 | 11 (79%) |
| Amputation | 15 | 9 (60%) |
| Total | 109 | 89 (82%) |

Abbreviations: NED, no evidence of disease.

concept of excisional therapy. Most series, however, have been reported either by surgeons[43,90,112,113] or pathologists,[19,100,110–117,126–130] and the possibility of bias could not be ruled out. In any event, the results obtained in the University of Illinois series of an overall five-year cure rate of 86 percent mostly following wide excision cannot be disregarded.

The end results based on the method of operative treatment at the University of Illinois series are shown in Table 7–7. The category of wide excisions also includes chest wall and abdominal wall resections. Amputation in this context refers only to limb ablative procedures. Major amputations have decreased in frequency, and the most commonly performed operation at the University of Illinois is wide excision or a variant thereof, resulting in limb salvage in most instances. Currently, the primary major amputation of an extremity is seldom required unless one encounters a neglected case or as a result of inadequate initial treatment (Fig. 7–18E).

In the present series, 15 patients required a limb ablative procedure, in each case for a locally recurrent tumor after failure of both local resection and/or radiation therapy.

Node dissection is seldom necessary. In the present series, only 14 patients had node dissection with wide soft tissue or muscle group resection. In most of these patients, the primary tumors were either in or adjacent to a node-bearing area, for example, axilla, groin, upper end of the thigh, or the breast.

From a study of the University of Illinois material, it appears that aggressive initial operative intervention along with adjuvant radiation therapy will provide most patients with liposarcoma a good to excellent prognosis. In general, operative intervention entails wide soft tissue resection or a variant. Infrequently, however, a major amputation becomes necessary, and, even in such circumstances, the salvage rate justifies these radical procedures. In 1966, Reszel and associates,[112] reviewing the Mayo Clinic experience of 55 years, stated as follows:

"Based on the data relative to recurrence, metastases, and death, it appears to us that, during the 55 years covered by this study, surgical treatment of liposarcomata has not been aggressive enough either at the Mayo Clinic or at other institutions. We think that greater effort should be made to eradicate the primary growth at the time of initial operation, since inadequate removal invites recurrence and, in all but grade I tumors, very possible metastases."

The only advance since the statement is the additional use of radiation therapy in the control of primary liposarcomas. It stands to reason that this bimodal therapy has reduced the necessity or indication for primary amputations.

In Table 7–8, the overall survival in all types of liposarcoma in the last four decades is summarized. From a 39 percent survival reported in 1958, there has been a gradual improvement, and currently it reaches about 86 percent. There is no question that the improvement is the result of many factors, including earlier diagnosis, better understanding of the relationship of the biologic behavior in relation to tumor phenotype, and aggressive initial surgical treatment complemented by supplemental radiation therapy using modern advanced technology.

**TABLE 7–8. FIVE-YEAR END RESULTS IN ELIGIBLE PATIENTS WITH LIPOSARCOMA IN FIVE SERIES**

| | Pack and Ariel,[17] 1958 | Enterline et al.,[110] 1960 | Brasfield and Das Gupta,[43] 1970 | Das Gupta,[32] 1981 | Present Series* 1996 |
|---|---|---|---|---|---|
| No. patients eligible | 64 | 40 | 184 (of 236) | 77 (of 95) | 221 (of 263) |
| No. patients living free of disease at five years | 2 (3%) | 5 (12.5%) | 92 (50%) | 63 (82%) | 189 (85.5%) |
| No. patients free of disease at five years with treatment for locally recurrent tumors in-between | 2 (3%) | 5 (12.5%) | 12 (6.5%) | 8 (10%) | 18 (8%) |
| Dead with liposarcoma | 39 (61%) | 18 (45%) | 76 (41%) | 14 (18%) | 10 (4.5%) |
| Dead of unrelated causes | — | 5 (12.5%) | 4 (2%) | 1 (1%) | 4 (2%)† |
| Overall five-year survival rate | 39% | 42.5% | 56.5% | 82% | 86% |

*Current series includes the patients described in our 1981 study.
†Two of the four patients died of another cancer: one from breast cancer, the other from squamous cell carcinoma of the oropharynx.

## Local Recurrence

Of the 189 liposarcoma patients eligible for appropriate staging and five-year end-result analysis in the University of Illinois series, 18 (8 percent) had local recurrence following initial treatment of the primary. Local recurrence rates for liposarcoma have been reported as 33.3 percent by Pack and Pierson,[20] 48 percent by Enterline and co-workers,[110] 70 percent by Reszel et al.,[112] and between 53 and 85 percent in the series reported by Enzinger and Winslow.[111] This marked reduction in the incidence of local recurrence in the University of Illinois series is largely due to an initial aggressive surgical approach in conjunction with supplemental radiation therapy where indicated.

Histologic prognostic criteria for patients with liposarcoma were developed by Enterline and his associates.[110] Later, Enzinger and Winslow[111] and Reszel and co-workers[112] analyzed their cases and tried to develop some general prognostic guidelines. SEER has developed a comprehensive staging system (Table 7–6).[126] Currently, various molecular markers are being used to estimate the prognosis of all types of liposarcomas (see Chapter 6 for details). In spite of these advances, it appears that a small, well-differentiated liposarcoma ($T_1G_1$ or $T_1G_2$) has less potential for local recurrence and distant metastases, and the patient thus has a better chance for cure. Therefore, it is logical to propose that an initial curative wide excision should be the therapy of choice. In contrast, dedifferentiated or pleomorphic forms of the tumor have a higher potential for local recurrence and metastases, with less chance for cure. Therefore, these tumors require not only aggressive initial resection, but adjuvant radiation therapy as well. The role of adjuvant chemotherapy in any type of liposarcoma remains unclear. However, in pleomorphic or round cell types, there might be a beneficial effect of use of adjuvant chemotherapy (see Chapter 18 for a detailed discussion).

## METASTATIC LIPOSARCOMA

Although the lungs remain the most common site of metastases in liposarcomas, along with other soft tissue sarcomas, more and more the incidence of extrapulmonary site metastases is being recognized. In our own institution, we have encountered a number of such instances. For example, there were six instances of distant soft tissue metastases: two in the liver, three in the colon, and one in the bone. One patient with intra-abdominal metastases is of extreme interest, and the clinical course is briefly described below.

A 45-year-old rather obese man was initially treated for a liposarcoma of the foot (both by excision and radiation therapy). Five years later, a mass in the pelvis was recognized and resected; it was a metastatic liposarcoma not attached to any of the viscus. The pelvis was radiated. Afterwards, he remained free of disease for two years, when another metastatic mass in the mesocolon (right) was identified and resected. One year later, he developed further metastases in the contralateral posterior thigh and buttock. This was resected and radiated. Two years later, he developed diffuse intra-abdominal disease, including metastases to the liver, and, 11 years after his original foot lesion was treated, he died of diffuse metastatic liposarcoma.

Recently, Cheng et al.[131] analyzed their experience and found that, in a series of 60 patients, an unusually high number of isolated extrapulmonary metastases were encountered. In our opinion, extrapulmonary metastases in liposarcoma is a distinct possibility, more so than in some other sarcomas. Thus, these tumors should be aggressively searched for, and aggressive excision frequently prolongs a productive life both with pulmonary and extrapulmonary metastases.

## RETROPERITONEAL LIPOSARCOMAS

Of all the lipomatous tumors, retroperitoneal liposarcomas have aroused the most interest, possibly because their location hampers both diagnosis and management.

Lipomatous tumors are one of the most common forms of retroperitoneal tumor. Only 4 of 30 retroperitoneal lipomatous tumors reported by Brasfield and Das Gupta[43] were histologically benign. Ockuly and Douglass[132] estimated that approximately 35 percent of retroperitoneal fatty tumors are of perirenal origin, which is logical since the largest amount of fat accumulates in the perirenal region.

Retroperitoneal fatty tumors occur more frequently in women than in men. Adair, Pack, and Farrow[88] reported the incidence in females to be 73 percent. In our present series of 19 patients, 11 were women. These tumors occur in patients of all ages, but most frequently in those between the ages of 40 and 60 years. The oldest patient in our group was 84 years of age.

Characteristically, retroperitoneal liposarcomas are "silent" during their early growth, and are capable of attaining tremendous size. Generally, their presence becomes known by reason of their increase in size, which causes progressive swelling of the abdomen, a palpable mass, and later, pain. Thirty of 35 patients in the series reported by Brasfield and Das Gupta[43] were first seen because of swelling of the abdomen. Enzinger and Winslow[111] found abdominal enlargement as the initial observation in 23 patients. The tumor may compress the adjacent structures, resulting in related symptoms. Larger and more highly malignant tumors cause weight loss, anorexia, and asthenia.

A preoperative diagnosis of retroperitoneal liposarcoma is difficult to make and frequently is possible only after an exploratory celiotomy. It has been suggested that retroperitoneal liposarcomas can be radiographically distinguished from other tumors in this location by their translucency in the roentgenogram. Although this suggestion is based on sound theoretical reasoning because of the low specific gravity of fat and water absorption coefficient, in practice the roentgenogram is rarely diagnostic. Recently, however, the accuracy rate of preoperative diagnosis has increased due to the increased use of MR imaging and computed axial tomography (CAT) scans (see Chapter 4). In most instances of large tumors, intravenous pyelogram, inferior venogram, and aortic angiogram help to define the extent of the tumor. These types of preoperative information are essential in the overall management of all retroperitoneal tumors, especially those which are unusually large in size.

The treatment of retroperitoneal liposarcoma is by excision. Every effort should be made to remove the entire tumor. Both preoperative and intraoperative radiation can play a significant role in the management of these tumors. As has been alluded to before, most retroperitoneal tumors (since, in general, they are at least 10 cm) should a priori be assumed at minimum to be dedifferentiated and aggressively treated. This statement implies that the assumption at the time of first operation should be that, in spite of our best efforts and extensive resection (including multiorgan resections), the margins of resection are inadequate and the need exists for supplemental radiation therapy either intraoperatively or postoperatively or a combination of both.

The end results of treatment of retroperitoneal liposarcomas are poor. Pack and Ariel[17] had 2 out of 17 patients (12 percent) living free of disease after five years. In a more recent series reported by McCormick et al.,[122] 16 of their retroperitoneal liposarcomas were dedifferentiated, and 13 (81 percent) recurred before five years. Only three patients are long-term survivors after multiple resections. Similarly, Lucas et al.,[128] in their series of six retroperitoneal liposarcomas, found that four recurred before five years. In our own series of 15 patients, because of our operational definition that all retroperitoneal liposarcomas are either high grade or at least dedifferentiated, we have taken a very aggressive approach surgically and, where indicated, added supplemental radiation therapy. Probably because of this, our success rate in reducing recurrence is somewhat better. Nine of 19 (47 percent) developed abdominal recurrence before five years. Of the 19, 15 are eligible for 10-year survival analysis, five of whom (33 percent) are living 10 years disease-free.

## ■ LIPOSARCOMAS IN UNUSUAL LOCATIONS

Although, theoretically, liposarcomas can be found in any part of the body, in certain sites they occur very rarely, if at all. The bone, the periorbital region, and the female breast are some examples. A brief review of acceptable cases of liposarcoma in these regions follows.

### LIPOSARCOMA OF THE BONE

Pack and Ariel[17] stated that Ewing, in 1928, described a patient with supposed liposarcoma of the bone marrow. Stewart[133] reported three additional cases in 1931. However, Stout,[134] in 1949, was reluctant to accept a diagnosis of primary liposarcoma of bone. This diagnosis has remained in doubt ever since. Goldman[135] reviewed the literature in 1964 and found 11 cases that could be accepted as true liposarcomas of the bone. To these, he added one of his own. Catto and Stevens[136] and Ross and Hadfield[137] added one case each. Ross and Hadfield's[137] case was unusual since it also produced neoplastic bone and was regarded as an osteoliposarcoma. In 1970, Schwartz and co-workers[138] reviewed the literature and reported an additional case of their own. We have not encountered a single instance of liposarcoma of the bone. Because of the extreme rarity of this entity, its biologic behavior is not well known.

### LIPOSARCOMA OF THE BREAST

Of the 263 patients in the University of Illinois series, only 3 women had liposarcomas of the breast. All three required not only mastectomies, but also excision of the underlying pectoralis major muscle and, in one instance, the chest wall as well. Recently, we were consulted on a case of low-grade liposarcoma in the breast tissue in a 51-year-old man. He has undergone a mastectomy elsewhere and apparently is doing well. Histologically, all of our three cases were well-differentiated liposarcomas, and all three patients are doing well 10 years since primary treatment. In the earlier reported series of 236 patients,[43,90] liposarcoma of the breast was found in two patients. In 1979, Rasmussen and Jensen[139] found 34 published cases of primary liposarcoma of the breast and added one of their own. These authors have described the clinical data in these 35 patients. The usual history is of a progressively enlarging tumor of the breast. Excision of the breast usually suffices; sometimes, the extent and local infiltration necessitate resection of the pectoral muscles and/or the underlying chest wall.

## LIPOSARCOMA OF THE PLEURA

In 1942, Ackerman and Wheeler[100] described a case of liposarcoma of the pleura. Gupta and Paolini[140] reported an additional case. In a review of the literature, they were unable to find any other case of primary liposarcoma of the pleura. We have not treated any such patient.

## INTRATHORACIC AND CARDIAC LIPOSARCOMAS

An intrathoracic liposarcoma is extremely rare. Currie,[141] in 1964, collected only 26 cases and added one of his own. In the same year, Cicciarelli and associates[142] reported eight cases from the Mayo Clinic. Razzuk and co-workers,[143] in 1971, reported one case and reviewed the literature. These authors found 44 cases of intrathoracic liposarcoma. The tumor originated in the mediastinum in 43 cases and in the pulmonary hilum in 1 case. All but two cases were in adult patients. The ages ranged from 13 to 63 years, with no significant sex predominance. Most patients were symptomatic. The onset and nature of the symptoms were related to the size and location of the tumors. Some patients remained relatively asymptomatic until the terminal stage. Symptoms included cough, chest pain, dyspnea, and, occasionally, symptoms of superior vena cava obstruction. Survival from the time of onset of symptoms in the 21 patients that were followed ranged from 2 months to 14 years. All but two patients were dead at the time of the original report. Five patients survived longer than five years: one was alive and well 6.5 years after operation, two lived for 9 years, and two for 14 years.

The clinical history of intrathoracic liposarcoma is not particularly characteristic. The diagnosis is usually confirmed by means of an exploratory thoracotomy and adequate biopsy. The results of therapy in 23 evaluable cases show that seven patients were treated by excision, and four of the seven lived for an average of 6.75 years.[143] Six patients were treated by both excision and irradiation. The average survival time in these six patients was three years. The remaining 10 patients were only palliated because of the extent of their disease. None of these patients lived for more than 18 months, the average survival time being 1 year. To the best of our knowledge, a documented case of primary liposarcoma of the heart has not been reported.

## LIPOSARCOMAS OF THE GASTROINTESTINAL TRACT AND OMENTUM

Liposarcomas of the gastrointestinal tract are exceptionally rare. Only one case of gastric liposarcoma[144] and one arising in the transverse colon[145] have been reported. Recently, McCormick et al.[122] reported one instance of a liposarcoma arising in the mesocolon. Omental sarcomas are extremely rare, despite the high fat content of the omentum. Only one such case has been encountered in the University of Illinois series. As with the patient reported by Robb,[146] our patient also had a hemoperitoneum due to rupture of the highly vascular tumor in the omentum. Hassan,[147] in 1970, reported a similar case of omental liposarcoma with a hemoperitoneum. This patient had a subcutaneous liposarcoma excised 5.5 years before the omental tumor.

## LIPOSARCOMA OF THE GENITOURINARY TRACT

Edson and associates[148] reported a case of perivesical liposarcoma. The presenting symptoms were prostatitis and frequent failure to respond to a brief course of antibiotic therapy. The patient was operated on with a presumptive diagnosis of prostatic abscess. The true nature of the tumor was discovered after the operation.

## LIPOSARCOMA OF THE SPERMATIC CORD AND SCROTUM

Liposarcomas of the spermatic cord are rare.[149] We have treated nine cases. These tumors appear either as a scrotal or inguinal mass. Most often, the enlarging inguinal mass mimics an incarcerated inguinal hernia. All our patients were referred to us after the urologist/surgeon operated on the presumptive diagnosis of an indirect inguinal hernia. In one patient, the inguinal mass extended proximally through the inguinal canal into the retroperitoneal region (Fig. 7–19). Wide excision entailing orchiectomy and high ligation of the cord is usually adequate. Currently, we recommend supplemental radiation therapy in all instances with moderate- or high-grade liposarcomas. Of the nine patients, one developed local recurrence within two years after what was presumed to be a wide soft tissue resection. Thus, the objective of initial therapy should be an aggressive wide excision. The prognosis is about the same as for a liposarcoma in other anatomic locations.

Waller[150] reported a case of liposarcoma of the scrotum, an uncommon tumor. If such a case is truly encountered, wide excision would be the therapy of choice.

## ■ DISEASES OF BROWN ADIPOSE TISSUE

In humans, disease of the brown adipose tissue is limited to occasional benign tumors or hibernomas. Although brown fat has a thermogenic property and can store either adrenal steroids or catecholamines, no systemic disease similar to the lipopathies of white adipose tissue has been described. It is indeed curious that tumors of the brown adipose tissue are usually benign, even though this apparently is a primitive type of adipose tissue. Rona[151] described two patients who died in shock following removal of a pheochromocytoma. One of these had a massive accumulation of brown fat 8 × 4.5 × 2 cm, weighing 18 gm. The other had similar masses of brown fat in the epicardium. Histologic examination showed that the transformed fatty tissue contained, in addition to adult fat cells, two other cell types: polygonal cells with central nuclei and pleurivacuolar cytoplasm that contained doubly retractile lipids; and cells with argentaffin and chromaffin properties. An extract prepared from the brown fat in one of the two patients exerted a pressor effect on injection into a cat. Hibernoma masquerading as a pheochromocytoma has also been described.[152]

## HIBERNOMAS

Hibernomas are found in the subcutaneous tissue of the neck, shoulder, axilla, interscapular region, and mediastinum. These are the areas in which immature fat or brown fat is found in mammals. Mesara and Batsakis[153] collected a total of 26 cases of hibernoma from the literature and reported one of their own. Twelve were in the interscapular region, four in the mediastinum, three in the axillae, four in the buttocks and thighs, two in the abdominal wall, and two in the neck. In 1973, Merlina and Pike[154] reported a case of hibernoma in the thigh of a 24-year-old man.

Hibernomas are slow-growing neoplasms. The subcutaneous variety is recognized only after excision of a tumor that appeared to be a solitary subcutaneous lipoma. On the other hand, hibernomas located in the neck or mediastinum may produce pressure symptoms, because of compression of the regional structures. Patients with mediastinal hibernomas occasionally present with symptoms of tracheal compression and cough. Leiphart and Nudelman[152] reported a case of hibernoma adjacent to both kidneys. This case was of particular interest since, by angiography, it had been diagnosed as a right-sided pheochromocytoma. An exploratory procedure revealed two masses of brown fat in the perirenal region with findings characteristic of hibernoma. Furthermore, at the bifurcation of the aorta, a 6 × 7 cm mass was found which was interpreted to be a pheochromocytoma. Lawson and Biller[155] found reports on 37 cases of hibernoma, of which 10 were interscapular, 6 were axillary, and 5 cervical or intrathoracic; the remaining 16 cases were distributed in the thigh, buttocks, popliteal region, chest wall, and abdominal wall. Hibernomas of the extremities are extremely rare.[154]

Recently, Meis and Enzinger[156] described the microscopic characteristics of 20 cases they termed *chondroid lipoma*, with unique features simulating liposarcoma and myxoid chondrosarcoma. However, these authors found the presence of glycogen in vacuolated cells reminiscent of brown fat, and these tumors were totally benign in their clinical course. Thus, it appears that, from a therapeutic standpoint, these tumors should be considered in the family of hibernomas and treated conservatively.

In 1967, Lowry and Halmos[157] published a report of a malignant hibernoma in the scapular region of a 24-year-old woman with Turner's syndrome. This tumor was considered to be malignant because of its infiltration into the surrounding muscles. Infiltration is not adequate evidence of malignancy, since the infiltrative qualities of benign intermuscular lipomas and angiolipomas are well established. A primary malignant hibernoma or malignant transformation of a benign hibernoma is still hard to document.[158] We have not encountered a single instance of malignant hibernoma.

## REFERENCES

1. Keys A, Brozek J: Body fat in adult man. Physiol Rev 33:235, 1953
2. Jeanrenaud B: Dynamic aspects of adipose tissue metabolism: A review. Metabolism 10:535, 1961
3. Hashim SA: Metabolism of body fat. NY J Med 16:1339, 1961
4. Steiner G, Cahill GF, Jr.: Adipose tissue physiology. Ann NY Acad Sci 110:749, 1963
5. Dercum FX: Three cases of a hitherto unclassified affliction resembling in its grosser aspects obesity, but associated with special nervous symptoms adiposis dolorosa. Am J Med Sci 104:521, 1892
6. Lynch HT, Harlan WL: Hereditary factors in adiposis dolorosa (Dercum's disease). Am J Human Genet 115:184, 1963
7. Wohl MG, Pastor N: Adiposis dolorosa (Dercum's disease). JAMA 110:1261, 1938
8. Pfeifer V: Ueber einen Fall von herdweiser Atrophie des subcutane Feitgewekes. Deutsch Arch Klin Med 1:438, 1892
9. Gilchrist TC, Ketron LW: A unique case of atrophy of the skin, preceded by large phagocytic cells (macrophages). Bull Johns Hopkins Hosp (Baltimore) 27:291, 1916
10. Weber FP: A case of relapsing nonsuppurative nodular panniculitis showing phagocytosis of subcutaneous fat-cells by macrophages. Br J Dermat 37:301, 1925
11. Christian HA: Relapsing febrile nodular nonsuppurative panniculites. Arch Int Med 42:338, 1928
12. Lever WF: Nodular nonsuppurative panniculitis (Weber-Christian disease). Arch Dermat Syph 59:31, 1949
13. Lever WF. The lipopathies. In Beeson PB, McDermott W (eds): Cecil-Loeb Textbook of Medicine, 11th ed. Philadelphia, WB Saunders, 1963, p 1336

14. Balzer F: Recherches sur la degenerescence granulo-graisseuse des tissues dans les maladies infectieuses; parasetisne du xanthelasma et de l'ictere grave. Rev de Med Par ii:307, 1882
15. Adair FE, Munzer TY: Fat necrosis of the female breast. Am J Surg 74:117, 1947
16. Weary PE, Graham GF, Selden RF: Subcutaneous fat necrosis of the newborn. South Med J 59:960, 1966
17. Pack GT, Ariel IM: Tumors of the Soft Somatic Tissues: A Clinical Treatise. New York, Hoeber-Harper, 1958, p 343
18. Ewing J: Fascial sarcoma and intermuscular myxoliposarcoma. Arch Surg 31:507, 1935
19. Stout AP: Liposarcoma—Malignant tumor of lipoblasts. Ann Surg 119:86, 1944
20. Pack GT, Pierson JC: Liposarcoma. A study of 105 cases. Surgery 36:687, 1954
21. Booher RJ: Lipoblastic tumors of the hands and feet. Review of the literature and report of thirty-three cases. J Bone Joint Surg 47A:727, 1965
22. Phalen GS, Kendrick JI, Rodriguez TM: Lipomas of the upper extremity. A series of fifteen tumors in the hand and wrist and six tumors causing nerve compression. Am J Surg 121:298, 1971
23. Paarlberg D, Linscheid RL, Soule EH: Lipomas of the hand including lipoblastomatosis in a child. Mayo Clin Proc 47:121, 1972
24. Howard WR, Helwig EB: Angiolipoma. Arch Dermat 82:126, 1960
25. Regan JM, Bickel WH, Broders AC: Infiltrating benign lipomas of the extremities. Western J Surg 54:87, 1946
26. Dionne G, Seemayer TA: Infiltrating lipomas and angiolipomas revisited. Cancer 33:732, 1974
27. Bradley RL, Klein MM: Angiolipoma. Am J Surg 108:887, 1964
28. Gonzalez-Crussi F, Enneking WF, Arean VM: Infiltrating angiolipoma. J Bone Joint Surg 48A:1111, 1966
29. Pearson J, Stellar S, Feigin I: Angiolipoma—Long-term cure following radical approach to malignant-appearing benign intraspinal tumor. J Neurosurg 33:466, 1970
30. Stimpson N: Infiltrating angiolipomata of skeletal muscle. Br J Surg 58:464, 1971
31. Lin JJ, Lin F: Two entities in angiolipoma: A study of 459 cases of lipoma with review of the literature on infiltrating angiolipoma. Cancer 34:720, 1973
32. Das Gupta TK: Tumors of the Soft Tissues. Norwalk, CT, Appleton-Century-Crofts, 1983, p 363
33. Kuttner H, Landors F: Die chirugie der Quergestrifleu Muskalatur. Dtsch Chir (A) 25:228, 1913
34. Greenberg SD, Isensee C, Gonzalez-Angulo A, Wallace SA: Infiltrating lipomas of the thigh. Am J Clin Pathol 39:66, 1963
35. Kindbloom LG, Angervall L, Stener B, Wickbom I: Intermuscular and intramuscular lipomas and hibernomas: A clinical, roentgenologic, histologic and prognostic study of 46 cases. Cancer 33:756, 1974
36. Davis C Jr., Gruhn JG: Giant lipoma of the thigh. Arch Surg 95:151, 1967
37. Calhoun NR: Lipoma of the buccal space. Oral Surg 16:246, 1963
38. Fothergill J: Medical and Philosophical Works. London, John Walker, 1781
39. Krause LB, Ross C: Intrathoracic lipomas. Arch Surg 84:444, 1962
40. Cicciarelli FE, Soule EH, McGoon DC: Lipoma and liposarcoma of the mediastinum: A report of 14 tumors including one lipoma of the thymus. J Thorac Cardiovasc Surg 47:411, 1964
41. Staub EW, Barker WL, Langston HT: Intrathoracic fatty tumors. Dis Chest 47:308, 1965
42. Elfving F, Hastbacka J: Primary solid tumors of the greater omentum. Acta Chir Scandinav 130:603, 1965
43. Brasfield RD, Das Gupta TK: Liposarcoma. CA Cancer J Clin 20 (Jan–Feb): 3, 1970
44. Delamater J: Mammoth tumor. Cleveland Gaz 1:31, 1859
45. DeWeerd JH, Dockerty MB: Lipomatous retroperitoneal tumors. Am J Surg 84:397, 1952
46. Seldin HM, Seldin SD, Rakower W, Jarrett WJ: Lipomas of the oral cavity: Report of 26 cases. J Oral Surg 25:270, 1967
47. Hatziotis JCH: Lipoma of the oral cavity. Oral Surg 31:511, 1971
48. Burzynski NJ, Sigman MD, Martin TH: Lipoma of the oral cavity: Literature review and case report. J Oral Med 26:37, 1971
49. Greer RO, Richardson JF: The nature of lipomas and their significance in the oral cavity: A review and report of cases. Oral Surg 36:551, 1973
50. Mayo CW, Pagtalunan RJG, Brown DJ: Lipoma of the alimentary tract. Surgery 53:598, 1963
51. Feldman M: An appraisal of associated conditions occurring in autopsied cases of lipoma of the gastrointestinal tracts. Am J Gastroenterol 36:413, 1961
52. Eliason EL, Wright VWM: Benign tumors of the stomach. Surg Gynecol Obstet 41:461, 1925
53. Rumold MJ: Submucous lipomas of the stomach. Surgery 10:242, 1941
54. Scott OB, Brunschwig A: Submucosal lipomas of the stomach. Arch Surg 52:254, 1946
55. Alvarez LF, Lastra JA, Leon P: Ulcerated gastric lipoma. Gastroenterology 11:746, 1948
56. Thompson HL, Oyster JO: Neoplasms of the stomach other than carcinoma. Gastroenterology 15:185, 1950
57. Furste W, Solt R Jr., Briggs W: The gastrointestinal submucosal lipoma: A cause of bleeding and pain. Am J Surg 106:903, 1963
58. Hart RJ: Submucous lipoma of the stomach presenting as pyloric obstruction. Br J Surg 54:157, 1967
59. Ling CS, Leagus C, Chahlgren LH: Intestinal lipomatosis. Surgery 46:1054, 1959
60. D'Jarid IF: Lipomas of the large intestine: Review of the literature and report of a case. J Int Coll Surg 33:639, 1960
61. Price EB Jr., Mostofi FK: Symptomatic angiomyolipoma of the kidney. Cancer 18:761, 1965
62. Kanter AE, Zummo BP: Lipomas of gynecologic interest. Am J Obstet Gynecol 71:376, 1956
63. Dede JA, Janovski NA: Lipoma of the uterine tube—A gynecologic rarity. Obstet Gynecol 22:461, 1963

64. Ashby BS, MacGillivray JB: Paratesticular lipoma. Br J Surg 53:828, 1966

65. Zakrewski A: Subglottic lipoma of the larynx. J Laryngol Otol 79:1039, 1965

66. Jonasson L, Soderlund S: Intrathoracic lipoma. Acta Chir Scand 126:558, 1963

67. Estevez JM, Thompson DS, Levinson JP: Lipoma of the heart: Review of the literature and report of two autopsied cases. Arch Pathol 77:638, 1964

68. Easler RE, Dowlin WM: Primary lipoma of the spleen. Arch Pathol 88:557, 1969

69. Rokitansky C: Lehbuch der pathologischen Anatomie, vol 2. Vienna, Braumuller, 1856, p 468

70. Ewing J: Neoplastic Disease, 4th ed. Philadelphia, WB Saunders, 1942

71. Manganiello LOJ, Daniel EF, Hair LQ: Lipoma of the corpus callosum. J Neurosurg 24:892, 1966

72. Ehni F, Love JG: Intraspinal lipomas. Report of cases, review of literature, and clinical and pathological study. Arch Neurol Psychiatr 53:1, 1945

73. Collins DH, Henderson WR: A case of intradural spinal lipoma. J Pathol Bact 61:277, 1949

74. Thomas JE, Miller RH: Lipomatous tumors of the spinal cord. A study of their clinical range. Mayo Clin Proc 48:393, 1973

75. Brooks D: Clinical presentation and treatment of peripheral nerve tumors. In Dyck PJ, Thomas PK, Lamber EH (eds): Peripheral Neuropathy. Philadelphia, WB Saunders, 1975, p 1354

76. Mikhail LK: Median nerve lipoma in the hand. J Bone Joint Surg 46B:726, 1964

77. Pulvertaft RC: Unusual tumors of the median nerve: Report of two cases. J Bone Joint Surg 46B:731, 1964

78. Seddon H: Surgical Disorders of the Peripheral Nerves. Edinburgh, Churchill Livingstone, 1972

79. Yeoman PM: Fatty infiltration of the median nerve. J Bone Joint Surg 46B:737, 1964

80. Callison JR, Thomas OJ, White WC: Fibrofatty proliferation of the median nerve. Plast Reconstr Surg 42:403, 1968

81. Rowland SA: Lipofibroma of the median nerve in the palm. J Bone Joint Surg 49A:1309, 1967

82. Watson-Jones R: Encapsulated lipoma of the median nerve of the wrist. J Bone Joint Surg 46B:736, 1964

83. Stout AP: Tumors of Peripheral Nerves. In Atlas of Tumor Pathology, Sect. 2, Fasc 6. Washington DC, AFIP, 1949

84. Bartlett EL: Periosteal lipoma. Arch Surg 21:1015, 1930

85. Dahlin DC: Bone Tumors, 3rd ed. Springfield, Ill., Thomas, 1978, p 149

86. Singewald ML: Sacroiliac lipomata—An often unrecognized cause of low back pain. Bull Johns Hopkins Hosp 118:492, 1966

87. Osment LS: Cutaneous lipomas and lipomatosis. Surg Gynecol Obstet 127:129, 1968

88. Adair FE, Pack CT, Farrow JH: Lipomas. Am J Cancer 16:1104, 1932

89. Ballard HS, Fame B, Hartsock RJ: Familial multiple endocrine adenomapeptide ulcer complex. Medicine 43:481, 1964

90. Das Gupta TK: Tumors and tumor-like conditions of the adipose tissue. In: Ravitch MM, Ellison EH, Julian OC, et al. Current Problems in Surgery. Chicago, Year Book Medical Publishers, 1970

91. Cameron AH, McMillan DH: Lipomatosis of skeletal muscle in Maffucci's syndrome. J Bone Joint Surg 38B:692, 1956

92. Nixon HH, Scobie WC: Congenital lipomatosis: A report of four cases. J Pediatric Surg 6:742, 1971

93. Fogg LB, Smyth WJ: Pelvic lipomatosis: Conditions simulating pelvic neoplasm. Radiology 90:558, 1968

94. Engels EP: Sigmoid colon and urinary bladder in high fixation: Roentgen changes simulating pelvic tumors. Radiology 72:419, 1959

95. Rosenberg B, Hurwitz A, Hermann H: Dercum's disease with unusual retroperitoneal and paravesical fatty infiltration. Surgery 54:451, 1963

96. Cook SA, Hayashi K, Lalli AF: Pelvic lipomatosis: Case report. Cleveland Clin Quart 40:36, 1973

97. Morettin LB, Wilson M: Pelvic lipomatosis. Am J Roentgenol Rad Ther Nucl Med 113:181, 1971

98. Grimmett CM, Hall MG Jr., Aird CC, Kurts LH: Pelvic lipomatosis. Am J Surg 125:347, 1973

99. Becker JA, Weiss RM, Schiff M Jr., Lytton B: Pelvic lipomatosis: A consideration in the diagnosis of intrapelvic neoplasms. Arch Surg 100:94, 1970

100. Ackerman LV, Wheeler PW: Liposarcoma. South Med J 35:156, 1942

101. Coffin CM, Dehner LP: Soft tissue tumors in first year of life: A report of 190 cases. Pediatr Pathol 10:509, 1990

102. Vellios F, Baez J, Schumacker HB: Lipoblastomatosis: A tumor of fetal fat different from hibernoma. Report of a case, with observations of the embryogenesis of human adipose tissue. Am J Pathol 34:1149, 1958

103. Sandberg AA, Gibas Z, Saren E, et al.: Chromosome abnormalities in two benign adipose tumors. Cancer Genet Cytogenet 22:55, 1986

104. Chung EB, Enzinger FM: Benign lipoblastomatosis. An analysis of 35 cases. Cancer 32:482, 1973

105. Kauffman SL, Stout AP: Lipoblastic tumors of children. Cancer 12:912, 1959

106. Mahour GH, Bryan BJ, Isaacs H: Lipoblastoma and lipoblastomatosis. A report of six cases. Surgery 104:577, 1988

107. Jimenez JF: Lipoblastoma in infancy and childhood. J Surg Oncol 32:238, 1986

108. Stringel G, Shandling B, Mancer K, Eln SH: Lipoblastoma in infants and children. J Pediatr Surg 17:277, 1982

109. Mentzel T, Calonje E, Fletcher CDM: Lipoblastoma and lipoblastomatosis: A clinicopathological study of 14 cases. Histopathology 23:527, 1993

110. Enterline HT, Culberson JD, Rochlin DB, Brady LW: Liposarcoma: A clinical and pathological study of 53 cases. Cancer 13:932, 1960

111. Enzinger FM, Winslow DJ: Liposarcoma: A study of 103 cases. Virchows Arch Pathol Anat 335:367, 1962

112. Reszel PA, Soule EH, Coventry MB: Liposarcoma of the extremities and limb girdles. J Bone Joint Surg 48A:229, 1966

113. Phelan JT, Perez-Mesa C: Liposarcoma of the superficial soft tissues. Surg Gynecol Obstet 115:609, 1962

114. Saunders JR, Jaques DA, Casterline PF, et al.: Liposarcoma of the head and neck: A review of the literature and addition of four cases. Cancer 43:162, 1979

115. Edland RW: Liposarcoma: A retrospective study of fifteen cases: A review of the literature and a discussion of radiosensitivity. Am J Roentgenol 103:778, 1968

116. McNeer GP, Cantin J, Chu F, Nickson J: Effectiveness of radiation therapy in the management of sarcoma of the soft somatic tissues. Cancer 22:391, 1968

117. Lindberg RD, Martin RG, Romsdahl MM, Barkley HT: Conservative surgery and postoperative radiotherapy in 300 adults with soft tissue sarcomas. Cancer 47:2391, 1981

118. Trojani M, Contesso G, Coindre JM, et al.: Soft tissue sarcomas of adults: Study of pathological prognostic variables and definition of a histopathological grading system. Int J Cancer 33:37, 1984

119. Enzinger FM, Weiss SW: Soft Tissue Tumors. 3rd ed., St. Louis, Mosby-Yearbook, 1995, p 431

120. Coindre JM, Trojani M, Contesso G, David M, et al.: Reproducibility of a histopathologic grading system for adult soft tissue sarcoma. Cancer 58:306, 1986

121. Evans HL: Liposarcoma: A study of 55 cases with a reassessment of its classification. Am J Surg Pathol 3:507, 1979

122. McCormick D, Mentzel T, Beham A, Fletcher CDM: Dedifferentiated liposarcoma. Am J Surg Pathol 18:1213, 1994

123. Weiss SW, Rao VK: Well-differentiated liposarcoma (atypical lipoma) of deep soft tissues of the extremities, retroperitoneum, and miscellaneous sites: A follow-up study of 92 cases with analysis of incidence of dedifferentiation. Am J Surg Pathol 16:1051, 1992

124. Hashimoto H, Enoji M: Liposarcoma: A clinicopathologic subtyping of 52 cases. Acta Pathol Jpn 32:933, 1982

125. Kindbloom LG, Angervall L, Svendsen P: Liposarcoma: A clinicopathological, radiographic, and prognostic study. Acta Pathol Microbiol Scand 253:1, 1975

126. Manual for Staging of Cancer. Chicago, American Joint Committee for Cancer Staging and End-Results Reporting, 1977

127. Bowden L, Booher RJ: Surgical treatment of sarcoma of the buttock. Cancer 6:89, 1953

128. Lucas DR, Nascimento AG, Sanjay BKS, Rock MG: Well-differentiated liposarcoma: The Mayo Clinic experience. Am J Clin Pathol 102:677, 1994

129. Suit HD, Proppe KH, Mankin HJ, Woods WC: Preoperative radiation therapy for sarcoma of soft tissue. Cancer 47:2269, 1981

130. Suit HD, Russell WO: Radiation therapy of soft tissue sarcomas. Cancer 36:759, 1975

131. Cheng EY, Springfield DS, Mankin HJ: Frequent incidence of extrapulmonary sites of initial metastasesin patients with liposarcomas. Cancer 75:1120, 1995

132. Ockuly EA, Douglass FM: Retroperitoneal perirenal lipomata. J Urol 37:619, 1937

133. Stewart FW: Primary liposarcoma of bone. Am J Clin Pathol 7:87, 1931

134. Stout AP: 1949 Tumor Seminar. J Missouri Med Assoc 46:259, 1949

135. Goldman RL: Primary liposarcoma of bone. Am J Clin Pathol 42:503, 1964

136. Catto M, Stevens J: Liposarcoma of bone. J Pathol Bact 86:248, 1963

137. Ross CF, Hadfield G: Primary osteoliposarcoma of bone (malignant mesenchymoma): Report of a case. J Bone Joint Surg 50B:639, 1968

138. Schwartz A, Shusters M, Becker SM: Liposarcoma of bone: Report of a case and review of the literature. J Bone Joint Surg 52A:171, 1970

139. Rasmussen J, Jensen H: Liposarcoma of the breast. Case report and review of the literature. Virchows Arch Pathol Anat Histol 385A:117, 1979

140. Gupta RK, Paolini FA: Liposarcoma of the pleura: Report of a case, with a review of literature and views on histogenesis. Am Rev Resp Dis 95:298, 1967

141. Currie RA: Mediastinal liposarcoma. Dis Chest 46:489, 1964

142. Cicciarelli FE, Soule EH, McGoon DCJ: Lipoma and liposarcoma of the mediastinum: A report of 14 tumors including one lipoma of the thymus. J Thorac Cardiovasc Surg 47:411, 1964

143. Razzuk MA, Urschel HC, Race GH: Liposarcoma of the mediastinum: Case report and review of the literature. J Thorac Cardiovasc Surg 61:819, 1971

144. Abrams MJ, Tuberville JS: Liposarcoma of the stomach. Southern Surg 10:891, 1941

145. Neel HB: Liposarcoma of the transverse mesocolon: Report of a case. Minn Med 35:867, 1952

146. Robb WAT: Liposarcoma of the greater omentum. Br J Surg 47:537, 1960

147. Hassan MA: Subcutaneous liposarcoma of forearm followed by liposarcoma of omentum. Br J Surg 57:393, 1970

148. Edson M, Friedman J, Richardson JF: Perivascular liposarcoma: A case report. J Urol 85:767, 1961

149. Datta NS, Singh SM, Bapna BC: Liposarcoma of the spermatic cord: Report of a case and review of the literature. J Urol 106:888, 1971

150. Waller JI: Liposarcoma of the scrotum. J Urol 87:139, 1962

151. Rona C: Changes in adipose tissue accompanying pheochromocytoma. Canad Med Assoc J 91:303, 1964

152. Leiphart CJ, Nudelman EJ: Hibernoma masquerading as a pheochromocytoma. Radiology 95:659, 1970

153. Mesara BW, Batsakis JG: Hibernoma of the neck. Arch Otolaryngol 85:199, 1967

154. Merfina AF, Pike RF: Hibernoma of the thigh. J Bone Joint Surg 55A:406, 1973

155. Lawson W, Biller HF: Cervical hibernoma. Laryngoscope 86:1258, 1976

156. Meis JM, Enzinger FM: Chondroid lipoma: A unique tumor simulating liposarcoma and myxoid liposarcoma. Am J Surg Pathol 17(11):1103, 1993

157. Lowry WSB, Halmos PB: Malignant tumors of brown fat in a patient with Turner's syndrome. Br Med J 4:720, 1967

158. Enterline HT, Lowry LD, Richman AVE: Does malignant hibernoma exist? Am J Surg Pathol 3:265, 1979

# 8

# Tumors of the Fibrous Tissue

Tumors and tumorlike conditions arising from the fibrous tissue have a protean manifestation. Seldom do these tumors have a clinically uniform pathognomonic presentation. Certain tumorlike conditions, strictly speaking, do not fall in the category of neoplasms, but they require classification and description, since they can mimic both benign and malignant neoplasms to such an extent that even the most experienced pathologist may have difficulty with diagnosis. These entities will be discussed under four broad headings: (1) benign fibrous proliferations (tumorlike conditions), (2) fibromatoses or histologically benign but clinically of intermediate type of malignancy tumors, (3) malignant fibrous tissue tumors (fibrosarcomas), and (4) fibrous tumors of infancy and childhood.

## ■ BENIGN FIBROUS PROLIFERATIONS (TUMORLIKE CONDITIONS)

Benign fibrous tissue proliferations consist of a heterogeneous group of entities. Their presenting features, natural history, and frequently clinical management are quite different. However, they are tied together essentially because they are all benign and their ontogeny is the peripatetic fibroblast. Thus, all these diverse tumorlike conditions are grouped under the heading of benign fibrous tissue proliferations.

## FIBROMA

True fibrous tissue proliferation leading to the formation of a so-called fibroma is indeed rare. This cuta-neous tumor occurs as a pedunculated polypoid structure and usually is excised for cosmetic reasons (Fig. 8–1). Fibromas rarely occur beneath the skin, despite abundant fibrous tissue. Most fibromas in the somatic tissues are of the mixed variety, for example, myofibroma, angiofibroma, or fibrolipoma, and occasionally osteofibroma or neurofibroma. Cutaneous fibromalike lesions sometimes accompany Gardner's syndrome and tuberous sclerosis. In contrast, the tumor in its pure form can occur in the kidney, liver, or ovary. A fibroma of the ovary is characterized by ascites and pleural effusion (Meigs' syndrome).

## NODULAR FASCITIS

This is a benign entity characterized by rapid proliferation of fibroblasts and is often mistaken for a sarcoma.[1] The exact cause and incidence of nodular fascitis is unknown, but these are indisputably benign. Other terms, such as pseudosarcomatous fascitis,[2,3] proliferative fascitis,[1] infiltrative fascitis,[1] and pseudosarcomatous fibromatosis,[4] have all been used; essentially, these all signify the same clinicopathologic entity.

These types of fascitis are usually encountered in adult patients of either sex. Hutter and co-workers,[5] however, had 9 patients below the age of 19 out of a total of 64 patients, and we have encountered 4 patients below the age of 16, one being a three-month-old infant.

This type of fascitis can occur in any anatomic site, but the most common sites are the extremities (Table 8–1).[6] The tumors can be present superficially or can be associated with deeper structures, such as the mus-

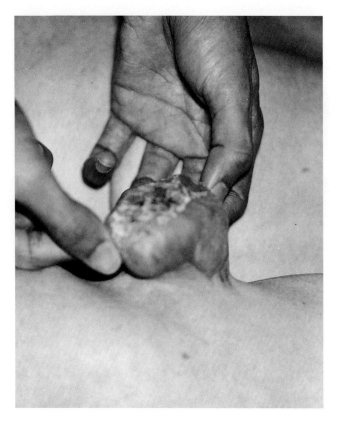

**Figure 8–1.** An unusually large pedunculated fibroma of the skin of the forearm.

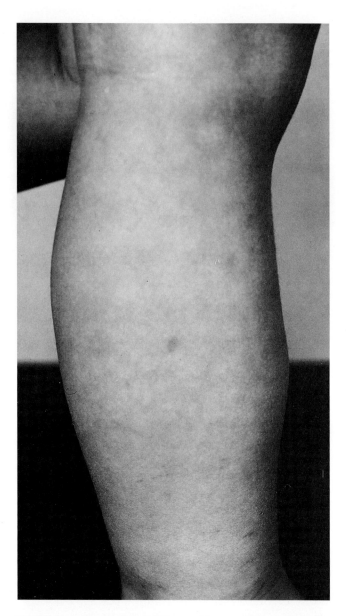

**Figure 8–2.** A case of nodular fascitis presenting as a diffuse swelling in the anterior leg of a 12-year-old girl. This tumor was locally excised in 1971. Twenty-five years later, she is doing well and there has been no evidence of local recurrence.

cles and tendons. In the extremities, these pseudotumors are frequently adherent to the underlying tendons, fascia, and/or muscles. Infrequently, these can be found as a solitary extension in a medium-sized vessel. Despite the intravascular growth, these tumors are benign. Hutter and associates[5,7] warned of the possibility of misdiagnosis of sarcoma in these cases of deep-seated fascitis, and this admonition should always be remembered.

Frequently, the patients give a history of only a few weeks' duration of the tumor. The tumor enlarges in size rather rapidly, reaching a plateau; subsequent growth is usually slow (Fig. 8–2).

Although the primary mode of therapy is excision, a major ablative procedure is contraindicated since

**TABLE 8–1. ANATOMIC DISTRIBUTION OF PSEUDOSARCOMATOUS FASCITIS IN TWO SERIES***

| Anatomic Site | Enzinger and Weiss[6] | University of Illinois |
|---|---|---|
| Head and neck | 20 | 18 |
| Trunk | 18 | 21 |
| Upper extremities | 46 | 39 |
| Lower extremities | 16 | 22 |

*From a review of more than 1,000 cases at AFIP. Numbers represent percentages.

these benign tumors are usually self-limiting. In a certain proportion of patients, recurrence might result, but even then, it is logical to limit the extent of reexcision, since some of these tumors regress spontaneously.

Hutter and associates,[7] in 1962, described four cases in which the pseudosarcomatous fascitis invaded and infiltrated the periosteum. The term *parosteal fascitis* was coined, and the entity was well described. These authors concluded that, like its soft tissue counterpart, parosteal fascitis is also self-limiting, and, even though the roentgenographic findings might appear to be ominous, the treatment should be conservative. Although

Toker[8] described another patient with bone infiltration, the benign interpretation of the tumor does not change, and any type of ablative operation is not indicated.

## PROLIFERATIVE FASCITIS

Proliferative fascitis is a lesion of the adult stage of life. About two-thirds of the lesions are located in the extremities. They are usually palpable subcutaneous nodules and seldom are larger than 5 cm in diameter. Frequently, they are tender, and this tenderness actually draws attention to the presence of these lesions. A deep counterpart of this entity, which is usually adherent to the underlying skeletal muscles, is termed intramuscular myositis.

## FIBROMA OF TENDON SHEATH

Fibroma of the tendon sheath is a slow-growing dense, fibrous nodule that is attached to the tendon sheath of origin. These tumors are mostly found in adults, usually involve the digits, and sometimes are associated with a history of trauma.[9] Since these tumors are benign, excision is only indicated either for cosmetic reasons of if the tumor is associated with tenderness.

## ELASTOFIBROMA

Elastofibroma is a rare benign tumor usually encountered in the deltoid region.[10,11] Mirra et al.[12] reviewed the literature up to and including 1974 and found a total of 56 cases, only two of which were outside the deltoid region. Older patients usually present with a swelling of short duration around the shoulder region, and histologic examination of the specimen provides the clue to the diagnosis. Since this is a benign degenerative process, a limited excision, mainly for histologic examination, is adequate therapy.

## NASOPHARYNGEAL ANGIOFIBROMA

Nasopharyngeal angiofibroma, which usually occurs in adolescent males, is an enigmatic tumor characterized by its unusual vascularity and its tendency to bleed (Figs. 4–11 & 5–20, Chapters 4 & 5). According to Martin and co-workers,[13] the tumor was first recognized by Chelius[14] in 1847. Subsequently, several case reports appeared in the literature.[15,16] Friedberg,[17] in 1940, reported three cases and first suggested the term *angiofibroma*. Martin and co-workers,[13] in 1948, reported 29 cases, all in males. The age at onset ranged from 7 to 10 years. In some cases, histologic confirmation was not obtained because of the threat of hemorrhage.

In 1950, Figi and Davis[18] published an additional 51 cases, all in males. About half of these were not diagnosed histologically; the age at onset generally ranged

from 9 to 17 years, but in one case was 23 years. Martin[19] described five patients, all of whom were treated with radiation therapy. In 1954, Sternberg[20] reviewed the material from 25 histologically proven cases, all in males. MacComb,[21] in 1963, described an additional nine cases, also all in males. Apostol and Frazell[22] made an exhaustive study of 40 cases, and Conley and co-workers,[23] in 1968, described 38 cases.

Today, it is generally agreed that nasopharyngeal angiofibroma is preponderantly a tumor of the male adolescent, although rare cases have been reported in older and younger male patients,[24] as well as in young women.[25] To what extent, if any, sex hormones play a role in the growth and development of this tumor is uncertain. A variety of theories have been forwarded,[18–23] none of which has yet been substantiated. The histologic features of this tumor, however, are extremely specific and provide a body of information about its clinical course.

The clinical behavior of the tumor depends largely upon the site of origin and its rate and direction of growth. As long as it remains localized in the nasopharynx, the tumor remains quiescent. Thus, many such tumors probably remain unrecognized, and their ultimate involution leaves their presence undetected. In contrast, the infiltrative tumors become symptomatic (Fig. 4–11 Chapter 4), the main presenting features being nasal obstruction, epistaxis, bulging cheek, bulging palate, exophthalmos, headache, and deafness. In Apostol and Frazell's[22] series, as well as in the series reported by Conley and associates,[23] nasal obstruction and epistaxis were the main presenting symptoms.

The best diagnostic aid is awareness that these tumors occur preponderantly in adolescent boys and produce the above-mentioned symptoms. Examination usually reveals a firm, rubbery, bulging mass in one or both sides of the nasopharynx, extending into the posterior portion of the nasal cavity. Occasionally, the surface of the tumor is ulcerated, especially if it has bled recently. Conley and associates[23] found tomography to be the best radiologic aid in defining the extent of the tumor. These authors[23] found 34 different sites of bone destruction in 18 of 38 patients: the pterygoid plate, 11 cases; the maxilla, 9 cases; the sphenoid, 6 cases; the base of the skull, 5 cases; and apex of the orbit, 3 cases. The number of sites highlights the potential local aggressiveness of the tumors. With the use of computed tomography (CT) and magnetic resonance (MR) scans, the radiologic diagnosis of these tumors has become much easier (see Chapter 4).

Microscopic diagnosis by means of preoperative incisional or wedge biopsy is not always required. In a juvenile male patient with all the characteristic clinical findings substantiated by CT or MR scans, the diagnosis is rather simple.

Surgical intervention constitutes the major treatment. Apostol and Frazell,[22] after reviewing all the operative methods used at Memorial Sloan-Kettering Cancer Center, concluded that the best approach is a modified Fergusson's incision through the anterior wall of the antrum, wide excision of the party wall, and thus into the nasopharynx. The exposure is adequate for visibility and removal of the tumor. Following removal, the nasopharynx and the antrum are packed. The end of the packing is brought out through the nostril for gradual removal.

Radiation therapy for these tumors is a viable alternative (Chapter 17). Recent improvement in cryosurgical techniques makes it likely that this method will be used increasingly in selected patients. Estrogens also have been tried; however, it is injudicious to use estrogen in adolescent males over a long period of time. Finally, the fact that these tumors can be self-limiting and can spontaneously regress must be taken into consideration before planning any aggressive form of therapeutic intervention.

## KELOID

Keloid commonly develops in susceptible persons, usually after trauma. The degree and extent of injury bear no relation to the keloid formation. A relatively minor trauma such as a needle prick can initiate the formation of a keloid. Keloidal diathesis is congenital, but whether it is hereditary is not known. The incidence of keloid is hard to establish, since most cases are not recorded. In certain parts of Africa, people are scarified to develop keloids in certain geometric formations.

The clinical appearance of keloids is so characteristic that the diagnosis of this lesion is never in any doubt. Keloids can occur in the skin in any location, but are more prone to occur on the ears and the presternal and intermammary areas (Fig. 8–3). These lesions are relatively fast-growing and have a tendency to spill outside the original site of trauma. Clinically, this growth pattern is one of the distinguishing features between a keloid and a hypertrophic scar.

The subjective symptoms are sometimes more annoying than the cosmetic blemish. Pain, itching, paresthesia, and increased epicritic sensibility are common. Of interest is the fact that the intensity of symptoms is not related to the size or location of the keloid.

Although Horton and his associates[26] described one case of malignant change in a keloid and cited a second case from the literature; we have never encountered any such instance.

The treatment of keloids has been an exercise in futility over the years. Excision usually results in another keloid formation. Fibrolytic agents have produced indifferent results, and radiotherapy, although it can sometimes be useful, is fraught with the inherent hazard of treating a benign lesion with radiation therapy. Therefore, before embarking on any treatment regimen, the patient should be made aware of the advantages and disadvantages of any therapy planned.

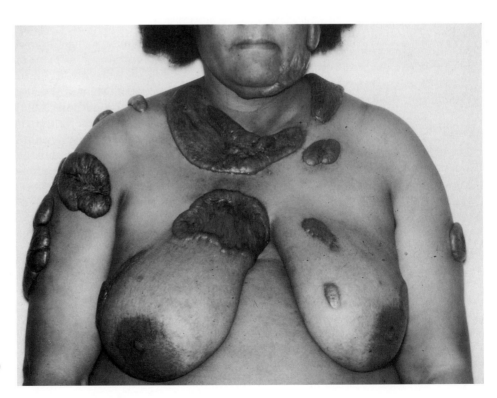

**Figure 8–3.** Woman with a tendency to develop keloids.

Considerable symptomatic relief is obtained by local injection of triamcinolone acetamide, 10 mg in 1 ml of saline (Kenalog 10 mg). The amount to be injected varies with the size of the lesion, and spraying with ethylchloride prior to injection frequently will prevent the temporary discomfort caused by the injection. In our hands, the best symptomatic results have been obtained when 1 to 1.5 cm segments of the keloid receive 1 to 2 mg of triamcinolone acetamide injected through a No. 25 needle. We repeat the course on a weekly basis for about three or four weeks. If there is no subjective improvement, we consider this mode of therapy a failure. In larger keloids, the best results seem to be provided by excision of the lesion with minimal trauma and the injection of Kenalog in the surrounding tissue, followed by careful skin approximation. In selected cases, immediate postoperative radiation therapy might be an effective means of controlling the recurrence of keloids.

# ■ FIBROMATOSES

The term *fibromatosis*, as proposed by Stout,[27] comprises a number of broad-based benign fibrous tissue proliferations, which appear benign histologically but biologically occupy an intermediate position between a benign lesion and fibrosarcoma. As has already been described (see Chapter 5), they infiltrate the surrounding structures and seldom if ever metastasize (aggressive fibromatoses/desmoids). From a clinical standpoint, these entities can be classified as follows:

Superficial Variants
1. Palmar and plantar fibromatosis
2. Penile fibromatosis

Deep Variants
1. Abdominal wall fibromatosis (abdominal wall desmoid)
2. Extra-abdominal fibromatosis (extra-abdominal desmoid)
3. Intra-abdominal fibromatosis with or without stigmata of Gardner's syndrome (intra-abdominal desmoid)
4. Intra-abdominal fibrosis (retroperitoneal fibrosis)
5. Desmoplastic fibroma

## PALMAR AND PLANTAR FIBROMATOSES (DUPUYTREN'S CONTRACTURE)

Dupuytren,[28] in 1839, described the palmar deformity that bears his name. This is a common deformity in the hand, often leading to flexion contractures of the metacarpophalangeal and interphalangeal joints of the fingers. Its incidence is presumed to be about 1 to 2

percent. The etiologic factors are unknown, but apparently trauma is not a cause.[29,30]

### Normal and Pathologic Anatomy

The palmar fascia, extending from the palmaris longus tendon at the base of the palm into the fingers and thumb to the level of the second phalanx, serve as a protective covering for the palm of the hand. Shortening or contracture of the fascial slips reaching into the fingers results in the characteristic flexion deformity of the metacarpophalangeal and the proximal interphalangeal joints. Palmar skin is firmly attached to the underlying fascia by numerous fasciculi, providing greater stability and accuracy in grasping objects. Subcutaneous fat is scant. The undersurface of the palmar fascia is connected with the deeper structures in the palm by perpendicular fascial septa, the most prominent of which is that to the third metacarpal, which divides the deep palm into the thenar and midpalmar spaces. Other minor septa compartmentalize the vital structures. The flexor digitorum superficialis and profundus tendons and sheaths course in an individual canal or compartment, whereas the neurovascular bundle and lumbrical muscles jointly occupy another.

The circulation of the subcutaneous tissue and skin arises from the superficial vascular arch, with tiny branches perforating the normal palmar fascia. As palmar fibromatosis develops, a skin pucker or dimple may appear, due to involvement of the tiny fasciculi attaching the skin to the palmar fascia. Contraction or shortening pulls the skin down into a dimple or pucker, which later becomes diffusely attached to the overlying skin, replacing the subcutaneous tissue and occluding the tiny perforating vessels. The attenuated circulation of this skin may result in delayed healing of dissected skin flaps, especially if large flaps are developed.

The fibromatous thickening also involves the perpendicular septa deep in the palm. Longitudinal bands or cords of hypertrophied fascia appear over the metacarpal bone and into the base of the finger. In the region of the web space, the main cord may branch out into the base of an adjacent finger, resulting in a flexion deformity of that metacarpophalangeal joint. When the thumb is involved, there is an adduction contracture and narrowed thumb cleft along with the flexion deformity of the thumb itself. All the fingers can be affected, but the third and fourth are the most commonly involved.

This disorder occurs in 1 to 2 percent of all people,[31] predominantly in males. Skoog[31] found 85 percent of the patients he studied were middle-aged males, and the age at onset is usually between 40 and 49 years.

The presenting symptom is a nodular subcutaneous enlargement, either in the palm or in one of the fingers. It tends to increase in size and gradually become more tender. The development of the flexion deformity may be so insidious that it escapes notice until it has progressed to a moderate degree. A well-developed case of Dupuytren's contracture is so characteristic that diagnosis is obvious.

## Treatment

The only satisfactory form of therapy is excision of the involved fascia. Although the principle of surgical therapy is simple and apparently uncomplicated, the pendulum of surgical technique has swung back and forth from the early practice of limited excision to the radical excision of the palmar fascia popularized in the 1960s; currently, it is back to some form of limited excision. The very number of proponents for each method demonstrates both the complexity of the problem and the fact that each technique has value only for certain selective situations.

The method of making the skin incision has been debated over the years. However, since Conway[32] showed that any horizontal incision, regardless of its relation to the normal palmar crease, will heal well with good functional results if proper surgical care is exerted, the argument over skin incisions has somewhat abated. A horizontal incision near the distal palmar crease, allowing access to the palmar aponeurosis with S-shaped and L-shaped finger incisions, permits exposure for resecting the digital fibrous bands where indicated. Asepsis, hemostasis, and thick skin flaps are the prerequisites for successful surgical therapy. If, during the operation, the overlying skin is found to be thin and infiltrated by the fibrous tissue, it is better to excise the damaged skin in toto and repair the skin defect. Rhode and Jennings, after reviewing their earlier experience with total excision of the palmar fascia, reverted to local excision. According to these authors, this method did not increase the incidence of recurrence, and the functional results were as good as those in patients receiving total excision of the fascia. Current dictum is to delay any surgical intervention as long as possible, preferably until the functional difficulty attains a magnitude that no options are left but to operate.

## PLANTAR FIBROMATOSIS

Plantar fibromatosis is the fibrous replacement of the plantar aponeurosis and is similar to Dupuytren's contracture of the hand. Compared with palmar fibromatosis, the plantar variety is indeed rare, although the exact incidence is not known, since a large number of these cases are not reported.

The etiologic factors again are obscure, but chronic trauma does not play an important role. The disease usually occurs in adult males after the age of 40 years. A relatively small number of cases are bilateral. Whether these tumors are familial is not clear, although cases have been recorded in multiple members of a family.[31]

A characteristic feature of plantar fibromatosis is subcutaneous nodular thickening, most frequently in the middle portion of the medial half of the sole of the foot (Fig. 8–4). These nodules are usually asymptomatic, but the chronic trauma of continuous standing induces tenderness, which frequently is the presenting symptom. Although the possibility of digital contracture similar to that seen in the hand does exist, the incidence of toe contracture is far less common. Skoog[31] suggested that the anatomic attachment of the plantar fascia is responsible for the low incidence of contracture.

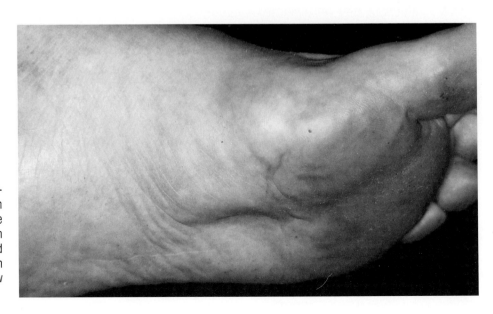

**Figure 8–4.** Plantar fibromatosis in a 60-year-old woman. Note the linear swelling in the medial plantar aspect. A conservative excision was resorted to after observation for eight years during which she functioned well. After excision, the results have been quite satisfactory. This patient is now 80 years old.

Plantar fibromatosis must be differentiated from fibrosarcoma. Clinically, either lesion can be a slow-growing, diffuse, and nonencapsulated nodular enlargement. Additionally, the age groups are similar. Histologically, the presence of mitoses with plump fibroblasts might lead to an erroneous diagnosis of fibrosarcoma. Pack and Ariel[29] described three cases in which the patients had been subjected to an amputation because of an incorrect diagnosis. However, today such instances are extremely rare.

The only satisfactory treatment of plantar fibromatosis is excision. Fortunately, excision of the plantar fascia is not accompanied by as many rehabilitation problems as for palmar fascia. Adequate excision, immobilization, and avoidance of weight-bearing for a short period produces good clinical results. However, the same admonition regarding treatment as in palmar fibromatoses holds true, and excision(s) should be delayed as long as possible. Occasionally, reexcisions are required, but these are not as complicated as in their palmar counterparts.

## PENILE FIBROMATOSES (PEYRONIE'S DISEASE)

Peyronie's disease represents a fibromatous infiltration of the sheath of the corpora cavernosa of the penis, frequently extending to Buck's fascia and the tunica albuginea. This form of fibromatosis can infiltrate the skin, producing multiple indurated skin nodules. According to Scott and Scardino,[33] Francois de la Peyronie should be credited with first describing this entity in 1743, although some believe that this disease was described earlier.[31]

The causative factors in the development of Peyronie's disease are unknown. In some instances, penile fibromatosis is associated with fibromatosis elsewhere; for example, 3 of 48 patients in the series of Burford et al.[34] had concomitant palmar fibromatosis. A similar association has been reported by other authors.[29,31,33]

Penile fibromatosis usually occurs between the ages of 45 and 60; however, younger and older patients have been encountered. The usual presenting feature is abnormal curvature of the penis, with single or multiple plaquelike nodules on the dorsum of the penis. Due to this penile deformity, erection and intercourse become difficult. Frequently, there is associated pain in the late stage of the disease.

Management of this condition is difficult. Although excision is probably the best treatment, local limited excisions have never provided a permanent control. In the past, various forms of irradiation were tried,[29,31] but none produced any tangible good result. Local infiltration with various agents ranging from vitamin E to steroids have all been tried, but not with consistent success. Administration of local steroids, as for keloids, with judicious excision of hard, plaquelike nodules, probably provides some relief.[33,34]

## ABDOMINAL FIBROMATOSES (ABDOMINAL WALL DESMOIDS)

In 1832, MacFarlane[35] of Glasgow described two tumors occurring between the layers of the abdominal muscles that resembled what we now call desmoid tumors. The term *desmoid* was first used in the English language in 1847.[36] However, Müller[37] is credited with coining the term in 1838. Paget,[38] in 1856, described a patient with a desmoid tumor of the abdominal wall and one of the arm. The phenomenon of local recurrence of these tumors following excision was stressed by both Paget[38] and Bennet.[39] Because of the high incidence of local recurrence, this tumor has occasionally been designated as recurring fibroid of Paget. Sanger[40] was the first to point out its predilection for the anterior abdominal wall. Since then, the term desmoid has been closely linked with this location.[41,42]

These tumors are rare. Pack and Ehrlich,[42] in 1944, found only 17 desmoid tumors in a series of 50,346 cases of neoplastic disease. Dahn and associates,[43] in 1963, commented on 24 abdominal desmoid tumors encountered during a period of 15 years at an institute of pathology serving approximately one million people. Brasfield and Das Gupta,[44] in 1969, reported 38 cases seen during the years 1931 to 1968 at Memorial Sloan-Kettering Cancer Center. These data should provide the reader with an idea of how infrequently this tumor occurs. Despite its relative rarity, however, there is no doubt that it is a distinct anatomic and clinical entity.

***Sex, Age, and Race.***    Most patients with anterior abdominal wall desmoids are women of childbearing age.[41–47] Twenty-one patients with abdominal wall desmoids have been treated by us at the University of Illinois Hospital. Of these, 16 (76 percent) were women of childbearing age. In the collected series of 38 patients from Memorial Sloan-Kettering Cancer Center,[44] the age distribution ranged from 1 to 81 years, with 26 (68.4 percent) between 20 and 40 years old. The median age was 30 years. In the present series, a similar age distribution was observed.

It appears that, in women, multiparity has some influence on the initiation of growth and progression of desmoid tumors of the anterior abdominal wall. In most studies dealing with large numbers of patients, a direct or indirect link with antecedent pregnancy could be demonstrated.[42–44] Our experience at the University of Illinois is similar in this respect.

Most patients have a painless tumor in the anterior abdominal wall, such as that seen in Fig. 8–5. Two male patients in our series were referred after multiple local recurrences following inadequate excisions. Brasfield

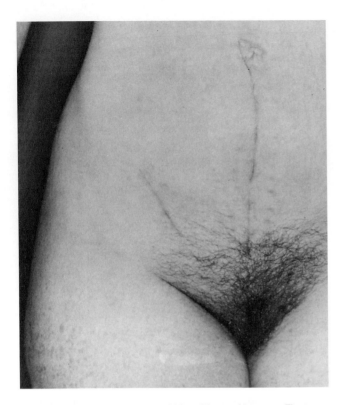

**Figure 8–5.** Abdominal wall desmoid in a 28-year-old woman. The tumor was predominantly in the right rectus abdominis muscle. After an attempted excision, she was referred to the University of Illinois. An abdominal wall resection was performed.

and Das Gupta[44] found 9 of 38 had locally recurrent tumors, 28 had untreated primary tumors, and one had had an incisional biopsy. If pain is present, it is usually due to the large volume of the tumor pressing on adjacent structures. Untreated tumors are frequently large. We have seen an unusually large tumor in a 40-year-old man (Fig. 8–6A and 8–6B). As expected, the size is directly proportional to the duration of the tumor.

Localization of these tumors follows a definite pattern. Most are located in the rectus abdominis muscle (Fig. 8–7) and the anterior layer of the rectus sheath and the linea alba (Table 8–2). The anatomic distribution of desmoid tumors in the anterior abdominal wall suggests that an unhealed injury of the midline musculature (Table 8–2) during repeated pregnancies might play a role in the etiogenesis. This preponderance of tumor occurrence in the rectus abdominis muscle and linea alba can be explained on the basis of the functions of these structures during pregnancy. During pregnancy, the fibers of all the abdominal muscles are repeatedly stretched, resulting in injury to the fibers. In the rectus abdominis, the fibers are parallel and, as a result, the stretching produces a long-standing injury and less opportunity for healing. Regarding the linea alba, a theoretic explanation could be forwarded that a

defect in the process of midline healing within the embryo results in these types of tumors.[45] In the two children in our previous group,[44] the desmoid tumors were in the midline. The midline desmoid tumors in adult female patients are most likely associated with diastases of the recti, an end result of more than one pregnancy.

***Diagnosis.*** In a multigravida, a midline anterior abdominal wall tumor with a history of relatively slow growth should be considered a desmoid tumor until proven otherwise by histologic examination of the biopsy specimen.

The treatment of an abdominal wall desmoid is radical excision.[46–48] Adequate surgical management may necessitate resection of a considerable portion of the abdominal musculature, underlying parietal peritoneum, and, under certain conditions, periosteum of the pelvic bones and parts of the small or large intestine. Successful resection of the parietal peritoneum for desmoid tumors was first performed by Sanger[40] in 1884. Although the neoplasm is histologically benign, local recurrences are frequent, so wide excision is mandatory. In case of doubt about the margins of resection in large tumors, histologic examination of the margins is indicated.

The effectiveness of radical excision was evident in the 21 patients treated by us at the University of Illinois. In none of our patients with intact abdominal wall desmoid did local recurrence occur after the type of wide three-dimensional excision we advocate. Furthermore, of the six patients who were referred to us after at least two excisions for locally recurrent tumor, it was possible to accomplish local control in three of them after the type of wide abdominal wall excisions described elsewhere in this book. Of the patients with intact primaries in Brasfield and Das Gupta's[44] series, only one had a recurrence. In this patient, the original tumor was approximately 20 cm in diameter. Three other patients who had recurrences were originally seen with recurrent disease and seeding of the operative site. This remarkably low incidence of recurrence, compared with the 10 to 40 percent reported by Musgrove and McDonald[49] or the 25 percent by Dahn and associates,[43] is justification enough for wide radical excision. Abdominal wall desmoids do not metastasize. Therefore, the only goal in therapy is local control of the primary tumor. The incidence of local recurrence reported by Enzinger and Weiss[50] only reflects the lack of aggressive surgical approach. As is described later in this chapter and elsewhere in this book, currently it is agreed that radiation therapy plays a distinct role in the management of abdominal wall desmoids, especially in large or recurrent tumors where the margins of resection appear compromised.

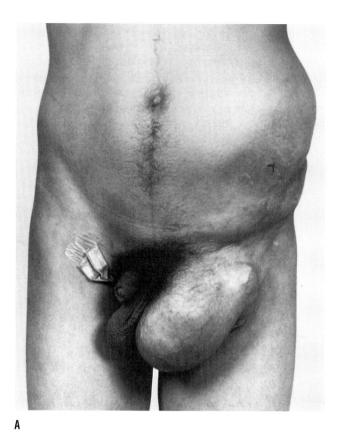

**A**

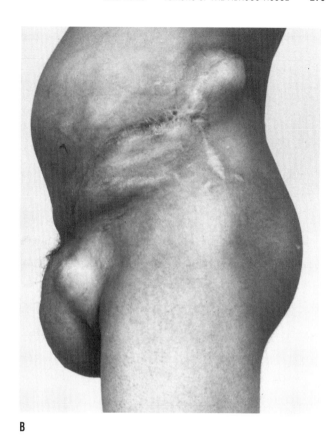

**B**

**Figure 8–6.** The anteroposterior (**A**) and lateral (**B**) views of an unusual neglected case of abdominal wall desmoid in a 40-year-old man. The tumor extended to the inguinal region.

It is suggested that aggressive fibromatosis of the anterior abdominal wall is hormone-dependent and probably can be treated by hormone manipulation. However, only fragmentary data exist to support this concept. Geschickter and Lewis[51] assayed various fibrous tissue tumors for estrogens and gonadotropins. In a desmoid tumor of the anterior wall, they found

13,000 rat units (RU) of gonadotropins per kilogram of tumor. Jadrijvic and colleagues[52] induced desmoid tumors experimentally in the abdominal wall by means of estrogens. The tumors apparently disappeared when hormone administration was interrupted. Testosterone, progesterone, and deoxycorticosterone acetate prevented development of these tumors. Pack and

**TABLE 8–2. RELATION OF DESMOIDS TO ABDOMINAL WALL MUSCULATURE**

| Muscle | Function | Number of Tumors* | |
| --- | --- | --- | --- |
| | | Brasfield and Das Gupta[44] (1969) | Present Series (1996) |
| External oblique | Compresses abdomen, flexes and laterally rotates spine, depresses ribs | 4 | 4 |
| Internal oblique | Compresses abdomen, flexes and laterally rotates spine, depresses ribs | 2[†] | 3 |
| Rectus abdominis | Compresses abdomen, flexes spine | 18 | 12 |
| Transversus abdominis | Compresses abdomen, depresses spine | 2[†] | — |
| Linea alba | Receives the attachments of the oblique and transverse abdominal muscles | 8 | 2 |

*Six patients had tumor in their surgical scar.
[†]Both the internal and transverse abdominis muscles involved.

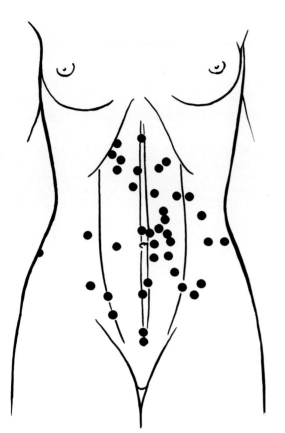

**Figure 8–7.** Scattergram showing the location of 38 desmoids of the anterior abdominal wall. *(Courtesy of* Surgery 65:241, 1969.)

Ehrlich[42] noted regression of a tumor after radiation castration. On the other hand, Strode[46] reported that some desmoid tumors subsided after menarche. Dahn and associates[43] described two patients in whom the tumor apparently subsided with menopause. In the series reported by Brasfield and Das Gupta,[44] there was no evidence that menarche or menopause induced any

appreciable regression. In 1986, we demonstrated the presence of tamoxifen receptors in both abdominal wall and extra-abdominal wall desmoids.[53] Thus, there appears some logic in treating some of these otherwise incurable patients with antiestrogens. In fact, some are being treated, but the results are not consistent enough to draw any sensible conclusions. Furthermore, in view of the available data on steroid hormone receptors,[54] in these types of tumors, it is quite likely that some form of adjuvant role of tamoxifen and/or other steroid hormones might prove to be of some value.

## EXTRA-ABDOMINAL WALL DESMOIDS

Nichols,[47] in 1923, was the first author to describe extra-abdominal wall desmoid tumors as an entity. He observed six patients in whom this tumor occurred in various sites: the thigh, popliteal space, gluteus maximus, adductor longus, pectoralis major, and the serratus anterior muscles, respectively. Musgrove and McDonald,[49] in 1948, analyzed 34 patients with this tumor and categorized the morphologic criteria. Since then, a number of relatively large series of reports have been published[43,49,55,56] (Table 8–3). An estimated 700 to 900 new cases are diagnosed annually in the United States.[57]

***Sex, Age, and Race.*** Thirty-eight of the 73 patients (52 percent) treated at the University of Illinois were women, and 35 (48 percent) were men. A similar sex incidence was found in our previous study.[58] In that group of 72 patients, 62 percent were women, and 38 percent were men.

The age at onset ranges from the neonatal period to old age. We have seen an extra-abdominal wall desmoid tumor in a child of eight months, and our oldest patient was 80 years old. However, the peak incidence is between the ages of 20 and 40 years. All races are equally afflicted by aggressive fibromatosis.

## TABLE 8–3. ANATOMIC LOCATION OF EXTRA-ABDOMINAL DESMOID TUMORS IN EIGHT SERIES

| Author(s) | Year of Publication | No. Patients | Head and Neck | Upper Extremities (including shoulder girdle) | Lower Extremities | Trunk | Miscellaneous |
|---|---|---|---|---|---|---|---|
| Nichols[47] | 1923 | 6 | — | — | 3 | 3 | — |
| Musgrove and McDonald[49] | 1948 | 34 | 5 | 7 | 9 | 13 | — |
| Ramsey[55] | 1955 | 8 | — | 3 | 2 | 3 | — |
| Hunt et al.[56] | 1960 | 22 | 4 | 9 | 2 | 6 | 1 (tongue) |
| Dahn et al.[43] | 1969 | 9 | 5 | 1 | 3 | — | — |
| Das Gupta et al.[58] | 1969 | 72 | 8 | 20 | 16 | 15 | 13 |
| Rock et al.[59] | 1984 | 194 | — | 71 | 96 | 19 | 8 |
| Present Series | 1996 | 73 | 9 | 27 | 12 | 14 | 11 |
| Total | | 418 | 31 | 138 | 143 | 73 | 33 |

***Anatomic Distribution.*** Extra-abdominal wall desmoid tumors may arise in any anatomic location. Table 8–3 shows the pattern of anatomic distribution of these tumors reported in major series since the time of proper recognition in 1923. However, there seems to be some predilection for the upper extremity, including the shoulder girdle. In our experience from our combined series with a total of 145 patients (Table 8–3), 12 percent were in the head and neck region, 32 percent in the upper extremities (including the shoulder girdle), 20 percent in the trunk, and 19 percent in the lower extremities. Twenty-four (17 percent) were located in miscellaneous sites: four in the retroperitoneal region, one in the broad ligament, three in the breast, three in the omentum, eight in the mesentery and small intestine, two in the pelvic floor, and three in the iliac fossa. The experience of Rock et al.[59] describing the anatomic sites of predilection in their 194 patients is similar to ours excepting the incidence of extra-abdominal sites encountered in our combined series of 145 patients.

Most of these patients are first seen with a painless tumor (Figure 8–8A), although, if in the extremities, the tumor, because of its location, might cause pain. One patient with a desmoid tumor of the arm was first seen with shooting pain because the tumor was located near and infiltrating the median nerve. Extra-abdominal desmoid tumors are slow-growing, and the size of the tumor at the time of initial presentation depends on duration. Frequently, the tumors are quiescent for a long period, thereby escaping recognition, especially if they are located in an unusual site, such as the retroperitoneum.

A history of antecedent trauma is rare. In only one case in the series of Das Gupta et al.[58] were the authors satisfied that some relationship might have existed. This was in a three-month-old child who was delivered with the help of forceps. Soon after birth, bilateral swelling of the temporal region was detected. The right-sided swelling completely subsided within a week, but the swelling on the left side, after an initial phase of regression, persisted. On examination at three months of age, the infant was found to have a preauricular tumor 2 × 2.5 cm. The lesion was excised, and histologic examination revealed the presence of aggressive fibromatosis. Unlike in aggressive fibromatosis of the anterior abdominal wall, which sometimes arises in scars, we have found only one patient in whom an extra-abdominal aggressive fibromatosis probably arose in a scar (Fig. 8–8A and 8–8B).

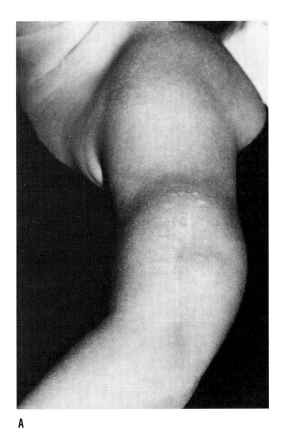

**A**

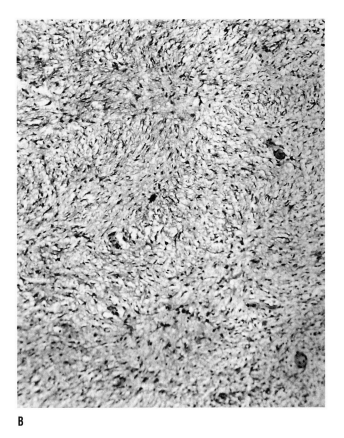

**B**

**Figure 8–8.** (**A**) A mass underneath the scar of a previous excision of an angiolipoma. (**B**) Micrograph of the excised tumor. Patient was treated by wide excision *(Courtesy of Annals of Surgery 170:109, 1969).*

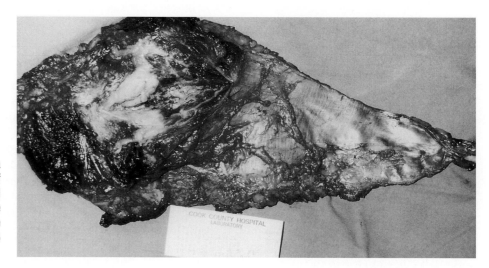

**Figure 8–9.** A specimen obtained by a wide soft tissue (muscle group) excision of a tumor in the lateral thigh of a 47-year-old man. Note white tumor in the center of the specimen surrounded by normal muscle tissue. The patient has remained well 15 years after this resection.

A correct clinical diagnosis of the primary tumor is almost impossible, but for a recurrent tumor it is not difficult, since most patients give a history of multiple excisions of a slow-growing tumor. The diagnosis of untreated primary tumor is made only after microscopic examination of the biopsy specimen.

Treatment of extra-abdominal wall desmoids consists of a wide, three-dimensional excision. The objective of optimum surgical treatment is to excise the tumor with an adequate margin of surrounding normal soft tissues (Fig. 8–9). Since the histologic structure does not reflect the growth potential of the tumors, after the diagnosis has been established, the therapy in all cases must be radical excision. To accomplish this objective, some patients require a muscle group excision or occasionally a major amputation. In our series of patients with extra-abdominal desmoid tumor, a wide excision including muscle group excision was curative in 80 percent of the patients (Fig. 8–10). A major amputation becomes a necessity in the extremity or shoulder girdle tumors when the tumor is recurrent after two or three rather conservative excisions. We

faced this type of problem in about 10 percent of our patients, where the patients were referred with massive recurrence(s) invariably after initial inadequate resection(s) (Fig. 8–11A and 8–11B). In most instances, a well-planned initial wide soft tissue excision will obviate the need for a major amputation.

There is a definite role for radiation therapy in the management of desmoid tumors (aggressive fibromatosis). In larger tumors where, due to anatomical reasons, it is not possible to accomplish a truly clear margin of resection, supplemental (adjuvant) radiation therapy plays a significant role in local control of the disease (see Chapter 17 for further details). It is important to note here that, in situations where the primary tumor is large or in patients with recurrent tumors following an adequate resection, supplemental radiation therapy should be the standard form of treatment. A major amputation should only be considered if this plan of management fails.

***End Results.*** Sixty of the 73 patients from the University of Illinois Hospital are eligible for 10-year follow-up.

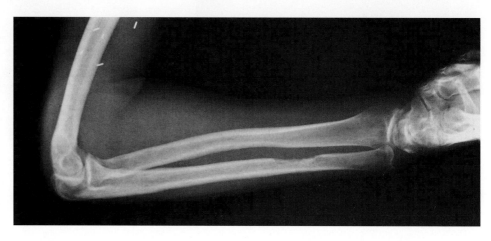

**Figure 8–10.** A 32-year-old man was referred for further therapy after three local recurrences of aggressive fibromatosis of the arm and forearm. The recurrent tumor of the forearm, which is seen infiltrating the ulna, was treated by wide excision of the ulna with a replacement bone graft. The patient has remained free of disease for 24 years. *(The replacement bone graft was performed by Dr. R. Baramada, Department of Orthopedics, University of Illinois.)*

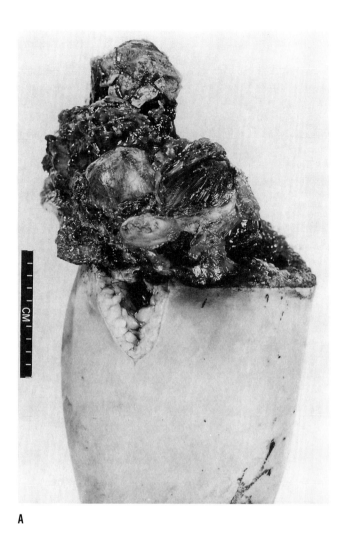

**A**

Of these 60 patients, 50 (83 percent) have been free of disease for ten years (Table 8–4). In the series reported by Das Gupta et al. in 1969,[58] of the 52 patients eligible for five-year analysis, only 33 (63 percent) had survived for five years or longer without any evidence of local recurrence. Enzinger and Shiraki[60] reported a 43 percent cure in their collected series of 30 patients with only shoulder girdle desmoids.

Seven (9.5 percent) of 73 patients in our series had local recurrence following resection of the initial tumor. In contrast, in Enzinger and Shiraki's[60] series, the local recurrence rate was 57 percent. A similar high incidence of local recurrence has been reported by other authors.[46,47,51,55,56,61–68] The primary consideration in the treatment of extra-abdominal tumors, as in their abdominal counterparts, is prevention of local recurrence. To avoid recurrence, an adequate excision of the lesion is mandatory. The low incidence in our series justifies an aggressive surgical approach. Frequently, the clinician is lulled into a false sense of security because the tumor is reported as microscopically benign. A review of several large series[46,47,55,58–64] shows that extra-abdominal desmoids can be a direct cause of death, although only rarely. One of 73 patients in our current series died postoperatively. This patient had a large tumor in the root of the mesentery, diagnosed during pregnancy. Of the remaining 72, one patient with a recurrent desmoid tumor of the neck had advanced local involvement that did not respond to any conventional form of treatment and expired of

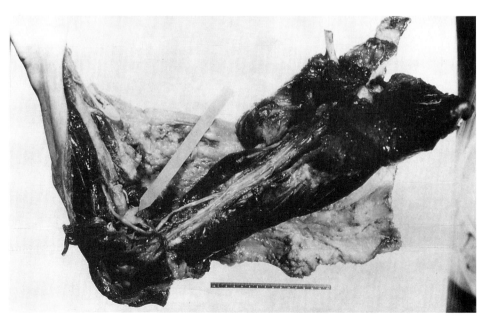

**B**

**Figure 8–11. (A)** This 28-year-old woman was found to have a large tumor during pregnancy. The pregnancy was allowed to reach full term, and she delivered a normal, healthy child. Following childbirth, she had a conservative excision and did not see her surgeons for three years, at which time she returned with a large right iliac fossa tumor. A diagnosis of aggressive fibromatosis was made, and a hemipelvectomy was performed. Note the large tumor with extensive infiltration of the surrounding tissue, even the ilium. **(B)** This 36-year-old man was seen with a large painful recurrent tumor involving the upper part of the forearm, elbow, and lower third of the arm. An interscapulothoracic amputation was performed.

**TABLE 8–4. ANATOMIC LOCATION OF 73 EXTRA-ABDOMINAL DESMOIDS (AGGRESSIVE FIBROMATOSES) WITH 10-YEAR FOLLOW-UP (1996)**

| Anatomic Location | No. Patients* | 10 Yr, NED |
|---|---|---|
| Head and neck region | 9 (8) | 7 |
| Upper extremities | 27 (24) | 21 |
| Trunk | 14 (10) | 7 |
| Lower extremities | 12 (9) | 7 |
| Miscellaneous sites | 11 (9) | 8 |

Abbreviations: NED, no evidence of disease.
*Numbers in parentheses represent patients eligible for 10-year survival analysis.

multiple complications. Death (albeit in a small number of patients) can be attributed to aggressive fibromatosis. It appears that, depending on the anatomic location and the number of recurrences, extra-abdominal wall desmoids can occasionally be lethal, and a complacent attitude regarding their management is not justifiable.

*Intra-Abdominal Desmoids or Aggressive Fibromatosis.* The intra-abdominal type of aggressive fibromatosis is rarer still, and the diagnosis can be established only after an exploratory celiotomy and open biopsy. Although most patients are initially seen because of a large intra-abdominal tumor without any discomfort, an occasional patient may complain of gastrointestinal symptoms. In one of our female patients, a palpable intra-abdominal mass was preceded by vague abdominal discomfort and chronic loss of weight. An upper gastrointestinal tract series was suggestive of a malabsorption syndrome. She was operated on, and a mesenteric desmoid tumor with extension to the small intestine was found.

The intra-abdominal sites of these tumors vary considerably. In the series reported from Memorial Sloan-Kettering Cancer Center,[58] 10 of 72 cases were found to arise from the mesentery. In our series of six intra-abdominal desmoids, three were mesenteric in origin, and the remaining three were pelvic in origin. Although retroperitoneal desmoids have been reported,[58] these are indeed rare. The management principle is similar to that for tumors encountered in other sites, namely, wide excision.

## GARDNER'S SYNDROME AND AGGRESSIVE FIBROMATOSIS (DESMOIDS)

The existence of an autosomal dominant syndrome comprised of colonic polyposis, soft tissue, and bone tumors was recognized originally by Gardner and Richards[69] in the early 1950s. Since then, a number of case reports have appeared that link the presence of aggressive fibromatosis or desmoids to Gardner's syndrome.[70–77] Although the exact genetic abnormality has not yet been clearly defined, it is assumed that karyotypic abnormalities of the Y-chromosome on 5q, similar to the findings in other types of fibromatosis, are present.[78,79] When Gardner[72] reviewed his cases in 1962, he added abnormal dentition and postoperative desmoids arising in surgical scars as part of the syndrome. In the interim, Smith,[71] and then Simpson, Harrison, and Mayo,[73] had included mesodermal tumors as part of Gardner's syndrome. They described fibrous tumors seen superficially on the skin, in the mesentery of the small or large intestine, and near or in a surgical scar after colectomy. The tumors usually developed within a year after surgery. Parks and associates,[75] in discussing desmoids of the extracolonic abnormalities of familial polyposis, stated, "Surgical trauma is the precipitating factor in their causation."

We have treated 11 patients with Gardner's syndrome. One patient had polyposis coli and a mesenteric tumor invading the head of the pancreas; a pancreaticoduodenectomy was performed (Fig. 8–12). In another patient, the concomitant mandibular osteomas, along with mesenteric desmoid, were so pronounced that, along with resection of the intra-abdominal desmoid, a partial resection of the mandible was also required.

Gardner's syndrome appears to be an abnormal proliferation of varying combinations of the three primary germ layers. Sebaceous and epidermoid cysts, and tumors of the central nervous system (Turcot syndrome) are abnormalities of the ectoderm.[78,79] Adenomas of the large bowel and rarely seen duodenal hamartomas and periampullary carcinomas are forms of entodermal proliferation.[76] Bone proliferations (in the form of osteomas, odontomas, and supernumerary teeth) and connective tissue proliferation represent disorders of the mesodermal element. The connective tissue forms include excessive postoperative intra-abdominal adhesions (approximately 20 percent of patients with Gardner's syndrome are reoperated on for adhesions), fibromas, and fibrosarcomas involving the mesentery, mesocolon, and retroperitoneum.[75,76,80] Of the reported cases of desmoids of the abdominal cavity associated with polyposis coli, more than half appear to occur after surgery; in the other cases, either this point is not clear or information is not available. Penn and co-workers[81] and Das Gupta et al.[58] found aggressive fibromatosis in patients in whom there was no history of antecedent operation. In our own material, we found that antecedent operative trauma has no role in the evolution of intra-abdominal fibrous tissue tumors. The polyps in Gardner's syndrome and those in familial polyposis are adenomas, and the roentgenographic picture is identical. The polyps are most prevalent in the rectum and descending colon. Although there are

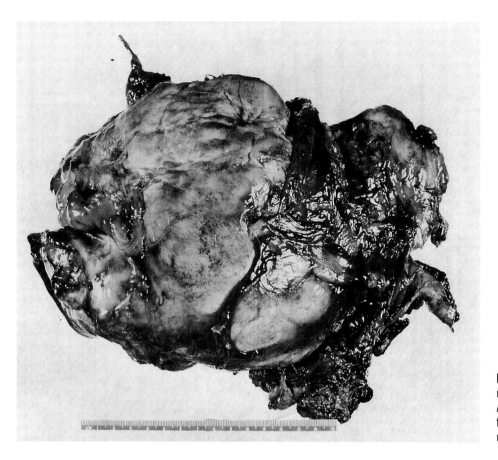

**Figure 8–12.** Operative specimen of a mesenteric desmoid in a 47-year-old man. A pancreaticoduodenectomy was performed, and he is doing well. See also Figure 5–30.

reports of polyps regressing,[70] eventually they regrow. Colonic polyps are usually manifest by the age of 20, and malignant transformation usually occurs about 15 years later.

## IDIOPATHIC RETROPERITONEAL FIBROSIS (ORMOND'S DISEASE)

Idiopathic retroperitoneal fibrosis is a disease of uncertain etiology and is characterized by proliferation of the retroperitoneal fibrous tissue. Apparently, the disease starts in the pelvic region and progresses cephalad.[82–85] Retroperitoneal fibrosis was first described in 1948 by Ormond.[86] Since then, a number of such cases have been reported. Today, retroperitoneal fibrosis is accepted as a valid clinical entity of unknown etiology.[87] Usually, the fibrous plaque is first seen over the sacral promontory, which then extends upward and laterally, encircling one or both ureters and resulting in obstructive uropathy (Fig. 8–13). Although idiopathic retroperitoneal fibrosis should always be considered in patients with urinary problems, frequently, underlying neoplasia (e.g., lymphoma) can be overlooked unless scrupulous attention is given to details, including multiple biopsies of the retroperitoneal fibrous tissue.

The treatment of idiopathic retroperitoneal fibrosis is directed to the urologic problem. The ureters are dissected free of their fibrous plaquelike encasement. This simple surgical maneuver relieves the ureteric obstruction and usually solves the urinary problems.

A fibrotic process similar to idiopathic retroperitoneal fibrosis has been recognized in the mediastinum,[88,89] and Barrett[90] suggested that Riedel's thyroiditis and pseudotumor of the orbit are further examples of the same disease. Tubbs[91] described a patient with both mediastinal and retroperitoneal fibrosis. Temperley[88] reported a case of multifocal fibrosclerosis that apparently was controlled with the use of steroids. However, steroids have not been useful in established cases of retroperitoneal fibrosis.

## DESMOPLASTIC FIBROMA

Jaffe[92] first described desmoplastic fibroma as an entity in 1958. In 1968, Rabhan and Rosai,[93] reviewed this entity in a total of 25 cases, 10 of which were from their own institution. These authors found that the tumor was distributed as follows: mandible, three; clavicle, one; humerus, five; radius, two; scapula, one; vertebra, two; ilium, three; femur, three; tibia, four; and calca-

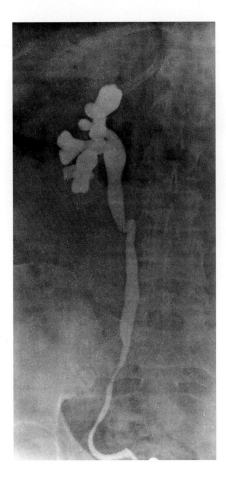

**Figure 8–13.** Intravenous pyelogram showing the narrowing of the right ureter near the pelvic brim. The diagnosis of retroperitoneal fibrosis was established by an exploratory celiotomy and biopsy.

neus, one. Although this is primarily a bone tumor, the anatomic sites of occurrence, as well as the macroscopic features, might easily confuse the examiner, and the tumor might be diagnosed as an aggressive fibromatosis. Microscopic examination can also pose a problem in distinguishing desmoids from desmoplastic fibromas. The biologic behavior of these tumors is similar to that of aggressive fibromatosis. Limited local excision results in recurrence. Wide three-dimensional excision of the tumor with surrounding normal soft and bony tissue usually results in cure.

## ■ FIBROSARCOMA

Paget,[63] in 1865, designated malignant tumors of fibrous tissue as recurrent fibroids. Cornil and Ranvier,[94] in 1880, considered them fasciculated sarcomas. Virchow[95] described them as fascial sarcomas (arising

from the fascia), usually in a lower extremity, slow-growing, with surgical removal resulting in cure. Birkett[96] and Billroth[97] recorded some of the earlier case histories. From these few case reports describing what apparently were sarcomas of the fibrous tissue, there came an avalanche of case reports, all purporting to describe fibrosarcomas. As mentioned in Chapter 5, after all tumors composed of cells capable of acting as facultative fibroblasts are excluded, the true incidence of fibrosarcoma will be found to be much lower than generally thought. The pioneering works of Ewing,[98] Stout,[99–104] Pack and Ariel,[29,105] and Stout and Lattes[106] provide excellent diagnostic criteria for the diagnosis of fibrosarcomas. Based on the original work of these authors, others[107–123] have reviewed their own material and published their experiences with the incidence and natural history of fibrosarcomas arising in various anatomic sites. There is no doubt that, with the recognition of malignant fibrous histiocytic tumors and variants of aggressive fibromatoses, the designation of any malignant tumor of fibrous tissue origin has declined. It is indeed difficult to calculate the exact incidence of fibrosarcoma. Pack and Ariel[29] found only 39 cases out of a total of 717 sarcomas (5.4 percent); the incidence of dermatofibrosarcoma protuberans in that series was about the same (5.9 percent). Fibrosarcomas, like most other soft tissue sarcomas, develop spontaneously, and no apparent etiologic agent has been identified. However, there are a number of documented cases developing in heavily irradiated tissues.

## ROLE OF IRRADIATION IN THE FORMATION OF FIBROSARCOMAS

Frequently, epidermoid carcinomas develop in irradiated tissues, and some areas show spindle cell metaplasia that microscopically can be confused with fibrosarcoma. Solway[124] found six cases of postirradiation fibrosarcoma in the files of the pathology department of the Columbia University College of Physicians and Surgeons. Only 11 such cases were documented up to 1970,[124–133] seven of which were the sequelae of treatment of retinoblastoma in children, and four of which were in adults. In 1979, Hajdu[134] reported five additional cases of postirradiation fibrosarcoma in adults. A comprehensive review of the literature shows that the true incidence of radiation-induced fibrosarcoma is indeed low.[132,135–138]

## CONGENITAL RELATIONSHIP

Congenital and infantile cases of fibrosarcoma have been reported.[100,107,108,116–118,139–142] There is still some controversy as to its true malignant potential. All the cases of congenital fibrosarcoma reported carry a much better prognosis than their adult counterparts and can be considered well-differentiated grade 1 type of fibrosarcoma.[112] Chung and Enzinger[107] found that 20 of 53 cases of infantile fibrosarcomas were present at birth. Including one case from our own experience, only a handful of such cases meet the histologic criteria of fibrosarcoma. Since these tumors have a better prognosis,[29,99,107,116–118,143–145] they should be treated only by local excision, and any form of mutilating procedure should be avoided.

## AGE, SEX, AND RACE

Fibrosarcoma is essentially a disease of adults. In our group of 103 patients (including 18 occurring in unusual sites), 43 (42 percent) were between the ages of 25 and 49 years, 8 percent of the patients were below 9 years of age, and 16 percent between 10 and 19 years. The remaining patients were all over 50 years of age. Fifty-seven percent of our patients were males, and 43 percent were females. Pritchard and associates[122] excluded 23 children from their study since, according to these authors, fibrosarcoma shows a benign behavior in children. However, in our study, we found that five of the 19 patients below the age of 19 died of metastatic fibrosarcoma. A more detailed description of childhood fibrosarcoma will be found in Chapter 21.

It appears that fibrosarcomas are found in all races in about equal incidence. In our series, the distribution was proportional. Crawford and associates[146] reported that fibrous tissue tumors probably have a higher incidence in American blacks than in whites, but this observation has not been substantiated.

## ANATOMIC DISTRIBUTION

Fibrosarcomas occur predominantly in the lower extremities. Pritchard and co-workers[122] found a 60 percent incidence in the lower extremities, and Werf-Messing and van Unnik,[123] a 32 percent incidence. Enzinger and Weiss[147] found 695 cases of fibrosarcomas in the Armed Forces Institute of Pathology (AFIP) files. Of these, 45 percent were in the lower extremity, 28 percent in the upper extremity, 17 percent in the trunk, and 10 percent in the head and neck region. Our experience with only 103 patients treated thus far is that the overall incidence of anatomic predilection corresponds to that reported by most of the authors, including Enzinger and Weiss.[147] The thighs and buttocks are the most common site of occurrence. Although fibrosarcomas are found most frequently in the

**TABLE 8–5. INCIDENCE OF 18 FIBROSARCOMAS IN UNUSUAL SITES (UNIVERSITY OF ILLINOIS SERIES)**

| Anatomic Site | No. Patients |
|---|---|
| Nasopharynx | 1 |
| Pharynx | 1 |
| Maxillary antrum | 1 |
| Buccal mucosa | 1 |
| Floor of mouth | 1 |
| Retroperitoneum | 4 |
| Mesentery | 1 |
| Breast | 4 |
| Diaphragm | 1 |
| Kidney | 1 |
| Ovary | 1 |
| Dura | 1 |
| Total | 18 |

extremities and torso, they can occur in any part of the body where fibrous tissue is present (e.g., in the alimentary tract, mesentery, omentum, retroperitoneal region, liver, kidney, urethra, vagina, lung, mediastinum, oral cavity, oropharynx, nasopharynx, orbit, and blood vessels). In our present series, 18 fibrosarcomas were encountered in various uncommon sites (Table 8–5). They are seldom located around major joints, although we did see one patient with fibrosarcoma around the knee joint.

## CLINICAL FEATURES

Fibrosarcomas do not present a characteristic symptom complex that could serve to differentiate this malignant neoplasm from benign tumors or other malignant tumors that involve the somatic tissues. Most commonly, the patient notices a painless mass that starts insidiously, grows slowly, and either reaches a huge size or, more rarely, causes the patient to seek treatment because of pressure against a nerve, producing pain or other disability (Fig. 8–14A to 8–14D). Infrequently, the patient complains of pain for a period before the neoplasm is actually identified. Eighty percent of our patients were initially seen because of a mass. In six patients, pain of a duration ranging from three months to five years preceded the actual discovery of the mass. The remaining patients were sent to us after local recurrence after initial therapy elsewhere. In patients with intact primary fibrosarcoma, the tumors measured less than 2 cm in only 16 patients; in the remaining patients, the tumors measured between 5 and 20 cm in maximum diameter.

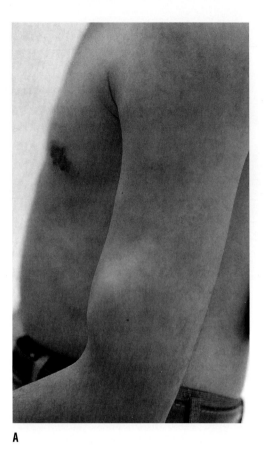

**A**

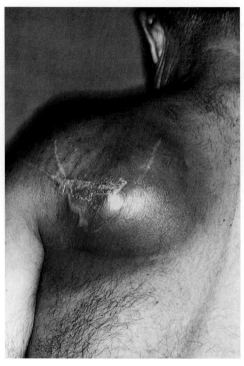

**B**

**Figure 8–14.** (**A**) Slow-growing tumor of the lower part of left arm in a 34-year-old man. This tumor was noticed about 12 months before attaining its present size. He came to our clinic not because of the tumor but because of associated pain and some muscle weakness. A muscle group excision was performed, and he has remained well for 12 years. (**B**) A fibrosarcoma of the back of long duration. The exact sequence of events was not known to the patient. After it attained considerable size, an inadequate excision was performed, and the tumor recurred. The patient was treated by irradiation before he was sent to us. At the time of this presentation, he already had lung metastases. *(Continued.)*

Involvement of regional lymph nodes in fibrosarcoma is extremely rare. We have not encountered any in our series. Stout[101] in 1948, reported an 8 percent incidence, but in the earlier series a number of cases were considered as fibrosarcomas when in fact they were not. Pack and Ariel[29] and Pritchard and associates[122] found only one instance each in their respective series of 39 and 199 patients. Bizer[148] also found no evidence of true nodal involvement in his series of 64 patients.

## TREATMENT

### Surgical

The principle in the management of fibrosarcomas is adequate radical excision of the soft tissues. The extent and type of excision will depend on the anatomic location of the tumor (Fig. 8–15A and 8–15B). The margins

of resection *must* be free of tumor cells on all sides. Adequacy of margin can be defined as the presence of at least one uninvolved fascial barrier between the tumor and the adjacent normal remaining structures. Determinants of this include the site and size of the tumor, histologic grading, neurovascular involvement, bone or joint involvement, and, finally, multicentricity of origin of some fibrosarcomas. The technical considerations for the specific types of operations are discussed in Chapter 16.

### Radiation Therapy for Fibrosarcoma

Radiation therapy alone has a limited role in the management of fibrosarcomas. However, as an adjuvant to resection, the role of radiation therapy is immense, and today the onus is to prove why postoperative radiation therapy in any tumor of 5 cm or larger is not required in a given situation (see Chapter 17 for details).

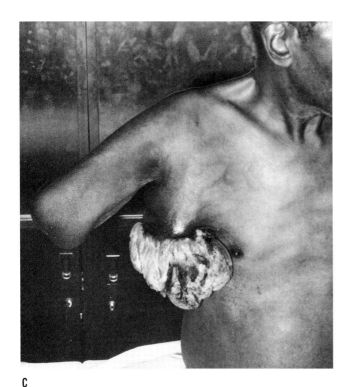

C

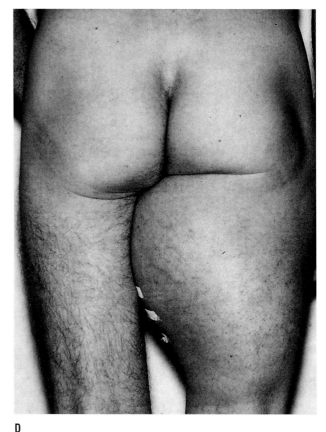

D

**Figure 8–14** *(continued).* (**C**) A neglected case of fibrosarcoma of the chest wall with fungation. There was no evidence of systemic disease at this time, and a regional resection was possible. Patient lived for one year, after which time he died of metastases. (**D**) Huge fibrosarcoma of the thigh, which, because of its location and size, was treated with major amputation. Patient lived only three-and-a-half years free of disease and died of massive lung and liver metastases.

## Chemotherapy

Although chemotherapy as a primary form of treatment of fibrosarcoma is not effective, it is being used increasingly as an adjuvant to primary surgical treatment. (See Chapter 18 for a detailed discussion.)

## End Results

In Table 8–6, the anatomic distribution of our 85 patients with tumors located in the head and neck, trunk, and the extremities are shown corresponding to their 5- and 10-year survival. Although this group contains primary tumors of all grades and sizes, the overall disease-free survival for 10 years was found to be 73 percent. An overall end result of 73 percent tumor-free survival for 10 years without any form of adjuvant therapy speaks well for radical excision. Similar results have been reported by Bizer,[148] Castro and associates,[149] and Pritchard et al.[122] Bizer[148] observed a 78 percent ab-

solute five-year survival for patients treated by radical excision. However, no data as to the number of patients treated by major amputation are available in his study. Castro and associates[149] found that, of 75 patients with lower extremity fibrosarcoma treated by muscle group excision, 43 (57 percent) survived free of disease for five years. Pritchard and co-workers[122] similarly observed that radical soft tissue resection provided a good to excellent five-year survival rate. The term *wide excision* in our series includes chest wall resection, abdominal wall resection, and other soft tissue resections. With advancing technology in the field of radiation oncology, a wide soft tissue resection in conjunction with postoperative radiation therapy has become the standard form of therapy, especially in all high-grade fibrosarcomas at the University of Illinois.

The natural history of fibrosarcomas can, to a large extent, be prognosticated by the type and degree of differentiation (histologic grading) of a given tumor. In our 85 patients with fibrosarcoma of the soft tissues, 66 were referred to us with intact primary tumor. The size and grade of these tumors, along with 5- and 10-year survival after primary treatment at University of Illinois is shown in Table 8–7. As has been alluded to, most primary tumors smaller than 5 cm of grade 1 or 2 were adequately treated with wide soft tissue resection. However, patients with primary tumors larger than 5 cm and of grades 3 or 4 (high grade) were all treated with postoperative radiation therapy. The technical considerations of these types of radiation are discussed in Chapter 17.

In our present series, 14 (16 percent) of the 85 patients had local recurrence after initial excision. Of the 66 patients seen initially with intact primary tumors, only 9 had local recurrence. Therefore, the true incidence of local recurrence after treatment of an intact primary in this series was 14 percent. The incidence of local recurrence was found to be 56 percent by Pack and Ariel,[29] 50 percent by Bizer,[148] 68 percent by Werf-Messing and Van Unnik,[123] 48 percent by Castro et al.,[149] and 76 percent by Pritchard et al.[122] However, in the Pritchard and co-workers' series,[122] if the 76 patients who were referred originally with recurrent tumors are excluded, then the true incidence of local recurrence is 18 percent. In a more recent review, Scott et al.[150] found that incidence of local recurrence is proportional to the adequacy of the original operation. Incidence was 79 percent with inadequate surgical mar-

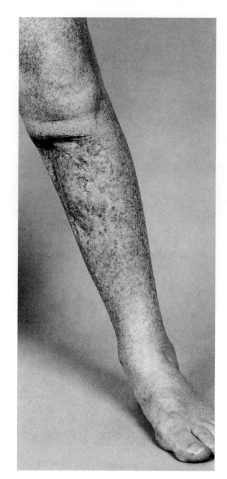

**A**

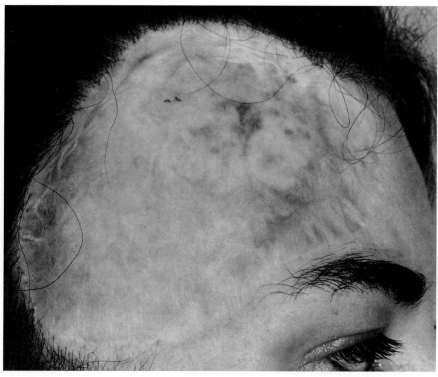

**B**

**Figure 8–15.** (**A**) Anteromedial aspect of the leg in a 56-year-old woman, showing the site of excision of low-grade fibrosarcoma from this area six years ago. At age 50, she was found to have a 3 × 3 cm grade 2 fibrosarcoma. The operation included resection of the surrounding soft tissue and a part of the tibia. She is still leading an active life 15 years later. (**B**) An area of wide excision of a 4 × 3 cm grade 2 fibrosarcoma in the scalp of a 19-year-old girl. She is doing well 17 years later. The outer table was excised. Defect was treated with split-thickness skin graft.

**TABLE 8–6. END RESULTS IN 85 PATIENTS WITH FIBROSARCOMA ACCORDING TO SITE (CURRENT SERIES)***

| Site of Primary Tumor | No. Patients[†] | Survival Free of Cancer | |
| --- | --- | --- | --- |
| | | 5 Yr | 10 Yr |
| Head and neck | 13 | 10 (77%) | 9 (69%) |
| Upper extremities | 18 | 12 (67%) | 12 (67%) |
| Trunk | 14 | 11 (78%) | 10 (71%) |
| Lower extremities | 40 | 32 (80%) | 31 (77%) |
| Total | 85 | 65 (76%) | 62 (73%) |

*18 patients with fibrosarcoma in unusual sites are excluded from this group.
[†]All grades and sizes of primary of tumors are included in this table.

gins and 18 percent with wide resection. Local recurrence of fibrosarcoma often reflects an inadequate primary excision. The most significant factor that influences local recurrence is adequacy of excision. Werf-Messing and Van Unnik[123] reported that, when the margins were not microscopically checked, the recurrence rate was 70 percent, whereas in cases in which microscopic examination was performed and the margins were apparently free of tumor, the recurrence rate was only 10 percent. In our series, 2 (14 percent) of the 14 patients with local recurrence had concomitant pulmonary metastases, and any form of locally directed therapy was useless. However, the remaining 12 patients were treated aggressively, 6 by a major amputation and 6 by radical soft tissue excision and additional radiation therapy. Two of the six in the amputation group, and two of the six in the soft tissue resection plus radiation therapy group, died with metastases within two years. It appears therefore that, even in patients with locally recurrent fibrosarcoma, a substantial proportion of patients can be salvaged with aggressive therapy, and this option should not be denied to the patients. Castro and associates[149] and Lindberg et al.[151] came to a similar conclusion from their studies. In sum, the salvage rate of primary fibrosarcoma depends on the size and histologic grade of the tumor and the aggressiveness of initial therapy (Table 8–7).

The most common site of metastasis is the lungs. Generally, these patients are treated with multi-agent chemotherapy. However, in selected cases, wedge resection(s) and sometimes lobectomy offer long-term palliation. We have several five-year survivors after wedge resection of pulmonary metastases.

## ■ FIBROSARCOMAS OF UNUSUAL LOCATIONS

### INTRAORAL AND PHARYNGEAL REGIONS

Fibrosarcomas of the oral region are extremely rare, as emphasized by the study of O'Day and associates.[152] These authors were able to find only 15 examples in the literature and added 6 additional cases from the files of the Mayo Clinic. In our files, there are five cases: one of the nasopharynx, one of the pharynx, one of the maxilla, one of the buccal mucosa, and one of the floor of the mouth (Fig. 8–16A and 8–16B). Treatment of these lesions entails wide excision with an adequate margin around the primary tumor. Although it is not possible to elaborate on the prognostic factors on the basis of so few case histories, adequate wide excision should be the primary goal of the initial treatment of fibrosarcomas in these locations.

### FIBROSARCOMA OF THE RETROPERITONEUM AND MESENTERY

Retroperitoneal fibrosarcomas occur only rarely (Table 8–5). Analysis of the data from comparatively larger series of fibrosarcomas shows that approximately 3 percent of fibrosarcomas occur in the retroperitoneal space.[29,101,123,151,153–157] There are no characteristic clinical features of retroperitoneal fibrosarcoma. Usually, the patients are first seen with a large retroperitoneal tumor, and the diagnosis is established after celiotomy. The accepted form of treatment is exploratory celiotomy followed by total excision of the tumor. It is almost impossible to obtain an adequate margin of normal soft tissue at the time of excision of the primary tumor. Consequently, excision does not yield as good a salvage as in fibrosarcomas of the trunk and extremities. Of the four patients in our series, only

**TABLE 8–7. ANALYSIS OF TUMOR SIZE AND TUMOR GRADE OF 66 PATIENTS SEEN INITIALLY WITH INTACT PRIMARY FIBROSARCOMAS***

| Tumor Size | No. Patients | Grades 1 and 2 | 10 Yr, NED | Grades 3 and 4[†] | 10 Yr, NED |
| --- | --- | --- | --- | --- | --- |
| Smaller than 5 cm | 25 | 16 | 16 | 9 | 5 |
| Larger than 5 cm | 31 | 14 | 12 | 17 | 13 |
| Larger than 5 cm and local infiltration to muscles and bone | 10 | 3 | 2 | 7 | 4 |
| Total | 66 | 33 | 30 (91%) | 33 | 22 (67%) |

Abbreviations: NED, no evidence of disease.
*These patients were treated by radical soft tissue excision and postoperative radiation therapy for high-grade tumors.
[†]All patients with high-grade primary tumor larger than 5 cm received postoperative radiation therapy.

one survived more than five years after excision of the tumor. Only 24 percent of eight patients in the series reported by Werf-Messing and Van Unnik[123] lived five years or more.

Fibrosarcoma of the mesentery that is not a part of Gardner's syndrome is extremely rare. Stout[101] found six such cases, and we have encountered only one. In our patient, the diagnosis was made at celiotomy, and the tumor could not be resected. The patient died with lung metastases within eight months of initial diagnosis.

## FIBROSARCOMA OF THE BREAST

Fibrosarcomas are the most common form of stromal sarcomas of the breast parenchyma. In the University of Illinois series, four patients had fibrosarcoma of the breast. Of these, two are living disease-free 10 years later. The prognosis of fibrosarcomas of the breast irrespective of their size and grade is comparatively worse than for their counterparts in the trunk and extremities. Quite likely, one reason for this reported bad end result is inadequate excision of the primary tumor,[157,158] though other factors might influence the prognosis. Controversy and confusion aside, these patients must be treated aggressively, and any operation less than a complete mastectomy is deemed inadequate.

## CYSTOSARCOMA PHYLLODES OF THE BREAST

In 1883, Mullee collected several cases of an unusual mammary tumor characterized chiefly by its large bulk, rapid growth following years of quiescence, benign nature, and peculiar gross and microscopic features.

He coined the term *cystosarcoma phyllodes* to designate these tumors (Fig. 8–17).

Cystosarcoma phyllodes is an uncommon neoplasm of the breast, composed of a cellular stroma and epithelial-lined duct. Although the tumor can arise de novo, a relationship with fibroadenomas (especially the intracanalicular types) of the breast has been reported by several authors.[157–163] A comprehensive review of the subject of cystosarcoma phyllodes, including our

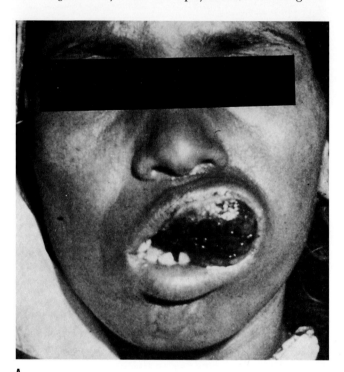

**A**

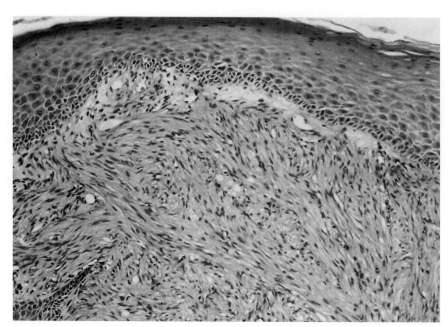

**Figure 8–16. (A)** Large fungating intraoral fibrosarcoma arising from the floor of the mouth. **(B)** Micrograph of the same tumor (H & E. Original magnification × 100).

**B**

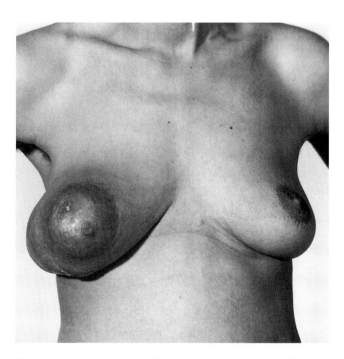

**Figure 8–17.** Cystosarcoma phyllodes of the right breast in a 38-year-old woman. A wide excision was performed, and she has remained well for 11 years.

own clinical experience, is not germane to this book. However, according to the criteria established by McDivitt and associates,[163] it is appropriate to differentiate between the benign and malignant varieties.[164] The malignant variant of this tumor must not be confused with the stromal fibrosarcoma of the breast described earlier. Malignant cystosarcoma phyllodes metastasizes to the regional nodes, as well as to other viscera. Kessinger et al.[165] reviewed the literature and found 66 cases of metastatic cystosarcoma phyllodes. To this series, they added one of their own.

The treatment of malignant cystosarcoma phyllodes is usually total mastectomy if there are no enlarged nodes. If the nodes are enlarged, then a radical mastectomy is indicated.[166] In only five of seven recorded cases was there histologic proof of ipsilateral nodal metastasis.[166]

## FIBROSARCOMA OF THE DIAPHRAGM

Fibrosarcoma arising in the diaphragm is also rare. We have only one such instance in our files. This patient, a 51-year-old woman, was referred with a large tumor in the left upper quadrant. An exploratory procedure revealed a localized tumor arising from the inferior leaf of the left diaphragm. The tumor, along with a portion of the diaphragm, was excised. The diaphragmatic defect was closed with Marlex mesh. She remained well for three years, after which retroperitoneal recurrence was noted with pulmonary metastases. The patient died within one year of recognition of the recurrent tumor.

## FIBROSARCOMA ARISING IN THE VISCERA

Fibrosarcomas can arise in any organ with a fibrous stroma. However, only a few documented cases of visceral fibrosarcomas have been reported. Since these cases are rare, a detailed analysis of the symptoms, signs, and natural history is not possible. From a therapeutic standpoint, these tumors should be excised whenever possible. Treatment with adjuvant radiation therapy and systemic chemotherapy might be of some value. In the following sections, fibrosarcomas in some of these viscera are described.

## PRIMARY FIBROSARCOMA OF THE LIVER

Eleven documented cases of fibrosarcoma of the liver were recorded until 1975 (Table 8–8),[167–177] only two of which were treated. One patient responded well to radiation therapy, and the second patient underwent resection of the fibrosarcoma. In four other cases, fibrosarcoma and carcinoma occurred as two separate tumors. These tumors usually are diagnosed at autopsy (Fig. 8–18A and 8–18B). Since the review of the literature by Alrenga,[177] we could not find any documented cases in the literature. Thus, it is not possible to define therapeutic guidelines for primary fibrosarcoma of the liver.

## PRIMARY FIBROSARCOMA OF KIDNEY

Primary fibrosarcoma of the kidney is also rare.[178–180] Unless several different areas of the tumor are microscopically examined, a diagnosis of sarcoma should not be made. In our files, we have only one instance of primary fibrosarcoma of the kidney. This female patient was sent to us after a recurrence of fibrosarcoma following simple nephrectomy. An angiogram showed massive retroperitoneal recurrence (Fig. 8–19A and 8–19B). She was operated on, but within six months metastatic involvement of the lungs, pleura, liver, and brain developed, and she expired.

## PRIMARY FIBROSARCOMA OF THE OVARY

Although fibromas of the ovary with concomitant pleural effusion are not uncommon, a true fibrosarcoma is indeed rare.[180] We have encountered only one such instance, and pulmonary metastases developed soon after resection of the primary ovarian tumor.

## PRIMARY FIBROSARCOMA OF THE THYROID

A fibrosarcoma of the thyroid, another rare tumor,[181] is difficult to distinguish from a spindle cell carcinoma. The treatment appears to be removal of the thyroid with an adequate margin of normal neck contents.

**TABLE 8–8. SUMMARY OF 11 CASES OF HEPATIC FIBROSARCOMA REPORTED IN THE LITERATURE**

| Author(s) | Year of Publication | Age/ Sex | Liver Weight (g) | Cirrhosis | Metastases | Gross Appearance of Tumor | End Results |
|---|---|---|---|---|---|---|---|
| Shallow and Wagner[167] | 1947 | 60/M | 5,200* | — | — | Massive, left lobe, solid, firm, central necrosis | Dead |
| Simpson et al.[168] | 1955 | 66/M | — | — | Lymph nodes, omentum and jejunum | Massive right lobe, cystic, grayish, satellite nodules | Dead |
| Steiner[169] | 1960 | 45/M | 4,100 | + | — | — | |
| Ojima et al.[170] | 1964 | 62/M | 3,190 | — | — | Massive, right lobe, solid, white | Dead |
| Snapper et al.[171] | 1964 | 60/M | 12,150 | — | Lungs | Massive, right lobe, solid, pinkish-white, satellite nodule | 5 yr, NED |
| Totzke and Hutcheson[172] | 1965 | 56/F | 650 | — | Lymph nodes | Massive, right lobe, solid, soft pinkish-yellow, satellite nodules | Dead |
| Belouet and Destombes[173] | 1967 | 38/M | — | — | — | — | |
| Cavallo et al.[174] | 1968 | 30/F | 2,820 | — | — | Two nodules, solid, yellowish-white central necrosis | Dead |
| Smith and Rele[175] | 1972 | 37/M | 7,325 | — | — | Massive, right lobe, solid, soft and fleshy | Dead |
| Walter et al.[176] | 1972 | 66/M | 1,780 | — | — | Multinodular lobe, solid, elastic | Living and well 1 yr after lobectomy |
| Alrenga[177] | 1975 | 51/M | 1,200 | — | — | Massive, right lobe, solid, grayish-white | Dead |

Abbreviations: NED, no evidence of disease.
*Weight of the operative specimen.

## PRIMARY FIBROSARCOMA OF THE SPERMATIC CORD

Arlen and co-workers[182] reviewed the world literature in 1969 and found 21 cases, including one of their own. This tumor presents as a firm, nontender, irregular mass that does not transilluminate and can be separated from the testicle. Orchiectomy with high ligation of the cord is the minimum therapy required. The patient described by Arlen and coworkers[182] was referred four months after orchiectomy with a large inguinal tumor, but died before therapy was instituted.

Fibrosarcomas are extremely rare in male genitalia. Dehner and Smith[183] made an exhaustive study of all soft tissue tumors of the penis in the files of the AFIP and found only 22 cases. Of these, two were fibrosarcomas, and one was a dermatofibrosarcoma protuberans. One of the two patients with fibrosarcoma died with pulmonary metastases within one year of therapy, and the other patient was lost to follow-up.

## FIBROSARCOMA OF THE BLOOD VESSELS

Primary sarcomas of the blood vessels are rare, and fibrosarcomas are rarer still.[184–200] Abell[201] described one case of fibrosarcoma of the inferior vena cava. Lunning[202] reported one of the femoral vein, and de Vries[203] reported a spindle cell sarcoma, probably a fibrosarcoma, of the small veins of the thigh. Fibrosarcomas of the systemic arteries are also extremely rare.[204–215] Salm,[204] in 1972, reported 13 cases of fibrosarcoma of the aorta, including one of his own. The cases reported by Sladden,[216] Bowles et al.[217] and Blenkinsopp and Hobbs[218] should be excluded from consideration, since they do not satisfy the histologic criteria for fibrosarcoma. Furthermore, in our opinion, the cases reported by Auffermann,[207] Detrie,[208] Karhoff,[211] and Kattus et al.[219] do not fulfill the criteria for fibrosarcoma and should also be excluded. There is no denial that these four cases represent sarcomas, but whether they can be considered fibrosarcomas is open to question. Therefore, only eight documented cases of fibrosarcoma of the aorta are recorded in the literature.

Salm,[204] in a superb analysis of the subject, described three main tumor types, namely, polypoidal and intraluminal, intimal, and adventitial. The intimal and polypoidal types frequently cause clinical vascular occlusions. However, the other types can produce myriad symptoms, and a clinical diagnosis is almost impossible. In the polypoidal types, if a preoperative diagnosis is made, these lesions can be removed. Resection of

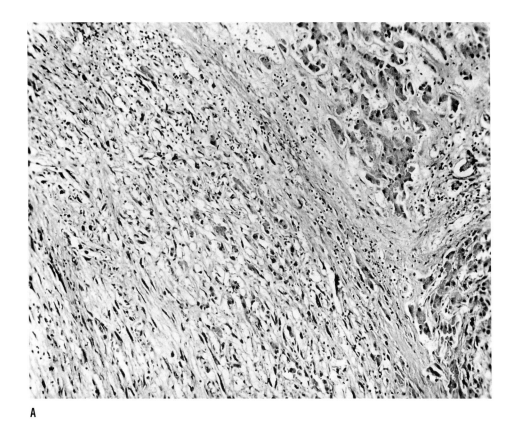

A

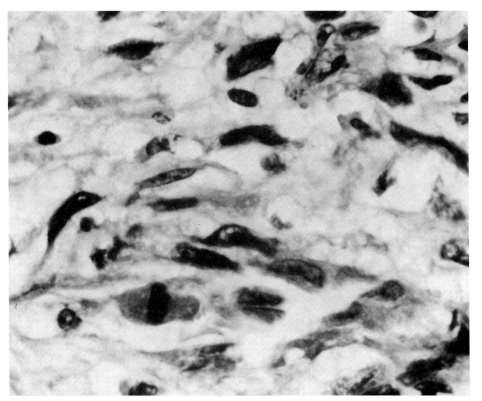

B

**Figure 8–18.** (**A**) Fibrosarcoma of liver. Diagnosis was made at autopsy. (H & E. Original magnification × 100.) (**B**) Higher magnification of malignant cells with a mitotic figure. (H & E. Original magnification × 500.) *(Courtesy of Dr. D. P. Alrenga, Department of Pathology, Cook County Hospital, and J. B. Lippincott.)*

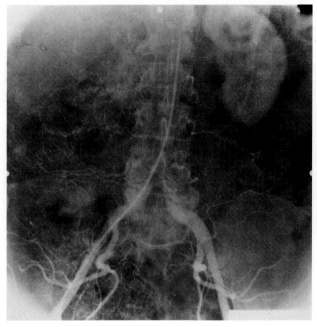

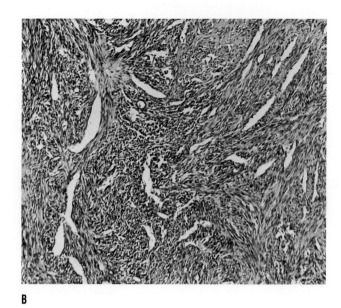

**Figure 8–19.** (**A**) Aortogram showing the recurrent renal fibrosarcoma on the right. Note the neovascularity in the right lumbar region. (**B**) Micrograph of the original renal fibrosarcoma. (H & E. Original magnification × 100.)

the segment of the artery containing the tumor, with replacement grafting, is the treatment of choice. Cure following this resection is rare, however.

In 1972, Burns and co-workers[220] reported a case in a 31-year-old man who had repair of a lacerated superficial femoral vessel by a woven Teflon-Dacron graft. Ten years later, he was admitted with an 8 × 10 cm mass in the left thigh that was found to be a fibrosarcoma. A wide soft tissue resection was performed, and 7 cm of the graft intimately adherent to the tumor was excised. This is probably the only documented case of fibrosarcoma developing after implantation of a vascular graft.

## FIBROSARCOMA OF THE BONE

Fibrosarcoma of the bone is a malignant fibroblastic tumor characterized by interlacing bundles of collagen fibers, lacking any tendency to form neoplastic bone, osteoid, or cartilage, either in its primary site or in its metastases. Until recently, there was some controversy regarding the nature of this tumor.[101,221,222] Today, it is generally agreed that fibrosarcoma of the bone is a distinct entity that can arise as a primary tumor of the skeletal system in either a medullary (central) or periosteal (peripheral) location.[222–224]

Dahlin and Ivins[223] found that fibrosarcomas of the bone constituted 23 percent of the primary bone sarcomas in the files of the Mayo Clinic. Huvos and Higginbotham[225] reported that primary fibrosarcomas of

the bone constituted 5 percent of all bony neoplasms treated at Memorial Sloan-Kettering Cancer Center.

Fibrosarcoma of the bone is found in all age groups and is about equally divided between the sexes. No racial predilection has been found in any of the larger series.[92,221–223,225] Any bone can be involved; however, Dahlin and Ivins[223] did not find any tumor in the hands or feet in their series. Usually there is a predilection for long tubular bones; for example, Huvos and Higginbotham[225] found 43 in the femur, 16 in the humerus, and 12 in the tibia in their series of 130 cases. The relative distribution of medullary and periosteal fibrosarcoma is similar. The tumor can be multifocal, and multiple separate areas of involvement can be found in the same bone.[225]

Pain and swelling are the most common symptoms, and associated roentgenologic findings of cystic lesions on the corresponding bone should arouse suspicion of a malignant lesion. The diagnosis can be established only by histologic examination of the biopsy specimen.

The treatment of fibrosarcoma of a long bone has primarily been amputation of the extremity.[222–225] However, when the lesions are located in areas in which an en bloc resection is possible, the tumors are treated accordingly. Huvos and Higginbotham[225] found that, when clinically feasible, an en bloc resection produced survival rates similar to those for major amputation.

Radiation therapy as a primary form of treatment has not been tried extensively. However, from limited trials to date, the results are not comparable to those achieved with resection.[223] From a theoretical standpoint, there is no reason to assume that the principle of wide resection and postoperative radiation therapy will not yield comparable end results as observed in the common type of soft tissue fibrosarcomas.

The end result of treatment of fibrosarcoma of the bone is better than that for osteogenic sarcoma. Cunningham and Arlen[222] reported a 29.6 percent five-year survival. Dahlin and Ivins[223] had an overall survival rate of 28.7 percent. In their series, patients with grade 2 tumors had a 40 percent five-year survival rate; grade 3, 30.8 percent; and grade 4, 13.6 percent. Huvos and Higginbotham[225] reported the overall five-year disease-free survival for fibrosarcoma of the bone as 34 percent. The 10-year, 15-year, and 20-year survival rates in their series were 28 percent, 27 percent, and 25 percent, respectively. According to these authors, it is more meaningful to use 10- and 15-year survival rates as indicators of cure.

## ■ FIBROUS TUMORS OF INFANCY AND CHILDHOOD

Fibrous tumors of infancy and childhood are usually benign. Although some of these tumors or tumorlike conditions microscopically resemble their adult counterparts, these entities are distinct and must be treated as such. Of all the fibrous tissue tumors encountered, the following are probably the most common.

### CONGENITAL FIBROMATOSIS

In its localized form, congenital fibromatosis is usually confined to an extremity and sometimes is erroneously designated as congenital fibrosarcoma.[29,99,100,106,107] But these tumors are definitely benign, and radical therapy must be avoided. In our experience, they are totally self-limiting and spontaneously regress. Nevertheless, the generalized form, as opposed to the localized, may have serious consequences. Occasionally an infant is born with multiple tumors all over the body, and this disease can be fatal. Teng and co-workers,[226] however, reported a case of the generalized form in which the tumors spontaneously regressed. Bartlett et al.[227] described a familial tendency to these tumors in one family.

### FIBROMATOSIS COLI (STERNOMASTOID TUMOR, CONGENITAL TORTICOLLIS)

Fibromatosis coli is a congenital fibrous replacement of the sternomastoid muscle. The replacement may represent a localized swelling (sternomastoid tumor), multiple small swellings, or diffuse involvement of the entire sternomastoid muscle.

The etiologic factors are unknown, but the association of the manifestation with difficult and prolonged labor in childbirth and its occasional relationship to forceps delivery has led to the assumption that probably torticollis (wryneck) is the result of some form of birth trauma. The entity is so rare that a definitive cause-and-effect relationship to trauma has not been proved. In 1948, Chandler[228] reviewed 101 cases of torticollis and suggested a hereditary relationship.

The mass usually becomes evident within one to two weeks after birth, gradually increases in size, and reaches its maximum growth by the end of the first month, after which regression sets in. It usually regresses slowly, but occasionally it disappears in a few weeks. An infant in whom the entire sternomastoid muscle is involved may, after a few months, hold its head toward the affected side, and torticollis may set in. Unless care is taken to avoid this postural deformity at the onset, concomitant asymmetry of the eyes, clavicle, and shoulder may develop. There may even be pain, requiring some form of therapy for the associated conditions.

The best treatment for fibromatosis coli of any intensity is to prevent the postural deformity that might occur. Therefore, parents must be instructed to observe the child closely, and any tendency toward wryneck must be checked by persuading the child not to hold his or her head on the affected side. Although attempts have been made to excise the localized lesions, this is not necessary, since almost all these tumors sooner or later regress.

### JUVENILE APONEUROTIC FIBROMA

Keasbey,[229] in 1953, first described juvenile aponeurotic fibroma as an entity arising in the hands and feet of children and called attention to its microscopic similarity to fibrosarcoma. Although it has a propensity for recurring after inadequate excision, it is benign and not life-threatening. It usually presents as a slow-growing tumor in the hands and feet of children, especially the palms or soles. Sometimes, these tumors are calcified, and roentgenograms show calcified nodules within the main tumor body. Keasbey,[229] Keasbey and Fanselau,[230] Lichtenstein and Goldman,[231] Goldman,[232] and Allen and Enzinger[233] reviewed the clinicopathologic features of a total of 59 such cases. There are four cases in the files of the University of Illinois: three in the upper extremities and one in the lower. About 70 percent of cases occur in the upper extremities. In this collected series of 63 cases, only one was in the head and neck region. Although the histologic features are of great interest and the tumors frequently infiltrate the surrounding subcutaneous tissue, tendons, and muscles, they actually are benign. Therefore, treatment should be conservative, and the major accent must be on obtaining a proper histologic diagnosis. A hurried misinterpretation of the histologic findings, especially when there is local recurrence, may lead to unnecessary radical therapy in these young patients.

## RECURRING DIGITAL FIBROMAS OF CHILDHOOD

Recurring digital fibroma is a rare form of juvenile fibromatosis characterized by the appearance of nodular tumors in the fingers and toes of young children. These tumors have a high propensity for recurring; instances are on record of multiple recurrences, even after apparently adequate local excision of the initial tumor.

Reye,[234] in 1965, first focused attention on this variant of fibromatosis by reporting six such cases in children. Similar case reports were published by Ahlquist and co-workers[235] and Shapiro.[236] Battifora and Hines[237] reported an additional case in 1971. It is conceivable that other cases have been found and probably have been reported without subclassification into the category of recurring digital fibromas. The treatment is local excision and, even in the presence of local recurrence or multicentricity, major excision is not warranted.

## PROGRESSIVE FIBROSING MYOSITIS (PROGRESSIVE MYOSITIS FIBROSA)

Progressive myositis fibrosa is a rare juvenile disorder in which fibrous tissue proliferation infiltrates the surrounding muscles and blood vessels, resulting in degeneration of muscle fibers and leading to various bizarre-shaped tumors. Stewart and MacGregor[238] found only 11 authenticated cases.

The child usually shows progressive and rapid involvement of numerous muscle groups, generally within the first five years of life. Despite the muscle involvement, the patient usually suffers little interference with normal health. There is complete absence of pain, tenderness, or any other systemic manifestation. Although this entity differs from progressive muscular dystrophy, the end result of both disease processes is the same. No known curative treatment exists, but the judicious use of physiotherapy and occupational therapy is indicated.

## INFANTILE DESMOID

Infantile desmoid was first identified by Stout.[99] These tumors are rare in infancy and childhood; however, in the few case reports published to date, they behave very much like their adult counterparts (i.e., they grow in size, infiltrate the surrounding structures, and, depending on the location, the symptoms vary from a solitary growing tumor to pain, tenderness, and inability to move the affected limb or the neck, which occurs in instances where these tumors arise in the head and neck region). Wide excision is the therapy of choice.

## ■ FIBROUS HISTIOCYTIC TUMORS

### BENIGN VARIETIES

#### Fibrous Histiocytomas

Fibrous histiocytomas are usually seen as small cutaneous or subcutaneous nodules covered by intact skin.[239] When located in the skin, these tumors have also been referred to as sclerosing angioma, dermatofibroma, and by a host of other names. They can remain localized over long periods without infiltration of the surrounding subcutaneous tissue. A conservative excision for histologic diagnosis is adequate therapy.

Fibrous histiocytomas have been reported in sites other than subcutaneous tissues, most commonly the lung. Grossman and associates[240] described one case and discussed other case reports in the literature. Although some authors have reported that pulmonary fibrous histiocytomas apparently behave like malignant tumors, unquestionable histologic and clinical proof of malignancy is lacking. Fibrous histiocytomas can occasionally be pigmented and can be clinically mistaken for a nodular malignant melanoma (Fig. 8–20A). The larger variety of these tumors can even mimic a dermatofibrosarcoma protuberans (Fig. 8–20B). Treatment consists of excision of the nodule.

#### Xanthogranuloma

Xanthogranulomas, like their counterparts, fibrous histiocytomas, exclusively occur in the skin and subcutis. These tumors frequently occur in children (juvenile xanthogranulomas). In most cases, these lesions regress (especially in children), and active intervention is not required. However, some are excised for cosmetic reasons.

#### Xanthoma

Xanthoma is a localized collection of lipid-filled histiocytes. It resembles a tumor and is usually associated with various hyperlipidimic states. Although, when seen in cutis or dermis, they appear as true neoplasms, once the diagnosis of the underlying cause is established, any form of excision is not indicated.

#### Rosai-Dorfman Disease

Since the original description by Rosai and Dorfman[241] of sinus histiocytes with massive lymphadenopathy, a number of extranodal cases resembling soft tissue sarcomas have been identified.[242] Patients with soft tissue

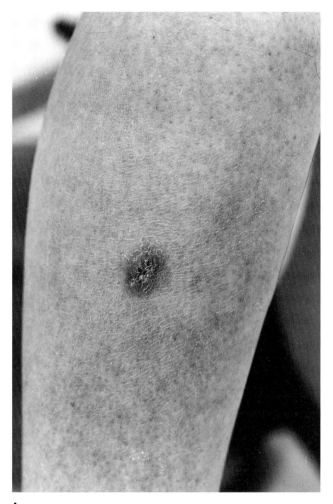

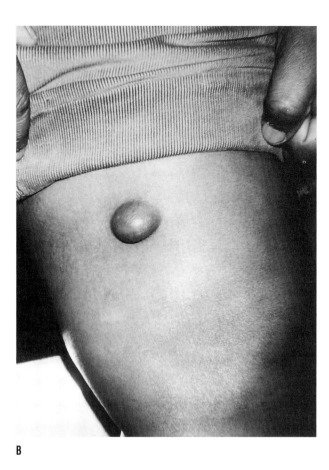

**Figure 8–20.** (**A**) Fibrous histiocytoma on the anterior aspect of the leg in a 40-year-old woman. She was referred to us with a presumptive diagnosis of malignant melanoma. (**B**) An umbilicated nodular lesion on the anteromedial aspect of the thigh of a 48-year-old woman. The umbilication and tense overlying skin mimic an early dermatofibrosarcoma protuberans.

Rosai-Dorfman disease are usually older and are usually cured after an adequate excision with histologically clear margins.

## FIBROUS HISTIOCYTIC TUMORS OF INDETERMINATE MALIGNANCY

### Dermatofibrosarcoma Protuberans

Darier and Ferrand[243] first described dermatofibrosarcoma protuberans, a relatively rare entity, in 1924. However, Hoffman,[244] in 1925, actually named the tumor *dermatofibrosarcoma protuberans*. Since these original descriptions, several case reports and series reports have appeared in the literature.[245–250] Although this is a relatively rare tumor, its clinical features have been adequately documented. McPeak and associates[249] reported that about two new patients are seen each year at Memorial Sloan-Kettering Cancer Center. The incidence in our institution is similar.

***Sex, Age, and Race.*** In our series of 28 patients, 16 were men and 12 were women. Taylor and Helwig[248] reported a fourfold higher incidence in males, probably because all their patients were from the files of the AFIP.

The tumor occurs in all age groups, but most frequently between the ages of 20 and 40 years. These tumors are rarely encountered in childhood.[251] The youngest patient reported by McPeak et al.[249] was seven years old. All races appear to be equally affected.

Although the tumor most commonly arises in the trunk (Fig. 8–21A and 8–21B), no anatomic location is spared (Fig. 8–22A to 8–22C). The tumor characteristically appears in early adult life as a small cutaneous nodule. It is rather firm and has a violaceous red color. Pressure on the surface on the nodule causes it to blanch. The periphery of the tumor infiltrates the adjacent skin and subcutaneous tissue, and other circumferentially located nodules may form. Coalescence of

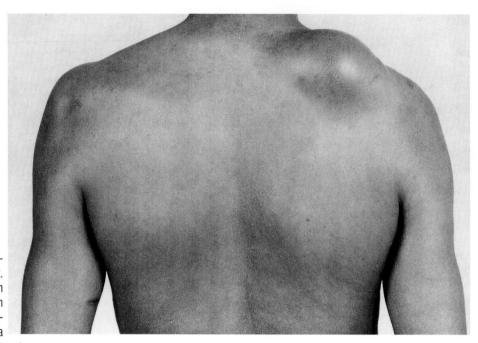

**Figure 8–21. (A)** Primary dermatofibroma protuberans on the posterior trunk. Patient stated the tumor grew to its size in four years. **(B)** A long-standing tumor in the scapular region showing the coalescence of a number of nodules, forming a plaque.

**A**

these nodules forms a fibrotic plaque in the dermis (Fig. 8–21B). After a few years, the nodular protrusions appear on the surface of the plaque, and at this stage, their growth frequently accelerates. The overlying skin is stretched and undergoes atrophic changes that lead to heightened susceptibility to trauma, resulting sometimes in superficial ulceration (Fig. 8–22C). In the initial stages, the rate of growth of these tumors is slow; consequently, a lesion on the back may have a history of onset ranging from a few months to several years. A well-developed dermatofibrosarcoma protuberans has such a characteristic appearance that, in most instances, a correct clinical diagnosis is possible.

Darier and Ferrand's[243] descriptive term *progressive and recurrent dermatofibroma* aptly describes the notorious tendency of these neoplasms to recur after excision. The local recurrence rate of the tumor stems from its infiltrative ability, which is not widely appreciated. Condensation of connective tissue at the periphery may give a false appearance of encapsulation, but actually the tumor may extend well beyond the apparent margins in fine microscopic projections. Usually this occurs in the adjacent subcutaneous fat, but deep fascia, muscle, and bone are similarly vulnerable. Inability to comprehend the infiltrative potential of this tumor results in local recurrence. McPeak et al.[249] reported that 21 of their patients had a collective total of 75 excisions prior to admission to Memorial Sloan-Kettering Cancer Center. Recurrences are probably a regrowth of residual disease following incomplete removal. Sometimes patients for whom an apparently total excision of the tumor had been performed have been sent to the Uni-

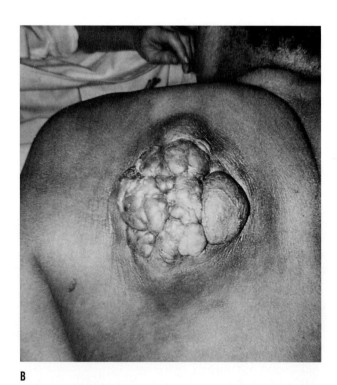

**B**

versity of Illinois, but on further elective excision, residual tumors were discovered. Similar experiences have been reported by other authors.[246,247,249]

The ideal treatment for dermatofibrosarcoma protuberans is wide excision. Although it is imprudent to try to define the parameters of excision in mathematical terms, upon review of the pertinent literature and from our own experience we would recommend a 4-cm

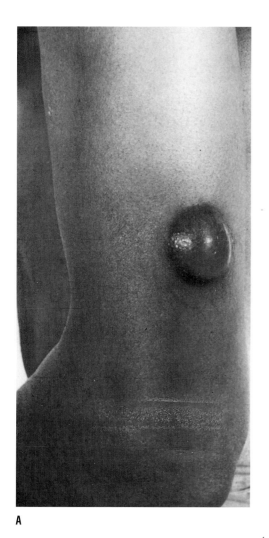

**A**

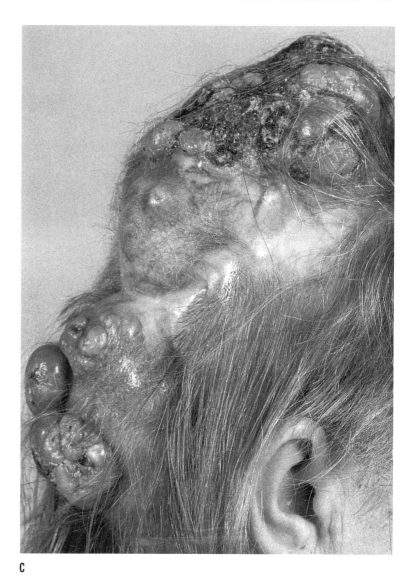

**C**

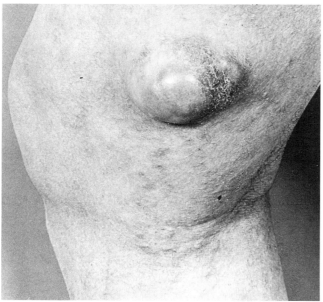

**B**

**Figure 8–22.** (**A**) Early tumor in the arm of a 29-year-old man, clinically thought to be a sclerosing angioma. (**B**) Dermatofibrosarcoma protuberans in the lower part of thigh in a 38-year-old woman. Note the umbilication of the primary tumor with a satellite nodule. (**C**) A neglected primary tumor of the scalp with ulceration and necrosis.

margin on all sides, including the deep fascia as well as part of the underlying muscle, if the location of the tumor necessitates such an excision. The skin closure in most cases would therefore require a skin graft. Based on this concept, even after apparent total excision of a primary tumor, if the margins of excision are not according to the guidelines described above, an elective reexcision is advised.

In general, dermatofibrosarcoma protuberans does not metastasize to the regional nodes, and therefore a routine node dissection is not indicated. However, rare instances of a malignant variant with the potential to metastasize to the regional nodes have been reported,[252] and in such instances node dissection might be required.

Of the 68 patients treated by us, 46 had an intact primary and the remaining 22 were seen with a locally recurrent tumor. Of the 46 patients treated for the primary tumor, one developed local recurrence (2 percent). Six of the 22 patients with locally recurrent tumor(s) required massive soft tissue resection for cure. McPeak and co-workers[249] reported 3 recurrences out of 27 primary tumors (11 percent), and Pack and Taba[246] had 8 (20.5 percent) local recurrences out of 39 primary tumors. Although these two groups recognized the need for adequate wide excision, neither performed as wide an excision as is recommended here. In contrast, in Taylor and Helwig's[248] collected series of 98 cases, the local recurrence rate after conservative excision was 49 percent. It appears that conservative excision has no place in the management of these tumors.

Local recurrence usually happens within the first two years after the primary excision, but recurrences have been noted as late as seven or eight years later. Local recurrence probably constitutes the only major problem in the management of dermatofibrosarcoma protuberans. It is not generally recognized that, with every local recurrence, the biologic behavior of this tumor changes,[248] and after several recurrences, the tumor can become lethal (Fig. 8–23). The primary objective, therefore, is to avoid local recurrence.

The question has often been posed as to whether there is a true malignant variant of a dermatofibrosarcoma protuberans that arises de novo. Although, in our opinion, the rare malignant variety is the result of multiple inadequate excisions of the primary tumors, we have three instances in our files in which the probability of primary malignant dermatofibrosarcoma protuberans can be assumed. One is a case in which the patient presented us with a neglected case of dermatofibrosarcoma protuberans of 15 years' duration. The case is briefly illustrated below.

***Case Report.***
A 64-year-old man was admitted with complaints of a rapidly growing swelling on the medial side of the right

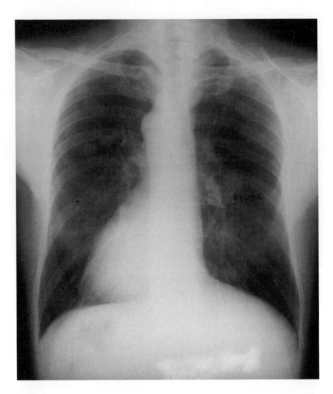

**Figure 8–23.** This 55-year-old man was inadequately operated on for a dermatofibrosarcoma of the skin of the forehead. This resulted in a locally recurrent tumor. He was referred to our clinic after three local excisions and a course of radiation therapy proved unsuccessful in treating the tumor, which had recurred for the fourth time. Although a review of the original histologic material showed it to be a dermatofibrosarcoma protuberans, by this time the patient had pulmonary metastases. He died six months later.

scapula and intermittent bleeding from the mass of several months' duration. The tumor on the back was 8 × 5 × 6 cm, protuberant, nodular, ulcerating, nontender, and firm. It was situated 2.5 cm medial to the inner border of the right scapula. The right axillary lymph nodes were enlarged (5 × 5 cm), hard, matted, and fixed to the chest wall. A chest roentgenogram revealed a right superior mediastinal mass and various nodular densities in both lung fields, suggestive of metastatic disease. Further investigation suggested metastatic disease into the vertebrae and sixth rib and infiltration of the left lobe of the liver. An incisional biopsy of the main mass and a biopsy of both axillary nodes were performed. The right axillary lymph nodes were totally replaced by metastatic tumor (Fig. 8–24A). The patient was treated with systemic chemotherapy but died within six months of initial diagnosis. An autopsy revealed diffuse involvement of the visceral system (Fig. 8–24B).

Brenner and associates[250] described a patient with inguinal node metastases synchronous with a primary intact tumor in the foot. Therefore, an ab initio development of malignant dermatofibrosarcoma protuberans is a possibility, albeit rare. For the present, however, it is more appropriate to consider that, in most cases,

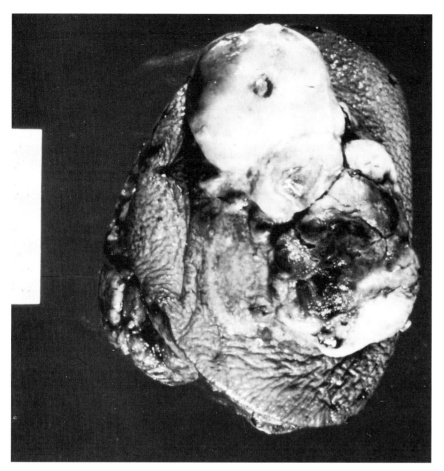

**A**

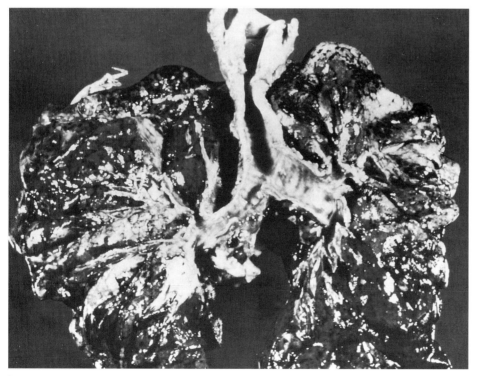

**B**

**Figure 8–24.** (**A**) Right axillary lymph node showing metastatic involvement with fungation. (**B**) Involvement of the lung is apparent.

multiple local recurrences probably initiate malignant transformation. The incidence of regional lymphatic metastases is so small that, even in patients with multiple local recurrences without obvious nodal enlargement, elective node dissection is not required.

Shmookler et al.[253] identified a juvenile analogue of adult dermatofibrosarcoma protuberans. The investigators termed this tumor *giant cell fibroblastoma.* It is an extremely rare form of tumor. If encountered, it should be managed like its adult counterpart.

### Bednar Tumor (Pigmented Dermatofibrosarcoma Protuberans)

Although the original description by Bednar presumed these tumors to be storiform neurofibroma with melanin pigment,[254] the current convention is to consider Bednar tumors as variants of dermatofibrosarcoma protuberans with melanin pigmentation. These tumors are uncommon,[255] and in general should be treated in a similar manner as the usual variety of dermatofibrosarcoma protuberans.

In recent years, two other fibrohistiocytic tumors have been described: angiomatoid fibrous histiocytoma[256] and plexiform fibrous histiocytic tumor.[257] Both appear to have some malignant potential (intermediate variety), and, when diagnosed, should be treated using the same general principles used in the treatment of dermatofibrosarcoma protuberans. In general, these tumors are found in young adults; thus, considerable attention should be given before the diagnosis is accepted.

### MALIGNANT FIBROUS HISTIOCYTOMA

Malignant fibrous histiocytoma is now a well-accepted clinicopathologic entity. The other terms commonly used to describe it are *malignant fibrous xanthoma* and *fibroxanthosarcoma.* Weiss and Enzinger[258] suggested that malignant fibrous histiocytoma is the most common soft tissue sarcoma of late adult life, and that, in the past, many of these tumors were erroneously diagnosed as liposarcoma, fibrosarcoma, or rhabdomyosarcoma. Histologically, malignant fibrous histiocytoma is currently subdivided into four types: (1) storiform-pleomorphic, (2) myxoid, (3) giant cell type, and (4) inflammatory type.[259–261] The histopathologic details of these subsets are discussed in detail in Chapter 5. The clinical features, however, are rather similar, and so, in this section, these features are collectively

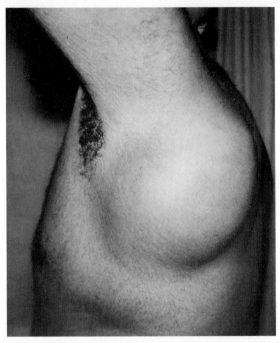

**A**

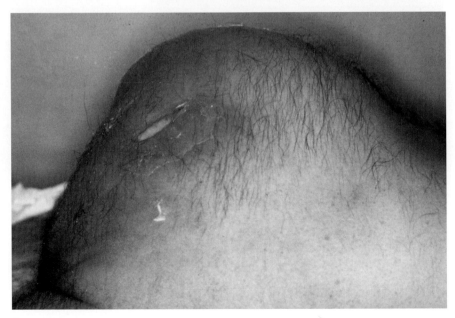

**Figure 8–25.** **(A)** Malignant fibrous histiocytoma of the left arm and trunk. Note the superficial location of the tumor. A wide excision with a skin graft provided local control. **(B)** Deep-seated malignant fibrous histiocytoma. This young man was treated for three to four months with heat and antibiotics on the presumptive diagnosis of a buttock abscess. When the swelling continued to increase in size, an attempted incision and drainage pointed to the true identity of the swelling. We attempted local control of the tumor by excising the buttock, but the tumor was extensive, and a hemipelvectomy with anterior flap was performed. The patient remained well for 16 months but died of massive intra-abdominal disease. *(Continued.)*

**B**

described. In instances where there are specific differences in the end results, they have been appropriately pointed out.

### Age, Sex, and Race

These tumors are seen in all age groups, but more commonly in patients between the ages of 50 and 70 years. Both sexes are about equally involved, and no racial predilection has been observed in any of the published series[114,258,262–265] or in our own clinical material.

### Location

Malignant fibrous histiocytomas can occur in all parts of the human body. However, they are more frequent in the skeletal muscles of the extremities and then the retroperitoneum. Occasionally, they arise in the subcutaneous tissues above the deep fascia (Fig. 8–25A). The anatomic location plays a role in the size of the initial tumor and has a distinct influence on the prognosis. Superficially located tumors are smaller, whereas the deep-seated ones are larger (Fig. 8–25B to 8–25D). Soule and Enriquez[264] suggested that the size at initial presentation has no prognostic significance. Weiss and Enzinger[258] analyzed the clinical behavior and size of the primary tumor in 151 of the 200 cases from the files of the AFIP to find a correlation between the size of the tumor and the incidence of local recurrence and metastases. Tumors smaller than 2.5 cm had a 50 percent

incidence of local recurrence and 21 percent of metastases. In contrast, for tumors larger than 5 cm, the local recurrence rate was 47 percent, and the incidence rate of metastasis was 34 percent. From a study of our patients, it appears that anatomic location and size play significant roles in the incidence of recurrence and metastases.

The presenting symptom in all our patients was the presence of a tumor of short duration. Weiss and Enzinger[258] also found that, in their collected series, the history usually was of less than six months' duration.

### Treatment

In all reported series,[114,258,262–265] including our own, these tumors have been primarily treated by excision. Currently, however, in most centers, including our own, supplemental radiation therapy is more a rule than exception after a wide soft tissue resection in extremity malignant fibrous histiocytomas that are larger than 5 cm in diameter. However, radiation therapy alone as the primary form of treatment is not advisable. In the past,[114,262,265] because of conservative excision, the incidence of local recurrence was high, in the range of 44 to 60 percent (Fig. 8–26A and 8–26B). However, today, with better understanding of the natural history of the disease and an initial aggressive surgical

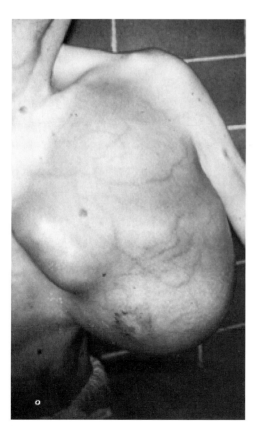

C

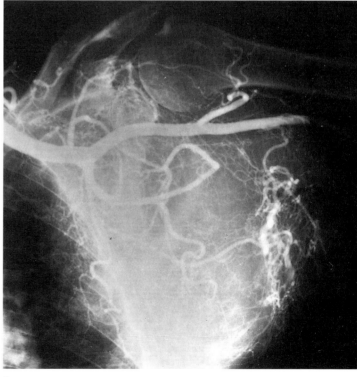

D

**Figure 8–25** *(continued).* (**C**) A neglected case of malignant fibrous histiocytoma of the chest wall. (**D**) Angiogram showing extensive neovascularity. No attempt was made to treat this patient, and he died of diffuse metastases three months later.

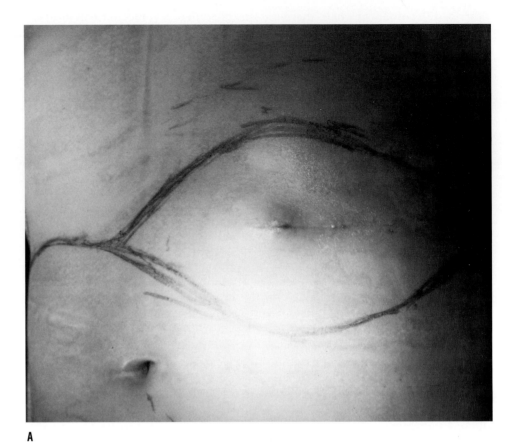

**A**

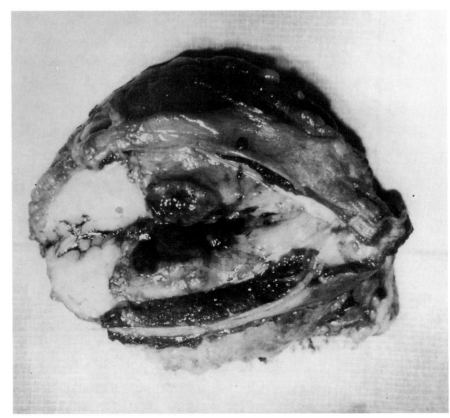

**Figure 8–26.** (**A**) Locally recurrent malignant fibrous histiocytoma of the anterior abdominal wall in a 48-year-old woman. Nine months previously, she had first noticed a small (3 × 2 cm) tumor. A conservative excision of the primary tumor was performed, but within six months the mass recurred. We performed a wide resection of the tumor, including the anterior abdominal wall. (**B**) Gross appearance of the tumor. Within six months of the second excision, she developed massive intra-abdominal disease and pulmonary metastases and died.

**B**

approach, the local recurrence rate is considerably lower. In our own material, when the patients were first treated with intact primary or with incisional biopsy, the local recurrence rate has been 6 percent.

A wide soft tissue excision and, when indicated, a regional node dissection is the therapy of choice. The incidence of regional node involvement is much less than what was previously thought. Based on the review of the literature[266] and our own experience, it appears that the incidence of regional node metastases in primary malignant fibrous histiocytoma of all subtypes probably varies between 10 and 12 percent.

## End Results

We have treated 92 patients with malignant fibrous histiocytoma; 75 are eligible for 10-year survival analysis. Forty-seven (63 percent) of these 75 are still free of tumor after ten years (Table 8–9). The incidence of local recurrence has been reported as ranging between 20 and 44 percent.[114,151,258,263] The recurrence rate of 6 percent (three patients) in our series shows the value of initial aggressive surgical therapy. Most reports with this entity have come from pathologists[114,258,262–265] who did not have the opportunity to plan therapy. Therefore, the term *wide resection*, as used by these authors, may not have the same meaning as used in this text. Wide soft tissue resection with preservation of functional limbs performed in our patients has consistently led to a lower incidence of local recurrence in all types of sarcoma, including malignant fibrous histiocytoma. Weiss and Enzinger[258] compared local recurrence rates between wide resection and amputation in two groups of 12 and 13 patients, respectively. In the first group, 58 percent had recurrence, and the other had none. However, as mentioned above, the validity of this comparison is open to question. Weiss and Enzinger[258] found a two-year survival rate of 60 percent and a local recurrence rate of 42 percent in their collected series of 200 patients. Soule and Enriquez[264] reported a 65 percent five-year survival rate and 38 per-

cent 10-year survival rate. It is difficult to calculate the exact survival rate in the series of Kempson and Kyriakos,[262] since their follow-up data were not complete. Lindberg and associates[151] reported that conservative surgery and postoperative radiation therapy yielded a survival rate of 65 percent and 56 percent for two and five years, respectively. Our clinical data suggest that an initial aggressive therapeutic approach reduces local recurrence and improves ultimate survival. Soule and Enriquez[264] emphasized that these tumors can recur or metastasize, or both, even after five years. We had similar experience with ten patients in whom metastases developed five years after initial therapy. Thus, our current 10-year survival rate is only 63 percent compared to a five-year survival of 76 percent.

## Prognostic Factors

Malignant fibrous histiocytoma is an aggressive form of sarcoma, and, unless adequately treated initially with wide excision and (if indicated) regional node dissection along with postoperative radiation therapy, the salvage rate from the standpoint of both local recurrence and metastases will be low.

Of the factors controlling the prognosis, the location in relation to the surrounding tissues, the size, and the histologic grading appear to be most significant. If the tumors are located superficially in the subcutaneous tissue or the deep fascia, and the size is smaller than 5 cm, the prognosis for patients with a low-grade tumor, after the therapy outlined above, is better than that for patients with a tumor larger than 5 cm that arises in an underlying muscle or the retroperitoneum, or is of a higher grade.

## Miscellaneous Sites

McCarthy and associates[267] described 35 primary cases of malignant fibrous histiocytoma of the bone. Spanier and co-workers[268] studied 11 cases and drew some general guidelines for management. In their opinion, a combination of chemotherapy and radiation therapy might be of value. The average survival time was 12 months in six of nine patients who had no secondary treatment of their metastases.

Like fibrosarcomas, malignant fibrous histiocytomas have been found to occur in the oral cavity and the mandible,[269] larynx,[270] genitourinary tract,[271–273] gastrointestinal tract,[274] and mediastinum.[275] Since these are rare locations, every case should be recorded in detail for better understanding of its natural history.

Fibrous histiocytoma of the lung[240,276] has also been reported. Grossman and co-workers[240] described such a case and reviewed the pertinent literature. Approximately eight cases have been documented. A review of these case reports suggests that probably the authors were describing either a benign or atypical

**TABLE 8–9. END RESULT ACCORDING TO ANATOMIC SITE OF THE PRIMARY TUMORS (MFH) SEEN IN 92 PATIENTS (CURRENT SERIES)***

| Anatomic Site | No. Patients | 10 Yr, NED |
|---|---|---|
| Head and neck | 6 (4) | 3 |
| Trunk | 12 (9) | 5 |
| Upper extremities | 24 (20) | 13 |
| Lower extremities | 38 (34) | 24 |
| Retroperitoneum | 12 (8) | 2 |
| Total | 92 (75) | 47 (63%) |

Abbreviations: MFH, malignant fibrous histiocytoma.
*Numbers in parentheses denote patients eligible for 10-year survival analysis.

kind of fibrous histiocytoma. Although microscopic diagnosis of these tumors might be in question, there is no denying that malignant fibrous histiocytoma of the pulmonary parenchyma is a distinct possibility.[276]

Inflammatory types of malignant fibrous histiocytoma[263] are the most aggressive varieties, and the prognosis is disproportionately worse than the other three types. Thus, extremely aggressive initial therapy is recommended when the pathologist renders this diagnosis.

## ATYPICAL FIBROXANTHOMA

Atypical fibroxanthoma is a pleomorphic tumor that usually occurs in actinic damaged skin of the elderly, and is most commonly seen in the head and neck region. Grossly, it appears like a basal cell carcinoma or a squamous cell carcinoma. The correct histologic diagnosis is only made after a microscopic examination. From a clinical standpoint, these tumors should be considered as a cutaneous variety of malignant fibrous histiocytoma and be treated with a wider margin than is currently practiced in the management of basal cell cancer.

## MALIGNANT GIANT CELL FIBROUS HISTIOCYTOMA

Malignant giant cell tumors of the tendon sheath are rare tumors originally described by Berger[277] in 1938. Since then, several small series have been reported.[278–281] Giant cell type malignant fibrous histiocytoma is synonymous with malignant giant cell tumor of soft parts. In 1972, Guccion and Enzinger[282] analyzed 32 cases and delineated the clinical and pathologic features of these types of tumors. The patient age is usually between 41 and 80 years. These tumors occur predominantly in males; pain and the presence of a mass are the two most common complaints. The most important laboratory finding is roentgenographic evidence of a soft tissue mass eroding the cortex of the adjacent bone. These tumors are classified as superficial or deep. The superficial tumors are usually less than 5 cm, while the deep ones can grow up to 30 cm. The tumor is commonly seen in adult males and frequently occurs in the extremities. It has a tendency for local infiltration, and involvement of adjacent bones is not uncommon. The primary treatment is wide soft tissue resection with negative margins.

## REFERENCES

1. Konwaler BJ, Keasbey L, Kaplan L: Subcutaneous pseudosarcomatous fibromatosis fascitis: Report of 8 cases. Am J Clin Pathol 25:241, 1955
2. Bono JA: Nodular pseudosarcomatous fascitis: Two case reports and review of the literature. Am Surg 40:601, 1974
3. Patchetsky AS, Enzinger FM: Intravascular fascitis: A report of 17 cases. Am J Surg Pathol 5:29, 1981
4. Sormann GW: The headbangers tumor. Br J Plast Surg 35:72, 1982
5. Hutter RVP, Stewart FW, Foote FW Jr.: Fascitis: A report of 70 cases with follow-up proving the benignity of the lesion. Cancer 15:992, 1962
6. Enzinger FM, Weiss SW: Benign fibrous tissue tumors, In Enzinger FM, Weiss SW (eds): Soft Tissue Tumors, 3rd ed. St. Louis, Mosby-Yearbook, 1995, p 168
7. Hutter RVP, Foote FW Jr., Francis KC, Higginbotham NL: Parosteal fascitis: A self-limited benign process that stimulates a malignant neoplasm. Am J Surg 104:800, 1962
8. Toker C: Pseudosarcomatous fascitis: Further observations indicating the aggressiveness capabilities of this lesion and justifying the inclusion of this entity within the category of the fibromatoses. Ann Surg 174:996, 1971
9. Pulitzer DR, Martin PC, Reed RJ: Fibroma of tendon sheath: A clinicopathologic study of 33 cases. Am J Surg Pathol 13:472, 1989
10. Jarvi OH, Saxen AE, Hopsu-Havu VK, et al.: Elastofibroma—A degenerative pseudotumor. Cancer 23:42, 1969
11. Renshaw TS, Simon MA: Elastofibroma. J Bone Joint Surg 55A:409, 1973
12. Mirra JM, Straub LR, Jarvi OH: Elastofibroma of the deltoid: A case report. Cancer 33:234, 1974
13. Martin H, Ehrlich HE, Abels JC: Juvenile nasopharyngeal angiofibroma. Ann Surg 127:513, 1948
14. Chelius JM: System of Surgery, vol. 2 (translated by John F. South). London, Henry Renshaw, 1847
15. Shaheen HB: Nasopharyngeal fibroma. J Laryngol Otol 45:259, 1930
16. New GB, Figi FA: Treatment of fibromas of the nasopahrynx: Report of 32 cases. Am J Roentgenol 12:340, 1924
17. Friedberg SA: Vascular fibroma of the nasopharynx (nasopharyngeal fibroma). Arch Otol 31:313, 1940
18. Figi FA, Davis RE: Management of nasopharyngeal fibromas. Laryngoscope 60:794, 1950
19. Martin JS: Nasopharyngeal fibroma and its treatment. J Laryngol Otol 68:39, 1954
20. Sternberg SS: Pathology of juvenile nasopharyngeal angiofibroma: A lesion of adolescent males. Cancer 7: 15, 1954
21. MacComb WS: Juvenile nasopharyngeal fibroma. Am J Surg 106:754, 1963
22. Apostol JV, Frazell EL: Juvenile nasopharyngeal fibroma: A clinical study. Cancer 15:869, 1965
23. Conley J, Healy WV, Blaugrund SM, Perkin HZ: Nasopharyngeal angiofibroma in the juvenile. Surg Gynecol Obstet 126:825, 1968
24. Acuna RT: Nasopharyngeal fibroma. Acta Otolaryngol 75:119, 1973
25. Svoboda DJ, Kirchner F: Ultrastructure of nasopharyngeal angiofibromas. Cancer 19:1949, 1966
26. Horton CE, Crawford J, Oakley RS: Malignant change in keloids. Plast Reconstr Surg 112:383, 1953

27. Stout AP: The fibromatoses. Clin Orthop 19:11, 1961
28. Dupuytren G: Lecons orales de clinique chirurgicale faites a L'Hotel Dieu Paris, Paris, 1832, vol. 1, chap. 1. Translated: Permanent retraction of the fingers produced by an affection of the palmar fascia. Lancet 2:222, 1934
29. Pack GT, Ariel IA: Tumors of the Soft Somatic Tissue: A Clinical Treatise. New York, Hoeber-Harper, 1958
30. Rhode CM, Jennings WD Jr.: Dupuytren's contracture. Am Surg 33:8555, 1967
31. Skoog T: Dupuytren's contraction: With special reference to etiology and improved surgical treatment: Its recurrence in epileptics; note on knuckle pads. Acta Chir Scand Suppl 96(139):1, 1948
32. Conway H: Dupuytren's contracture. Am J Surg 87:101, 1954
33. Scott WW, Scardino PL: A new concept in the treatment of Peyronie's disease. South Med J 41:173, 1948
34. Burford EH, Glenn JE, Burford CE: Therapy of Peyronie's disease. Urol Cutan Rev 55:337, 1951
35. MacFarlane J: In Robertson D (ed): Clinical Reports of the Surgical Practice of the Glasgow Royal Infirmary, 1832, Robertson, p 32
36. Onion CT (ed): The Shorter Oxford English Dictionary on Historical Principles, 3rd ed. London, Oxford University Press, 1967
37. Müller J: Uber den fienern Bau und die Formen der Krankhaften Grechwulste. Berlin, G Reimer, 1838, p 80
38. Paget J: Fibronucleated tumor of the abdomen of fourteen years' growth: Removal. Lancet 1:625, 1856
39. Bennet JH: On Cancerous and Canceroid Growths. Edinburgh, Southerland & Knox, 1849, p 176
40. Sanger M: Uber desmoide Greschwulste der Bauchwand und deren operation mit resection des peritoneum parietale. Arch Gynak 24:1, 1884
41. Stone HB: Desmoid tumors of the abdominal wall. Ann Surg 48:175, 1908
42. Pack GT, Ehrlich HE: Neoplasms of the anterior abdominal wall with special consideration of desmoid tumors. Int Abst Surg 79:177, 1944
43. Dahn I, Jonsson N, Lundh G: Desmoid tumors, a series of 33 cases. Acta Chir Scandi 126:305, 1963
44. Brasfield RD, Das Gupta TK: Desmoid tumors of the anterior abdominal wall. Surgery 65:241, 1969
45. Keith A: Human Embryology and Morphology. London, Edward Arnold Ltd., 1948, p 50
46. Strode JE: Desmoid tumors, particularly as related to their surgical principles. Ann Surg 139:335, 1954
47. Nichols RW: Desmoid tumors: A report of thirty-one cases. Arch Surg 7:227, 1923
48. Mason JB: Desmoid tumors. Ann Surg 92:444, 1930
49. Musgrove JE, McDonald JR: Extra-abdominal desmoid tumors. Arch Pathol 45:513, 1948
50. Enzinger FM, Weiss SW: Fibrous tumors of infancy and childhood. In Enzinger FM, Weiss SW (eds): Soft Tissue Tumors, 3rd ed. St. Louis: Mosby-Yearbook, 1995, p 219
51. Geshickter EF, Lewis D: Tumors of connective tissue. Am J Cancer 25:630, 1935
52. Jardijvic D, Mardones E, Lipschutz A: Antifibromato-

genic activity of 19-Nor-α-ethinyltestosterone in the guinea pig. Proc Soc Exp Biol Med 91:38, 1956
53. Lim CL, Walker MJ, Mehta RR, Das Gupta TK: Estrogen and antiestrogen binding sites in desmoid tumors. Eur J Cancer Clin Oncol 22(5):583, 1986
54. Chaudhuri PK, Walker MJ, Beattie CW, Das Gupta TK: Presence of steroid receptors in human soft tissue sarcomas of diverse histological origin. Cancer Res 40:861, 1980
55. Ramsey RH: The pathology, diagnosis and treatment of extra-abdominal desmoid tumors. J Bone Joint Surg 37B:1012, 1955
56. Hunt RN, Morgan HC, Ackerman LV: Principles in the management of extra-abdominal desmoids. Cancer 13:285, 1960
57. Reitano JJ, Hayry P, Nykyri E, et al.: The desmoid tumors. I. Incidence, age, sex, and anatomical distribution in the Finnish population. Am J Clin Pathol 77:665, 1982
58. Das Gupta TK, Brasfield RD, O'Hara J: Extra-abdominal desmoids: A clinicopathologic study. Ann Surg 170(1):109, 1969
59. Rock MG, Pritchard DJ, Reiman HM, et al.: Extra-abdominal desmoid tumors. J Bone Joint Surg 66A:1369, 1984
60. Enzinger FM, Shiraki M: Musculo-aponeurotic fibromatosis of the shoulder girdle (extra-abdominal desmoid): Analysis of thirty cases followed up for ten or more years. Cancer 20:1131, 1967
61. Gonatas NK: Extra-abdominal desmoid tumors. Arch Pathol 71:217, 1961
62. Bowden L, Booher RJ: The principles and technique of resection of soft parts for sarcoma. Surgery 44:963, 1958
63. Paget J: Lectures on Surgical Pathology, 3rd ed. Philadelphia, Lindsay & Blakiston, 1865
64. Masson JK, Soule EH: Desmoid tumors of the head and neck. Am J Surg 112:615, 1966
65. Brodsky JT, Gordon MS, Hajdu SI, et al.: Desmoid tumors of the chest wall: A locally recurrent problem. J Thorac Cardiovasc Surg 104:900, 1992
66. Easter DW, Halasz NA: Recent trends in the management of desmoid tumors: Summary of 19 cases and review of the literature. Ann Surg 210:765, 1989
67. Markheda G, Lundgren L, Bjurstam N, et al.: Extra-abdominal desmoid tumor. Acta Orthop Scand 57:1, 1986
68. Lopez R, Kemalyan N, Mosely HS, et al.: Problems in diagnosis and management of desmoid tumors. Am J Surg 159:450, 1990
69. Gardner EJ, Richards RC: Multiple cutaneous and subcutaneous lesions occurring simultaneously with hereditary polyposis and osteomatosis. Am J Hum Genet 5:139, 1953
70. Hubbard TB Jr: Familial polyposis of the colon: The fate of the retained rectum after colectomy in children. Ann Surg 23:577, 1957
71. Smith WG: Desmoid tumors in familial multiple polyposis. Proc Staff Meet Mayo Clin 34:31, 1959
72. Gardner E: Follow-up study of Gardner's syndrome. Am J Hum Genet 14:376, 1962
73. Simpson RD, Harrison EG, Mayo CW: Mesenteric fibromatosis in familial polyposis. Cancer 17:526, 1964

74. Thomas KE, Watne AL, Johnson JG, et al.: Natural history of Gardner's syndrome. Am J Surg 115:218, 1968

75. Parks TG, Bussey HJR, Lockhart-Mummery HE: Familial polyposis of coli associated with extracolonic abnormalities. Gut 11:323, 1970

76. Jones TR, Nance FC: Periampullary malignancy in Gardner's syndrome. Ann Surg 185:565, 1977

77. Gold RS, Mucha SJ: Unique case of mesenteric fibrosis in multiple polyposis. Am J Surg 130:366, 1975

78. Okamoto M, Sato C, Kohno Y, et al.: Molecular nature of chromosome 5Q loss in colorectal tumors and desmoids from patients with familial adenomatous polyposis. Hum Genet 85:595, 1990

79. Pierce ER, Weisbord T, Mekusick VA: Gardner's syndrome: Formal genetics and statistical analysis of a large Canadian kindred. Clin Genet 1:65, 1970

80. Haggitt RC, Booth JL: Bilateral fibromatosis of the breast in Gardner's syndrome. Cancer 25:161, 1970

81. Penn D, Federman Q, Finkel M: Fibromatosis in Gardner's syndrome. Am J Gastroenterol 59:174, 1973

82. Mende S, Volpel M, Rotthauwe I: Idiopathic retroperitoneal fibrosis (Ormond's disease) with unusual extension involving the brain. Beitr Pathol 153:80, 1974

83. Skeel DA, Shols GW, Sullivan MJ, Witherington R: Retroperitoneal fibrosis with intrinsic ureteral involvement. J Urol 113:166, 1975

84. Cauble WG: Retroperitoneal fibrosis with bowel obstruction: Presentation of one case. Am J Proctol 25:75, 1974

85. Rothman D, Kendall AB: Bilateral ureteral entrapment by perianeurysmal fibrosis: Case reports. Vasc Surg 8:259, 1974

86. Ormond JK: Bilateral ureteral obstruction due to envelopment and compression by inflammatory retroperitoneal process. J Urol 59:1072, 1948

87. Ormond JK: Idiopathic retroperitoneal fibrosis: An established clinical entity. JAMA 174:1561, 1960

88. Temperley JM: Multifocal fibrosclerosis. Br J Clin Pract 28:217, 1974

89. Yacoub MH, Thompson VC: Chronic idiopathic pulmonary hilar fibrosis—A clinical pathologic entity. Thorax 26:365, 1971

90. Barrett NR: Idiopathic mediastinal fibrosis. Br J Surg 46:207, 1958

91. Tubbs OS: Superior vena caval obstruction due to chronic mediastinitis. Thorax 1:247, 1946

92. Jaffe HL: Tumors and Tumorous Conditions of Bones and Joints. Philadelphia, Lea & Febiger, 1958, p 298

93. Rabhan WN, Rosai J: Desmoplastic fibroma: Report of ten cases and review of the literature. J Bone Joint Surg 50:487, 1968

94. Cornil V, Ranvier L: A Manual of Pathological History. Philadelphia, Henry C Lea, 1880

95. Virchow R: Die Krankhafter Geschwulste. Berlin, Hirschwald, 1864–65

96. Birkett J: Contributions to the practical surgery of new growths or tumors. II. Fibroplastic growths. Guy's Hospital Reports 4(3):231, 1858

97. Billroth T: Lectures on Surgical Pathology and Therapeutics. London, The New Sydenham Society, 1877–78

98. Ewing J: Neoplastic Disease, 4th ed. Philadelphia, WB Saunders, 1942, p 164

99. Stout AP: Juvenile fibromatoses. Cancer 7:953, 1954

100. Stout AP: Fibrosarcoma in infants and children. Cancer 15:1028, 1962

101. Stout AP: Fibrosarcoma: The malignant tumor of fibroblasts. Cancer 1:30, 1948

102. Stout AP: The fibromatoses. Clin Orthop 19:11, 1961

103. Stout AP: Mesenchymal tumors of the soft tissues. Trans Stud Coll Physicians Phila 31:91, 1963

104. Stout AP: Recent observations on mesenchymal tumors in adults and children. Canad Med Assoc J 88:453, 1963

105. Pack GT, Ariel IA: Fibrosarcoma of the soft somatic tissues: A clinical and pathologic study. Surgery 31:443, 1952

106. Stout AP, Lattes R: Tumors of the soft tissues. Atlas of Tumor Pathology, Sec. 2, Fasc 1. Washington DC, AFIP, 1967

107. Chung EB, Enzinger FM: Infantile fibrosarcoma. Cancer 38:729, 1976

108. Kauffman SL, Stout AP: Congenital mesenchymal tumors. Cancer 18:460, 1965

109. Bruce KW, Royer RQ: Central fibromyxoma of the maxilla. Oral Surg 5:1277, 1952

110. da Silva Neto JB: Results of 22 cases of breast sarcoma over five years after surgery. Tumori 56:39, 1970

111. Malek RS, Utz DC, Farrow GM: Malignant tumors of the spermatic cord. Cancer 29:1108, 1972

112. Soft Tissue Tumors: Case 14, contributed by Hartney TX, discussed by Lattes R. Proc Annu Meet Am Soc Clin Pathol, Chicago, 1973, p 75

113. Hajdu SI, Shiu MH, Fortner JG: Tendosynovial sarcoma: A clinicopathological study of 136 cases. Cancer 39:1201, 1977

114. O'Brien JE, Stout AP: Malignant fibrous xanthomas. Cancer 17:1446, 1964

115. Schwartz DT, Alpert M: The malignant transformation of fibrous dysplasia. Am J Med Sci 247:1, 1964

116. Balsaver AM, Butler JJ, Martin RG: Congenital fibrosarcoma. Cancer 20:1607, 1967

117. Exelby PR, Knapper WH, Huvos AG, Beattie EJ Jr.: Soft-tissue fibrosarcoma in children. J Pediatr Surg 8:415, 1973

118. Dahl I, Save-Soderbergh J, Angervall L: Fibrosarcoma in early infancy. Pathol Eur 8:193, 1973

119. Seel DJ, Booher RJ, Joel R: Fibrous tumors of musculoaponeurotic origin. Surgery 56:497, 1964

120. Mackenzie DH: Fibroma: A dangerous diagnosis. A review of 205 cases of fibrosarcoma of soft tissues. Br J Surg 51:607, 1964

121. Gould SE, Hinerman DL, Batsakis JG, Beamer PR: Diagnostic patterns: Lesions of fibrous tissue. Am J Clin Pathol 40:411, 1963

122. Pritchard DJ, Soule EH, Taylor WF, Ivins JE: Fibrosarcoma. A clinicopathological and statistical study of 199 tumors of soft tissues and trunk. Cancer 33:88, 1974

123. Werf-Messing BV, van Unnik JAM: Fibrosarcoma of the soft parts. Cancer 18:1113, 1965

124. Solway HB: Radiation-induced neoplasms following curative therapy for retinoblastoma. Cancer 19:1984, 1966

125. Schoenberg MJ: Report on a case of bilateral glioma of the retina, cured in the non-enucleated eye by radium treatment. Arch Ophthalmol 56:221, 1927

126. Pettit VD, Chamness JT, Ackerman LV: Fibromatosis: A fibrosarcoma following irradiation therapy. Cancer 7:149, 1954
127. Forrest AW: Tumors following radiation about the eye. Trans Am Acad Ophthalmol Otol 65:694, 1961
128. Frezzotti R, Guerra R: Sarcoma following irradiated retinoblastoma. Arch Ophthalmol 70:461, 1973
129. Fabrikant JI, Dickson RJ, Fetter BF: Mechanisms of radiation carcinogenesis at the clinical level. Br J Cancer 18:459, 1964
130. Regalson W, Bross ID, Hananiau J, Goryum N: The incidence of second primary tumor in children with cancer and leukemia: A 7-year survey of 150 consecutive autopsied cases. Cancer 18:58, 1965
131. Schwartz EF, Rothstein JD: Fibrosarcoma following radiation therapy. JAMA 203:296, 1968
132. Oberman HA, O'Neal RM: Fibrosarcoma of the chest wall following resection and irradiation of carcinoma of the breast. Am J Clin Pathol 53:407, 1970
133. Hatfield PM, Schultz MD: Post-irradiation sarcoma including 5 cases after x-ray therapy of breast carcinoma. Radiology 96:593, 1970
134. Hajdu SI: Pathology of Soft Tissue Tumors. Philadelphia, Lea & Febiger, 1979, p 526
135. Donaldson I: Fibrosarcoma in a previously irradiated larynx. J Laryngol Otol 92:425, 1978
136. Gray GR: Fibrosarcoma: A complication of interstitial irradiation therapy for benign hemangioma occurring after 18 years. Br J Radiol 47:60, 1974
137. Laskin WB, Silverman TA, Enzinger FM: Postradiation soft tissue sarcomas. Cancer 62:2330, 1988
138. Wiklund TA, Blomquist CP, Raety J, et al.: Postirradiation sarcoma analysis cancer registry material. Cancer 68:524, 1991
139. Grub RL, Dehner LP: Congenital fibrosarcoma of the thoracolumbar region. J Pediatr Surg 9:785, 1974
140. Hays DM, Mirabal VQ, Karlan MS, et al.: Fibrosarcoma in infants and children. J Pediatr Surg 5:176, 1979
141. Salloum E, Calland JM, Flamant F, et al.: Poor prognosis infantile fibrosarcoma with pathologic features of malignant fibrous histiocytoma after local recurrence. Med Pediatr Oncol 18:295, 1990
142. Soule EH, Pritchard DJ: Fibrosarcoma in infants and children: A review of 110 cases. Cancer 40:1711, 1977
143. Vink M, Altman DA: Congenital malignant tumors. Cancer 19:967, 1966
144. Anderson DH: Tumors of infancy and childhood. I. In a survey of those seen in the pathology laboratory of the Babies Hospital during the years 1935–50. Cancer 4:890, 1951
145. Enzinger FM: Fibrous hamartoma of infancy. Cancer 18:241, 1965
146. Crawford M, Chung EB, Leffall LD, White JE: Soft part sarcoma in Negroes. Cancer 26:503, 1970
147. Enzinger FM, Weiss SW: Fibrosarcoma. In Enzinger FM, Weiss SW (eds): Soft Tissue Tumors, 3rd ed. St. Louis: Mosby-Yearbook, 1995, p 270
148. Bizer LS: Fibrosarcoma: Report of 64 cases. Am J Surg 121:586, 1971
149. Castro B, Hajdu SI, Fortner JG: Surgical therapy of fibrosarcoma of the extremities: A reappraisal. Arch Surg 107:284, 1973
150. Scott SM, Reiman HM, Pritchard DJ, et al.: Soft tissue fibrosarcoma: A clinicopathologic study of 132 cases. Cancer 64:925, 1989
151. Lindberg RD, Martin RG, Romsdahl NW, Barkley HT: Conservative surgery and postoperative radiotherapy in 300 adults with soft tissue sarcomas. Cancer 47:2391, 1981
152. O'Day RA, Soule EH, Gores RJ: Soft tissue sarcoma of the oral cavity. Mayo Clin Proc 39:169, 1964
153. Andrews CF: Primary retroperitoneal sarcoma: Report of 28 cases. Surg Gynecol Obstet 30:480, 1923
154. Frank RJ: Primary retroperitoneal tumors: Report of 3 cases and 107 cases from literature. Surgery 4:562, 1938
155. McNamara WL, Smith HD, Boswell CS: Retroperitoneal tumors: Report of 8 cases. Am J Cancer 38:63, 1940
156. Donnelly BA: Primary retroperitoneal tumors. Report of 95 cases and review of literature. Surg Gynecol Obstet 83:705, 1946
157. Oberman HA: Sarcoma of the breast. Cancer 18:1233, 1965
158. Rissanen PM, Holsti P: A retrospective study of sarcoma of the breast and the results of treatment. Oncology 22:258, 1963
159. Treves N, Sunderland DA: Cystosarcoma phyllodes of breast, malignant and benign tumor—Clinicopathological study of 77 cases. Cancer 4:1286, 1951
160. Lester J, Stout AP: Cystosarcoma phyllodes. Cancer 7:335, 1954
161. Rix DB, Tredwell JJ, Forward AD: Cystosarcoma phyllodes (cellular intracanalicular fibroadenoma)—Clinicopathological relationship. Canad J Surg 14:31, 1974
162. Norris HJ, Taylor HB: Relationships of histologic features to behavior of cystosarcoma phyllodes. Cancer 20:2090, 1967
163. McDivitt RW, Urban JA, Farrow JH: Cystosarcoma phyllodes. Johns Hopkins Med J 120:33, 1967
164. Hajdu SI, Espinosa MH, Robbins GF: Recurrent cystosarcoma phyllodes: A clinicopathologic study of 32 cases. Cancer 38:1402, 1976
165. Kessinger A, Foley JF, Lemon HM, Miller DM: Metastatic cystosarcoma phyllodes: A case report and review of the literature. J Surg Oncol 4:131, 1972
166. Faraci RP, Schour L: Radical treatment of recurrent cystosarcoma phyllodes. Ann Surg 180:796, 1974
167. Shallow TA, Wagner FB: Primary fibrosarcoma of the liver. Ann Surg 125:439, 1947
168. Simpson HM, Baggenstoss AH, Stauffer MH: Primary sarcoma of the liver—A report of three cases. South Med J 48:1177, 1955
169. Steiner PE: Cancer of the liver and cirrhosis in Trans-Saharan Africa and the United States of America. Cancer 13:1085, 1960
170. Ojima A, Sugiyama T, Takeda T, et al.: Six cases of rare malignant tumors of the liver. Acta Pathol Jpn 14:95, 1964
171. Snapper I, Schraft WC, Ginsberg DM: Severe hypoglycemia due to fibrosarcoma of the liver. Maandschr Kindergeneeskd 32:337, 1964

172. Totzke HA, Hutcheson JB: Primary fibrosarcoma of the liver—Case report. South Med J 58:236, 1965
173. Balouet G, Destombes P: Apropos of several apparently primary hepatic mesenchymal tumors—Trial classification and diagnosis of spindle cell tumors of the liver. Ann Anat Pathol (Paris) 12:273, 1967
174. Cavallo T, Lichewtiz B, Rozov T: Primary fibrosarcoma of the liver—Report of a case. Rev Hosp Clin Fac Med Sao Paulo 23:44, 1968
175. Smith D, Rele SR: A case of primary fibrosarcoma of the liver. Postgrad Med J 48:62, 1972
176. Walter VE, Bodner E, Lederer, B: Primary fibrosarcoma of the liver. Wien Klin Wochenschr 84:808, 1972
177. Alrenga DP: Primary fibrosarcoma of the liver. Cancer 36:446, 1975
178. Ali MY, Muir CS: Malignant renal neoplasms in Singapore. Br J Urol 77:792, 1964
179. Ashley DB: In Evans RW (ed): Histological Appearance of Tumor, vol. 2, 3rd ed. Edinburgh, Churchill Livingstone, 1978, p 813
180. Willis RA: The Borderland of Embryology and Pathology. London, Butterworth, 1958, p 506
181. Chesky VE, Hellwig CA, Welch JW: Fibrosarcoma of the thyroid gland. Surg Gynecol Obstet 111:767, 1960
182. Arlen M, Grabstald H, Whitmore WF: Malignant tumors of the spermatic cord. Cancer 23:525, 1969
183. Dehner LP, Smith BH: Soft tissue tumors of the penis. Cancer 25:1431, 1970
184. Bailey RV, Stribling J, Weitzner S, Hardy JD: Leiomyosarcoma of the inferior vena cava: Report of a case and review of the literature. Ann Surg 184:169, 1976
185. Melchior E: Sarcom der Vana Cava Inferior. Dtsch Z Chir 213:135, 1928
186. Cope JS, Hunt CJ: Leiomyosarcoma of the inferior vena cava. Arch Surg 68:752, 1954
187. Ornerheim WO, Tesluk H: Leiomyosarcoma of the inferior vena cava. Arch Surg 82:395, 1961
188. Allen J, Burnett W, Lee FD: Leiomyosarcoma of the inferior vena cava. Scot Med J 9:352, 1964
189. Staley CJ, Valaitis J, Trippel OH, Franzblau SA: Leiomyosarcoma of the inferior vena cava. Am J Surg 113:211, 1967
190. Couinaud C: Tumerus de la Veine Cave Inferieure. J Chir (Paris) 105:411, 1973
191. Demoulin JC, Sambon Y, Bandinet V, et al.: Leiomyosarcoma of the inferior vena cava: An unusual cause of pulmonary emboli. Chest 66:597, 1974
192. Dube VE, Carlquist JH: Surgical treatment of leiomyosarcoma of the inferior vena cava: Report of a case. Am J Surg 37:87, 1971
193. Gue'don J, Mesnard J, Poisson J, Kuss R: Hypertension renovasculaire par leiomyosarcoma de la Veine Cava Inferieure, Guerison de l'Hypertension et Survie de 2 ans apres Intervention Chirurgicale. Ann Med Interne (Paris) 121:905, 1970
194. Hivet M, Poilleux J, Gastard J, Hernandez C: Sarcome de la Veine Cave Inferieure. Nouv Presse Med 2:569, 1973
195. Johansen JK, Nielsen R: Leiomyosarcoma of the inferior vena cava. Acta Chir Scand 137:181, 1971
196. Juraj MN, Midell AL, Bederman S, et al.: Primary leiomyosarcoma of the inferior vena cava. Report of a case and review of the literature. Cancer 26:1349, 1970
197. Kalsbeek HL: Leiomyosarcoma of the inferior vena cava. Arch Chir Neerl 26:35, 1974
198. Kevorkian J, Cento DP: Leiomyosarcoma of the large arteries and veins. Surgery 73:390, 1973
199. Stuart FP, Barker WH: Palliative surgery for leiomyosarcoma of the inferior vena cava. Ann Surg 177:237, 1973
200. Wray RC, Dawkins H: Primary smooth muscle tumors of the inferior vena cava. Ann Surg 174:1009, 1971
201. Abell MR: Leiomyosarcoma of the inferior vena cava. Review of the literature and report of two cases. Am J Clin Pathol 28:272, 1957
202. Lunning P: Flebosarcoom van de vena femoralis. Ned Tijdschr Geneeskd 112:713, 1968
203. de Vries WM: Primary sarcoma of the veins of left leg. Atlas of Selected Cases of Pathological Anatomy. Amsterdam, JG de Bussy Ltd., 1933, p 16
204. Salm R: Primary fibrosarcoma of aorta. Cancer 29:73, 1972
205. Brodowski W: Primares sarcom der Aorta thoracica mit Verbreitung des Neugebildes in der unteren Korperhalfte. Jahresber Leistung Fortschr Ges Med 8:213, 1873
206. Ali MY, Lee GS: Sarcoma of the pulmonary artery. Cancer 17:1220, 1964
207. Auffermann H: Primare Aortengeschwulst eigentumlichen Riesenzellen. Z Krebsforshc 11:298, 1912
208. Detrie P: Tumeur primitive intravasculaire de l'aorte. J Chir (Paris) 80:666, 1960
209. Miura M: Das primare Riesenzellsarcoma der Aorta thoracica. Int Beitr Wissensch Med Festschr R Virchow 2:249, 1891
210. Nencki L: Zur Kenntnis der Primartumoren der gorssen Gefasstamme. Ueber einen Fall von Primarem Sarcom der Aorta abdominalis. Cardiologica 10:1, 1946
211. Karhoff B: Primartumor der aorta. Zentralbl Allg Pathol 89:46, 1952
212. Kovaleva AN, Press BO: A case of primary sarcoma of the intima of the aorta (in Russian). Arkh Patol 21:62, 1959
213. Kaignodova PE, Berezovskaya EK: Endothelioma of the thoracic aorta (in Russian). Grudn Khun 5:88, 1963
214. Zeitlhofer J, Holzner JH, Krepler P: Primares fibromyxosarkom der aorta. Krebsarzt 18:259, 1963
215. Smeloff EA, Reece JM, Masters JH: Primary intraluminal malignant tumor of the aorta. Am J Cardiol 15:107, 1965
216. Sladden RA: Neoplasia of aortic intima. J Clin Pathol 17:602, 1964
217. Bowles LT, Ring EM, Hill WT, Cooley DA: Haemangiopericytoma in a resected thoracic aortic aneurysm. Ann Thorac Surg 1:746, 1965
218. Blenkinsopp WK, Hobbs JT: Pedunculated hemangiopericytoma attached to the thoracic aorta. Thorax 21:193, 1966
219. Kattus AA, Longmire WP, Cannon JA, et al.: Primary intraluminal tumors of the aorta producing malignant hypertension. N Engl J Med 262:694, 1960
220. Burns WA, Kanhonwa S, Tillman L, et al.: Fibrosarcoma occurring at the site of a plastic vascular graft. Cancer 29:66, 1972
221. Geschieter CF, Copeland MM: Tumors of Bone, 3rd ed. Philadelphia, J. B. Lippincott, 1949

222. Cunningham MP, Arlen M: Medullary fibrosarcoma of bone cancer. Cancer 21:31, 1968

223. Dahlin DC, Ivins JC: Fibrosarcoma of bone. Cancer 23:35, 1969

224. Jaffe HL: Tumors and Tumorous Conditions of the Bones and Joints. Philadelphia, Lea & Febiger, 1958, p 298

225. Huvos AG, Higgenbotham NL: Primary fibrosarcoma of bone: A clinicopathologic study of 130 patients. Cancer 35:837, 1975

226. Teng P, Warden MN, Cogen WL: Congenital generalized fibromatosis (renal and skeletal) with complete spontaneous regression. J Pediatr 62:748, 1963

227. Bartlett RE, Otis RD, Laasko AO: Multiple congenital neoplasms of soft tissues: Report of four cases in one family. Cancer 14:913, 1961

228. Chandler FA: Muscular torticollis. J Bone Joint Surg 30A:566, 1948

229. Keasbey LE: Juvenile aponeurotic fibroma (calcifying fibroma). A distinctive tumor arising in the palms and soles of young children. Cancer 6:338, 1953

230. Keasbey LE, Fanselau HA: The aponeurotic fibroma. Clin Orthop 19:115, 1961

231. Lichtenstein L, Goldman RL: The cartilaginous analogue of fibromatosis: A reinterpretation of the condition called "juvenile aponeurotic." Cancer 17:810, 1964

232. Goldman RL: The cartilage analogue of fibromatosis (aponeurotic fibroma): Further observations based on seven new cases. Cancer 26:1325, 1970

233. Allen PW, Enzinger FM: Juvenile aponeurotic fibroma. Cancer 26:857, 1970

234. Reye RDK: Recurring digital fibrous tumors of childhood. Arch Pathol 80:228, 1965

235. Ahlquist J, Pohjanpelto P, Hjelt L, Hurme K: Recurrent digital fibrous tumor of childhood: Clinical and morphological aspects of a case. Acta Pathol Microbiol Scand 70:291, 1967

236. Shapiro L: Infantile digital fibromatosis and aponeurotic fibroma: Case reports of two rare pseudosarcomas and review of the literature. Arch Dermatol 99:237, 1969

237. Battifora H, Hines JR: Recurrent digital fibrous tumors of childhood: An electron microscope study. Cancer 27:1530, 1971

238. Stewart AM, MacGregor AR: Myositis fibrosa generalisata. Arch Dis Child 26:515, 1951

239. Fretzin DF, Helwig EB: A typical fibroxanthoma of the skin: A clinicopathologic study of 140 cases. Cancer 31:1541, 1973

240. Grossman RE, Bemis EL, Pemberton AH, Narodick BG: Fibrous histiocytoma or xanthoma of the lung with bronchial involvement. J Thorac Cardiovasc Surg 65:653, 1973

241. Rosai J, Dorfman RF: Sinus histiocytosis with massive lymphadenopathy: A pseudolymphomatous benign disorder: Analysis of 234 cases. Cancer 30:1174, 1972

242. Enzinger FM, Weiss SW: Benign fibrohistiocytic tumors. In Enzinger FM, Weiss SW (eds): Soft Tissue Tumors, 3rd ed. St. Louis, Mosby-Yearbook, 1995, p 293

243. Darier J, Ferrand M: Dermatofibrosarcomes progresifs et recidivants, on fibrosarcomes de la peau. Ann Dermatol Syph 5:545, 1924

244. Hoffmann E: Knobby fibrosarcoma of the skin. Dermatol 43:1, 1925

245. Michelson HE: Dermatofibrosarcoma protuberans (Darier, Hoffmann). Arch Dermatol Syph 25:1127, 1932

246. Pack GT, Taba EJ: Dermatofibrosarcoma protuberans: Report of 39 cases. Arch Surg 62:391, 1951

247. Woolridge WE: Dermatofibrosarcoma protuberans: A tumor too lightly considered. Arch Dermatol 75:132, 1957

248. Taylor HH, Helwig EB: Dermatofibrosarcoma protuberans. Cancer 15:717, 1962

249. McPeak CJ, Cruz T, Nicastri AD: Dermatofibrosarcoma protuberans: An analysis of 86 cases—Five with metastasis. Ann Surg 166:805, 1967

250. Brenner W, Schaefler K, Chhabra H, Postel A: Dermatofibrosarcoma protuberans metastatic to the regional lymph node: Report of a case and review. Cancer 36:1897, 1975

251. McKee PH, Fletcher CD: Dermatofibrosarcoma presenting in infancy and childhood. J Cutan Pathol 18:241, 1991

252. Kahn LB, Saxe N, Gordon W: Dermatofibrosarcoma protuberans with lymph node and pulmonary metastases. Arch Dermatol 114:599, 1978

253. Shmookler BM, Enzinger FM, Weiss SW: Giant cell fibroblastoma: A juvenile form of dermatofibrosarcoma protuberans. Cancer 15:2154, 1989

254. Bednar B: Storiform neurofibroma in core of a naevocellular nevi. J Pathol 101:199, 1970

255. Dupree WB, Langless JM, Weiss SW: Pigmented dermatofibrosarcoma protuberans (Bednar tumor): A pathologic, ultrastructural, and immunohistochemical study. Am J Surg Pathol 9:630, 1985

256. Enzinger FM: Angiomatoid malignant fibrous histiocytoma: A distinct fibrohistiocytic tumor of children and young adults simulating a vascular neoplasm. Cancer 44:2147, 1979

257. Enzinger FM, Zhang RY: Plexiform fibrohistiocytic tumors presenting in children and young adults. Am J Surg Pathol 12:818, 1988

258. Weiss SW, Enzinger FM: Malignant fibrous histiocytoma. An analysis of 200 cases. Cancer 41:2250, 1978

259. Enzinger FM: Malignant fibrous histiocytoma 20 years after Stout. Am J Surg Pathol 10 (suppl 1):43, 1986

260. Enzinger FM: Recent developments in the classification of soft tissue sarcomas. In Management of Primary Bone and Soft Tissue Sarcomas. Chicago, Year Book Medical Publishers, 1976

261. Weiss SW: Malignant fibrous histiocytoma: A reaffirmation. Am J Surg Pathol 6:773, 1982

262. Kempson RL, Kyriakos M: Fibroxanthosarcoma of the soft tissues: A type of malignant fibrous histiocytoma. Cancer 29:961, 1972

263. Kyriakos M, Kempson RL: Inflammatory fibrous histiocytoma, malignant fibrous histiocytoma, malignant histiocytoma, and epithelioid sarcoma: A comparative study of 65 tumors. Cancer 37:1584, 1976

264. Soule EH, Enriquez P: Atypical fibrous histiocytoma, malignant fibrous histiocytoma, malignant histiocytoma, and epithelioid sarcoma: A comparative study of 65 tumors. Cancer 30:128, 1972

265. Weiss SW, Enzinger FM: Myxoid variant of malignant fibrous histiocytoma. Cancer 39:1672, 1977

266. Bertoni F, Capanna R, Biagini R, et al.: Malignant fibrous histiocytoma of soft tissues: An analysis of 78 cases located and deeply seated in the extremities. Cancer 56:365, 1985

267. McCarthy EF, Matsuno T, Dorfman HD: Primary malignant fibrous histiocytoma of bone: A study of 35 cases. Hum Pathol 10:57, 1979

268. Spanier SS, Enneking WF, Enriquez P: Primary malignant fibrous histiocytoma of bone. Cancer 36:2084, 1975

269. Solomon MP, Sutton AL: Malignant fibrous histiocytoma of the soft tissues of the mandible. Oral Surg 35:653, 1973

270. Ferlito A, Recher G, Polidro F, Rossi M: Malignant pleomorphic fibrous histiocytoma of the larynx (further observation). J Laryngol Otol 93:1021, 1979

271. Usher SM, Beckley S, Merrin CE: Malignant fibrous histiocytoma of the retroperitoneum and genitourinary tract: A clinicopathological correlation and review of the literature. J Urol 122:105, 1979

272. Raghavaiah NV, Mayer RF, Hagitt R, Soloway MS: Malignant fibrous histiocytoma of the kidney. J Urol 123:951, 1980

273. Williamson JC, Johnson JD, Lamm DL, Tio F: Malignant fibrous histiocytoma of the spermatic cord. J Urol 123: 785, 1980

274. Sewell R, Levine BA, Harrison GK, et al.: Primary malignant fibrous histiocytoma of the intestine—Intussusception of a rare neoplasm. Dis Colon Rectum 23:198, 1980

275. Chen W, Chan CW, Mok CK: Malignant fibrous histiocytoma of the mediastinum. Cancer 50:797, 1982

276. Kern WH, Hughes PK, Myer BW, Harley DP: Malignant fibrous histiocytoma of the lung. Cancer 44:1793, 1979

277. Berger L: Synovial sarcomas in serous bursae and tendon sheaths. Am J Cancer 34:501, 1938

278. Black WC: Synovioma of the hand: Report of a case. Am J Cancer 28:481, 1936

279. De Santo DA, Tennant R, Rosahn PD: Synovial sarcomas in joints, bursae and tendon sheaths. Surg Gynecol Obstet 72:951, 1941

280. Bliss BO, Reed RJ: Large cell sarcomas of tendon sheath: Malignant giant cell tumors of tendon sheath. Am J Clin Path 49:776, 1968

281. Eisenstein R: Giant-cell tumor of tendon sheath: Its histogenesis as studied in the electron microscope. J Bone Joint Surg 50A:476, 1968

282. Guccion JG, Enzinger FM: Malignant giant cell tumor of soft parts: An analysis of 32 cases. Cancer 29:1518, 1972

# 9

# Tumors of the Muscle Tissue

## ■ LEIOMYOMAS

### CUTANEOUS (SUPERFICIAL) LEIOMYOMAS

Superficial or cutaneous leiomyomas are rare, and they can be divided into two distinct anatomical types. In one, leiomyomas are presumed to arise from the arrectorum piloris muscle of the skin. Although most of these tumors are solitary, multiple types have been reported. For solitary types, a conservative excision is usually curative (Fig. 9–1). Some multiple cutaneous leiomyomas are familial[1] and can be found along the course of a nerve supplying a specific dermatome. Management of these lesions can be vexing.

Superficial leiomyomas are also encountered in the genital region. Although these tumors can occur in areola, nipple, penis, labia, and vulva, they are most frequently encountered in the labia.[2,3] The tumors are usually asymptomatic, and, like in their counterparts elsewhere, a simple excision is usually curative.

### VASCULAR LEIOMYOMA

Vascular leiomyomas are far more common than the cutaneous or subcutaneous varieties. As pointed out in Chapter 5, it is sometimes difficult microscopically to distinguish these tumors from angiomatous tumors. They are usually painful. Local excision is adequate, and recurrence following adequate excision is uncommon.

### LEIOMYOMA OF THE DEEP SOFT TISSUES

Leiomyomas of the deep soft tissues are extremely rare, and only sporadic cases have been reported. Like their superficial counterparts, they are mostly solitary, and the diagnosis is generally established after excision of a given tumor. Infrequently, a leiomyoma may occur in the retroperitoneum.[4–6] Pack and Ariel[7] reported one such instance in which the tumor was successfully excised. We recently encountered a case of benign retroperitoneal leiomyoma, in an 82-year-old woman (Fig. 5–44). Vaginal leiomyomas occasionally appear to be hormone-dependent,[8–10] and there have been a number of case reports[8,9] describing a change in size and appearance of these polypoid lesions during pregnancy or under the influence of exogenous hormones.

Rarely, leiomyomas occur as primary intraocular neoplasms,[11] and they have often been mistaken for ocular malignant melanomas. Meyer and co-authors,[11] however, described seven cases of leiomyomas of the ciliary body from the Armed Forces Institute Registry of Ophthalmic Pathology, providing confirmatory data from their ultrastructural studies.

### VISCERAL LEIOMYOMAS

Visceral leiomyomas are common, especially those of the uterus and gastrointestinal tract; in fact, *uterine leiomyomas* are one of the most common benign tumors encountered in women. Although only about 1 percent undergo malignant transformation, the possibility should be kept in mind. Aaron and associates,[12] in a review of Mayo Clinic material, found that, of 105 leiomyosarcomas, 22 (21 percent) showed definite evidence of origin in a preexisting leiomyoma. This high incidence is probably skewed because the Mayo Clinic is a referral center, but it emphasizes the possibility of malignant transformation. Occasionally, some uterine

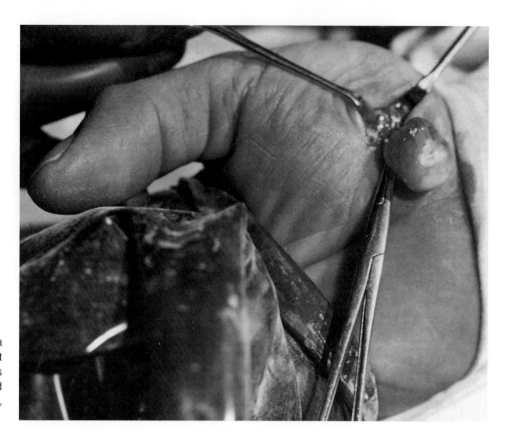

**Figure 9–1.** Operative specimen of a subcutaneous leiomyoma of the right hand in a 41-year-old man. Tumor was locally excised, and patient has remained well for 17 years (see also Fig. 5–45, Chapter 5).

leiomyomas metastasize, in spite of all the histologic criteria defining the tumor as benign.[13] Steiner[14] first used the term *metastasizing fibroleiomyoma* in a case report of a 36-year-old woman who died with bilateral lung involvement from an apparently benign tumor of the uterus. Spiro and McPeak[15] reviewed the literature and described seven additional cases of metastasizing leiomyoma, including one in the files of the Memorial Sloan-Kettering Cancer Center. In 1976, Pocock and co-workers[16] found a total of nine cases (Table 9–1).[14–21] Since then, similar case reports have not appeared in the literature. Obviously, the diagnosis of

so-called metastasizing leiomyoma is retrospective and currently is viewed with considerable skepticism.

*Intravenous leiomyomatosis* is a term used to describe a type of benign-appearing smooth muscle growth beyond the confines of the uterus. It is characterized by intravascular extension of cords and strands of benign myomatous tissue into the venous channels draining the pelvis. With the publications of Marshall and Morris,[22] Harper and Scully,[23] Thompson and co-workers,[24] and Steiner et al.,[25] the existence of this entity was established. Marshall and Morris[22] cited two instances in which death resulted from direct extension of the

**TABLE 9–1. PULMONARY LEIOMYOMA ASSOCIATED WITH UTERINE LEIOMYOMA**

| Author | Patient Age | Duration of Chest X-Ray Changes | Solitary | Multiple | End Result |
|---|---|---|---|---|---|
| Steiner[14] (1939) | 36 | 1.5 yr | | 5 cm | Died of respiratory failure (autopsy) |
| Spiro and McPeak[15] (1966) | 41 | 1 + yr | + | | Alive and well at 10+ yr |
| Ariel and Trinidad[17] (1966) | 40 | 2.5 yr | | | Alive at 3 yr, but two new small pulmonary nodules |
| Konis and Belsky[18] (1966) | 36 | 1 mo. | + | | No follow-up after thoracic surgery (1966) |
| Piccaluga and Capelli[19] (1967) | 50 | 3 yr | | | Died of cardiac failure (autopsy) |
| Lefebvre et al.[20] (1971) | 48 | 16 yr | | 4 cm | Died with lung adenocarcinoma (autopsy) |
| Lefebvre et al.[20] (1971) | 41 | 21 yr | | 4 cm 5 cm | Died of acute hemorrhagic pancreatitis (autopsy) |
| Barnes and Richardson[21] (1973) | 25 | 1 yr | + | | Omental leiomyoma noted 4 yr before chest x-ray changes noted |
| Pocock et al.[16] (1976) | 41 | 21 yr | + | | Further details not available |

tumor up the inferior vena cava and into the right atrium, but, more recently, several authors[26,27] have described the natural history of this unusual entity. In general, it is seen in premenopausal women; bleeding and pain are the accompanying symptoms. The extension into the veins is mostly confined to the wall of the uterus or immediately beyond[26,28] and can, in about 70 percent of the cases, be cured by hysterectomy; whereas, in 30 percent of the cases, the disease may persist but without any permanent damage. However, in some instances, intravascular extension goes much beyond (i.e., hepatic veins, the heart, or lungs); in these cases, unless the lesions are removed, it might prove fatal.[26–29]

## LEIOMYOMAS OF THE GASTROINTESTINAL TRACT

### Esophagus

Leiomyoma is the most common form of benign tumor found in the esophagus (Fig. 9–2), although compared to carcinoma it is still rare. Serematis and co-workers[30] reviewed the world literature and found 838 cases up to 1971, including 19 of their own. It occurs more frequently in men than in women, the ratio being 1.9 to 1.0. Over 50 percent of patients with leiomyoma of the esophagus are asymptomatic. Dysphagia and vague pain are the most common symptoms. Pyrosis is mentioned in the literature as being present in about 40 percent of cases, but it is considered mainly a symptom of coexistent hiatal hernia. Diagnostic problems often arise, since smooth muscle tumors may mimic mediastinal neoplasms, cysts, or even aneurysms, or may complicate coexisting hiatal hernia and esophageal diverticulum. Transthoracic enucleation is the procedure of choice, although resection of the esophagus may be required in a few cases. Postoperative morbidity is minimal and results are excellent.

### Stomach

Leiomyomas of the stomach usually are submucosal and mostly located in the posterior wall. Most patients are 50 years or older. Both sexes and all races are affected. With the advent of endoscopy, diagnosis of leiomyoma of the stomach is usually incidental; however, as the tumor grows, it can give rise to mucosal ulceration leading to either occult bleeding or overt hemorrhage. Sometimes, it produces other gastric symptoms, and the diagnosis is made by means of endoscopy and endoscopic biopsy or by upper gastrointestinal x-rays. The treatment is local excision. If the tumor is large, partial gastrectomy might become necessary.

### Small Intestine

Among benign intestinal neoplasms, leiomyomas are second in frequency to adenomas. Skandalakis and associates[31] comprehensively reviewed the subject in

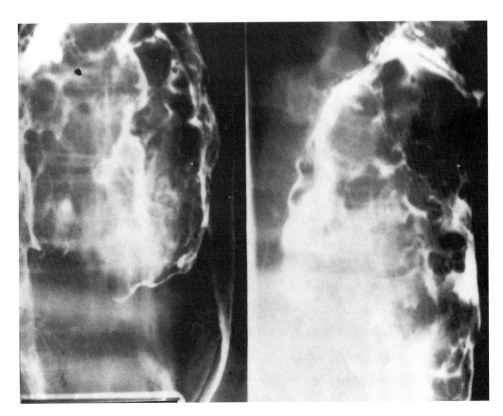

**Figure 9–2.** Preoperative roentgenogram (barium swallow) in a 59-year-old woman showing massive involvement of the intrathoracic esophagus with a polypoid mass consisting of both leiomyoma and leiomyosarcoma. A total esophagectomy was performed, and the gastrointestinal continuity was accomplished by a left colon interposition. Patient refused any form of adjuvant treatment. One year later, she was seen with metastatic leiomyosarcoma. (See also Fig. 5–48, Chapter 5 for operative specimen.)

1964 and found 713 cases of smooth muscle tumors of the small intestine. Leiomyomas are found in the duodenum, jejunum, and ileum, most occurring in the jejunum. These tumors are usually diagnosed by a long history of occult bleeding. Skandalakis and his co-workers[31] found that 72.6 percent of such patients had a history of gastrointestinal tract bleeding and 54.4 percent had pain as the predominant symptom. Occasionally, the tumors were palpable. The treatment is excision of the tumor-bearing segment of the small intestine, with an end-to-end anastomosis.

Infrequently, leiomyomas occur in other viscera. However, their rarity and the absence of symptoms frequently allow them to go unnoticed during the patient's lifetime.

## ■ LEIOMYOBLASTOMA (EPITHELIOID LEIOMYOMA, BIZARRE LEIOMYOBLASTOMA)

Martin and co-workers[32] are credited with the first description of leiomyoblastoma as a clinicopathologic entity in 1960. In 1962, Stout[33] described a series of 69 cases of gastric leiomyoblastoma. Since Stout's paper, additional cases arising in the stomach and elsewhere have been reported.[34–38] In recent years, considerable controversy has been generated as to the histogenesis of these tumors, especially since morphologically similar tumors are seldom found in soft tissues elsewhere outside the gastrointestinal tract. Although the term *gastrointestinal mixed tumor*, engulfing various types of tumors including smooth muscle tumor, is being used, the World Health Organization Committee for the Classification of Soft Tissue Tumors prefers to use the term *epithelioid smooth muscle tumor* to designate these types of gastrointestinal tract neoplasms. Although these tumors can be malignant, most are benign. Lavin and associates[34] described 44 cases in the files of Memorial Sloan-Kettering Cancer Center. Table 9–2 shows the anatomic locations in these 44 patients, along with the survival data.

The stomach is the most common site of origin. In 1973, Abramson[38] collected over 190 cases of gastric leiomyoblastoma and added three of his own. Males are more often affected than females. About 75 percent of these tumors are both histologically and biologically benign; the remaining 25 percent are malignant.[39] We have treated six cases at the University of Illinois and the West Side Veterans Administration Hospital. Gastric leiomyoblastoma is usually seen in patients over age 40 and is rarely encountered in adolescents. Gastric symptoms are similar to those of leiomyomas or any other gastric polypoid tumor. Endoscopic examination with biopsy of the lesion should provide an accurate preoperative diagnosis. About 70 percent of the tumors

**TABLE 9–2. ANATOMIC LOCATION OF LEIOMYOBLASTOMAS AND SURVIVAL DATA ON PATIENTS AT MEMORIAL SLOAN-KETTERING CANCER CENTER\***

| Primary Site | No. Patients | Alive or Died of Other Disease | Died with Disease |
|---|---|---|---|
| Esophagus | 1 | — | — |
| Neck | 1 | 1 | — |
| Stomach | 26 | 16 | 10 |
| Duodenum | 1 | — | 1 |
| Jejunum | 2 | — | 2 |
| Ileum | 2 | 1 | 1 |
| Colon | 2 | 1 | 1 |
| Rectum | 1 | 1 | — |
| Retroperitoneum | 1 | — | 1 |
| Uterus | 6 | 3 | 3 |
| Vulva | 1 | 1 | — |
| Total | 44 | 24 | 19 (43%) |

\*Adapted from Lavin et al.[34]

are located in the antrum of the stomach. Roentgenologic examination should visualize a polypoid defect. Leiomyoblastomas are locally infiltrating lesions, a fact which should be taken into account when planning treatment. Partial or subtotal gastrectomy is the minimal acceptable form of therapy.

Abramson[38] described 23 cases of malignant gastric leiomyoblastoma (epithelioid leiomyosarcoma). Lavin and co-workers[34] reported 10 cases; in 9, the patients died with metastatic disease an average of three years after initial treatment and one year after clinical evidence of recurrence. Cornog[36] found 1 out of 10 cases of gastric leiomyoblastoma to be malignant. We have treated four cases of the malignant variety. Three of the four patients are living free of clinically detectable disease eight years after subtotal gastrectomy, and one died within two years of diagnosis. A rare form of the disease was originally described by Carney (Carney's triad),[40] in which the malignant tumor of the stomach is associated with adrenal or extra-adrenal paraganglioma and pulmonary chondroma.

Among the rare extragastric sites of leiomyoblastoma, the uterus appears to be the most common. Lavin et al.[34] found 6 such instances (14 percent) in a total series of 44 patients. Kurman and Norris[35] described the clinicopathologic features of 26 cases of uterine leiomyoblastoma in the files of the Armed Forces Institute of Pathology (AFIP). Like their gastric counterparts, most of these tumors are benign, but on rare occasions they metastasize.[35] In the series described by Lavin and co-workers,[34] three of six patients with uterine leiomyoblastoma died of metastatic disease at 1, 3, and 3.5 years, respectively, after undergoing abdominal hysterectomy. The three remaining patients were alive without evidence of disease 1, 21, and 40 years, respectively, after operation. In Kurman and Norris's[35] series of 26 patients, 25 were treated by hysterectomy. Follow-up information was available on 24 patients. Nineteen of the 24 were free of disease at the time of the report in April, 1976, the survival time ranging from 1 year, 9 months to 17 years, 8 months. Recurrence developed in three patients, and one died; the other two were treated successfully.

Pizzimbono et al.[41] analyzed the collective experience from the literature and found that 90 percent of these malignant tumors are gastric in origin, and about 17 percent of them ultimately metastasized and the patients succumbed to their disease. The commonest site of metastases was the liver. Ten-year survival rate in malignant gastric leiomyoblastoma is about 48 percent.[42]

Leiomyoblastomas in other sites are so rare that general guidelines regarding their biologic behavior and principles of management are difficult to establish. Lavin, Hajdu, and Foote[34] found 12 patients with these tumors in unusual locations. The tumors in the two patients who died of the disease were located in the esophagus and retroperitoneum. Both tumors measured 10 cm. The patient with the esophageal primary survived nine years, and the one with retroperitoneal tumor died two years after palliative surgery. A leiomyoblastoma of the neck recurred locally six months after excision. Another patient with a vulvar primary was free of disease one year after wide local excision.

# ■ LEIOMYOSARCOMAS

Leiomyosarcomas of the soft tissue are rare and account for only 5 to 10 percent of all adult soft tissue sarcomas.[43–45] However, they are far more common in the gastrointestinal tract[31,45–48] and uterus[12,49,50] than any other sarcomas.[51–57] In general, leiomyosarcomas are more common in women than men, and 66 percent of retroperitoneal leiomyosarcomas and 75 percent of vena cava leiomyosarcomas occur in women.[58,59]

Although all leiomyosarcomas exhibit similar histologic feature(s), from an operational standpoint, it is advantageous to divide them clinically into the following categories: (1) superficial (cutaneous and subcutaneous) leiomyosarcoma, (2) leiomyosarcoma of the deep soft tissues, (3) leiomyosarcoma of the viscera, and (4) vascular leiomyosarcoma.

## SUPERFICIAL OR CUTANEOUS LEIOMYOSARCOMA

Superficial (cutaneous or subcutaneous) leiomyosarcomas account for 2 to 3 percent of all superficial soft tis-

sue sarcomas.[60] They are more common in men than in women, the ratio being 2 to 1 or 3 to 1.[61] These tumors are usually solitary and can be found in all anatomic sites. However, they usually occur in the extremities. These tumors rarely metastasize.[62] We have treated nine patients with cutaneous leiomyosarcomas. In our experience, once the diagnosis is established, wide excision is the therapy of choice. The incidence of recurrence reported by Fields and Helwig[61] is rather high and possibly reflects inadequate initial resection (Fig. 9–3A). Of the nine patients we have initially treated, there has been no incidence of local recurrence. The involvement of regional lymph nodes is extremely rare; thus, elective node dissection is not advocated. However, in patients with locally recurrent leiomyosarcomas, the possibility of nodal metastases increases, and sometimes treatment requires a simultaneous regional node dissection.

## LEIOMYOSARCOMAS OF THE DEEP SOFT SOMATIC TISSUE

In our series of 44 patients with leiomyosarcoma of the deep soft somatic tissues, 20 were women. Eighteen of the 44 tumors were in the extremities (Table 9–3)—a high incidence, since only occasional cases of leiomyosarcomas of the extremities have been encountered by most authors.[63–65] Most patients were women.[60] Rarely, this tumor has been reported in children.[63] Yannopoulos and Stout[63] described three female children with leiomyosarcomas of the superficial soft tissues and commented on two more from the literature. Botting, Soule, and Brown,[66] reviewing the files of Mayo Clinic, found five cases in children, three of whom were girls. The youngest of the 18 patients with extremity leiomyosarcoma treated by us at the University of Illinois Hospital was a 15-year-old girl. Because of the rarity of leiomyosarcomas in the extremities (Figs. 9–3B to 9–3D), the data on all 18 patients are briefly presented in Table 9–4.

Leiomyosarcomas of the deep tissues are principally encountered in the retroperitoneal space and abdominal cavity.[5,44] Our experience is essentially simi-

**TABLE 9–3. DISTRIBUTION OF LEIOMYOSARCOMA OF DEEP SOFT TISSUES ACCORDING TO SITE OF ORIGIN**

| Anatomic Site | No. of Cases |
|---|---|
| Soft tissues of head and neck region | 3 |
| Upper extremity | 7 |
| Trunk | 2 |
| Lower extremity | 11 |
| Retroperitoneum and pelvis | 21 |
| Total | 44 |

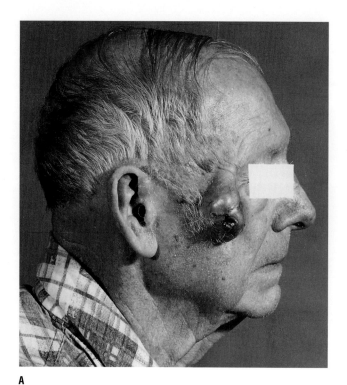

**A**

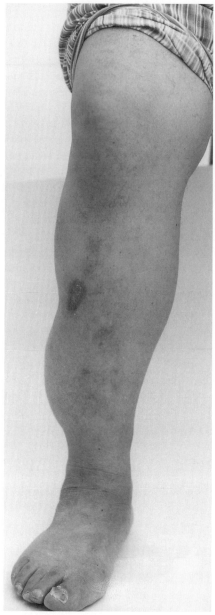

**B**

**Figure 9–3.** (**A**) Recurrent leiomyosarcoma of the skin of face of a 78-year-old man. Following wide excision, he was treated with radiation therapy. Although the local disease was controlled, he died with pulmonary metastases 18 months later. (**B**) Leiomyosarcoma of the lateral aspect of right leg of a 56-year-old man (Patient 1, Table 9–4). *(Continued.)*

lar to those encountered by other authors:[59] about half (21 of 44, see Table 9–3) were found in the retroperitoneum and pelvis. The presenting signs and symptoms are similar to all other retroperitoneal sarcomas. Preoperative diagnosis is most often impossible. The diagnosis therefore is usually made after resection of the tumor. At the University of Illinois Hospital, whenever possible, especially in large tumors, a computed tomography (CT)-guided needle biopsy is attempted. If an adequate sample can be provided, frequently the pathologist can provide a reasonable idea as to the histologic type of the tumor. If it appears to be a leiomyosarcoma, we treat the patient with preoperative systemic chemotherapy, and, if indicated, with radiation therapy too. After this, the patient is operated on. In our experience of these 23 patients, in no instance did we have to leave behind gross tumors within the abdominal cavity; however, in certain instances, resection of part or whole organ (e.g., kidney, spleen, parts of liver, gastrointestinal tract, uterus, etc.) has been necessary.

From our own experience and the information gleaned from the published reports,[60,63–66] it appears that, although difficult and to some extent inexact, some guidelines can still be developed regarding the management of leiomyosarcomas of the deep somatic tissues. It is appropriate to suggest that primary therapy of leiomyosarcomas of the deep somatic tissues is wide soft tissue resection. To aid this endeavor, preoperative chemotherapy, and radiation therapy in certain instances, are useful adjuncts and should be seriously considered. However, the role of adjuvant chemotherapy still remains to be elucidated. Further, where indicated, the regional node-bearing areas should be taken into consideration when planning primary therapy. Patient 2 (Table 9–4), refused a radical groin dissection, and inguinofemoral node metastases developed 14 months after an above-the-knee amputation. The 11 patients who survived five years or more without recur-

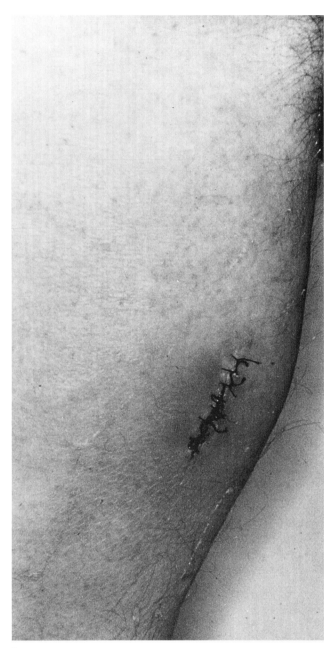

C

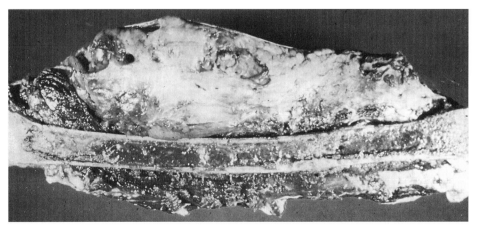

D

**Figure 9–3** *(continued).* (**C**) Tumor of the right medial thigh in a 57-year-old man (Patient 2, Table 9–4). (**D**) Operative specimen of the thigh in same patient.

**TABLE 9–4. CLINICAL SUMMARY OF 18 PATIENTS WITH LEIOMYOSARCOMA OF THE EXTREMITIES (UNIVERSITY OF ILLINOIS SERIES, 1996)**

| Patient No. | Age/ Sex | Location and Size of Primary Tumor | Status of Primary Tumor When First Seen at U of I | Regional Node Status | Type of Treatment | Recurrence (Local) | Metastases | End Result |
|---|---|---|---|---|---|---|---|---|
| Lower Extremity |||||||||
| 1 | 56/M | Right leg, 8-cm ovoid mass (Fig. 9–4B) | Intact primary | Not enlarged at time of primary | Above-the-knee amputation | — | Regional node | 2 yr, Dead |
| 2 | 57/F | Right medial thigh (Fig. 9–4D), 10 × 8 cm | Referred after a wedge biopsy | Not palpable | Radical groin dissection with hip joint disarticulation | — | Microscopic nodes in groin | 6 yr, NED |
| 3 | 55/F | Right thigh, 6 × 5 cm | Referred after excision, radiated 6,500 rads | + | Muscle group excision with node dissection | — | Nodes, liver, brain | 2 yr, Dead |
| 4 | 48/F | Right groin, original size of tumor, 5 × 4 cm, enucleated | Intact primary | – | Hemipelvectomy | — | — | 9 yr, NED |
| 5 | 48/F | Left posterior thigh, 5 × 6 cm | Recurrent tumor | – | Muscle group excision with groin dissection | None | 2 Positive nodes | 3 yr, NED |
| 6 | 74/F | Left thigh, 6 × 6 cm | Primary enucleated | – | Wide excision; postop radiation therapy | None | None | 2 yr, NED since last local recurrence |
| 7 | 38/M | Right posterior thigh, 8 × 8 cm | Intact primary | – | Preop chemotherapy; muscle group excision; postop radiation therapy | Local; 18 mos. postop | None | Resection of recurrent tumor; 8 yr, NED |
| 8 | 39/F | Left calf, 3 × 3 cm | Intact primary | – | Wide muscle group excision; postop radiation therapy | None | None | 5 yr, NED |
| 9 | 27/F | Left thigh, 5 × 5 cm | Intact primary | – | Preop chemotherapy; muscle group excision; postop radiation therapy with node dissection | Local & nodal mets; reoperation | Nodal | 7 yr, NED |
| 10 | 19/M | Right leg, 4 × 5 cm | Intact primary | – | Preop chemotherapy; muscle group excision; postop radiation therapy | None | None | 3 yr, NED |
| 11 | 15/F | Left leg | Intact primary | – | Preop chemotherapy; muscle group excision; postop radiation therapy | None | None | 4 yr, NED |
| Upper Extremity |||||||||
| 12 | 15/F | Left upper arm, 4-cm ovoid tumor biopsy | Referred after excision | – | Forequarter amputation | — | — | 18 yr, NED |
| 13 | 56/M | Right upper arm, 6 × 5 cm | Intact primary | – | Muscle group excision with axillary dissection | — | — | 5 yr, NED |
| 14 | 46/M | Right palm, 3 × 4 cm | Intact primary | – | Wide excision with axillary node dissection | — | 1 positive node | 7 yr, NED |
| 15 | 52/F | Right medial arm, 8 × 12 cm | Intact primary | – | Intra-arterial infusion preop radiation therapy, muscle group excision with axillary dissection | None | None | 21 yr, NED |
| 16 | 28/F | Left upper arm, 10 × 9 cm | Recurrent tumor after enucleation | – | Preop i.v. chemotherapy × 3; muscle group excision; postop radiation therapy | None | None | 7 yr, NED |
| 17 | 74/F | Right medial arm, 5 × 5 cm | Intact primary | – | Preop chemotherapy not tolerated after first course; muscle group excision; postop radiation therapy | None | Lung and Liver | 3 yr, DOD |
| 18 | 36/M | Right medial arm, 4 × 4 cm | Recurrent tumor | – | Preop chemotherapy; muscle group excision; postop radiation therapy | None | None | 8 yr, NED |

Abbreviations: DOD, died of disease; i.v., intravenous; NED, no evidence of disease.

rence underwent regional node dissection at the time of primary therapy. Recently, one other patient was referred to us after the development of axillary node metastases from a primary tumor in the lateral trunk. Weingrad and Rosenberg[67] analyzed the incidence of regional lymph node metastases in leiomyosarcomas and found that, in a collected series of cases, in all sites and at all stages, the overall incidence was 11 percent. However, the major problem arises when operating on patients with leiomyosarcoma of the retroperitoneum. Although it is not possible to plan a node dissection in retroperitoneal tumors, we suggest that all enlarged nodes encountered be excised. Although it is difficult to quantify the true incidence of regional node metastases in other locations in the deep soft tissues, unless otherwise contraindicated, if it is anatomically feasible, a regional node dissection in the extremity and truncal leiomyosarcomas of the soft tissues is prudent primary surgical therapy.

With the increasing use of preoperative chemotherapy and radiation therapy, the need for amputation in leiomyosarcomas of the extremities has diminished considerably. Today, Patient 1 in our series would not be subjected to a forequarter amputation without a trial of the above-mentioned treatment program.

### End Results

Stout and Hill[60] found that, in a series of 34 determinant cases, only 12 (35 percent) survived with no evidence of tumor. Eleven (32 percent) died with tumor, and another 11 (32 percent) were alive after either local recurrence or metastases, or both. Primary therapy failed in 22 (65 percent) of the patients in that collected series. More recently, Gustafson et al.[43] reported a 64 percent five-year survival rate. The major problem in assessing the end result following treatment of leiomyosarcoma is the fact that most authors report on retroperitoneal tumors, interspersed with a few instances of leiomyosarcomas of other locations.[59,68,69] In our experience, after aggressive initial therapy (as described in Table 9–4), the five-year disease-free survival of leiomyosarcomas of the extremities and trunk is comparable to other types of sarcomas of comparable TNM staging. In contrast, leiomyosarcomas of the retroperitoneum carry a grave prognosis.[6,59,68,69] In spite of this, wherever we have been able to be aggressive as mentioned previously, we have been able to provide effective palliation, sometimes extending to two to three years and, in ten patients (56 percent), an apparently disease-free and symptom-free survival for five years or more. Based on our experience, we believe that, if a CT-guided core biopsy provides a tentative diagnosis of leiomyosarcoma, wherever possible these patients should receive preoperative systemic chemotherapy and radiation therapy followed by aggressive

resection in which all the gross tumors and enlarged nodes are removed, even if it requires a multiorgan resection.

## LEIOMYOSARCOMA OF THE VISCERA

### Gastrointestinal Tract

Twenty-eight cases of leiomyosarcoma of the gastrointestinal tract constitute our present series, 11 being in the stomach, 1 in the duodenum, 6 in the jejunum, 5 in the ileum, and 5 in the colon and rectum.

***Stomach.***   Berg and McNeer[70] assessed the incidence of gastric leiomyosarcoma to be 1.3 percent of all gastric neoplasms. The clinical presentation of these tumors is similar to that of all other submucosal tumors. In large lesions, a preoperative diagnosis is possible either radiographically or by means of endoscopy and biopsy (Fig. 9–4). These tumors are commonly located in the posterior wall of the greater curvature of the stomach. The ideal treatment is partial or subtotal gastrectomy. Berg and McNeer[70] found that tumors smaller than 10 cm had a low incidence of regional metastases. Recurrence or regional node metastasis is usually found in the omentum, mesentery, or liver. Regional node metastasis is less frequent than with leiomyosarcomas of the small intestine.

The results of treatment of gastric leiomyosarcoma are relatively good. In the 24 cases reported by Berg and McNeer,[70] 11 (46 percent) patients died, the crude survival rate being 54 percent. In 1971, Bergis and coworkers[71] found a five-year survival rate of 50 percent and a ten-year rate of 35 percent. In their study of 52 patients, those treated with a curative gastric resection had a 62 percent five-year survival rate. It appears that high histologic grade, large tumor size (larger than 5 cm diameter), and invasion of adjacent organs adversely affect the prognosis. Of our 11 patients, six had lower grade tumors which were smaller than 5 cm in diameter, and all six have remained free of disease for 10 years.

Leiomyosarcoma of the stomach is also seen in children. Yannopoulos and Stout[63] found one case in the literature and described two cases of their own. One of these three patients died of metastases to the liver, and the other two were alive and well at two and seven years, respectively. Botting et al.[66] had four childhood cases in their files at the Mayo Clinic. Two patients were long-term survivors following gastric resection. The third patient died 39 months after initial resection, with two instances of recurrence between initial operation and death. The fourth patient died of massive recurrence within three months.

***Small Intestine.***   In 1955, Starr and Dockerty[72] reviewed the Mayo Clinic experience with 76 myomatous tumors

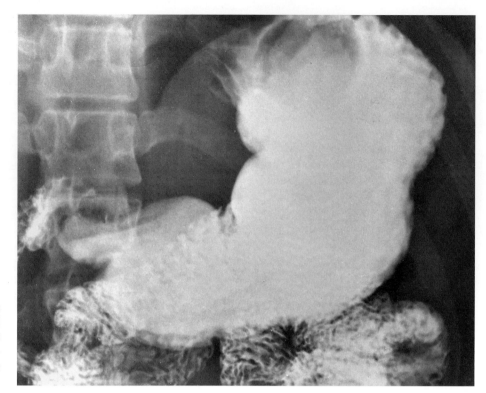

**Figure 9–4.** Leiomyosarcoma of the gastric fundus in a 44-year-old man. A radical subtotal gastrectomy was performed. All the nodes were negative. Patient received adjuvant chemotherapy and is still disease-free after 12 years.

of the small intestine, and an additional 230 cases reported elsewhere. In more than 60 percent of the Mayo Clinic patients, the tumors were leiomyosarcomas. In 1964, Skandalakis et al.[31] reviewed the location of 259 reported cases of leiomyosarcomas in the small intestine and found the incidence to be as follows: duodenum, 66; jejunum, 77; ileum, 84. In eight cases, the tumors involved both the jejunum and ileum, and in the remaining 24, the exact location could not be ascertained. Infrequently, these tumors are multicentric.[72] Leiomyosarcomas of the duodenum and small intestines are usually found in adults of both sexes. Neither Yannopoulos and Stout[63] nor Botting et al.[66] found any instance in children. Skandalakis and associates[31] reported that, in their 259 cases, fewer than 10 patients were under the age of 10. Of the 12 patients with leiomyosarcoma of the duodenum and small intestine in our series, one was a 13-year-old boy with leiomyosarcoma of the jejunum.

The clinical presentation of small bowel leiomyosarcomas is not characterized by any particular symptom or constellation of symptoms. Melena or hematemesis is probably the most common associated symptom. Palpable tumors or pain due to intussusception are rarely encountered. Radiographic findings are positive in about 60 percent of patients and, when positive, confirm the presence of a small intestine tumor characterized either by filling defects or by outlining the contour of a polypoid tumor.

Leiomyosarcomas of the small intestine metastasize to surrounding viscera, omentum, mesentery, liver, lung, and, in some cases, to the regional nodes.[31,73,74] About one-third of all leiomyosarcomas have metastasized by the time they are operated on.[31,72,73]

The ideal treatment is resection. Segmental resection should be performed in jejunal and ileal tumors, but a duodenal leiomyosarcoma might require a pancreaticoduodenectomy. We have treated one patient with duodenal leiomyosarcoma who successfully underwent pancreaticoduodenectomy at age 66, but died five years later of a cardiovascular accident. However, in instances where the primary tumor is large, postoperative radiation therapy might play a role in the overall management of these tumors. In their review, Skandalakis and associates[31] found that only 23 of their 259 patients (9 percent) were followed-up for five years or longer. Of those for whom end-result data were available, 82 percent had died of metastatic disease. In 1967, McPeak[73] reported that, of the 16 patients treated at Memorial Sloan-Kettering Cancer Center, 5 (31 percent) survived for five years. Of our 12 patients, five have been free of disease for five years, and one patient, as mentioned above, died after five years from unrelated causes, giving an overall tumor-free survival rate of 50 percent. The remaining six patients died with metastases within 24 to 36 months of initial surgery. In one, solitary metastasis to the right lung was found 14 months after resection, and a right lower lobe lobectomy was performed. The patient remained clinically free of disease for 18 months, then succumbed to massive metastatic disease within three months.

***Colon and Rectum.***   Leiomyosarcomas of the colon and rectum are rare. The most common symptoms are constipation, localized rectal pain, and rectal bleeding.[74] Quan and Berg[74] found that leiomyosarcomas constituted 0.1 percent of all malignant tumors of the colon and rectum. The pattern of metastatic spread is similar to that of small intestine leiomyosarcomas. The treatment of choice for rectal lesions is still abdominoperineal resection,[74] although lesser procedures have been tried in some patients, with apparently good results.[48,74] Our patients with rectal leiomyosarcoma were primarily treated by abdominoperineal resection, mostly because of size (larger than 5 cm) of the tumor. In the past, the selection of the type of operation has not been based on any specific guideline. However, with increasing information on this disease, it appears that the small-sized tumors of the rectum can be adequately treated with local resection and postoperative radiation therapy. However, in patients who fail this multimodal therapy program, an extensive abdominoperineal resection is indicated, and under no circumstances should the extent of excision be curtailed for the sake of better or more rapid ambulation and/or avoidance of a permanent colostomy.

## LEIOMYOSARCOMA OF THE MESENTERY

Yannopoulos and Stout[64] reported two cases of leiomyosarcoma and five cases of nonmalignant smooth muscle tumors of the mesentery. Paul and colleagues,[75] in 1968, reported an additional case. We have not come across any smooth muscle tumors in the mesentery or omentum, either benign or malignant.

## LEIOMYOSARCOMAS OF THE GENITOURINARY TRACT

Leiomyosarcomas of the genitourinary tract are also rare. Occasional cases of prostatic leiomyosarcomas have been reported in children.[51] Similarly, leiomyosarcomas of the kidney, bladder, spermatic cord, epididymis, and penis have also been described.[52,76–80] However, these instances are rare, and most reports are solitary case histories.

### Male Prostate and Genital Tract

We have treated two adults with leiomyosarcoma of the prostate. In both patients, the tumors were large and produced urinary obstruction. After transurethral resection to open the urinary flow, both patients were treated with three cycles of preoperative chemotherapy (MAID regimen) and radiation therapy. These treatments were followed by radical prostatectomy and three cycles of postoperative chemotherapy and radiation therapy. One is free of disease for four years and is totally functional in his profession. The other died after 2 years. Although he was clinically free of disease, autopsy showed multiple minute metastatic lesions in the pleura and liver.

Yannopoulos and Stout[63] described one instance of a five-year-old boy with leiomyosarcoma of the prostate. We have also treated one such case in an eight-year-old boy, who was first seen with dysuria and a palpable suprapubic mass. The urologist in charge of the case performed a suprapubic cystostomy and intracystic removal of the tumor. When the histologic diagnosis was rendered, the child was referred to us for further management. After discussion with the operating surgeon, we treated the patient with irradiation. The family refused any further treatment, and no follow-up data are available.

### Spermatic Cord

Arlen, Grabstald, and Whitmore,[79] on reviewing the malignant tumors of the spermatic cord in the files of Memorial Sloan-Kettering Cancer Center, found only one case of leiomyosarcoma. They reported that only 18 such instances had appeared in the literature up to 1969. Buckley and Tolley[80] found a later case in the literature and added one of their own. Most patients are seen first with a palpable tumor in the groin along the course of the spermatic cord, which is frequently mistaken as an indirect inguinal hernia. Diagnosis is established while exploring during presumed repair of the hernia. Although no definitive guidelines for management are possible, it is recommended that these tumors, like leiomyosarcomas elsewhere, be treated by a multimodal management program.

### Penis

Dehner and Smith[78] found three cases of leiomyosarcoma of the shaft of the penis in the files of the AFIP. One of the three patients had multiple local recurrences finally extending to the anterior abdominal wall, and the other two were living at the time the report was published.

Leiomyosarcoma of the scrotum is indeed rare. Recently, Johnson et al.[81] reported one case and, upon review of the literature, found only four additional cases.

### Female Genital Tract

Leiomyosarcomas of the female genital tract are not uncommon. Uterine leiomyosarcomas[22,50,82–84] are the most frequent, but involvement of other parts has also been reported.[85–87] We have treated 11 cases of leiomyosarcoma of the uterus, 1 of the fallopian tube, 1 of the vagina, and 1 of the round ligament.

***Uterus.*** Leiomyomas, or fibroids, are the most common tumors encountered in the human uterus. Whereas the bulk of smooth muscle tumors occurring in other locations are malignant, those in the uterine musculature are benign in 99 percent of the cases. Aaron, Symmonds, and Dockerty[12] reviewed the Mayo Clinic experience over a period of 26 years and found 105 cases of uterine leiomyosarcoma, constituting 59 percent of all the uterine sarcomas.

Most patients with uterine leiomyosarcomas are over age 40, and there is no apparent relation to parity.[12,50,82,84] Aaron and co-workers[12] commented on the role of radiation therapy in the development of leiomyosarcomas. Instances have been reported in which uterine sarcomas developed years after irradiation for benign uterine bleeding. Of the 105 patients in the Mayo Clinic series,[12] 7 had a history of previous roentgen or radium therapy to the pelvis for benign disease. Periods varying from 14 months to 33 years after irradiation elapsed before symptoms of malignancy developed. In recent years, however, such drastic treatment for functional uterine bleeding has been abandoned, and radiation-induced leiomyosarcomas are not seen. We have no instance in the files of the University of Illinois Hospital.

Abnormal vaginal bleeding and abdominal or pelvic pain, along with a palpable tumor, constitute the most common presenting symptoms. In most instances, physical examinations of a pelvic mass with uterine localization is possible. Aaron and co-workers[12] found that 3 (2.9 percent) of 105 patients had an antecedent history of rapid growth of an apparent uterine fibroid. Montague et al.[84] documented a similar case of leiomyosarcoma arising in a leiomyoma of the uterus. We have not encountered among our patients any case of malignant transformation of benign leiomyoma of the uterus.

The patterns of metastatic spread in uterine leiomyosarcoma are similar to those in other anatomic sites. Metastases to the lung and regional pelvic involvement are the most common forms of metastatic spread. Involvement of the liver, vagina, and other sites is less common.

The clinical data on our 11 patients are summarized in Table 9–5. In the Mayo Clinic series, of the 95 determinant patients, 30 (31.5 percent) survived for five years or longer. Of the 11 patients in our series, three (27 percent) are disease-free after ten years, and one patient died of unrelated causes within five years of the initial therapy. An overall survival rate of 30 percent has been reported by authors reviewing much larger series.[12,49,50]

The outcome of the uterine leiomyosarcoma depends on the grade of tumor and extension of tumor in the intestinal wall. Sixty of the 105 patients (57 percent) in the series reported by Aaron et al.[12] could be evaluated for correlation of the grade of the primary tumor's malignancy and the results of treatment. Of the 18 patients with a grade 1 lesion, 13 survived for five years or more, as did 7 of 17 with grade 2, 3 of 12 with grade 3, and 2 of 13 with grade 4. When the gross anatomic extent of the lesion was correlated, these authors[12] found that, of 20 patients with malignancy limited to the myometrium, 14 survived five years. When the lesion involved the endometrium or the endocervix, 9 of 19 patients lived five years or more. However, only 1 of 9 survived five years when uterine serosa were involved, and only 1 of 12 when the primary tumor showed extension beyond the uterus. It should be noted that these data were generated when routine use of multimodal therapy was not in vogue. The end-result data will likely be substantially improved with combined therapy.

***Fallopian Tubes.*** Leiomyosarcoma of the fallopian tubes is indeed rare, as are all malignant tumors of this anatomic site. Because of its rarity,[88] no general guidelines regarding therapy can be devised. Only one such instance, in a 23-year-old woman, appears in our files. This patient was seen with a large tumor on the left side of the pelvis. A total abdominal hysterectomy and bilateral salpingo-oophorectomy was performed. The patient died with metastatic tumor within three years of diagnosis of the tumor.

***Vagina.*** Like those of the fallopian tubes, leiomyosarcomas of the vagina are rare.[85,86] The largest series published was from the Mayo Clinic,[85] where eight cases were encountered from 1908 through 1961. No leiomyosarcomas of the vagina were reported in a 1971 study of vaginal cancers by Underwood and Smith.[87] Yannopoulos and Stout[63] reported one personal case of vaginal leiomyosarcoma in a 13-year-old girl and reviewed a case of vulvar leiomyosarcoma reported by Kelly.[89] The 13-year-old had a 7.5 × 5 × 4 cm lesion in the vagina, which was treated by local excision and irradiation. She has remained well for 17 years. Kelly's patient was 16 months old. After treatment by local excision and irradiation, local recurrence developed. The patient died 32 months after initial resection of the primary.

We have treated one patient with leiomyosarcoma of the vagina. She was a 71-year-old woman who was first seen with a polypoid mass in the posterior wall of the vagina about 4 cm from the outlet. A histologic diagnosis of leiomyosarcoma grade 3 was rendered, and she was treated by posterior pelvic exenteration and vaginectomy. She lived disease-free for nine years and died of a stroke.

**TABLE 9–5. SUMMARY OF CLINICAL FINDINGS IN ELEVEN PATIENTS WITH UTERINE LEIOMYOSARCOMA TREATED AT THE UNIVERSITY OF ILLINOIS HOSPITAL**

| Patient No. | Age | Type of Treatment | Pelvic Recurrence | Metastasis | End Result | Remarks |
|---|---|---|---|---|---|---|
| 1 | 56 | Total abdominal hysterectomy and bilateral salpingo-oophorectomy | 10 mo., mass in pelvis | Lung | Dead in 1 yr | Received radiation therapy and actinomycin-D |
| 2 | 58 | Total abdominal hysterectomy, bilateral salpingo-oophorectomy | 4 mo., mass in pelvis | Diffuse | Dead in 4 mo. | Received actinomycin-D |
| 3 | 56 | Total abdominal hysterectomy and bilateral salpingo-oophorectomy | Multiple pelvic and abdominal masses | Ascites | Died 9 mo. later | Received postop irradiation when disease far advanced |
| 4 | 66 | Total abdominal hysterectomy and bilateral salpingo-oophorectomy | None | Liver and small intestine | Dead in 1 yr | Received postop radiation therapy |
| 5 | 41 | Total abdominal hysterectomy and bilateral salpingo-oophorectomy | None | None | Alive and well at 10 yr | Primary tumor was small |
| 6 | 59 | Total abdominal hysterectomy and bilateral salpingo-oophorectomy; resection of abdominal wall | None | Lung, adrenals | Dead in 1.5 yr with disease | Tumor was large |
| 7 | 62 | Total abdominal hysterectomy and bilateral salpingo-oophorectomy (palliative) | None | Lung | Dead in 3 mo. | Received adriamycin |
| 8 | 55 | Total abdominal hysterectomy and bilateral salpingo-oophorectomy | Regional nodes | Lung and liver | Dead in 11 mo. | None |
| 9 | 62 | Total abdominal hysterectomy and bilateral salpingo-oophorectomy | None | None | Died of other causes | None |
| 10 | 46 | Total abdominal hysterectomy and bilateral salpingo-oophorectomy | None | None | Alive and well at 10 yr | None |
| 11 | 61 | Total abdominal hysterectomy and bilateral salpingo-oophorectomy | None | None | Alive and well at 6 yr | None |

*Round Ligament.* Leiomyosarcoma of the round ligament of the uterus is extremely uncommon. The same general guidelines can be used as for uterine or vaginal leiomyosarcomas. We have treated one such patient. She was first seen with a painful mass in the right groin. The tumor penetrated the periosteum of the pubis. A hemipelvectomy was performed, and she lived disease-free for five years, after which she developed multiple lung metastases and ultimately expired of metastatic leiomyosarcoma.

*Kidney.* We have treated two patients with primary leiomyosarcoma of the kidney, and both were treated by radical nephrectomy (Fig. 9–5). However, within two years, both patients developed intra-abdominal recurrences, and one of them also developed a cutaneous

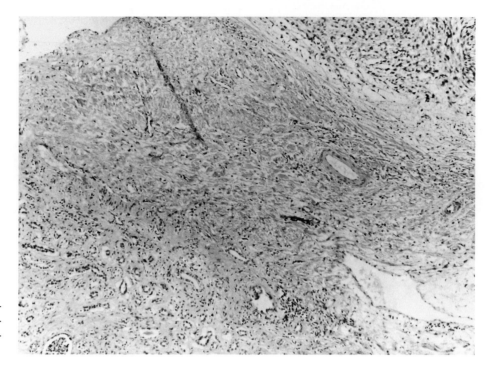

**Figure 9–5.** Micrograph of a leiomyosarcoma of kidney (H & E. Original magnification × 100). Patient died of massive intra-abdominal recurrence.

metastatic ulcerating tumor of the buttock. Both died within one year of diagnosis of intra-abdominal recurrence. Usually, the most common symptom is pain on the side of the lesion, followed by hematuria and weight loss. Although the preoperative diagnosis of a renal neoplasm is straightforward, the histologic diagnosis is usually made after operation. Most patients described in the literature were found to have local recurrence or metastases, or both, following resection.[90–92] In none of these cases, though, was there an adequate trial of adjuvant chemotherapy and radiotherapy.

**Urinary Bladder.** Leiomyosarcoma of the bladder is an extremely rare entity.[52,93] We have treated one such case, in a 32-year-old woman. She was treated by total cystectomy and construction of an ileal conduit. She refused any form of chemotherapy and/or radiation therapy. She remained well for three years, then developed both lung and liver metastases and died of diffuse metastases within six months of first appearance of metastases.

## LEIOMYOSARCOMA OF THE RETROPERITONEUM

Retroperitoneal leiomyosarcomas can reach large sizes (Fig. 9–6A&B), in contradistinction to the smaller lesions elsewhere, such as the superficial tissues or gastrointestinal tract. All our patients were seen initially because of abdominal pain and large intra-abdominal tumors. Because of their unimpeded growth potential, these tumors are difficult to dissect anatomically, and in some instances are almost impossible. Retroperitoneal leiomyosarcomas can locally infiltrate the surrounding viscera or metastasize to the regional nodes and the liver. All our patients had visceral involvement. The incidence of lung metastases is similar to that for leiomyosarcomas in other sites.

The treatment of retroperitoneal leiomyosarcoma is complete excision with adjuvant chemotherapy and, when indicated, radiation therapy. However, the results of treatment will not substantially improve until the diagnosis of these tumors is made much earlier. Only two of our five patients remained well for three years, but later all had recurrent disease.

## VASCULAR LEIOMYOSARCOMA

Smooth muscle tumors arising from the vasculature are relatively rare, although a number of instances of leiomyosarcoma have been reported arising from either large arteries[94–98] or veins.[98–151] There appear to be more case reports of venous leiomyosarcoma than of their arterial counterparts. The reason is unknown.

### Major Arteries

Leiomyosarcomas originating in the major arteries are indeed rare.[94–98,152] Most reported cases have been in the pulmonary vasculature.[94–98] Even in this site, often the diagnosis is made at the operating table during thoracotomy performed for a suspected pulmonary embolus, or at postmortem examination. Because of the rarity of the tumor and absence of any characteristic clinical findings, guidelines for management cannot be drawn.

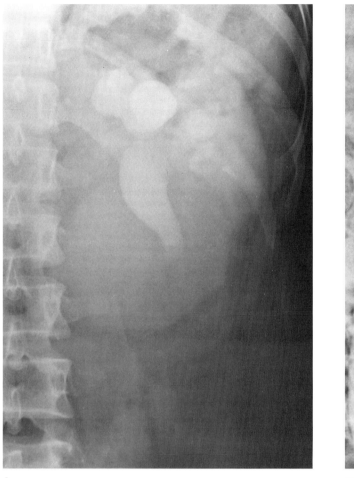

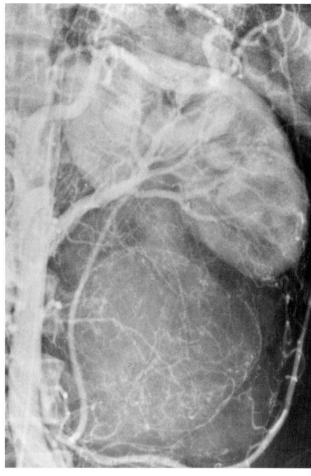

**A**

**B**

**Figure 9–6.** (**A**) Intravenous pyelogram showing the hydronephrotic displaced left kidney with a retroperitoneal tumor located inferiorily. (**B**) Angiogram outlining the retroperitoneal tumor.

## Veins

The rarity of leiomyosarcomas of the veins is evident by the fact that, in 1957, Abell,[102] in reporting two cases of leiomyosarcoma of the inferior vena cava, could cull only six other cases, either benign or malignant, arising from the inferior vena cava. Nineteen years later, in 1976, Bailey and co-workers,[122] reviewing the literature on leiomyosarcomas of the inferior vena cava, found 46 cases, including two of Abell's and one of their own. Of interest is that 22 of the 46 were not diagnosed until autopsy. The reported incidence of tumors arising from other major veins is still rare. Stout and Hill[60] found only one instance in the superficial veins. In 1960, Thomas and Fine[126] found five cases of leiomyosarcomas of other veins, including one case of their own of the internal jugular vein, and also the case of the femoral vein already reported by Stout and Hill.[60] Szasz et al.[99] reviewed the literature in 1969 and found 19 cases of venous sarcoma, some of which probably did not represent true leiomyosarcomas. However, Hashimoto et al.[45] commented that at least one-quarter of

the leiomyosarcomas of the peripheral soft tissues arose from or involved a vessel. This might be accurate insofar as smaller unnamed veins or arteries are concerned. Still, the incidence in larger, named vessels are indeed rare.

*Inferior Vena Cava.* Of all the veins, the inferior vena cava is the most common site for the development of this rare tumor. We have treated two such cases. After a preoperative diagnosis of a leiomyosarcoma of the inferior vena cava, both patients were operated on, and the retroperitoneal tumors, including the vena cavae, were excised. In one patient, the left kidney had to be removed. In one, the azygos system was so well-developed that vena cava reconstruction was not necessary; in the other, a segment of inferior vena cava was reconstructed with prosthetic material. The first patient remained well for two years and then developed a solitary chest wall metastasis. This was excised. She remained well six months, then developed a spinal cord metastasis and died three years after her initial opera-

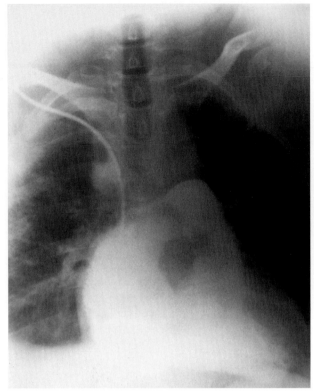

**A**

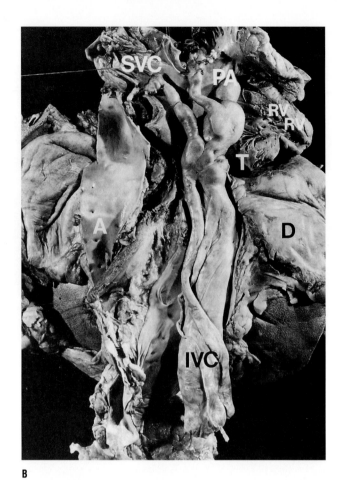

**B**

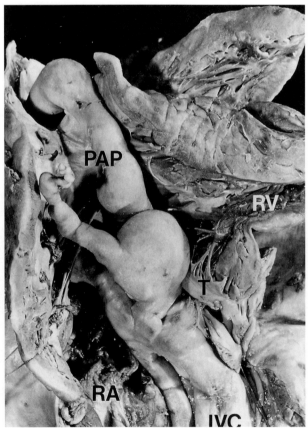

**C**

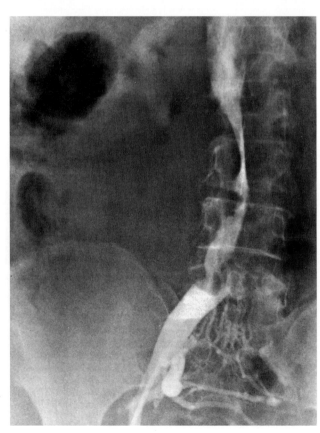

**D**

tion. The second patient has remained well for two years and currently is clinically disease-free. Both these patients refused postoperative radiation and chemotherapy.

In 1966, Jonasson and co-workers,[123] from the University of Illinois, reported a case in which the extent of the disease was discovered only at autopsy (Fig. 9–7A to 9–7C).

Leiomyosarcoma of the inferior vena cava is primarily a disease of women, usually occurring in their sixties, although cases in younger patients have been reported.[103–111] Most frequently, the tumor involves the middle-third of the inferior vena cava,[103,109,112,113] and both local spread and distant metastases are common.[111,123,124] Extensive local spread, with involvement of more than one segment of the inferior vena cava, the hepatic veins,[122,127] the right atrium,[107] and the renal veins,[144,146] is not unusual. The most common sites of metastatic disease are the lung and liver. Associated leiomyomas of the uterus and esophagus have been reported,[111] as have primary carcinomas of the colon, breast, and lung.

Symptoms vary from those of our patients with palpable tumor, to those with rapidly progressive hepatic failure or massive edema from venous obstruction.[111,122–124,127] The signs and symptoms vary with the location of the tumor, the Budd-Chiari syndrome being found with the upper-third lesions,[127] renal vein thrombosis with the middle-third,[121] and isolated lower extremity edema with the lower-third.[121,145] In patients with no venous obstruction, the growth of the tumor is primarily extraluminal. Relatively few cases are operated on with the hope of control of the primary tumor.

Preoperative angiography, both arterial and venous, is of utmost importance (Fig. 9–7D). The local recurrence rate following surgery for the primary lesion has been reported to be 36 percent.[111] This high rate of local failure probably represents a lack of aggressiveness on the part of the operating surgeon at the time of initial operation. It appears that aggressive initial therapy might improve the overall disease-free survival; however, in such a rare disease, any specific guidelines cannot be developed.

***Veins Other Than Vena Cava.***   In a 1960 review of primary leiomyosarcomas of the veins, Thomas and Fine[126] found 13 cases, only five of which were in veins other than the inferior vena cava: one each in the femoral, inferior colic, internal jugular, antecubital, and saphenous.[126] Since then, only a few such case reports have appeared. In 1969, Szasz and associates[99] found a total of 19 cases. In our review of the literature until 1981, 30 such cases could be found. Since then, similar case reports have occasionally appeared in the literature; however, none of these added anything new other than cataloguing the signs and symptoms of given patients. Our patient had a leiomyosarcoma of the saphenous system of the left leg. Following an attempted vein stripping for what was erroneously thought to be varicosity of the long saphenous vein of the left lower extremity, this 63-year-old woman was referred for further management. The segment of the saphenous vein excised elsewhere showed leiomyosarcoma. Multiple subcutaneous nodules were still palpable along the course of the long saphenous vein. An en bloc wide soft tissue resection was performed, beginning at the medial malleolus and ending at the saphenofemoral junction, with in-continuity superficial groin dissection. The nodes were negative. The patient remained disease-free 10 years after excision of the primary leiomyosarcoma. She died 20 years after her initial operation from unrelated causes.

The major point to be emphasized in superficially located venous leiomyosarcomas is that, with proper excision, most patients can be salvaged. Furthermore, with addition of radiation therapy, long-term survival might be achieved.

Recently, primary leiomyosarcomas have been found to occur in various unusual anatomic sites.[54–57,153–155] Because of the rarity of this tumor in these locations, no guidelines regarding treatment can be developed. For the present, these cases should be recorded in detail so that further clinical data can be generated.

## ■ STRIATED MUSCLE TUMORS

### BENIGN

#### Rhabdomyoma

An occasional benign tumor has been described in the striated muscles of the somatic tissues, larynx, vulva, vagina, tongue, or nasal cavity.[156–159] Moran and Enter-

**Figure 9–7. (A)** Venus angiocardiogram. Note filling defect in venous outflow tract. **(B)** Autopsy specimen. Posterior aspect of viscera; vena cava has been opened to show the intraluminal extension of the tumor. *IVC* = inferior vena cava; *D* = diaphragm; *A* = aorta; *SVC* = superior vena cava; *PA* = pulmonary artery; *RV* = right ventricle; and *T* = tricuspid valve. **(C)** Close-up of right heart chambers opened to demonstrate tumor coming from inferior vena cava *(IVC)* into right atrium *(RA)*, crossing triscuspid valve *(T)* into right ventricle *(RV)* and protruding out the pulmonary artery *(PA)*. *(Courtesy of O. Jonasson, M.D., Cancer 19:1311, 1966.)* **(D)** Inferior venacavogram showing the sarcomatous involvement of the inferior vena cava. The tumor was diagnosed preoperatively—one of the unusual instances of a preoperative cavogram outlining a leiomyosarcoma originating in the inferior vena cava.

line[159] found only 11 acceptable cases and added one of their own. These tumors are benign and seldom grow to a large size. The symptom usually depends on the location; for example, in the vulva, a protruding grapelike mass spurs concern, and in the larynx, patients become hoarse. A diagnosis of rhabdomyoma is usually made after excision of the tumor. Excision is usually adequate.

Rhabdomyoma of the heart is found most often in neonates and children (Fig. 5–52A and 5–52B, Chapter 5). In 1939, LaBate[160] collected 51 cases, 46 of which were in children younger than 15 years. Batchelor and Maun[161] found that 52 percent died in the first year of life. Most likely, these tumors represent a developmental malformation.[162] Burke and Virmani[163] found that cardiac rhabdomyosarcomas usually occur in children, are mostly multifocal, and involve the myocardium of both ventricles and interventricular septum. Pack and Ariel[7] noted that cardiac rhabdomyomas were frequently associated with other congenital anomalies, such as harelip, cleft palate, cystic kidneys, sebaceous adenomas, and tuberosclerosis. However, this observation has not been reproduced.

Fetal rhabdomyoma[164–166] is an extremely rare tumor, rarer than its adult counterpart. The only importance of this is the recognition that, in rare instances, it is mistaken for a rhabdomyosarcoma, resulting in unnecessary radical therapy and considerable heartache to the child and parents.

## MALIGNANT

### Rhabdomyosarcoma

Rhabdomyosarcomas are the most common soft tissue sarcomas in children under age 15 and are also frequently encountered in adolescents and young adults. Rhabdomyosarcomas are usually classified into four different histologic types: embryonal, botryoid, pleomorphic, and alveolar. Although there is considerable overlapping among the various categories, when possible, the histologic distinction should be adhered to, because the clinical behavior of these tumors indeed differs. The clinical features of each type are described in this section.

### *Embryonal Rhabdomyosarcoma.*

Embryonal rhabdomyosarcomas account for 50 to 60 percent of all the four categories and are mostly found in children. These tumors are encountered in all parts of the human body, including some viscera.[7,65,167] A detailed discussion of embryonal rhabdomyosarcomas in children will be found in Chapter 21 dealing with childhood sarcomas. However, as these tumors do occasionally arise in young adults and adults, they will also be alluded to in this section.

### *Head and Neck Region.*

The head and neck region is the most common site of embryonal rhabdomyosarcomas occurring in children and young adults (i.e., 19 to 21 years). These tumors are usually subgrouped into those arising in the region of the orbit and those arising elsewhere within the head and neck region. Although the orbit is the most common site in children,[167–176] we have encountered several instances in young adults and even a few in patients older than 40 years. Masson and Soule,[172] reviewing the Mayo Clinic material, found that these tumors most often originate in the upper inner quadrant and frequently involve the upper eyelid early in their clinical course (Fig. 9–8). Sutow et al.,[177] in their review of the M.D. Anderson Hospital material, found the orbital variety in 15 of 78 patients (19 percent) with head and neck rhabdomyosarcomas. More recently, Sutow et al.[178] found that, in a series of 202 head and neck rhabdomyosarcomas, 26 percent affected the orbit and eye, and 46 percent affected the parameningeal sites. Our experience is similar: the primary tumor was in the orbit in 9 of 33 such patients (27 percent).

Exophthalmos is probably the most characteristic sign of true orbital rhabdomyosarcoma (Fig. 9–8). The rapid progression of the exophthalmos is a striking feature. If the lesion starts in the eyelid, swelling and ptosis are frequently the presenting clinical features. Occasionally, children are first brought to the physician with a discrete mass.

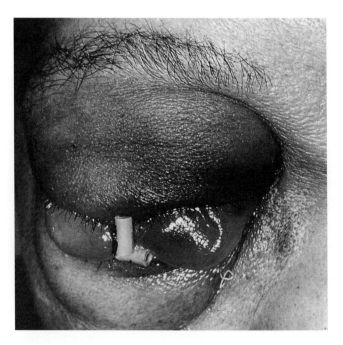

**Figure 9–8.** Embryonal rhabdomyosarcoma arising in right upper eyelid. The tumor progressed rapidly, and the exuberant growth soon prevented vision. A tarsorraphy was performed to prevent corneal ulceration.

The management of orbital rhabdomyosarcoma has undergone considerable modification in the last decade. It is generally agreed[177,179–187] that orbital exenteration, customarily resorted to in the past in all patients,[169–176,188] can be avoided in most instances without sacrificing the reported excellent end result. Liebner[179] has published good results with radiation therapy, even with apparently unresectable tumors. Recent data on the results of treatment with a combination of surgery, chemotherapy, and radiation therapy[181–183,188] show that, in most instances, exenterative operations should be confined only to multimodal treatment failures. For a more comprehensive discussion of the treatment of these tumors, see Chapter 21.

The end result following appropriate management indicates that tumors of the orbit have the best prognosis among all types of rhabdomyosarcomas.[170–175,177,179–187] The primary tumors of the orbit and eyelids usually are recognized early and treated at an early stage. This satisfactory end result is even true in adults. Orbital tumors studied in the Intergroup Rhabdomyosarcoma Study II (IRS-2) had a 92 percent five-year survival rate.[189–193] Seven of our nine patients (78 percent) with orbital rhabdomyosarcoma had a 10-year disease-free survival. Three of the nine (33 percent) had clinically positive regional nodes at the time of initial therapy, and in one, a positive neck node subsequently developed. Two of the three with regional node involvement have survived for 10 years. Only one of these patients required an orbital exenteration for a locally recurrent tumor.

Embryonal rhabdomyosarcomas in any other site in the head and neck region are often designated as parameningeal rhabdomyosarcomas because of their potential intracranial extension and seeding, resulting in less favorable prognosis.[194,195] Masson and Soule[172] found that, after the orbit, the sites in decreasing order of frequency were the nasopharynx, nose, antrum, parotid area, mandible, tongue, soft palate, tonsil, larynx, temple, external auditory canal, mastoid, submaxillary area, cheek, and forehead. Thirty-one cases of extraorbital embryonal rhabdomyosarcoma in the head and neck region have been treated by one of us.

The patients were predominantly male, and the peak incidence was between the ages of 2 and 8 and 13 and 15.[168,170–175,181,184–188,196,197] The initial symptom is the presence of a painless tumor, usually of short duration. Patients with nasal or nasopharyngeal tumors frequently complain of nasal congestion, breathing difficulty, and nosebleeds. Diplopia might be the only early symptom in some patients. Tumors in the parotid area even infiltrate the facial nerve and give rise to facial nerve palsy. These tumors can be so infiltrative that, without computed tomography (CT) scans or magnetic resonance imaging (MRI), the extent of the involvement can never be accurately determined. Thus, these two investigative methods are musts for management of rhabdomyosarcomas of the head and neck region. In some instances, the initial presentation is nodal enlargement alone. Although it is never possible to pinpoint the exact duration of the symptoms, in most instances, the onset is sudden and the progression of symptoms rapid.

The incidence of regional node involvement in embryonal rhabdomyosarcoma of the head and neck region is high.[172,179,196] In our experience, the incidence was 22 percent; however, of the 40 patients, 12 (30 percent) were first sent to us with locally recurrent tumor after inadequate therapy. Weingrad and Rosenberg[67] found that, in a combined total of 888 published cases of all types of rhabdomyosarcomas located in all anatomic sites, 108 patients (12.2 percent) had metastatic regional nodes. Initial treatment planning should, therefore, include the regional node-bearing area.

The current dogma in the management of rhabdomyosarcomas of the head and neck regions is the judicious use of conservative excision, local radiation therapy, and systemic chemotherapy. The role of each mode of therapy has been more clearly identified, and pessimism has given way to considerable optimism.[179–195]

*Trunk and Extremities.* Although embryonal rhabdomyosarcomas (in adults) in the trunk and extremities are not encountered as commonly as in the orbit or elsewhere in the head and neck region, the incidence of these groups of tumors found in IRS-1 and IRS-2 was 18 percent occurring in the lower extremity and 12 percent in the upper extremity.[198]

We have managed 45 adult patients with embryonal rhabdomyosarcoma of the trunk and extremities. The primary sites were as follows: superficial trunk, 8; retroperitoneum and pelvis, 9; perineal area, 3; upper extremities, 11; and 14 in the lower extremities, including groin and buttocks. Eleven of these patients were seen in consultation; however, they were treated as recommended, and follow-up data were provided so that these cases could be included in the present description.

Nineteen of the 45 patients in this series were older adults (i.e., between the ages of 40 and 50). The remaining 26 patients were young adults (i.e, between the ages of 17 and 23). It is noteworthy that, even in adults, the male preponderance was similar to that reported in the pediatric literature.[7,65,171–174,181,188,197,199–202]

*Regional Node Metastases.* In 18 of our 45 patients, the primary tumor was in the retroperitoneum and pelvis;

therefore, clinical evaluation of the regional nodes was possible in only 27 patients. Seven of the 27 (26 percent) had both clinically and histologically positive node involvement at the time of initial therapy. Masson and Soule[172] found that regional nodes were affected in 37.5 percent of their cases. Lawrence and co-workers[173] had 8 (16.6 percent) of 48 patients with regional node involvement. In 1977, Lawrence and associates[203] reviewed the incidence of regional node metastasis in 264 eligible entries in the Intergroup Rhabdomyosarcoma Study. These authors found the incidence as follows: extremities (17 percent), genitourinary sites (19 percent), head and neck region (3 percent), trunk (10 percent), and orbit (0 percent).

The extent of the disease at diagnosis has a profound influence on the prognosis. Survival is longer with localized resectable tumors and no regional extension. Therefore, a staging system has been developed to accurately assess the end results following various methods of management. It is important to note here that the staging system used for adult rhabdomyosarcomas essentially corresponds to that used in classification and staging of pediatric rhabdomyosarcomas.

Treatment.  In the superficial trunk and extremities, if the primary tumor can be completely excised and, when indicated, coupled with concomitant regional node dissection, this should be considered the successful form of primary therapy. Amputation of an extremity for embryonal rhabdomyosarcoma is generally not required, since in most instances a wide soft tissue excision can control the primary tumor. For retroperitoneal tumors, removal of the tumor and of the accessible nodes is the ideal form of therapy, but in most instances, the size of these tumors precludes such a regional node dissection. As with embryonal rhabdomyosarcomas of the head and neck region, a judicious combination of excision, radiation therapy, and systemic chemotherapy provides the best chance of cure.

End Results.  The overall prognosis of embryonal rhabdomyosarcoma has considerably improved during the last 30 years.[172,177,199,204,205] With the continued use of multimodal therapy regimen(s) and better staging and/or grouping of these patients, it has been found that prognosis in IRS-1 and IRS-2 is excellent.[192] In our own series of 76 patients (Table 9–6), when the patients were grouped, 5-year and 10-year survival rates in group I patients were respectively 87 percent and 77 percent. Similarly, in group II, the 5-year and 10-year survival rates were respectively 82 percent and 71 percent. The end result in this and similar studies[206,207] using any type of reasonable staging system shows that, in localized disease, a well-thought out multimodal regimen

**TABLE 9–6. END RESULT IN EMBRYONAL RHABDOMYOSARCOMAS ACCORDING TO INTERGROUP RHABDOMYOSARCOMAS STUDY (UIC, DEPARTMENT OF SURGICAL ONCOLOGY; 76 PATIENTS)***

|  | No. Patients | 5-year NED | 10-year NED |
|---|---|---|---|
| Group I | 30 | 26 (87%) | 23 (77%) |
| Group II | 34 | 28 (82%) | 24 (71%) |
| Group III | 12[†] | — | — |

Abbreviations: NED, no evidence of disease.
*Excludes nine patients with orbital rhabdomyosarcoma.
[†]Group III patients were referred after initial treatment elsewhere; most received treatment for recurrent tumor elsewhere as well.

has improved the overall prognosis in all cases. However, the overall plan of therapy might need to be altered depending on the anatomic location and, sometimes, on the histologic type of the primary tumor.

Botryoid Embryonal Sarcoma.  Botryoid embryonal sarcoma is a variant of embryonal rhabdomyosarcoma. It accounts for about 5 percent of all rhabdomyosarcomas and is characterized by a polypoid grapelike growth pattern, paucity of cells, and abundance of richly mucoid, myxomalike stroma. These tumors are usually encountered in mucosa-lined hollow visceral organs, such as the vagina, genitourinary tract, and other abdominal viscera.[180,201]

Embryonal Rhabdomyosarcoma (Botryoid Sarcoma) of the Genitourinary Tract.  Lesions of the genitourinary tract, commonly seen in children, should be further subclassified according to the patient's sex. In general, the tumors arising in the female genital tract carry a better prognosis than those in the male counterpart, with the urinary bladder occupying a middle position. Although, in Chapter 21, the overall management of botyroid sarcoma has been dealt with, Table 9–7 presents a summary of our experience with this entity.

Embryonal Rhabdomyosarcomas of the Urinary Bladder.  Embryonal rhabdomyosarcomas of the urinary bladder are relatively common in children of both sexes and, when localized to the urinary bladder, the results of treatment are good.

Patients with vesical rhabdomyosarcoma commonly complain of frequent urination, straining to void, acute urinary retention, and hematuria. Hydronephrosis and renal deterioration eventually ensue, owing to rapidly progressing urinary obstruction from tumor growth. The diagnosis usually is confirmed by excretory urography, cystoscopy, and cystography. Rarely, a polypoid tumor may be observed protruding through the urethral meatus (Fig. 9–9). The tumor usually arises from the trigone or bladder base.

**TABLE 9–7. CLINICAL SUMMARY OF SEVEN PATIENTS WITH EMBRYONAL RHABDOMYOSARCOMA OF THE GENITOURINARY TRACT (UNIVERSITY OF ILLINOIS [AUTHOR'S] SERIES)**

| Patient No. | Age/ Sex | Primary Site | Status of Primary Tumor | Stage | Regional Extension | Regional Nodes | Surgery | Chemotherapy | Radiation Therapy | Survival | Comments |
|---|---|---|---|---|---|---|---|---|---|---|---|
| 1 | 4 mo./F | Bladder | Recurrent tumor | IIA | Urethra and vagina | + | Anterior exenteration | VAC regimen | 800 rads preop | 21 yr, NED | — |
| 2 | 4 yr/M | Prostate | Recurrent after radiation therapy; palpable suprapubic mass | IIB | Bladder | + | Anterior exenteration | VAC regimen | — | 14 yr, NED | Received curative course of radiation therapy and 22 mo. of chemotherapy (see text) |
| 3 | 9 yr/M | Spermatic cord | Untreated, 2 × 2 cm | IIA | — | + | Orchiectomy excision of cord and retroperitoneal node dissection | VAC regimen | 5,000 rads | 11 yr | — |
| 4 | 4 yr/M | Spermatic cord | Recurrent tumors, 6 × 6 cm | IIB | Surrounds soft tissue | + | Excision of bulk of the tumor | VAC regimen | 6,000 rads | 14 yr | — |
| 5 | 19 yr/M | Testis | Untreated, 6 × 6 cm | IIB | Extension to spinal cord | − | Radical inguinoscrotal excision | Adriamycin and DTIC | — | 15 yr, NED | Adriamycin and DTIC protocol is being used in adults |
| 6 | 11 mo./F | Vagina | Untreated, 2 × 2 cm | IIA | — | − | Hysterectomy and vaginectomy | VAC regimen | 5,000 rads | 12 yr, NED | — |
| 7 | 14 yr/F | Vaginal tumor, filling vagina | Recurrent | IIB | Urethra and bladder | + | Anterior exenteration | VAC regimen | 5,000 rads | 1.5 yr | Dead of disease |

Abbreviations: DTIC, dimethyltriazenoimidazole carboxamide dacarbazine; NED, no evidence of disease; VAC, vincristine, adriamycin, cyclophosphamide.

329

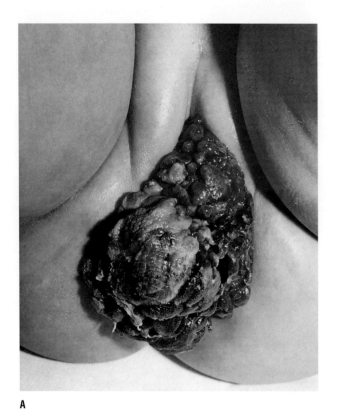
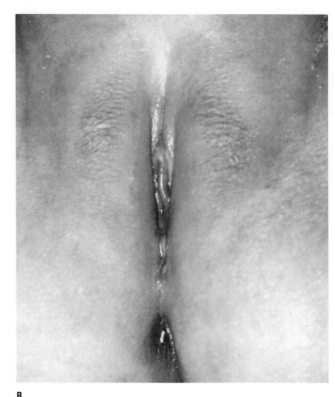

A

B

**Figure 9–9.** (**A**) Botryoid sarcoma of the vagina in a 13-month-old infant. (**B**) Following preoperative course of actinomycin-D and radiation therapy, the protruding tumor dramatically subsided. *(Courtesy of H. Firor, M.D.).*

Extensive local tumor invasion early in the evolution of these tumors may occur prior to the onset of symptoms.[200] Thus, radical cystectomy, prostatectomy, pelvic lymphadenectomy (since rhabdomyosarcoma frequently metastasizes to the lymph nodes), and urinary diversion in the form of an ileal conduit might be required for total eradication of gross tumor. However, with judicious use of multimodal therapy protocols, every attempt should be made to avoid such a radical procedure. Since the bulbomembranous urethra is a common site of involvement and recurrence, resection of this area is also indicated.[200] However, as mentioned above, today, with earlier diagnosis and use of combined modality treatment, such major resectional procedures are seldom, if ever, indicated.

**Embryonal Rhabdomyosarcoma of the Prostate.** Prostatic rhabdomyosarcoma occurs at all ages; however, 50 percent are found during infancy and childhood,[208,209] and the median age of occurrence is five years.[209] In the past, the average life expectancy after appearance of the first symptom was only seven months.[208–210] Prostatic sarcomas cause relatively late-appearing obstructive symptoms by displacing the urinary bladder, distorting the urethra, or compressing the rectum. Unlike the vesical rhabdomyosarcomas, the prostatic variety is aggressive, and regional node metastasis occurs early, as does metastasis to the lung. Local extension to the pubic bones and other pelvic bones is relatively common, even in the early stages of the tumor. Lemmon et al.[209] found that, of the 46 published cases of prostatic rhabdomyosarcoma, 39 (85 percent) had local extension to the bones. This early local involvement of the bone is a major reason for the high local recurrence rate reported in the past.[209]

Adult prostatic rhabdomyosarcoma is extremely rare. Waring et al.,[211] in 1992, reported on nine cases, including three of their own. The clinicopathologic details of these 9 patients are shown in Table 9–8. We have treated two adults with prostatic rhabdomyosarcoma.

The cure of prostatic rhabdomyosarcoma requires early diagnosis. Rectal examination of the prostate with ultrasound at the earliest hint of difficulty with micturition or defecation is the most informative diagnostic procedure. Cystography may demonstrate bladder displacement by a prostatic neoplasm. An ultrasound-guided rectal or perineal biopsy can most often be adequate to obtain a microscopic diagnosis. A transurethral biopsy is sometimes impossible because it is extremely difficult to perform cystoscopy with prostatic sarcoma displacing the urethra and the urinary bladder. In 1966, Lemmon and colleagues[209] reviewed the literature on rhabdomyosarcoma of the prostate and found a total of 46 cases, including one of their own, and only one instance of cure. Radical surgery was tried in only 7 of these 46 cases. Reviewing the state of the art until the mid-1960s, these authors concluded that rhabdomyosarcomas were resistant to chemotherapy and radiation therapy, and the authors stressed early diagnosis and radical operation for cure of localized tumors. Grosfeld, Smith, and Clatworthy,[210] reviewing their experience with six childhood prostatic rhabdomyosarcomas, found that, with aggressive radical surgery coupled with radiation therapy and chemotherapy, three of six patients with stage I disease could be salvaged. Pratt et al.[181] also described one patient with a stage IIb tumor who, after a perineal needle biopsy of the prostate, was treated only with radiation therapy to the perineum and para-aortic nodes. This treatment was combined with chemotherapy (vincristine, cyclophosphamide, and dactinomycin), with a resultant 23-month disease-free survival at the time of their report. In adult rhabdomyosarcoma of the prostate, the same general principle of multimodal management is applicable. However, the prognosis is rather dismal. In Waring's review of nine patients (Table 9–8), all of them were dead within two years of diagnosis. Of our two patients, one is living two years, and the other died within 18 months of diagnosis. It is difficult to develop management guidelines based on individual case reports. However, it appears that, in prostatic rhabdomyosarcoma, neoadjuvant chemotherapy followed by radical prostatectomy and postoperative radiation therapy probably provides the best opportunity for control of the disease in adults.

### Testicular and Paratesticular Embryonal Rhabdomyosarcoma.
A groin or scrotal mass calls attention to testicular and paratesticular embryonal rhabdomyosarcomas, which most commonly arise from the structures of the spermatic cord.[79,210,212] Metastases to the lymph nodes are known to occur and appear to follow the spermatic vessels in patients with noninfiltrating lesions.[213–215] The para-aortic chain was positive in 3 of 11 boys who had routine retroperitoneal node dissection.[212] Of the three patients in our own series, two had positive retroperitoneal nodes. The inguinal and external iliac chains can be affected when the sarcoma invades adjacent structures of the scrotum or inguinal canal.

Treatment consists of inguinal orchiectomy, with high ligation of the spermatic cord, and retroperitoneal lymph node dissection. The removal of the iliac nodes is restricted to the ipsilateral side.[202] Preservation of the branches of the contralateral sacral plexus avoids retrograde ejaculation, a troublesome complication that occurs following bilateral pelvic surgery. The margins

of resection should be identified to assist the radiation therapist in planning treatment. The transscrotal route for biopsy or removal is contraindicated because of possible tumor implantation in the incision, as may occur with testicular cancers. In such cases, hemiscrotectomy is performed to avoid local recurrence.

All patients should be treated with adjuvant chemotherapy, and those with stage IIb tumors with microscopic disease should also be treated with postoperative radiation therapy. Patients with node involvement are treated with 4,000 to 6,000 rads in four to six weeks. Both kidneys should be shielded when the ipsilateral inguinal nodes, pelvic lymph nodes, and para-aortic nodes are irradiated. A biopsy of the scalene node is sometimes indicated and, if positive, the mediastinum should also be treated with radiation therapy.

The prognosis for patients with testicular or paratesticular rhabdomyosarcoma has been discouraging in the past.[212,216] In recent years, the prognosis has improved, as it has for embryonal types in other sites. Pratt et al.[181] provided a more optimistic picture. Although the prognosis in testicular and paratesticular rhabdomyosarcoma is probably worse than for all other sites in the genitourinary tract, certainly this tumor is by no means beyond cure if properly diagnosed and treated while in stage I or II.

### Embryonal Rhabdomyosarcoma of the Uterus and Vagina.
These tumors present as fleshy outgrowths from the introitus.[7,181,214,215,217–219] The tumors become manifest because of a bloody, often foul-smelling discharge. In children, they arise from the vagina rather than from the cervix, as is the case in adults,[217,219] and they infiltrate adjacent structures. Metastases to lymph nodes or more distant sites occur relatively late.

Hilgers et al.[217] reviewed the files from the Mayo Clinic and found 10 instances of botryoid sarcoma of the vagina. These authors, after an extensive general review of the literature, described the results of treatment in these patients. From their own clinical material and other published cases, they developed the following general guidelines for management: (1) Every genital tract lesion or episode of vaginal bleeding occurring in a young girl should be considered potentially malignant until proved otherwise. (2) Once the diagnosis has been established, a reasonable effort should be made to ascertain the extent of the disease. These authors[217] found that no patient with locally recurrent tumor due to inadequate initial treatment had ever been cured. (3) An initial radical pelvic surgery provides the patient with maximum opportunity for a cure, and an anterior exenteration is the best initial radical procedure. A similar opinion regarding treatment has been expressed by Grosfeld et al.[200] Although Pratt and co-workers[181] advocated a somewhat less radical proce-

**TABLE 9–8. SUMMARY OF CLINICAL FEATURES OF REPORTED CASES OF PROSTATIC EMBRYONAL RHABDOMYOSARCOMA IN ADULTS**

| Authors | Year | Age | Presenting Symptoms | Stage | Treatment | Course | Outcome | Survival |
|---|---|---|---|---|---|---|---|---|
| Patton and Horn[247] | 1962 | 29 | 9 mo.; not stated | Large, pelvic tumor | Partial resection, $^{60}$Co, streptovitacin | Lung metastases | Died | 11 mo. |
| King and Finney[248] | 1977 | 54 | 4 mo.; urinary difficulty; low back pain | Local spread to pelvic side walls and pelvic and para-aortic lymph nodes (III) | Palliative radiation therapy | Uremia | Died | 9 wk |
| Dupree and Fisher[249] | 1982 | 31 | Incidental findings of prostatic nodule | Stage I | None | Represented 4 and 6 yr later, subsequently disseminated | Died | 7 yr |
| Keenan and Graham[250] | 1985 | 68 | 4 mo.; prostatism | Tumor protruding into bladder | Local resection, radiation therapy, chemotherapy | Recurrence at 8 mo.; disseminated | Died | 10 mo. |
| Henkes and Stine[251] | 1987 | 22 | 1 mo.; left leg pain, dysuria | Not stated | Not stated | Not stated | Not Stated | Unknown |
| Miettinen[252] | 1988 | 63 | 6 mo.; dysuria, urinary retention | Not stated | Cystostomy | Paraurethral fistula, large pelvic tumor and peritoneal metastases | Died, pulmonary embolus | 2 mo. |
| Waring[253] | 1992 | 46 (Pt. 1) | 1 mo.; dysuria at hematuria | Infiltrating bladder wall, pelvic and para-aortic lymph nodes (III) | TUR, radiation therapy, chemotherapy | Uremia, disseminated | Died | 13 mo. |
| | | 20 (Pt. 2) | 2 mo.; prostatism | Pelvic and para-aortic lymph nodes (III) | TUR, chemotherapy (refused additional treatment) | Massive pelvic/abdominal mass; uremia disseminated | Died | 16 mo. |
| | | 18 (Pt. 3) | Dysuria, acute retention | Disseminated (IV) | None | Paraplegia, uremia, disseminated | Died | 2 wk |

Abbreviations: TUR, transurethral resection.

dure, they agreed with the premise of adequate extirpation of the primary tumor.

### Embryonal Rhabdomyosarcoma of Unusual Sites.

Embryonal rhabdomyosarcoma has been reported in various unusual sites.[7,65,220–228] Their rarity in these sites arouses more interest in the embryogenesis of striated muscle fibers in these unusual locations than in the development of any logical management program. Hays and Snyder[220] reported two cases of rhabdomyosarcoma of the extrahepatic bile ducts. Both children were treated with resection and radiation therapy, but both died shortly after operation. In their review of the literature, these authors found only six such cases. All the patients died shortly after operative intervention. Goldman and Friedman[227] described two patients with embryonal rhabdomyosarcoma of the hepatic parenchyma. Mihara and colleagues[229] described a case of rhabdomyosarcoma in the gallbladder of a six-year-old girl. After an extensive review of the literature, they concluded that there were 26 established and 7 probable cases of rhabdomyosarcoma of the liver and the biliary system. These cases exemplify the rarity of this type of tumor. The presence of muscle tumors in the liver parenchyma or in the extrahepatic biliary system, where normally skeletal muscles are not observed, supports the concept that the normal hepatic blastema is derived from both endodermal and mesodermal elements (Chapter 2). The presence of rhabdomyosarcoma in the gastrointestinal tract also raises the intriguing question of the origin of skeletal muscle.

### Pleomorphic Rhabdomyosarcoma.

Pleomorphic rhabdomyosarcoma is a rare variant of rhabdomyosarcoma (see Chapter 5 for details) and is predominantly a tumor of adult males (Fig. 9–10A to 9–10E). We have treated 36 patients in whom a diagnosis of pleomorphic rhabdomyosarcoma was made, and only 3 of 36 (8 percent) were below the age of 20 years, and 2 were older than 70 years; the remaining patients were between the ages of 20 and 60 years. A similar observation regarding the distribution of age and sex has been made by other authors.[230,231]

These tumors are found in all parts of the human body, but the predominant site of origin is the lower extremities. In our series, 19 of 36 (53 percent) were found in a lower extremity and only one in the retroperitoneum. These tumors have also been reported in many other sites, such as those of apparent pulmonary origin,[225] the gastrointestinal tract,[220,221] the ovaries,[226] and the uterus.[232] However, some of these reports must be viewed with reservation, since absolute documentation has not been provided that these tumors were indeed pleomorphic rhabdomyosarcomas. Weiss and

Enzinger[233] have expressed doubt that some of the case reports published before might not even be pleomorphic rhabdomyosarcomas but actually malignant fibrous histiocytomas.

The presenting complaint in most patients is a painless mass of relatively short duration (Fig. 9–10A and 9–10B). In some instances, the patient becomes aware of the tumor after minor trauma. Pain and discomfort are the presenting symptoms in about 25 percent of patients. Pain in the sciatic nerve distribution, as in other sarcomas of the buttock, is a relatively common symptom for tumors arising in that location.

The treatment of primary pleomorphic rhabdomyosarcoma is mainly operative. In contrast to treatment of the embryonal variety, radical excision has a better role. The type of radical excision, however, depends on the location of the primary tumor. In the present series, all 36 patients were treated with radical surgery, and 30 of 36 (83 percent) also received postoperative radiation therapy. In the series reported by Linscheid and associates,[231] 84 of 87 patients (97 percent) were treated by surgery and three by radiation therapy. Of the 36, 12 (33 percent) received adjuvant chemotherapy, mostly because of the size of the tumor. It is our present practice to treat all primary pleomorphic rhabdomyosarcomas with supplemental radiation therapy. Although, in line with embryonal rhabdomyosarcoma, the treatment of pleomorphic type probably should use some type of multimodal regimen, the exact role of adjuvant chemotherapy has not yet been properly defined.

The results of treatment in our 36 patients show that, of 30 patients who received postoperative radiation therapy, only 4 (13 percent) developed local recurrence. Of the remaining six who were treated with only resection, two had major amputation for locally recurrent tumor, and the other four had major muscle group excision with considerable difficulty in ambulation. However, in two (33 percent) of the six patients, there was local recurrence along with distant metastases. Overall, five-year disease-free survival in the group of 36 patients was 61 percent (i.e., 22 of 36 survived disease-free for five years).

The end result reported here is better than the results reported by earlier authors.[230,231] However, it is difficult to actually compare results published more recently,[234–236] especially due to refinement of diagnostic criteria, improvement of radiation therapy technology, and introduction of doxorubicin-based chemotherapy protocols. However, from our experience at the University of Illinois and from a review of the data from other larger series,[7,197,199,233–239] it appears that radical operation should still be considered the mainstay for local control of primary pleomorphic rhabdomyosarcoma.

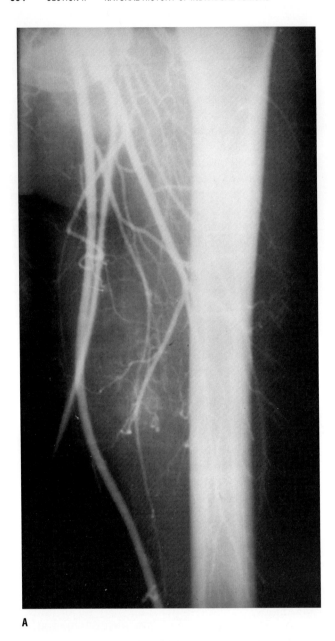
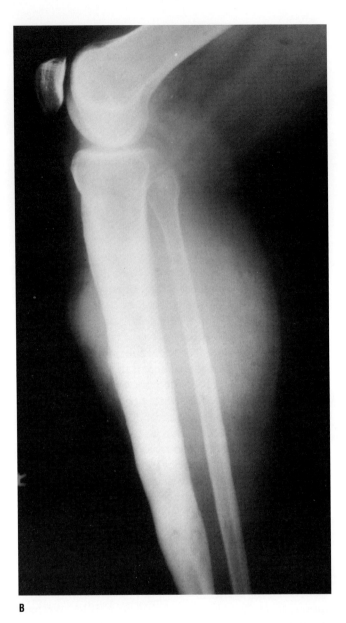

A

B

**Figure 9–10.** **(A)** Angiogram outlining a pleomorphic rhabdomyosarcoma in the left thigh of a 44-year-old man. This tumor was treated with our protocol of pre-operative intra-arterial infusion with adriamycin, and by radiation therapy followed by a muscle group excision and groin dissection. After the wound healed, radiation therapy was completed, and adjuvant therapy continued for one year. Patient is still disease-free after 14 years. **(B)** Pleomorphic rhabdomyosarcoma of the leg. Note secondary involvement of the bone. Tibia was extensively involved. Patient underwent an above-the-knee amputation. *(Continued.)*

*Pleomorphic Rhabdomyosarcoma of Unusual Sites.* Pleomorphic rhabdomyosarcomas have been reported in various sites outside the body somite.[221–232] All are case reports of one or two patients. Consequently, no general guidelines regarding the natural history or management can be provided. Pleomorphic rhabdomyosarcomas have been reported in the esophagus, stomach, and duodenum,[221,223] as well as the gin-

giva,[240] uterus,[240] and ovaries.[226] If the case reports are any guide, these patients should be treated by excision of the primary tumor. The results of treatment, however, have not been very satisfactory.

Pleomorphic rhabdomyosarcomas of the heart are extremely rare, with only about 33 such cases on record.[224,225] These tumors are rarely diagnosed ante-mortem. Matloff and co-workers[224] reported one such

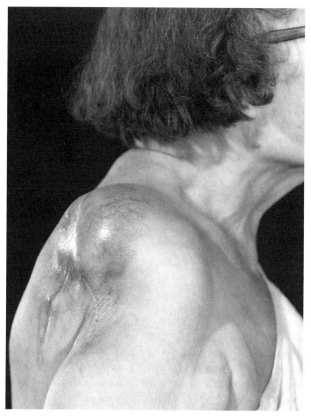

C

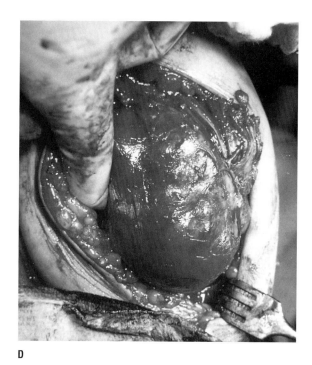

D

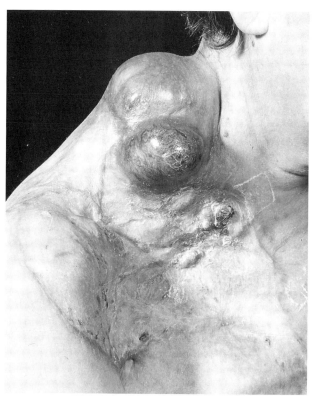

E

**Figure 9–10** *(continued)*. (**C**) Locally recurrent tumor of the shoulder. The extensiveness of the tumor necessitated a forequarter amputation. Patient refused adjuvant chemotherapy and died of metastatic disease within two years. (**D**) Pseudocapsule in a tumor. As in most other malignant mesenchymal tumors, this pseudocapsule frequently confuses the operating surgeon and an inadequate excision is performed. (**E**) Fungating metastatic cervical nodes; primary was located in the arm.

case in which the diagnosis was made and the patient was operated on. Following a second excision of the recurrence, she lived for a total of 34 months.

### Alveolar Rhabdomyosarcoma.
In 1956, a significant contribution toward the recognition of a sizable group of these neoplasms was provided by Riopelle and Theriault,[241] who demonstrated that certain "round cell sarcomas" with a peculiar pseudoglandular or pseudoalveolar pattern are actually malignant tumors of the rhabdomyoblasts. Today, alveolar rhabdomyosarcoma as an entity has become widely accepted.[242] The alveolar variant of rhabdomyosarcoma is a relatively frequent malignant neoplasm affecting patients under the age of 20. Enzinger and Shiraki[243] found that alveolar and embryonal rhabdomyosarcomas were the two most common soft tissue tumors in patients 20 years or younger in the files of the AFIP.

In 1969, Enzinger and Shiraki[243] reported the largest series on record of patients with alveolar rhabdomyosarcoma (110 patients from the files of the AFIP) and actually defined the general principles in the histologic diagnosis and the natural history of these tumors. We have treated 18 such patients.

The age at initial onset can range from a few months after birth to the sixth decade, although, as stated above, most occur in patients under 20 years. The median age in Enzinger and Shiraki's group[243] was 15 years. In our series, the median was 18 years. There were nine males and six females in our group, and a similar ratio has been found by other authors.[243–245]

These tumors, like other rhabdomyosarcomas, can arise in any part of the human body. In the University of Illinois group of 18 patients, three tumors were in the neck, four were in the trunk, six in the upper extremities, and five in the lower extremities. In Enzinger and Shiraki's[243] series of 110 patients, the primary site could be determined in 109. The tumors were distributed as follows: head and neck, 20; trunk, 30; upper extremities, 29; and lower extremities, 30.

The presenting feature usually is a tumor of relatively short duration. Associated pain or tenderness is rare. The diagnosis is usually reached after an adequate biopsy examination.

The treatment of primary alveolar rhabdomyosarcoma is mainly along the same lines as that of the embryonal type. The treatment plan should include judicious use of radiation therapy, excision of the primary with regional node dissection when indicated, and adjuvant chemotherapy.

Hays and associates[246] reviewed the end-result data from the IRS. The period of follow-up ranged from 2.5 to 7.5 years after treatment of the primary tumor in all anatomic sites with the multimodal treatment protocols in operation. These authors observed an increased incidence of recurrence in extremity tumors as opposed to tumors arising in the head and neck or in the trunk. Further analysis of their data, based on histologic types, shows that the incidence of relapse is highest with alveolar rhabdomyosarcoma.[246] In clinical group 1, the recurrence rate with the alveolar subtype was five of eight, compared to one of seven in embryonal and one of six in all other types. Similarly, in clinical group 2, the relapse rate in the alveolar type was 6 of 12, whereas in the embryonal it was 5 of 11, and 3 of 10 in all other types. These authors concluded that, in their group of patients, a cluster of the alveolar type of rhabdomyosarcomas occurred in the extremities, and hence the worsening of the prognosis. The reason for this, however, is not immediately apparent.

Our experience with this histologic subtype of tumors is not as desolate as that of the IRS. Of the 18 patients in our series, 11 (61 percent) have been free of disease for seven years or longer, and 8 died with widespread metastases. These survival data, compared with the report by Enzinger and Shiraki[243] of a median survival of nine months before institution of a well-designed plan of treatment, are certainly more favorable. Although the number of patients treated and followed by us is only 18, an overall long-term disease-free survival rate of 61 percent is certainly gratifying. The end result after radical operation followed by adjuvant chemotherapy certainly provides a better outlook than previously reported.[243–245]

Our own observations of embryonal, pleomorphic, and alveolar rhabdomyosarcomas have led us to conclude that, in spite of histologic variations among these three types, all myogenic tumors arising from the skeletal muscles are responsive to both radiation therapy and chemotherapy, although the pleomorphic and alveolar types are not as sensitive as the embryonal type.

## REFERENCES

1. Fisher WC, Helwig EB: Leiomyomas of the skin. Arch Dermatol 88:510, 1963
2. Tavassoli FA, Norris HJ: Smooth muscle tumors of the vulva. Obstet Gynecol 53:213, 1979
3. Yokoyama R, Hashimoto H, Daimura Y, et al.: Superficial leiomyomas: A clinicopathologic study of 34 cases. Acta Pathol Jpn 37:1415, 1987
4. Willis RA: The Borderland of Embryology and Pathology, London, Butterworth, 1958, p 411
5. Golden T, Stout AP: Smooth muscle tumors of the gastrointestinal tract and retroperitoneal tissue. Surg Gynecol Obstet 73:784, 1941
6. Ranchod M, Kempson RL: Smooth muscle tumors of the gastrointestinal tract and retroperitoneum. Cancer 39:255, 1977
7. Pack GT, Ariel IA: Tumors of the Soft Somatic Tissue. New York, Hoeber-Harper, 1958, p 535

8. Rywlin AM, Simmons RJ, Robinson MJ: Leiomyoma of vagina recurrent in pregnancy. South Med J 62:1449, 1969

9. Elliott GB, Reymonds HA, Fidler HK: Pseudosarcoma botryoides of cervix and vagina in pregnancy. J Obstet Gynecol Br Commonw 74:728, 1967

10. Norris HJ, Taylor HB: Polyps of vagina. A benign lesion resembling sarcoma botryoides. Cancer 19:227, 1966

11. Meyer SL, Fine BS, Font RL, Zimmerman L: Leiomyoma of the ciliary body: Electron microscopic verification. Am J Ophthalmol 66:1061, 1968

12. Aaron LA, Symmonds RE, Dockerty MB: Sarcoma of the uterus: A clinical and pathologic study of 177 cases. Am J Obstet Gynecol 94:101, 1966

13. Edelson MG, Davids AM: Metastasis of uterine fibroleimyomata. Obstet Gynecol 21:78, 1963

14. Steiner P: Metastasizing fibroleiomyoma of the uterus. Am J Pathol 15:98, 1939

15. Spiro R, McPeak CT: On the so-called metastasizing leiomyoma. Cancer 19:544, 1966

16. Pocock E, Craig JR, Bullock WR: Metastatic uterine leiomyomata. Cancer 38:2096, 1976

17. Ariel IM, Trinidad S: Pulmonary metastases from a uterine "leiomyoma." Report of a case: Evaluation of differential diagnosis and treatment policies. Am J Obstet Gynecol 94:110, 1966

18. Konis EE, Belsky RD: Metastasizing leiomyoma of the uterus: Report of a case. Obstet Gynecol 27:442, 1966

19. Piccaluga A, Capelli A: Metastasizing fibroleiomyomatosis of the uterus. A morphologic, histochemical and histomechanical study. Arch Ital Anat Istol Pathol 41:99, 1967

20. Lefebvre R, Nawar T, Fortin R, et al.: Leiomyoma of the uterus with bilateral pulmonary metastases. Can Med Assoc J 105:501, 1971

21. Barnes HM, Richardson RJ: Benign metastasizing fibroleiomyoma—A case report. J Obstet Gynecol Br Commonw 80:569, 1973

22. Marshall JF, Morris DS: Intravenous leiomyomatosis of the uterus and pelvis—Case report. Ann Surg 149:126, 1959

23. Harper RS, Scully RE: Intravenous leiomyomatosis of the uterus: A report of four cases. Obstet Gynecol 18:519, 1961

24. Thompson JW, Symmonds RE, Dockerty MB: Benign uterine leiomyoma with vascular involvement. Am J Obstet Gynecol 84:182, 1962

25. Steiner G, Warren JW, Judd AS: Intravenous leiomyomatosis—A case report. Am J Obstet Gynecol 87:166, 1963

26. Clement PH: Intravenous leiomyomatas of the uterus. Pathol Ann 23:153, 1988

27. Clement PH, Yong RH, Scully RE: Intravenous leiomyomatosis of the uterus: A clinicopathological analysis of 16 cases with unusual histologic features. Am J Surg Pathol 12:932, 1988

28. Scurry JP, Carcy MP, Targett CS, et al.: Soft tissues lipoleiomyoma. Pathology 23:360, 1991

29. Suguinami H, Kaura R, Ochi H, et al.: Intravenous leiomyomatosis with cardiac extension: Successful surgical management and histopathologic study. Obstet Gynecol 76:527, 1990

30. Serematis MG, Lyons WS, deGuzman VC, Peabody JW Jr.: Leiomyomata of the esophagus: An analysis of 838 cases. Cancer 38:2166, 1976

31. Skandalakis JE, Gray SW, Shepard D: Smooth muscle tumors of the small intestine. Am J Gastroenterol 42:172, 1964

32. Martin JF, Bazin P, Feroldi J, Cabanne F: Tumeurs myoides intramurales de l'estomac—Considerations microscopiques a propos de 6 cas. Ann Anat Pathol (Paris) 5:484, 1960

33. Stout AP: Bizarre smooth muscle tumors of the stomach. Cancer 15:400, 1962

34. Lavin P, Hajdu SI, Foote FW Jr.: Gastric and extragastric leiomyoblastomas. Cancer 29:305, 1972

35. Kurman RJ, Norris HG: Mesenchymal tumors of the uterus. VI. Epithelioid smooth muscle tumors including leiomyoblastoma and clear-cell leiomyoma: A clinical and pathologic analysis of 26 cases. Cancer 37:1853, 1976

36. Cornog JL Jr.: Gastric leiomyoblastoma: A clinical and ultrastructural study. Cancer 34:711, 1974

37. Abramson DJ: Gastric leiomyoblastoma: Report of three cases, one malignant. Ann Surg 179:625, 1973

38. Abramson DJ: Gastric leiomyoblastoma: Collective review. Surg Gynecol Obstet 136:118, 1973

39. Appleman HD, Helwig EB: Gastric epithelioid leiomyoma and meiomyosarcoma (leiomyoblastoma). Cancer 38:708, 1976

40. Carney JA: The triad of gastric epithelioid leiomyosarcoma, pulmonary chondroma, and functioning extra-adrenal paraganglioma. Cancer 43:374, 1979

41. Pizzimbono CA, Higa E, Wise L: Leiomyoblastoma of the lesser sac: Case report and review of the literature. Am Surg 39:692, 1973

42. Ueyama T, Guo K-J, Hashimoto H, et al.: A clinicopathologic and immunohistochemical study of gastrointestinal stromal tumors. Cancer 69:947, 1992

43. Gustafson P, Willen H, Baldentorp B, et al.: Soft tissue leiomyosarcoma: A population-based epidemiologic and prognostic study of 48 patients, including cellular DNA content. Cancer 70:114, 1992

44. Russel WO, Cohen J, Enzinger FM, et al.: A clinical and pathological staging system for soft tissue sarcomas. Cancer 40:1562, 1977

45. Hashimoto H, Daimaru Y, Tsuneyoshi M, et al.: Leiomyosarcoma of the external soft tissues. Cancer 57:2077, 1986

46. Stout AP: Tumors of the stomach. In Atlas of Tumor Pathology, Sect. 6 Fasc 21. Washington DC, AFIP, 1953

47. Somervell JL, Mayer PF: Leiomyosarcoma of the rectum. Br J Surg 58:144, 1974

48. Stavorovsky M, Jaffa AJ, Papo J, Baratz M: Leiomyosarcoma of the colon and rectum. Dis Colon Rectum 23:249, 1980

49. Christopherson WM, Williamson EO, Gray LA: Leiomyosarcoma of the uterus. Cancer 29:1512, 1972

50. Vardi JR, Tovell HM: Leiomyosarcoma of the uterus: Clinicopathologic study. Obstet Gynecol 56(4):428, 1980

51. Smith BH, Dehner LP: Sarcoma of the prostate gland. Am J Clin Pathol 58:43, 1972

52. Weitzner S: Leiomyosarcoma of urinary bladder in children. Urology 12:450, 1978

53. Pritchett PS, Fu YS, Kay S: Unusual ultrastructural features of a leiomyosarcoma of the lung. Am J Clin Pathol 63:901, 1975

54. Schanher PW Jr.: Primary pulmonary leiomyosarcoma: Case report and review of literature. Ann Surg 181:20, 1975

55. Morgan PG, Ball J: Pulmonary leiomyosarcomas. Br J Dis Chest 74(3):245, 1980

56. Overgaard J, Frederiksen P, Helmig O, Jensen OM: Primary leiomyosarcoma of bone. Cancer 39:1664, 1977

57. Shamsuddin AK, Reyes F, Harvey JW, Toker C: Primary leiomyosarcoma of bone. Hum Pathol 11(5):S581, 1980

58. Hashimoto H, Tsuneyoshi M, Enjoji M: Malignant smooth muscle tumors of the retroperitoneum and mesentery: A clinicopathologic analysis of 44 cases. J Surg Oncol 28:177, 1985

59. Shmookler BM, Lauer DH: Retroperitoneal leiomyosarcoma: A clinicopathologic analysis of 36 cases. Am J Surg Pathol 7:269, 1983

60. Stout AP, Hill WT: Leiomyosarcoma of the superficial soft tissues. Cancer 11:844, 1958

61. Fields JP, Helwig EB: Leiomyosarcoma of the skin and subcutaneous tissue. Cancer 47:156, 1981

62. Dahl I, Angervall L: Cutaneous and subcutaneous leiomyosarcoma: A clinicopathologic study of 47 patients. Pathologica 9:307, 1974

63. Yannopoulos K, Stout AP: Smooth muscle tumors in children. Cancer 15:958, 1962

64. Yannopoulos K, Stout AP: Primary solid tumors of the mesentery. Cancer 16:915, 1963

65. Stout AP, Lattes R: Tumors of the soft tissues. In Atlas of Tumor Pathology. Fasc 1. Washington DC, AFIP, 1967

66. Botting AJ, Soule EH, Brown AL: Smooth muscle tumors in children. Cancer 18:711, 1965

67. Weingrad DN, Rosenberg SA: Early lymphatic spread of osteogenic and soft-tissue sarcomas. Surgery 84:231, 1978

68. Kay S, McNeill DD: Leiomyosarcoma of the retroperitoneum. Surg Gynecol Obstet 129:285, 1969

69. Wile AG, Evans HL, Romsdahl MM: Leiomyosarcoma of soft tissue: A clinicopathologic study. Cancer 48:1022, 1981

70. Berg J, McNeer G: Leiomyosarcoma of the stomach: A clinical and pathological study. Cancer 13:25, 1960

71. Bergis JN, Dockerty MB, Re Mino MT: Sarcomatous lesions of the stomach. Ann Surg 173:758, 1971

72. Starr GF, Dockerty MB: Leiomyomas and leiomyosarcoma of the small intestine. Cancer 8:101, 1955

73. McPeak CJ: Malignant tumors of the small intestine. Am J Surg 114:402, 1967

74. Quan SHQ, Berg JW: Leiomyoma and leiomyosarcoma of the rectum. Dis Colon Rectum 5:415, 1962

75. Paul M, Attygalle D, Thambirajah M: The origins of leiomyomas. Br J Surg 55:9, 1968

76. Clinton-Thomas CL: A giant leiomyoma of the kidney. Br J Surg 43:497, 1956

77. Hutcheson JB, Wittaker WW, Fronstin MH: Leiomyosarcoma of the penis: Case report and review of literature. J Urol 101:874, 1969

78. Dehner LP, Smith BH: Soft tissue tumors of the penis: A clinicopathologic study of 46 cases. Cancer 25:1431, 1970

79. Arlen M, Grabstald H, Whitmore WF Jr.: Malignant tumors of the spermatic cord. Cancer 23:525, 1969

80. Buckley PM, Tolley DA: Leiomyosarcoma of the spermatic cord. Br J Urol 53:193, 1981

81. Johnson S, Rondell M, Platt W: Leiomyosarcoma of the scrotum. Cancer 41:1830, 1978

82. Bartsich EG, Bowe ET, Morre JG: Leiomyosarcoma of the uterus. A 50-year review of 42 cases. Obstet Gynecol 32:101, 1968

83. Hannigan EV: Uterine leiomyosarcoma. A review of prognostic clinical and pathological features. Am J Obstet Gynecol 134:557, 1979

84. Montague ACW, Swartz DP, Woodruff JD: Sarcoma arising in a leiomyoma of uterus. Am J Obstet Gynecol 92:421, 1965

85. Malkasian GD, Welch JS, Soule EH: Primary leiomyosarcoma of the vagina. Am J Obstet Gynecol 86:730, 1963

86. Tobon H, Murphy AI, Salazar H: Primary leiomyosarcoma of the vagina. Cancer 32:450, 1973

87. Underwood PB Jr., Smith RT: Carcinoma of the vagina. JAMA 217:46, 1971

88. Chalmers JA: Fibromyoma of the fallopian tube. J Obstet Gynecol Br Emp 55:156, 1948

89. Kelly JA: Gynecologic cancer in children. Pediatrics 15:354, 1939

90. Islam MU, Tablibi MA, Boyd PF, Laughlin VC: Leiomyosarcoma of kidney. JAMA 212:2266, 1970

91. Weisel W, Dockerty MD, Priestly JT: Sarcoma of the kidney. J Urol 50:564, 1963

92. Bazaz-Malid C, Gupta DN: Leiomyosarcoma of kidney: Report of case with review of literature. J Urol 95:754, 1966

93. Papacharalambous AN, Pavlakis AJ: Leiomyosarcoma of the bladder. Br J Urol 51:321, 1979

94. Henrichs KJ, Wenisch JH, Hofmann W, Klein F: Leiomyosarcoma of the pulmonary artery: A light and electron microscopical study. Virchows Arch [A] 383:207, 1979

95. Munk J, Giffel B, Kogan J: Primary mesenchymoma of pulmonary artery: Radiologic features. Br J Radiol 38:104, 1965

96. Jacques JE, Barclay R: Solid sarcomatous pulmonary artery. Br J Dis Chest 54:217, 1960

97. Wolf PL, Kirsenman RC, Langston JD: Fibrosarcoma of the pulmonary artery masquerading as a pheochromocytoma. Am J Clin Pathol 34:146, 1960

98. Kevorkian J, Cento DP: Leiomyosarcoma of large arteries and veins. Surgery 73:390, 1973

99. Szasz IJ, Baff R, Scobie TK: Leiomyosarcoma arising from veins: Two cases and a review of the literature on venous neoplasms. Can J Surg 170:415, 1969

100. Cope JS, Hunt CJ: Leiomyosarcoma of the inferior vena cava. Arch Surg 68:752, 1954

101. Font AJ, Noer HR: Primary leiomyosarcoma of antecubital vein: Report of case with review of literature. Grace Hosp Bull (Detroit) 33:35, 1955

102. Abell JR: Leiomyosarcoma of inferior vena cava: Review

of literature and report of two cases. Am J Clin Pathol 28:272, 1957

103. Harland WA, Clamen M, Rodriguez VM: Leiomyosarcoma of inferior vena cava with clinical feature of Chiari's syndrome. Can Med Assoc J 83:1964, 1960

104. Melchior E: Sarcom der Vana Cava Inerior. Dtsch Zentralbl Chir 213:135, 1928

105. Allan J, Burnett W, Lee FD: Leiomyosarcoma of the inferior vena cava. Scott Med J 9:352, 1964

106. Caplan BB, Halasz NA, Bloomer WE: Resection and ligation of the suprarenal inferior vena cava. J Urol 92:25, 1966

107. Gariepy JA, Pope RH: Leiomyosarcoma of the inferior vena cava. Conn Med 31:102, 1967

108. Nartowicz E, Domaniewaki J, Wiecko W: Leiomyosarcome de la Veine Cava Inferieure Traitement Errone de Cholecystite. Maroc Med 47:339, 1967

109. Staley CJ, Valaitis J, Trippel OH, Franzblau SA: Leiomyosarcoma of the inferior vena cava. Am J Surg 113:221, 1967

110. Hopson WB, Burlison PE, Sherman RT: Leiomyosarcoma of the inferior vena cava. Ann Surg 168:290, 1968

111. Gue'don J, Mesnard J, Poisson J, Kuss R: Hypertension renovasculaire par leiomyosarcoma de la veine cava Inferieure, Guerison del' hypertension et Survie de 2 ans apres intervention chirurgicale. Ann Med Interne (Paris) 121:905, 1970

112. Jurayj NM, Midell Al, Bederinan S, et al.: Primary leiomyosarcoma of the inferior vena cava: Report of a case and review of the literature. Cancer 26:1349, 1970

113. Dube VE, Carlquist JH: Surgical treatment of leiomyosarcoma of the inferior vena cava: Report of a case. Am Surg 37:87, 1971

114. Wray RC, Dawkins H: Primary smooth muscle tumors of the inferior vena cava. Ann Surg 174:1009, 1971

115. Johansen JK, Nielsen R: Leiomyosarcoma of the inferior vena cava. Acta Chir Scand 137:181, 1971

116. Couinaud C: Tumerus de la Veine Cave Inferieure. J Chir (Paris) 105:411, 1973

117. Hivet M, Poffleux J, Gastard J, Hernandez C: Sarcome de la Veine Cave Inferieure. Nouv Presse Med 2:569, 1973

118. Stuart FP, Barker WH: Palliative surgery for leiomyosarcoma of the inferior vena cava. Ann Surg 177:237, 1973

119. Demoulin JC, Sambon Y, Bandinet V, et al.: Leiomyosarcoma of the inferior vena cava: An unusual cause of pulmonary embolism. Chest 66:597, 1974

120. Kapsinow R, Brierre JT: Leiomyosarcoma of the inferior vena cava. J Louisiana State Med Soc 126:400, 1974

121. Kalsbeek HD: Leiomyosarcoma of the inferior vena cava. Arch Chir Neerl 26:35, 1974

122. Bailey RV, Stribling J, Weitzner S, Hardy JD: Leiomyosarcoma of the inferior vena cava: Report of a case and review of literature. Ann Surg 184:169, 1976

123. Jonasson O, Pritchard J, Lond D: Intraluminal leiomyosarcoma of the inferior vena cava: Report of a case. Cancer 19:1311, 1966

124. Light HG, Peskin GW, Ravdin IS: Primary tumors of the venous system. Cancer 13:818, 1960

125. Smout MS, Fisher JH: Leiomyosarcoma of saphenous vein. Can Med Assoc J 83:1066, 1960

126. Thomas NM, Fine G: Leiomyosarcoma of veins: Report of two cases and review of the literature. Cancer 13:96, 1960

127. Beaird JB, Scofield GF: Budd-Chiara syndrome: Hepatic vein occlusion due to leiomyosarcoma primary in the inferior vena cava. Arch Intern Med 110:435, 1962

128. Brohl H: Sarcoma wenae femoralis dextra ligatura venae femoralis (abstr). Dtsch Wochenschr (Vereins-Beilage) 23:30, 1897

129. Borchard: Ueber einc von Varicen des Unter-schenkels ausgehende eigenthunifiche Gesch-wulstdung (Angiosarkom). Arch Klin Chir 80:675, 1906

130. Ehrenberg L: Zwei Falle von Tumor in Herzen: ein Beitrag zur Kenntnis der Pathologie und symptomatologie der Herztumorch. Dtsch Arch Klin Med 103:293, 1911

131. van Ree A: Phlebosarcoma racemosum. Ned Tijdschr Geneeskd 1:759, 1919

132. Razzaboni G: Sarcoma primitivo defla vena safena interna (trombizzata). Arch Ital Chir 2:483, 1920

133. Ausbüttel F: Primares Lungensarkom. Frankfurt Ztschr f Pathol 53:303, 1939

134. Puig-Sureda J, Gallart-Esquerdo A, Roca de Vinals R, Salleras V: Leiomiosarcoma de la vena colica izquierda inferior. Med Clin 8:104, 1947

135. Haug WA, Losli EJ: Primary leiomyosarcoma within the femoral vein. Cancer 7:159, 1954

136. Johnston JH Jr., Shands WC: Primary leiomyosarcoma of the femoral vein. Surgery 38:410, 1955

137. DeWeese JA, Terry R, Schwartz SI: Leiomyoma of the greater saphenous vein with preoperative localization by phlebography. Ann Surg 148:859, 1958

138. Stout AP: Sarcomas of the soft tissue. Cancer 11:210, 1961

139. Dorfman HD, Fishel ER: Leiomyosarcoma of greater saphenous vein. Am J Clin Pathol 39:73, 1963

140. Allison NE: Leiomyosarcoma of the femoral vein: Report of a case in a child. Clin Pediatr 4:28, 1965

141. Cheek JH, Nickey WM: Leiomyosarcoma of venous origin. Arch Surg 90:396, 1965

142. Lawrence MS, Crosby VG, Ehrenhaft JL: Leiomyosarcoma of the right iliac vein: Case report. Ann Surg 164:924, 1966

143. Sakura O, Toda A, Morimoto K: Primary leiomyosarcoma within the femoral vein. Clin Orthop 44:197, 1966

144. Lopez-Varela EA, Peveira-Garro C: Leiomyosarcoma of the renal vein. Intl Surg 47:340, 1967

145. Leu HJ, Nipkow P: Malignant primary vein tumors. Angiologica 6:302, 1969

146. Bhathena D, Vasquez M: Primary renal vein leiomyosarcoma. Cancer 30:542, 1972

147. Larmi TKI, Ninimaki T: Leiomyosarcoma of the femoral vein. J Cardiovasc Surg 15:602, 1974

148. Nesbit RR Jr., Rob C: Leiomyosarcoma of a vein: Survival for six years. Arch Surg 110:118, 1975

149. Gross E, Horton MA: Leiomyosarcoma of the saphenous vein. J Pathol 116:37, 1975

150. Jemstrom P, Gowdy RA: Leiomyosarcoma of the long saphenous vein Am J Clin Pathol 63:25, 1975

151. Gierson ED, Rowe JG: Renal vein leiomyosarcoma. Am Surg 42:594, 1976

152. Hernandez FJ, Stanley TM, Ranganath KA, Rubinstein AI: Primary leiomyosarcoma of the aorta. Am J Surg Pathol 3:251, 1979

153. Bloustein PA: Hepatic leiomyosarcoma: Ultra-structural study and review of the differential diagnosis. Hum Pathol 9:713, 1978

154. Kullman GL: Intranasal leiomyosarcoma. J Fla Med Assoc 67:931, 1980

155. Anderson WR, Cameron JD, Tsai SH: Primary intracranial leiomyosarcoma. Case Report with ultrastructural study. J Neurosurg 53(3):401, 1980

156. Cermsak RJ: Benign rhabdomyoma of the vagina. Am J Clin Pathol 52:604, 1969

157. Hanbury WJ: Rhabdomyomatous tumors of the urinary bladder and prostate. J Pathol Bacteriol 64:763, 1952

158. Misch KA: Rhabdomyoma purum: A benign rhabdomyoma of tongue. J Pathol Bacteriol 75:105, 1958

159. Moran JJ, Enterline HT: Benign rhabdomyoma of the pharynx. A case report and review of the literature and comparison with cardiac rhabdomyoma. Am J Clin Pathol 42:174, 1964

160. LaBate JS: Congenital rhabdomyoma of the heart. Am J Pathol 15:137, 1939

161. Batchelor TM, Maun ME: Congenital glycogenic tumors of the heart. Arch Pathol 39:67, 1945

162. Winstanley DP: Sudden death from multiple rhabdomyoma of the heart. J Pathol Bacteriol 81:249, 1961

163. Burke AP, Virmani R: Cardiac rhabdomyoma: A clinicopathologic study. Mod Pathol 4:70, 1991

164. Crotty PL, Nakleh RE, Dehner LP: Juvenile rhabdomyosarcoma: An intermediate form of skeletal muscle tumor in children. Arch Pathol Lab Med 117:43, 1993

165. Di Sant Agnese PA, Knowles DM: Extracardiac rhabdomyoma: A clinicopathologic study and review of the literature. Cancer 46:780, 1980

166. Kapadia SB, Meis JM, Frisman DM, et al.: Fetal rhabdomyosarcoma of the head and neck: A clinicopathologic and immunophenotypic study of 24 cases. Hum Pathol 24:754, 1993

167. Bizer LS: Rhabdomyosarcoma. Am J Surg 140:687, 1980

168. Sessions DG, Ragab AH, Vietti TJ, et al.: Embryonal rhabdomyosarcoma of the neck in children. Laryngoscope 83:890, 1973

169. Jones IS, Reese AB, Kraut MD: Orbital rhabdomyosarcoma: An analysis of 62 cases. Am J Ophthalmol 62:203, 1959

170. Frayer WC, Enterline HT: Embryonal rhabdomyosarcoma of the orbit in children and young adults. Arch Ophthalmol 62:203, 1959

171. Pinkel D, Pickren J: Rhabdomyosarcoma in children. JAMA 174:293, 1961

172. Masson JK, Soule ED: Embryonal rhabdomyosarcoma of the head and neck: Report on eighty-eight cases. Am J Surg 110:585, 1965

173. Lawrence W Jr., Gegge G, Foote FW Jr.: Embryonal rhabdomyosarcoma: A clinicopathological study. Cancer 17:361, 1964

174. Koop CE, Tewarson IP: Rhabdomyosarcoma of the head and neck in children. Ann Surg 160:95, 1964

175. Grossi C, Moore O: Embryonal rhabdomyosarcoma of head and neck. Cancer 12:69, 1962

176. Porterfield JF, Zimmerman LE: Rhabdomyosarcoma of the orbit. A clinicopathologic study of 55 cases. Virchows Arch Path [A] 335:329, 1962

177. Sutow WW, Sullivan MP, Reid HL, et al.: Prognosis in childhood rhabdomyosarcoma. Cancer 25:1384, 1970

178. Sutow WW, Lindberg RD, Gehan EA, et al.: Three year relapse free survival rates in childhood rhabdomyosarcoma of the head and neck: Report from the Intergroup Rhabdomyosarcoma Study (IRS). Cancer 49:2217, 1982

179. Liebner EJ: Embryonal rhabdomyosarcoma of the head and neck in children. Cancer 37:2777, 1976

180. Horn RC, Enterline HT: Rhabdomyosarcoma: A clinicopathological study and classification of 39 cases. Cancer 11:181, 1958

181. Pratt CB, Hustu HO, Fleming ID, Pinkel D: Co-ordinated treatment of childhood rhabdomyosarcoma with surgery, radiotherapy, and combination chemotherapy. Cancer Res 32:606, 1972

182. Cassady RJ, Sagerman RW, Trelter P, Ellsworth RM: Radiation therapy for rhabdomyosarcoma. Radiology 91:116, 1968

183. Heyn RN, Holland R, Rewton WA, et al.: The role of combined chemotherapy in the treatment of rhabdomyosarcoma in children. Cancer 34:2128, 1974

184. Maurer HM: Current concepts in cancer. N Engl J Med 299:1345, 1978

185. Jaffe BF: Pediatric head and neck tumors. Laryngoscope 83:1644, 1973

186. Donaldson SS, Castro JR, Wilburn JR, Jesse RJ: Rhabdomyosarcoma of the head and neck in children: Combination treatment by surgery, irradiation, and chemotherapy. Cancer 31:26, 1973

187. Jaffe N, Fitler RM, Farber S, et al.: Rhabdomyosarcoma in children. Am J Surg 125:482, 1973

188. Heyn RN: The role of chemotherapy in the management of soft tissue sarcomas. Cancer 35:921, 1975

189. Bale PM, Parsons RE, Stevens MM: Diagnosis and behavior of juvenile rhabdomyosarcoma. Hum Pathol 14:596, 1983

190. Crist WM, Garnsey L, Beltangady MS, et al.: Prognosis in children with rhabdomyosarcoma: A report of Intergroup Rhabdomyosarcoma studies I and II. J Clin Oncol 8:443, 1990

191. Ghavimi F, Mandell LR, Heller G, et al.: Prognosis in childhood rhabdomyosarcoma of the extremity. Cancer 64:2233, 1989

192. Maurer HM, Gehan EA, Beltangady M, et al.: The Intergroup Rhabdomyosarcoma study II. Cancer 71:1904, 1993

193. Raney RB Jr., Crist WM, Maurer HM, et al.: Prognosis of children with soft tissue sarcoma who relapse after achieving a complete response: A report from the Intergroup Rhabdomyosarcoma study I. Cancer 52:44, 1983

194. Berry MP, Jenkin RDT: Parameningeal rhabdomyosarcoma in the young. Cancer 48:281, 1981

195. Raney RB Jr., Teft M, Newton WA, et al.: Improved prognosis with intensive treatment of children with cranial soft tissue sarcomas arising in nonorbital parameningeal sites. Cancer 59:147, 1987

196. Pack GT, Eberhart WF: Rhabdomyosarcoma of skeletal muscle. Report of 100 cases. Surgery 32:1023, 1952
197. Stout AP: Rhabdomyosarcoma of skeletal muscle. Ann Surg 123:447, 1946
198. Hays DM: Rhabdomyosarcoma. Clin Orthop 289:36, 1993
199. Ehrlich FF, Haas JE, Kieswelter WB: Rhabdomyosarcoma in infants and children—Factors affecting long-term survival. J Pediatr Surg 6:571, 1971
200. Grosfeld JL, Clatworthy HW Jr., Newton WA Jr.: Combined therapy in childhood rhabdomyosarcoma: An analysis of 42 cases. J Pediatr Surg 4:637, 1969
201. Albores-Saavedra J, Martin RG, Smith JL: Rhabdomyosarcoma: A study of 35 cases. Ann Surg 157:186, 1963
202. Ghavimi F, Exelby PR, D'Angio, et al.: Combination therapy of urogenital embryonal rhabdomyosarcoma in children. Cancer 32:1178, 1973
203. Lawrence W Jr., Hays DM, Moon TE: Lymphatic metastasis with childhood rhabdomyosarcoma. Cancer 39:556, 1977
204. Dito WR, Batsakis JG: Rhabdomyosarcoma of the head and neck: Appraisal of biologic behavior in 170 cases. Arch Surg 84:582, 1962
205. Enzinger FM, Lattes R, Torloni H: Histological typing of soft tissue tumors. In: International Histological Classification of Tumors, no. 3. Geneva, WHO, 1969
206. Flamant F, Hill C: The improvement is survival associated with combined chemotherapy in childhood rhabdomyosarcoma: A historical comparison of 345 patients in the same centers. Cancer 53:2417, 1984
207. Rodery C, Flamant F, Donaldson SS: An attempt to use a common staging system in rhabdomyosarcoma: A report of an international workshop initiated by the International Society of Pediatric Oncology (SIOP). Med Pediatr Oncol 17:210, 1989
208. McDougal WS, Persky L: Rhabdomyosarcoma of the bladder and prostate in children. J Urol 124:882, 1980
209. Lemmon WT Jr., Holland JM, Ketcham AS: Rhabdomyosarcoma of the prostate. Surgery 59:736, 1966
210. Grosfeld JL, Smith JP, Clatworthy HW Jr.: Pelvic rhabdomyosarcoma in infants and children. J Urol 107:673, 1972
211. Waring PM, Newland RC: Prostatic embryonal rhabdomyosarcoma in adults. Cancer 69:755, 1992
212. Alexander F: Pure testicular rhabdomyosarcoma. Br J Cancer 22:498, 1968
213. Littmann R, Tessler AN, Valensi Q: Paratesticular rhabdomyosarcoma: A case presentation and review of the literature. J Urol 108:190, 1972
214. Tank ES: Treatment of urogenital tract rhabdomyosarcoma in infants and children. J Urol 107:324, 1972
215. Ghazali S: Embryonic rhabdomyosarcoma of the urogenital tract. Br J Surg 60:124, 1973
216. Tanimura H, Matsuhiro F: Rhabdomyosarcoma of the spermatic cord. Cancer 22:1215, 1968
217. Hilgers RD, Malkasian GD Jr., Soule EH: Embryonal rhabdomyosarcoma (botryoid type) in the vagina: A clinicopathologic review. Am J Obstet Gynecol 107:485, 1970
218. D'Angio GJ, Teft M: Radiation therapy in the management of children with gynecologic cancers. Ann NY Acad Sci 142:675, 1967
219. El-Mahdi AM, Marks R, Thornton WN, Constable WC: Twenty-five-year survival of sarcoma botryoides treated by irradiation. Cancer 33:653, 1974
220. Hays DM, Snyder WH Jr.: Botryoid sarcoma (rhabdomyosarcoma) of the bile ducts. Am J Dis Child 110:595, 1965
221. Yartid T, Nickels J, Hockerstedt K, Scheinin TM: Rhabdomyosarcoma of the esophagus. Light and electron microscopic study of a rare tumor. Virchows Arch Path [A] 386:357, 1980
222. Moses I, Coodley EL: Rhabdomyosarcoma of duodenum. Am J Gastroenterol 51:48, 1969
223. Templeton AW, Heslin DI: Primary rhabdomyosarcoma of stomach and esophagus. Am J Roentgenol 86:896, 1961
224. Matloff JM, Bas H, Dalen JE: Rhabdomyosarcoma of the left atrium. J Thorac Cardiovasc Surg 61:451, 1971
225. Makela V, Sjogren AL, Eisalo A: Rhabdomyosarcoma of the heart: A case report. Acta Pathol Microbiol Scand, 78A:71, 1970
226. Payan H: Rhabdomyosarcoma of the ovary: Report of a case. Obstet Gynecol 26:373, 1965
227. Goldman RL, Friedman NB: Rhabdomyosarcohepatoma in an adult and embryonal hepatoma in a child. Am J Clin Pathol 51:137, 1969
228. Conquest HF, Thornton JL, Massie JR, Coxe JW: Primary pulmonary rhabdomyosarcoma: Report of three cases and literature review. Ann Surg 161:688, 1965
229. Mihara S, Matsumoto H, Tokunaga F, et al.: Botryoid rhabdomyosarcoma of the gallbladder in a child. Cancer 49:812, 1982
230. Keyhani A, Booher RJ: Pleomorphic rhabdomyosarcoma. Cancer 22:956, 1968
231. Linscheid RL, Soule EH, Henderson ED: Pleomorphic rhabdomyosarcomata of the extremities and limb girdles: A clinicopathologic study. J Bone Joint Surg 47B:715, 1965
232. Middlebrook LF, Tennant R: Rhabdomyosarcoma of uterine corpus. Obstet Gynecol 32:537, 1968
233. Enzinger FM, Weiss SW: Soft Tissue Tumors 3rd ed. Mosby, St. Louis, 1995, p 563
234. deJong AS, van Kessel-van Mark M, Albus Lutter CE: Pleomorphic rhabdomyosarcoma in adults: Immunohistochemistry as a tool for its diagnosis. Hum Pathol 18:298, 1987
235. Gaffney EF, Dervan PA, Fletcher CD: Pleomorphic rhabdomyosarcomas in adulthood: Analysis of 11 cases with definition of diagnostic criteria. Am J Surg Pathol 17:601, 1993
236. Lloyd RV, Hajdu SI, Knapper WH: Embryonal rhabdomyosarcoma in adults. Cancer 51:557, 1983
237. Thompson GCV: Rhabdomyosarcoma of skeletal muscle. Clin Orthop 19:29, 1961
238. Phelan JT, Juardo J: Rhabdomyosarcoma. Surgery 52:585, 1962
239. Purry H, Chu FCH: Radiation therapy in the palliative management of soft tissue sarcomas. Cancer 15:179, 1962

240. Kaloyannides TM: Pleomorphic rhabdomyosarcoma. Surg 27:150, 1969

241. Riopelle JS, Thierault JP: Sur une forme meconnue de sarcome des parties molies: Le rhabdomyosarcoma alve-olaire. Ann Anat Pathol (Paris) 1:88, 1956

242. Enzinger FM: Recent trends in soft tissue pathology. In: Tumors of Bone and Soft Tissue. Clinical Conference on Cancer, 1963. Chicago, Year Book Medical Publishers, 1965, p 315

243. Enzinger FM, Shiraki M: Alveolar rhabdomyosarcoma: An analysis of 110 cases. Cancer 24:18, 1969

244. Enterline HT, Hom RC: Alveolar rhabdomyosarcoma. A distinctive tumor type. Am J Clin Pathol 29:356, 1958

245. Mikulowski P, Thorbjorn B: Alveolar rhabdomyosar-coma. Acta Pathol Microbiol Scand 74:282, 1969

246. Hays DM, Soule EH, Lawrence W Jr, et al.: Extremity lesions in the Intergroup Rhabdomyosarcoma Study (IRS-1): A preliminary report. Cancer 49:1, 1982

247. Patton RB, Horn RC Jr.: Rhabdomyosarcoma: Clinical and pathological features and comparison with human fetal and embryonal skeletal muscle. Surgery 52:572, 1961

248. King DG, Finney RP: Embryonal rhabdomyosarcoma of the prostate. J Urol 117:88, 1977

249. Dupree WB, Fisher C: Rhabdomyosarcoma of prostate in adult. Long-term survival and problem of histologic diagnosis. Urology 19:80, 1982

250. Keenan DJ, Graham WH: Embryonal rhabdomyosar-coma of the prostatic-urethral region in an adult. Br J Urol 57:241, 1985

251. Henkes DN, Stein N: Fine-needle aspiration cytology of prostatic embryonal rhabdomyosarcoma: A case report. Diagn Cytopathol 3:163, 1987

252. Miettinen M: Rhabdomyosarcoma in patients older than 40 years of age. Cancer 62:2060, 1988

253. Waring PM, Newland RC: Prostatic embryonal rhab-domyosarcoma in adults: A clinicopathologic review. Cancer 69:755, 1992

# 10

# Tumors of the Peripheral Nerves

## ■ BENIGN TUMORS

Though morphologic classification of peripheral nerve tumors is clouded with considerable controversy (see Chapter 5), the principles of management of these tumors or tumorlike conditions remain unaffected. Thus, in this chapter, the subsets of benign tumors of Schwannian origin and those arising from the nerve sheath have been combined into a single clinical entity—*schwannoma*. However, we will allude to situations in which a specific histologic subset needs to be emphasized for better planning of the management of these entities; otherwise, the terms *neurofibroma* and *neurilemoma* are used interchangeably in this chapter. For detailed discussion of the histogenetic difference of these terms, see pages 129–139, Chapter 5.

### SOLITARY SCHWANNOMA

A benign solitary schwannoma (neurilemoma, perineural fibroblastoma), usually an encapsulated tumor, may occur in any part of the body.[1-3] If the tumor arises from a large peripheral nerve, it can easily be seen; but if it arises from an unnamed small nerve twig, it is clinically indistinguishable from other types of soft tissue tumors.

#### Anatomic Distribution

Table 10–1 shows the general anatomic distribution of benign solitary schwannomas encountered in clinical practice. Clearly, these tumors have a predilection for the head and neck region.

Although the symptoms and signs vary according to anatomic location, most patients are first seen with a painless mass of relatively long duration (Figure 10–1).

### TABLE 10–1. ANATOMIC DISTRIBUTION OF BENIGN SOLITARY SCHWANNOMAS

| Anatomic Site | Das Gupta et al.[4] (1969) | Present Series |
|---|---|---|
| Head and neck | 136 | 35 |
| Upper extremities | 58 | 27 |
| Trunk | 26 | 12 |
| Lower extremities | 41 | 26 |
| Mediastinum | 28 | 3 |
| Miscellaneous sites | 14* | 6[†] |
| Total | 303 | 109 |

*Miscellaneous sites (Memorial Sloan-Kettering Cancer Center) include breast, 8; hernial sac, 1; pelvis, 1; inguinal canal, 1; retroperitoneal region, 1; and sciatic nerve, 1.
[†]Miscellaneous sites (University of Illinois) include retroperitoneum, 3; inguinal region, 2; and breast, 1.

If the tumor arises from a peripheral nerve, the patient may have pain along the course of the nerve before the mass is discovered. Some patients are initially seen solely because of pain along the radial, median, ulnar, or sciatic nerve.

Of the 303 patients in our original series,[4] 56.7 percent were female and 43.3 percent were male; 63 percent of the tumors occurred in patients between the ages of 30 and 60 years. A similar sex and age distribution was observed in our patients in our current series. No racial predilection was apparent in either series.

***Head and Neck Region.*** Most commonly, this tumor is seen as a fusiform mass in the lateral portion of the neck (Table 10–2), and frequently it poses a diagnostic and therapeutic problem (Fig. 10–2A to 10–2F).

**TABLE 10–2. BENIGN SCHWANNOMAS OF THE HEAD AND NECK REGION**

| Anatomic Site | Das Gupta et al.[4] (1969) | Present Series |
|---|---|---|
| Scalp | 7 | 3 |
| Forehead | 1 | 1 |
| Face | 2 | 2 |
| Nose | 4 | 1 |
| Cheek | 9 | 1 |
| Tongue | 8 | 1 |
| Lip | 3 | — |
| Neck (lateral) | 60 | 18 |
| Parotid gland | 10 | 1 |
| Pharynx | 8 | — |
| Submaxillary gland | 4 | — |
| Hard palate | 3 | 1 |
| Soft palate | 3 | 1 |
| Miscellaneous sites | 14* | 5† |
| Total | 136 | 35 |

*Miscellaneous sites include eyelid, 1; auditory canal, 1; gum, 1; floor of mouth, 1; supraorbital region, 2; infraorbital region, 1; vagus nerve, 2; vocal cord, 1; pterygoid, 1; preauricular area, 2; and mastoid region, 1.
†Miscellaneous sites include eyelid, 1; vagus nerve, 1; and behind the ear over the mastoid region, 3.

**TABLE 10–3. ANATOMIC DISTRIBUTION OF BENIGN SCHWANNOMAS IN THE EXTREMITIES**

| Anatomic Site | Das Gupta et al.[4] (1969) | Present Series |
|---|---|---|
| **Upper extremities** | | |
| Hand | 20 | 4 |
| Wrist | 5 | 4 |
| Forearm | 8 | 8 |
| Elbow | 2 | — |
| Arm | 13 | 9 |
| Shoulder girdle | 10 | 2 |
| **Lower extremities** | | |
| Sole | — | 1 |
| Dorsum | — | 3 |
| Ankle | 11 | 4 |
| Leg | 6 | 4 |
| Calf | 3 | 2 |
| Knee | 10 | 2 |
| Thigh | 6 | 5 |
| Buttock | 2 | 5 |
| Groin | 3 | — |
| Total | 99 | 53 |

Although the primary surgical objective for schwannomas of the neck should be a simple excision, occasionally a modified form of neck dissection is required. However, the guiding principle of surgical therapy is conservatism. In all other areas of the head and neck region, enucleation is usually adequate.[4–9] Lesions in the scalp sometimes require sequential excision (Fig. 10–2A), depending on the extent and local infiltration. Total extirpation of scalp lesions is often fraught with considerable blood loss. Lesions of the face and parotid region require exposure of the facial nerve.

Benign schwannoma of the vagus nerve is a rare and interesting clinical entity.[5,7,10,11] Only 63 cases were published until 1979.[11] These tumors do not produce any symptoms of vagal insufficiency, and diagnosis is usually made at the time of operation.

***Upper Extremities.*** Table 10–3 shows the anatomic distribution of benign schwannomas of the extremities. Most patients seek medical advice because of a mass along the course of a nerve. Usually this mass enlarges slowly, creating a cosmetic defect. In a smaller number of patients, pain along the nerve is the initial symptom. Rarely, there may be pain because of pressure of the mass on a bone: for example, a neurofibroma pressing on a phalanx (Fig. 10–3A and 10–3B).[4,9] In our series of 27 patients (Table 10–3) at the University of Illinois, 18 were initially seen because of a mass and 9 because of

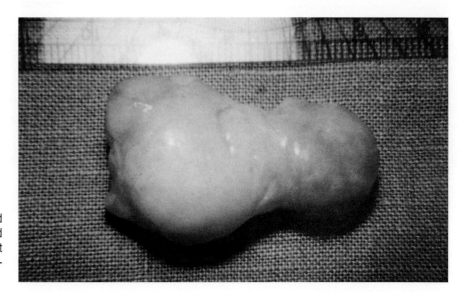

**Figure 10–1.** Benign schwannoma enucleated from the radial nerve. This patient, a 36-year-old woman, presented with an asymptomatic tumor at the posterolateral aspect of the right arm, requesting tumor be removed for cosmetic reasons.

referred pain along the course of a major nerve. These tumors can be enucleated from the nerve of origin with relative ease.

***Lower Extremities.***   Table 10–3 shows the distribution of these tumors in the lower extremities. In our series of 26 patients, 5 had pain along the course of the sciatic nerve as the initial complaint. The pain occurred three to four months before recognition of the tumor. These tumors, like those in the upper extremities that are associated with a major nerve, can usually be enucleated from that nerve.

***Trunk.***   Usually a mass is the presenting symptom in schwannomas of the trunk.[3,6,8] In our series of 12 cases, 8 tumors were encountered in various parts of the anterior, lateral, or posterior chest wall, and the remaining 4 were in the anterior abdominal wall or lumbosacral region.[4] These tumors can be easily and successfully excised (Fig. 10–4).

***Miscellaneous Sites.***   Benign solitary schwannomas usually occur in the mediastinum[12,13] and various other miscellaneous sites.[8,9,14–21] These patients are essentially asymptomatic, and diagnosis is often made after a routine chest roentgenogram.

Retroperitoneal benign schwannomas can also be encountered. In one, a large (21 × 20 × 12 cm) tumor was found at operation, lying posterior to the gastrocolic omentum (Fig. 10–5). It was removed without difficulty. The specimen weighed 2.5 kg and had a dense fibrous capsule. The patient remained well for three years, at which time a carcinoma of the left breast was diagnosed. She underwent a radical mastectomy elsewhere and died two years later, apparently of metastatic breast cancer. An autopsy was not performed.

A benign solitary schwannoma is easily excised. Since the chance of malignant transformation is extremely rare (see Chapter 5 for detailed discussion), wide excisions are not advocated. When the tumor arises from a major nerve, it should be enucleated from the nerve trunk. Resection of the nerve is seldom required (Fig. 10–6). Benign peripheral nerve tumors are easily separated from the nerve trunk, which can and must be left intact.[22] Likewise, in the mediastinum and the peritoneal and pelvic cavities, the benign tumor can be enucleated.

Cellular schwannoma was originally described by Harkin and Reed[23] and Woodruff et al.[24] This tumor is now accepted as a distinct clinical entity and a variant of schwannomas.[25] Because of their cellularity, mitotic activity, and destruction of surrounding tissues (e.g., bone), these tumors are frequently mistaken for low-grade malignant schwannomas. However, several studies[25,26] have shown that these tumors are indeed benign, and the method(s) of management are exactly those for benign schwannomas (neurofibromas) (i.e., conservative excision).

## SOLITARY SCHWANNOMAS AND ASSOCIATED TUMORS

In 1969, Das Gupta et al.[4] reported that 49 (16 percent) of 303 patients with benign solitary neurogenic tumors had an associated malignant tumor of some kind. Twenty-two had been treated for a malignancy before developing schwannoma, and 16 were found to have a simultaneous carcinoma. Seven were first seen because of the benign tumor and nine because of the malignancy. In 11 patients, cancer developed after excision of the benign tumor.

The associated cancers seen most frequently in this study were epidermoid cancers of the skin (15), carcinoma of the breast (12), and carcinoma of the gastrointestinal tract (8). There were also carcinomas of the thyroid, uterine cervix, endometrium, and larynx, and three malignant melanomas. Of particular interest is the development of malignant melanoma and gastrointestinal tract cancers. In our present series of 109 patients, 18 were treated for an associated cancer: six had cancer of the breast; seven of the colon and rectum; three malignant melanoma; and one each of the cervix and ovary.

## MELANOTIC SCHWANNOMA

Melanotic schwannoma is a rare form of pigmented neural tumor that is usually associated with the sympathetic nervous system. These tumors are usually laden with melanin pigment, circumscribed, and occur anywhere in the body, but, as mentioned above, they are usually found where sympathetic trunk is most prominent (e.g., posterior mediastinum).[27–29] The rarity of these tumors does not allow any specific information as to their natural history or method(s) of management.

## MUCOSAL NEUROMA

Mucosal neuroma involves the mucous membranes of the oral cavity, lips, and intestine of patients with multiple endocrine neoplasia, type 2b characterized by bilateral pheochromocytoma, C-cell hyperplasia, medullary carcinoma of the thyroid, and parathyroid hyperplasia.[30] In most instances, the neuromas do not cause any specific symptoms, and they seldom require any excision. In those associated with endocrine neoplasia, treatment is directed towards that disorder.

## ■ TRAUMATIC NEUROMAS (AMPUTATION NEUROMAS)

The term *amputation neuroma* was first proposed in 1811 by Odier,[31] who believed these tumors to be of peripheral nerve origin. An accurate description of this entity, however, was first provided by Wood[32] in 1829.

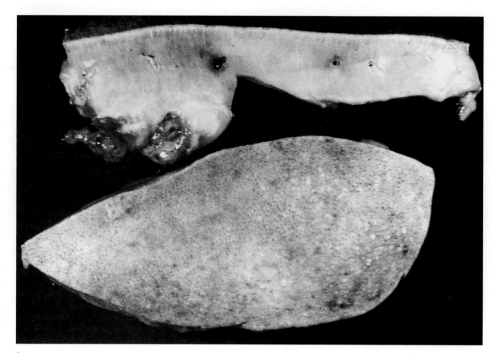

**Figure 10–2. (A)** Benign solitary schwannoma of the scalp. Cut section shows infiltration of thickness of the scalp by glistening white neoplastic tissue. **(B)** Solitary schwannoma of the face, excised without residual deformity. **(C)** Benign schwannoma of the tongue. Patient complained of gradually increasing feeling of "heaviness" in the tongue. The tumor was excised with a rim of tongue tissue.

*(Continued.)*    **A**

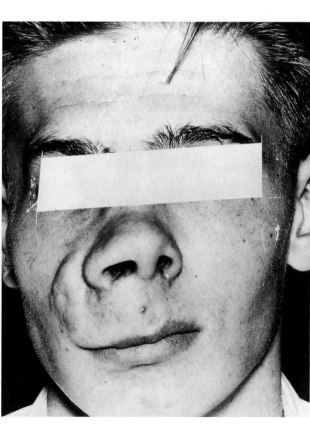

**B**

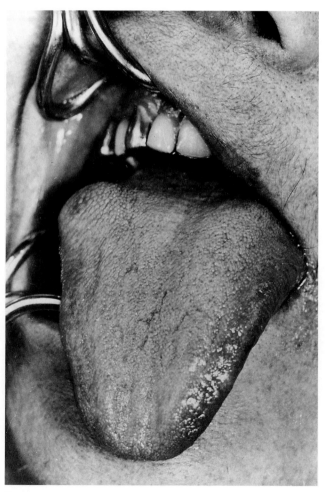

**C**

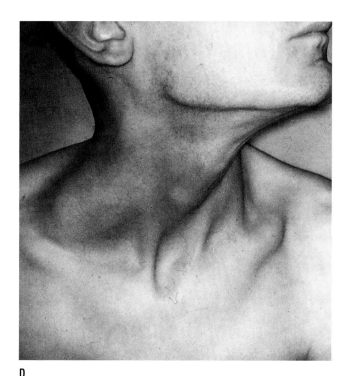

D

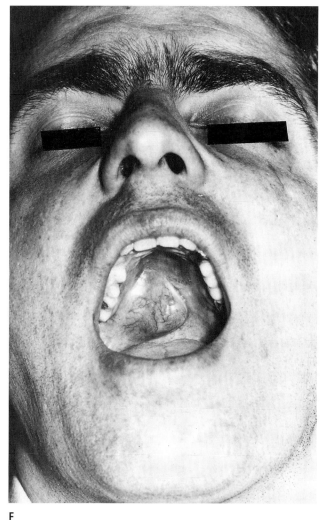

E

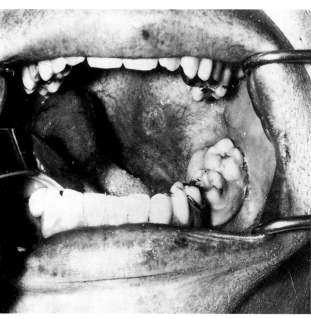

F

**Figure 10–2** *(continued).* **(D)** Solitary schwannoma of the right side of the neck. Tumor arose from brachial plexus and was enucleated. **(E)** Benign schwannoma enucleated from soft palate of a 31-year-old man. **(F)** Benign schwannoma of the hard palate, left side. Note central ulceration (pressure necrosis) of the mucosa. This large mass required a subtotal maxillectomy. The orbital floor, however, could be saved.

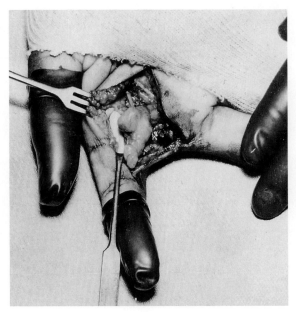

**A**

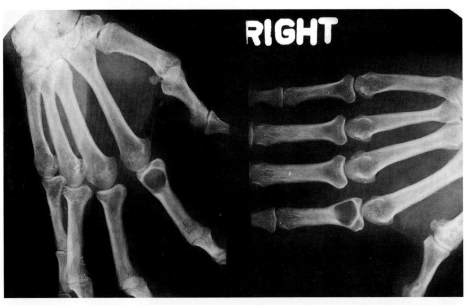

**Figure 10–3. (A)** Multilobulated neurofibroma being excised from the base of the index finger. **(B)** Roentgenographic appearance of the base of the index finger as a result of bone absorption *(Courtesy of Cancer 24:355, 1969).*

**B**

Although there was a definite lack of interest concerning this entity among the investigators of the early and middle nineteenth century, it was established that scar tissue was one of the contributing factors in the formation of amputation neuromas. In 1920, Huber and Lewis,[33] using rabbit peripheral nerves as their experimental system, described the histogenesis of amputation neuromas and popularized this term. A comprehensive clinical report of this entity in a large number of patients was reported by Cieslak and Stout[34] in 1946. At present, the terms *amputation neuroma* and *traumatic neuroma* are used interchangeably. Since the report by

Cieslak and Stout,[34] several other studies dealing with the clinical and histopathologic features have been published.[35–38]

Neuromas arising at the end of a bisected peripheral nerve following amputation for a benign disease, or after traumatic amputations, have been well described.[38,39] In 1969, Das Gupta and Brasfield[40] analyzed the clinicopathologic features of traumatic neuromas in 67 cancer patients in whom a neuroma developed after radical operation for a primary malignant tumor. They found that traumatic neuromas occurred at all ages, in both sexes, and in all anatomic sites.

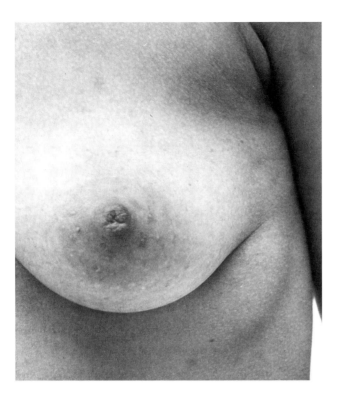

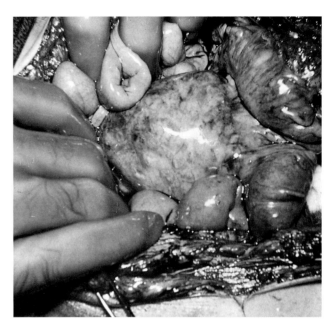

**Figure 10–5.** Intraoperative view of retroperitoneal benign schwannoma. The entire tumor could be enucleated with little difficulty.

**Figure 10–4.** Benign solitary schwannoma arising from the sixth intercostal nerve. The lesion was excised with a free margin of intercostal nerve on both sides of the fusiform tumor. It was necessary to enter the chest cavity. Patient is still well 15 years later.

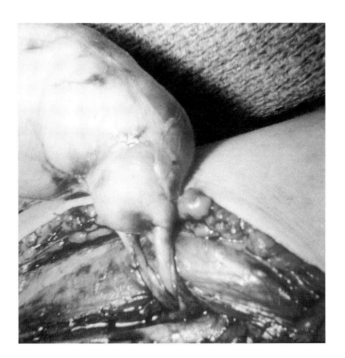

**Figure 10–6.** A relatively large schwannoma of the median nerve. A segmental excision of the nerve was considered; however, a diagnosis of malignancy was not forthcoming. The tumor was thus dissected out from the main trunk of the median nerve. Final histologic diagnosis of a benign neurogenic tumor justified the time-consuming dissection. Patient is well 14 years later, without any functional deformity.

Almost all types of surgical procedures lead to the development of traumatic neuromas. However, traumatic neuromas appear more frequently in the lateral portion of the neck, after a radical neck dissection or a forequarter amputation.

A swelling or mass of varying diameter in the surgical area is a common sign of a traumatic neuroma. Distinguishing a traumatic neuroma at the site of operation from local recurrence of the malignant tumor is often almost impossible (Fig. 10–7). In our previous study,[40] 7.5 percent of the neuromas were observed concomitantly with local recurrence. Furthermore, in 33 percent of the patients, local recurrence appeared after one or more traumatic neuromas were excised. A diagnosis of traumatic neuroma in cancer patients must therefore be substantiated by histologic examination.

There is no known method of preventing the development of traumatic neuroma, especially in regions where a surgical procedure necessarily leads to the resection of a number of peripheral nerves. The plan of treatment of a traumatic neuroma is to identify the nerve stump, free it from the surrounding scar tissue, resect it at a higher plane, and direct it away from the line of scar formation. During the initial operation, sharply resecting the nerve trunk and directing it away from the site of scar formation probably provides the best known protection against the development of neuromas.

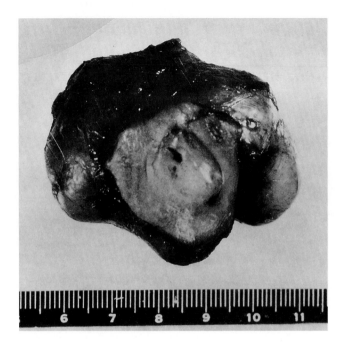

**Figure 10–7.** Traumatic neuroma removed from the lateral neck following radical neck dissection. Preoperatively, tumor was considered to be local recurrence.

## TRITON TUMORS

Triton tumors are extremely rare hamartomous conditions in which both skeletal muscles and neural elements are intertwined. A more common occurrence is a malignant variant where a malignant schwannoma is seen with rhabdomyoblastic differentiation (see page 143, Chapter 5 for further details). Treatment is usually conservative excision.

## ■ VON RECKLINGHAUSEN'S NEUROFIBROMATOSIS (MULTIPLE NEUROFIBROMATOSIS)

Multiple neurofibromatosis has been observed in all races and in every part of the world.[41-43] The incidence was estimated by Prieser and Davenport[44] in 1918 at approximately 1 in 2,000 persons. Crowe and associates[42] estimated the incidence in the state of Michigan to be 1 in every 2,500 to 3,000 live births. Brasfield and Das Gupta[45] encountered an average of only five patients a year at Memorial Sloan-Kettering Cancer Center over a period of 20 years. At the University of Illinois, there are approximately 10 new patients a year with von Recklinghausen's neurofibromatosis out of about 17,000 admissions.[46] Sexual distribution is probably equal, although early reports indicated a predilection for males. Crowe and associates[42] found that male patients constituted 52 percent of their series of 149. Fisher[47] reviewed the 466 cases reported up to 1927 and found that 64 percent of the patients were male. In a series of 110 patients from the Memorial Sloan-

Kettering Cancer Center, combined with 60 patients from the University of Illinois Hospital, the percentage was 53 percent female.[45,46] Sergeyev[48] found a 52 percent female predominance in his series of 195 patients. The gender ratio has remained the same even in our current enlarged series of patients.

This disease is currently divided into two distinct types: type 1 (formerly peripheral type) and type 2 (formerly central type). Type 1 (peripheral form) is more common. In a consensus conference held in 1987, certain diagnostic criteria were established for type 1 neurofibromatosis.[49] The presence of two or more of the following signs would confirm the diagnosis: (1) six or more café-au-lait spots larger than 5 mm in diameter in prepubescent individuals and 15 mm in postpubertal individuals; (2) two or more neurofibromas of any type or one plexiform neurofibroma; (3) freckling in the axillary or inguinal region; (4) optic glioma; (5) two or more Lisch nodules; (6) a distinctive osseous lesion, such as sphenoid dysplasia or thinning of long bone cortex with or without pseudoarthrosis; and (7) a first-degree relative (parent, sibling, or offspring) with neurofibromatosis as defined by the above criteria.

Because of the association of von Recklinghausen's neurofibromatosis with various benign and malignant soft tissue tumors and other cancers (Table 10–4),[45] some of the intriguing facets of the disease will be described in detail.

## GENETIC ASPECTS

The occurrence of this disease in multiple family members was reported by Virchow[50] as early as 1847, and again in 1862 by Hitchcock.[51] However, Thomson,[52] in 1900, was the first to point out that the condition was clearly hereditary. A year later, Adrian[53] reported that 20 percent of patients exhibited direct transmission. In 1918, Prieser and Davenport[44] established that the condition was not sex-linked and that it followed the Mendelian law as a dominant trait.

**TABLE 10–4. INCIDENCE OF ASSOCIATED COMPLICATIONS IN PATIENTS WITH VON RECKLINGHAUSEN'S NEUROFIBROMATOSIS**

| Associated Complications | No. Patients* | Percentage |
|---|---|---|
| Benign schwannomas (neurofibromas, neurilemmomas) | 65 | 58.0 |
| Osseous involvement | 52 | 47.2 |
| Other types of cancer | 16 | 14.5 |
| Central nervous system involvement | 13 | 12.0 |
| Gastrointestinal tract involvement | 12 | 11.0 |
| Vascular lesion involvement | 4 | 3.6 |
| Miscellaneous cancers | 5 | 4.5 |

*Total number of patients studied is 110. Some patients had more than one system involved.
Adapted from Brasfield and Das Gupta.[45]

Prieser and Davenport[44] noted that penetrance of the dominant gene is greater than 80 percent, which has been recently confirmed in other studies.[41,42,45] The penetrance of the gene in children of persons with sporadic cases is likewise greater than 80 percent, as attested to by the fact that approximately 40 percent of the children are affected. The expression of specific manifestations in multiple generations has been reported frequently, but, as a rule, the manifestations in a particular family vary (Fig. 10–8).

The sporadic cases make up approximately half of those reported in the literature, and it is impossible to distinguish them clinically from the familial types. It has not yet been established whether a sporadic case appears as the result of a new mutation or occurs in the child of a person possessing a nonpenetrant gene. Fifty percent of the patients are found to have affected relatives.[45,46] We have previously reported that, in five families, the disease could be traced through four generations.[45]

In monozygotic twins, concordance of clinical manifestations has been reported far more frequently than discordance.[54] As a rule, there is marked phenotypic variation of the disease in a family, although Crowe and co-workers[42] found palmar and plantar neurofibromas to be an exception to this rule (Fig. 10–9). Type 1 neurofibromatosis is associated with deletions, insertions, or mutations in the neurofibromatosis 1 gene, a tumor suppressor gene located in the pericentric region of Chromosome 17.[55,56] It is one of the longest human genes identified to date (300 kb) and contains within it three additional genes. It encodes a protein known as neurofibromin and can be found in all tissues. Neurofibromin probably plays an important role in cell growth through down-regulation of the ras gene product.

## CLINICAL MANIFESTATIONS

Most patients manifest the physical signs before the age of 20 years.[45,46] In a study conducted at a pediatric hospital, Feinman and Yakovac[57] reported that 43 percent of their 46 patients had the stigmata at birth. The most common manifestation leading to diagnosis is multiple café-au-lait spots, along with subcutaneous and cutaneous neurofibromas.

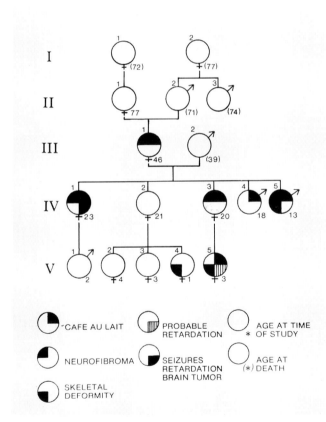

**Figure 10–8.** Pedigree of a family with von Recklinghausen's neurofibromatosis. Symbol III-1 is a patient with a sporadic case, representing either mutation or an instance in which one of the parents (II-1 and II-2) possessed a nonpenetrant gene. Symbol V-4 represents a patient with congenital bowed tibia; in this case, either the mother (IV-2) possessed a nonpenetrant gene or the disease is late in being expressed and will become evident later in life *(Courtesy of Ravich MM et al. (eds):* Current Problems in Surgery, *vol. 14, Chicago, Year Book Medical Publishers, 1977).*

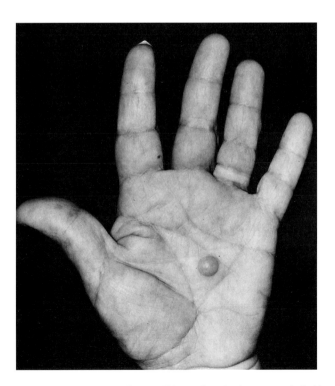

**Figure 10–9.** Palmar neurofibroma. This manifestation is rare even in florid cases of von Recklinghausen's neurofibromatosis, but is expressed frequently in families in whom it does occur. Patient had long family history of relatively uniform florid manifestations of von Recklinghausen's neurofibromatosis *(Courtesy of* Current Problems in Surgery, *1977.)*

## Pigmentary Changes

The lesion classically identified with von Recklinghausen's neurofibromatosis is a brown macular pigmentation of the skin with definite, circumscribed geographic borders. This characteristic appearance has led to the use of the descriptive term *café-au-lait spot*. These spots may be located anywhere on the body and vary in size, configuration, and number (Fig. 10–10).

After Crowe and co-workers[42] investigated the genetic and clinical significance of these macular pigmentations, there was no question that these lesions were very much part of the disease. Their report in 1956 concluded that café-au-lait spots are pathognomonic findings of generalized neurofibromatosis. They suggested that any person with more than six café-au-lait spots larger than 1.5 cm must be presumed to have neurofibromatosis, even in the absence of a positive family history. In a number of patients, the only initial evidence of neurofibromatosis is macular pigmentation, with cutaneous tumors developing later in life.

Until 1987, these characteristics were the benchmarks for diagnosing neurofibromatosis. However, the consensus conference held in 1987 modified the criteria (see page 350 for details).

A variation of the café-au-lait spots consists of numerous small spots in the axilla. This is referred to as *axillary freckling* (Fig. 10–11) and is probably diagnostic of neurofibromatosis. Crowe[58] found this pigmentation present in 20 percent of 523 neurofibromatosis patients he examined. He observed that axillary freckling is a pathognomonic sign of von Recklinghausen's neurofibromatosis. Hyperpigmentation may also be associated with neurofibromas, especially the plexiform type. The affected area assumes grotesque shapes and sizes and frequently becomes elephantoid, with thick, loose, redundant hyperpigmented skin (Fig. 10–12A and 10–12B). Giant pigmented nevi (bathing trunk nevi) are sometimes associated with either underlying plexiform neurofibromatosis (Fig. 10–13)[42,45,59] and/or with malignant melanoma (Fig. 10–14).[60] We encountered a similar case. An 11-year-old girl was referred to the University of Illinois with a history of metastatic brain tumor. The parents informed us she had been born with a bathing trunk nevus and had been seen by

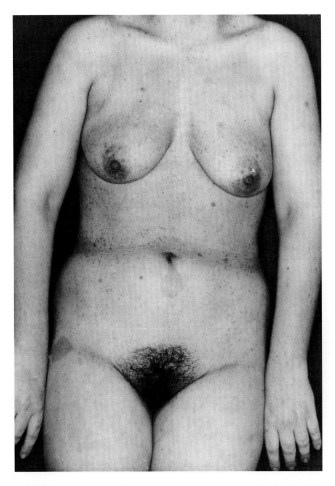

**Figure 10–10.** A 37-year-old woman with a large café-au-lait spot in the periumbilical region and in the inguinal crease. Also manifests small cutaneous neurofibromas.

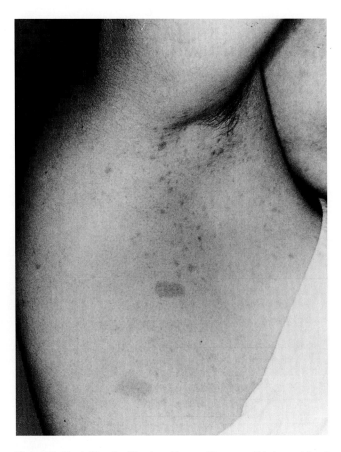

**Figure 10–11.** Axillary freckling in a 41-year-old woman. This is considered a pathognomonic sign of neurofibromatosis.

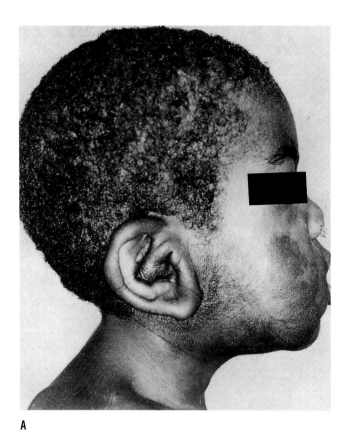

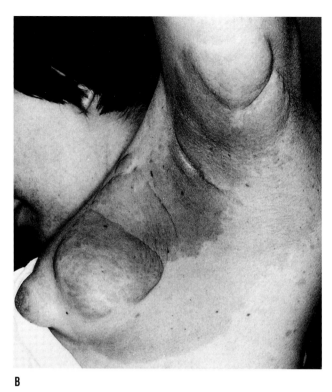

**Figure 10–12.** **(A)** A 7-year-old boy with area of hyperpigmentation of right side of face and hypertrophy of right ear. **(B)** Left axilla of 16-year-old girl with plexiform neurofibroma of breast and large area of hyperpigmentation *(Courtesy of* Current Problems in Surgery, *1977).*

several dermatologists, only some of whom recommended sequential excision of the lesion. Because of the controversy regarding excision, the parents delayed until the child was nine years old, at which time sequential excision was begun. However, after only three excisions in two years, she was admitted to the University of Illinois Hospital with evidence of a brain tumor. On exploratory craniotomy, a left parietal lobe metastatic melanoma was noted. She received radiation therapy but died within three months. The primary site of the melanoma was never found, either in the excised skin or in the remainder of the integument. The possibility of a primary leptomeningeal melanoma was ruled out.

Sequential excision during childhood is recommended for all giant nevi (Fig. 10–15). The major reason for early excision is to eliminate the 10 percent chance of transformation into malignant melanoma or malignant transformation of the underlying plexiform neuroma. Early excision may also decrease the secondary psychological effects of these cosmetically objectionable lesions. If melanoma supervenes, then the general principles of treatment for deep-level melanoma should be adhered to, that is, a careful workup followed by primary excision with in-continuity node dissection.

## BENIGN NERVE SHEATH TUMORS ASSOCIATED WITH VON RECKLINGHAUSEN'S NEUROFIBROMATOSIS

Cutaneous or subcutaneous peripheral nerve tumors (neurofibromas, schwannomas, or neurilemmomas) vary in size from a few millimeters to about 20 cm and may be scattered over the body. Feinman and Yakovac[57] had 14 patients with cutaneous tumors at birth, although in Brasfield and Das Gupta's series,[45] most initially appeared at puberty, the earliest occurrence being at six months of age and the latest at 18 years. The usual sequence is as follows.

The neurofibromas are small, palpable, subcutaneous tumors; they can be found at birth or at infancy but usually become visible in the second and third decades of life (Fig. 10–16A and 10–16B). Some become pedunculated by the fourth decade (Fig. 10–16C), with an increasing number involving most of the body, including the areola in women, by the fifth decade (Fig. 10–16D). The plexiform neurofibroma (Fig. 10–17A to 17E), the characteristic feature of neurofibromatosis, is known to harbor a potential for malignant transformation. Even with this consideration aside, the plexiform neurofibroma still presents myriad difficult therapeutic problems.

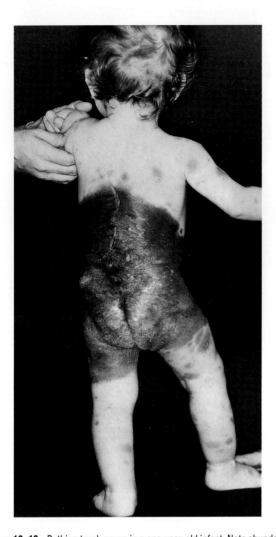

**Figure 10–13.** Bathing trunk nevus in a one-year-old infant. Note abundance of hair, a characteristic feature. Nodular growths within the nevus are evident. Biopsy of these nodules showed them to be plexiform neurofibromas *(Courtesy of* Current Problems in Surgery, *1977).*

Clinically, the extent of this lesion is difficult if not impossible to assess; thus, resection is frequently incomplete and leads to recurrence. Whether the problem is cosmetic or whether it is an obstruction in the urinary, alimentary, or respiratory tract, radical treatment may be required to obtain a satisfactory result. Figure 10–18A to 10–18E demonstrates the frustration that occurs with attempts at cosmetic excision of subcutaneous plexiform neurofibromas. Similar, apparently insurmountable cosmetic and orthopedic problems directly caused by the plexiform neurofibroma are frequently encountered. Figure 10–19 shows the effect of a large plexiform neuroma of the left thigh in a 23-year-old man with von Recklinghausen's neurofibromatosis. Local gigantism associated with elephantoid, hyperpigmented skin overlying a plexiform neurofibroma (neurilemoma) is relatively common.

In Brasfield and Das Gupta's[45] series, 75 percent occurred in persons younger than 19, and 15 percent in those between the ages of 20 and 29 years. In patients with type 1 neurofibromatosis, solitary neurofibromas can usually be dissected out of major peripheral nerves. However, in areas where the relation of the tumor to a named peripheral nerve cannot be demonstrated, a simple wide excision is adequate. Although attempts at total extirpation should always be made in patients with plexiform neurofibroma, a degree of conservatism should be used in the young of both sexes. It is extremely unusual to observe malignant transformation in a plexiform neurofibroma in children, adolescents, or young adults, and a major soft tissue resection is therefore seldom required.

**Figure 10–14.** This 17-year-old girl was referred with a large nodular mass in the gluteal region of her bathing trunk nevus. Biopsy of the mass showed it to be malignant melanoma. Wide excision and incontinuity radical groin dissection were performed; the nodes contained both benign neval cells and metastatic malignant melanoma. She died of the metastatic melanoma within one year. Parents stated that while the girl was prepubertal they received conflicting opinions regarding the advisability of excising the nevus *(Courtesy of the late GP McNeer, MD, and* Current Problems in Surgery, *1977).*

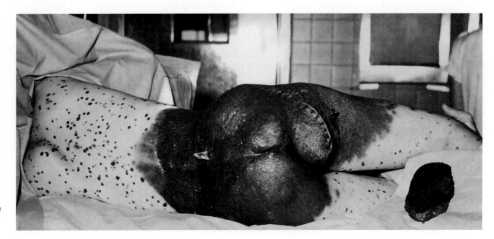

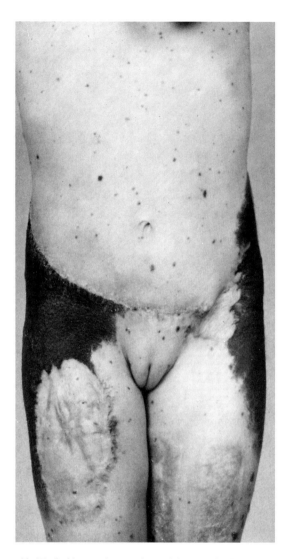

**Figure 10–15.** Bathing trunk nevus in an eight-year-old girl who has been treated by segmental excision. She was referred to us after several excisions were performed elsewhere. She is now 25 years old, and, after several cosmetic procedures, she is leading a relatively normal life.

## ASSOCIATED CLINICAL MANIFESTATIONS OF NEUROFIBROMATOSIS

The multifaceted clinical manifestations associated with von Recklinghausen's neurofibromatosis are extremely interesting, and a comprehensive study of these manifestations is of far-reaching clinical importance. Although detailed analysis of all these manifestations is beyond the scope of this book, a brief description of the more common associated conditions follows.

### Alimentary Tract

Recognition of involvement of the alimentary tract did not have to await sophisticated diagnostic studies to be appreciated as part of the disease. In his original paper,

von Recklinghausen[61] described a patient with neurofibromas and malignant transformation in the stomach and jejunum. Most patients with neurofibromas of the gastrointestinal tract do not have associated von Recklinghausen's neurofibromatosis. River, Silverstein, and Topel[62] found that tumors of nerve sheath origin constituted 6 percent of the benign small bowel neoplasms in their series. They also found that 15 percent of the patients with neurofibromas of the gastrointestinal tract had von Recklinghausen's neurofibromatosis. Only 12 percent of the patients with von Recklinghausen's neurofibromatosis had gastrointestinal involvement.[45,63,64] Hochberg and associates,[64] however, hypothesized that 50 percent of von Recklinghausen patients may show hyperplasia of Auerbach's plexus throughout the entire gastrointestinal tract.

Involvement of the oral cavity is rare. Rappaport[65] found only seven cases reported between 1893 and 1946, but subsequent reports by Baden and co-workers,[66] Borberg,[41] Preston and associates,[67] and Chen and Miller[68] indicated an incidence in the range of 6 percent. The oral cavity is distinct from the remainder of the alimentary tract, in that the mucosa is derived from the neuroectoderm. The oral area most commonly involved with neurofibroma is the tongue. As early as 1849, Smith[69] reported a case of multiple neurofibromatosis with oral manifestations, describing a tumor the size of a walnut on the left side of the tongue.

Isolated neurofibromas lend themselves to local excision; multiple lesions present a more difficult management problem. The teeth do not appear to be primarily involved, except as part of congenital hemifacial hypertrophy in which there is uniform enlargement of the whole side or part of the face and similar enlargement of the underlying bone. Mandibular involvement is usually the result of a subperiosteal neurofibroma that has caused cortical erosion, or there may be irregular distortion by an adjacent plexiform neurofibroma.[70] One of the most distressing manifestations is secondary to cranial nerve involvement, with impairment of the gustatory senses, coordination in swallowing, or the gag reflex.

The most frequently involved sites in von Recklinghausen's neurofibromatosis are the jejunum and the stomach, followed by the ileum and duodenum.[71] Only rarely are the esophagus[72] or colon[73] affected (Fig. 10–20). This is contrary to the predominantly ileal location in isolated neurofibromas of the intestine not associated with the systemic disease. Hochberg et al.[64] reviewed 32 cases of gastrointestinal involvement in the literature and added 7 cases of their own. The average age at diagnosis was 46 years. About one-third of the patients were asymptomatic, but others presented with bleeding, obstruction, intussusception, volvulus, or a mass. In some patients, large segments of the jejunum

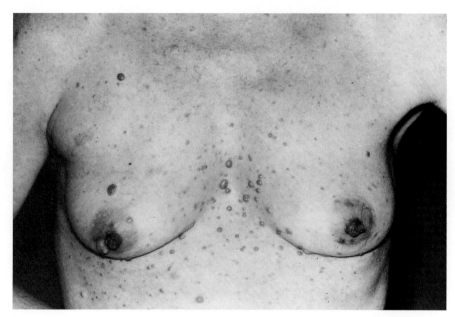

**Figure 10–16. (A)** A 23-year-old woman with cutaneous and subcutaneous nodules, not as yet unsightly *(Courtesy of Current Problems in Surgery, 1977).* **(B)** Cutaneous and subcutaneous nodules are apparent in this 32-year-old man.
*(Continued.)*   **A**

required excision to control bleeding.[45] The most common origin of the neurofibromas is extraluminally in the subserosa, but submucosal and intramural locations are also encountered. Approximately 15 percent of the gastrointestinal tumors appear to be malignant, usually occurring in patients over the age of 40 years (Fig. 10–21). Ulcerations, if present, are small and discrete in benign lesions; in malignant lesions, they tend to be large and irregular. Multiplicity of gastrointestinal tumors occurs in approximately a third of those so affected.

Excision of these intestinal tumors, if possible, is favored. Malignant lesions require an en bloc resection with adjacent mesentery and may include other viscera or adjacent structures.

### Genitourinary Tract

Involvement of the urinary tract with generalized neurofibromatosis was first reported by Gerhardt[74] in 1878. A 30-year-old patient had neurofibromas of the bladder neck, as well as cutaneous, intraspinal, intraabdominal, and intrathoracic lesions. In 1932, Kass[75] first reported bladder involvement in a child. So far, fewer than 40 cases of urinary tract involvement have been reported in patients with neurofibromatosis.[46]

One-third of all cases are reported in children, with involvement of males being twice as common. In general, the patients are either totally asymptomatic or complain of serious symptoms such as incontinence, retention, pain, or hematuria. Most male patients with urinary tract involvement are found to have a palpable mass above the prostate, and, in a few instances, a su-

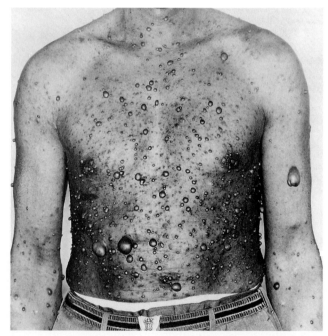

**B**

prapubic mass can be felt. A submucosal mass may be visible on cystoscopy. The involvement may be localized and nodular; however, the usual picture is one of diffuse disease with ill-defined borders (Fig. 10–22).

The origin of the tumor appears to be the pelvic autonomic plexi,[76] which are located along the lateral aspects of the pelvic viscera, forming an extensive network of nerve fibers. The vesical and prostatic plexi are associated with the lower ureters and the bladder neck.

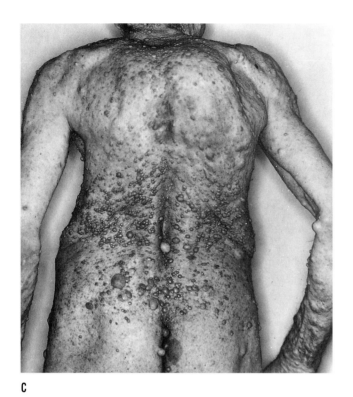

C

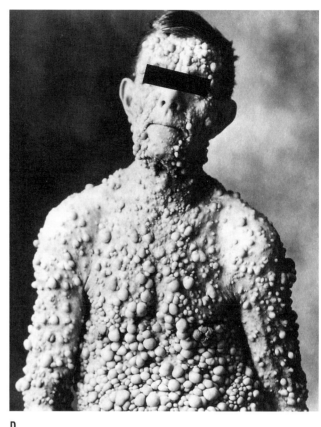

D

**Figure 10–16** *(continued).* **(C)** Same patient as in Figure 10–16B, at age 49. Note progression of nodules and spinal deformity. **(D)** A 57-year-old man with extensive cutaneous involvement over entire body *(Courtesy of L. Solomon, and* Current Problems in Surgery, *1977).*

This critical location accounts for the combined ureteral and vesical obstruction that occurs when the urinary tract is involved (Fig. 10–23A and 10–23B).

Treatment of plexiform neuromas of the bladder or other parts of the genitourinary tract depends on the symptoms produced by the tumor. Although limited excision should initially be attempted, frequently the local extension of the tumor necessitates a radical operation, as described above.

Malignant transformation in the urinary bladder is rare. Ross's[77] case in 1957 probably represents the only undisputed case of neurofibrosarcoma of the urinary bladder in a patient with von Recklinghausen's neurofibromatosis.

Ravich[78] reported a case of localized involvement of the ureter with neurofibroma, but none of the stigmata of generalized neurofibromatosis. To our knowledge, genital involvement has never been reported in a male patient, and only rarely in a female patient. Brasfield and Das Gupta[45] reported one patient with vulvar involvement, and one other such patient was seen by us at the University of Illinois.

### Skeletal Involvement

The following assortment of skeletal involvement has come to be considered as part of neurofibromatosis: scoliosis, kyphosis, scalloping of vertebral bodies, enlarged vertebral foramina, long bone erosion, cysts, bowing, pseudoarthrosis, hypertrophy, and hypoplasia. Hunt and Pugh,[79] Brasfield and Das Gupta,[45] and Heard and Payne[80] in their large series found bony changes in about 50 percent of patients. About one-half of those so affected had vertebral abnormalities. Table 10–5 shows the clinical features of the common forms of osseous involvement and their treatments (Fig. 10–24A to 10–24C).

### Central Nervous System

von Recklinghausen's neurofibromatosis type-2 is a much rarer form of the syndrome and is generally characterized by bilateral acoustic neuromas along with other central nervous system tumors (Table 10–6). As in type 1, the consensus conference held in 1987[49] developed a set of diagnostic criteria for neurofibromatosis type-2. These are (1) bilateral eighth nerve

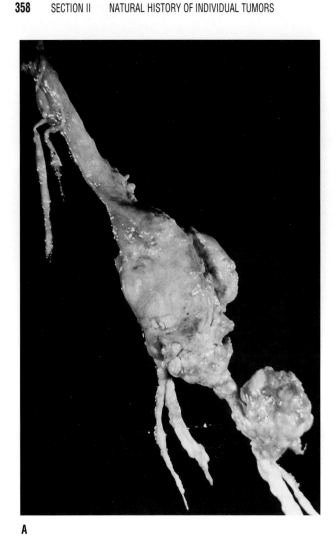

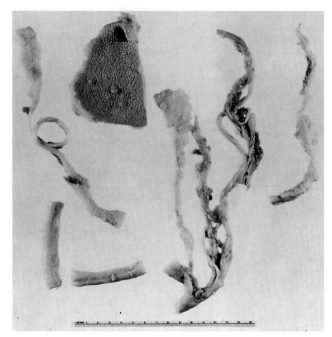

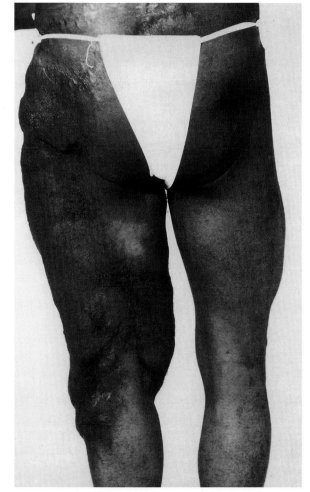

**Figure 10–17. (A)** Dissected sciatic nerve from a 28-year-old woman with malignant schwannoma arising in the lower part of the nerve, prior to division. The larger mass was malignant. Note smaller pedunculated plexiform neuroma and the beaded appearance of the lower branches. She was treated by a major amputation (Dissection of sciatic nerve was performed by J. Wander, M.D.). **(B)** A composite of an elephantoid skin with a small neurofibroma and dissected cutaneous nerves showing the beading characteristic of plexiform neurofibroma of von Recklinghausen's neurofibromatosis. **(C)** Hyperpigmentation and redundancy of skin overlying a plexiform neurofibroma of long duration. *(Continued.)*

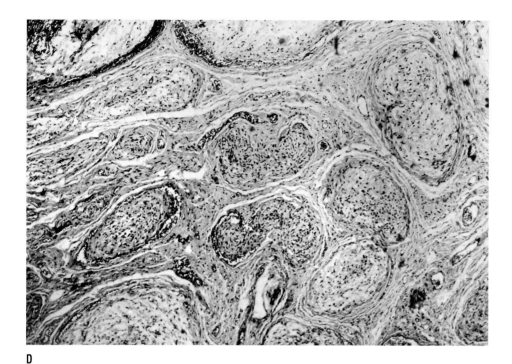

D

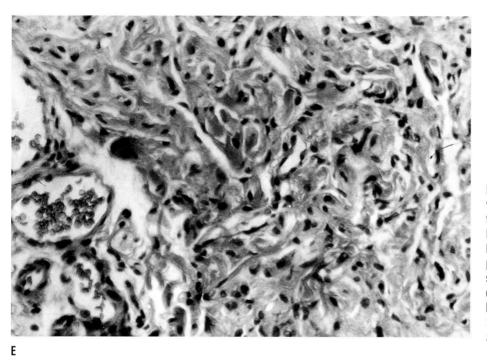

E

**Figure 10–17** *(continued).* **(D)** Low-power view of a plexiform neurofibroma showing the proliferating Schwann cells arranged in bundles separated by fibrous tissue. (H & E. Original magnification × 80.) **(E)** High-power view of sciatic nerve showing preserved myelinated fibers and plump spindle cells embedded in a fibrillary myxomatous background. (H & E. Original magnification × 250.) *(Figs. 10–17A and 10–17D courtesy of* Current Problems of Surgery, *1977.)*

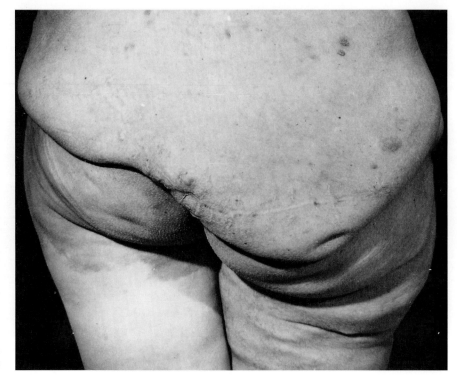

**Figure 10–18. (A)** to **(E)** shows the long-term effort required to obtain the semblance of a cosmetic result. This patient was 32 years old when she was referred with this huge plexiform neuroma of the lower back and buttock. Lateral view **(E)** is 11 operations and three-and-a-half years later. One of the major problems encountered was the extensive microscopic involvement of the surrounding peripheral tissue, which is not usually recognized until recurrence in the margins of sequential excision.

**A**

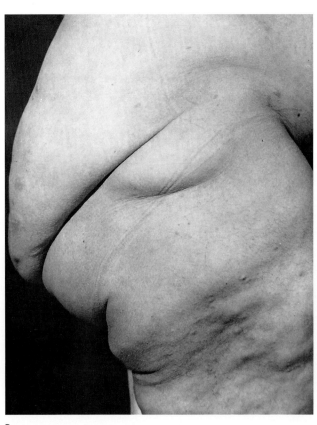

**B**

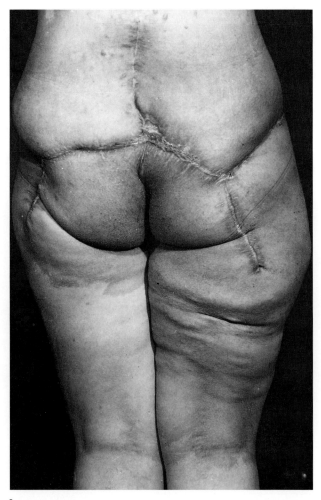

**C**

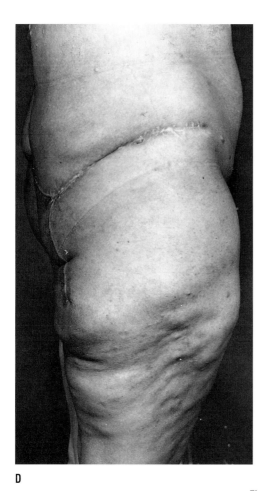

D

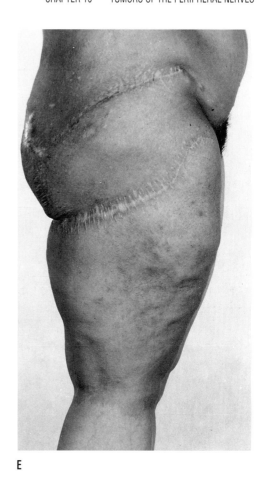

E

**Figure 10–18** *(continued).*

**TABLE 10–5. COMMON SKELETAL INVOLVEMENT**

| Histologic Type | Age at Clinical Onset | Symptoms | Treatment |
|---|---|---|---|
| Kyphoscoliosis | 7–17 | Deformity, back pain, dyspnea, paralysis | Milwaukee brace, skeletal traction, spinal fusion (Harrington rod) |
| Hypertrophy | 2–20 | Overgrowth usually associated with an adjacent plexiform neurofibroma | Resection of the plexiform neurofibroma is unlikely to be complete. Stapling of epiphysis at appropriate times may equalize growth |
| Vertebral scalloping | 10–40 | Usually none | None; may occur with no adjacent lesion causing erosion |
| Erosions | 5–40 | Usually none; however, any bone is subject to deformity due to an adjacent neurofibroma | None, unless function or deformity dictates the need for therapy |
| Bowed tibia with pseudoarthrosis | Birth–5 | Bowed tibia, spontaneous fracture that does not heal | Long grafts spanning almost the entire diaphysis; casting very rarely successful |
| Cysts | 10–40 | Usually none; may palpate mass or sustain pathologic fracture | Usually none. If fracture occurs, removal of the offending neurofibroma in the bone is followed by a cast |
| Sphenoid bone dysplasia | Birth–15 | Usually none; exophthalmos, orbital neurofibromas, pulsatile exophthalmos | No treatment to the bone defect; associated plexiform neurofibroma may be partially excised |

*Courtesy of Ravich MM et al. (eds):* Current Problems in Surgery, *Vol 14. Chicago, Year Book Medical Publishers, 1977.*

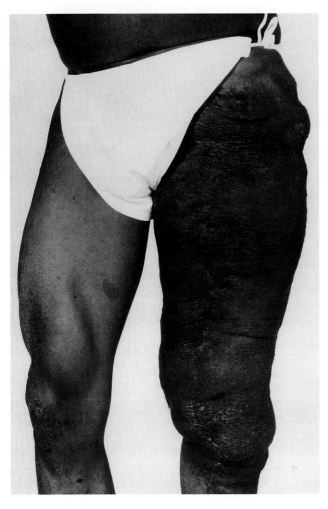

**Figure 10–19.** This 23-year-old man with known von Recklinghausen's neurofibromatosis came to our clinic with a history of café-au-lait spots present at birth and cutaneous neurofibromas developing at the age of 3 years. The plexiform neurofibroma that eventually involved his entire left thigh first became evident at the age of 7 years. It progressively enlarged, with the overlying skin becoming more pigmented, redundant, and thickened, and with concurrent overgrowth of the length and width of the femur. To retard growth of the bone, the distal femoral epiphysis was stapled when the patient was 10 years old, and the proximal epiphysis of the left tibia and fibula was stapled at age 15. This resulted in the legs being nearly equal in length at the completion of growth. By age 15, the patient had a thoracolumbar scoliosis and required spinal fusion. Pseudoarthrosis of the fusion developed, and, because of continued pain, a second fusion was performed when the patient was 22, by use of a Harrington rod. From age 10 until the present, he has had numerous subcutaneous and cutaneous masses removed, all of which have been benign plexiform neurofibromas *(Courtesy of* Current Problems in Surgery, *1977).*

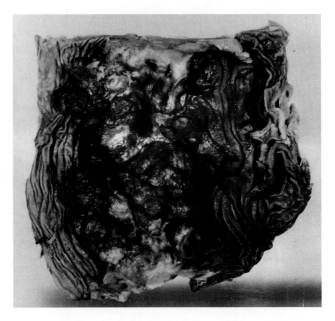

**Figure 10–20.** Unusual rectal involvement in a patient who died of pulmonary metastasis from a primary malignant schwannoma of a lower extremity. The only symptom the patient had of a rectal neurofibroma was occasional bleeding from the anus *(Courtesy of* Current Problems in Surgery, *1977).*

terior subcapsular lenticular opacity. A brief description of the more common central nervous system involvement is given below and has been summarized in Table 10–6.

***Acoustic Neuroma.*** For the past 50 years, bilateral acoustic neuroma has been considered to be associated with von Recklinghausen's neurofibromatosis. In Rodriguez and Berthong's[81] report, there were 40 cases of bilateral and 9 cases of unilateral acoustic neuroma. In 1916, Henschen[82] collected 245 cases of unilateral acoustic neuroma, of which only 5 were associated with von Recklinghausen's neurofibromatosis. But, of the 24 cases of bilateral acoustic neuroma, 19 were associated with this syndrome. Gardner and Frazier[83] reviewed 18 additional cases of bilateral acoustic neuroma reported between the years 1915 and 1930, and von Recklinghausen's neurofibromatosis was present in all of them. Crowe et al.[42] found a 4.5 percent incidence of acoustic neuroma in his large group of neurofibromatosis patients. Rarely are the symptoms manifest before the third decade of life; most commonly, they are noted during the fifth decade. The tumors grow slowly with focal symptoms for years before increased intracranial pressure. Tinnitus is the usual presenting symptom, although some patients may first complain of progressive deafness or vertigo. If the tumor is small, it may be difficult to identify the expansion radiographically, but in late stages, the destruction of the walls of the inter-

tumors (visualized with appropriate imaging techniques) or (2) a first-degree relative with neurofibromatosis type-2 and either a unilateral eighth nerve tumor or two of the following: neurofibroma(s), meningioma(s), glioma, schwannoma, or juvenile pos-

**TABLE 10–6.  COMMON INVOLVEMENT(S) OF THE CENTRAL NERVOUS SYSTEM IN VON RECKLINGHAUSEN'S NEUROFIBROMATOSIS**

| Histologic Type | Age at Clinical Onset | Symptoms | Treatment |
|---|---|---|---|
| Schwannoma | | | |
|    Tumor of cranial nerves VIII (acoustic neuroma) | 30–50 | Tinnitus, vertigo, deafness, facial nerve paralysis, ataxia | Observation for very early lesions, subcapsular or total excision for all other lesions |
| Astrocytoma | 10–30 | Increased intracranial pressure or focal paralysis | Total or partial excision if possible; post-operative radiation if excision is partial |
| Glioma | | | |
|    Optic nerve and chiasmal glioma | 1–15 | Diminished visual field, proptosis, blindness | None (surgery and radiation no longer recommended) |
| Meningioma | | | |
|    Orbital | 20–40 | Extremely variable symptoms dependent upon location (all meningiomas) | Excision; treatment augmented by radiation if excision is incomplete |
|    Intracranial | 20–50 | | |
|    Intraspinal | 20–40 | | |
| Tumor of fifth (trigeminal) nerve | 30–50 | Facial pain | Chemical or radiofrequency lesion of ganglion |
| Spinal nerve roots | 20–50 | Dermatone pain or paresthesia, cord compression with eventual paralysis | Excision of tumor and decompression of the nerve or cord |
| Neurofibroma | | | |
|    Spinal nerve roots | 20–50 | As in schwannoma | As in schwannoma |
| Ependymoma | 10–50 | Cord compression. If intracranial, symptoms are of increased intracranial pressure | Excision rarely possible; decompression followed by radiation is the usual therapy |
| Syringomyelia | 15–40 | Slowly progressive sensory and motor loss with a bizarre pattern distribution | Radiotherapy may result in some pain relief, surgery is usually harmful; no therapy is probably best |
| Heterotopia of cortical architecture | Birth | Mental retardation | None |

nal auditory canal becomes obvious (Fig. 10–25). Diagnostic accuracy of small tumors has increased considerably with routine use of magnetic resonance imaging (MRI) in these patients.

The treatment of an acoustic neuroma is excision. Although intracapsular enucleation of the tumor is probably therapeutic, in about two-thirds of all cases it is advisable to attempt total excision, because it is more definitive, and recurrence is unusual.[46,84] Unfortunately, operative injury to the facial nerve can be expected in about 50 percent of cases and is directly proportional to the size of the tumor. The five-year recurrence-free rate is twice as high with total removal as with partial resection.[84]

***Gliomas.***    One of the more common lesions is glioma of the optic nerve and the chiasma. In contrast to gliomas, medulloblastomas are uncommon.[85] These tumors are usually found in younger patients, many in their second and third decades.[86] The gliomas described by Rubinstein[86] are the juvenile type of pilocytic astrocytomas of the third ventricle and ependymomas. The ependymomas are often multiple and are usually in the spinal cord. Exceptionally diffuse gliomas have been reported involving large areas of the central nervous system in about 45 percent of patients with

von Recklinghausen's neurofibromatosis.[81] In gliomas affecting the optic nerve or the chiasma, gradual visual impairment is the rule. Radiographically, the usual finding is enlargement of the optic canal with retention of distinct cortical margins. Advanced cases may result in proptosis and blindness (Fig. 10–26A and 10–26B).

***Meningioma.***    The occurrence of multiple intracranial tumors in this entity has been widely reported. In 1956, David and co-workers[87] reviewed 84 cases of multiple meningiomas and found that 42 of the patients had von Recklinghausen's neurofibromatosis, acoustic neuromas, or both. In 1966, Rodriguez and Berthong[81] reviewed the published cases and found 49 instances of multiple meningioma in the following distribution: intracranial, 54 percent; intraspinal, 4 percent; intraspinal and intracranial, 42 percent; and orbital, 6 percent.

Multiple intracranial and spinal meningiomas associated with other tumors of the central nervous system are thought to be characteristic of neurofibromatosis type-2.[86] Radiographs show that intracranial meningiomas frequently cause localized hyperostosis, erosion, increased vascularity, or calcification (Fig. 10–27A and 10–27B).

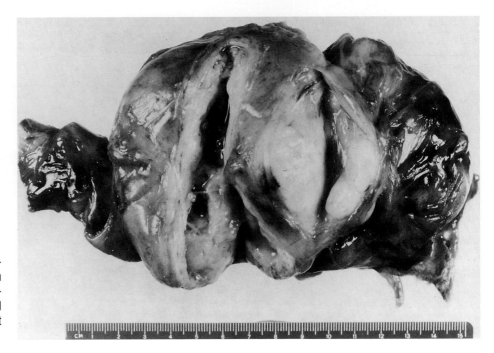

**Figure 10–21.** A polypoid neurofibrosarcoma in the jejunum of a 31-year-old man with neurofibromatosis. This tumor produced intussusception, causing small bowel obstruction (*Courtesy of* Current Problems in Surgery, *1977*).

***Spinal Lesions.*** In plain x-ray, intraspinal meningiomas produce radiographic changes in only about 10 percent of cases, compared with 45 percent in patients with intraspinal neurofibromas.[54] However, with increased use of MRI, these abnormalities are being routinely identified. In the group reported by Brasfield and Das Gupta,[45] there was spinal cord involvement only in those patients in whom the stigmata of multiple neurofibromatosis were observed after six years of age, with symptoms appearing between the ages of 20 and 25 years.

***Syringomyelia.*** Syringomyelia was present in 20.5 percent of Rodriguez and Berthong's[81] patients with multiple intracranial tumors. The cavities were distributed throughout the spinal cord and the medulla oblongata. Poser,[88] in 1956, reviewed 234 cases of central nervous system neoplasms associated with syringomyelia. In 17 of his cases, syringomyelia was associated with von Recklinghausen's neurofibromatosis, and in 9, both von Recklinghausen's neurofibromatosis and meningioma were present.

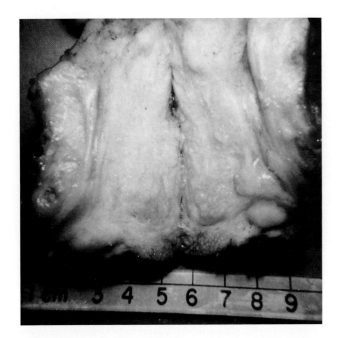

**Figure 10–22.** Urinary bladder; bisected specimen shows extensive involvement of the bladder wall with plexiform neuroma. Note thickness of the wall.

# ■ GRANULAR CELL TUMORS

Granular cell tumors are encountered in all age groups. The histogenesis of this tumor has gone through several interpretations (see Chapter 5). Currently, it is considered to be of neural origin and hence is included in this section. Strong et al.,[89] reviewing the Memorial Sloan-Kettering experience, found that their youngest patient was 11 months old and the oldest 68 years, the average age being 38.1 years. Vance and Hudson,[90] in their series, found the average age to be 29 years, the youngest being 10 years old and the oldest 72 years old.

In the University of Illinois material, the tumor occurred predominantly in women. Similar observations have been made by Strong et al.[89] and by Vance

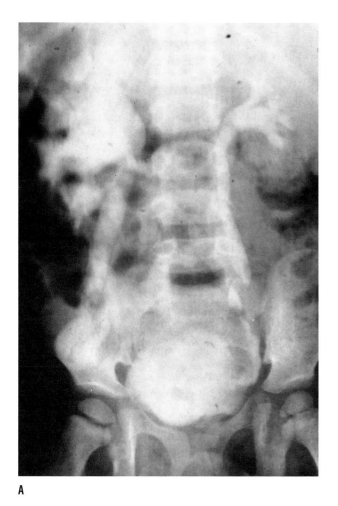

A

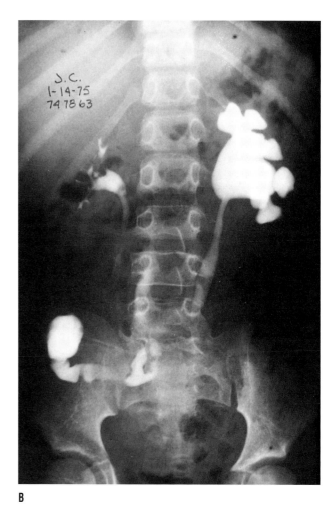

B

**Figure 10–23. (A)** Intravenous pyelogram of a four-year-old boy with massive involvement of the urinary bladder. There is marked dilation of the pelvis and ureter of the left side, with resultant thinning of the cortex *(Courtesy of* Current Problems in Surgery, *1977).* **(B)** Same child seven years after a cystectomy and ileal conduit formation.

and Hudson.[90] Although Vance and Hudson suggested a greater propensity for these tumors to grow in American blacks, our own observations, as well as those of others,[89–95] do not seem to substantiate this. In our series of 52 patients, no racial or ethnic predilection was noted.

Granular cell tumor occurs in all parts of the human body. In the published reports, the tongue is overwhelmingly cited as the predominant location for this neoplasm.[89,91,95–97] The incidence was 28.2 percent in the series reported from Memorial Sloan-Kettering Cancer Center[89] and 25 percent in the series reported by Vance and Hudson.[90] However, in our own experience with 52 patients, the tumor was encountered in the tongue in only five (9.6 percent). In Vance and Hudson's series,[90] there were 50 tumors in 42 patients. In the series reported by Strong and co-authors,[89] there were 110 tumors in 95 patients, and in our series, there

were 60 tumors in 52 patients. No organ or tissue of the body is free from developing this entity.[89,90] Various reports have included origin in the middle and external ear,[98] breast,[95,99] larynx,[100] parotid,[101] esophagus,[102,103] tracheobronchial tree,[104–106] gastrointestinal tract (including cystic duct, pancreas, and common bile duct),[107–112] urinary bladder,[113] and female reproductive tract.[114–116] Stout and Lattes[117] considered congenital epulis as a congenital granular cell tumor.

Most of our patients sought medical opinion for a slow-growing, asymptomatic tumor (Fig. 10–28). Only six patients complained of associated pain or a tingling sensation. In most scrics,[89–92] the initial presentation was an asymptomatic lump. However, in some instances, certain specific symptoms have been noted, depending on the location of the tumor. For example, patients with tumors in the vocal cords complained of hoarseness,[100] those with tumors in the gastrointestinal tract were seen for bleeding,[107,108] and those with tumors of the biliary tract have had symptoms of acute cholecystitis.[111,112]

In a number of instances, the tumor has been identified only at autopsy.[102,110] These unusual locations of granular cell tumors are interesting and provide an insight into the histogenesis of the tumor. However, from a clinical viewpoint, preoperative or antemortem diagnosis of these tumors in locations such as the biliary tract or the pancreas is impossible. These tumors are usually small, nonulcerated, nodular lesions arising from the dermis or subdermal or submucosal tissue. Rarely, larger tumors have occurred deeper in the somatic tissues.[89,90]

The treatment of granular cell tumors is wide local excision. In the past, owing to lack of information concerning the histogenesis and natural history of these tumors, various other forms of treatment were tried,[89,90] resulting in less than optimum results. There is no place for radiation therapy or chemotherapy in the treatment of these benign tumors. Most of the local recurrences directly relate to inadequate excision. Based on our experience and a review of the literature, a 2- to 3-cm margin on all sides is sufficient in most instances. In lesions located in the viscera, excision sometimes must be radical because of the location. For example, granular cell tumors of the stomach or cecum might require a partial gastrectomy or right hemicolectomy.

The patients in our series have all been followed up for at least five years, and all have remained free of the problem for which they were initially treated. In our series, 8 of 52 patients (15 percent) had multiple primary tumors. Early reports implied that multiplicity is a rare occurrence; however, with increasing information, it appears that multiple primary granular cell tumors are not uncommon. Various theories regarding this multiplicity have been forwarded,[93,108] but none have been substantiated.

## MALIGNANT GRANULAR CELL TUMOR

The malignant variant of granular cell tumors is indeed rare.[118] Some authors consider that the organoid type is similar to an alveolar soft part sarcoma.[117] However, there is a nonorganoid type that probably can be classified as a malignant variant. In 1952, Ross, Miller, and Foote[119] could find only four unequivocal cases of malignant granular cell tumor, to which they added three of their own. In 1955, Gamboa[120] reviewed the literature and added one case of his own, bringing the total to 11. Cadotte[121] reviewed the literature in 1974 and concluded that there were only 22 documented cases.[119,121–137] We have treated only one such case. In our patient, the primary tumor was in the interscapular region, and the ipsilateral axilla contained metastatic

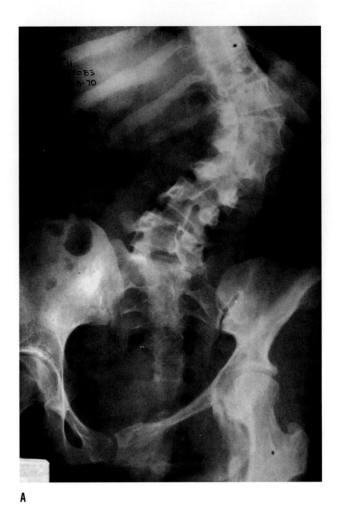

**A**

**Figure 10–24. (A)** An example of severe kyphoscoliosis in a young adult. This patient also had pseudoarthrosis of the tibia and fibula, which ultimately resulted in a below-the-knee amputation. Note dysplasia of hemipelvis.

*(Continued.)*

tumor. The patient died within six months, and autopsy showed diffuse metastatic involvement of the viscera.

Based on the scanty information on a small numbers of patients[119,121–137] and on observation of our own patient, it appears that these neoplasms are aggressive. Primary treatment should consist of radical excision and, when indicated, lymph node dissection. Adjuvant systemic chemotherapy may play a role. However, the types of agents and the program that might yield the best end result are not yet known.

## MALIGNANT TUMORS OF THE PERIPHERAL NERVES

A malignant tumor of the peripheral nerves can arise from Schwann cells, perineural fibroblasts, or simple fibroblasts. Thus, purely from a histogenetic standpoint, each of the tumors should be subclassified based

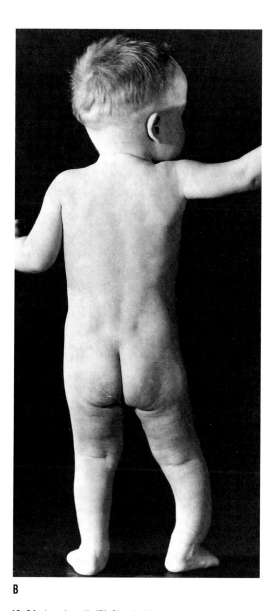

B

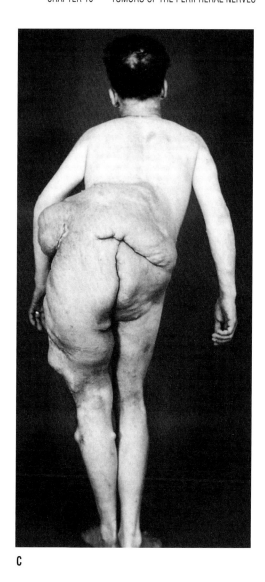

C

**Figure 10–24** *(continued).* **(B)** Classical bowing of tibia with pseudoarthrosis in a three-year-old patient. **(C)** An advanced case of von Recklinghausen's neurofibromatosis. Note the kyphoscoliosis, elephantiasis of localized skin, plexiform neurofibroma of the left gluteal area, and multiple cutaneous or subcutaneous neurofibromas. This 54-year-old man died of metastatic malignant schwannoma (see Figure 10–36).

on the cell of origin. However, from a therapeutic standpoint, it is neither possible nor necessary. As a result, in recent years, an all-inclusive term, *malignant peripheral nerve sheath tumor* (MPNST), has been coined. This term essentially supersedes the conventional designation "malignant schwannoma," which for many years described these tumors. We are not convinced that this new nomenclature of MPNST is any improvement over malignant schwannoma, but for the sake of uniformity, the malignant tumors described as malignant schwannoma in the previous edition will be designated here as malignant peripheral nerve sheath tumors.

## ■ SOLITARY MALIGNANT PERIPHERAL NERVE SHEATH TUMORS (SCHWANNOMA)

### SEX, AGE, AND RACIAL DISTRIBUTION

Solitary malignant peripheral nerve sheath tumors are about equally divided between the sexes.[138–141] In our series of 76 patients, 41 (54 percent) were men, and 35 (46 percent) were women. In our earlier series, 56 percent were men, and 44 percent were women.[140] The tumor occurs in all ages; however, in one study,[140] 42 percent of patients were between 30 and 50 years of age, and 15 percent were between 20

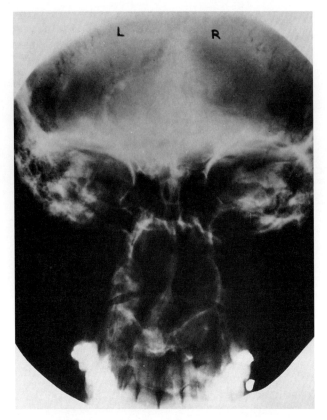

**Figure 10–25.** Skull film of a 53-year-old woman demonstrating erosion of left internal auditory canal by a large acoustic neuroma. She was known to have von Recklinghausen's neurofibromatosis and was seen because of pain in the tongue.

and 29 years of age. No racial predilection has been observed.

## ANATOMIC DISTRIBUTION

Solitary malignant peripheral nerve sheath tumors can arise in the peripheral nerves in practically every anatomic region.[139–141] The anatomic distribution in the present group of 76 patients is shown in Table 10–7.

Patients with MPNST are usually seen with a mass. In some instances, as in its benign counterpart, pain along the course of a peripheral nerve is the initial symptom (between 6 and 7 percent of patients). The size of the primary tumor usually depends on the duration of the tumor. In the present group of 76 patients, the largest tumor had a diameter of 20 cm and was located in the retroperitoneum.

### Head and Neck Region

A diagnosis of malignant schwannoma and/or MPNST in the head and neck region is primarily based on microscopic examination of the mass. The propensity of benign schwannomas to grow in the lateral portion of the neck has already been described. In contrast,

**TABLE 10–7.  ANATOMIC DISTRIBUTION OF MPNST OR SOLITARY MALIGNANT SCHWANNOMA**

| Anatomic Site | Present Series |
|---|---|
| Head and neck | 13 (17%) |
| Upper extremities | 19 (25%) |
| Trunk | 11 (14%) |
| Lower extremities | 25 (33%) |
| Miscellaneous sites* | 8 (11%) |
| Total | 76 |

Abbreviations: MPNST, malignant peripheral nerve sheath tumor.
*This category includes retroperitoneum, 4; pelvic wall, 2; and perineum, 2.

solitary malignant schwannomas of the head and neck region are infrequent.[1–3,139,140,142] In the present series of 13 patients, the distribution was four in the antero-lateral neck, two in the posterior neck, one in the cheek, and six in the scalp (Fig. 10–29A to 10–29C). A fusiform solid tumor in the lateral portion of the neck, which is movable from side to side but relatively immobile vertically, should be considered a tumor arising from a peripheral nerve until proved otherwise. Microscopic examination will ascertain the malignancy or benignity of the lesion.

### Upper Extremities

In our previous study of 69 patients,[140] 23 had tumors in the shoulder and axillae, 22 in the upper arm, 18 in the forearm, and 1 in the palm. In the remaining five, the tumor arose directly from the brachial plexus. In the present group of 19, six had tumors in the shoulder, eight in the upper arm, four in the forearm, and one in the palm. In 11 of 19, the primary tumor could be identified as arising from unknown peripheral nerve (Fig. 10–30A and 10–30B).

### Trunk

For MPNST patients, the trunk is a relatively rare site, especially for those patients who do not have von Recklinghausen's neurofibromatosis. However, in our 1970 report,[140] 38 patients were found to have this tumor in the soft tissue of the trunk. Eleven were in the anterior chest, nine in the lumbosacral region, and five in the anterior abdominal wall. The remaining 13 were distributed in the posterior and lateral trunk. In only 10 patients was the tumor associated with pain. In the present group of 11 patients, the tumor was located in the posterior trunk in 7 patients and in the anterior trunk in 4 patients.

### Lower Extremities

The most frequent sites of origin of this tumor are the thigh and the buttocks (Fig. 10–31). Of the 25 patients in the present group, six tumors (24 percent) were in

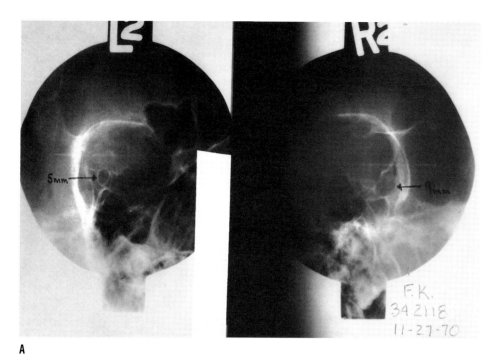

A

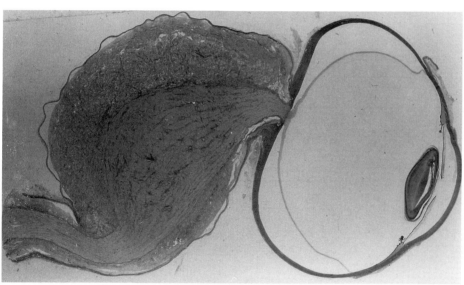

B

**Figure 10–26. (A)** Views of optic canals demonstrating a normal optic canal on the right with the left canal almost twice the diameter. **(B)** A large optic glioma that resulted in severe proptosis and blindness. Compression of the posterior globe is evident *(Courtesy of D. Apple, M.D., and* Current Problems in Surgery, *1977).*

the buttocks and ten (40 percent) in the anterior and posterior thigh. The remaining nine tumors were located in the leg and region of the ankle. Das Gupta and Brasfield[140] described a series of 89 patients with tumor in the lower extremities: 42 were in the thigh, 17 in the legs, 10 in the buttocks, 9 in the area of the knee joints, 6 on the feet and ankles, and 5 in the groin. The lesions in the buttocks frequently produce pain along the sciatic distribution resembling the pain of sciatica.

### Miscellaneous Sites

In our present series, eight tumors (11 percent) were in miscellaneous sites: four in the retroperitoneum, two in

the pelvis, and two in the perineum. A similar distribution was observed in our previous report.[140] An accurate diagnosis can be made only after histologic examination of the specimen.

### TREATMENT

Management of MPNSTs is radical excision, based on location, shape, size, and local spread. The tumor plus its bed and any attached muscle, bone, fascia, or blood vessel, should be resected en bloc. If the nerve of origin is identified, it should be resected through a normal segment. The proximal margin of the resected nerve

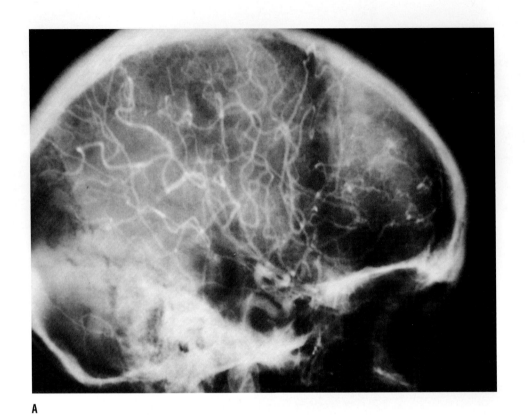

**A**

**B**

**Figure 10–27.** **(A)** Carotid angiogram showing a falx meningioma. **(B)** Line drawing of feeding vessels. *CS* = carotid sypnon; *PA* = pericalosal artery; *FB* = frontal branch of superficial temporal; *AM* = anterior meningeal artery; *FP* = frontopolar artery; *OA* = ophthalmic artery. *(Courtesy of* Current Problems in Surgery, *1977).*

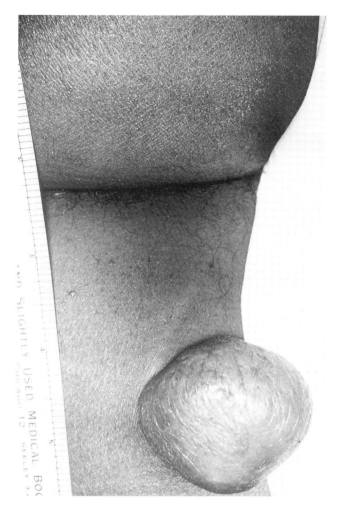

**Figure 10–28.** A slow-growing pedunculated granular cell tumor of five years' duration in the posterior thigh of a 48-year-old woman. Following excision, she has remained well.

should be examined histologically at the time of the operation. Regional node dissection is not indicated, since hematogenous spread is the primary route of metastases. When radical local excision is performed, restoration of nerve continuity is not always feasible. Since 68 percent of solitary malignant schwannomas arise in the peripheral nerves of the extremities, the feasibility of peripheral nerve grafting should be determined.

If the tumor is near the shoulder or hip joints, or if there is nodular enlargement along the course of the affected major peripheral nerve, the logical primary treatment is an amputation. Limited local excisions are associated with local recurrences.

Radiation therapy alone as a curative form of management for primary MPNSTs has been tried in the past.[142,143] McNeer and co-workers[143] reported that three of their four patients were long-term survivors. In our previous study,[140] 22 of 48 patients (46 percent) treated with radiation therapy alone survived for at least

**TABLE 10–8. SOLITARY MALIGNANT SCHWANNOMA (MPNST) LOCAL CONTROL IN 76 PATIENTS ACCORDING TO TREATMENT***

| Type of Treatment | No. Patients | 5 Yrs | 10 Yrs |
|---|---|---|---|
| Radical surgery only | 44 | 34 (77.3%) | 31 (70%) |
| Surgery and postop radiation therapy | 32 | 26 (81%) | 17 (53%) |
| Total | 76 | 60 (79%) | 48 (63%) |

Abbreviations: MPNST, malignant peripheral nerve sheath tumor.
*Local control signifies that there was no evidence of recurrence in the primary site during the period of follow-up.

five years. Suit and co-workers[144] and Lindberg and associates[145] argued in favor of radiation therapy as a major mode of treatment (see Chapter 17). There is as yet no evidence that adjuvant chemotherapy plays a significant role in the treatment of malignant schwannomas (Chapter 18).

## END RESULTS

In our present series of 76 patients, 44 (58 percent) were treated by radical excision alone, and 32 (42 percent) by surgery and postoperative radiation therapy. Local control was achieved in 79 percent of the patients for five years and 63 percent for ten years (Table 10–8). Of the 60 in whom the disease was locally controlled for five years, metastatic involvement was noted in 12 (20 percent). However, after five years, the incidence of distant metastasis was extremely low: only one patient was seen with lung metastases 11 years after the original operation.

In an attempt to define the type of excision most suitable for management of these tumors, the results of resection in our 1970 report[140] have been compared with those in our present series (Table 10–9). Local limited excision alone[140] salvaged only 30 percent of the

**TABLE 10–9. SOLITARY MALIGNANT SCHWANNOMA: 5-YEAR END RESULT ACCORDING TO TYPE OF RESECTION***

| Type of Operation | Das Gupta and Brasfield (1970)[143] | Present Series (1996) |
|---|---|---|
| Local excision | 15/51 (29.4%) | Not performed |
| Soft tissue resection (including muscle group resection) | 12/45 (26.6%) | 50/54 (93%) |
| Minor amputation | 7/15 (46.6%) | Not performed |
| Hemipelvectomy | 1/2 (50%) | 5/8 (63%) |
| Hip joint disarticulation | 1/5 (20%) | 6/10 (60%) |
| Forequarter amputation | 1/5 (20%) | 3/4 (75%) |
| Pelvic exenteration | 0/1 | |
| Total | 37/124 (30%) | 64/76 (84%) |

*Numbers in the numerator represent 5-year survivors; those in the denominator represent total number of patients.

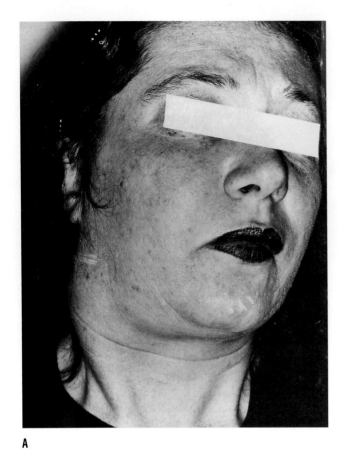

**A**

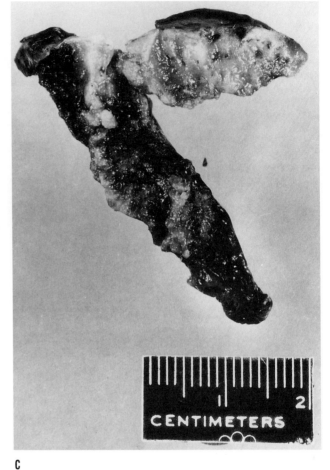

**C**

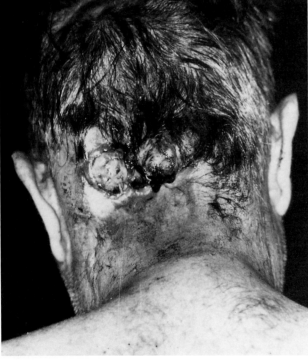

**B**

**Figure 10–29.** **(A)** Malignant schwannoma of the right side of neck. The nerve of origin could not be detected. Patient was treated with a standard radical neck dissection. **(B)** Recurrent malignant schwannoma of the scalp *(Courtesy of* Ann Surg *171:419, 1970).* **(C)** Excised scalp showing extensive infiltration of the entire thickness.

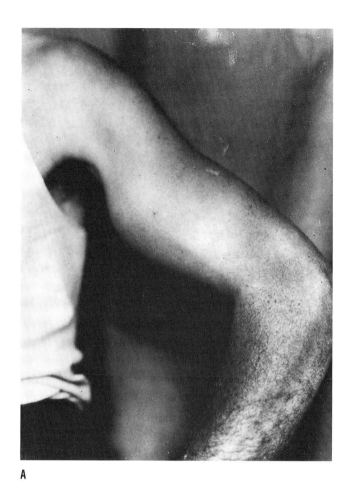

A

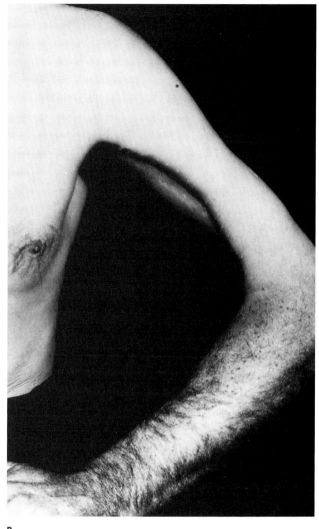

B

**Figure 10–30. (A)** A solitary malignant schwannoma of the arm. The tumor arose from the median nerve. The segment of nerve containing the tumor was excised. **(B)** Postoperative appearance of arm and forearm *(Courtesy of* Ann Surg *171:419, 1970).*

patients; therefore, its continued use has been abandoned. Comparison of soft tissue resection results between the two series is startling. In the 1970 report,[140] there was a 27 percent five-year disease-free survival, whereas in the present series it is 92 percent. This vastly superior end result in the current series cannot be explained solely on the basis of technical considerations. In our opinion, the improvement of the result during those 25 years is due to better and earlier diagnoses, resulting in primary tumors being smaller with lower grade and less local tissue involvement. In addition, the anatomic concept of soft tissue resection (muscle group excision) has been better understood, especially in relation to MPNSTs.

The necessity and indications for major amputation have decreased considerably, except in certain spe-

cific anatomic sites (i.e., MPNST of the sacral plexus or upper end of the sciatic nerve). Major amputations such as hemipelvectomy or hip-joint articulations are usually indicated for locally recurrent tumors of the upper thigh and/or buttock. Theoretically, if the original resection is done properly and supplemental radiation therapy is used appropriately, the incidence of local failure will be so low that such mutilating operations will become rarer still.

Combined radical resection and postoperative radiation therapy provided excellent local control and prolonged disease-free survival in our series (Table 10–8). Based on our experience, our current practice is to use both modes of therapy in most cases. The only exception is tumors which are $T_1G_1$ and are superficially located, wherein adequate resection is usually

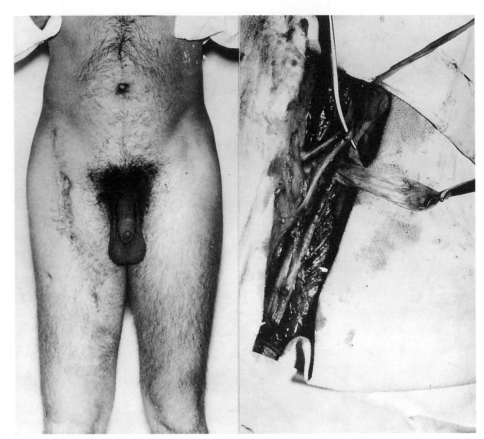

**Figure 10–31.** Recurrent malignant schwannoma of the anterior thigh in a 50-year-old man. The recurrence under the scar *(left)* can be easily appreciated. The operative field *(right)* shows the branches of the femoral nerve entering the tumor. Femoral vessels retracted laterally with a Penrose drain *(Courtesy of Ann Surg 171: 419, 1970).*

curative. In our experience, adjuvant chemotherapy has not been found to be useful; thus, chemotherapy as an adjuvant therapy for MPNSTs (malignant schwannomas) should only be used in a clinical trial setting.

Based on our current experience, it is logical to propose that the prognosis of MPNSTs (malignant schwannomas) depends on tumor size, grade, and location (Table 10–10). Adequate local control of the disease provides a reasonably satisfactory disease-free survival. Thus, the current practice of wide soft tissue resection and postoperative radiation therapy should remain as the standard form of management of these tumors.

### ■ MALIGNANT SCHWANNOMAS (MPNSTs) ASSOCIATED WITH VON RECKLINGHAUSEN'S NEUROFIBROMATOSIS

The association of MPNST with von Recklinghausen's neurofibromatosis (Figs. 10–32 to 10–36) is well known.[43,46] Harkin and Reed,[3] D'Agostino et al.,[138] and Hope and Mulvihill[85] found it impossible to establish the true incidence. Brasfield and Das Gupta[45] reported an overall incidence of 29 percent. Their conclusion was based on long-term observation of a large number of hospital-based patients. This incidence is based primarily on patients who are cared for in a tertiary hospital; thus, the true incidence of MPNST in all patients

**TABLE 10–10. ANALYSIS OF TUMOR SIZE AND TUMOR GRADE IN 76 PATIENTS WITH MALIGNANT SCHWANNOMA (MPNST) (UNIVERSITY OF ILLINOIS SERIES, 1996)**

| Tumor Size | No. Patients | Grades 1 and 2 | 5 Yr, NED | Grades 3 and 4 | 10 Yr, NED |
|---|---|---|---|---|---|
| Less than 5 cm | 44 | 30 | 25 (83%) | 14 | 10 (71%) |
| Greater than 5 cm | 21 | 8 | 5 (63%) | 13 | 5 (38%) |
| Greater than 5 cm and local infiltration to muscles and/or bones | 11 | 3 | 1 (33%) | 8 | 0 |
| Total | 76 | 41 | 31 (76%) | 35 | 15 (43%) |

Abbreviations: MPNST, malignant peripheral nerve sheath tumor; NED, no evidence of disease.

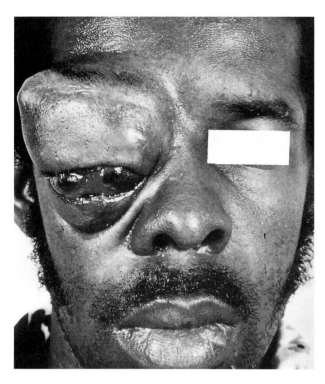

**Figure 10–32.** A 17-year-old boy with malignant schwannoma of the right upper eyelid, which had developed on a plexiform neurofibroma that had been partially excised when the patient was eight years old. In the intervening four years between the first excision and development of malignant schwannoma, several other procedures were performed *(Courtesy of* Current Problems in Surgery, *1977).*

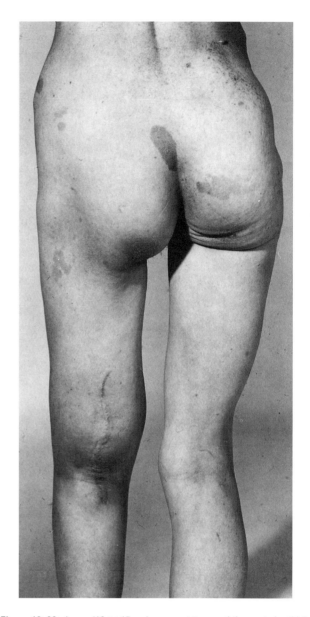

**Figure 10–33.** Large (12 × 15 cm) recurrent tumor of the posterior thigh and popliteal space in a 28-year-old woman. Dissected sciatic nerve specimen from this patient is shown in Figure 10–17A. *(Courtesy of* Current Problems in Surgery, *1977).*

with any form of stigmata of von Recklinghausen's neurofibromatosis can never be ascertained because most of these individuals do not seek medical attention. Suffice it to point out that all florid cases of von Recklinghausen's neurofibromatosis are at risk of developing MPNST. Of 18 patients observed until they were older than 50 years of age, 9 developed MPNST. In other age categories, the incidence was smaller. In a more recent study of 60 patients at the University of Illinois,[46] we found a similar high incidence of MPNSTs. An increased incidence with advancing age is noted when the patients with the florid form of the disease are followed-up over a long period.

Whether the MPNST arises ab initio or is the product of malignant transformation of a preexisting benign nerve sheath tumor is a moot point.[146] D'Agostino et al.[138] found only 2 of 21 patients in whom there was actual intermingling of the sarcomatous and neurofibromatous tissues. Harkin and Reed[3] argued that transformation of a benign schwannoma into a malignant variety rarely, if ever, occurs. In contrast, MPNSTs often are closely associated with a plexiform neurofibroma, and transition to malignancy can be demonstrated (Fig. 10–24C). A positive conclusion to this controversy

may never be reached. This controversy, however, does not affect patient management, since therapy is not planned on the basis of whether the tumor arises ab initio or appears as a malignant transformation.

Malignant peripheral nerve sheath tumors develop in relatively older patients. The peak age incidence in Heard's[147] series was between the ages of 20 and 30 years. D'Agostino and co-workers[138] reported a median age of 28 years. In Brasfield and Das Gupta's report,[45] 27 of 32 patients were over the age of 30 years. In Guccion and Enzinger's[146] review of cases, the median was

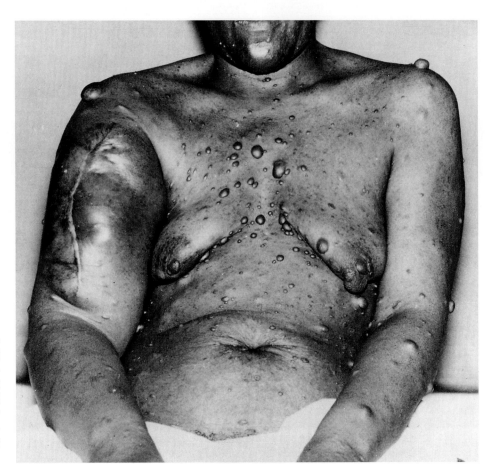

**Figure 10–34.** Obvious stigmata of neurofibromatosis with recurrent malignant schwannoma in right arm following inadequate local excision. Patient underwent muscle group excision, and the local tumor was controlled at the time of her death, which was due to distant metastases. *(Courtesy of* Current Problems in Surgery, *1977).*

34 years. This information, combined with the knowledge that MPNSTs are uncommon before the age of 20 years, suggests that nerve sheath tumors in the first two decades of life should be considered benign, unless there is convincing pathologic evidence to the contrary.

The natural history of malignant schwannomas (MPNSTs) is similar, irrespective of when the stigmata of von Recklinghausen's neurofibromatosis are first observed. Pain, sudden enlargement of a preexisting mass, or the occurrence and rapid growth of a new tumor in an adult patient suggests malignancy. The mass should be biopsied to determine malignancy. More than a single malignant primary lesion may occur in a patient with von Recklinghausen's neurofibromatosis.

The management of MPNSTs associated with von Recklinghausen's neurofibromatosis is similar to that for the solitary variety. However, the prognosis is relatively poorer than with their solitary counterparts.[138,140,146,147] Of the 76 patients with solitary malignant schwannoma in the present study, 63 percent survived 10 years free of disease (Table 10–8); whereas, in 18 patients with full-fledged stigmata of von Recklinghausen's neurofibromatosis, only 22 percent had a disease-free five-year survival.

## MALIGNANT TUMORS ASSOCIATED WITH VON RECKLINGHAUSEN'S NEUROFIBROMATOSIS

Patients with von Recklinghausen's neurofibromatosis have a higher than normal incidence of associated malignant tumors. A review of the published works[138,139] shows that about half the malignancies of peripheral nerve sheath origin occur in patients with neurofibromatosis. Although the most common form encountered is a malignant tumor of peripheral nerve origin, several other apparently unrelated epithelial cancers are seen as well. This association of epithelial tumors, however, is of considerable interest.

Brasfield and Das Gupta[45] found that, in their series of 110 patients with von Recklinghausen's neurofibromatosis, 16 (14.5 percent) had nonneurogenic malignant tumors. Five of the 54 female patients (9 percent) were treated for carcinoma of the breast, 6 for malignant melanoma (Fig. 10–37), 4 for carcinoma of the thyroid, and 1 for cancer of the lung. Although there is one published case report of melanoma arising in a café-au-lait spot,[148] we have never encountered such a case. An estimation of the true incidence of epithelial cancer in von Recklinghausen's neurofibromatosis is not available at this time.[85] To what extent

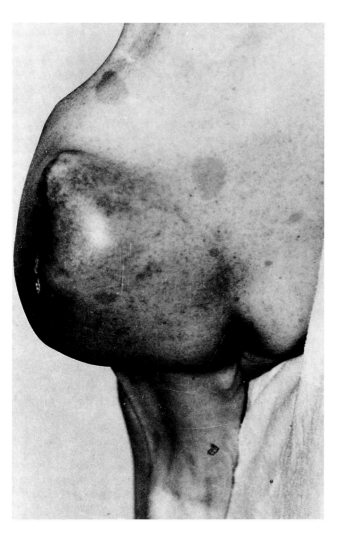

**Figure 10–35.** Large neurofibrosarcoma of the buttock *(Courtesy of* Current Problems in Surgery, *1977).*

the underlying neurofibromatosis influences the prognosis is uncertain.

## MALIGNANT TRITON TUMORS

Although any tumor containing both neural and skeletal components can be considered a triton tumor, by convention only those MPNSTs or schwannomas that contain rhabdomyosarcomatous elements are designated *malignant triton tumors.* This neoplasm was first described by Masson and Martin.[149] However, from a clinical standpoint, these tumors are usually seen in patients with MPNST associated with von Recklinghausen's neurofibromatosis and carry a poor prognosis.[150–152] Principles of management are essentially the same as malignant schwannomas with or without generalized neurofibromatosis.

Recently, a number of cases of MPNST with glandular differentiation and other morphologic cellular heterogeneity (e.g., epithelioid type of schwannoma) have been described by pathologists. Although these morphologic peculiarities arouse considerable interest from the standpoint of phylogeny and homology of neural crest derivations,[153] the clinical management of the variants are exactly the same as solitary schwannomas (MPNSTs). In general, the prognosis is not as good as in solitary MPNST, however. The incidence of these morphologic variants is not large enough for making a definitive statement regarding either the best method(s) of management or the overall prognosis.

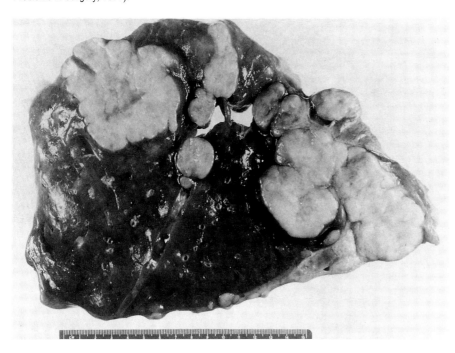

**Figure 10–36.** Metastatic malignant schwannoma to the liver. The primary site was on the back. The clinical photograph is shown in Figure 10–24C.

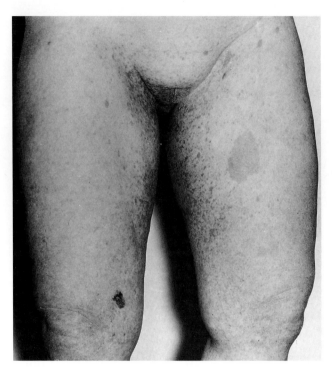

**Figure 10–37.** Large café-au-lait spot on left thigh, with melanoma in right distal thigh *(Courtesy of* Current Problems in Surgery, *1977).*

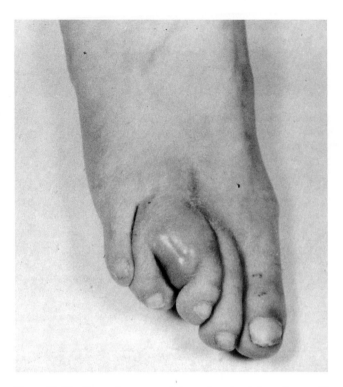

**Figure 10–38.** Clear cell sarcoma of the tendon sheath in a 47-year-old woman. Apparently, this tumor had been growing for three or four years before its present appearance.

## CLEAR CELL SARCOMA OF TENDON SHEATH OR MELANOMA OF SOFT PARTS

Clear cell sarcoma was originally described by Enzinger in 1965.[154] Since that time, it has been accepted as a distinct clinicopathologic entity. Although it produces melanin[155–160] and, like melanoma, is probably neuro-dermal in origin, the natural histories of these tumors are not akin to cutaneous or mucosal melanomas. Therefore, the general principles of treatment should be tailored to these unique tumors.

Clear cell sarcoma (Fig. 10–38) is a tumor of the extremities occurring in young adults, with some pre-ponderance in women. Enzinger[154] concluded that, in civilian personnel, the tumor occurs probably twice as frequently in women as in men. No racial predilection has been reported.

The tumors are usually slow-growing and most commonly encountered in the extremities, especially in the region of the foot, ankle, and occasionally the knee joint. In most instances, they adhere to the underlying tendons and consequently are movable in only one axis. These tumors have a firm consistency. In our series of 12 patients, the primary tumors were located in the lower extremity in seven instances and in the upper extremity in five instances. Most of these were located distal to the knee and elbow joints.

Clear cell sarcomas are usually deep-seated and do metastasize to the regional nodes. However, the exact incidence of nodal metastases is unknown. Enzinger[154] found 4 of 21 patients (19 percent) and Mackenzie[157] reported 4 of 6 (66 percent) that had regional node metastases. Of the 12 cases treated by us, 3 had metas-tases to the regional nodes.

It is not possible to develop guidelines for treat-ment on the basis of experience with so few patients. From an operational viewpoint, it is logical to consider these tumors as having the potential to develop lym-phatic metastases and to treat them accordingly. This would imply a wide excision with concomitant regional node dissection. The location of a clear cell sarcoma near a tendon or joint frequently poses a problem as to the extent of wide excision, and sometimes an amputa-tion becomes necessary. The role of curative radiation therapy for primary clear cell sarcoma and the efficacy of adjuvant chemotherapy in such tumors is unknown and needs assessment.

The overall five-year survival in patients with clear cell sarcoma is difficult to evaluate. From their col-lected material, Chung and Enzinger[160] found that 62 of 115 (54 percent) were alive and 50 of 115 (43 per-cent) died of metastatic disease. They also found that the incidence of local recurrence was 48 percent. How-ever, these data, though valuable, must be viewed with caution because therapy in these 115 patients was not uniform and the technical aspects of the operation were not standardized. In our series of 12 patients, only one (8 percent) developed local recurrence, which was in conjunction with systemic metastases. Of the 12 patients, nine (75 percent) have lived disease-free for five years or more.

## ■ TUMORS OF THE SYMPATHOCHROMAFFIN SYSTEM

### GANGLIONEUROMA

Ganglioneuromas can occur along the entire sympathochromaffin axis (Fig. 10–39). Although a benign ganglioneuroma is a relatively rare tumor, it is encountered often enough to merit discussion.

The sites in which these tumors most commonly develop are the posterior mediastinum, retroperitoneum, pelvis, adrenal medulla, and neck, in order of decreasing frequency.[1,161] Multiple ganglioneuromas are uncommon and may be associated with the stigmata of von Recklinghausen's neurofibromatosis.[162–166] The symmetrical distribution of ganglioneuromas, as well as cutaneous presentation of these tumors, has also been described.[162,165,167,168] However, it appears that such presentations should be regarded as unusual manifestations of a neurocutaneous syndrome.[45,46,167,168]

These tumors are seen in all races and in both sexes. The incidence in females apparently predominates in a ratio of three to two.[169] They are seldom encountered in infants, but 75 percent of these tumors appear before the age of 20 years.[170]

Ganglioneuromas are usually recognized incidentally to some other ailment or on routine physical examination. Hamilton and Koop[171] found 12 of their 17 patients were asymptomatic. In the other five, the symptoms consisted of diarrhea, chest pain, abdominal distention, ptosis, and an altered gait. Occasional instances of diarrhea, sweating, and hypertension, along with other sundry symptoms have been described.[172–174] Diarrheal symptoms have been attributed to the presence of vasoactive intestinal peptides, which can be immunocytochemically localized in ganglion cell cytoplasm.[172] In our series of only six patients, the diagnosis was made on routine physical examination. Four of the six tumors were located in the mediastinum and two in the retroperitoneum. These are slow-growing tumors and often become quite large before detection. The symptoms are caused by pressure upon contiguous structures. In the mediastinum, the enlarging tumors might produce pressure on the trachea, resulting in persistent cough, dyspnea, or stridor.

Benign ganglioneuromas seldom are hormonally active.[171] Hamilton and Koop[171] found that, in a relatively small number of patients, there is an increase in homovanillic (HVA) and vanillylmandelic (VMA) acid excretion levels. In those patients where these metabolites are elevated, serial determination of the levels,

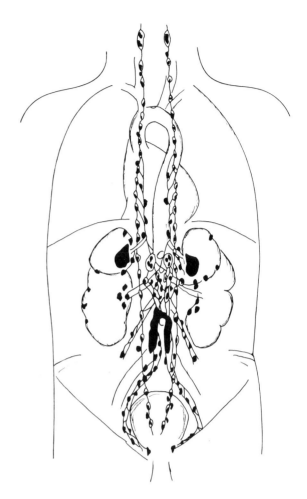

**Figure 10–39.** Diagram of the distribution of chromaffin tissue in the newborn infant.

both preoperatively and postoperatively, might be of value as a biologic marker.

Since the most common site is the posterior mediastinum in children and young adults, the roentgenographic appearance of the chest is of clinical interest. A well-circumscribed mass may be evident, and the adjacent vertebrae and ribs may show thinning and erosion. When the ganglioneuroma is of the so-called dumbbell or hourglass shape, x-rays may show a paravertebral mass, erosion of the pedicles, and enlargement of the paravertebral foramen. Calcification, when present, helps to distinguish a posterior mediastinal ganglioneuroma from congenital problems, such as duplication of the foregut or bronchogenic cysts. Retroperitoneal ganglioneuromas have no specific x-ray findings. Abdominal computed axial tomography (CAT) scans and ultrasonograms might provide some clues but are never diagnostic.

### Treatment

The treatment of ganglioneuroma is excision. These tumors are well encapsulated and can be separated from their beds with remarkable ease. In the neck, careful dissection is needed from the surrounding structures. Frequently, the tumor will arise from a sympathetic ganglion, resection of which might lead to Horner's syndrome. In the hourglass variety, exploration of the vertebral canal is required as well.

## PHEOCHROMOCYTOMA

Pheochromocytomas are rare tumors that produce a remediable form of hypertension, together with a wide spectrum of associated clinical manifestations. The location of these tumors within the body follows the embryonic distribution of chromaffin tissue derived from the primitive neuroectoderm. Many of the unique features of the disease are attributable to the pharmacologic effects of catecholamines, which the chromaffin tumors produce. Approximately 60 percent of pheochromocytomas occur in the adrenal glands, and more than 90 percent lie between the diaphragm and pelvic floor.

***Physiologic Considerations.*** In most respects, the symptoms of pheochromocytoma stem directly from the excess production of catecholamines. In past decades, many important advances were made toward understanding the pathways of biosynthesis and degradation of these compounds and the mechanisms that govern their storage and release.[175–177] These advances will be reviewed briefly, but the reader is referred elsewhere for more comprehensive reviews.

The scheme of biosynthesis was first proposed in 1939[178] and has been confirmed by several workers in recent years.[175–177] The parent compound, tyrosine, is concentrated in body tissues by an active transport system and subsequently finds its way into several important metabolic pathways. The biosynthesis of catecholamines occurs in the adrenal medulla, in sympathetic nerve endings, in parts of the brain, and in enterochromaffinlike cells found in various parts of the gastrointestinal tract, lung, and various other organs.[177–179] The conversion of tyrosine to dihydroxyphenylalinine (DOPA), catalyzed by the enzyme tyrosine hydroxylase, takes place in the mitochondria of the cell. DOPA is subsequently converted to dopamine, which is then converted to norepinephrine in specialized granules within the sympathetic nerve endings and in the adrenal medulla.

Most of the norepinephrine thus synthesized remains in situ until released by the action of sympathetic nerves. Norepinephrine is the principal catecholamine released by the sympathetic nerves.[177] The conversion of norepinephrine to epinephrine results from the action of an enzyme (phenylethanolamine N-methyl transferase) normally located only in certain cells of the adrenal medulla. This gland normally synthesizes and stores both norepinephrine and epinephrine.

In pheochromocytomas, the biosynthesis of catecholamines proceeds along the same pathways as in normal tissue, although the rate of synthesis is more rapid. In many pheochromocytomas, only norepinephrine is formed. Others produce both norepinephrine and epinephrine. Those tumors that produce epinephrine usually arise within the adrenal medulla. Tumors that exclusively produce epinephrine are extremely rare.

Catecholamines and other forms of biogenic amines are stored in the cells derived from the sympathochromaffin tissue. These intracytoplasmic storage sites have received considerable attention in recent years. The granules are specialized subcellular particles, identifiable in adrenergic nerves and chromaffin cells by electron microscopy. Similar granules have been identified in pheochromocytomas and in neuroblastoma tissue.[165,177,180]

Norepinephrine and epinephrine are inactive as long as they remain within granules, but their full activity is manifested on release. The mechanisms by which the catecholamines are released from the granules have been extensively investigated.[178,179] Normally, small amounts of norepinephrine are released continuously and larger amounts in spurts, possibly representing phasic alterations in sympathetic nerve impulses. Following release at the effector site as a result of sympathetic stimulation, norepinephrine, which remains free, is again taken up by the granules, and its physiologic action is terminated.

In patients with a pheochromocytoma, circulating catecholamines released from the tumor are taken up and stored in sympathetic nerve granules. Thus, even after removal of the tumor, these patients may have increased stores of pressor amines and an increased excretion of norepinephrine and epinephrine, and their catabolites may occur in the urine for several days following successful surgery.

Inactivation or degradation of catecholamines is largely effected by the enzyme catechol-O-methyltransferase (COMT). This enzyme is present in high concentrations in the liver and kidney and is principally responsible for inactivating released or circulating catecholamines, since the O-methylated catecholamine derivatives metanephrine (M) and normetanephrine (NM) are no longer physiologically active. The other enzyme principally involved in the metabolic destruction of the catecholamines is monoamine oxidase (MAO). This enzyme, which is present in most tissues, seems to play a major role in disposing of excessive stores of catecholamines by deamination in situ. The principal end products of catecholamine catabolism are those which are O-methylated (M and NM), and the final product of both O-methylation and deamination is 4-hydroxy-3-methoxymandelic acid (or vanillylmandelic acid [VMA]). The measurement of the urinary excretion of the catecholamines or their major catabolites is now recognized as a major means of establishing the diagnosis of pheochromocytoma.

*Clinical Features.*  The initial manifestation of a pheochromocytoma may be a complicating vascular accident. The principal complications of an untreated pheochromocytoma stem from arterial hypertension, with findings similar to those in patients with sustained hypertension of comparable severity and duration. These include retinopathy, a cerebral vascular accident, myocardial infarction, congestive heart failure, or full-fledged malignant hypertension.[181–187] In addition, persistently high circulating catecholamine levels may result in cardiac arrhythmias, particularly those of ventricular origin.[188] Pheochromocytomas occurring during pregnancy have sometimes produced symptoms of eclampsia.[189] Hyperglycemia and glycosuria often simulate diabetes mellitus.[181,186] The major cause is thought to be the catecholamine-induced inhibition of insulin secretion. Thomas and associates[182] found that patients with a pheochromocytoma have multiple symptoms: headaches (80 percent) and palpitation without tachycardia (64 percent) were among the major symptoms in a series of 100 patients.

*Pharmacologic Tests.*  The histamine provocative test, the benzodioxane adrenolytic test, and the phentolamine test are rarely used for the diagnosis of pheochromocytomas. A provocative test with histamine has its chief value in patients having paroxysms of hypertension with intermittent normal pressure. This test has the hazard of being complicated by a cerebral vascular accident or myocardial infarction. Although a provocative test with tyramine[190] is supposedly free of side effects,[181] it is safer to rely on chemical methods of diagnosis.

*Chemical Tests.*  The diagnosis of pheochromocytoma is generally made by chemical measurement of catecholamines and their degradation products.[181,186,191] Serum catecholamines can be measured accurately, and the standardized methods for measuring urinary catecholamines are widely available. Over 90 percent of pheochromocytoma patients are identifiable by a single accurate determination of 24-hour urinary catecholamines. Interference may be caused by agents containing sympathomimetic amines. Therefore, extreme care should be used in the collection of 24-hour urinary specimens. Methods for measurement of epinephrine and norepinephrine have been adequately developed and are routinely used in conjunction with examination of urinary catecholamines in the diagnosis of pheochromocytomas. Furthermore, the use of vena cava blood sampling at different levels with estimation of the levels of biogenic amines has been suggested as an aid in localizing these pheochromocytomas. However, such sampling is seldom necessary. History, physical examination, and chemical tests will usually confirm a diagnosis of pheochromocytoma. However, in some unusual cases, confusion with an intracranial tumor might occur.

Pheochromocytomas can be radiologically localized by means of MRI and CAT scan. Angiography can detect thin tumors accurately, but this is almost never used due to associated hazards of catastrophic hyperplastic crisis. Recently, radionuclide scans, such as using radioiodinated mIGB (metaiodobenzylguanidine) or octneorrdi scan, have been shown to be an extremely valuable adjunct in localization of pheochromocytoma.

*Treatment.*  The treatment of pheochromocytoma is excision, irrespective of its location or the associated complicating factors. It is mandatory that preoperative evaluation be complete, and judicious preparation with α-blockade, adequate hydration, and, if necessary, β-blockade should be performed preoperatively. During the operation, the patient should be well monitored. The operative approach must take into consideration the fact that 10 to 15 percent of pheochromocytomas are bilateral. Since these tumors can occur anywhere within the sympathochromaffin axis, all patients should have an exploratory procedure.

### Pheochromocytoma in Children

Pheochromocytomas have also been reported in children.[181,192] The ratio of males to females before puberty is 2 to 1. However, with puberty, there is a marked increase in incidence in females. The youngest patient on record with a symptomatic pheochromocytoma was one month old. The average age at diagnosis is 9.8 years.[181]

A high incidence of bilateral, multiple, and ectopic tumors, and a severe and stormy course, are characteristic of this disease. In one series, 140 tumors were found in 100 children, including many in extra-adrenal locations.[192] In five children, a second tumor developed after initial surgery.

Common symptoms in children are headache, sweating, nausea, vomiting, weight loss, visual disturbance, seizures, weakness, and fatigue.[181,186,192] A peculiar reddish-blue mottling of the skin has also been reported. Polydipsia and polyuria are more common in children than in adults. Occasionally, obstructive uropathy or obstruction of a renal artery is the initial manifestation. Catecholamine excretion in children usually is predominantly norepinephrine, and sustained hyperexcretion is present in about 90 percent of patients. Since hypertension in children is uncommon, pheochromocytoma should always be considered.

The association of pheochromocytoma with cyanotic congenital heart disease has been reported in children.[183] It has been postulated that persistent hypoxemia could produce adrenal medullary hyperplasia and, eventually, an autonomously functioning pheochromocytoma. Hypertension and other signs and symptoms of catecholamine excess should be carefully considered when evaluating patients with congenital heart disease because of the risks associated with cardiac catheterization, angiography, and surgery. Some neuroblastomas and ganglioneuromas of childhood can produce catecholamines and thereby create confusion in the diagnosis. However, the natural histories of these tumors are entirely different and a diagnosis should not be difficult.

### Familial Pheochromocytoma

Familial occurrence of pheochromocytoma has been known since the report of Calkins and Howard in 1947.[184] At least 16 kindreds have been studied and described. The mode of inheritance was autosomal dominant with a high degree of penetrance. Several features set these cases apart from the more common sporadic type. The incidence of multiple tumors in familial patients is approximately 50 percent. The range of age at the time of onset of symptoms varies widely. Sustained hypertension has been more common than the paroxysmal type. Increased occurrence of familial thyroid neoplasms in patients with familial pheochromocytomas has also been reported,[193] as has the triad of familial bilateral pheochromocytomas, medullary carcinoma of the thyroid, and hyperparathyroidism (multiple endocrine neoplasia).[185,194]

### Pheochromocytoma and Neurofibromatosis

The relationship between pheochromocytoma and neurofibromatosis was first noted by Suzuki[195] in 1910. MacKeith[196] reviewed the literature in 1944 and found that 165 cases of pheochromocytomas had been reported and that neurofibromatosis was present in nine. Davis and his co-workers[197] reviewed the literature up to 1950 and estimated the incidence of neurofibromatosis in patients with pheochromocytoma to be about 5 percent (10 of 203 patients).

In the two large series reported by Crowe and associates[42] and Brasfield and Das Gupta,[45] there was a low incidence of pheochromocytoma in patients with von Recklinghausen's neurofibromatosis (only one in each study). In the series reported by Wander and Das Gupta,[46] there were no instances of pheochromocytoma in a series of 60 patients with von Recklinghausen's neurofibromatosis. Lynch and associates,[198] whose findings were similar, estimated the incidence of pheochromocytoma in von Recklinghausen's neurofibromatosis to be less than 1 percent. Tilford and Kelsch,[199] in 1973, reported a collected series of 57 neurofibromatosis patients with pheochromocytoma. The mean age of these patients was 41 years, and only three patients were under the age of 18 years. In adults with neurofibromatosis, hypertension is seven times more likely to be caused by pheochromocytoma than by renal artery stenosis. In children, however, the ratio is reversed, with renal artery stenosis being the more common cause.

In 1953, Glushien and co-workers[200] estimated that as many as 10 percent of patients with pheochromocytoma might have "neurocutaneous syndromes" and suggested that pheochromocytoma, neurofibromatosis, tuberous sclerosis, Sturge-Weber syndrome, and von Hippel-Lindau syndrome were all of common neuroectodermal origin and likely to appear in combination with significant frequency. These authors presented three cases—one of neurofibromatosis and pheochromocytoma, and two of neurofibromatosis and von Hippel-Lindau syndrome. In recent years, an association has been observed between pheochromocytoma, the so-called neurocutaneous syndromes, and other disorders such as medullary thyroid carcinoma. Today, many agree that a 5 percent overall incidence of pheochromocytoma probably represents a reasonable estimate[201] in patients with all types of neurocutaneous syndromes.

### Multiple Endocrine Neoplasia II

A relationship between Sipple's syndrome and neurofibromatosis has been proposed because of the occurrence of pheochromocytomas and mucosal neuromas in Sipple's syndrome.[202] Since Sipple's report in 1961, the syndrome has undergone further clarification.[203,204] The mucosal tumor that occurs primarily in the lip should be classified as a true neuroma rather than a nerve sheath tumor characteristic of von Recklinghausen's neurofibromatosis. Patients with these neuromas are now classified as having multiple endocrine neoplasia (MEN), type IIb, which is characterized by medullary carcinoma of the thyroid, pheochromocytomas, multiple mucosal neuromas of the lips, tongue, and upper eyelids, plus marfanoid habitus. The only true overlap clinically with neurofibromatosis is the occurrence of pheochromocytoma. The C cell, which makes up the medullary carcinoma, belongs to the amine precursor uptake and decarboxylation (APUD) series.[205] It is possible to attribute to the neural crest all the changes in Sipple's syndrome except for hyperparathyroidism, which only rarely occurs in the MEN IIb form.

### Pheochromocytoma of the Bladder

The location of a pheochromocytoma in the bladder wall produces a distinct syndrome.[206] The unique situation of the tumor in a structure that changes dimensions in the physiologic process of micturition accounts for its different behavioral pattern. Typically, severe paroxysmal symptoms, especially throbbing headaches, occur with or shortly after micturition. Painless hematuria occurs in approximately 50 percent of cases.

In some cases, urinary metabolites of catecholamines have been normal, possibly because bladder tumors are symptomatic early in their existence, when hyperexcretion of catecholamines is present for very brief periods during contraction of the bladder. It is therefore important that the possibility of a pheochromocytoma of the bladder not be dismissed because of the absence of the usual biochemical findings, if this diagnosis is suggested from clinical evaluation.

Bladder pheochromocytomas are usually small and located in the muscular wall of the organ; therefore, cystoscopic findings and cystograms may be normal. The behavior of blood pressure during massage of the bladder and the adrenal region, and during distention of the bladder, may be of critical importance in confirming clinical suspicion.

# ■ NEUROBLASTOMA

Neuroblastomas are highly malignant tumors occurring predominantly in infancy and early childhood. In the California Tumor Registry, neuroblastomas constitute 5 percent of all childhood malignancies.[207] Several children's centers have reported the rate to be 10 to 12 percent.[167,208] These tumors are considered the third most common in children.[209]

## AGE, SEX, AND RACE

This tumor occurs primarily in infancy;[210] it is suggested that about one-fourth of neuroblastomas are congenital.[211–214] In any large series, about 40 percent of the patients are between the ages of 2 and 6 years (Table 10–11). In about 17 percent, the tumors occur between the ages of 7 and 19 years.[207,215–218] Neuroblastomas are found with almost equal frequency in both sexes, and no racial predilection has been recorded.

## ANATOMIC DISTRIBUTION

Neuroblastoma characteristically arises in any area along the distribution of the sympathetic chain, including the cranial ganglia. Primary intraspinal, intracranial, bone, and soft tissue tumors have also been described.[165] Most, however, are located in the retroperitoneum, with the mediastinum the next most likely site of occurrence. Recently, Haase et al.[219] analyzed the children's cancer group experience with neuroblastomas and found that, out of a combined total of 945 cases, 41 (4.3 percent) were located in the pelvis. This subset they considered separate from their cohort of 945 located elsewhere.

The early and widespread metastases resulting from the deep-seated primary tumor result in bizarre clinical expressions. The initial symptoms may be fever and anemia, with no localizing signs, but, more frequently, these symptoms accompany an abdominal mass. A common clinical presentation is enlarged metastatic cervical lymph nodes. An accurate diagnosis is established only after microscopic examination of the tissue with corroborative chemical examination.

The increasing abdominal girth that is frequently a presenting symptom must be differentiated from other space-occupying lesions. Wilms' tumor is probably the most common neoplasm from which neuroblastomas must be differentiated. The characteristic feature of an intra-abdominal mass containing calcific deposits suggests neuroblastoma. Typically, the calcification consists of finely stippled densities in the central portion of the tumor. CAT scans and/or MRI adds to the accuracy of preoperative diagnosis. The presence of osteolytic lesions along with a retroperitoneal tumor is almost diagnostic of neuroblastoma. Mediastinal lesions are usually diagnosed by means of routine chest x-rays.

Elevated urinary excretion of dopamine, VMA, HVA, and MHPG (3-methoxy-4-hydroxyphenylglycol) in neuroblastomas has been adequately demonstrated.[208,220–224] Therefore, these chemical diagnostic tests should be routinely used. If the levels of the biogenic amines and their breakdown products are lower after excision of the tumor, these data can be used as

**TABLE 10–11. COMPARATIVE AGE DISTRIBUTION OF NEUROBLASTOMA IN FIVE LARGE SERIES***

| Age Distribution | Hospital for Sick Children, London[216] (129 cases) | Children's Hospital Columbus[215] (90 cases) | Children's Medical Center, Boston[217] (217 cases) | Tumor Registry California[207] (212 cases) | Memorial Sloan-Kettering Cancer Center[218] (133 cases) |
|---|---|---|---|---|---|
| 0–11 mo | 38 | 30 | 23 | 32 | 17 |
| 12–23 mo | 16 | 20 | 24 | 14 | 14 |
| 2–6 yr | 38 | 38 | 41 | 37 | 48 |
| 7–19 yr | 8 | 12 | 13 | 17 | 21 |

*Numbers represent percentages.

prognostic guides, since subsequent elevation might herald either local recurrence or metastases.

## TREATMENT

Neuroblastoma must be diagnosed early and treated by radical excision and radiation therapy. Although the addition of chemotherapy was championed in the last decade, it is probably of little or no value in the ultimate outcome.[225,226]

### End Results

The reported overall cure rate in the past varied between 9.7 and 36 percent.[210] The California Tumor Registry[207] found the overall cure rate to be directly related to age at diagnosis. For patients under one year of age, it was 60 percent; for one-year-olds it was 21 percent; between two and six years old, 10 percent; and between 7 and 19 years old, 8 percent.[207,208,211–213,215–218,220–223,225–227]

Survival of children with neuroblastoma is influenced by numerous factors: the extent or stage of the disease at diagnosis, the age of the patient, the site of the primary tumor, histologic evidence of tumor maturation (grading), and the presence or absence of lymphocytes in the tumor, bone marrow, or peripheral blood.[225–230] Evans et al.[231] summarized the prognostic factors in two-year survival in neuroblastoma (Table 10–12).

The prognostic aspects of the clinical staging and different forms of therapy have been studied in a prospective fashion by the Children's Cancer Study Group (CCSG).[226] From their studies, it appears that the staging of the tumor as proposed by Evans and co-workers[229,231] is of considerable prognostic import. In this clinical staging system, stage I tumors are confined to the organ or structure of origin. Stage II tumors extend in-continuity beyond the organ structure of origin but do not cross the midline (regional lymph nodes on the homolateral side may be involved). The tumor is also stage II if it extends intradurally. Stage III tumors extend in-continuity beyond the midline (regional nodes may be involved bilaterally). Stage IV remote disease involves skeleton, organs, soft tissues, distant lymph nodes, or other structures. Stage IV-S are patients who would otherwise be Stage I and II but who have remote disease contained to one or more of the following sites: liver, skin, or bone marrow.

The age of the patient at the time of diagnosis also influences the overall prognosis. According to the CCSG therapeutic protocols, all eligible patients were treated by curative surgery, radiation therapy, or both, for localized stage I, II, and III tumors. On a randomized basis, half of these patients received cyclophosphamide for one year.[229] The results of treatment in 134 such patients showed that there were no relapses in stage I. In stages II and III, the relapse rate was 13 per-

**TABLE 10–12. TWO-YEAR SURVIVAL RATES IN NEUROBLASTOMA BY PROGNOSTIC FACTORS***

| Prognostic Factors | No. patients | Survival (%) |
|---|---|---|
| **Age** | | |
| 2 years or younger | 73 | 77 |
| Older than 2 years | 51 | 38 |
| **Neuron-Specific Enolase** | | |
| Normal (1–100 ng/ml) | 60 | 76 |
| Abnormal (> 100 ng/ml) | 23 | 17 |
| **Ferritin** | | |
| Normal (0–150 ng/ml) | 64 | 83 |
| Abnormal (> 150 ng/ml) | 27 | 54 |
| **VMA/VHA** | | |
| High (> 1) | 28 | 84 |
| Low (< 1) | 22 | 44 |
| **Stage** | | |
| I | 15 | 100 |
| II | 27 | 82 |
| III | 18 | 42 |
| IV | 51 | 30 |
| IV-S | 13 | 100 |
| **Pathology (Shimada System)**** | | |
| Favorable type | 52 | 94 |
| Unfavorable type | 36 | 39 |

*Total number of patients studied is 124; total percentage of survival is 60 percent. Adapted from Evans et al.[231]
**Shimada H, Chatten J, Newton WH Jr., et al. Histopathologic prognostic factors in neuroblastic tumors: Definition of subtypes of ganglioneuroblastoma and an age-linked classification of neuroblastoma. J Natl Cancer Inst 73:405, 1984.

cent and 38 percent, respectively. Use of adjuvant cyclophosphamide for one year did not influence the prognosis either way. When computed according to age, the survival was found to be 90 percent for children in the first and second years of life, falling to 47 percent for children two years of age or older. Similar aggregated survival data have been published in the past from retrospective studies as well.[207,215–218]

To what extent regional node involvement influences the prognosis is hard to define, since very few of the published reports have dealt with this facet adequately. The paucity of data is evident even in the CCSG Study,[229] since information was available to the authors in only 46 of 134 patients. Twenty-seven of 32 patients with stage II and 12 of 14 with stage III tumors had positive nodes. Eleven of 39 (28 percent) with positive nodes developed local recurrence and metastatic disease. There were no relapses in the six patients with no nodal metastases.

The prognostic influence of the site of the primary has been dealt with at length by various authors.[215–217] Whether above or below the diaphragm, it has little influence on the rate of recurrence or metastases, assuming that the tumor is adequately staged and is categorized according to the age of the patient.

It appears that the use of chemotherapy in an adjuvant setting has little or no influence on the overall prognosis. From all the available information, it seems that better staging, more aggressive resection, and radiation therapy are the causes of this improved end result. The aggressive attitude toward therapy is observed even in the management of metastatic neuroblastoma. Although most of these patients are treated by chemotherapy or radiation therapy (or both), in selected instances excision of the metastatic tumor is possible and is advocated.[171]

Finally, in recent years, numerous studies[232–236] have shown that N-myc amplification influences the prognosis in neuroblastoma. Thus, when all the clinical, histologic, metabolic, and molecular factors are taken together, the following stand out as favorable prognostic factors in neuroblastoma: (1) young age (< 2 yrs); (2) favorable histologic type; (3) low stage (I, II, IV-S); (4) no N-myc amplification; (5) low serum ferritin; (6) hyperploidy; and (7) high expression of TRK gene.

## MATURATION OF NEUROBLASTOMA

Although relatively rare, neuroblastomas and undifferentiated ganglioneuromas are known to mature into ganglioneuromas.[237–241] Cushing and Wolback,[238] in 1927, first reported the maturation of a neuroblastoma. Fox et al.[239] studied a patient 46 years after partial treatment and found no evidence of recurrence of the tumor. Since then, several such cases have been reported.[227,237,240–242] All these case reports show the unique potential of an undifferentiated tumor in rare instances to become differentiated and spontaneously grow into mature ganglion cells. However, the factors responsible for such maturation still remain puzzling.

## RELATION TO VON RECKLINGHAUSEN'S NEUROFIBROMATOSIS

A possible relationship between familial neuroblastoma and von Recklinghausen's neurofibromatosis was suggested by Knudson and Amromin[162] and Chatten and Voorhees,[243] who noted a high incidence of café-au-lait spots in their patients' families. Bolande and Towler[164] noted maturation of cutaneous lesions in familial neuroblastoma into ganglioneuromas and, finally, into lesions that closely resembled neurofibromas. After an extensive morphologic review, they were able to identify ganglion cells or ganglioneuromatous elements in von Recklinghausen's neurofibromas (i.e., isolated ganglioneuroma resulting from the maturation of cutaneous lesions in familial neuroblastoma). According to Bolande and Towler,[164] the simultaneous occurrence of these two diseases in a single patient has been reported only twice in the literature. The common neural crest origin of both the Schwann cell and the neuroblast led them to speculate on the embryologic and genetic relationships that may be shared by the two diseases. Additional embryologic information or greater evidence of a clinical association is necessary to consider their relationship significant.

## NEUROBLASTOMA IN UNUSUAL SITES

Primary neuroblastoma can occur in many unusual sites: for example, in the intraspinal space, intracranial locations, orbit, buttock, leg (Fig. 5–76A and 5–76B, Chapter 5), and the nares.[165] However, olfactory neuroblastoma (esthesioneuroblastoma) constitutes a truly unusual entity and therefore is briefly discussed below.

### Esthesioneuroblastoma

Olfactory esthesioneuroblastoma is a rare malignant tumor arising in the region of the roof of the nasal cavity. Since Berger et al.[244] described the first case in 1924, about 105 additional cases have been reported.[245] In the files of the University of Illinois Hospital, there are only two such cases, both occurring in males. Hutter et al.[246] reviewed the experience with 18 patients at Memorial Sloan-Kettering Cancer Center and concluded that esthesioneuroblastoma is a low-grade neuroblastoma; 3 of their 18 patients (17 percent) showed regional node metastases. Skolnick et al.[247] found cervical node metastases in 11 of 97 (11 percent) collected cases. These tumors are usually seen in the second decade and probably are more common in males. Multiple recurrences after excision or irradiation have been reported,[246,247] usually because adequate excision was not possible. However, with the combined craniofacial approach standardized in recent years, adequate excision can now be achieved and, combined with postoperative radiation therapy, should provide good salvage.[246–248]

## ■ GANGLIONEUROBLASTOMA

Ganglioneuroblastoma probably occupies an intermediate position in the degree of histologic differentiation among the tumors designated as neuroblastomas and ganglioneuromas. By common acceptance, ganglioneuroblastomas are those primary tumors that arise outside the retroperitoneum but histologically resemble neuroblastoma. Depending on the extent of neuroblastoma or differential ganglioneuromas, an entity such as malignant ganglioneuroma can be visualized. But even if such an entity is possible, it is extremely infrequent. It usually occurs in the lateral portion of the neck and, rarely, in the perineal region. Priebe and Clatworthy[215] found 3 of 92 (3 percent) consecutive cases of neuroblastoma in the neck, and all were in the one-year-or-under age group. Rosenfeld and Graves[6] reported that, of 32 primary neurogenic tumors of the lateral portion of the neck, only one (3 percent) was a malignant ganglioneuroma and three (9 percent) were benign ganglioneuromas. Oberman and Sullenger,[7] reviewing neurogenic tumors of the head and neck region at the University of Michigan, found that, over a period of 21 years, there had been 43 cases, of which two (4.6 percent) were neuroblastomas (malignant ganglioneuromas) of the neck.

The clinical presentation of these tumors is like that of any other lateral neck mass. Diagnosis is established by means of either an excision or an incision biopsy. In one of our patients (a two-year-old child), the diagnosis was established after excision of an enlarged node. In children and young adults in whom there is difficulty in interpretation of the biopsy material from a neck tumor, chemical diagnostic tests for neuroblastoma are recommended.

The treatment of ganglioneuroblastoma and/or malignant ganglioneuroma is radical excision. Oberman and Sullenger[7] reported that one of their patients survived six years after partial excision and irradiation. In view of the rarity of these tumors, it is not possible to arrive at average survival figures. However, it is conjectured that, if these tumors are treated as neuroblastomas, the results in the favorable age group would probably match those for neuroblastoma.

## ■ MALIGNANT PHEOCHROMOCYTOMA

Malignant pheochromocytomas are rare tumors, and only a handful of cases have ever been documented.[165,249,250] It is almost impossible to clinically diagnose either a benign or malignant pheochromocytoma. If, at the time the tumor is excised, there is regional nodal metastases and these nodes are found to be chromaffin-positive, then a tentative diagnosis of malignant pheochromocytoma can be made. Otherwise, the diagnosis should be based on the natural history of the tumor. If the patient dies of widespread metastases and the metastatic deposits are chromaffin-positive, then the diagnosis, of course, is certain.

### EXTRASKELETAL EWING'S SARCOMA

In 1975, Angervall and Enzinger[251] described the pathologic features and clinical behavior of 39 small, round, or oval sarcomas occurring in the soft tissues. These tumors are histologically indistinguishable from Ewing's sarcoma of the bone. Although, clinically and morphologically, skeletal and extraskeletal Ewing's sarcoma represent two different entities, most authors favor that both these tumors are of neural origin and are closely related to peripheral malignant neuroepithelioma.[252–255] In fact, it has been suggested that peripheral neuroepithelioma and Ewing's sarcoma occupy opposite ends of the spectrum of primitive neural tumors.[252–255]

These tumors chiefly affect young adults (median age 20 years) and most commonly involve the soft tissues of the lower extremities and the paravertebral region. Follow-up data ranging from 1 month to 14 years were available in 35 of the 39 patients (90 percent). Of these, 13 (33 percent) were alive at the time of the report.[251] In most of the fatal cases, the clinical course was rapid, with metastatic lesions developing within a few months after excision of the primary tumor. From this study,[251] guidelines regarding therapy are impossible. A number of these patients were treated with different types of excision, radiation therapy, and, finally, a variety of chemotherapeutic agents. However, based on the histologic features, which resembled those of Ewing's sarcoma of the bone, it is appropriate to assume that this tumor should show a good response to combination radiation therapy and sequential chemotherapy, as reported for Ewing's sarcoma of the bone.[256,257]

We have treated 14 adults with this tumor. All were males between the ages of 22 and 40 years. Although most (nine) of the tumors were located in the pelvis, especially in the rectosacral space, these were also found in the extremities: three in the lower and two in the upper. Unfortunately, the sacral tumors are usually diagnosed after several months delay. The initial symptom is pain, and in most instances the pain is attributed to sciatica or some other unrelated cause. Thus, a delay in diagnosis inevitably results. In all our nine patients with rectosacral extraskeletal Ewing's tumor, the patients were referred to us after several months of conservative therapy, by which time the prognosis is grave even after the most aggressive form of therapy. In our series, after multimodal management, only four patients (29 percent) are long-term survivors.

The prognosis in children is better than in adults. In a preliminary review of 26 cases encountered in the Intergroup Rhabdomyosarcoma Study, Soule et al.[258] found that these lesions were more common in the extremities, and that 17 (65 percent) of 26 patients were apparently disease-free at the time of their report. All 26 patients were treated by wide local excision, radiation therapy, and systemic chemotherapy. More recently, Schmidt et al.[259] reported a 66 percent five-year survival in children with extraskeletal Ewing's sarcoma.

## ■ PARAGANGLIOMAS

### CAROTID BODY TUMORS

Carotid body tumors are among the rarest of the neoplasms in the cervical region.[260–262] Diagnosis can be established by biopsy, and once the diagnosis is established, the treatment depends entirely on the symptoms produced by the tumor. Excision must be undertaken with great caution. Small tumors can easily be dissected from the carotid vessels. Resection of the carotid artery is certainly not indicated in otherwise asymptomatic patients; but in symptomatic patients, if dissection of the tumor from the surrounding arteries is not possible, resection of the carotid vessels with reconstruction should be performed.

The simultaneous occurrence of a carotid body tumor and a pheochromocytoma is extremely rare.

## CHEMODECTOMAS

### Benign Chemodectoma

Benign chemodectomas (nonchromaffin paragangliomas) have been demonstrated to originate in the glomus jugulare,[263–266] the ganglion nodosum of the vagus nerve,[267–268] the auricular branches of the vagus nerve,[269] the tympanic ganglia of the glossopharyngeal nerve,[269] the ciliary ganglia,[269] the orbit,[270] the aortic bodies,[268–273] the mediastinum,[273,274] the retroperitoneum,[275,276] the lower extremities,[277,278] the cauda equina,[279] the muscular wall of the small intestine,[280,281] in rare instances in the pineal organ,[282] and in the lung.[283–285]

Most are benign, showing only hyperplasia on microscopic examination, and usually occur in adults between the ages of 40 to 60 years.[170] It is suggested that these tumors are found more frequently in women. Brown[158] and Brown and Freyer[286] estimated that the occurrence in females is five times greater than in males. There is no outstanding racial incidence.

The symptoms produced depend entirely on the location of the tumor. In the glomus jugulare tumors, when the eardrum is still intact, the most common presenting symptom is a conductive hearing loss accompanied by tinnitus and a feeling of fullness in the ear. As the tumor continues to grow, it becomes visible as a dark mass through the lower part of the drum. In advanced cases, bloodstained discharge from the ear and deafness are common findings. As its growth progresses, the tumor extends through the jugular foramen and spreads to the base of the skull. In about 40 percent of these patients, the seventh cranial nerve is involved.[264]

In the ganglion nodosum of the vagal nerve, a cervical tumor is usually the presenting feature. In the mediastinum or in the retroperitoneum, the mass produces all the symptoms of a space-occupying lesion, and

the histologic diagnosis is usually made after excision of the tumor. Smithers and Gowing[272] collected 28 cases of chemodectoma in the region of the aortic arch, including one of their own. They found that, in all these cases, the tumors were of long duration, and the mediastinal component with classic roentgenographic findings made preoperative diagnosis possible. Chemodectomas of the gastrointestinal tract can be diagnosed only after excision.

Smith, Hughes, and Ermocilla[282] reported a case of chemodectoma of the pineal body. Infrequently, chemodectomas may be hormonally active.[1,263,287–290] Instances of catecholamine-secreting nonchromaffin paragangliomas of the glomus jugulare, carotid body, and retroperitoneum are on record.[1,263–293] Levit and co-workers[265] suggested that, until the true frequency of functioning tumors is known, all patients with paragangliomas or chemodectomas should have routine preoperative determination of urinary catecholamines and their metabolites to decrease surgical morbidity and mortality.

### Malignant Chemodectoma

Malignant chemodectomas are extremely rare, and most authors have personal experience with only one or two cases.[294–299] Frey and Karoll[293] described malignant chemodectomas in three patients, all of whom died. One had brain metastases, and the other two had locally untreatable tumors. Approximately 32 cases have been reported in which there was metastasis to the regional lymph nodes or to distant sites proven by microscopic examination.[294–301] Reported sites of distant metastases include lung, bone, liver, pancreas, thyroid, heart, trachea, orbit, and extradural space.[300–305]

Malignant chemodectomas, like their benign counterparts, occur in the aortic bodies,[271–273] the ganglion nodosum of the vagus nerve,[247–249] glomus jugulare,[263–266] the ciliary ganglion,[269] the lungs,[284] the duodenum,[280,281] the middle ear,[264] and the retroperitoneum.[275] Olson and Abell[275] found the highest incidence of metastases in retroperitoneal chemodectomas (35 percent); next in order was the vagal body (20 percent) (Table 10–13). In all other sites, the incidence of

**TABLE 10–13. CLINICOPATHOLOGIC COMPARISON OF CHEMODECTOMAS (NONCHROMAFFIN PARAGANGLIOMAS) ARISING IN VARIOUS SITES**

| Anatomic Site | No. Cases | Average Age | No. Patients with Metastases | No. Patients with Metastases (%) |
|---|---|---|---|---|
| Carotid body[302] | 500 | 41 | 32 | 6 |
| Glomus jugulare[303] | 316 | 49 | 6 | 2 |
| Vagal Body[267] | 20 | 44 | 4 | 20 |
| Mediastinum[272,304] | 20 | 40 | — | — |
| Lung[284,305] | 25 | 68 | — | — |
| Duodenum[281] | 9 | 52 | — | — |
| Retroperitoneum[275] | 23 | 33 | 8 | 35 |

distant metastases was negligible. Experience shows that, of all the malignant chemodectomas (paragangliomas), the retroperitoneal variety is the most lethal.[275] Our experience is limited to two male patients, and both succumbed within three years of excision of the primary.

## Treatment

The treatment of choice for all chemodectomas is excision.[262,263,292,293] In certain instances, because of the location and extension of the tumor, adequate excision is difficult. In such cases, partial excision might be attempted, since these are extremely slow-growing tumors. Radical excision should be considered in treating malignant chemodectomas, whenever possible. Excision should include the carotid vessels with replacement by a prosthesis.

## REFERENCES

1. Pack GT, Ariel I: Tumors of the Soft Somatic Tissues. New York, Hoeber-Harper, 1958
2. Russell DS, Rubinstein LJ: Pathology of Tumors of the Nervous System, 3rd ed. Baltimore, Williams & Wilkins, 1971
3. Harkin JC, Reed RJ: Tumors of the peripheral nervous system. In Atlas of Tumor Pathology. Sect. 2, Fasc 3. Washington DC, AFIP, 1969
4. Das Gupta TK, Brasfield RD, Strong EW, Hajdu SI: Benign solitary schwannomas (neurilemomas). Cancer 24:355, 1969
5. Putney FJ, Moran JJ, Thomas GK: Neurogenic tumors of the head and neck. Trans Am Laryngol Rhin Otol Soc, p 465, 1964
6. Rosenfeld L, Graves H Jr.: Primary neurogenic tumors of the lateral neck. Ann Surg 167:847, 1968
7. Oberman HA, Sullenger G: Neurogenous tumors of the head and neck. Cancer 20:1994, 1967
8. Robitaille Y, Seemayer TA, El Deiry A: Peripheral nerve tumors involving paranasal sinuses: A case report and review of the literature. Cancer 35:1254, 1975
9. Das Gupta TK, Brasfield RD: Tumors of peripheral nerve origin: Benign and malignant solitary schwannomas. CA 20:229, 1970
10. Holland GW: Neurilemoma of the vagus nerve in the neck. Aust N Z J Surg 38:146, 1968
11. Pesavento G, Ferlito A, Recher G: Benign solitary schwannoma of the cervical vagus nerve: A case report with a review of the literature. J Laryngol Otol 93:307, 1979
12. Oberman HA, Abell MR: Neurogenous neoplasms of the mediastinum. Cancer 13:882, 1960
13. Ackerman LV, Taylor EF: Neurogenous tumours within the thorax: A clinicopathological evaluation of forty-eight cases. Cancer 13:669, 1959
14. Sarot IA, Schwinner D, Schechter DC: Primary neurilemmoma of diaphragm. NY State J Med 69:837, 1969
15. Gore DO, Rankow R, Hanford JM: Parapharyngeal neurilemoma. Surg Gynecol Obstet 103:193, 1956
16. Dragh LV, Soule EH, Masson JK: Benign and malignant neurilemomas of the head and neck. Surg Gynecol Obstet 111:211, 1960
17. Lane N, Murray MR, Fraser GC: Neurilemoma of the lung confirmed by tissue culture. Report of a case. Cancer 6:780, 1953
18. Collins R, Gan G: Neurilemoma presenting as a lump in the breast. Br J Surg 60:242, 1973
19. Hart MS, Bason WC: Neurilemoma involving bone. J Bone Joint Surg 49A:465, 1958
20. Fawcet JK, Dahlin DC: Neurilemoma of bone. Am J Clin Pathol 47:759, 1967
21. Ashley DJB: Tumours of the nerve sheath. In Ashley DJB (ed): Evans' Histological Appearance of Tumors, 3rd ed. Edinburgh, London, Churchill Livingstone, 1978
22. Cutler EC, Gross RE: Neurofibroma and neurofibrosarcoma of peripheral nerves unassociated with von Recklinghausen's disease. Arch Surg 33:733, 1936
23. Harkin JC, Reed RJ: Tumors of the peripheral nervous system. In Atlas of Tumor Pathology. Sect. 2, Fasc. 3, Washington, DC, Armed Forces Institute of Pathology, 1969
24. Woodruff JM, Marshall ML, Erlandson RA, et al.: Cellular schwannoma: A variety of schwannoma sometimes mistaken for a malignant tumor. Am J Surg Pathol 5:733, 1981
25. Fletcher CDM, Davies SE, McKee PH: Cellular schwannoma: A distinct pseudosarcomatous entity. Histopathology 11:21, 1987
26. White W, Shiu MH, Rosenblum MK, et al.: Cellular schwannoma: A clinicopathologic study of 57 patients and 58 tumors. Cancer 66:1266, 1990
27. Miller WG: A malignant melanotic tumor of ganglion cells arising from thoracic sympathetic ganglion. J Pathol Bacteriol 35:351, 1932
28. Fu YS, Kaye GI, Lattes R: Primary malignant melanocytic tumors of the sympathetic ganglia with an ultrastructural study of one. Cancer 36:2029, 1975
29. Carney JA: Psammomatous melanotic schwannoma: A distinctive heritable tumor with special associations including cardiac myxoma and the Cushing syndrome. Am J Surg Pathol 14:206, 1990
30. Carney JA, Hayles AB: Alimentary tract manifestations of multiple endocrine neoplasia type 2b. Mayo Clinic Proc 52:543, 1977
31. Odier L: Mannual de Medicine practique. Geneva, JJ Paschond, 1811
32. Wood W: Observations on neuromas, with cases and histories of the disease. Trans Med Chir Soc Edinburgh 3:68, 1829
33. Huber GC, Lewis D: Amputation neuromas, their development and prevention. Arch Surg 1:85, 1920
34. Cieslak AK, Stout AP: Traumatic and amputation neuromas. Arch Surg 53:646, 1946
35. Farley NH: Painful stump neuroma—Treatment of. Minn Med 48:347, 1965
36. Klintworth GK: Axon regeneration in the human spinal

cord with formation of neuromata. J Neuropathol Exp Neurol 23:123, 1964

37. Tulenko JF: Cicatricial neuromas following neck dissection. Plast Reconst Surg 35:419, 1965

38. Gillesby WJ, Wu KH: Amputation neuromas of vagus nerves. Am J Surg 110:673, 1965

39. Swanson HH: Traumatic neuromas. A review of the literature. Oral Surg 14:317, 1961

40. Das Gupta TK, Brasfield RD: Amputation neuroma in cancer patients. NY State J Med 69:2129, 1969

41. Borberg A: Clinical and genetic investigation into tuberous sclerosis and Recklinghausen's neurofibromatosis: Contribution to elucidation of interrelationship and eugenics of the syndromes. Acta Psychiatr Neurol (Suppl) 71:11, 1951

42. Crowe FW, Schull WJ, Neel JV: A clinical, pathological, and genetic study of multiple neurofibromatosis. Springfield, Ill., Thomas, 1956

43. Thannhauser SJ: Neurofibromatosis (von Recklinghausen's) and osteitis fibrosa cystica localistata et disseminate (von Recklinghausen's). Medicine 23:105, 1944

44. Prieser SA, Davenport CB: Multiple neurofibromatosis (von Recklinghausen's disease) and its inheritance. Am J Med Sci 156:507, 1918

45. Brasfield RD, Das Gupta TK: von Recklinghausen's disease: A clinicopathological study. Ann Surg 175:86, 1972

46. Wander JV, Das Gupta TK: Neurofibromatosis. In: Current Problems in Surgery, vol. 14, no. 2. Chicago, Year Book Medical Publishers, 1977

47. Fisher GA: Recklinghausenshe krankheit und huttermaeler. Dermatol Wchnshr 84:89, 1927

48. Sergeyev AS: On mutation rate of neurofibromatosis. Hum Genet 28:129, 1975

49. National Institutes of Health Consensus Development Conference Statement, vol. 6, July 13–15, 1987

50. Virchow R: Uber die reform der Pathologischen und therapeutischen anschanngen durch die microskopischen untersuchungen. Virchows Arch [B] 1:207, 1847

51. Hitchcock A: Some remarks on neuroma, with brief account of three cases of anomalous cutaneous tumors in one family. Am J Med Sci 43:320, 1862

52. Thomson A: On Neuroma and Neurofibromatosis. Edinburgh, Turnbull & Spear, 1900

53. Adrian C: Uber Neurofibromatose und ihre Komplikationen. Beitr Klin Chir 31:1, 1901

54. Vinken PJ, Bruyn GW: The Phakomatoses. In Vinken PJ, Bruyn GW, eds. Handbook of Clinical Neurology, vol. 14. New York, Elsevier, 1972

55. Barker D, Wright E, Nguyen L, et al.: Gene for von Recklinghausen's neurofibromatosis is in the pericentromeric region of chromosome 17. Science 236:1100, 1987

56. Gutmann DH, Collins FS: Recent progress toward understanding the molecular biology of von Recklinghausen's neurofibromatosis. Ann Neurol 31:555, 1992

57. Feinman NL, Yakovac WC: Neurofibromatosis in childhood. J Pediatr 76:339, 1970

58. Crowe FW: Axillary freckling as a diagnostic aid in neurofibromatosis. Ann Intern Med 61:1142, 1964

59. Pack GT, Davis J: Nevus giganticus pigmentosus with malignant transformation. Surgery 49:347, 1961

60. McNeer GP: Treatment of melanoma (panel discussion) in "The Pigment Cell"—Molecular, Biological and Clinical Aspects. Ann NY Acad Sci 100:166, 1963

61. von Recklinghausen FD: Ein herz von einem neugebornen welches mehrere theirs nach aussen, theils nach den hohlen prominierende tumoren (Myomen) turg. Verh Ges Geburtsch 15, 1863

62. River L, Silverstein J, Topel JW: Collective review. Benign neoplasms of the small intestine. Int Abstr Surg 102:1, 1956

63. Ghrist TD: Gastrointestinal involvement in neurofibromatosis. Arch Intern Med 112:357, 1962

64. Hochberg FH, DaSilva AB, Goldabine J, Richardson EP Jr.: Gastrointestinal involvement in von Recklinghausen's neurofibromatosis. Neurology 24:1144, 1974

65. Rappaport HM: Neurofibromatosis of the oral cavity. Oral Surg 6:559, 1946

66. Baden E, Pierce HE, Jackson WF: Multiple neurofibromatosis with oral lesions. Oral Surg 8:263, 1955

67. Preston FW, Walsh WS, Clarke TH: Cutaneous neurofibromatosis (von Recklinghausen's disease): Clinical manifestations and incidence of sarcoma in 61 male patients. Arch Surg 64:813, 1952

68. Chen AU, Miller AS: Neurofibroma and schwannoma of the oral cavity: A clinical and ultrastructural study. Oral Surg 4:522, 1979

69. Smith RW: A Treatise on the Pathology. Diagnosis and Treatment of Neuroma. Dublin, Hodges & Smith, 1849

70. Prescott GH, White RE: Solitary central neurofibroma of the mandible: Report of a case and review of the literature. J Oral Surg 28:305, 1970

71. Logan PJ: Visceral neurofibromatosis. Br J Surg 31:3060, 1964

72. Sturdy DE: Neurofibroma of the esophagus. Br J Surg 54:315, 1967

73. Raszkowski HJ, Hufner RF: Neurofibromatosis of the colon: An unique manifestation of von Recklinghausen's disease. Cancer 27:34, 1971

74. Gerhardt G: Zur diagnostk multiple neurobildung. Dtsch Arch Klin Med 21:268, 1878

75. Kass IH: Neurofibromatosis of the bladder. Am J Dis Child 44:1040, 1932

76. Pessin JL, Bodian M: Neurofibromatosis of the pelvic autonomic plexuses. Br J Urol 36:510, 1964

77. Ross JA: A case of sarcoma of the urinary bladder in von Recklinghausen's disease. Br J Urol 29:121, 1957

78. Ravich A: Neurofibroma of the ureter: Report of a case with operation and recovery. Arch Surg 30:442, 1935

79. Hunt JC, Pugh DG: Skeletal lesions in neurofibromatosis. Radiology 76:1, 1961

80. Heard GE, Payne EE: Scalloping of vertebral bodies in von Recklinghausen's disease of the nervous system (neurofibromatosis). Neurol Surg Psychiatr 25:345, 1962

81. Rodriguez HA, Berthong M: Multiple primary intracranial tumors in von Recklinghausen's neurofibromatosis. Arch Neurol 14:467, 1966

82. Henschen F: Zur histologic unit Pathogense der Kleinhimbrichen winkletumoven. Arch Psychiatr Nervekr 56: 21, 1916

83. Gardner WJ, Frazier GH: Bilateral acoustic neurofibromas: A clinical study and field survey of a family of five generations with bilateral deafness in 28 members. Arch Neurol Psychiatr 23:266, 1930

84. Olivecrona H: Acoustic tumors. J Neurosurg 26:6, 1967

85. Hope DG, Mulvihill JJ: Malignancy in neurofibromatosis. In Riccardi VM, Mulvihill JJ (eds): Advances in Neurology, vol. 19. Neurofibromatosis (von Recklinghausen's Disease). New York, Raven Press, 1981, p 39

86. Rubinstein LJ: Tumors of the central nervous system. In Atlas of Tumor Pathology. Fasc. 6. Washington DC, AFIP, 1972

87. David M, Hecaen J, Bonis A, cited by Wertheimer P, et al.: Reflexions sur la Coexistence de neurinomes multiples, de miningiomes et de gliomes encephaliques dans la maladie nerveusede Recklinghausen: A propos deckitoneuromes. Neurochirugie 3:145, 1957

88. Poser CN: The Relationship between Syringomyelia and Neoplasm. Springfield, Ill, Thomas, 1956

89. Strong EW, McDivitt RW, Brasfield RD: Granular cell myoblastoma. Cancer 25:415, 1970

90. Vance SF III, Hudson RP Jr.: Granular cell myoblastoma: Clinicopathologic study of forty-two patients. Am J Clin Pathol 52:208, 1969

91. Horn RC Jr., Stout AP: Granular cell myoblastoma. Surg Gynecol Obstet 76:315, 1943

92. Moscovic EA, Azar HA: Multiple granular cell tumors ("myoblastomas"). Cancer 20:2032, 1967

93. Papageorgiou S, Litt JZ, Pomeranz JR: Multiple granular cell myoblastomas in children. Arch Dermatol 96:168, 1967

94. Powell EB: Granular cell myoblastoma. Arch Pathol 42:517, 1946

95. Kirschner H: Uber einen Fall von maligne entartetem Myoblastenmyon der Mamma. Bruns Beitr Klin Chir 204:87, 1962

96. Hagen JO, Soule EH, Gores JF: Granular cell myoblastoma of the oral cavity. Oral Surg 14:454, 1961

97. Rafel SS: Granular cell myoblastoma. Oral Surg 15:192, 1962

98. Gray SH, Gruenfeld GE: Myoblastoma. Am J Cancer 30:699, 1937

99. Friedman RM, Hurwitt ES: Granular cell myoblastoma of the breast. Am J Surg 112:75, 1966

100. Pope TA: Laryngeal myoblastoma. Arch Otolaryngol 81:80, 1965

101. Nussbaum M, Haselkom A: Granular cell myoblastoma in parotid gland. NY State J Med 72:2887, 1972

102. De Gouveici OF, Pereira AA, Netto BM, et al.: Granular cell myoblastoma of the esophagus. Gastroenterology 54:805, 1960

103. Keshishian JM, Alford TC: Granular cell myoblastoma of the esophagus. Am Surg 30:263, 1964

104. Archer FL, Harrison RW, Moulder PV: Granular cell myoblastoma of the trachea and carina treated by resection and reconstruction. J Thorac Cardiovasc Surg 45: 539, 1963

105. Rojer CL: Multicentric endobronchial myoblastoma. Arch Otolaryngol 82:652, 1965

106. Weitzner S, Oser JF: Granular cell myoblastoma of bronchus. Am Rev Respir Dis 97:923, 1968

107. Goldman ML, Gottlieg LS, Zamchek N: Granular cell myoblastoma of the stomach and colon. Am J Dig Dis 7:432, 1962

108. Schwartz DT, Gaetz HP: Multiple granular cell myoblastomas of the stomach. Am J Clin Pathol 44:453, 1965

109. Winne BE, Bacon HE: Myoblastoma of the anal canal. Dis Colon Rectum 4:206, 1961

110. Wellmann KF, Tsai CY, Reyes FB: Granular cell myoblastoma in pancreas. NY State J Med 78:1270, 1975

111. LiVolsi VA, Perzin KH, Badder EM, et al.: Granular cell tumor of the bilary tract. Arch Pathol 95:13, 1973

112. Reul GH, Rubio PA, Berkman NL: Granular cell myoblastoma of the cystic duct. A case associated with hydrops of the gall bladder. Am J Surg 129:583, 1975

113. Ravich A, Stout AP, Ravich RA: Malignant granular cell myoblastoma involving the urinary bladder. Ann Surg 121:361, 1945

114. Svesko VS: Granular cell myoblastoma of the vulva. Am J Obstet Gynecol 87:143, 1963

115. Wolfe DS, Mackles A: Uncommon myogenic tumors of the female genital tract. Obstet Gynecol 22:199, 1963

116. Doyle WF, Hutchinson JR: Granular cell myoblastoma of the clitoris. Am J Obstet Gynecol 100:589, 1968

117. Stout AP, Lattes R: Tumors of the soft tissues. In Atlas of Tumor Pathology. Sect. 2, Fasc 3, Washington DC, AFIP, 1967

118. Hunter DT Jr., Dewar JP: Malignant granular cell myoblastoma: Report of a case and review of the literature. Am Surg 26:554, 1960

119. Ross RC, Miller TR, Foote FW Jr.: Malignant granular cell myoblastoma. Cancer 5:112, 1952

120. Gamboa LG: Malignant granular cell myoblastoma. Arch Pathol 60:663, 1955

121. Cadotte M: Malignant granular cell myoblastoma. Cancer 33:1417, 1974

122. Powell EB: Granular cell myoblastoma. Arch Pathol 42:517, 1946

123. Ravich A, Stout AP, Ravich RA: Malignant granular cell myoblastoma involving the urinary bladder. Ann Surg 121:361, 1945

124. Dunnington JH: Granular cell myoblastoma of the orbit. Arch Ophthalmol 40:1422, 1948

125. Ceelen W: Uber die Natur der sog. Myoblastome (zugleich ein Bericht uber eine maligne Myoblastengeschwulst). Zentralbl Allg Pathol 85:289, 1949

126. Schwidde JT, Meyers R, Sweeney DB: Intracerebral metastatic granular cell myoblastoma. J Neuropathol Exp Neurol 10:303, 1951

127. Crawford ES, De Bakey ME: Granular cell myoblastoma: Two unusual cases. Cancer 6:786, 1953

128. Svejda J, Horn V: Disseminated granular cell pseudotumor, so-called metastasizing granular cell myoblastoma. J Pathol Bacteriol 75:343, 1958

129. Busanny-Caspari W, Hammer CH: Zur Malignitat der sogenanntem Myoblastenmyome. Zantralbl Allg Pathol 98:401, 1958

130. Caby F, Duperrat B, Eoochard JC: Un cas de tumeur

dabrikoffof a evolution maligne. Mem Acad Chir 86: 585, 1960

131. Obiditsch-Mayer I, Salzer-Kuntschik M: Malignant granular cell neuroma, so-called "myoblastoma" of the esophagus. Beitr Pathol Anat 125:357, 1961

132. Krieg AF: Malignant granular cell myoblastoma: Case report. Arch Pathol 74:251, 1962

133. Nitze von H: Das sogenannte Myoblastenmyom und weine maligne Verlaufsform. Z Laryngol Rhinol Otol 45:740, 1966

134. Mackenzie DH: Malignant granular cell myoblastoma. J Clin Pathol 20:739, 1967

135. McCabe MM, Harman JW: Malignant myoblastoma: A case report. J Irish Med Assoc 62:284, 1969

136. Al-Sarraf M, Loud AV, Vaitkevicius VM: Malignant granular cell tumor. Arch Pathol 91:550, 1971

137. Kuchemann von K: Malignes granulates Neurom (Granularzell-myoblastom) Fallbericht und Literaturubersicht. Zentralbl Allg Pathol 114:426, 1971

138. D'Agostino AN, Soule EH, Miller RH: Sarcomas of peripheral nerves and somatic tissues associated with multiple neurofibromatosis (von Recklinghausen's disease). Cancer 16:1015, 1963

139. D'Agostino AN, Soule EH, Miller RH: Primary malignant neoplasms of nerves (malignant neurilemomas) in patients without manifestations of multiple neurofibromatosis (von Recklinghausen's disease). Cancer 16:1003, 1963

140. Das Gupta TK, Brasfield RD: Solitary malignant schwannoma. Ann Surg 171:419, 1970

141. Ghosh BC, Ghosh L, Huvos AG, Fortner JG: Malignant schwannoma: A clinicopathologic study. Cancer 31:184, 1973

142. Hammond HL, Calderwood RG: Malignant peripheral nerve sheath tumors of the oral cavity. Oral Surg Oral Med Oral Pathol 28:97, 1969

143. McNeer GP, Cartin J, Chu F, Nickson J: Effectiveness of radiation therapy in the management of sarcoma of the soft somatic tissues. Cancer 22:391, 1968

144. Suit HD, Russel WO, Martin RG: Sarcoma of soft tissues: Clinical and histopathological parameters and response to treatment. Cancer 35:1478, 1973

145. Lindberg RD, Martin RD, Romsdahl MM, Barkley HT: Conservative surgery and postoperative radiotherapy in 300 adults with soft tissue sarcomas. Cancer 47:2391, 1981

146. Guccion JG, Enzinger FM: Malignant schwannoma associated with von Recklinghausen's neurofibromatosis. Virchow's Arch [A] 383:43, 1979

147. Heard G: Nerve sheath tumors and von Recklinghausen's disease of the nervous system. Ann R Coll Surg 31:229, 1962

148. Perkinson NG: Melanoma arising in a café-au-lait spot of neurofibromatosis. Am J Surg 93:1018, 1957

149. Masson P, Martin JF: Rhabdomyomes des niefs. Bull Cancer 27:751, 1938

150. Ducatman BS, Scheitthauer BW: Malignant peripheral nerve sheath tumors with divergent differentiation. Cancer 54:1049, 1984

151. Woodruff JM, Chernik NL, Smith MC, et al.: Peripheral nerve tumors with rhabdomyosarcomatous differentiation (malignant triton tumors). Cancer 32:426, 1973

152. Brooks JS, Freeman M, Enterline HT: Malignant triton tumors: Natural history and immunohistochemistry of nine new cases with literature review. Cancer 55:2543, 1985

153. Weston JA: The migration and differentiation of neural crest cells. Adv Morphogen 8:41, 1970

154. Enzinger FM: Clear cell sarcoma of tendons and aponeuroses—An analysis of 21 cases. Cancer 18:1163, 1965

155. Bearman RM, Noe J, Kempson R: Clear cell sarcoma with melanin pigment. Cancer 36:977, 1975

156. Boudreaux D, Waisman J: Clear cell sarcoma with melanogenesis. Cancer 41:1387, 1978

157. Mackenzie DH: Clear-cell sarcoma of tendon and aponeuroses with melanin production. J Pathol 114:231, 1974

158. Tsuneyoshi M, Enjoji M, Kubo T: Clear cell sarcoma of tendon and aponeuroses: A comparative study of 13 cases with a provisional subgrouping into the melanotic and synovial types. Cancer 42(1):243, 1978

159. Bridge JA, Sreekantaiah C, Neff JR, et al.: Cytogenetic findings in clear cell sarcoma of tendons and aponeurosis: Malignant melanoma of soft parts. Cancer Genet Cytogenet 52:101, 1991

160. Chung EB, Enzinger FM: Malignant melanoma of soft parts: A reassessment of clear cell sarcoma. Am J Surg Pathol 7:405, 1983

161. Stout AP: Ganglioneuromata of the sympathetic nervous system. Surg Gynecol Obstet 84:101, 1947

162. Knudson AG Jr., Amromin GD: Neuroblastoma and ganglioneuroma in a child with multiple neurofibromatosis: Implications for the mutational origin of neuroblastoma. Cancer 19:1032, 1966

163. Smith J: A case of adrenal neuroblastoma. Lancet 2:1214, 1932

164. Bolande RP, Towler WF: A possible relationship in neuroblastoma to von Recklinghausen's disease. Cancer 26:162, 1970

165. Stowens D: Neuroblastoma and related tumors. Arch Pathol (Berlin) 63:451, 1957

166. Weller RO, Cervos-Navarro J: Pathology of Peripheral Nerves. London, Butterworth, 1977

167. Dargeon MW: Tumors of Childhood. New York, Hoeber-Harper, 1960

168. Ashley DJB: Tumors of chromaffin tissue. In Ashley DJB (ed.): Evans' Histological Appearance of Tumors, 3rd ed. Edinburgh, Churchill Livingstone, 1978

169. Carpenter WB, Kernohan JW: Retroperitoneal ganglioneuromas and neurofibromas: A clinical pathological study. Cancer 16:788, 1963

170. Hauer GT, Andrews WD: The surgery of mediastinal tumors. Am J Surg 50:146, 1940

171. Hamilton JP, Koop CE: Ganglioneuromas in children. Surg Gynecol Obstet 121:803, 1965

172. Mendelsohn G, Eggleston JC, Olson JL, et al.: Vasoactive intestinal peptide and its relationship to ganglion cell differentiation in neuroblastic tumors. Lab Invest 41:44, 1979

173. Nagashima F, Hayashi J, Araki Y, et al.: Silent mixed ganglioneuroma/pheochromocytoma which produces a vasoactive intestinal polypeptide. Intern Med 32:63, 1993

174. Trump DL, Livingston JN, Baylin SB: Watery diarrhea syndrome in an adult with ganglioneuroma-pheochromocytoma. Cancer 40:1526, 1977

175. Iverson LL: The catecholamines. Nature 214:8, 1967

176. Wurtman RJ: Catecholamines. N Engl J Med 273:637, 1965

177. Paton DM (ed): The Mechanism of Neuronal and Extraneuronal Transport of Catecholamines. New York, Raven Press, 1976

178. Polashko H: Specific action of L-Dopadecarboxylase. J Physiol 96:50, 1939

179. Pearse AGE: The APUD Concept: Embryology, cytochemistry, and ultrastructure of the diffuse neuroendocrine system. In Friesen SR (ed): Surgical Endocrinology. Philadelphia, J.B. Lippincott, 1978

180. Page LB, Jacoby GA: Catecholamine metabolism and storage granules in pheochromocytoma and neuroblastoma. Medicine 43:379, 1964

181. Page LB, Coopeland RB: Pheochromocytoma. Dis Mon, pp. 1–40 January 1968

182. Thomas JE, Rooke ED, Kvale WF: The neurologist's experience with pheochromocytoma. JAMA 197:754, 1966

183. Reynolds JL, Gilchrist TF: Congenital heart disease and pheochromocytoma. Am J Dis Child 112:251, 1966

184. Calkins E, Howard JE: Bilateral familial pheochromocytoma with paroxysmal hypertension: Successful surgical removal of tumors in two cases, with discussion of certain diagnostic procedures and physiological considerations. J Clin Endocrinol 7:475, 1947

185. O'Brien D: Pheochromocytoma with endocrinopathy. N Engl J Med 268:1365, 1963

186. Gifford RW, Kvale WF, Maher FT, et al.: Clinical features, diagnosis, and treatment of pheochromocytoma: A review of 76 cases. Mayo Clin Proc 39:281, 1964

187. Maier HC: Intrathoracic pheochromocytoma with hypertension. Ann Surg 130:1059, 1949

188. Samaan HA: Risk of operation in a patient with unsuspected pheochromocytoma. Br J Surg 57:462, 1970

189. El-Minawa MF, Paulino E, Cuesto M, Ceballos J: Pheochromocytoma masquerading as preeclamptic toxemia. Am J Obstet Gynecol 109:389, 1971

190. Engleman K: A new test for pheochromocytoma. JAMA 189:107, 1964

191. Gitlow SE, Mendlowitz M, Bertani LM: The biochemical techniques for detecting and establishing the presence of pheochromocytoma. Am J Cardiol 26:270, 1970

192. Stackpole RH, Myer NM, Uson AC: Pheochromocytoma in children. J Pediatr 63:315, 1963

193. Nourok DS: Familial pheochromocytoma and thyroid carcinoma. Ann Intern Med 60:1028, 1964

194. Schinke RN, Startmen WH: Familial amyloid producing medullary thyroid carcinoma and pheochromocytoma. Ann Intern Med 63:1027, 1965

195. Suzuki S: Ueber zwei tumoren aus nebennier-enmarkgewebe. Berl Klin Wschr 47:1623, 1910

196. MacKeith R: Adrenal-sympathetic syndrome: Chromaffin tissue tumor with paroxysmal hypertension. Br Heart J 6:1, 1944

197. Davis FW Jr., Hull JG, Vardell JC Jr.: Pheochromocytoma with neurofibromatosis. Am J Med 8:131, 1950

198. Lynch JD, Sheps SG, Bematz PE, et al.: Neurofibromatosis and hypertension. Minn Med 55:25, 1972

199. Tilford DL, Kelsch RC: Renal artery stenosis in childhood neurofibromatosis. Am J Dis Child 126:665, 1973

200. Glushien PS, Mansuy MM, Littman DS: Pheochromocytoma: Its relationship to the neurocutaneous syndromes. Am J Med 14:318, 1953

201. Modlin IM, Famdon JR, Shepherd A, et al.: Pheochromocytomas in 72 patients: Clinical and diagnostic features, treatment and long-term results. Br J Surg 66:456, 1979

202. Sipple JH: The association of pheochromocytoma with carcinoma of the thyroid gland. Am J Med 31:163, 1961

203. Kairi MRA, Dexter RN, Burznyski NJ, Johston CC: Mucosal neuroma, pheochromocytoma, and medullary thyroid carcinoma: Multiple endocrine neoplasia. Type 3. Medicine 54:89, 1975

204. Harrison TS, Thompson NW: Multiple endocrine adenomatosis, I and II. In Ravitch MM, et al. (eds): Current Problems in Surgery. Chicago, Year Book Medical Publishers, 1975, pp 1–51

205. Pearse AGE, Polak JM: Cytochemical evidence for the neural crest origin of mammalian ultimobranchial cells. Histochemistry 27:96, 1971

206. Higgins PM, Tresidder GC: Pheochromocytoma of the urinary bladder. Br Med J 2:274, 1966

207. deLorimier AA, Bragg KJ, Linden G: Neuroblastoma in childhood. Am J Dis Child 118:441, 1969

208. Bill AH, Hartmann JR, Beckwith JB: The unique biology of childhood tumors with special reference to the biology of neuroblastoma. Pacific Med Surg 75:281, 1967

209. Beckwith JB, Martin RF: In situ neuroblastomas: A contribution to the natural history of neural crest tumors. Am J Pathol 43:1089, 1963

210. Miller RW, Fraumeni JF Jr., Hill JA: Neuroblastoma: Epidemiologic approach to its origins. J Pediatr Surg 3:141, 1968

211. Vinik M, Altman DH: Congenital malignant tumors. Cancer 19:967, 1966

212. Wells HG: Occurrence and significance of congenital malignant neoplasms. Arch Pathol 30:535, 1940

213. Simpson TE, Lynn HB, Mills SD: Congenital neuroblastoma in the scrotum. Clin Pediatr 8:174, 1969

214. Reynolds CP, Seeger RC, Vo DD, et al.: Model system for removing neuroblastoma cells from bone marrow monoclonal antibodies and magnetic immunobeads. Cancer Res 46:5882, 1986

215. Priebe CJ, Clatworthy HWJ: Neuroblastoma: Evaluation of treatment of ninety children. Arch Surg 95:538, 1967

216. Bodian M: Neuroblastoma. Pediatr Clin North Am 6:449, 1959

217. Gross RE, Farber S, Martin LW: Neuroblastoma sympathicum. A study and report of 217 cases. Pediatrics 23:951, 1959

218. Fortner J, Nicastri A, Murphy ML: Neuroblastoma: Nat-

ural history and results of treating 133 cases. Ann Surg 167:132, 1968

219.. Haase GM, O'Leary MC, Stram DO, et al.: Pelvic neuroblastoma—Implications for a new favorable subgroup: A Children's Cancer Group experience. Ann Surg Oncol 2:516, 1995

220. Hinterberger H, Bartholomew EJ: Catecholamines and their acidic metabolites in urine and in tumor tissue in neuroblastoma, ganglioneuroma, and pheochromocytoma. Clin Chim Acta 23:169, 1969

221. Voorhess ML: The catecholamines in tumor and urine from patients with neuroblastoma, ganglioneuroblastoma, and pheochromocytoma. J Pediatr Surg 3:147, 1968

222. LaBrosse EH: 3-methoxy-4-hydroxyphanylglycol in neuroblastoma. J Pediatr Surg 3:148, 1968

223. Gitlow S, Bertani LM, Rausen A, et al.: Diagnosis of neuroblastoma by qualitative and quantitative determination of catecholamine metabolites in urine. Cancer 25: 1377, 1970

224. Lopez-Ibop B, Schwartz AD: Neuroblastoma. Pediatr Clin North Am 32:755, 1985

225. Maurer HM: Current concepts in cancer: Solid tumors in children. N Engl J Med 299:1345, 1978

226. Evans AE, Albo V, Bangio GJ, et al.: Factors influencing survival of childhood neuroblastoma. Cancer 38:661, 1976

227. Swaen GJV, Sloof JL, Stoelinga GRA: A differentiating neuroblastoma. J Pathol Bacteriol 90:333, 1965

228. Beckurth JB, Martin RF: Observations on the histopathology of neuroblastoma. J Pediatr Surg 3:106, 1968

229. Evans AE, D'Angio GJ, Randolph J: A proposed staging system for children with neuroblastoma. Cancer 27:374, 1971

230. Lauder I, Aherne W: The significance of lymphocytic infiltration in neuroblastoma. Br J Cancer 26:321, 1972

231. Evans AE, Angio GJ, Propert K, et al.: Prognostic factors in neuroblastoma. Cancer 59:1853, 1987

232. Brodeur GM, Azar C, Brother M, et al.: Neuroblastoma: Effect of genetic factors on prognosis and treatment. Cancer 70:1685, 1992

233. Brodeur GM, Green AA, Hayes FA: Cytogenetic studies of primary human neuroblastoma. In: Evans AE (ed.) Advances in Neuroblastoma Research. New York, Raven, 1980

234. Favrot MC, Combaret V, Goillot E, et al.: Expression of integrin receptors in 45 clinical neuroblastoma specimens. Int J Cancer 49:347, 1991

235. Knudson AG Jr., Meadows AT: Regression of neuroblastoma IV-S: A genetic hypothesis. N Engl J Med 302:1254, 1980

236. Seeger RC, Brodeur GM, Sather H: Association of multiple copies of the N-myc oncogene with rapid progression of neuroblastoma. N Engl J Med 313:111, 1985

237. Dyke PC, Mulkcy DA: Maturation of ganglioneuroblastoma to ganglioneuroma. Cancer 20:1343, 1967

238. Cushing H, Wolback SB: The transformation of a malignant paravertebral sympathicoblastoma into a benign ganglioneuroma. Am J Pathol 3:62, 1927

239. Fox F, Davidson J, Thomas LB: Maturation of sympathicoblastoma into ganglioneuroma. Cancer 12:108, 1959

240. Kissane JM, Ackerman LV: Maturation of tumours of sympathetic nervous system. J Fac Radiol (London) 7: 109, 1955

241. Stewart FW: Experiences in spontaneous regression of neoplastic disease in man. Tex Rep Biol Med 10:239, 1952

242. Visfeldt J: Transformation of sympathicoblastoma into ganglioneuroma. Acta Pathol Microbiol Scand 58:44, 1963

243. Chatten JE, Voorhees ML: Familial neuroblastoma. Report of a kindred with multiple disorders. N Engl J Med 277:1230, 1967

244. Berger L, Richard L: L'esthesioneuroepithelioma olfactif. Bull Cancer 13:410, 1924

245. Kahn LB: Esthesioneuroblastoma: A light and electron microscopic study. Hum Pathol 5:364, 1974

246. Hutter RVP, Lewis JS, Foote FW Jr., Tollefsen HR: Esthesioneuroblastoma: A clinical and pathological study. Am J Surg 106, 1963

247. Skolnick EM, Massari FS, Tenta LT: Olfactory neuroepithelioma: Review of the world literature and presentation of 2 cases. Arch Otolaryngol 84:644, 1966

248. Castro L, de la Paya S, Webster JH: Esthesioneuroblastoma: A report of seven cases. Am J Roentgenol 105:7, 1969

249. Sellwood RA, Wapnick S, Breckenridge A, et al.: Recurrent pheochromocytoma. Br J Surg 57:309, 1970

250. Campbell CB, Mortimer RH: A functioning malignant phaeochromocytoma occurring in a patient with neurofibromatosis. Aust Ann Med 17:331, 1968

251. Angervall I, Enzinger FM: Extraskeletal neoplasm resembling Ewing's sarcoma. Cancer 36:240, 1975

252. Jaffe R, Santamaria M, Yunis EJ, et al.: The neuroectodermal tumor of bone. Am J Surg Pathol 8:885, 1984

253. Cavazzana AO, Miser JS, Jefferson J, et al.: Experimental evidence for a neural origin of Ewing's sarcoma of bone. Am J Pathol 127:507, 1987

254. Shimada H, Newton WA Jr., Soule EH, et al.: Pathologic features of extraosseous Ewing's sarcoma: A report from the intergroup rhabdomyosarcoma study. Hum Pathol 19:442, 1988

255. Dehner LP: Primitive neuroectodermal tumor and Ewing's sarcoma. Am J Surg Pathol 17:1, 1993

256. Dahlin DC: Ewing's sarcoma and malignant lymphoma (reticulum cell sarcoma) of bone. In Dahlin DC (ed.) Tumors of Bone and Soft Tissue. Chicago, Year Book Medical Publishers, 1965, p 179

257. Rosen G, Wollner N, Tan C, et al.: Disease-free survival in children with Ewing's sarcoma treated with radiation therapy and adjuvant four-drug sequential chemotherapy. Cancer 33:384, 1974

258. Soule EH, Newton W, Moor TE, Teffi M: Extraskeletal Ewing's sarcoma. A preliminary review of 26 cases encountered in the Intergroup Rhabdomyosarcoma Study. Cancer 42:259, 1978

259. Schmidt D, Herrmann C, Jurgens H, et al.: Malignant peripheral neuroectodermal tumor and its necessary distinction from Ewing's sarcoma: A report from the Kiel Pediatric Tumor Registry. Cancer 68:2251, 1991

260. Krupski WC, Effeney DJ, Ehrenfeld WK, Stoney RJ: Cervical chemodectoma: Technical considerations and management options. Am J Surg 144:215 1982

261. Shamblin WR, ReMine WH, Sheps SG, Harrison EG: Carotid body tumor (chemodectoma). Clinicopathological analysis of ninety cases. Am J Surg 122:732, 1971

262. Faff HW: Carotid body tumors: A thirty-year experience at Memorial Hospital. Am J Surg 114:614, 1967

263. Brown JS: Glomus jugulare tumors. Methods and difficulties of diagnosis and surgical treatment. Laryngoscope 77:26, 1967

264. Lattes R, Waltner JG: Nonchromaffin paraganglioma of the middle ear (carotid body-like tumor; glomus-jugulare tumor). Cancer 2:447, 1949

265. Levit SA, Sheps SG, Espinosa RE, et al.: Catecholamine-secreting paraganglioma of glomus-jugulare region resembling pheochromocytoma. N Engl J Med 281:805, 1969

266. Duke WW, Roshell BR, Soteres P, et al.: A norepinephrine-secreting glomus jugulare tumor presenting as a pheochromocytoma. Ann Intern Med 60:1040, 1964

267. Burman SO: The vagal body tumor. Ann Surg 141:488, 1955

268. Johnson WS, Beaher OH, Harrison EG: Chemodectoma of the glomus intravagale (vagal-body tumor). Am J Surg 104:812, 1962

269. Byme JJ: Carotid body and allied tumors. Am J Surg 95:351, 1958

270. Fisher ER, Hazard JB: Nonchromaffin paraganglioma of the orbit. Cancer 5:521, 1952

271. Sixnons JN, Beahrs OH, Woolmer LB: Chemodectoma of an aortic body. Am J Surg 117:363, 1969

272. Smithers DW, Gowing NFC: Chemodectomas in the region of the aortic arch. Thorax 20:182, 1965

273. Olson JD, Salyer WR: Mediastinal paragangliomas (aortic body tumors). Cancer 41:2405, 1978

274. Mapp EM, Krouse TB, Fox EF, Voci G: Chemodectoma of the anterior mediastinum. Report of a case of probable aortic body origin with arteriographic findings. Radiology 92:547, 1969

275. Olson JR, Abell MR: Nonfunctional nonchromaffin paragangliomas of the retroperitoneum. Cancer 23:1358, 1969

276. Shimazaki M, Ueda G, Kurimoto H, et al.: Retroperitoneal nonchromaffin paraganglioma with hormonal activity. Acta Pathol Jpn 15:145, 1965

277. Johnson RWP, Somerville PG: A malignant soft-tissue paraganglioma of the leg. Br J Surg 44:605, 1957

278. Carey JP, Bradley RL: Chemodectoma: A review with two new cases. Arch Surg 87:897, 1963

279. Horoupian DS, Kerson LA, Saiontz H, Valsamis M: Paraganglioma of cauda equina: Clinicopathologic and ultrastructural studies of an unusual case. Cancer 33:1337, 1974

280. Lukash WM, Hyams VJ, Nielsen OF: Neurogenic neoplasms of the small bowel: Benign non-chromaffin paraganglioma of the duodenum: Report of a case. Am J Dig Dis 11:575, 1966

281. Taylor HB, Helwig EB: Bengin nonchromaffin paragangliomas of the duodenum. Arch Pathol Anat 335, 1962

282. Smith WT, Hughes B, Ermocilla R: Chemodectoma of the pineal region, with observations on the pineal body and chemoreceptor tissue. J Pathol Bacteriol 92:69, 1966

283. Korn D, Bensch K, Liebow AA, Castleman B: Multiple minute pulmonary tumors resembling chemodectomas. Am J Pathol 37:641, 1960

284. Fawcett EJ, Husband FM: Chemodectoma of lung. J Clin Pathol 20:260, 1967

285. Ichinose H, Hewitt RL, Drapana T: Acute pulmonary chemodectoma. Cancer 28:692, 1971

286. Brown JB, Freyer MP: Carotid body tumors: Report of removal of tumor thought to be largest recorded. Surgery 32:997, 1952

287. Pryse-Davies J, Dawson IMP, Westbury G: Some morphologic, histochemical, and chemical observations on chemodectomas and the normal carotid body, including a study of the chromaffin reaction and possible ganglion cell elements. Cancer 17:185, 1964

288. Glenner GG, Crout JR, Robers WC: A functional carotid body-like tumor secreting levarterenol. Arch Pathol 73:230, 1962

289. Hamberger B, Ritzen M, Wersafl J: Demonstration of catecholamines and 5-hydroxytryptamine in the human carotid body. J Pharmacol Exp Ther 152:1966

290. Berdal P, Braaten M, Cappelan C Jr., et al.: Non-adrenaline-adrenaline producing nonchromaffin paraganglioma. Acta Med Scand 172:249, 1962

291. Duke WW, Bashell BR, Soters P, Carr JH: A norepinephrine-secreting glomus jugulare tumor presenting as a pheochromocytoma. Ann Intern Med 60:1040, 1964

292. Salyer KE, Ketchum LD, Robinson DW, Masters PW: Surgical management of cervical paragangliomata. Arch Surg 98:572, 1969

293. Frey CF, Karoll RP: Management of chemodectomas. Am J Surg 111:536, 1966

294. Hamberger CA, Hamberger CB, Wersal J, et al.: Malignant catecholamine-producing tumor of the carotid body. Acta Pathol Microbiol Scand 69:439, 1967

295. Cohen SM, Persky L: Malignant non-chromaffin paraganglioma with metastasis to the kidney. J Urol 96:122, 1966

296. Tu H, Bottomley RH: Malignant chemodectoma presenting as a military pulmonary infiltrate. Cancer 33:248, 1974

297. Coulson WF: A metastasizing carotid body tumor. J Bone Joint Surg 52A:752, 1969

298. Pendergrass EP, Kirsch D: Roentgen manifestations in the skull of metastatic carotid body tumor (paraganglioma) of meningioma and of mucocoele—A report of three unusual cases. Am J Roentgenol 57:417, 1947

299. Romanski R: Chemodectoma (nonchromaffin paraganglioma) of the carotid body with distant metastases. Am J Pathol 30:1, 1954

300. Rangwala AF, Sylvia LG, Becker SM: Soft tissue metastasis of a chemodectoma. A case report and review of the literature. Cancer 42:2865, 1978

301. Say CC, Hori J, Spratt J Jr.: Chemodectoma with distant metastases. Case report and review of literature. Am Surg 39:333, 1973

302. Staats EF, Brown RL, Smith RR: Carotid body tumor: Benign and malignant. Laryngoscope 76:907, 1966

303. Alford BR, Guilford FR: A comprehensive study of the tumors of the glomus jugulare. Laryngoscope 72:765, 1962

304. Patcher MR: Mediastinal nonchromaffin paragranuloma. J Thorac Cardiovasc Surg 45:152, 1963

305. Zak FG, Chaber A: Pulmonary chemodectomatosis. JAMA 813:887, 1963

# 11

# Tumors of the Synovial Tissue

## ■ BENIGN TUMORS AND TUMORLIKE CONDITIONS OF THE SYNOVIAL TISSUE

### GIANT CELL TUMOR OF THE TENDON SHEATH

Giant cell tumor of the tendon sheath is the most common benign tumor and is frequently encountered in the small joints of the extremities. Occasionally, these tumors are also referred to as *synovioma* (Fig. 11–1). Most commonly, they are found in women in their forties. They occur predominantly in the hands and feet, especially the digits, on both the flexor and extensor aspects of the tendon sheaths (Fig. 11–2A and 11–2B). These tumors may produce pressure erosion in the underlying bones; such an x-ray finding should not be taken as a sign of malignant transformation. There may be associated lipodystrophies, and, although various theories regarding etiology have been postulated,[1] none has yet been confirmed.

These tumors tend to grow as nodular overgrowths, and their size is frequently determined by their location. Those of the fingers usually remain small and nodular, varying in size from 1 to 2 cm, whereas those occurring more proximally may grow as large as 6 to 7 cm. In the fingers, the expanding tumor sometimes ruptures the tendon sheath and extends subcutaneously. Rarely do these tumors infiltrate the overlying skin.

Benign giant cell tumors of the tendon sheath are treated by conservative excision, although there is a possibility of recurrence. Pack and Ariel[1] found that the recurrence rate reported in the literature varied from 7 to 44 percent. More recently, Schwartz et al.[2] reported the recurrence rate to be 25 percent. A meticulous dissection of the primary lesion reduces the incidence of local recurrence. Radical excision of the surrounding tendons or curettage of the underlying bone should be avoided. Amputation certainly cannot be justified.

### VILLONODULAR SYNOVITIS (TENOSYNOVIAL GIANT CELL TUMORS OR PIGMENTED VILLONODULAR BURSITIS)

Villonodular synovitis is frequently seen in and around the flexor tendons of the fingers, wrist, and toes (Fig. 11–3), and sometimes around the weight-bearing joints. In rare instances, this tumor is found completely outside any joint.[3,4] It usually occurs in middle-aged persons of both sexes, but instances have been reported in children.[5] Bobechko and associates[5] reported pigmented villonodular synovitis in three children with cavernous hemangioma of the knee joint. Usually, it is painless, although in some cases pain may be the presenting clinical feature. In general, the tumors are small and take the shape of the tendon over the joint around which they occur. Compared to localized giant cell tumor, this form is rather rare. The most common site for this disease is the knee, followed by the ankle and wrist. Treatment of these cystlike swellings consists of excision. Prior to excision, the extent of the tumor

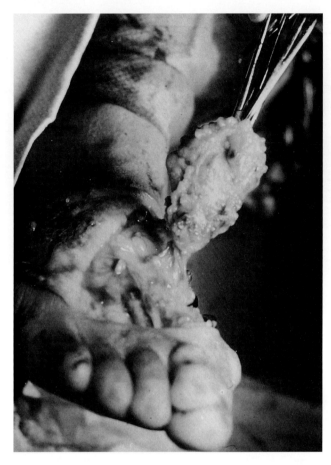

**Figure 11–1.** Synovioma of the dorsum of the foot in a 36-year-old man. The lesion was asymptomatic but was excised for cosmetic reasons. This lesion was incorrectly diagnosed as a neurofibroma in 1978.

and the presence or absence of any associated systemic disease and local degenerative arthritic problems should be assessed.[6]

## GANGLION

Ganglions are cystic swellings in and around joint cavities and are not true neoplasms. The incidence is unknown, since most of them are not reported either by the physician or by the patient. Ganglions occur most frequently in the dorsum of the wrist (Fig. 11–4), arising from the tendon sheaths of the extensor tendons. Other sites of origin are the palmar aspect of the wrist, fingers, ankle, dorsum of the foot, and, occasionally, the popliteal region. This is usually a disease occurring in adults and is seldom encountered in children.[1,7]

A ganglion forms a smooth round or ovoid mass over the affected joint. The cystic consistency and mobility along the course of the tendon sheath makes clinical diagnosis relatively simple. These benign cystic

lesions usually do not necessitate any active therapy. If, however, these lesions are large and produce cosmetic problems, they should be dissected from the tendon sheaths. Most local recurrences following excision are the result of inadequate excision through a small incision.

## ■ MALIGNANT TUMORS OF THE SYNOVIAL TISSUE

### SYNOVIAL SARCOMA (MALIGNANT SYNOVIOMA)

Sarcomas arising from synovial membrane were described in unillustrated communications by Hardie and Salter,[8] Marsh,[9] and Lockwood,[10] but the tumor was first adequately described in 1910 by Lejars and Rubens-Duvall.[11] However, the term *synovioma* was first coined by Smith in 1927[12] and *synovial sarcoma* by Knox in 1936.[13] Some authors still use different nomenclature to designate the same entity as *tenosynovial sarcoma*.[14] By 1965, Cadman, Soule, and Kelly[15] estimated that a total of 519 cases existed in the literature. In 1966, Mackenzie[16] reported an additional 58 cases, bringing the total to 577. Rissanen and Holsti[17] added 13 cases in 1970. Van Andel,[18] reviewing the literature on treated cases, accepted a total of 450 and added 28 of his own. Gerner and Moore[19] found 34 cases in the files of Roswell Park Memorial Institute in 1975. Several other cases have also been documented.[20–34] Currently, synovial sarcoma incidence is estimated to comprise 5 to 6 percent of all sarcomas.[35,36] Although this type of sarcoma is relatively rare, enough data have been generated, making it possible to define the natural history and develop general guidelines regarding its management.

### Sex, Age, and Race

There is no predilection for either sex, although some authors have found a slight preponderance in males. Of the 93 patients in our current series, 48 were men and 45 were women.

Synovial sarcoma is essentially a disease of young adults. Pack and Ariel[1,23] found that 60 percent of their patients were between the ages of 15 and 40 years. In our series of 93 patients, the youngest was 14 years old and the oldest 79, the average age being 39 years.

### Anatomic Location

Pack and Ariel[1] reported that synovial sarcoma occurs most frequently in the extremities. Most authors,[15–19,22,23,29–34,37,38] including us, have found that these tumors indeed occur predominantly in the extremities, especially near large joints (e.g., knee, elbow, etc.). However, Cadman et al.[15] observed that only rarely is an obvious relationship found between the

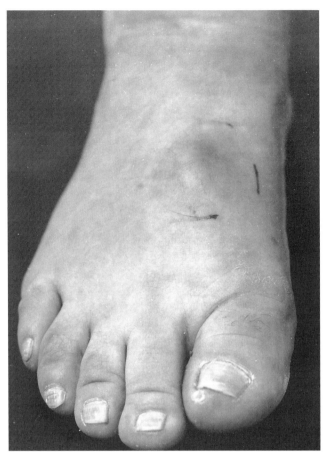

**A**

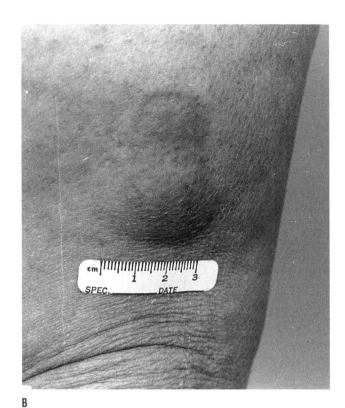

**B**

**Figure 11–2. (A)** Giant cell tumor in the dorsum of the foot. The lesion was deceptive, extending much further than could be seen or palpated. **(B)** Giant cell tumor of the tendon sheath around the knee joint.

tumor and the synovial membrane. Instances of the tumor arising in the neck and trunk are also on record.[25–31] Table 11–1 shows the anatomic distribution in our series of cases, along with that in five other series.

Synovial sarcoma is encountered frequently in and around the knee joint: 48 percent in our series, and 49.5 percent in the series reported by Enzinger and Weiss.[39] In the remainder of cases in the lower extremities, the tumors seem to have no specific anatomic

**TABLE 11–1. ANATOMIC LOCATIONS OF SYNOVIAL SARCOMAS IN SIX SERIES**

| Anatomic Site | Haagensen and Stout[31] (1944) | Pack and Ariel[1] (1958) | Cadman et al.[15] (1965) | Mackenzie[16] (1966) | Enzinger and Weiss[39] (1995) | Present Series (1996) |
|---|---|---|---|---|---|---|
| Head and neck | — | — | 1 | — | 31 | 8 |
| Trunk | — | 2 | 6 | — | 28 | 5 |
| Upper extremities | 22 | 24 | 32 | 22 | 80 | 30 |
| Lower extremities | 82 | 34 | 95 | 36 | 206 | 50 |
| Unknown | — | — | — | 1 | — | — |
| Total cases | 104 | 60 | 134 | 59 | 345 | 93 |

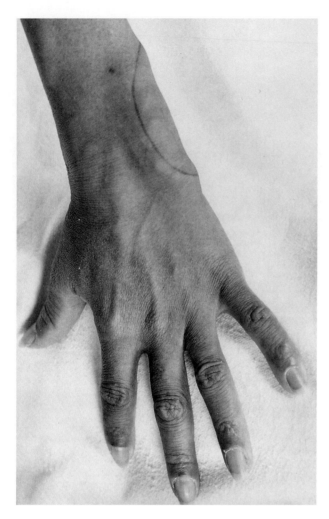

**Figure 11–3.** Villonodular synovitis in the wrist of a 51-year-old woman.

predilection (Fig. 11–5A and 11–5B). In the upper extremities, most cases occur in the wrist and hands. In our series, 60 percent occurred below the elbow (Fig. 11–5C). The synovial sarcomas that arise in the tendons and bursae adjacent to the articular surfaces of a joint seldom involve the articular surfaces.

Synovial sarcomas rarely occur in the head and neck region (Table 11–1). In the series reported from the Armed Forces Institute of Pathology (AFIP)[39] 9 percent of the cases were encountered in the head and neck region, and in our current study, only 8 percent were found in the head and neck region. Because of this rarity, several authors have published case reports.[25–28] Golomb et al.,[26] in 1975, reported one case and found an additional 15 in the literature. Recently, Enzinger and Weiss[39] reported that, in the files of the AFIP, they came across seven cases in the pharynx and seven in the larynx; previously, Shmookler et al.[40] pointed out that these tumors can also be found in the face and oral cavity.

In support of the hypothesis that synovial cell sarcoma most likely arises from undifferentiated mesenchymal tissue rather than from synovial tissue, numerous cases of these tumors in unusual anatomic locations have been reported. Synovial cell sarcoma has also been reported in the esophagus.[41] Zeren et al.[42] from the AFIP reported 25 cases of primary synovial cell sarcoma arising from the lung. Most of these lesions were monophasic synovial cell sarcoma. Again, the sex and age distribution were quite similar to reported series of synovial cell sarcoma in other locations. Most patients presented with chest pain, cough, shortness of breath, and hemoptysis. Tumor size varied from less than 1 cm in size to more than 20 cm in diameter, with

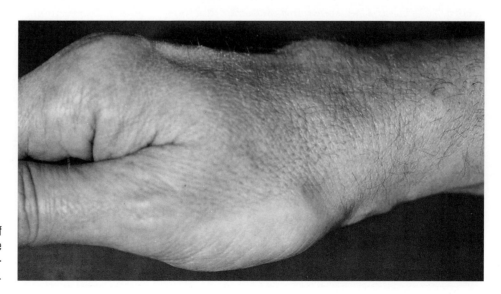

**Figure 11–4.** Ganglion of the dorsum of the wrist. This was excised only because the patient complained of various symptoms associated with this cystic swelling.

areas of hemorrhage and necrosis. Out of these 25 cases, four patients were found to be alive and well without evidence of recurrence or metastasis after 2 to 20 years follow-up.[42]

There have been reported cases of synovial cell sarcoma arising from the heart. The evaluation of these lesions showed the typical translocation of chromosomes that is usually noted in cases of synovial cell sarcoma.[43,44] Tak et al.[45] also reported another case of synovial cell sarcoma of the right ventricle. LeMarc'hadour[46] reported mediastinal synovial cell sarcoma with typical translocation of the chromosome that this tumor is noted for.

The anterior abdominal wall is an uncommon site for synovial cell sarcoma, but several authors have reported synovial cell sarcoma involving the anterior abdominal wall. In 1980, Katenkamp reported a case of synovial cell sarcoma of the abdominal wall in a 56-year-old female patient. This tumor has a characteristic biphasic appearance and electron microscopic appearance of synovial cell sarcoma.[47] Al-Dewachi et al.[48] also reported synovial cell sarcoma of the anterior abdominal wall in a 50-year-old female patient. Reviewing the English literature up to 1978, he also reported eight other cases of synovial cell sarcoma involving the anterior abdominal wall. These lesions in the abdominal wall tend to occur more frequently in females, in contrast to synovial tumors in the extremity and neck which have no specific sex predilection.

Later, in 1993, Fetsch and Meis[49] from the AFIP reported a relatively large series of 27 patients with synovial cell sarcoma of the anterior abdominal wall, and they reviewed the clinical features and prognosis in this group of patients. There were 12 male and 15 female patients, ranging from 8 to 58 years of age. Fifty percent of the patients were younger than 23 years. These tumors were either biphasic or monophasic, and in some cases poorly differentiated. Seventeen of the 27 patients had tumors greater than 5 cm in size. Follow-up was available in 18 cases, and nine patients were alive and well in the period from 1 to 264 months of follow-up. Nine patients died with the disease, with a median follow-up of 26 months. We have treated one abdominal wall biphasic synovial cell sarcoma in a 15-year-old female patient. She received postoperative radiation therapy and has remained well for three years. Patients with tumors greater than 5 cm had a higher mortality rate, and patients with poorly differentiated tumors had 100 percent mortality rate in this group.

Helliwell et al.[50] reported a case of a 46-year-old man with polyarthralgia and mass in the ileal mesentery, which subsequently was found to be a biphasic synovial cell sarcoma with characteristic chromo-somal translocation t(X;18). Interestingly, though this patient had anemia and polyarthralgia, after resection of the tumor, the polyarthralgia resolved. Shmookler[51] reported four cases of retroperitoneal synovial cell sarcoma, and all four patients had the typical biphasic pattern. In a short follow-up, two of these four patients died from metastatic disease as a result of peritoneal sarcomatosis. Adam et al.,[52] among a group of 12 retroperitoneal sarcoma patients, reported one case of synovial cell sarcoma. Later, Miyashita et al.[53] reported a case of primary retroperitoneal synovial sarcoma with monophasic pattern. They also compiled a list of 16 other reported cases in the literature and found that 1 out of the 16 cases survived more than five years.

Sarcomas of the vagina are extremely rare in adult patients. However, Schiffman and Chong[54] reported a case of an adult female who was seen with history of vaginal bleeding, and subsequent workup showed the lesion to be a synovial cell sarcoma.

## Clinical Features

Most patients with a synovial sarcoma present with a slow-growing, painless mass. Pack and Ariel[1] reported that 58 percent of their patients had this initial symptom. In our series of 93 patients, 60 percent were initially seen with a painless mass. Although pain is not usually associated with synovial cell sarcoma,[55,56] about 9 percent of our patients stated that a dull, aching pain preceded the appearance of a mass. Because of the mistaken notion that the pain is usually associated with an arthritic or other degenerative disease, the diagnosis of sarcoma frequently is missed for several months, particularly in older patients. One of our patients, a 74-year-old man, had had pain around the left knee joint and the popliteal space for more than nine months before being referred to our clinic. He had been treated only with analgesics, and a slow-growing swelling in the popliteal space was missed. After the tumor became large enough to cause concern to the family, an aggressive diagnostic approach was undertaken.

Roentgenographic examination of the affected area might provide a clue to the diagnosis of synovial sarcoma. In a substantial number of instances, the roentgenogram of a soft tissue mass appears as a rounded, lobulated swelling of moderate density. Destruction of an underlying bone and/or joint is quite unusual, but periosteal reaction of an adjacent bone is not uncommon. In about 15 to 20 percent of the cases, multiple areas of focal calcification and occasionally bone formation are observed in soft tissue roentgenograms.[57,58] These findings, along with computed tomography scan and magnetic resonance images of the affected area, provide an indication as to the presumed diagnosis and extent of the disease,[59] but the only way that an accurate diagnosis can be made is by microscopic examination of the specimen.

## Regional Metastases

Synovial sarcomas have some tendency to metastasize to the regional nodes. In our series, the incidence was 12 percent. Pack and Ariel[1] reported a 16 percent incidence in their series, and Haagensen and Stout[31] reported an 11 percent incidence. Gerner and Moore[19] found about a 12 percent incidence. Weingrad and Rosenberg[60] found no instance of node metastases in their analysis of five cases from the files of the National Cancer Institute, but reported an overall incidence of 17 percent in a total of 535 published cases. The published incidence (Table 11–2) is difficult to interpret and even more difficult to apply in developing therapeutic guidelines. The true incidence of regional node metastases in stage I tumors is hard to define, but for high-grade tumors (grades 3 and 4), we recommend regional node dissection along with resection of the primary. In locally advanced cases, the incidence is usually much higher, and treatment should incorporate the regional node-bearing area.

## Treatment

The treatment of primary synovial sarcoma is wide soft tissue excision (Chapter 16). Synovial sarcomas are also sensitive to radiotherapy. Infrequently, amputation of an extremity is indicated. However, according to our present multimodal treatment protocol,[61] there has seldom been a need to amputate an extremity. For synovial sarcomas located elsewhere in the body, we perform a wide excision of the primary tumor with adjuvant radiation therapy. The question of adjuvant chemotherapy still remains unclarified. If the regional node-bearing area is near the primary site, it should be included in the therapeutic planning. If the primary tumor is larger than 5 cm and is pleomorphic, then a

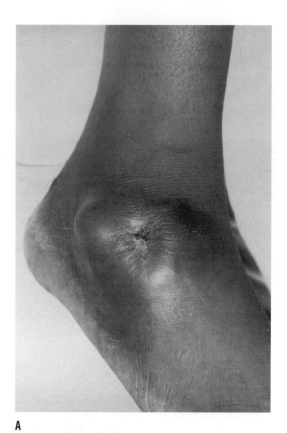

**A**

**Figure 11–5. (A)** Synovial sarcoma around the ankle joint in a 44-year-old man. The patient underwent a below-the-knee amputation and regional node dissection. One of 18 nodes contained a metastatic tumor. *(Continued.)*

regional node dissection is advocated, irrespective of its distance from the tumor.

## End Results

Of the 93 patients in our series, 31 were treated by operation alone. The 62 remaining patients received postoperative radiation therapy for control of the primary tumor; of these, 18 were treated by our multimodal limb salvage protocol. Of the 93 patients, 75 are eligible for five-year survival analysis: 55 (73 percent) remained disease-free, and, of the 60 eligible for 10-year analysis, 51 have lived for 10 years or more. Our results appear somewhat better than the currently reported end results for mostly adult patients.[62–67]

In the past, the overall five-year survival rate in synovial sarcoma was described as poor by most authors.[1,15,16,19–23,30,32] However, with meticulous staging and consistent therapy protocols, the end results have improved,[62–64] and our data of 73 percent five-year survival and 85 percent 10-year survival certainly substantiate this observation.

Varela-Duran and Enzinger[65] recently described a group of patients with synovial sarcoma in whom the

## TABLE 11–2. COMPARATIVE INCIDENCE OF REGIONAL NODE METASTASES IN SYNOVIAL SARCOMA

| Author(s) | Year of Publication | Total No. Cases Reported | No. Cases with Nodal Metastases |
|---|---|---|---|
| Haagensen and Stout[31] | 1944 | 104 | 11 (10.6%) |
| Pack and Ariel[1] | 1958 | 60 | 10 (16.7%) |
| Cadman et al.[15] | 1965 | 17 (134)* | 4 (23.5%) |
| Rissanen and Holsti[17] | 1970 | 13 | 0 |
| Gerner and Moore[19] | 1975 | 34 | 4 (11.8%) |
| Roth et al.[25] | 1975 | 8 (24)† | 1 (4.2 %) |
| Present Series | 1996 | 93 | 11 (11.8%) |

*Only 17 of 134 cases had node dissection.
†All 24 cases were in the neck; only 8 had neck dissection.

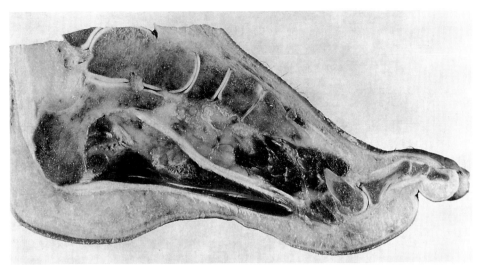

B

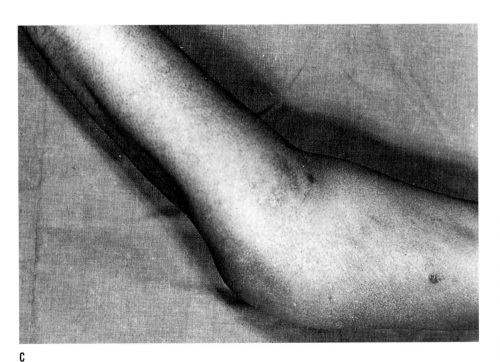

C

**Figure 11–5** *(continued).* **(B)** Sagittal view of the bisected specimen of synovial sarcoma of the left foot. The tumor has extended to several compartments. *(Courtesy of Drs. R. M. Barone and S. Saltzstein, San Diego, CA)* **(C)** Synovial sarcoma in the ulnar aspect below the elbow. Patient was treated with wide soft tissue resection and postoperative radiation therapy, and has been disease-free for nine years.

primary tumor showed extensive calcification. Analysis of the histologic criteria and the natural history of 32 calcifying synovial sarcomas from the files of the AFIP led these authors to conclude that, in this subset of patients, the prognosis is better than with the most common variety of synovial sarcomas. Of the 26 patients with follow-up information (average 8.9 years), 17 were alive and well and 6 died of disease. The five-year disease-free survival rate was 82.6 percent.

Data on the treatment of synovial sarcoma by means of curative radiation therapy alone are sparse,

and no definitive statement as to its efficacy can yet be made.[1,15,19,22,23,30,32] Roth et al.,[25] reviewing 24 cases in the files of the AFIP, found that four patients received either preoperative or postoperative radiation therapy. Of these, only one was living without evidence of disease after two years. McNeer et al.[38] found that two of five patients (40 percent) treated by radiation therapy alone survived for five years and that the addition of postoperative irradiation was useful in 47 percent of the cases, whereas preoperative radiation therapy was unsatisfactory. The data on the role of radiation therapy found in the literature up to 1970 usually consisted of retrospective analyses of clinical material; in most of these, the technical aspects were not sufficiently sophisticated, and the conclusions should be viewed with caution. Shiu and colleagues,[66] after a planned use of modern technology, obtained a 66 percent two-year salvage rate after local excision and radical radiation therapy. Lindberg et al.[37] obtained absolute two- and five-year salvages of 75 percent and 58 percent, respectively. This series was further updated in 1994 by Mullin and Zagars,[67] and, out of 85 patients treated mostly with postoperative radiation therapy and a smaller number with preoperative radiation therapy, the 5-, 10-, and 15-year survival rates were 76 percent, 63 percent, and 57 percent, respectively. The local recurrence rate overall was 14 percent in this group of patients. A more detailed discussion on the role of radiation therapy in the management of soft tissue sarcomas will be found in Chapter 17.

Pack and Ariel[1] attempted to develop some prognostic criteria for patients with synovial sarcoma. From their series of 60 patients, they concluded that the overall prognosis is better for younger women with tumors arising in the fingers. Cadman and co-workers[15] found the incidence in fingers to be extremely low in their series of 164 cases. There are no definitive guidelines regarding sex or anatomic location in making a prognosis for synovial sarcoma patients. As with most other patients, if the diagnosis is made when the tumor is small and less pleomorphic, and all the treatment principles outlined above are applied, the prognosis will be improved. However, in recent years, most authors consider better prognostic markers to be young age, distal location, small tumor size, biphasic histopathologic pattern, euploidy, and marked calcification and/or ossification of the primary tumor.

Shiu,[66] of Memorial Sloan-Kettering, reported on the survival of 109 patients with synovial cell sarcoma and found a 70 percent five-year survival among the patients who initially presented without any evidence of previous local recurrence. In the group of patients who were treated following local recurrence, the survival was 61 percent. The local recurrence rate in this group of patients was 18 percent after wide radical resection and 4 percent after amputation. Mullen et al.[67] reported the outcome of 85 patients with a median follow-up of 8.4 years. Their five-year survival was 76 percent, 10-year survival was 63 percent, and 15-year survival was 57 percent. The overall local recurrence in this group of patients was 14 percent at five years, and, in patients who did not have any evidence of metastasis, the local recurrence rate was 9 percent. Tumor size and patient's age were the most important prognostic variables in this group of patients.

In an analysis of 18 patients, Yokoyama et al.[68] also found that tumor size is one of the most important prognostic variables in patients with synovial sarcoma. Similarly, Oda et al.,[69] in analyzing a group of 56 patients, found size of the tumor, grade of the lesion, stage of the lesion, and presence of rhabdoid cells to be prognostic variables. In multivariate analysis, the stage of the tumors was the most important prognostic variable in this report.

Recently, tumor suppressor gene p53 has also been correlated to the outcome in patients with soft tissue sarcoma.[70] In an analysis of 96 patients with all different types of soft tissue sarcoma, Kawai et al.[70] found that 50 percent of synovial cell sarcomas expressed p53 gene. As a whole, the group of patients who overexpress p53 gene have significantly poorer outcome than patients who do not express p53 gene. However, a much larger series of patients is needed to evaluate the independent prognostic influence of p53 (see Chapter 6).

## REFERENCES

1. Pack GT, Ariel IR: Tumors of the Soft Somatic Tissues. New York, Hoeber-Harper, 1958, p 494
2. Schwartz HS, Unii KK, Pritchard DJ: Pigmented villonodular sinuvitis: A retrospective review of affected large joints. Clin Orthop 247:243, 1989
3. Arthaud JB: Pigmented nodular synovitis: Report of 11 lesions in nonarticular locations. Am J Clin Pathol 58:511, 1972
4. Probst FP: Extra-articular pigmented villonodular synovitis affecting bone: The role of angiography as an aid in its differentiation from similar bone-destroying conditions. Radiology 13:436, 1979
5. Bobechko WP, Kostuik JP: Childhood villonodular synovitis. Can J Surg 11:480, 1968
6. Docken WP: Pigmented villonodular synovitis: A review with illustrative case reports. Semin Athritis Rheum 9:1, 1979
7. Stout AP, Lattes R: Tumors of the soft tissues. In Atlas of Tumor Pathology. Washington, DC, AFIP, 1967
8. Hardie J, Salter SC: Primary sarcoma of the knee joint. Lancet 1:1619, 1894
9. Marsh HA: A case of sarcoma of knee joint. Lancet 2:1330, 1898
10. Lockwood CB: A case of sarcoma of synovial membrane of the knee joint. Lancet 2:1398, 1902
11. Lejars F, Rubens-Duvall H: Les Sarcomas primitifs des Synoviales articularies. Rev Chir 41:751, 1910
12. Smith LW: Synoviomata. Am J Pathol 3:355, 1927
13. Knox LC: Synovial sarcoma: Report of three cases. Am J Cancer 28:461, 1936
14. Shiu MH, McCormack PM, Hajdu SI, et al.: Surgical treatment of tenosynovial sarcoma. Cancer 43:889, 1979
15. Cadman NL, Soule EH, Kelly PJ: Synovial sarcoma: An analysis of 134 tumors. Cancer 18:613, 1965

16. Mackenzie DH: Synovial sarcoma: A review of 58 cases. Cancer 19:169, 1966

17. Rissanen PM, Holsti P: Synovial sarcoma and its treatment. Oncology 24:108, 1970

18. Van Andel JG: Synovial sarcoma—A review and analysis of treated cases. Radiol Clin Biol 41:145, 1972

19. Gerner RE, Moore GE: Synovial sarcoma. Ann Surg 181:22, 1975

20. Aurich Von G: Uber mahgne synovialome. Archiv fur Geschwulstforsch 26:156, 1965

21. Wright CJE: Malignant synovioma. J Pathol Bact 64:585, 1952

22. Vincent RG: Malignant synovioma. Ann Surg 152:777, 1960

23. Ariel IM, Pack GT: Synovial sarcoma: Review of 25 cases. N Engl J Med 168:1272, 1963

24. Shiu MH, Castro EB, Hajdu SI, et al.: Surgical treatment of 297 soft tissue sarcomas of the lower extremity. Ann Surg 182:597, 1975

25. Roth JA, Enzinger FM, Tannenbaum M: Synovial sarcoma of the neck: A follow-up study of 24 cases. Cancer 35:1243, 1975

26. Golomb HM, Gorny J, Powell W, et al.: Cervical synovial sarcoma at the bifurcation of the carotid artery. Cancer 35:483, 1975

27. Batsakis JH, Nishiyama RH, Sullinger GD: Synovial sarcomas of the neck. Arch Otolaryngol 85:327, 1967

28. Kurgman ME, Rosin HD, Toker C: Synovial sarcoma of the head and neck. Arch Otolaryngol 98:53, 1973

29. Anderson KJ, Wildermuth O: Synovial sarcoma. In DePalma AE (ed) Clin Orthop, 19:55, 1961

30. Jacobs LA, Weaver AW: Synovial sarcoma of the head and neck. Am J Surg 128:527, 1974

31. Haagensen CD, Stout AP: Synovial sarcoma. Ann Surg 120:826, 1944

32. Kogstad O: Malignant synovioma. Acta Rheum Scand 16:81, 1970

33. Murray JA: Synovial sarcoma. Orthop Clin North Am 8:963, 1977

34. Schiffman R, Chong TW: Vaginal bleeding as a presenting symptom of synovial sarcoma. Cancer 45:2428, 1980

35. Tsuneyoshi M, Yokoyamak K, Enjoji M: Synovial sarcoma: A clinicopathological and ultrastructural study of 42 cases. Acta Pathol Jpn 33:23, 1983

36. Russel WO, Cohen J, Enzinger F, et al.: A clinical and pathological staging system for soft tissue sarcomas. Cancer 40:1562, 1977

37. Lindberg RD, Martin RG, Romsdahl MM, Barkley HT: Conservative surgery and postoperative radiotherapy in 300 adult soft tissue sarcomas. Cancer 47:2397, 1981

38. McNeer GP, Cantin J, Chu F, Nickson J: Effectiveness of radiation therapy in the management of sarcoma of the soft tissues. Cancer 22:391, 1968

39 Enzinger FM, Weiss SW: Synovial sarcoma. In Enzinger FM, Weiss SW (eds): Soft Tissue Tumors, 3rd ed. St Louis, Mosby-Yearbook, 1995, p 759

40. Shmookler BM, Enzinger FM, Brannon RB: Oro-facial synovial sarcoma: A clinicopathologic study of 11 new cases and review of the literature. Cancer 50:269, 1982

41. Perch SJ, Sofen EM, Whittington R, Brooks JJ: Esophageal sarcomas. J Surg Oncol 48(3):194, 1991

42. Zeren H, Moran CA, Suster S, et al.: Primary pulmonary sarcomas with features of monophasic synovial sarcoma: A clinicopathological, immunohistochemical, and ultrastructural study of 25 cases. Human Pathol 26(5):474, 1995

43. Karn CM, Socinski MA, Fletcher JA, et al.: Cardiac synovial sarcoma with translocation (X;18) associated with asbestos exposure. Cancer 73(1):74, 1994

44. LeMarc'hadour F, Peoc'h M, Pasquier B, Leroux D: Cardiac synovial sarcoma with translocation (X;18) associated with asbestos exposure. Cancer 74(3):986, 1994

45. Tak T, Goel S, Chandrasoma P, et al.: Synovial sarcoma of the right ventricle. Am Heart J 121(Pt 1):933, 1991

46. LeMarc'hadour F, Pasquier B, Leroux D, Jacrot M: Mediastinal synovial sarcoma with translocation (X;18). Cancer Genet Cytogenet 55(2):265, 1991

47. Katenkamp D, Stiller D: Synovial sarcoma of the abdominal wall. Light microscopic, histochemical and electron microscopic investigations. Virchows Archiv 388(3):349, 1980

48. Al-Dewachi HS, Sangal BC, Zakaria MA: Synovial sarcoma of the abdominal wall: A case report and study of its fine structure. J Surg Oncol 18(4):335, 1981

49. Fetsch JF, Meis JM: Synovial sarcoma of the abdominal wall. Cancer 72(2):469, 1993

50. Helliwell TR, King AP, Raraty M, et al.: Biphasic synovial sarcoma in the small intestinal mesentery. Cancer 75(12):2862, 1995

51. Shmookler BM: Retroperitoneal synovial sarcoma. A report of four cases. Am J Clin Pathol 77(6):686, 1982

52. Adam YG, Oland J, Halevy A, Reif R: Primary retroperitoneal soft-tissue sarcomas. J Surg Oncol 25(1):8, 1984

53. Miyashita T, Imamura T, Ishikawa Y, et al.: Primary retroperitoneal synovial sarcoma. Internal Medicine. 33(11):692, 1994

549. Schiffman R, Chong TW: Vaginal bleeding as a presenting symptom of synovial sarcoma. Cancer 45(9):2428, 1980

55. Kaempffe FA: Neoplasm as a cause of shoulder pain. J Fam Pract 40(5):480, 1995

56. Ichinose H, Wickstrom JK, Hoerner HE, Derbes VL: The early clinical presentation of synovial sarcoma. Clin Orthop 142:185, 1979.

57. Mendez LR, Brien E, Brien WW: Synovial sarcoma: A clinicopathologic study. Orthop Rev 21:465, 1992

58. Wright PH, Sim FH, Soule EH, et al.: Synovial sarcoma. J Bone Joint Surg 64A:112, 1982

59. Morton MJ, Berquist TH, McLeod RA, et al.: MR imaging of synovial sarcoma. Am J Roentgenol 156:337, 1991

60. Weingrad DN, Rosenberg SA: Early lymphatic spread of osteogenic and soft tissue sarcomas. Surgery 84:231, 1978

61. Levine EA, Trippon MJ, Das Gupta TK: Preoperative multimodality treatment for soft tissue sarcomas Cancer 71(11):3685, 1993

62. Goluh R, Vuzevski V, Braco M, et al.: Synovial sarcoma: A clinicopathologic study of 36 cases. J Surg Oncol 45:20, 1990

63. Oda Y, Hashimoto H, Tsuneyoshi M, et al.: Survival in synovial sarcoma: A multivariate study of prognostic factors with special emphasis on the comparison between early death and long-term survival. Am J Surg Pathol 17:35, 1993

64. Soule EH: Synovial Sarcoma. Am J Surg Pathol 10(suppl. 1):78, 1986

65. Varela-Duran J, Enzinger FM: Calcifying synovial sarcoma. Cancer 50:345, 1982

66. Shiu MH, McCormack PM, Hajdu SI, Fortner JG: Surgical treatment of tendosynovial sarcoma. Cancer 43(3):889, 1979

67. Mullen JR, Zagars GJ: Synovial sarcoma outcome following conservation surgery and radiotherapy. Radiother Oncol 33(1):23, 1994

68. Yokoyama K, Shinohara N, Kondo M, Mashima T: Prognostic factors in synovial sarcoma: A clinicopathologic study of 18 cases. Jpn J Clin Oncol 25(4):131, 1995

69. Oda Y, Hashimoto H, Tsuneyoshi M, Takeshita S: Survival in synovial sarcoma. A multivariate study of prognostic factors with special emphasis on the comparison between early death and long-term survival. Am J Surg Pathol 17(1):35, 1993

70. Kawai A, Noguchi M, Beppu Y, et al.: Nuclear immunoreaction of p53 protein in soft tissue sarcomas. A possible prognostic factor. Cancer 73(10):2499, 1994

# 12

# Tumors of Vascular and Perivascular Tissue

Tumors and tumorlike conditions of the vascular tissue comprise one of the most common groups of neoplasms of the soft somatic tissue. Although, strictly speaking, most hemangiomas are hamartomas rather than tumors, operationally it is reasonable to consider them as tumors. A strict categorization of vascular hamartomas, congenital malformations, and tumors is not always possible; however, a practical classification—useful in clinical management—is provided (Table 12–1).

## ■ HEMANGIOMA

The growth of hemangiomas is, in general, inconsistent. They may remain constant in size or may grow pari passu with the child. The tumor inherits a certain momentum of growth that is usually uncertain but self-limited. Once the patient has achieved full size, the hemangioma generally stops growing, with the exception of the cirsoid or racemose type. The growth of vessels comprising the neoplasm is markedly affected by the element of mechanical pressure of the circulation. Therefore, the rate of growth and the architecture of the tumor depend somewhat on the factor of blood supply to the vessels of the hemangiomas.

The hemangioma is the most common tumor of infancy and childhood.[1] About 75 percent of these tumors are evident at birth, and the greater part of the remainder appear in early infancy. In about one out of five patients, the hemangiomas are multiple, with as many as 25 observed in a single patient. No explanation is available for the preponderance in females, usually in

a ratio of two to one. On occasion, hemangiomas have exhibited a startling acceleration in growth rate during pregnancy and, less frequently, at the onset of menstruation. There is no racial predilection. Hemangiomas can occur in all parts of the body; however, most are found in the skin and subcutaneous tissues, and at least 50 percent are located in the head and neck region. The location of the tumor in certain special regions such as the retro-orbital space, breast, scrotum, and so forth, calls for special consideration of treatment, which will be discussed later. Other hemangiomas, developing primarily in the central nervous system (CNS), tongue, liver, brain, retina, bone, and skeletal muscle, will also be separately reviewed.

### CAPILLARY HEMANGIOMA

Capillary hemangioma is the most common of all hemangiomas and occurs in the skin and mucous membranes. It is congenital, although it may not be recognizable until variable periods after birth. The capillary hemangioma may grow rapidly, ranging in size from the minute De Morgan's spots to the large, flat, port-wine stain. The common type, however, is a circumscribed, sessile, lobulated, and bright red tumor. The lumens of the vessels that comprise this tumor are either empty or contain a few immature-to-degenerate red blood corpuscles.

#### Port-wine Stain (Nevus Venosus; Nevus Flammeus)

The port-wine stain, a pink-to-purplish, flat, and superficial hemangioma, is a congenital defect evident at birth and grows pari passu with the child. The superfi-

**TABLE 12–1. CLASSIFICATION OF VASCULAR AND PERIVASCULAR HAMARTOMAS AND NEOPLASMS**

**Vascular Tissue**

Benign
    Capillary hemangiomas
        Simple
        Port-wine stain
        Spider angioma (nevus araneus, De Morgan's spots)
    Infectious hemangioma—pyogenic granuloma
    Cavernous hemangioma
        Superficial
        Hypertrophic
        Visceral
    Cirsoid or racemose hemangioma—arteriovenous fistula
    Special regional hemangiomas
        Orbit and eye
        Brain
        Tongue
        Gastrointestinal tract
        Liver
        Skeletal muscle
        Bone
    Systemic hemangiomatosis
        Congenital
        Acquired
    Hereditary hemorrhagic telangiectasis (Rendu-Osler-Weber disease)
    Congenital neurocutaneous syndromes associated with angiomatosis
        von Recklinghausen's neurofibromatosis and angiomas of the skin
        Tuberous sclerosis (Bourneville's disease)
        Pringle's disease and regional angiomas
        Encephalofacial angiomatosis (Sturge-Weber syndrome)
        Retinocerebral angiomatosis (von Hippel-Lindau disease)
Malignant
    Angiosarcoma (malignant hemangioendothelioma)
    All forms of Kaposi's sarcoma

**Perivascular Tissue**

Benign
    Glomus tumors
    Hemangiopericytoma
Malignant
    Hemangiopericytoma

cial vessels of the dermis exhibit diffuse telangiectasia, but there are no proliferative masses such as are found with other hemangiomas. The purple patch blanches on pressure. In some cases, as the child grows older, the color darkens rather than fades. Unfortunately, the face is the most common site, and the mucosa of the lip, cheek, and oral cavity may be involved in continuity.

Treatment is disappointing and requires infinite patience and caution. It is important to emphasize to the parents that most port-wine stains disappear with age and that patience is essential. The feeding vessels are not large enough for sclerotherapy. Dermabrasion of the facial port-wine stain provides excellent results. Sometimes tattooing of the stain is recommended. Tattooing, however, is a cosmetic maneuver and should not be indiscriminately used in children. In adults, the technique might be useful in instances where the port-wine stain is persistent and creates an embarrassment for the patient.

### Spider Angioma (Nevus Araneus)

The cutaneous arterial spider is a tiny red angioma that owes its descriptive name to its resemblance to a small red spider. It has been known by several synonyms, namely, spider nevus, vascular spider, spider angioma, spider telangiectasia, stellate hemangioma, nevus araneus, and nevus arachnoideus.

The arterial spider has a central point, bulb, or eminence from which many fine, hairlike, wavy strands radiate for 0.5 to 1.0 cm. The central point, or body, of the lesion may be so small as to be seen only by magnification, or it may be a few millimeters wide, elevated, and palpable. The central point is often surrounded by a circular or star-shaped area of erythema, peripheral to which a contrasting halo may be seen. The fiery red color of the spider nevus is due to two factors: arterial blood and the thinness of the vascular walls. Spider angiomas are commonly located on the face, arms, fingers, upper trunk, and, less frequently, on the lower trunk and legs. Spiders of similar structure have been reported in the mucous membranes of the conjunctiva, tongue, lips, nasal mucosa, and gastrointestinal and genitourinary tracts. A congenital analog may also be found in Rendu-Osler-Weber disease. Spider angiomas seldom occur in hairy skin such as the scalp, axilla, or pubis; in the elderly male, they are sometimes related to underlying hepatic cirrhosis.[2,3] Cutaneous spiders are also encountered in patients with gynecomastia; they do not need any active treatment.

### Pyogenic Granuloma

Pyogenic granuloma is an exuberant proud flesh that consists of multiple new capillaries, usually under the intact dermis or mucous membrane. Although the cause is obscure, it is usually seen after a small penetrating wound. It can arise anywhere in the body and usually is pedunculated. It appears infected and bleeds easily. The term *pyogenic granuloma* is a misnomer, since infection is seldom present. Excision results in cure.

### CAVERNOUS HEMANGIOMA

The blood vessels become much more dilated in cavernous hemangioma than in the capillary type. This physical characteristic is due to an expanding connection between the general circulation and the channels of the fundamental capillary hemangioma, so that the capillaries become distended and form pools or sinuses. These spaces are limited by thin septa and form spherical sacculations or culs-de-sac in which the circulation is sluggish. The efferent vessels are larger than in the capillary hemangioma. These tumors are soft and readily compressible, frequently extending into the subcutaneous tissues and presenting as grotesque-appearing masses. Depending on their vascular connections and location, visceral hemangiomas of the liver and gastrointestinal tract may reach an enormous size and exhibit aggressive growth.

Cavernous hemangiomas of the subcutaneous tissues are frequently encountered in the extremities (Fig. 12–1A to 12–1C). In these anatomic locations, the angiomas may be totally devoid of any cutaneous manifestation. McNeill and Ray[4] found that, of 35 patients with hemangioma of the extremities seen by the orthopedic department at the University of Illinois Hospital, only 12 (34 percent) had associated skin involvement. Most patients seek medical advice because of the painful swelling (Fig. 12–1D). Occasionally, large cavernous hemangiomas result in platelet consumption, due to mechanical trapping of platelets or congestive heart failure (Kasabach-Merritt syndrome).[5] Fortunately, these are rare clinical manifestations. Patients with this type of hematologic manifestation require active intervention; otherwise, these cases of Kasabach-Merritt syndrome might be lethal. Local gigantism is also encountered, but unilateral extremity enlargement in the absence of systemic angiomatosis is rare (Fig. 12–2). In the series reported by McNeill and Ray,[4] 6 of 29 patients had systemic angiomatosis, and all had extremity enlargement; in the remaining 23 patients, swelling and tenderness were the major complaints. Atrophy was noted in 12 patients.

## HYPERTROPHIC HEMANGIOMA

Hypertrophic hemangioma is a solid, noncompressible tumor of variable hue, usually purplish-red (Fig. 12–3). The endothelial cell is the neoplastic unit, and the overgrowth of these endothelial cells tends to obliterate the lumens of the blood vessels. These neoplasms are often locally aggressive and tend to recur after inadequate excision. Although they are of hemangiomatous origin, they are solid tumors and never undergo spontaneous regression. The injection of sclerosing fluids is futile; complete excision is the treatment of choice.

## RACEMOSE HEMANGIOMA (CIRSOID ANEURYSM OR ARTERIOVENOUS HEMANGIOMA)

The arterial racemose hemangioma develops de novo or through transformation of a preexisting quiescent hemangioma, such as the port-wine stain. The essential or distinguishing feature is the size of the arteriovenous fistula, which may gradually become evident or have a surprisingly sudden onset, chiefly in adults. Most cirsoid hemangiomas are located on the face or neck and have close vascular connections with branches of the

carotid artery. The tumor frequently resembles a pulsating mass of earthworms, due to the clinical appearance of the dilated, tortuous, throbbing vessels. As with aneurysms, the constant pulsation of the tumor can erode adjacent bone. It may extend over the scalp, erode the skull, penetrate the cranium, and even communicate with the meningeal vessels. Excision after preliminary ligation of the arterial supply (in severe cases the external carotid artery) may be feasible. If the hemangioma is inoperable, the communicating artery must be ligated before attempting conservative therapy. Although arteriovenous hemangiomas are more common in the head and neck region, sometimes they are also encountered deep in the muscles of the extremities; they frequently resemble sarcomas. Principles of surgical management are essentially the same (i.e., resection and, when indicated, ligation of the vessels in the first stage and, at a later date, excision of the residual tumor).

## Spontaneous Regression of Hemangioma

Spontaneous cure of hemangiomas is possible and follows progressive diminution in the blood supply to the tumor by a stenosis of the afferent vessels, supplemented by progressive fibrous hyperplasia of the stroma. This retrogression of hemangiomas without any treatment is often accelerated at the period of first or second dentition. Although the exact incidence of spontaneous regression is unknown, the frequency is high enough to justify a conservative attitude on the part of both the parents and the pediatrician.

## Treatment of Hemangiomas

Hemangiomas that ultimately require intervention can generally be treated by conservative methods. Although the role of steroids in hemangiomas is unclear, systemic administration of prednisone during the active growth phase of these lesions results in arrest of this process in 90 percent of patients.[6] A recommended therapeutic regimen is 40 mg (for a 15-pound baby) orally every alternate day for eight doses, with gradual tapering during a 60-day or 90-day period. Response to steroids becomes evident within 3 to 21 days. Once the accelerated growth phase is reversed, a plan for future therapy can be developed without any pressure.

Freezing or producing artificial frostbite with cryoprobes is still an effective method of treating superficial hemangiomas. In larger hemangiomas, the appropriate areas are sequentially treated with cryoprobes for 10 to 20 seconds. Several such applications at two-to-three-week intervals are frequently required before the effectiveness of this therapy is appreciated. Goldwin and Rosoff[7] concluded that cryosurgery is most useful in small, circumscribed saccular and superficial cavernous hemangiomas. Our experience is similar to that of

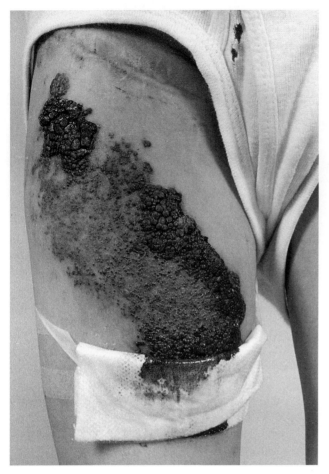

**A**

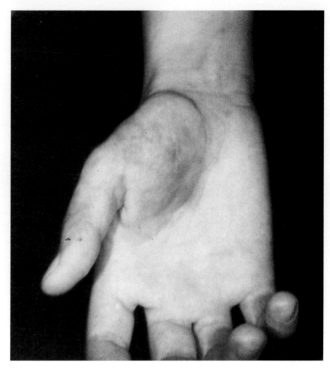

**B**

**Figure 12–1.** **(A)** Superficial spreading cavernous angioma of the right thigh in a five-year-old boy. In certain areas, capillary elements were also present. Apparently, an excision was attempted (see scar in inguinal crease). The lesion was ulcerated and bleeding and was treated by wide excision 14 years ago; the child has grown into a normally functioning young man. **(B)** Cavernous angioma of the thumb and thenar space in an 18-year-old boy. Note pigmentary change spreading through the skin of the thumb. He was treated conservatively with ligation of the feeding vessels and injection of sclerosing fluid with excellent cosmetic and functional end results. *(Continued.)*

Goldwin and Rosoff.[7] For extensive hemangiomas with multiple arteriovenous shunts involving the oral cavity, pharynx, and larynx, cryosurgery is not usually successful.[6] However, before proceeding to any other more radical methods, an attempt with sequential use of cryoprobes is strongly recommended.

The intravascular injection of sclerosing solutions is designed to cause thrombosis of the constituent vessels. This in turn produces sclerosis, atrophy, and absorption of the blood vessels with consequent regression and disappearance of the tumors. The needle must be introduced with great care and blood drawn prior to injection of any sclerosing fluid. The incidence of complications such as embolism are rare and usually not of any significant consideration. Nor is the type of sclerosing agent of any major import. Pack and Miller[2] used

hot water, urethane, and morrhuate sodium with satisfactory results. In large hemangiomas with identifiable efferent vessels, the use of sclerosing fluid has been replaced with intravascular clots or plugs. The role of interventional radiology in managing these vexing problems cannot be overemphasized. In large hemangiomas or in cirsoid aneurysms affecting an extremity or the head and neck region, a combination of ligation of the feeding vessels with clotting is useful (Fig. 12–4).

Many hemangiomas of the skin and subcutaneous tissues are so well encapsulated and redundant that excision is the quickest and simplest method of treatment (Fig. 12–5). The fine linear scar is less conspicuous than the appearance of flat white skin that follows more conservative procedures. The exposure and double ligature of the entering vessels is easily accom-

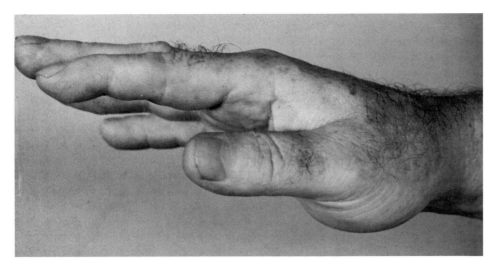

C

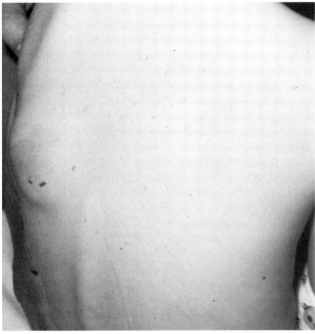

D

**Figure 12–1** *(continued).* **(C)** Cavernous hemangioma of the thenar space extending to the remainder of the palm in a 44-year-old man. The hemangioma was tender and interfered with his livelihood (auto mechanic). However, extensive excision would have resulted in a nonfunctional hand. He has been treated by sequential excision and coagulation with cryotherapy. Although all the hemangioma has not been eradicated, he has a symptomless, functional, and cosmetically acceptable hand. **(D)** Cavernous angioma of the trunk in a five-year-old boy. The child complained of pain and tenderness. The lesion was excised, with cure.

The end results of treatment of hemangiomas are usually excellent. Their effective control frequently requires prolonged periods of treatment, taxing the patience of the clinician, the patient, and the family. Before treatment is initiated, it is advisable to have a conference with all parties concerned regarding the protracted nature of the disease and the chronicity of the management program. The judicious, unhurried use of one method, or a combination of the methods outlined above, will result in satisfactory end results in most instances.

## SPECIALIZED REGIONAL HEMANGIOMAS

Hemangiomas may occur anywhere in the body. A few distinctive hemangiomas occurring in locations that present specific clinical challenges are described below.

### Hemangiomas of the Head and Neck Region

Orbital hemangiomas in extreme cases may involve either the eyelid or conjunctiva or may develop in the retrobulbar fat, causing unilateral exophthalmos (Fig. 12–6). Although it may be possible to dissect these tumors out, the operation is often uncertain, bloody, incomplete, and mutilating. Pack and Miller[2] and Pack and Ariel[8] suggested the use of nonoperative methods for the control of hemangiomas in this location. These are the locations where selective use of cryoprobes, vascular embolization, and all other nonoperative methods *must* be tried before an attempted excision.

### Hemangiomas of the Brain

Hemangiomas of the brain can be solitary or part of more generalized manifestations. The symptoms pro-

plished by traction on the tumor after the circumferential incision has been made, making the operation relatively bloodless. McNeill and Ray[4] obtained good results by complete excision of the tumors. In seven (20 percent) of their 35 patients, amputations were required (Table 12–2). From their analysis of treatment of extremity hemangiomas, these authors concluded that end results are poor in cases of overgrowth of the affected extremity. Amputation of an extremity should be resorted to only in patients in whom conservative means of therapy, including several attempts at excision, have failed.

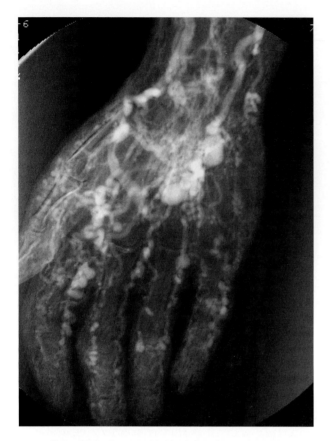

**Figure 12–2.** An example of local gigantism of the hand.

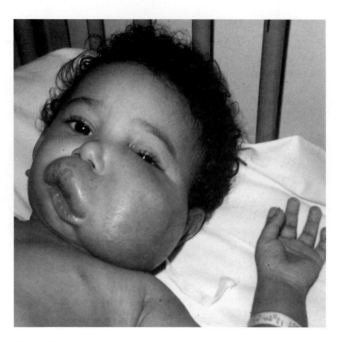

**Figure 12–4.** Large expanding hemangioma of the left cheek and neck in a male infant. This mass produced some respiratory distress and was infected. He was treated conservatively after ligation of the ipsilateral facial artery and vein with excellent results.

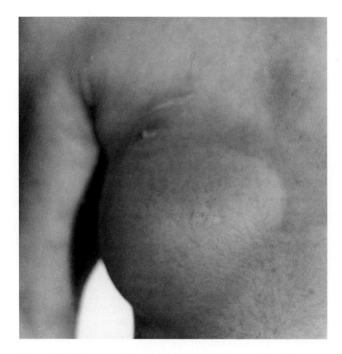

**Figure 12–3.** Hypertrophic hemangioma of the chest wall in a 24-year-old man. This tumor had to be widely excised before all margins were found to be free of extension of the exuberative overgrowth of endothelial lining.

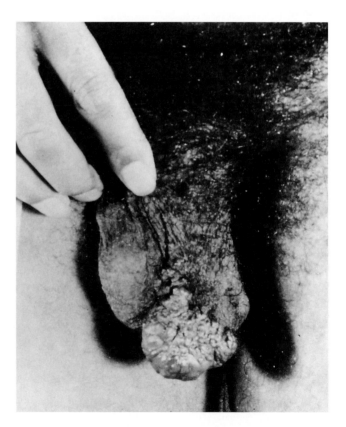

**Figure 12–5.** Scrotal hemangioma. The lesion was excised with excellent end results *(Courtesy of Ray B, Clark SS:* Hemangioma of the scrotum. *Urology 8:502, 1976).*

**TABLE 12–2. AMPUTATION FOR EXTREMITY HEMANGIOMAS IN SEVEN PATIENTS (UNIVERSITY OF ILLINOIS SERIES)**

| Patient No. | Age/Sex | Location | Complaint | Angiogram | End Result | Remarks |
|---|---|---|---|---|---|---|
| 1 | 15/M | Calf | Pain and limp | No | Good with prosthesis | Apparently no recurrences |
| 2 | Birth/F | Right lower extremity | Deformity and limp (diffuse) | No | Poor, recurrence in stump | Multiple local excisions; no evidence of disease |
| 3 | 12/M | Arm (diffuse) | Pain and tender mass | No | Good after amputation | Results poor before amputation |
| 4 | Birth/M | Lower half body (diffuse) | Multiple masses | No | Good after hip disarticulation | Good results with prosthesis; received radiation therapy in infancy |
| 5 | Birth/M | Overgrowth | Mass and pain | Yes | Poor, even after amputation | Recurrence |
| 6 | Birth/M | Hypertrophy of foot | Enlarged foot | No | Transmetatarsal amputation | |
| 7 | Birth/M | Arm | Swelling | No | Recurrence in amputated stump | Second amputation required |

Courtesy of *Clin Orthop* 101:154, 1974.

duced may not be solely due to the extent of involvement of the angioma, but perhaps are caused in part by hemorrhage within the tumor. Treatment of these lesions is based on the same general principles used for all other intracranial neoplasms.

### Hemangiomas of the Mediastinum

Hemangiomas of the mediastinum are rare and are usually cavernous.[9] The clinical presentation can be that of any space-occupying tumor in the mediastinum, without any specific radiographic clue. The diagnosis is made after exploratory thoracotomy and excision of the tumor.

### Hemangiomas of the Tongue

Lingual hemangiomas are usually the cavernous type and congenital in origin (Fig. 12–7A and 12–7B). The tip of the tongue is the most common site, but the entire tongue may be involved. With arterial communications, it may become an erectile organ of enormous dimensions—macroglossia angiomatosa. Profuse hemorrhage can follow the slightest trauma from a minor bite or rough food. The bulk of the tumor may interfere with mastication and speech. In most instances, repeated injection of sclerosing agents in small doses will produce fibrosis; occasionally, local fibrotic areas can be excised with an acceptable result.

### Hemangiomas of the Gastrointestinal Tract

Hemangiomas of the stomach are rare. Pack[10] described 16 cases in a collected series, but adequately documented cases are few. Probably, gastric hemangiomas are all congenital, although signs in newborns

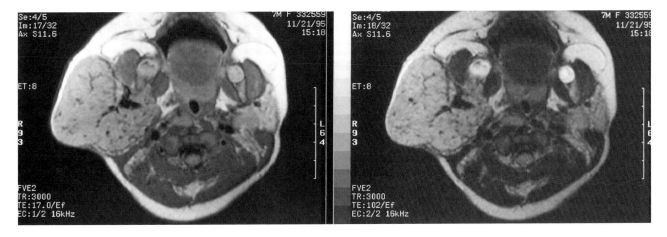

**Figure 12–6.** A CT scan of massive angiomatosis in a one-year-old male infant. The patient was treated with steroids, and after three months, the mass shrank to 25 percent of its size. He is still under observation at the time of this report.

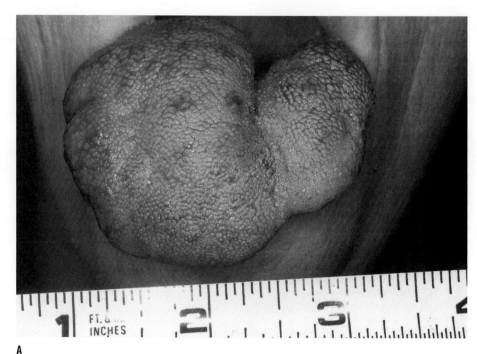

**Figure 12–7.** **(A)** Hemangioma of tongue in a 29-year-old woman. **(B)** Lateral view of the same patient. Note the prominent cavernous area. Chewing chronically traumatized this area. Patient allowed injection of sclerosing fluid only. Although macroglossia has been a major problem, she refused any treatment. Size of tongue did not change for five years, but patient was lost to follow-up.

**A**

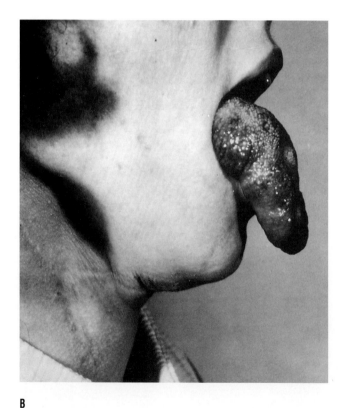

**B**

are rare. The symptoms and signs are similar to those in all other gastric neoplasms, and the treatment is excision.

The small intestine and colon (Fig. 12–8) are occasionally the sites of multiple hemangiomas, usually associated with known superficial tumors. Cryptic intestinal

hemorrhages herald the presence of these neoplasms. Intervention with resection and anastomosis is sometimes necessary, because repeated hemorrhage may be almost exsanguinating.

## Hemangiomas of the Liver

Hemangiomas of the liver are quite common, and the vast majority are small, presenting no clinical problems. In unusual instances, they may attain large proportions and excision is indicated. These hemangiomas are usually of the cavernous type and may be single or multiple, usually lying just beneath or projecting from the surface of the liver. Niemann and Penitschka,[11] in their review of 103 cases collected from the literature, found that 81 percent of the patients were women, 11 percent men, and 8 percent infants and neonates. A similar observation has been made by other authors.[12–22]

A patient with a large hepatic angioma usually complains of an abdominal mass and nonspecific pressure symptoms such as abdominal pain, fullness, nausea, and vomiting. Infrequently, attention is directed to the upper abdomen due to rupture and bleeding from the hemangioma following blunt trauma. The operative mortality in such patients is high.[16,18,22]

In the past, preoperative diagnosis of hepatic hemangiomas was difficult. Schumacker[12] reported that in only 2 of 67 cases was a preoperative diagnosis possible. In hepatic angiograms, the characteristic features are areas of "cotton-wool-like" scattered pooling, which persists for a period, even in the venous phase (Fig. 12–9). Some authors[22] have found laparoscopy useful for preoperative diagnosis, but it is difficult to ascertain the extent of liver involvement or the

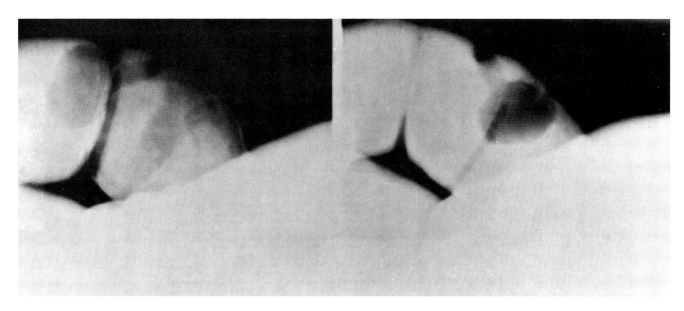

**Figure 12–8.** Polypoid hemangioma of the sigmoid colon. The lesion was treated by sleeve resection of the colon.

resectability of the tumor by means of laparoscopy alone.

Now, fairly accurate diagnosis of hepatic hemangioma can be made by dynamic computed tomography (CT) scan, which has become the preferred method of diagnosis. However, some patients still may require exploratory laparotomy for diagnosis, though most of the diagnostic tests should be performed and all possible information should be obtained before an exploratory celiotomy. Although most patients may be managed conservatively, some will require exploratory celiotomy for appropriate management.

The treatment of large symptomatic hepatic hemangiomas, if technically possible, is excision. The resectability rate of hepatic angiomas cannot be accurately described, because most authors' experience is limited to only a handful of cases. A review of the literature[8,14,15,17,19,22] shows that the only curative form of treatment is excision, including right or left lobectomies, even in children and neonates.[21] We have operated on a handful of cases of massive hemangioma of the right lobe of the liver with good results (Fig. 12–9). The technical considerations for hepatic lobectomy for hemangiomas have already been described.[11,14,19]

## Hemangiomas of the Skeletal Muscles

Hemangioma of the skeletal muscle may occur de novo as an isolated tumor in one muscle belly or group of muscles, or it may be part of a systemic hemangiomatosis involving an entire extremity.[23–26] In the former case, it is difficult to diagnose and to distinguish from other deeply situated somatic tumors, benign or malignant. The following six diagnostic points are perhaps helpful: (1) diffuse tumefaction within the muscle proper; (2) temporary enlargement of the lesion after the application of a tourniquet above; (3) decreased size of the tumor after elevation of the extremity; (4) pain and functional disability; (5) an aspiration biopsy that secures blood instead of identifiable solid tissue; and (6) roentgenographic localization of calcium deposits or phleboliths within the tumor.[27,28]

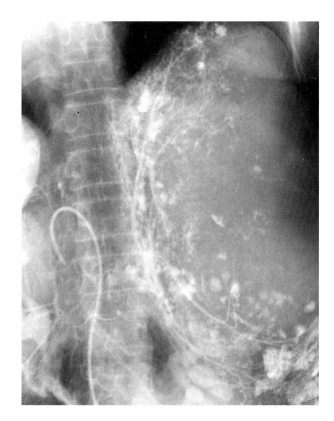

**Figure 12–9.** Hemangioma of right lobe of liver of a 57-year-old woman who was referred because of an expanding mass. Right lobectomy was performed, and she is still well 19 years later.

The patients are generally under age 30, and the upper extremities appear to be the most common site. With the advent of preoperative magnetic resonance imaging (MRI), preoperative diagnosis has become simpler, resulting in better end results. The treatment of intermuscular hemangiomas consists of judicious use of the techniques of cryotherapy, embolization, and, if indicated, sequential excision. The incidence of recurrence of 50 percent reported by Behan and Fletcher[26] is too high and has not been our experience with intramuscular hemangiomas.

## Hemangiomas of the Bone

Although a primary hemangioma of the bone is rare,[2,4,8,28,29] many such tumors likely remain undetected throughout life because most are slow-growing and asymptomatic. They may be discovered coincidentally at the time of radiographic examination for other lesions. The bones of the skull are most frequently involved, but other bones, namely, the vertebral column (especially the lumbar vertebrae), scapula, pelvic bones, rib, and phalanges, may be sites of origin. The radiographic appearance of primary bone hemangiomas is usually characterized by their anatomic location.[30] For example, in the vertebral column, the vertical striations are characteristic and diagnostic; in the flat bone, sunburst trabeculations of unusual size radiate usually from a common center and chiefly from the plane of the bone; in the cylindrical long bones, the usual loculations of the tumor are small and interspersed with a fine fibrillary framework. The cortex is usually destroyed but may extend into the center of the tumor. The periosteum may be elevated or expanded but is seldom ruptured. The x-ray appearance of a hemangioma of the bone may closely simulate giant cell tumor, fibrous dysplasia, or eosinophilic granuloma. A biopsy is necessary to establish the correct diagnosis. Hemangioma of the calvaria often erodes through the inner and outer tables and is difficult to distinguish from a dural endothelioma.

A cavernous hemangioma of a vertebra may provoke persistent backache and thereby lead to discovery through roentgenologic examination. The inaccessibility of this tumor and its intimate incorporation into an irremovable structure prohibit any attempt at complete excision. Occasionally, the hemangioma progresses and destroys the body of the vertebra, resulting in its collapse, with a protruding tumor compressing the spinal cord. Whenever symptoms of spinal cord compression occur, laminectomy is indicated.

Accessible hemangiomas of the bone may be suitable for a direct surgical attack. Curettage of the lesions in long bones with the help of cryoprobes, the implantation of bone chips, rib resection, trephine and removal of a table of calvaria, partial scapulectomy, segmental resection, and bone grafting are all feasible measures under certain conditions.

Bone changes secondary to hemangioma in closely adjacent soft tissues follow four common patterns:

1. Local erosion and destruction of the bone: The hemangioma, by constant pressure and, in the case of cirsoid or arterial hemangiomas, by pulsating pressure, destroys the adjacent bone, leaving an irregular roentgenographic finding of combined destruction and regeneration.
2. Exostosis or osteoma: Bony outgrowths can develop at sites on the bones overlapped by deep hemangiomas. The similarity of sites of these two lesions speaks against coincidental occurrence. Probably the increased vascularity of the part causes the abnormality.
3. Local overgrowth or hypertrophy of the bone: The diameter of the bone is locally expanded, thickened, and hypertrophied.
4. Elongation of long bones of the extremity: In the presence of a systemic hemangioma involving an entire extremity, it is not uncommon for the long bones of the affected site to lengthen sufficiently to cause a limp, because of the disparity in length with the normal side.

## MAFFUCCI'S SYNDROME

Maffucci's syndrome is a rare developmental disorder characterized by multiple hemangiomas and enchondromas. The vascular tumors are cavernous hemangiomas and are usually noticeable at birth. The cartilaginous abnormality is marked by overgrowth of cartilage plates. Treatment is purely symptomatic. Occasional malignant transformation to chondrosarcoma or angiosarcoma has been described.

## SYSTEMIC HEMANGIOMATOSIS

Systemic hemangiomas are those diffuse vascular tumors that usually occupy an entire extremity or portion of the head or trunk (Fig. 12–10). As much as the entire half of the body may be involved in this congenital process (Fig. 12–11). In the head and neck region, the hemangioma may follow the cutaneous distribution of some major nerve (e.g., the trigeminal). In the extremities, the anlage of this tumor probably begins at the time of limb budding so that, as the arm or leg is formed, all of the tissues (skin, muscle, bone, etc.) become infiltrated by the tortuous vessels of the hemangioma. This is often associated with lymphangiomatous involvement; often these two anomalies are so intertwined that a given condition cannot be classified based on a single diagnostic entity. The extremity from the shoulder to the nail beds or from the pelvis

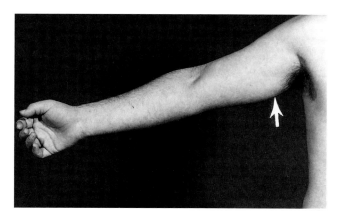

**Figure 12–10.** Overall involvement in the left arm of a 40-year-old man, extending from the palm (note the thenar eminence) to the axilla. A bulge in the upper medial aspect of the arm is obvious. Patient was treated with segmental resections.

be multiple communications between the arteries and veins. Blood vessels of all types take part in the process. The tumor may be partly capillary and partly cavernous in structure; or it may be, as mentioned above, a mixed hemolymphangioma. Other angiomatous lesions of visceral distribution (e.g., in the liver, kidney, or brain) may coexist with these systemic hemangiomas.

The systemic hemangiomatosis is usually associated with some disturbance of the sympathetic nervous system of the portion of the body or the extremity involved. This is manifested either by hyperhidrosis or vasoconstriction. The extent of the arteriovenous shunt in systemic hemangiomas varies greatly, depending on the size and number of the fistulous communications. In a few of our advanced cases, the lesion was predominantly an arteriovenous communication. Various types

to the toes may be completely involved. With this increased blood supply, all the tissues of the extremity become hypertrophied, and the long bones increase in length and diameter. The leg or arm is sometimes so heavy, bulky, and cumbersome that the unfortunate patient is functionally handicapped in addition to being disfigured (Fig. 12–12).

Fundamentally, the systemic hemangioma is a congenital arteriovenous aneurysmal anomaly. There may

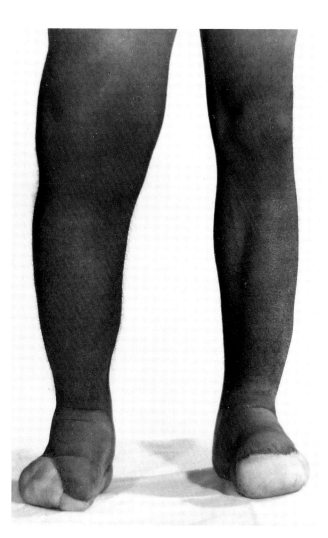

**Figure 12–12.** This 24-year-old man was born with systemic angiomatosis of both lower extremities. The diameter of the right leg and lower thigh is almost double that of the left. Involvement of the foot was so extensive that local hypertrophy (gigantism) interfered with walking. Tarsometatarsal amputation had to be performed on both sides.

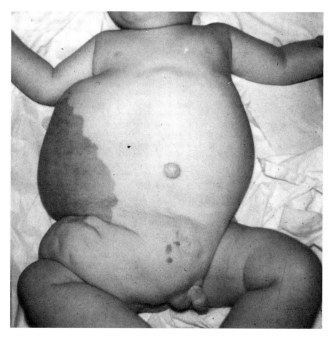

**Figure 12–11.** Angiomatosis of the right half of the body. Infant survived only two years after this photograph was taken. Angiomatosus malformation extended to the opposite side, and ulceration of the overlying skin with concomitant sepsis was the cause of death.

of cardiovascular problems may be associated with angiomatosis. In patients in whom the arteriovenous fistula could be identified, pressure proximal to the fistula resulted in the elevation of blood pressure and lowering of the pulse rate.

Treatment of systemic hemangiomatosis is difficult and unsatisfactory. Dissection of the main artery and vein, with ligation, sometimes provides reasonably good results. If the exact location of the fistula is identified, then the task becomes simple. Attempts have been made to ligate the subcutaneous vessels. A modified Kondoleon operation has also been attempted, but the results have been far from satisfactory. Amputation of the extremity is occasionally performed as a last resort.[4]

Systemic hemangiomatosis in some infants perhaps represents a basic defect in organization and development. It is frequently associated with neuroectodermal defects of diverse types, often identified by curious syndromes and symptom complexes bearing eponyms. A description of some of these will be given in detail.

### Hereditary Hemorrhagic Telangiectasia

Hereditary hemorrhagic telangiectasia (Rendu-Osler-Weber Disease) is an inherited maldevelopment of the minute blood vessels in localized areas, predisposing them to injury and serious bleeding.[31] The requisite triad fulfilling the definition of this disease are (1) mucosal hemorrhages, usually epistaxis; (2) familial occurrence; and (3) the presence of telangiectatic small angiomas of the skin and mucosa, commonly in the oral and nasal cavities.

The disease is transmitted as a simple dominant gene, affecting both sexes and transmitted either through the male or female with the atavistic skipping of individuals or generations. Although the anlage of the angiomas may be congenital, the minute tumors appear relatively late in the development of the individual. The onset of the disease may be heralded in children by nosebleeds, but the severe hemorrhages and clinically evident telangiectases usually start in the fourth or fifth decade of life.

The source of the epistaxis is usually in Kiesselbach's vascular plexus situated in the lower anterior segment of the nasal septum. Although the hemorrhages have been known to occur from the upper respiratory passages, the gastrointestinal tract, and even the kidney (hematuria), epistaxis is the most frequent expression and can follow simple sneezing. The intermittence and severity of the bleeding may require repeated blood transfusions. The angiomas are usually tiny telangiectatic reddish-purple dots, seldom larger than 5 mm. It is a serious and crippling disease, and spontaneous remission is not known to occur.

### Congenital Neurocutaneous Syndromes Associated with Angiomatosis

Certain neuroectodermal defects involving the central nervous system and peripheral nerves are also frequently found in association with hemangiomatous lesions that may be intracranial, dermal, and visceral in distribution. Attempts have been made to lump many of these disorders under the headings of *phakomatoses, neurocutaneous syndromes,* or *neuroectodermal dysplasias.* The phakomatoses are tied together because they are congenital conditions of nonsex-linked dominant inheritance, with skin lesions, multiple tumors, and involvement of the central nervous system. They have variable widespread manifestations that occasionally overlap. Many of the reasons for forming such a group of diseases are artificial. The term *phakomatoses* is purely descriptive, and has no pathologic basis.[32] Bielschowsky[33] was the first to associate tuberous sclerosis with neurofibromatosis as dysplasia with a tendency toward the formation of blastema. In 1923, Van der Hoeve[34] coined the term *phakomatosis* to characterize the two disorders. He then added the terms *cerebral angiomatosis*[35] and *encephalotrigeminal angiomatosis.*[36] Since these original four maladies were grouped together under the term *phakomatoses,* several other entities have been added. The following better-known entities in the group of phakomatoses will be briefly described: (1) tuberous sclerosis (Bourneville's disease), (2) regional angiomas (Pringle's disease), (3) encephalotrigeminal angiomatosis (Sturge-Weber syndrome), and (4) retinocerebral angiomatosis (von Hippel-Lindau syndrome).

*Tuberous Sclerosis (Bourneville's Disease).* Although one of the early reports of this entity was by von Recklinghausen,[37] tuberous sclerosis was first associated with neurofibromatosis in 1919. It is characterized by sebaceous adenomas, cutaneous angiomas, mental deficiency, and epilepsy. Hyperpigmentation may occur in the form of a single café-au-lait spot; however, multiple white maculae are far more characteristic, histologically appearing to be secondary to a decreased amount of melanin in a normal number of melanocytes. Visceral organs are commonly involved with benign dysplasias, hamartomas, or cystic changes. These malformations most commonly occur in the kidney, heart, and lung and are usually asymptomatic, but in later life, progression may result in symptoms. The pulmonary cystic changes are very similar to those found in neurofibromatosis and may progress to respiratory failure. The brain characteristically has focal areas of disorganized cortical architecture (tubers) against a background of a distorted cortical pattern. Radiographically, intracerebral calcifications may be present after puberty. Retinal tumors and subungual fibromas occur in about 10 percent of these patients. Life expectancy in patients with significant cerebral involvement is less than two decades, but those with only cutaneous manifestations can expect near-normal longevity.

***Regional Angiomas (Pringle's Disease).*** Regional angiomas appear as numerous nodules—pink, yellow, brown, and red, varying from1 mm to 1 cm in size—that are scattered in a butterfly distribution over the skin of the nose, nasolabial folds, and cheeks. This specific and symmetrical predilection has been explained as due to the distribution along the terminal filaments of the fifth cranial nerve. The terms *sebaceous adenoma* or *nevus multiplex of Pringle* have been found to be incorrect.[2] The nodules in fact are angiofibromas and analogous in many ways to von Recklinghausen's neurofibromatosis.

***Encephalotrigeminal Angiomatosis (Sturge-Weber Syndrome).*** Encephalotrigeminal angiomatosis was classified as one of the phakomatoses in 1936.[36] It is usually present at birth and is characterized by a cutaneous telangiectatic hemangioma (port-wine stain) in the distribution of the trigeminal nerve. On the ipsilateral side, meningeal angiomatosis extends into the depths of the sulci, with underlying cortical atrophy. After infancy, calcification develops in the affected cortex, resulting in epilepsy and mental retardation, with longevity greatly decreased. Rarely, pheochromocytoma has been reported to occur in these patients.

***Retinocerebral Angiomatosis (von Hippel-Lindau Syndrome).*** Von Hippel described the retinal changes in retinocerebral angiomatosis in 1911, but it was not until 1926 that Lindau[32] made an extensive report of the visceral and central nervous system pathology. The most important lesion in this disease is the cerebellar hemangioblastoma, which can be either highly vascular or cystic. Angiomatosis may occur throughout the central nervous system and is especially diagnostic when present in the retina. The embryologic origin of most of the manifestations of this disease is primarily mesodermal. Pheochromocytoma is frequently associated with von Hippel-Lindau syndrome and neurofibromatosis, the incidence being higher in von Hippel-Lindau syndrome. The onset of symptoms of this disease is usually in middle age, being either neurologic or visual. No cases have been reported prior to puberty, and no particular skin lesion is characteristic. Both Sturge-Weber syndrome and von Recklinghausen's neurofibromatosis have been reported to occur in patients and families with von Hippel-Lindau syndrome, resulting in a confusing picture but leading to interesting genetic speculation. It is doubtful that these reports represent any more than the chance synchronous occurrence of two distinct syndromes.

# ■ MALIGNANT TUMORS

## HEMANGIOENDOTHELIOMA

Hemangioendothelioma is an empiric term applied to a spectrum of vascular tumors that occupy, both in morphologic appearance and biologic behavior, an intermediate position between a benign angioma and its malignant counterpart, angiosarcoma. In general, these tumors carry a much better prognosis than angiosarcomas. Currently, hemangioendotheliomas are histologically distinguished into the following types: epithelioid, spindle cell, Kaposiform, and endovascular papillary. Of these, the epithelioid type is the most frequently encountered entity.

Epithelioid hemangioendothelioma can occur in any location, including a viscus. In mesenchymal tissues, it develops as a solitary painful mass, and, in at least half of the cases, a close relationship with an adjacent identifiable vessel can be demonstrated. If the site of origin is a major vein and has associated edema, thrombophlebitis is the initial symptom.

Microscopic differential diagnosis frequently poses some problems and necessitates differentiation from metastatic carcinoma, melanoma, and other sarcomas that have a preponderance of epithelioid cells.

Hemangioendotheliomas are slow-growing and have much better prognoses than angiosarcomas.[38,39] Weiss et al.,[39] in 1986, analyzed 46 cases from the Armed Forces Institute of Pathology (AFIP) files and reported on the indolent course of the disease. Our own experience consists of a handful of cases (six in the last 10 years) and in general tends to support the findings reported by Weiss et al.[39] Of interest is the fact that, in three of these six cases, regional lymph node involvement occurred within three years after excision of the primary tumors. However, therapeutic regional node dissection controlled the progression of the disease, and patients have remained disease-free over five years. Epithelioid hemangioendothelioma has been reported in many viscera and in long bones.[40–42] Our own experience is limited to primary tumors of the liver. A resection is usually the therapy of choice. In one of our patients, a trisegmentectomy was performed, and the patient has remained disease-free for 10 years. Of the six, two (33 percent) died of metastatic disease within five years after diagnosis of the primary tumors.

In recent years, a spindle cell variety[43] and a Kaposiform variety[44] have been described. From a therapeutic standpoint, there is little or no difference between all these varieties. Kaposilike hemangioendothelioma occurs mostly in children. The management principles and overall prognosis in all these varieties are similar.

Juvenile angiosarcoma of the liver is rarer still. Blumenfeld et al.[45] found only 36 cases in the literature up to 1969 and added one of their own. Of these 37 patients, 32 had multiple lesions, and 5 had solitary. Thirty of the patients with multiple tumors died. In one patient, the tumor metastasized to the lung and lymph nodes. Apparently, two of the patients with multiple lesions survived.[45] All the patients with solitary lesions were living at the time of Blumenfeld and co-workers' report in 1969. Of interest is the statement that in one child the tumor spontaneously regressed, resulting in cure.[45]

## ANGIOSARCOMA

Angiosarcomas are rare neoplasms. McCarthy and Pack[46] suggested that the true incidence was probably higher than the reported incidence. Pack and Ariel[8] reported that, in a 10-year period, 1,056 cases of benign angiomas were seen at Memorial Sloan-Kettering Cancer Center, but during that same period, there were only 20 (1.8 percent) cases of angiosarcomas. During the same 10 years, the Pathology Department of Memorial Sloan-Kettering Cancer Center reviewed the microscopic materials from an additional 27 cases from all over the country.[8] Angiosarcomas of the skin,[47] head and neck region,[48,49] omentum,[50,51] trunk,[8,46–52] breast,[53–63] and viscera[8,64–72] have been described. Most of these represent reports of a few cases, and adequate guidelines for clinical management are not possible. Table 12–3 shows the anatomic distribution of 42 cases of angiosarcoma encountered at the University of Illinois Medical Center.

Angiosarcomas tend to behave differently based on their anatomic location. Most of these tumors start in the skin (cutaneous angiosarcoma); then, they infiltrate the surrounding and underlying fat and muscle, resembling a soft tissue sarcoma. Thus, the true incidence of deep-seated angiosarcomas of the mesenchyma is hard to determine. Some authors[73] have combined angiosarcoma associated with lymphedema as a single entity. However, in this chapter, we have included only those instances which are not associated with lymphedema; thus, the description of the cutaneous variety described herein has no etiologic relationship with lymphedema.

Although primary angiosarcomas of the liver have been associated with polyvinyl chloride (PVC) and other agents,[74–87] little is known regarding their etiology in general. However, there are some reports[88–91] that radiation might induce the development of angiosarcoma. Although this is a distinct possibility,

**TABLE 12–3. ANATOMIC DISTRIBUTION OF ANGIOSARCOMAS (UNIVERSITY OF ILLINOIS SERIES, 1996)**

| Anatomic Site | No. Cases |
| --- | --- |
| Head and neck | 8 |
| Upper extremities | 6 |
| Lower extremities | 7 |
| Trunk | 3 |
| Breast | 8 |
| Retroperitoneum | 1 |
| Viscera | 9 |
| Total | 42 |

before considering a given case as being radiation-induced, the data should be carefully reviewed. In general, these tumors arise 10 to 12 years after radiation therapy. Angiosarcomas are found in all ages, both sexes, and all races. The youngest patient in our group was 12, and the oldest 84 years old.

### Angiosarcoma of the Extremities

Patients with angiosarcoma usually present with a moderately rapid-growing mass in the extremities (Fig. 12–13A and 12–13B). The rapidity of the progression of the disease is sometimes the clue to the correct diagnosis of a given tumor. Pack and Ariel[8] considered that the incidence rate of regional node metastases was as high as 45 percent. In the 11 patients in their series with extremity tumors, nine tumors were locally recurrent, and the patients had been referred after a delay of more than a year. Weingrad and Rosenberg,[92] in their survey of the literature, did not come across any significant series other than that of Pack and Ariel's[8] for analysis of the incidence of regional node metastases. In our own series of 13 patients with extremity tumors, five had primary tumors, three of whom were sent to us after a wedge biopsy. Five (38 percent) had metastatic disease to the regional nodes at the time of their initial operation at the University of Illinois.

***Treatment.*** The treatment of angiosarcomas of the extremities has been unsatisfactory over the years.[8,46–49,93] In our series of 13 patients with extremity angiosarcomas, seven (54 percent) remained disease-free five years or more after the primary operation. The other six patients developed recurrence either locally and/or extraregionally within five years of the treatment of the original tumors (Table 12–4). Our end results are somewhat better than those reported by Fletcher et al.[94] Apparently, initial radical excision with or without supplemental radiation therapy (as is our practice) improves overall end result. McNeer et al.[95] found that, of seven patients with angiosarcoma, three

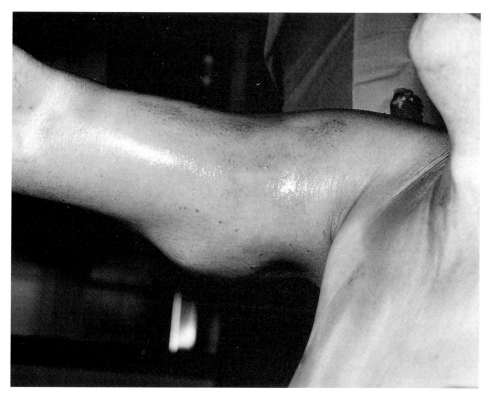

**Figure 12–13. (A)** An angiosarcoma of the upper arm in a 56-year-old man. **(B)** Angiosarcoma of the buttock of a 24-year-old basketball player. A diagnosis of gluteal abscess was made and the tumor incised. The drainage was sanguinous, with blood clots. When the drainage continued after five weeks, a biopsy was performed, which showed angiosarcoma. A hemipelvectomy was performed, and he survived for one-and-a-half years (Patient 12, Table 12–4).

A

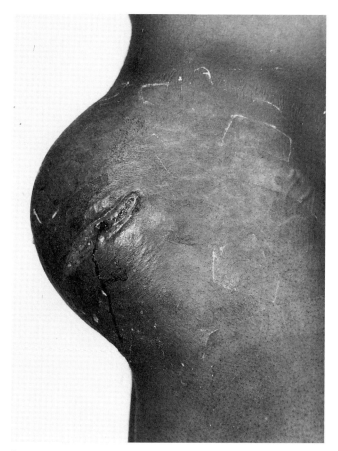

B

treated with surgery alone survived for five years, as did two who received postoperative irradiation.

Systemic chemotherapy as an adjuvant to surgery was used in three of our patients with extremity angiosarcomas (Table 12–4). All three have survived five years free of tumor. However, there are no substantive data that adjuvant chemotherapy plays a significant role in the management of these tumors.

## Angiosarcoma of the Breast

Angiosarcoma of the breast was first described by Schmidt.[96] However, Borrman[97] is credited with an adequate description of this entity in 1907. In 1969, Gulesserian and Lawton[60] presented a collective review of 42 cases of primary angiosarcoma of the breast. Since then, several other case reports have been published.[58,59,61–63] We have encountered four additional cases.

Of the four patients, three were initially seen with localized tumors of the breast and were treated by modified radical mastectomy. In only one did the regional axillary nodes contain any metastatic tumor. All four patients received adjuvant chemotherapy. One has remained disease-free for eight years, one is disease-free after four years, and another died of diffuse metastases two-and-a-half years later. The fourth patient was initially referred with advanced disease (Fig. 12–14)

**TABLE 12–4. CLINICAL SUMMARY OF 13 PATIENTS WITH ANGIOSARCOMAS OF THE EXTREMITIES**

| Patient No. | Age/ Sex | Location | Status of Primary Tumor | Regional Nodes | Type of Treatment | Metastases | End Result (Length of Survival) | Remarks |
|---|---|---|---|---|---|---|---|---|
| 1 | 65/F | Right upper arm | 3 × 4 cm | − | Forequarter amputation | Lung, liver, neck nodes | 6 months, DOD | Had widespread metastases prior to death |
| 2 | 46/F | Left forearm | 2 × 2 cm | − | Wide excision | | 7 yrs, NED | Tumor apparently was of six months' duration, biopsied elsewhere. Treated with adjuvant chemotherapy |
| 3 | 54/F | Left hand | 3 × 2 cm | − | Midarm amputation with axillary dissection | — | 5, yrs, NED | Referred with local recurrence following conservative excision |
| 4 | 61/F | Left upper arm | 5 × 5 cm | − | Wide soft tissue resection with postop radiation therapy | — | 18 yrs, alive with internal recurrence | Developed local recurrence; was reexcised; has remained well to date |
| 5 | 32/M | Right forearm | 3 × 2 cm | − | Wide soft tissue resection with postop radiation therapy | — | 7 yrs, NED | |
| 6 | 76/M | Right medial arm | 5 × 8 cm | − | Wide soft tissue resection with postop radiation therapy | — | 1 yr, DOD | |
| 7 | 58/M | Right buttock | 8 × 8 cm | − | Wide soft tissue resection with postop radiation therapy | Widespread | 9 mos, DOD | Autopsy showed extensive metastases |
| 8 | 65/F | Left upper thigh | 5 × 4 cm | − | Wide soft tissue resection with postop radiation therapy | Lung | Wedge excision | Treated with chemotherapy, but died of metastatic disease within two years of wedge resection |
| 9 | 40/M | Right lateral thigh | 3 × 3 cm | − | Wide soft tissue resection with postop radiation therapy | — | 2.5 yrs, NED | |
| 10 | 36/F | Right leg | 2 × 2 cm | − | Wide soft tissue resection with postop radiation therapy | — | 5 yrs, NED | |
| 11 | 57/M | Right thigh | 4 × 5 cm | − | Hip joint disarticulation | | 6 yrs, NED | Mass persisted for one-and-a-half years before patient sought medical advice (treated with adjuvant chemotherapy) |
| 12 | 24/M | Left buttock | 15 × 10 cm | + | Hemipelvectomy with axillary dissection | Widespread | 1.5 yrs, dead | Patient seen after an incision biopsy of the lesion (five weeks' duration) |
| 13 | 34/M | Left leg | 2 × 2 cm | − | Above-the-knee amputation | — | 5 yrs, NED | Treated with adjuvant chemotherapy |

Abbreviations: DOD, dead of disease; NED, no evidence of disease.

and did not receive any treatment. She died within two months of her first visit.

Angiosarcoma of the breast usually occurs in relatively young multiparous women. In 4 of the 51 cases, the patient was pregnant at the time of diagnosis.[54,63,64] In eight, the angiosarcoma developed after menopause.[63] Involvement of both breasts occurred in three patients.[56,63] However, in two,[63] the tumor probably was metastatic from the opposite breast.

The treatment is primarily excision, and, for all practical purposes, a total mastectomy is adequate; however, in recurrent tumors, since there is some possibil-

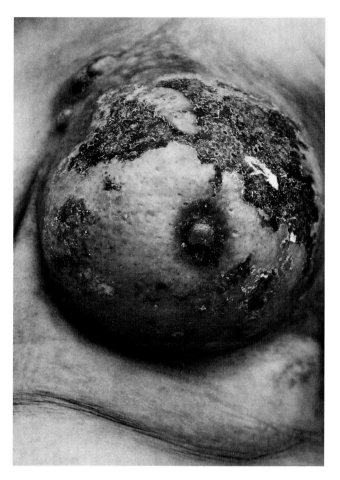

**Figure 12–14.** Angiosarcoma of the left breast of a 43-year-old woman. Note skin involvement. She was seen with far-advanced disease and was deemed incurable.

ity of regional node metastases, a modified radical mastectomy is in order. Although the role of postoperative radiation therapy and chemotherapy is still being evaluated, it appears that use of a multimodal program in the management of the angiosarcomas of breast is a logical and rational approach to managing these tumors.[61]

### Angiosarcoma of the Head and Neck Region

Angiosarcomas of the head and neck region are primarily cutaneous and are not associated with any regional lymphedema. Considering the unusual frequency of hemangiomas in this region,[8,46,48,49,98] the incidence is curiously rare. Pack and Ariel[8] treated seven cases in the head and neck region. In 1968, Bardwil and co-workers[48] described 10 cases of hemangiosarcoma from the M.D. Anderson Tumor Institute, and in 1970 Farr et al.[49] published 10 cases from the files of the Memorial Sloan-Kettering Cancer Center. Since then, only a few case reports have been published.[90,99,100] Only seven cases have been encountered at the University of Illinois Hospital, all in the scalp (Fig. 12–15A and 12–15B). It appears that this is the

most common site in the head and neck region. Most cases occur in the fifth decade, although these tumors have been reported in children. Four of our five patients were older than 60 years.

In general, patients are first seen with an umbilicated dark lesion of the scalp. In untreated cases, satellite nodules are found surrounding the primary tumor. Initially, the tumors appear vascular and often give the impression of a granuloma. Wide excision with adjuvant radiation therapy in this initial stage might provide up to 50 percent incidence of control of the primary tumor. However, untreated or inadequately treated cases have a relatively high incidence of regional node metastases; at this stage, the results of treatment are unsatisfactory. Of the seven patients in our group, three were seen with relatively localized disease. Two of these are living disease-free for over seven years; one died of disease within a year. Four of the seven presented with advanced disease. Two died within a year, and, in the other two, the disease has been controlled for three and four years, respectively.

In the primary treatment of angiosarcomas of the scalp, it is essential to recognize that there are deceptive horizontal and vertical extensions of the lesion that can only be discerned by microscopic examination of all the margins of the resected specimen. The primary excision of the scalp should be full-thickness, including the pericranium and, if indicated, the outer table of the cranial vault. The margins should be wide (at least 5 cm) on all sides. Furthermore, supplemental radiation is essential if the prognosis is to be improved.

### Angiosarcoma of the Viscera

Angiosarcomas of the intra-abdominal viscera, namely of the spleen and the liver, have been reported, but angiosarcomas of other viscera are extremely rare.

### Angiosarcoma of the Heart

Of the 53 cases of angiosarcoma of the heart analyzed by Rossi and associates,[71] 34 were in males. The tumors most commonly originate in the right atrium. Most of the patients are adults, but a few cases have been reported in adolescents. Various treatment programs have been tried, consisting of excision, radiation therapy, and chemotherapy. The median survival time from onset of symptoms is approximately three months. Bennett and co-workers[101] emphasized that patients with primary angiosarcoma of the heart typically have signs of right-sided congestive heart failure. These authors suggested that an earlier diagnosis can be made by a nuclear cardiac scan which would show any filling defect.

### Angiosarcoma of the Lungs

Angiosarcoma of the lungs is extremely rare, the first case being reported in 1931 by Wollstein.[64] Since then,

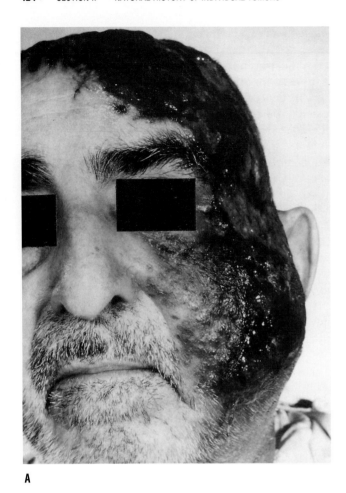

**A**

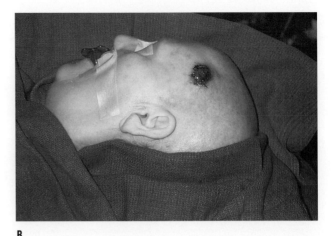

**B**

**Figure 12–15. (A)** Angiosarcoma of the scalp extending to the face. Treated with radiation therapy and systemic chemotherapy. The disease progressed relentlessly, and, within four months, the patient died of diffuse metastases (Courtesy of *Surg Ann*, 1975[323]). **(B)** Angiosarcoma of the scalp in a 55-year-old white woman. The lesion was resected with a 5-cm margin. Although the margins were microscopically clear, she received radiation to the entire scalp. She is living free of disease two years.

occasional case reports have appeared in the literature, but it is difficult to establish whether the lung was the primary site in these reports. It is not possible to make any generalization concerning pulmonary angiosarcomas.

### Angiosarcoma of the Liver

Alrenga[102] estimated that, up to 1975, 165 cases of angiosarcoma of the liver, with an autopsy frequency of 6 in 100,000, had appeared in the literature. Heath and co-authors[80] stated that the expected annual incidence of the tumor is 0.014 in 100,000, or 25 to 30 cases a year in the United States. Eight cases in 40,000 autopsies were encountered in Holland.[87] In contrast, 14 cases were noted in the population of 5,000 workers in PVC polymerization plants in the United States in a 15-year period.[79] Based on these data, it is suggested that PVC is an etiologic agent in the development of hepatic angiosarcoma. However, Fiechtner and Reyes[86] described four patients with hemangiosarcoma of the liver, and all were from rural areas of Wisconsin with no known exposure to industrial pollutants.

The clinical manifestation of angiosarcoma of the liver in adult patients is not characterized by any spe-

cific presentation. In most patients, there is evidence of a hepatic tumor associated with liver failure of varying degrees. The diagnosis is established by angiography and finally by exploratory celiotomy (Fig. 12–16). Fiechtner and Reyes[86] noted that all their patients had symptoms of advanced liver disease: abdominal pain and distention of short duration. In adults, sudden unexplained enlargement of the liver with rapid liver failure should lead to a working diagnosis of angiosarcoma of the liver.

The rarity of the tumors and the advanced stage at which diagnosis is made have resulted in a dismal prognosis after any form of therapy. Nagasue et al.[72] reported an eight-month control of a patient with angiosarcoma, using hepatic artery ligation and infusion of 5-fluorouracil through the portal vein for 27 days. These and other forms of innovative therapy must be attempted to control angiosarcoma of the liver in adults.

We have treated only five patients with angiosarcoma of the liver. In only one was a hepatic resection for cure possible. This patient is living six years after hepatic resection. In another patient, both lobes were involved, and she was treated with intra-arterial infusion and radiation therapy. She died nine months after diagnosis (Fig. 12–16). The remaining two patients had lobectomies and adjuvant chemotherapy. Of these, only one survived three years; then, she died of disease. The other died within 18 months of the resection.

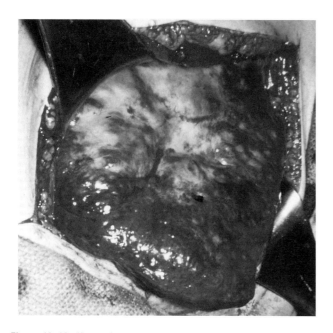

**Figure 12–16.** Hemangiosarcoma of the right lobe of the liver. Although involvement of the right lobe was known preoperatively, at operation it was also found to involve both lobes. Patient was treated with intra-arterial infusion and radiation therapy but died of extensive disease nine months after diagnosis was established.

### Angiosarcoma of the Spleen

Angiosarcoma of the spleen is rare,[67,103] and only about 50 cases have been reported. Three of these 50 were encountered in children (two girls and one boy).[104] Of the three, one was 13,[105] and the other two were 15 years old.[106,107] Of these three cases of childhood angiosarcoma, details are available only from the one reported by Garlock.[105] This child had a splenectomy for an intact tumor and lived for two years, after which the child was not followed.

Angiosarcoma of the spleen has been recorded in 47 adult patients.[67,103,108–114] Das Gupta, Coombes, and Brasfield[67] reported one of the first cases of an adult splenic angiosarcoma treated electively by splenectomy. This was in a 52-year-old woman who was admitted with a diagnosis of anemia and splenomegaly. At laparotomy, the spleen weighed 2,400 g and measured 7 × 8 × 9 cm. A diagnosis of angiosarcoma of the spleen was made from the specimen. After splenectomy was done, the patient recovered and was discharged. She was readmitted four months later with diffuse metastatic involvement of the abdomen. She died within a month. A review of the published case reports in adults shows that, in 23 (49 percent) of the 47 cases, splenectomy was performed, and the remaining cases were diagnosed at autopsy. Sixteen of the 23 (70 percent) required emergency splenectomy because of rupture of the spleen. None of the patients who were operated on were long-term survivors.

Angiosarcoma of the spleen in adults is uncommon; however, the true incidence is probably not reflected in these 47 patients. Thus, when the cause of splenic enlargement from disorders such as leukemia, lymphoma, and other hematologic abnormalities is ruled out, the possibility of angiosarcoma of the spleen should be considered. The prognosis for these patients is poor, and currently the only possible method of salvage is early diagnosis followed by splenectomy.

Primary angiosarcomas have been reported in other intra-abdominal locations.[50,51] Kalisher and co-workers[50] reported a case in the greater omentum. They concluded that tumors located in the mesentery, omentum, and retroperitoneum all had a similar clinical presentation and natural history and could be treated in a similar fashion. One retroperitoneal angiosarcoma has been treated by the author. This was excised, and the patient remained well for three years but died before five years. Ongkasuwan and associates[115] found only eight instances of angiosarcoma of the uterus and only two in the ovary.

Angiosarcomas arising in peripheral nerves have always generated considerable interest, but the incidence is indeed rare.[116] In 1977, Bricklin and Rushton[117] reported a case in the radial nerve and found only one other such instance in the literature. Recently, however, angiosarcoma in association with schwannomas in von Recklinghausen's neurofibromatosis has been described.[118–120] Because of the rarity of these tumors, no management guidelines can be provided. In fact, they are more of interest to the embryologist and morphologist than to the clinician.

### KAPOSI'S SARCOMA

Kaposi's sarcoma was first described as a clinical entity in 1872.[121] Kaposi's original description of the entity is worth repeating: "There develops on the skin, without known cause, either general or local, brown-red to blue-red nodules of the size of a grain of wheat, a pea, or a hazelnut. Their surface is smooth, their consistency densely elastic. Often they are swollen like a sponge filled with blood. . . ." This accurate description of the initial presentation of this entity has not been bettered during the last 125 years.

The classic type of Kaposi's sarcoma is most frequently encountered in patients from Eastern and Central Europe and certain parts of Northern Italy.[8,122,123] In the United States, most patients belong to these ethnic groups. With the increased immigration from Eastern Europe, Greece, and the Middle East, the frequency with which the chronic form of this disease is encountered has increased. In the University of Illinois series of 35 patients with chronic Kaposi's sarcoma, only two patient were black, and both were women. Only 1 of 35 was of Northern European descent.

It is difficult to assess the actual incidence of Kaposi's sarcoma, since a number of these cases remain unrecognized and thus unreported. Although the disease is relatively rare in American blacks, it occurs with some frequency among African blacks,[124–130] ranging from 0.8 percent in Ghana to 4 percent in Tanzania.[127,129–136] This entity is more frequently encountered as one approaches the equator. The disease is infrequent in dry, sandy areas, the highest incidence being in moist, tropical areas.[128–130] Taylor and co-workers[126] found that Kaposi's sarcoma in the equatorial region can be clinically divided into nodular, aggressive, and generalized types, with the clinical behavior varying from indolent (occasionally showing spontaneous regression) to fulminant (resulting in death). Because of the geographic and clinical similarities between Kaposi's sarcoma and Burkitt's lymphoma, the possibility of immune deficiency states as an etiologic factor in the development of Kaposi's sarcoma has been suggested.[125,137,138] The variable course of the disease and the emergence of Kaposi's sarcoma within certain groups of patients with acquired immunodeficiency syndrome (AIDS) known to be coinfected with other viruses has reinforced the concept that Kaposi's sarcoma is not only associated with immunodeficiency but is indeed a virally induced malignant tumor.

In the past, the most notable evidence in favor of an immune deficiency state was provided by the de novo appearance of Kaposi's sarcoma in renal transplant patients receiving prolonged immunosuppressive therapy.[139–143] Hardy and co-workers[139] reported one such case and reviewed the findings in five other patients. Two of the six eventually had visceral involvement, and one had reticulum cell sarcoma of the brain.[139] In the first case, diagnosis was made at autopsy. In two cases,[142] discontinuation of all immunosuppressive agents led to complete regression of the skin nodules. In another case,[140] in which both prednisone and azathioprine were reduced but not discontinued, the lesions recurred and progressed without apparent visceral involvement. In one patient,[139] discontinuation of azathioprine led to the virtual disappearance of the skin nodules, leaving scars and persistent edema. Among the recipients of transplant, the incidence of Kaposi's sarcoma is highest in patients receiving liver transplant. The incidence of Kaposi's sarcoma among liver transplant patients is approximately 1.24 percent; among renal transplant patients, 0.45 percent; and among heart transplant patients, 0.41 percent. Chronic hepatitis-B surface antigen carriers were more frequently involved with Kaposi's sarcoma among transplant recipients. Also, among the

transplant recipients, the patients treated with cyclosporin were thought to have a more fulminant course and a shorter time interval from time of transplant to development of Kaposi's sarcoma.[144–150]

Reynolds, Winkelman, and Soule[150] pointed out that Kaposi's sarcoma not only is correlated with lymphoid and plasmacytic dyscrasias, but also becomes manifest in patients with collagen disease treated with corticosteroids. Serial immunologic studies, both in vitro and in vivo, have shown that normal blastogenic response to various mitogens and a positive reaction to purified protein derivative (PPD) are altered with the progression of the disease.[138,140,141–143,151,152]

The significance of the immune deficiency, demonstrated either in vitro by lymphocyte responses or in vivo by cutaneous anergy when there is clinical progression of the disease, is unclear and does not offer any etiologic explanation. However, if it is argued that, with immunosuppression, latent oncogenic viruses are activated,[153] leading to the development of Kaposi's sarcoma, then a clear role of a virus in the development of the disease can be hypothesized. Patients with Kaposi's sarcoma have been examined from the virologic viewpoint by Giraldo and co-workers.[153] These authors found herpes virus with the antigenicity of the Epstein-Barr virus (EBV) in cultures derived from Kaposi's tumors. Hardy et al.[139] reported that four of six allografted patients with Kaposi's sarcoma had documented herpes simplex infections prior to the onset of the tumor. In their own patients, Hardy et al.[139] found no apparent viral infection, but they were able to demonstrate an elevated titer of EBV antibody in the serum.

Kaposi's sarcoma syndrome observed in certain groups of AIDS patients[154] known to be coinfected with other viruses continues to provide credibility to the viral etiology of this entity.[155] However, it is noteworthy that, as yet, identifiable causative agents have not been isolated. Furthermore, from the available data, it does not appear that human immunodeficiency virus (HIV) can be solely imputed in the genesis of AIDS-related Kaposi's sarcoma. This presumption is based on three major reasons: (1) Kaposi's sarcoma occurs preferentially within some AIDS risk groups, (2) there is no seroepidemiologic association between the classic (chronic) form of Kaposi's sarcoma and AIDS infection, and (3) HIV-1 sequences have not yet been identified within Kaposi's sarcoma cells.

The issue of causative agent(s) has been further complicated by the apparent finding of human papilloma virus (HPV)-16-like sequences and HPV-related neoplasms.[156,157] An enormous amount of investigation is in progress, and the results obtained therein are beyond the scope of this chapter. However, it seems clear that Kaposi's sarcoma cells produce a number of cytokines that may stimulate their growth,[158,159] and that HIV-infected T cells release substances that also enhance the growth of Kaposi's sarcoma cells.[160,161]

Clinically, Kaposi's sarcoma occurs in four distinct clinical types: (1) classic or chronic, (2) lymphadenopathic, (3) posttransplantation, and (4) AIDS-related.

### Classic or Chronic Kaposi's Sarcoma

In the United States, the classic form accounts for only 0.02 percent of all cancer, and most patients are older. The mean age at the time of diagnosis in the series reported by O'Brien and Brasfield was 70 years.[122] In the University of Illinois group, the mean age was 60 years, the youngest patient being 45 years old. Oettle[128] found that Kaposi's sarcoma is encountered in younger patients in Africa: all his patients were between the ages of 35 and 44 years. Slavin and co-workers[129] found that 8 cases (7 percent) in a series of 117 were in children below the age of 16 years. Males predominate in all series. In Africa, Gordon[127] found 128 men in a total of 136 patients, and Slavin et al.[129] reported 108 males and 9 females. A similar male preponderance is found in Europe and North America.[122,151,162–164] In the series reported by O'Brien and Brasfield,[122] 81 percent were men, and 19 percent were women. In our series of 35 patients, 32 were men, and 3 were women.

The classic form of Kaposi's sarcoma is often associated with either a second malignant tumor or an immune deficiency state not associated with AIDS infection.[155,165] The initial presentation of a classic bluish-red macule can occur in the skin of all parts of the human body. However, the lower extremity constitutes the most common site (33 of 35 in our series). The lesions are usually small, 0.2 mm to 1 mm in diameter, lying in the dermis or subcutis and bulging the overlying epidermis (Fig. 12–17A to 12–17D). Closely continuous lesions sometimes coalesce and produce large conglomerate lesions (Fig. 12–17A). The more diffuse lesions give rise to plaquelike nodules (Fig. 12–17B). Although the lesions are principally in the subcutis or dermis, superficial ulceration frequently accompanies Kaposi's sarcoma of long duration (Fig. 12–17C).

The disease frequently involves symmetrical areas in the other extremity in a "stocking" or "glove" fashion and later extends centripetally to the trunk. As the subcutaneous tissues are diffusely infiltrated by the hemorrhagic, verrucous plaques, edema of the extremity ensues, and the tumors ulcerate and bleed. Pain is not associated with this disease process, with the exception of tumors on the soles of the feet and of the penis. Variations to the classic macule, nodule, plaque, ulceration, and edema can also be encountered. In some patients, the disease involves intense fibrous tissue reaction and

resembles some type of fibrous tissue tumor. Sometimes the lesions resemble a lymphangioma.

Regional lymphadenopathy is common in all phases of tumor growth. However, most patients with Kaposi's sarcoma do not have lymph node biopsies, and the extent to which the lymphadenopathy is due to associated infection, edema, or actual node involvement is hard to evaluate. Bhana et al.[166] suggested that regional node involvement from a locally aggressive tumor is more common in older patients.

The clinical presentation of Kaposi's sarcoma can be described as follows: the *nodular* variety is usually indolent, and there is seldom regional node involvement; the *florid* form is locally aggressive and tends to fungate and ulcerate; the *infiltrative* type invades muscles and bones; and the *lymphadenopathic* type is disseminated and virulent.

In the natural progression of the disease, about half of the patients ultimately have involvement of the submucosa of the gastrointestinal tract (Fig. 12–18A to 12–18C). From the gastrointestinal tract, the disease progresses to both lungs, retroperitoneal nodes, thoracic nodes, and bones, in the terminal stages of the disease. Rarely, there is neurologic involvement in the terminal stages of Kaposi's sarcoma.[167]

Deviations from typical cutaneous onset are known to occur. However, before Dorffel's[168] monograph in 1932, it was generally believed that all extracutaneous lesions were metastatic, inasmuch as, up to that time, few cases had been described in which skin lesions were absent or had been preceded by visceral lesions. Since then, several cases have been reported, apparently of primary tumors in the viscera[122,169–174] or other unusual locations.[122,164,174–179] Today, the trend of evidence suggests that Kaposi's sarcoma is a slow-growing, systemic, multicentric disease with long intervals between clinical manifestations in different sites.

Although the multicentricity of Kaposi's sarcoma is generally acknowledged, certain sites of clinical presentation have always aroused considerable clinical interest. These will be briefly elaborated upon.

### *Anatomic Sites*

*Kaposi's Sarcoma of the Head and Neck.*    Kaposi's sarcoma may occur in the head and neck region, usually in conjunction with cutaneous lesions of the extremities.[122,127,129,162] However, in rare instances, the initial manifestation of the disease might be a solitary lesion in the head and neck region. Table 12–5, developed from published reports,[122,151,152,163,176,180,181] shows the involvement of various anatomic sites within the head and neck region. In this series of 77 patients, only in 14 (18 percent) was the head and neck region the initial

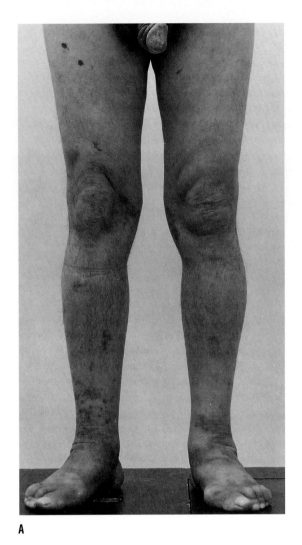

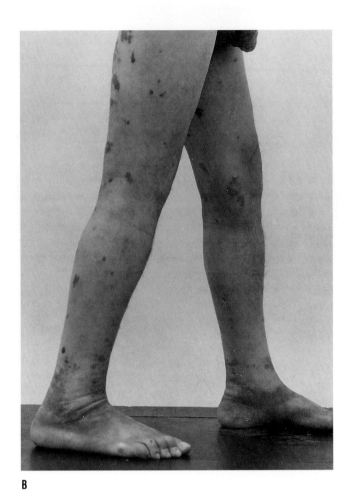

**Figure 12–17. (A)** Kaposi's sarcoma in a 69-year-old man. Note confluence on the anterior aspect of the leg in the ankle region. Several small umbilicated nodules can be seen in the thigh. **(B)** Same patient; the lesions are progressing proximally. In the lateral aspect, several small lesions have coalesced to form plaques. *(Continued.)*

site of clinical presentation. In the remaining 82 percent, concomitant lesions elsewhere were present. Slavin et al.[129] found five head and neck cases in their series of 117 (4.3 percent). However, these authors cautioned that the incidence in their series might be underestimated because in African patients the only available method of diagnosis was biopsy of the cutaneous lesions. In the present series of 35 patients treated by us, only two (6 percent) had lesions in the head and neck region at the time of initial diagnosis. Both lesions were in the scalp, and both patients had cutaneous manifestations elsewhere.

Intraoral primary Kaposi's sarcoma is extremely rare.[176] In 1975, Farman and Uys[176] reviewed the published reports and found eight cases and added one of their own. The locations included the palate, tongue, alveolar ridge, and lower lip. These authors[176] operated

on their patient, who died six months later, apparently of unrelated causes. At autopsy, there was no evidence of Kaposi's sarcoma anywhere in the body.

*Kaposi's Sarcoma of the Lymph Nodes.* In 1962, Ecklund and Valaitis[178] reviewed eight cases of apparent primary Kaposi's sarcoma of the lymph nodes and described one case of their own. Lee and Moore[179] added one more case from the Memorial Sloan-Kettering Cancer Center. Bhana et al.[166] found that 16 (33 percent) of their 48 African patients had nodal disease. Dutz and Stout,[182] in 1960, reviewed 1,256 cases of so-called Kaposi's sarcoma in children under the age of 16; they accepted 36 cases and added four of their own. In 9 (22.5 percent) of these 40 cases, the patients presented with lymph node involvement. The known duration of disease in these nine cases varied from 6 months to

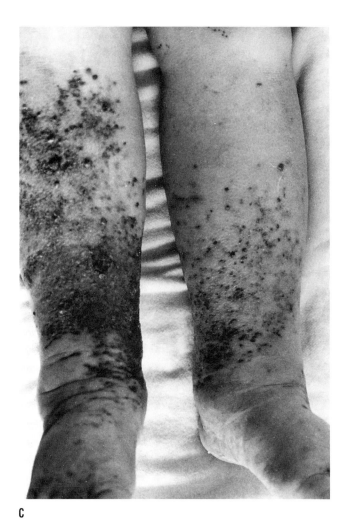

C

27 years. Bhana et al.[166] concluded that there are probably two main types of nodal involvement. One (lymphadenopathic type) occurs predominantly in younger patients and involves many groups of lymph nodes. This is a fulminant type, where skin manifestations are rather rare, and the incidence of internal involvement is high, with a higher mortality rate.[183] The sarcoma probably develops in situ and is associated with a poor prognosis.[183] The other form is the result of metastases to nodes from an apparently aggressive tumor in the regional area. This variety is rare and in the classic form occurs more frequently in older patients and carries a better prognosis than the lymphadenopathic type of Kaposi's sarcoma.

*Kaposi's Sarcoma of the Gastrointestinal Tract.*   Although, in the late stage of the disease, Kaposi's sarcoma involves the submucosa of the gastrointestinal tract in about 50 percent of patients,[122,130,163,169,174] abdominal symptoms due to relatively localized segmental disease are rare. White and King,[169] in 1964, described two patients who were seen for intra-abdominal pain and intestinal obstruction. During operation, only segmental involvement with Kaposi's sarcoma was noted, and these segments were resected. Both patients required right hemicolectomy. They were apparently well and free of any obvious disease at the time of the report. Adlersberg,[170] in 1970, reported a case of Kaposi's sarcoma associated with ulcerative colitis and found only one other such case in the literature.[171] In our series, one

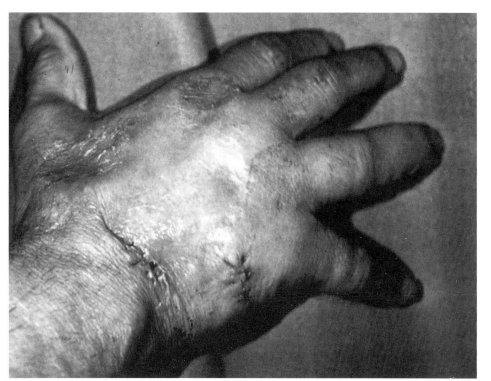

D

**Figure 12–17** *(continued).* **(C)** Kaposi's sarcoma in a 65-year-old patient, with extensive confluence of the cutancous lesions producing "brawny" legs and skin ulcerations. **(D)** Unusual instance of Kaposi's sarcoma involving the upper extremity. Note the flat pigmented lesion at the base of the thumb and index finger. Similar lesions were excised (incisions are seen) and provided the diagnosis.

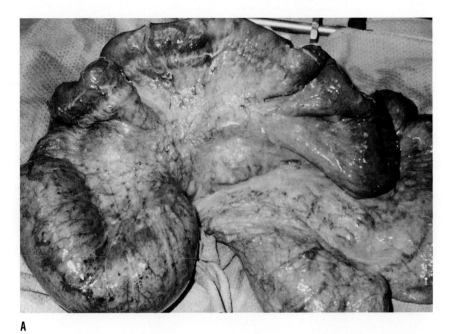

A

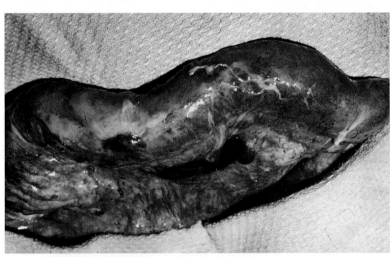

B

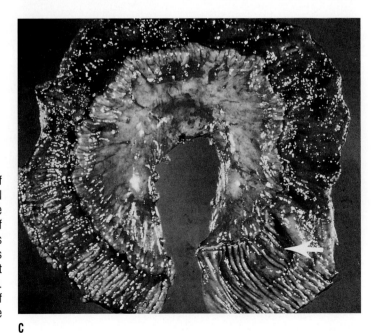

C

**Figure 12–18.** This 66-year-old man was admitted to the Division of Surgical Oncology of the Veterans Administration West Side Hospital (Chicago) with evidence of lower gastrointestinal bleeding. Because he was being followed in our clinics for Kaposi's sarcoma, a diagnosis of gastrointestinal tract involvement was made preoperatively, and he was operated on. **(A)** Note the multiple punctate hemorrhagelike spots involving the serosa and the mesentery of the small intestine. A segment of the ileum appears to be dark with submucosal hemorrhage *(right).* **(B)** This segment was excised. The extensive plaquelike involvement of the mesentery is obvious. **(C)** Segment was cut open, showing the extensive segmental involvement of the mucosa and submucosa.

**TABLE 12–5. KAPOSI'S SARCOMA OF THE HEAD AND NECK\***

| Site | No. Cases | Head and Neck Lesions Only | Coexistent Cutaneous Lesions of the Extremities | Involvement of the Extremity Lesion |
|---|---|---|---|---|
| Skin of head and neck | 13 | — | 13 | 100% |
| Cervical lymph nodes | 4 | 2 | 2 | 50% |
| Oral cavity and oropharynx | 15 | 1 | 14 | 93% |
| Tongue | 4 | 2 | 2 | 50% |
| Tonsils | 2 | 1 | 1 | 50% |
| Ear | 12 | 4 | 8 | 66% |
| Nose | 8 | 1 | 7 | 87% |
| Larynx | 13 | — | 13 | 100% |
| Generalized lymphadenopathy | 6 | 3 | 3 | 50% |
| Total | 77 | 14 | 63 | 83% |

\* This table was developed from the following published reports: references 122, 142, 143, 154, 173, 177, 178.

patient required resection for segmental Kaposi's sarcoma of the ileum and the cecum (Fig. 12–18A to 12–18C).

It is not appropriate to either recommend or perform an exploratory celiotomy in all patients with Kaposi's sarcoma who complain of abdominal symptoms. However, in patients in whom the disease is in remission, long-term palliation can be provided by a segmental resection of the involved portion of the intestine. Preoperative diagnosis of visceral involvement with Kaposi's sarcoma in the absence of any cutaneous manifestation is impossible.

Infrequently, Kaposi's sarcoma is encountered in the spleen,[168] heart,[180] adrenal,[168] and other unusual sites, but it seldom poses a clinical problem, as it does when occurring in the gastrointestinal tract.

*Kaposi's Sarcoma Associated with Other Neoplasms.* Since the original description of this entity,[121] reviews on the subject have clearly established that Kaposi's sarcoma is frequently associated with other neoplasms, among which lymphomas are the most common.[122,123,127,128,151,162,165,177,179,180,184]

In our series of 35 patients, three (9 percent) had associated lymphoma, two had Hodgkin's disease, and the third had lymphoma of the stomach. Although association with lymphoma is relatively well established, association with multiple myeloma is extremely rare.[151,172] Mazzaferri and Penn[185] argued that the low incidence of reported cases probably does not represent the true incidence of multiple myeloma in association with Kaposi's sarcoma. In support of their contention, these authors cited the reported description of moderate bone marrow plasmacytosis by a number of authors.

Primary cutaneous lesions in Kaposi's sarcoma frequently resemble malignant melanoma, but the con-

comitant appearance of melanoma and Kaposi's sarcoma is rare.[122] We have two instances in which Kaposi's sarcoma was diagnosed during the follow-up observation after treatment of primary cutaneous melanoma. Rarely, thymomas have been reported in association with Kaposi's sarcoma.[186]

The incidence of posttransplantation Kaposi's sarcoma is less than 1 percent, whereas, in the near East, it is estimated to be about 4 percent.[187,188] There are conflicting data as to whether the type of immunosuppression affects this risk.[189] The clinical course of this disease depends on both the stage of the disease and the ability to successfully manipulate the dosage of immunosuppressives. In patients in whom the disease is restricted to the skin, the intensity can be controlled by modulating the dose of immunosuppressive agents. In patients in whom the disease is internally manifested, the incidence of mortality is rather high.

*Treatment.* The classic or chronic type of Kaposi's sarcoma in initial stages is extremely radiosensitive, and radiation therapy is the choice of treatment. In most instances, the superficial macular lesions completely regress with a dosage of 1,000 to 2,000 rads. Radiation therapy is also effective in recurrent and/or confluent cutaneous lesions.

Systemic chemotherapy has been found to be useful in locally advanced cases of Kaposi's sarcoma and in patients with multiple site involvement.[186,190–193] Several instances are on record in which the use of systemic chemotherapy has produced long-term remission of the disease.

The prognosis in Kaposi's sarcoma is usually based on the stage of the disease:[194] (1) stage I, the disease is localized to the skin (indolent); (2) stage II, cutaneous but locally aggressive with or without regional node involvement; (3) stage III, generalized mucocutaneous or lymphadenopathic involvement or both; and (4) stage IV, visceral involvement with or without symptoms.

The prognosis for patients with the classic type of Kaposi's sarcoma, which are usually found in stages I and II, is good, because most of these are slow-growing and the disease remains localized for long periods of time. However, in some patients, the tumor can grow aggressively, centripetally, and quickly, and proves fatal.

In our series of 35 patients, all of whom were of classic chronic type, the longest follow-up has been for 20 years. Of the 16 suitable for 15-year analysis, 11 are living apparently free of disease, and three are living with disease. Two patients died of a second primary cancer, one of a cancer of the pancreas five years after diagnosis of Kaposi's sarcoma, and the other of cancer of the prostate six years after diagnosis of Kaposi's sarcoma. It is not possible to estimate accurately the life expectancy in the chronic form of Kaposi's sarcoma. From all available data, it can be presumed to be an indolent malignancy, whereas those arising in an immune deficient state have an aggressive behavior, progress inexorably, and are in general fatal.

### AIDS-related Kaposi's Sarcoma

The recent increase in the incidence of soft tissue sarcoma is mostly related to an increase in the number of Kaposi's sarcoma in AIDS patients. This occurs in various well-defined risk populations with known risk factors. There is increasing epidemiological evidence that HIV-related Kaposi's sarcoma may be a sexually transmitted disease.[195]

Biggar et al.,[196] using the data from the Surveillance, Epidemiology, and End-Result (SEER) program of the National Cancer Institute for the years 1973 to 1990, reported that there were 4,946 cases of Kaposi's sarcoma observed from 1980 to 1990. This contrasted with the 169 cases to be expected before the epidemic of AIDS. Among these 4,946 Kaposi's sarcoma patients, the risks of developing malignancies like non-Hodgkin's lymphoma increased 198-fold, while the risk of other cancers increased only marginally.[196]

The incidence of Kaposi's sarcoma among HIV-1 infected patients increased an estimated 7,000-fold.[197] Patients with long-term survival after HIV infection also show markedly high incidences of Kaposi's sarcoma.[198] Of 4,073 reported patients diagnosed with AIDS from 1978 through 1983, after at least four years follow-up, 119 (3 percent) were alive and another 186 (4.5 percent) were lost to follow-up. Among the 119 patients definitely alive with HIV infection and followed long-term, 41 were positive for continued HIV infection, and 6 had no laboratory evidence specific for human deficiency virus infection (negative antibody, negative antigen, and no viral isolation or polymerase chain reaction

assay). Of the 41 patients who had positive HIV tests, 25 (61 percent) developed Kaposi's sarcoma.

In another study reported by Geddes et al.[199] from Italy, the authors studied the changing incidence of Kaposi's sarcoma from 1976 to 1990. In the period before the AIDS epidemic, the incidence of Kaposi's sarcoma was 1.05 per 100,000 men and 0.27 per 100,000 women. Although this incidence of classical type Kaposi's sarcoma in this Italian population is approximately two- to threefold higher than in the United States and Sweden, in the same region during 1985 to 1990, the incidence of Kaposi's sarcoma increased nearly twofold in Italian men below age 50 (from 0.15 in 1976–1984, to 0.47 in 1985–1990). Conversely, a decline was recorded in Kaposi's sarcoma incidence in older men in this same time period.

Another study, by Reynolds et al.,[200] reported from population-based disease registries for AIDS patients developing cancer in the San Francisco area from 1980 to 1987; 1,756 newly diagnosed malignancies were identified among members of AIDS cohorts. Of these, 1,752 malignancies occurred among AIDS patients, 99.7 percent in males. The breakdown of the malignancies was as follows: Kaposi's sarcoma, 83 percent; non-Hodgkin's lymphoma, 13 percent; and Hodgkin's disease, 1 percent. In this study's population, malignancies known to be associated with AIDS (e.g., Kaposi's sarcoma and non-Hodgkin's lymphoma) were dramatically more prevalent among AIDS patients; however, non-HIV associated cancers, such as nonmelanoma skin cancer, and carcinoma of the rectum, anus, and nasal cavity, were only slightly increased. Also, AIDS-related malignancies were more apt to be diagnosed during or after first AIDS diagnosis.

Among the overall AIDS population, 10 percent of the patients develop Kaposi's sarcoma.[201] Several epidemiologic studies attempted to outline the risks and risk factors and incidence of Kaposi's sarcoma in AIDS patients. In a study reported from Johns Hopkins University, Hoover et al.[202] studied the epidemiology of Kaposi's sarcoma in a cohort of 2,591 gay men infected with HIV-1 in a multicenter AIDS Cohort Study between 1984 and 1992. Among 844 AIDS cases, 202 patients presented with early Kaposi's sarcoma, 101 developed Kaposi's sarcoma at a later stage of the AIDS, and 541 were not diagnosed with Kaposi's sarcoma. Overall, 37.4 percent of the AIDS cases were diagnosed with Kaposi's sarcoma before death.[202] In this study, early Kaposi's sarcoma diagnosed at an early stage of AIDS was significantly more common than Kaposi's sarcoma diagnosed at the later stage of AIDS. In another study from the same institution, Armenian et al.[203] reported a composite risk score for Kaposi's sarcoma based on case-control and longitudinal study in the multicenter AIDS Cohort Study population. In this study, more Kaposi's sarcomas were found among patients from the west coast or patients with sexual partners from the west coast. Also, incidence of Kaposi's sarcoma increased with more sexually active populations and higher numbers of sexual partners. Certain infections, such as hepatitis and gonorrhea, also increased the incidence of Kaposi's sarcoma. However, immunosuppression resulting from HIV infection does not explain the full spectrum of distribution of Kaposi's sarcoma across the risk group.[204]

In a study reported by Bernstein et al.,[204] most cases occurred among homosexual men, particularly those with oral-anal contact and those with sexual contact in high-risk cities and among populations with frequent use of nitrite inhalants ("poppers"), suggesting an unidentified etiologic cofactor. Haverkos et al.[205] also found nitrite inhalant use as a variable often associated with Kaposi's sarcoma among AIDS patients. Other authors have also suggested that persons can reduce their risk of Kaposi's sarcoma by avoiding nitrite inhalants and changing behavior to reduce the risk of sexually transmitted infection.[206] Patients who develop AIDS from intravenous drug abuse have a much lower incidence of Kaposi's sarcoma.

In a study reported by the Italian Cooperative Group on AIDS and Tumors, a distinct difference was found in the incidence of Kaposi's sarcoma according to the etiology for AIDS. Among intravenous drug users, the incidence of Kaposi's sarcoma was only 3 percent; among homosexual men, the incidence was 25 percent. In this study, increased numbers of Kaposi's sarcomas have been observed since 1982.[207] Authors in this study also noted an actual decrease of the percentage of incidence of Kaposi's sarcoma among AIDS patients: 18 percent in 1984 to 6 percent in 1989. A similar decrease has been noted by others.[208] Lundgren et al.[208] reported a correlation between CD4 cell count and development of Kaposi's sarcoma among AIDS patients. When the CD4 cell count was less than $200 \times 10^{-6}$ per liter of blood at the time of AIDS diagnosis, there was an increased incidence of developing Kaposi's sarcoma. Age of the patient, antiretroviral therapy, and primary *Pneumocystis carinii* prophylaxis failed to influence the development of Kaposi's sarcoma. Thus, the occurrence of Kaposi's sarcoma remained constant over time, but developed later in the course of AIDS and was associated with more severe immunosuppression.[208]

Other authors have reported an apparent decline in the incidence of Kaposi's sarcoma among AIDS patients.[209] Schechter et al.[209] reported 677 cases of Kaposi's sarcoma among 3,047 AIDS patients (homosexual/bisexual men) diagnosed in Canada between 1980 and 1989. The proportion of Kaposi's sarcoma declined from 32.2 percent, during the years 1980 to

1985, to 15 percent, during 1989. However, this suggested decline in incidence among AIDS patients should be viewed with caution,[210] because this decrease is found over the years following seroconversion, but not over the calendar time.

Several authors have reported differences in the incidence of Kaposi's sarcoma among AIDS patients based on the etiology of their disease. Patients who develop AIDS secondary to sexually transmitted routes (for example, homosexual male patients and heterosexual patients with multiple sexual partners), have a much higher incidence of Kaposi's sarcoma than do those who acquired HIV by intravenous drug abuse. Thus, the role of a sexually transmitted cofactor is strongly suspected. The influence of oral-anal sex with fecal contamination has been reported in detail by Beral et al.[211] These authors found a strong correlation between frequency of oral-anal sex to the incidence of Kaposi's sarcoma among AIDS patients. Besides infection with HIV-1, other factors believed to be strongly correlated to development of Kaposi's sarcoma include HPV, cytomegalovirus (CMV), herpesvirus, and HIV-1 Tat protein, which promotes the growth of spindle cells derived from AIDS-associated Kaposi's sarcoma.

Herpesviruslike DNA sequences have been reported to be associated with various forms of Kaposi's sarcomas in HIV-1 infected patients.[212–215] Recently, a new herpesvirus has also been implicated in the genesis of Kaposi's sarcoma in HIV-infected patients.[216–219] Various other growth factors and cytokines have also been implicated in the etiology of Kaposi's sarcoma in AIDS patients. These include HIV Tat gene, some oncogenes, and cytokines like interleukin-6, basic fibroblast growth factor, transforming growth factor-beta, oncostatin M, platelet-derived growth factor, and so forth.[220]

***Clinical Presentation.*** Clinical presentation of AIDS-related Kaposi's sarcoma is somewhat different from the de novo Kaposi's sarcoma found in elderly patients. The head and neck region remains the most dominant site for involvement, and several authors have reported involvement in over 60 percent of the cases. Intraoral lesions can mimic a number of other clinical entities, including atrophic candidiasis, erythroplakia, pyogenic granuloma, bacillary angiomatosis, and hemangioma or lymphoma.[221]

Among patients presenting with Kaposi's sarcoma, lesions are usually multifocal with the head and neck as the dominant primary site.[222] In this region, cutaneous lesions are most commonly seen (in approximately 70 percent of the cases), followed by mucosal lesions in 56 percent, and involvement of the deeper tissue in 14 percent. Most patients (80 percent) with AIDS-related Kaposi's sarcoma involving the head and neck area are asymptomatic. Mucosal lesions are associated with symptoms about 30 percent of the time, whereas cutaneous lesions had symptoms only about 5 percent of the time. Occasionally, head and neck involvement may be due to involvement of the intraparotid lymph node, giving the appearance of a parotid mass.[223] The lesions in the head and neck region are rarely the cause of death in these patients, although they can cause significant morbidity including pain, bleeding, dysphagia, airway obstruction, and severe disfigurement, and as such, consideration should be given for treatment in the early stages.[224]

There is a much higher incidence of diffuse involvement of the body, including intra-abdominal and thoracic viscera. The frequency of gastrointestinal tract involvement is higher than in classic Kaposi's sarcoma.[225,226] Among patients with gastrointestinal tract involvement, upper gastrointestinal involvement is more common than lower gastrointestinal involvement.[227] Although most of the involvement in the gastrointestinal tract can be multicentric, diffuse involvement of the stomach, like linitis plastica, has also been described.[228] At times, the intra-abdominal involvement may be the only presentation of Kaposi's sarcoma, with no clinical cutaneous or mucocutaneous lesion. Often, Kaposi's sarcoma with intra-abdominal involvement presents with features similar to acute appendicitis due to appendiceal involvement or massive gastrointestinal bleeding.[229–233]

Involvement of the skin of the extremities is encountered less often than in classic Kaposi's sarcoma; however, the patient may present with lymphedema and lower extremity involvement (Fig. 12–19). Such lymphangiomalike variants of Kaposi's sarcoma could produce extensive lymphedema formation involving the legs, face, or hands. Early recognition of this lymphedema involving the extremities in Kaposi's sarcoma patients will allow proper treatment to avoid a limb-threatening situation.[234,235] In other cases, extensive plaque formation and edema of the lower extremity may take the appearance of cellulitis.[236] Involvement of the intra-abdominal visceral organs and chest may also result in presentation of a patient with ascites, chylothorax, or chylous ascites.[237–239] Male genital involvement of Kaposi's sarcoma has also been reported by various authors. However, involvement of the vulva in Kaposi's sarcoma patients is very rare.[240]

Primary Kaposi's sarcoma of the lung has been reported by several authors, and patients may present with pulmonary symptoms including advanced symptoms of respiratory failure. Diffuse pulmonary involvement may make diagnosis of lung involvement difficult in AIDS patients with opportunistic infections. In other cases, solitary involvement of the pulmonary tissue makes diagnosis easy.[241–244]

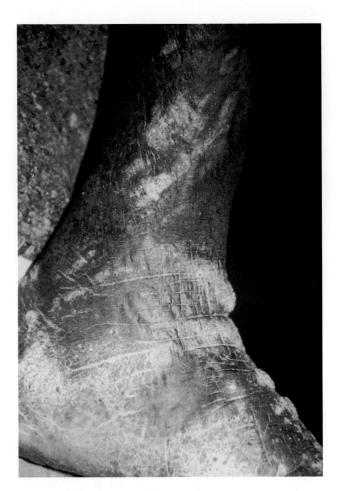

**Figure 12–19.** Plaque-like involvement of the lower leg in Kaposi's sarcoma in a patient with AIDS.

Involvement of unusual organs like the heart or thyroid has also been described.[245–246] Bone and bone marrow involvement is relatively rare in this group of patients; however, patients may present with either involvement of the bone marrow or osteolytic lesion in the bone. This primary intraosseous occurrence of Kaposi's sarcoma has been reported by several authors.[247–248]

**Treatment.** Kaposi's sarcoma is the most common malignant lesion among AIDS patients. Presentation varies considerably, from a small cutaneous nodule to aggressive disseminated disease. Hence, the treatment plan for this group of patients will have to be individualized depending on the presentation and symptoms.

The current goal in the treatment of AIDS-associated Kaposi's sarcoma patients is mostly palliative. Kaposi's sarcoma in this group of patients can seldom be cured; thus, treatment should be oriented towards palliation of various bothersome symptoms and morbidity resulting from the presence of the lesion. The treatment of Kaposi's sarcoma can vary from observation to surgical excision, radiation therapy, intra-lesional chemotherapy, sclerotherapy, cryotherapy, photodynamic therapy, and multi-agent systemic chemotherapy or treatment with cytokines.[249–251] Typically, limited local disease is amenable to a variety of local treatment measures. Extensive symptomatic AIDS-related Kaposi's sarcoma requires more extensive systemic chemotherapy or cytokine therapy. Multi-agent chemotherapy is usually reserved for treatment of patients most severely affected by AIDS cases. Judicious use of radiation therapy can also result in excellent palliation.

The underlying degree of immune suppression is an important consideration in the management of AIDS patients.[251] Kahn et al.[251] made a reasonable correlation between the CD4$^+$ T-lymphocyte count and requirement of treatment in AIDS patients. Patients with CD4$^+$ T-lymphocyte count greater than 500/mm$^3$ usually have more localized disease and require only local therapy. Patients with CD4$^+$ T-lymphocyte count between 200 to 500/mm$^3$ are usually good candidates for treatment with recombinant interferon, since such cytokine therapy results in excellent response. Cytokines combined with zidovudine, which has anti-HIV properties, has been found to be quite useful. Patients with CD4$^+$ T-lymphocyte count less than 200/mm$^3$ usually have more extensive and symptomatic Kaposi's sarcoma, and usually require systemic multi-agent chemotherapy along with antiretroviral therapy.

AIDS-related Kaposi's sarcoma per se is rarely life-threatening; most patients die of their underlying AIDS. Thus, a treatment plan based on the underlying immune deficiency state is of paramount importance. For smaller lesions, intralesional injection using bleomycin, interferon, or vinblastine has shown good-to-excellent results.[252–255] Small cutaneous or mucocutaneous lesions can be excised and closed primarily; however, a surgical approach to control this disease should be restricted only to small mucocutaneous lesions. Other local therapy such as the use of infra-red coagulator or sclerotherapy using 3 percent sodium tetradecyl sulfate (Sotradecol) has been used with limited success. Photodynamic therapy using Photofrin and 630 nm laser light, although showing good response, has severe side effects, and the treatment is considered unsatisfactory.[256] Similar to the chronic type, AIDS-related Kaposi's sarcoma in the localized form is very effectively treated by radiation therapy. However, the recurrence rate is relatively high. Radiation therapy is usually well-tolerated, except to the oral cavity, which has a relatively high rate of side effects due to mucositis. A recommended dose is 15 Gy for oral lesions, or 20 Gy for lesions involving conjunctiva, eyelids, lips, hands, feet, genitalia, or the anal region. These doses were sufficient to shrink tumor and pro-

vide good palliation of symptoms. For cutaneous lesions on other sites, a 30 Gy dose could be given safely. The overall regression rate was over 85 percent.

The complete regression rate for cutaneous lesions is also very high; however, unlike the chronic or classic variety, in a follow-up period of just under eight months, the recurrence rate is approximately 70 percent.[257,258] In a prospective randomized trial to evaluate the dose-dependent response of Kaposi's sarcoma to radiation, Stelzer et al.[259] used three separate radiation doses to treat Kaposi's sarcoma. The first dose was 8 Gy in one fraction, the second was 20 Gy in 10 fractions, and the third was 40 Gy in 20 fractions. Following the treatment, they evaluated the response rate and recurrence rate. The complete response rate was higher with higher doses of radiation: approximately 80 percent for 40 Gy and 20 Gy, compared to 50 percent for 8 Gy. Also, the median time to failure was much longer with higher doses of radiation: 43 weeks for 40 Gy, 26 weeks for 20 Gy, and 13 weeks for 8 Gy. From this study, they concluded that fractionated radiation therapy to a higher total dose resulted in improved response and better control of cutaneous Kaposi's sarcoma in AIDS patients.[259]

In a study reported from San Francisco, Meyer[260] outlined the role of whole-lung radiation in diffuse involvement of the lung in patients with Kaposi's sarcoma. Low-dose radiation varying from 100 cGy to 150 cGy resulted in good symptomatic relief in 78 percent of the patients, but only approximately 30 percent of the patients showed marked improvement in the chest x-ray infiltrate. The response was transient, and median duration of response was a little over 12 weeks.

LeBourgeois et al.,[261] from France, also reported good response of Kaposi's sarcoma to radiation. However, patients with cutaneous lesions tolerated the treatment far better than patients with mucosal lesions, who had far greater side effects, even at lower doses of radiation. In their studies, the objective remission rate was 96 percent for cutaneous lesions with a dose of 10 to 20 Gy of radiation. Penile and scrotal lesions showed a good response rate: approximately 70 percent. In their opinion, the toxicity due to mucositis from radiation severely restricts the use of radiation as a mode of treatment in large intraoral lesions.[261]

Extensive involvement by Kaposi's sarcoma is usually treated with systemic therapy. Recently, cytokine treatment has shown to be fairly effective in treating AIDS-related Kaposi's sarcoma. In a prospective study of efficacy of cytokine in the treatment of malignant lesions, Garbe reported[262] approximately 30 to 50 percent response to systemic interferon-alpha treatment. The effectiveness of Kaposi's sarcoma's treatment was further improved by combining interferon-alpha and zidovudine. In another study reported by Mauss et al.,[263] in a prospective nonrandomized study using low-dose interferon-alpha 2b (IFN-α 2b) given at a dose of 3 mU three times per week in combination with 250 mg of zidovudine given twice daily, the complete and partial response rate was approximately 65 percent. In some patients, the response rate lasted up to 24 months. The response to the treatment depended strongly on pretreatment values of $CD4^+$ T-lymphocyte count, and the complete and partial responses occurred only in patients with pretreatment $CD4^+$ T-lymphocyte counts higher than 250/mm[3]. In general, the treatment was very well-tolerated, and this study suggested that a combination of low-dose interferon-alpha and zidovudine is therapeutically effective and well-tolerated in the early stages of progressive Kaposi's sarcoma.[263]

Various single-agent and multi-agent chemotherapy has been attempted with moderate success in AIDS-related Kaposi's sarcoma, including the use of etoposide, Taxel (paclitaxel), and foscarnet. The response rate to etoposide was only 36 percent, whereas it was 65 percent to paclitaxel, and 60 percent to foscarnet in a small group of patients.[264–266] In poor prognostic patients, multi-agent chemotherapy using doxorubicin, bleomycin, and vindesine was found to be effective. However, this kind of treatment has severe side effects, and neutropenia remains the dose-limiting factor. A dose of doxorubicin using more than 15 mg/m[2] was associated with severe neutropenia.[267,268] The most common cause of death in this group was opportunistic infection. Although doxorubicin in AIDS-related Kaposi's sarcoma gives high response rates, its toxicity limits the clinical efficacy. Several investigators used liposomally entrapped doxorubicin and achieved relatively high response rates (74 percent). However, almost all responses were only partial, and the median duration of response was short.[269–271] Use of granulocyte-macrophage colony-stimulating factor (GM-CSF) improved the tolerance in a group of 27 patients with mostly poor prognosis. The overall response rate was 70 percent, with mean duration of response of 18 weeks and median survival of 30 weeks.[272]

Systemic hyperthermia over 42°C was also found to have a high partial response rate (70 percent) and occasional complete response rate (10 percent). The hyperthermia also resulted in a significant rise in $CD4^+$ T-lymphocyte count in some patients.[273,274] All-trans-retinoic acid alone or in combination with interferon-alpha 2a has been tried in AIDS-related Kaposi's sarcoma with minimal success.[275]

Recently, some new approaches for the treatment of Kaposi's sarcoma have been used. In an experimental model, human chorionic gonadotropin was found to be beneficial,[276] and such therapy has been attempted in humans[277] with mixed results. An occasional case report[278] of the efficacy of immunoglobulins has also been investigated. The various treatment options outlined above should be judiciously used to achieve palliation. Aggressive systemic multi-agent therapy is usually reserved for rapidly progressive systemic disease.

***Prognosis.*** In a cluster analysis using a new data structure called a *dendrogram*, Lee et al.[279] showed three patterns of metastasis involving skin, upper gastrointestinal tract, and midgastrointestinal tract. These three distinct patterns of metastasis suggest different etiology and mechanism of dissemination of AIDS-associated Kaposi's sarcoma. The prognosis of Kaposi's sarcoma in AIDS patients depends on a number of factors. In a study of prognostic variables in this group of patients using the Cox proportional hazard regression model, Miles et al.[280] demonstrated that $CD4^+$ cell count, hematocrit, number of Kaposi's lesions, and body mass index are the most important predictors of Kaposi's sarcoma. Others have reported an association of opportunistic infection as an important prognostic variable.[281]

In another study, Tambussi et al.[282] correlated the prognosis to the TNM-TIS classification as suggested by the Center for Disease Control. In this staging system, *T* represents the anatomical extent of lesion, *I* represents the immune system status, and *S* represents HIV-related systemic illness, such as opportunistic infection. Of the parameters considered, the anatomic extent was not a prognostic factor; however, immune status and concomitant systemic illness were important prognostic variables. In a report of cause of death in patients with AIDS, McKenzie et al.[283] found less than 7 percent of patients dying as a direct cause of Kaposi's sarcoma, although about 60 percent of patients had Kaposi's sarcoma at the time of death.

# ■ PERIVASCULAR TUMORS

Recent classification of soft tissue tumors adopted by the World Health Organization[284] included tumors like glomus tumors and hemangiopericytomas as arising from cells that support blood vessels (i.e., pericytes and glomus cells) rather than cells which feature endothelial differentiation. Conceptually, it appears to be more logical; thus, these tumors are included in this chapter under the subheading of perivascular tumors.

## GLOMUS TUMOR

Glomus tumors are distinctive tumors, the cells of which resemble modified smooth muscle cells of the glomus jugulare. These are usually small tumors (3 to

5 mm) and are frequently encountered in the subungual region.[285–289] Although glomus tumors are encountered in both sexes, there is a 3:1 female preponderance in lesions located in the subungual region.[290]

Glomus tumors are usually single, but several instances of multiple tumors have been reported.[1,289] We have encountered six such instances. The tumor is found in adults of both sexes and has no specific racial predilection. Although most of the glomus tumors are superficial (i.e., in the trunk or extremities), a few cases have been reported in several unusual locations where normal glomus bodies are usually sparse or absent.[291–298]

The color of the visible tumors ranges from deep red to purple or blue, with blue being the most prominent color. The tumor is usually well demarcated from the surrounding tissues. Pack and Ariel[8] described 20 patients with glomus tumors, the anatomic distribution being as follows: temple, one; thoracic wall, one; scapular region, one; hand, one; knee, two; arm, two; forearm, five; fingers, seven. We have treated 16 patients with superficially located glomus tumors: nine were in the upper extremities, two in the lower, and five in the trunk. Of the nine in the upper extremities, seven were in the subungual region. Tsuneyoshi and Enjoji[299] recently reviewed 63 cases of glomus tumors. These authors found that these tumors were more common in young women and the most common anatomic location was the fingers; 74 percent occurred in the subungual region. All patients but one complained of pain. These authors histologically classified glomus tumors into three types: vascular (29 cases), myxoid (23 cases), and solid (11 cases). In keeping with recent observations, the presence of smooth muscle cells in these tumors was also observed.

The characteristic symptom of glomus tumor is pain, which occasionally is associated with localized vasomotor disturbance. The diagnosis of glomus tumor is made by the location and the accompanying pain. Infrequently, the pulsatile nature of the tumor can erode the terminal phalanx, and a clear-cut destruction of the cortex of the terminal phalanx is seen. Clinical diagnosis is usually satisfactory, and treatment can be initiated.

In most other locations, a glomus tumor produces symptoms characteristic of the site at which it arises. For example, Appelman and Helwig[292] reviewed the clinical features of 12 glomus tumors of the stomach from the files of the AFIP, plus 17 cases from the literature. They found that, of 29 patients, 11 were seen for ulcer symptoms and 12 for upper gastrointestinal bleeding. In the remaining patients, the glomus tumor was an incidental finding. These observations have been substantiated in more recent literature. The ideal treatment of a glomus tumor is excision.

The existence of glomangiosarcoma has been alluded to;[300,301] however, even if they exist, the incidence is so low that the only statement that can be made regarding their management is conservative excision and observation.

## ■ HEMANGIOPERICYTOMA

### BENIGN HEMANGIOPERICYTOMA

Hemangiopericytoma is considered benign if mitosis is absent microscopically. In tumors in which only occasional mitotic activity is observed, the general tendency has been to consider them more or less benign; however, on a long-term basis, their malignant potential becomes obvious with the development of local recurrence. Therefore, the treatment should be wide excision of the normal soft tissues surrounding the tumor. In our present group of patients, six had tumors that were classified as benign hemangiopericytoma. All six patients had subcutaneous tumors in the extremities, and in none was the primary tumor larger than 3 cm. Unlike the situation with glomus tumors, none of the patients presented with unusual pain or tenderness related to the primary tumor. They all have remained free of disease for at least ten years.

### MALIGNANT HEMANGIOPERICYTOMA

Malignant hemangiopericytoma was first described by Stout and Murray[302] in 1942. In 1949, Stout[303] described the natural history of 25 cases, thus firmly establishing the clinicopathologic features of this relatively new neoplasm. Although the etiologic factors of hemangiopericytoma are generally unclear, polyvinyl alcohol has been alluded to as a causative agent.[304] Prout and Davis[305] reported a case of hemangiopericytoma of the urinary bladder following exposure to polyvinyl alcohol. Hemangiopericytoma may occur in any part of the human body.[306–311] It has been described in the thorax,[312] a number of viscera,[305,313] the pelvis,[314,315] and several unusual sites.[316,317]

Of the 32 patients in our present series, 17 were women and 15 were men. A similar ratio has been reported by other authors.[306–308] The peak incidence appears to be between the ages of 30 and 45 years.[306–310]

The tumor usually presents as a painless, slow-growing mass, which is often nodular and circumscribed. In some patients, the presenting symptom is due to pressure on the adjoining structures (Fig. 12–20). In one of our patients with a presacral hemangiopericytoma, the pressure on the rectum simulated the symptoms of a cancer of the rectum.

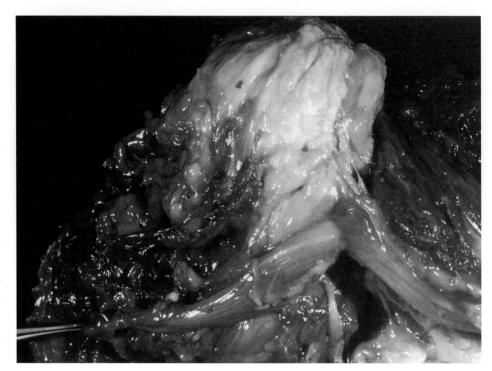

**Figure 12–20.** Resected hemipelvectomy specimen. Note the tumor is pressing on the sacral plexi. The plexi are separated in a V-shaped manner to show the relation of the tumor to the nerve roots. This 56-year-old woman complained of tense pain along the course of the sciatic nerve for one year before a pelvic and rectal examination was performed. Following hemipelvectomy, she remained well for 15 years and died of unrelated causes.

Of the 32 hemangiopericytoma patients in this series, only 12 were seen with intact primary tumors or after a wedge biopsy, and the remaining 20 patients were seen with locally recurrent tumors. The presenting size of the primary tumors varied: less than 5 cm, four patients; between 6 and 9 cm, four patients; and 10 cm in maximum diameter, four patients. In the recurrent group, the size of the tumors varied from 10 to 25 cm in maximum diameter. Cellular pleomorphisms and mitotic activity vary considerably depending on the location of the tumor. From a histopathologic standpoint, the differential diagnosis usually has to be made from malignant fibrous histiocytoma, synovial sarcoma, and mesenchymal chondrosarcoma. The difficulty in rendering an accurate diagnosis and predicting clinical behavior has been stressed by all who manage these tumors. From all available evidence, it appears that tumors with large size, a mitotic rate of 4/10 to 6/10 high-powered fields (HPF), a high degree of cellularity, and foci of hemorrhage and/or necrosis should be considered malignant, and these tumors carry a worse prognosis.

Malignant hemangiopericytoma metastasizes via both the lymphatics and the bloodstream. Regional node metastasis in primary low-grade tumors is rare, but may be encountered either in high-grade primary tumors or in tumors recurring locally after initial excisions. In our series of 12 primary tumors, only three had metastatic regional nodes. Of the 20 patients with recurrent tumors, 12 had regional node involvement.

The ideal treatment of malignant hemangiopericytoma is wide excision with clear margins of at least 2 cm wherever it is anatomically feasible. In our series of 32 patients, four underwent major amputation (Fig. 12–20). All four had local recurrences after initial excision(s) elsewhere. Unfortunately, because of lack of appreciation of the malignant potential of this type of neoplasm, most patients are initially treated with less than adequate excision. This results in repeated local recurrences and ultimately systemic extension and death. The following two case reports exemplify the existing confusion in the management of these patients.

### CASE REPORT 1

A 24-year-old woman was referred to the University of Illinois Hospital with a diagnosis of recurrent hemangiopericytoma of the right groin. At the age of 23, she had noticed a "walnut-shaped" painless lump in the inner part of her right groin. Her physician recommended observation for three months. The size of the mass did not change. Although the physician wanted to continue observation, she insisted on excision. The tumor was excised, and a diagnosis of hemangiopericytoma was made. She was told that the tumor had been adequately removed, that such tumors do not recur or metastasize, and that no further excision was indicated. The mass reappeared within three months, and another "wide" excision was performed. The tumor reappeared within six months, resulting in another excision. This time, the tumor recurred within two months, and the patient started having pain in the anterior aspect of the thigh. Because of three recurrences within one year of primary excision, she was sent to the University of Illinois. Examination showed a 4 × 3 cm mass, located on the lateral margin of the femoral triangle about 2.5 cm below the anterior superior iliac spine. A muscle group excision of the anterolateral compartment of the thigh and excision of the anterior superior iliac spine with 3 cm of the anterior aspect of the iliac crest was then performed. The specimen showed the recurrent tumor infiltrating the anterior cutaneous nerve of the thigh. She has remained well for 20 years. At age 43, she is active and has no residual deformity.

### CASE REPORT 2

A 26-year-old man was referred with a diagnosis of recurrent hemangiopericytoma of the anterior abdominal wall and a bleeding duodenal ulcer. Three years previously, he had noticed a small, painless mass about two inches above the umbilicus on the right side of the abdominal wall. The tumor was locally excised and a diagnosis of hemangiopericytoma was made. The tumor recurred in three months, and a second excision was performed. The tumor was then radiated. He remained well for one-and-a-half years and completed his college studies. The tumor reappeared 20 months later, and he was treated with multi-agent chemotherapy. The tumor did not shrink, and the patient started to have upper gastrointestinal hemorrhage, complicated by gastric outlet obstruction. At this time, he was transferred to the University of Illinois.

On admission, a large epigastric mass was readily palpable, with skin changes over the mass. After appropriate supportive care and investigation, he underwent an extensive resection with excision of the anterior abdominal wall, partial gastrectomy, pancreaticoduodenectomy, and wedge excision of both lobes of the liver (Fig. 12–21). Reconstruction of the gastrointestinal continuity was performed on classical lines. The anterior abdominal wall was repaired. He remained free of tumor for four years. However, in the fifth year, he developed intra-abdominal recurrence with extension to the posterior mediastinum. Another attempt at a massive excision was considered, but celiotomy showed the abdominal cavity to be replaced with tumor. He died soon after his last operation.

These two case reports illustrate the commonly held misconceptions regarding the management of patients with malignant hemangiopericytoma: (1) that they are slow-growing tumors of low-grade malignancy and (2) that they can be adequately controlled either by conservative local excision or by just using primary radiation therapy. Long-term control of malignant hemangiopericytoma in any anatomic location can be accomplished only if the tumor is widely excised. *Wide excision* means a margin of normal soft tissue surround-

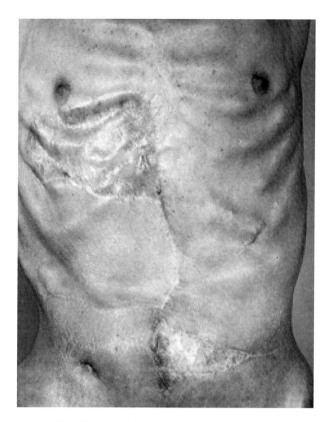

**Figure 12–21.** Three years after resection of anterior abdominal wall for hemangiopericytoma. Patient had no disability.

ing the tumor. However, in locations where an adequate margin is either not possible or is limited due to anatomical barriers (for example, in the pelvic space), postoperative radiation therapy is helpful.[318,319] Mira and co-workers[319] reported a relatively good response in large tumors after radiation therapy. Whenever there is doubt as to the adequacy of margin or if the tumor is large (both with intact primary and locally recurrent tumor), postoperative radiation therapy is strongly recommended.

### End Results

In our present series of 32 patients with malignant hemangiopericytoma, 25 patients are eligible for five-year follow-up analysis. Twenty-one (84 percent) of the 25 patients are free of local recurrence and/or metastases. Of the 14 patients eligible for ten-year analysis, all of them are still free of disease.

Backwinkle and Diddams[309] reviewed the literature in 1970 and found that, of the combined series of 177 cases treated by surgery alone, 95 patients (53.6 percent) survived for five years or more. Enzinger and Smith[306] found of 106 patients (67 percent) collected from various sources were alive and 60 percent were without evidence of tumor at the time of their report in 1976. McMaster and co-workers[307] computed the results of treatment according to whether the tumors were histologically of borderline malignancy or were frankly malignant. In the borderline group of 16 patients, six (38 percent) were free of disease for five years or more. In the frankly malignant group, 5 (15.6 percent) of 32 patients survived without evidence of cancer. This striking difference in results of treatment reported in the collected series[307–309] can probably be explained on the basis of differences in the concept of wide excision. In any retrospective analysis spanning a long period and in which a number of surgeons participate, frequently the same operation is performed differently by different authors and the results cannot be compared.

The recurrence rate after primary operation is directly proportional to the inadequacy of the operation. Our two case reports show the problem of inadequate operation. In the present group of 12 patients with primary tumors where the same tenet of wide excision was applied to all patients, in only one (8 percent) was local recurrence encountered after initial operation. In the series reported by McMaster et al.,[307] 6 of 16 (37.5 percent) in the borderline group and 15 of 32 (47 percent) in the frankly malignant group had local recurrence. Therefore, it is logical to suggest that all hemangiopericytomas be considered as potentially malignant, and those with any degree of cellular pleomorphism or 4–6 mitotic figures per 10 HPF should be presumed to be highly malignant, because the true malignant potential of these supposedly indolent tumors becomes evident only after some time has elapsed. The best treatment for malignant hemangiopericytomas is wide excision with wide margins of free soft tissues along with postoperative radiation.

### Pelvic Hemangiopericytoma

Hemangiopericytoma of the pelvis is relatively infrequent. In 1964, Spiro and associates[314] found 24 cases, 18 uterine and 6 extrauterine. In 1975, Wilbanks et al.[315] found 24 additional patients with the uterine variety and three with the extrauterine pelvic variety.

These tumors may present as a pelvic mass simulating either ovarian cancer or uterine enlargement, with menometrorrhagia-simulating fibroids. Patients with uterine hemangiopericytomas have a better prognosis than those with the extrauterine variety. Wilbanks and co-workers[315] reviewed the literature and found that, in the 43 determinant cases of uterine hemangiopericytoma, four patients (9 percent) either died of their disease or had recurrence following primary excision. In contrast, of the seven patients with extrauterine hemangiopericytoma, only three survived. We have treated four patients with pelvic hemangiopericytoma arising from corpus uteri. All the patients were referred to us after hysterectomy. In two, pelvic exenteration was required to obtain adequate margins.

## REFERENCES

1. Matthews DN: Hemangiomata. Plast Reconstr Surg 41: 528, 1968
2. Pack GT, Miller TR: Hemangiomas: Classification, diagnosis and treatment. Angiology 1:405, 1950
3. Patek AF Jr., Post J, Victor JC: The vascular spider associated with cirrhosis of the liver. Am J Med Sci 200:3417, 1940
4. McNeill TW, Ray RD: Hemangioma of the extremities: Review of 35 cases. Clin Orthop 101:154, 1974
5. Kasabach HH, Meritt KK: Capillary hemangioma with extensive purpura: Report of a case. Am J Dis Child 59: 1063, 1961
6. Edgerton MT, Hiebert JM: Vascular and lymphatic tumors in infancy, childhood and adulthood: Challenge of diagnosis and treatment. In Current Problems in Cancer, vol. 11, no. 7. Chicago, Year Book Medical Publishers, 1978
7. Goldwin RM, Rosoff CB: Cryosurgery for large hemangioma in adults. Plast Reconstr Surg 43:605, 1969
8. Pack GT, Ariel IR. Tumors of the Soft Somatic Tissues, Chap. 19. New York, Hoeber-Harper, 1958, p 384
9. Attar S, Cowley A: Hemangioma of the mediastinum: Collective review and case report. Am Surg 30:141, 1964
10. Pack GT: Unusual tumors of the stomach. Ann NY Acad Sci 114:985, 1964
11. Niemann F, Penitschka W: Die kavemosen Haemangiome "Kavernoma" der Leber. Bruns Beitr Klin Chir 195:257, 1957
12. Shumacker HB Jr: Hemangioma of the liver. Surgery 11: 209, 1942
13. Hendrick JG: Hemangioma of the liver causing death in newborn infant. J Pediatr 32:309, 1948
14. Brunschwig A, Smith RR: Large hemangioma of the liver: Successful excision. Ann Surg 135:124, 1952
15. Wilson H, Tyson WT: Massive hemangioma of the liver. Ann Surg 135:766, 1952
16. Matsuo I: Hemangioma of the liver, complicated with massive intra-abdominal hemorrhage. Tokyo Med J 70: 104, 1953
17. Henson SW Jr., Gray HK, Dockerty MB: Benign tumor of the liver. Surg Gynecol Obstet 103:327, 1956
18. Sewell JH, Weiss K: Spontaneous rupture of hemangiomata of the liver. Arch Surg 83:729, 1961
19. Krippaehne WW, Herr RH: Resection of massive hemangiomas of the liver. Surg Gynecol Obstet 116:761, 1963
20. Muehlbauer MA, Farber MG: Hemangioma of the liver. Am J Gastroenterol 45:355, 1966
21. Stone HH, Nielson IC: Hemangioma of the liver in the newborn: Report of a successful outcome following hepatic lobectomy. Arch Surg 90:319, 1965
22. Kato M, Sugawara I, Okada A, et al.: Hemangioma of the

liver: Diagnosis with combined use of laparoscopy and hepatic arteriography. Am Surg 129:698, 1975

23. Backman L, Ohman U: Hemangioma of striated muscle: Report of a case. Acta Chir Scand 134:160, 1968

24. Watson WL, McCarthy WD: Blood and lymph vessel tumors. Surg Gynecol Obstet 71:569, 1940

25. Allen PW, Enzinger FM: Hemangioma of the skeletal muscle: An analysis of 89 cases. Cancer 29:8, 1972

26. Behan A, Fletcher CDM: Intramuscular angioma: A clinicopathologic analysis of 74 cases. Histopathology 18:53, 1991

27. Jones KG: Cavernous hemangioma of striated muscle. J Bone Joint Surg 35A:717, 1953

28. Heitzman E Jr., Jones B: Roentgen characteristics of cavernous hemangioma of striated muscle. Radiology 74: 420, 1960

29. Unnik K, Ivins JC, Beabout JW, Dahlin DC: Hemangioma: Hemangiopericytoma and hemangioendothelioma (angiosarcoma) of bone. Cancer 27:1403, 1971

30. Dahlin DC: Benign vascular tumors. In: Bone Tumors. Springfield, Ill., Thomas, 1978, p 137

31. Osler W: A family form of recurring epistaxis associated with multiple telangiectases of the skin and mucous membranes. Bull Johns Hopkins Hosp 12:333, 1901

32. Lindau A: Studien uber Kleinhimcysten. Bau, Pathogenese und Beziehungen zur angiomatosis retinue. Acta Pathol Microbiol Scand (suppl) 1:1, 1926

33. Bielschowsky M: Entwurf eines Systems der Heyredodegene rationen des Zentrolnervens systems einsch liesslich der zugehorigen Striaturner Krankungen. J Physchol Neurol Leipz 24:48, 1918

34. Van der Hoeve T: Eye disease in tuberous sclerosis of the brain and in Recklinghausen's disease. Trans Ophthalmol Soc UK 43:534, 1923

35. Van der Hoeve T: Eye symptoms in phakomatoses: The Doyne Memorial Lecture. Trans Ophthalmol Soc UK 52:380, 1932

36. Van der Hoeve T: Eine vierte phakomatoses. Ber Keutsch Ophthalmol Ges 51:136, 1936

37. Von Recklinghausen FD: Ein herz von einem neugebornen welches mehrere thefls nach aussen, theirs nach den hohlen prominierende tumoren (Myomen) trug Ver handl. Ges Geburtsch 15, 1863

38. Weiss SW, Enzinger FM: Epithelioid hemangioendothelioma: A vascular tumor often mistaken for a carcinoma. Cancer 50:970, 1982

39. Weiss SW, Ishak KG, Dail DH, et al.: Epithelioid hemangioendothelioma and related lesions. Semin Diagn Pathol 3:259, 1986

40. Dean PJ, Haggitt RC, O'Hara CJ: Malignant epithelioid hemangioendothelioma of the liver in young women: Relationship to oral contraceptive use. Am J Surg Pathol 9:695, 1985

41. Ishak KG, Sesterhenn IA, Goodman ZD, et al.: Epithelioid hemangioendothelioma of the liver: A clinicopathologic and follow-up study of 32 cases. Hum Pathol 15:839, 1984

42. Mira JM, Kameda N: Myxoid angioblastoma of bones: A case report of rare, multifocal entity with light ultrami-

croscopic and immunopathologic correlation. Am J Surg Pathol 9:450, 1985

43. Perkins P, Weiss SW: Spindle cell hemangioendothelioma: A clinicopathologic study of 78 cases. Mod Pathol 7:9A, 1994

44. Tsang WYW, Chang JKC: Kaposi-like infantile hemangioendothelioma: A distinctive vascular neoplasm of the retroperitoneum. Am J Surg Pathol 15:982, 1991

45. Blumenfeld TA, Fleming ID, Johnson WW: Juvenile hemangioendothelioma of the liver: Report of a case and review of the literature. Cancer 24:853, 1969

46. McCarthy WD, Pack GT. Malignant blood vessel tumors: A report of 56 cases of angiosarcoma and Kaposi's sarcoma. Surg Gynecol Obstet 91:465, 1950

47. Girard C, Hohnson WC, Graham IH: Cutaneous angiosarcoma. Cancer 26:868, 1970

48. Bardwil JM, Mocega EE, Butler JJ, Russin DJ: Angiosarcoma of the head and neck region. Am J Surg 116:548, 1968

49. Farr HW, Carandang CM, Huvos AG: Malignant vascular tumors of head and neck. Am J Surg 120:501, 1970

50. Kalisher L, Straatsma GW, Rosenberg BF, Vaitkevicius VK: Primary malignant hemangioendothelioma of the greater omentum. A case report. Cancer 22:1126, 1968

51. Stout APO, Hendry J, Purdie J: Primary solid tumors of the great omentum. Cancer 16:231, 1963

52. Gill W, McGregor JD: Malignant haemangioendothelioma. J R Coll Surg Edinb 365:155, 1968

53. Stout AP: Hemangioendothelioma of the breast. Ann Surg 118:445, 1943

54. Enticknap JB: Angioblastoma of the breast complicating pregnancy. Br Med J 2:51, 1946

55. Mallory TB, Castleman B, Parris EE: Hemangiosarcoma of the breast. N Engl J Med 241:241, 1949

56. Batchelor GB: Haemangioblastoma of the breast. Br J Surg 46:647, 1959

57. Steingaszner LC, Enzinger FM, Taylor HB: Hemangiosarcoma of the breast. Cancer 18:352, 1965

58. Chen K, Kirkegaard D, Bocian J: Angiosarcoma of the breast. Cancer 46:368, 1980

59. Migliori E: Angiosarcoma of the breast. Tumori 63:199, 1977

60. Gulesserian HP, Lawton RL: Angiosarcoma of the breast. Cancer 24:1021, 1969

61. Antman KH, Corson J, Greenberger J, Wilson R: Multimodality therapy in the management of angiosarcoma of the breast. Cancer 50:2000, 1982

62. Kessler E, Kozenitsky IL: Haemangiosarcoma of the breast. J Clin Pathol 24:530, 1971

63. Dunegan LJ, Tobon H, Watson CG: Angiosarcoma of the breast: A report of two cases and a review of the literature. Surgery 79:57, 1976

64. Wollstein M· Malignant hemangioma of the lung with multiple visceral foci. Arch Pathol 12:562, 1931

65. Packard GB, Palmer HD: Primary neoplasms of the liver in infants and children. Ann Surg 142:214, 1955

66. Edmonton HA: Differential diagnosis of tumors and tumorlike lesions of the liver in infancy and childhood. Am J Dis Child 91:168, 1956

67. Das Gupta TK, Coombes B, Brasfield RD: Primary malignant neoplasms of the spleen. Surg Gynecol Obstet 120: 947, 1965

68. Alpert LI, Benisch B: Hemangioendothelioma of the liver associated with microangiopathic hemolytic anemia: Report of four cases. Am J Med 48:624, 1970

69. Truell JE, Peck SD, Reiquam CW: Hemangiosarcoma of the liver complicated by disseminated intravascular coagulation. Gastroenterology 65:936, 1973

70. Strohl KP: Angiosarcoma of the heart. Arch Intern Med 136:928, 1976

71. Rossi NP, Kioschos JM, Achenbrener CA, Ehrenhaft JL: Primary angiosarcoma of the heart. Cancer 37:891, 1976

72. Nagasue N, Ogawa Y, Inokuchi K: Hemangiosarcoma of liver and spleen treated by hepatic artery ligation, intraportal infusion chemotherapy, and splenectomy. Cancer 38:1386, 1976

73. Enzinger FM, Weiss SW: Malignant vascular tumors. In: Soft Tissue Tumors, 3rd ed., 1995, St. Louis, Mosby-Yearbook, p 641

74. McMahon HE, Murphy AS, Bates M: Endothelial cell sarcoma of the liver following Thorotrast injection. Am J Pathol 23:585, 1947

75. da Silva HJ, Abbott JD, Cayolla da Mott L, et al.: Malignancy and other late effects following administration of Thorotrast. Lancet 2:201, 1965

76. Regelson W, Kim U, Ospina J, et al.: Hemangioendothelial sarcoma of liver from chronic arsenic intoxication by Fowler's solution. Cancer 21:514, 1968

77. Creech JL Jr., Johnson MN: Angiosarcoma of the liver in the manufacture of polyvinyl chloride. J Occup Med 16: 150, 1974

78. Block JB: Angiosarcoma of the liver following vinyl chloride exposure. JAMA 229:53, 1974

79. Lloyd JW: Angiosarcoma of the liver in vinyl chloride/polyvinyl chloride workers. J Occup Med 16:809, 1974

80. Heath CW, Falk H, Creech JL: Characteristics of cases of angiosarcoma of the liver among vinyl chloride workers in the United States. Ann NY Acad Sci 246, 231:1975

81. Lander JJ, Stanley RJ, Sumner HW, et al.: Angiosarcoma of the liver associated with Fowler's solution (potassium arsenite). Gastroenterology 68:1582, 1975

82. Popper H: The heuristic importance of environmental pathology: Lessons from the vinyl chloride program. Arch Pathol 99:71, 1975

83. Thomas LB, Popper H, Berk PD, et al.: Vinyl-chloride-induced liver disease: From idiopathic portal hypertension (Banti's syndrome) to angiosarcomas. N Engl J Med 292:17, 1975

84. Doll R: Discussion, toxicity of vinyl chloride-polyvinyl chloride. Ann NY Acad Sci 246:320, 1975

85. Vinyl chloride and cancer (editorial). Can Med Assoc J 112:269, 1975

86. Fiechtner JJ, Reyes CN Jr: Angiosarcoma of the liver in a rural population: Four cases diagnosed in a 29-month period. JAMA 236:1704, 1976

87. Dalderup LM, Freni SC, Bras G, et al.: Angiosarcoma of the liver. Lancet 1:246, 1976

88. Chen KTK, Hoffman KD, Hendricks EJ: Angiosarcoma following irradiation. Cancer 44:2044, 1979

89. Davies JD, Rees GIG, Mefra SL: Angiosarcoma in irradiated postmastectomy chest wall. Histopathology 7:947, 1983

90. Hodgkinson DJ, Soule EH, Wood JE: Cutaneous angiosarcoma of the head and neck. Cancer 44:1106, 1979

91. Paik HH, Komorowski R: Hemangiosarcoma of the abdominal wall following radiation therapy of endometrial carcinoma. Am J Clin Pathol 66:810, 1976

92. Weingrad DN, Rosenberg SA: Early lymphatic spread of osteogenic and soft tissue sarcomas. Surgery 231, 1978

93. Theile FS: Uber Angiome und sarkomatose Angiome der Milz. Virchows Arch [A] 178:296, 1904

94. Fletcher CDM, Behan A, Bekir S, et al.: Epithelioid angiosarcoma of the soft tissues: A distinctive tumor readily mistaken for an epithelial neoplasm. Am J Surg Pathol 15:915, 1991

95. McNeer GP, Cantin J, Chu F, Nickson JJ: Effectiveness of radiation therapy in the management of sarcoma of the soft somatic tissues. Cancer 22:391, 1968

96. Schmidt GB. Uber das Angiosarkom der Manima. Arch Klin Chir 26:121, 1887

97. Borrman R: Metastasenaildung bei histologisch gutartign Geschwiilsten. Beitr Pathol Anat 40: 372, 1907

98. Topuzlu C, Andrews WE, Trainer TK, Caccavo FA: Angiosarcoma of the carotid body. Am J Surg 117:400, 1969

99. Holden CA, Jones EW: Angiosarcoma of the face and scalp. J R Soc Med (suppl 11) 78:30, 1985

100. Holden CA, Spittle M, Jones EW: Angiosarcoma of the face and scalp: Prognosis and treatment. Cancer 59: 1046, 1987

101. Bennett MT, Weber PM, Killebrew ET: Primary angiosarcoma of the heart detected by technetium-labeled erythrocyte cardiac imaging. Cancer 49:2587, 1982

102. Alrenga DP: Primary angiosarcoma of the liver. Int J Surg 60:198, 1975

103. Aranha GV, Gold J, Grage TB: Hemangiosarcoma of the spleen: Report of a case and review of previously reported cases. J Surg Oncol 8:481, 1976

104. Autry JR, Weitzner S: Hemangiosarcoma of spleen with spontaneous rupture. Cancer 35:534, 1975

105. Garlock JH: Primary angiosarcoma of the spleen. Mt Sinai J Med 6:319, 1940

106. Smith C, Rusk G: Endothelioma of the spleen. Arch Surg 7:371, 1923

107. Ferrara G, Shione R: L'Angiosarcoma primitive della milza. Rass Fisiopat Chn 27:759, 1955

108. Boume M, Cook T, Williams G: Hemangiosarcomatosis—Two cases presenting as hematologic problems. Br Med J 213:275, 1965

109. Wilkinson H, Lucas J, Foote T: Primary splenic angiosarcoma. Arch Pathol 85:213, 1968

110. Castrup HJ, Lennartz KJ: Haemangiosarkom der Milz. Zentralbl Allg Pathol 113:395, 1970

111. Donald D, Dawson D: Microangiopathic hemolytic anemia associated with hemangioendothelioma. J Clin Pathol 24:456, 1971

112. Toghill PJ, Rigby C, Hall G: Hemangiosarcoma of the spleen. Br J Surg 59:406, 1972

113. Stutz F, Tormey PC, Blom J: Hemangiosarcoma and pathologic rupture of the spleen. Cancer 31:1213, 1973

114. Hopfner C, Dufour M, Bluot M, Caulet T: Hemangioendotheliosarcoma splenique avec erythrophagocytose et angiopathie thrombotique. Virchows Arch [A] 356:66, 1975

115. Ongkasuwan C, Taylor JE, Tang C, Prempree T: Angiosarcomas of the uterus and ovary: A clinicopathologic report. Cancer 49:1469, 1982

116. Conway JD, Smith MB: Hemangioendothelioma originating in a peripheral nerve. Ann Surg 134:138, 1951

117. Bricklin AS, Rushton HW: Angiosarcoma of venous origin in radial nerve. Cancer 39:1556, 1977

118. Brown RW, Toronos C, Evans HL: Angiosarcoma arising from malignant schwannoma in a patient with neurofibromatosis. Cancer 48:1141, 1992

119. Chaudhuri B, Ronan SGR, Manaligod JR: Angiosarcoma arising in a plexiform neurofibroma. Cancer 46:605, 1980

120. Meis JM, Kindblom LG, Enzinger FM: Angiosarcoma arising in von Recklinghausen's disease (NF-1): Report of 5 additional cases. Mol Pathol 7:8A, 1994

121. Kaposi M: Idiopathisches multiples pigmet Sarkom der Haut. Arch Dermatol Syph 4:265, 1872

122. O'Brien PH, Brasfield RD: Kaposi's sarcoma. Cancer 19:1497, 1966

123. Rothman S: Some clinical aspects of Kaposi's sarcoma in the European population. Acta Univ Int Cancer 18:382, 1962

124. Lee FD: A comparative study of Kaposi's sarcoma and granuloma pyogenicum in Uganda. J Clin Pathol 21:119, 1966

125. Taylor JF, Smith PG, Bull D, Pike MC: Kaposi's sarcoma in Uganda—Geographic and ethnic distribution. Br J Cancer 26:483, 1972

126. Taylor JF, Templeton AC, Bogel CL, et al.: Kaposi's sarcoma in Uganda—A clinical pathological study. Int J Cancer 22:122, 1971

127. Gordon JA: Kaposi's sarcoma: A review of 136 Rhodesian African cases. Postgrad Med J 43:513, 1967

128. Oettle AG: Geographical and racial differences in the frequency of Kaposi's sarcoma as evidence of environmental or genetic causes. Acta Univ Int Cancer 18:331, 1962

129. Slavin G, Cameron HM, Singh H: Kaposi's sarcoma in mainland Tanzania: A report of 117 cases. Br J Cancer 23:349, 1969

130. Oettle AG: Geographical and racial differences in the frequency of Kaposi's sarcoma as evidence of environmental or genetic causes. In Symposium on Kaposi's Sarcoma. Monograph No. 2, African Cancer Committee of the International Union Against Cancer. New York, Karger, 1963, p 17

131. Elmes BG, Baldwin RBJ: Malignant disease in Nigeria: An analysis of a thousand tumors. Ann Trop Med Parasitol 41:321, 1944

132. Edington GM: Malignant disease in the Gold Coast. Br J Cancer 10:595, 1956

133. Thijs A: Considerations sur les tumeurs malignes des indigenes du Congo Belge et du Ruande-Urundi. A propos de 2536 cas. Ann Soc Beig Med Trop 37:295, 1957

134. Higginson J, Oettle A: Cancer incidence in the Bantu and "Cape Colored" races of South Africa: Report of a cancer survey in the Transvaal (1953 to 1955). J Natl Cancer Inst 24:589, 1960

135. Timms GL: Personal communication (1961) quoted by Oettle AG, 1962

136. Lothe F: Kaposi's sarcoma in Ugandan Africans. Acta Pathol Microbiol Scand (Suppl. 161)1:1, 1963

137. Gilbert TT, Evjy JT, Edelstein L: Hodgkin's disease associated with Kaposi's sarcoma and malignant melanoma: Case report of multiple primary malignancies. Cancer 28:293, 1971

138. Master SP, Taylor JF, Kyalwazi SK, Ziegler JL: Immunological studies in Kaposi's sarcoma and malignant melanoma: Case report of multiple primary malignancies. Cancer 28:293, 1971

139. Hardy MA, Goldfarb P, Levine S, et al.: De novo Kaposi's sarcoma in renal transplantation: Case report and brief review. Cancer 38:144, 1976

140. Dobozy B: Immune deficiencies and Kaposi's sarcoma (letter). Lancet 1:625, 1973

141. Haim S, Shafir A, Better DS, et al.: Kaposi's sarcoma in association with immunosuppressive therapy. Ir J Med Sci 8:1993, 1972

142. Myers BD, Kessler E, Levi J, et al.: Kaposi's sarcoma in kidney transplant recipients. Arch Intern Med 133:370, 1974

143. Taylor JF: Lymphocyte transformation in Kaposi's sarcoma (letter). Lancet 2:883, 1973

144. Trattner A, Hodak E, David M, et al.: Kaposi's sarcoma with visceral involvement after intra-articular and epidural injections of corticosteroids. J Am Acad Dermatol 29(5 Pt 2):890, 1993

145. Farge D: Kaposi's sarcoma in organ transplant recipients. The Collaborative Transplantation Research Group of Ile de France. Eur J Med 2(6):339, 1993

146. Pedagogos E, Nicholls K, Dowling J, Becker G: Kaposi's sarcoma postrenal transplantation. Aust NZ J Med 24(6):722, 1994

147. Helg C, Adatto M, Salomon D, et al.: Kaposi's sarcoma following allogeneic bone marrow transplantation. Bone Marrow Transplant 14(6):999, 1994

148. Margolius L, Stein M, Spencer D, Bezwoda WR: Kaposi's sarcoma in renal transplant recipients. Experience at Johannesburg Hospital, 1966–1989. South Afr Med J 84(1):16, 1994

149. Hertzler G, Gordon SM, Piratzky J, et al.: Case report: Fulminant Kaposi's sarcoma after orthotopic liver transplantation. Am J Med Sci 309(5)278, 1995

150. Lopez-Rubio F, Anguita M, Arizon JM, et al.: Visceral Kaposi's sarcoma without mucocutaneous involvement in a heart transplant recipient. J Heart Lung Transplant 13(5):913, 1994

151. Reynolds WA, Winkelman RK, Soule EH: Kaposi's sarcoma. Medicine 44:419, 1965

152. Mazzaferri EL, Penn GM: Kaposi's sarcoma associated with multiple myeloma. Arch Intern Med 122:521, 1968

153. Giraldo G, Beth E, Coeur P, et al.: A new model in

search for viruses associated with human malignancies. J Natl Cancer Inst 49:1496, 1972

154. Friedman-Kien AE: Disseminated Kaposi's sarcoma in young homosexual men. J Am Acad Dermatol 5(4–6): 468, 1981

155. Bigger RJ, Melbye M, Kesten SL, et al.: Kaposi's sarcoma in Zaire is not associated with HLTV-III infection. N Engl J Med 311:1051, 1984

156. Huang YQ, Li JJ, Rush MG, et al.: HPV-16 related DNA sequences in Kaposi's sarcoma. Lancet 339:515, 1992

157. Nickoloft BJ, Huang YQ, Li JJ et al.: Immunohistochemical detection of papillomavirus antigens in Kaposi's sarcoma. Lancet 339:548, 1992

158. Ensoli B, Barillari G, Salahuddin SZ, et al.: Tat proteins of HIV-I stimulates growth of cells derived from Kaposi's sarcoma: Lesions of AIDS patients. Nature 345:84, 1990

159. Ensoli B, Nakamura S, Salahuddin SZ: AIDS-Kaposi's cells long-term culture with growth factor from retrovirus infected CD4+ T cells. Science 242:430, 1988

160. Mohaz JH, Zelickson AS: Electron microscopic observations of Kaposi's sarcoma. Acta Derm Venereol 46:195, 1966

161. Nakamura S, Salahuddin SZ, Biberfeld P, et al.: Kaposi's sarcoma cells long term culture with growth factor from retrovirus infected CD4+ T cells. Science 242:426, 1988

162. Cook J: Kaposi's sarcoma. J R Coll Surg Edinb 2:519, 1966

163. Bluefarb SM: Kaposi's Sarcoma: Multiple Idiopathic Hemorrhagic Sarcoma. Springfield, Ill., Thomas, 1957, p 123

164. Ackerman LV, Murray JF: Symposium en Kaposi's sarcoma. Acta Univ Intern Cancer 18:311, 1962

165. Safai B, Johnson KG, Myskowski PL, et al.: The natural history of Kaposi's sarcoma in the acquired immunohistodeficiency syndrome. Ann Intern Med 103:744, 1985

166. Bhana D, Templeton AC, Master SP, Kyalwazj SK: Kaposi's sarcoma of lymph nodes. Br J Cancer 15:464, 1970

167. Gonzalez-Crussi F, Mossemen A, Robertson DM: Neurological involvement in Kaposi's sarcoma. Can Med Assoc J 100:481, 1969

168. Dorffel J: Histogenesis of multiple idiopathic hemorrhagic sarcoma of Kaposi's sarcoma. Arch Dermatol Syph 26:608, 1932

169. White JAM, King MJ: Kaposi's sarcoma presenting with abdominal symptoms. Gastroenterology 46:197, 1964

170. Adlersberg R: Kaposi's sarcoma complicating ulcerative colitis: Report of a case. Am J Clin Pathol 54:143, 1970

171. Gordon HW, Rywlin AM: Kaposi's sarcoma of the large intestine associated with ulcerative colitis. A hitherto unreported occurrence. Gastroenterology 50:248, 1966

172. Gellin GA: Kaposi's sarcoma: Three cases of which two have unusual findings in association. Arch Dermatol 94:92, 1966

173. Stats D: Visceral manifestations of Kaposi's sarcoma. J Mt Sinai Hosp 12:971, 1946

174. Siegel JH, Janis R, Alper JC, et al.: Disseminated visceral Kaposi's sarcoma: Appearance after human renal homograft operation. JAMA 207:1493, 1969

175. Gibbs RC, Hyman AB: Kaposi's sarcoma at the base of a cutaneous horn. Arch Dermatol 98:37, 1968

176. Farman AG, Uys PB: Oral Kaposi's sarcoma. Oral Surg 39:288, 1975

177. Rajka G: Kaposi's sarcoma associated with Hodgkin's disease. Acta Derm Venereol 45:40, 1965

178. Ecklund RE, Valaitis J: Kaposi's sarcoma of lymph nodes: A case report. Arch Pathol 74:244, 1962

179. Lee SCH, Moore OS: Kaposi's sarcoma of lymph nodes. Arch Pathol 80:651, 1965

180. Cox FH, Helwig EB: Kaposi's sarcoma. Cancer 12:289, 1959

181. Gibbs R: Kaposi's sarcoma involving ears. Arch Dermatol 98:104, 1968

182. Dutz W, Stout AP: Kaposi's sarcoma in infants and children. Cancer 13:684, 1960

183. Dorfman RF: Kaposi's sarcoma with special reference to its manifestation in infants and children and to concepts of Arthur Purdy Stout. Am J Surg Pathol (suppl) 10:68, 1986

184. Mortel CC: Multiple primary malignant neoplasms, their incidence and significance. In: Recent Results in Cancer Research, vol 7. New York, Springer-Verlag, 1966, p 34

185. Mazzaferri EL, Penn GM: Kaposi's sarcoma associated with multiple myeloma. Arch Intern Med 122:521, 1968

186. Maberry JD, Stone OJ: Kaposi's sarcoma with thymoma. Arch Dermatol 95:210, 1967

187. Harwood A: Kaposi's sarcoma in renal transplant patients. In: AIDS: The Epidemic of Kaposi's Sarcoma and Opportunistic Infections. New York, Masson, 1984

188. Qurubi WY, Barri Y, Alfurayh O, et al.: Kaposi's sarcoma in renal transplant recipients: A report of 26 cases from a single institution. Transplant Proc 25:1402, 1993

189. Shmueli D, Shapira Z, Yussim A, et al.: The incidence of Kaposi's sarcoma in renal transplantation patients and its relation to immunosuppression. Transplant Proc 21:3209, 1989

190. Scott WP, Voight JA: Kaposi's sarcoma: Management with vincaleucoblastine. Cancer 19:557, 1966

191. Vogel CL, Templeton CJ, Templeton AC, et al.: Treatment of Kaposi's sarcoma with actinomycin-D and cyclophosphamide: Results of a randomized clinical trial. Int J Cancer 8:136, 1971

192. Vogel CL, Primack A, Dhru D, et al.: Treatment of a Kaposi's sarcoma with a combination of actinomycin-D and vincristine: Results of a randomized clinical trial. Cancer 51:1382, 1973

193. Vogel CL, Clements D, Wanume DK, et al.: Phase II clinical trials of BCNU (NSC-409962) and bleomycin (NSC-125066) in the treatment of Kaposi's sarcoma. Cancer Chemother Rep 57:325, 1973

194. Shmueli D, Shapira Z, Yussim A, et al.: The incidence of Kaposi's sarcoma in renal transplantation patients and its relation to immunosuppression. Transplant Proc 21:3209, 1989

195. Buchbinder A, Friedman-Kien AE: Clinical aspects of epidemic Kaposi's sarcoma. Cancer Surv 10:39, 1991

196. Biggar RJ, Curtis RE, Cote TR, et al.: Risk of other cancers following Kaposi's sarcoma: Relation to acquired immunodeficiency syndrome. Am J Epidemiol 139:362, 1994

197. Miles SA: Pathogenesis of HIV-related Kaposi's sarcoma. Cur Opin Oncol 6:497, 1994

198. Hardy AM: Characterization of long-term survivors of acquired immunodeficiency syndrome. The Long-term Survivor Collaborative Study Group. J Acquir Immune Defic Syndr 4:386, 1991

199. Geddes M, Francheschi S, Banchielli A, et al.: Kaposi's sarcoma in Italy before and after the AIDS epidemic. Br J Cancer, 69:333, 1994

200. Reynolds P, Saunders LD, Layefsky ME, Lemp GF: The spectrum of acquired immunodeficiency syndrome (AIDS)-associated malignancies in San Francisco, 1980–1987. Am J Epidemiol 137:19, 1993

201. Nichols CM, Flaitz CM, Hicks MJ: Treating Kaposi's lesions in the HIV-infected patient. J Am Dent Assoc 124(11):78, 1993

202. Hoover DR, Black C, Jacobson LP, et al.: Epidemiologic analysis of Kaposi's sarcoma as an early and later AIDS outcome in homosexual men. Am J Epidemiol 138(4): 266, 1993

203. Armenian HK, Hoover DR, Rubb S, et al.: Composite risk score for Kaposi's sarcoma based on a case-control and longitudinal study in the Multicenter AIDS Cohort Study (MACS) population. Am J Epidemiol 138(4):256, 1993

204. Bernstein L, Hamilton AS: The epidemiology of AIDS-related malignancies. Cur Opin Oncol 5(5):822, 1993

205. Haverkos HW, Drotman DP: Measuring inhalant nitrite exposure in gay men: Implications for elucidating the etiology of AIDS-related Kaposi's sarcoma. Genetica 95(1–3):157, 1995

206. Drotman DP, Peterman TA, Friedman-Kien AE: Kaposi's sarcoma. How can epidemiology help find the cause? Dermatol Clin 13(3):575, 1995

207. Tirelli U, Vaccher E, Lazzanin A, et al.: Epidemic Kaposi's sarcoma in Italy, a country with intravenous drug users as the main group affected by HIV infection. Ann Oncol 2(5):373, 1991

208. Lundgren JD, Melbye M, Pederson C, et al.: Changing patterns of Kaposi's sarcoma in Danish acquired immunodeficiency syndrome patients with complete follow-up. The Danish Study Group for HIV Infection (DASHI). Am J Epidemiol 141(7):652, 1995

209. Schechter MT, Marion SA, Elmslie KD, et al.: Geographic and birth cohort associations of Kaposi's sarcoma among homosexual men in Canada. Am J Epidemiol 134(5):485, 1991

210. Veugelers PJ, Strathdee SA, Moss AR, et al.: Is the human immunodeficiency virus related Kaposi's sarcoma epidemic coming to an end? Insight from the tricontinental seroconversion study. Epidemiology 6(4): 382, 1995

211. Beral V, Bull D, Darby S, et al.: Risk of Kaposi's sarcoma and sexual practices associated with faecal contact in homosexual or bisexual men with AIDS. Lancet 339(8794):632, 1992

212. Rady PL, Yen A, Rollefson JL, et al.: Herpesvirus-like DNA sequences in non-Kaposi's sarcoma skin lesions of transplant patients. Lancet 345(8961):1339, 1995

213. Kempf W, Adams V, Pfaltz M, et al.: Human herpesvirus type 6 and cytomegalovirus in AIDS-associated Kaposi's sarcoma: No evidence for an etiological association. Hum Pathol 26(8):914, 1995

214. Albini A, Barillari G, Benelli R, et al.: Angiogenic properties of human immunodeficiency virus type 1 Tat protein. Proc Natl Acad Sci U S A 92(11):4838, 1995

215. Adams V, Kempf W, Hassam S, et al.: Detection of several types of human papilloma viruses in AIDS-associated Kaposi's sarcoma. J Med Virol 46(3):189, 1995

216. Cohen J: Controversy: Is KS really caused by new herpesvirus? Science 268(5219):1847, 1995

217. Anonymous: New research suggests herpes virus may cause Kaposi's sarcoma. Infect Control Hosp Epidemiol 16(3):186, 1995

218. Huang YQ, Li JJ, Kaplan MH, et al.: Human herpesvirus-like nucleic acid in various forms of Kaposi's sarcoma. Lancet 345(8952):759, 1995

219. Dupin N, Grandadam M, Calvez V, et al.: Herpesvirus-like DNA sequences in patients with Mediterranean Kaposi's sarcoma. Lancet 345(8952):761, 1995

220. Montagnino G, Bencini PL, Tarantino A, et al.: Clinical features and course of Kaposi's sarcoma in kidney transplant patients: Report of 13 cases. Am J Nephrol 14(2): 121, 1994

221. Flaitz CM, Nichols CM, Hicks MJ: An overview of the oral manifestations of AIDS-related Kaposi's sarcoma. Compendium 16(2):136, 1995

222. Singh B, Har-el G, Lucente FE: Kaposi's sarcoma of the head and neck in patients with acquired immunodeficiency syndrome. Otolaryngol Head Neck Surg 111(5): 618, 1994

223. Mongiardo FD, Tewfik TL: Kaposi's sarcoma of the intra-parotid lymph nodes in AIDS. J Otolaryngol 20(4): 243, 1991

224. Goldberg AN: Kaposi's sarcoma of the head and neck in acquired immunodeficiency syndrome. Am J Otolaryngol 14(1):5, 1993

225. Ravera M, Reggiori A, Cocozza E, et al.: Kaposi's sarcoma and AIDS in Uganda: Its frequency and gastrointestinal distribution. Ital J Gastroenterol 26(7):329, 1994

226. Danzig JB, Brandt LJ, Reinus JF, Klein RS: Gastrointestinal malignancy in patients with AIDS. Am J Gastroenterol 86(6):715, 1991

227. Parente F, Cernuschi M, Orlando G, et al.: Kaposi's sarcoma and AIDS: Frequency of gastrointestinal involvement and its effect on survival. A prospective study in a heterogeneous population. Scand J Gastroenterol 26(10):1007, 1991

228. Hadjiyane C, Lee YH, Stein L, et al.: Kaposi's sarcoma presenting as linitis plastica. Am J Gastroenterol 86(12): 1823, 1991

229. Sarode VR, Datta BN, Savitri K, et al.: Kaposi's sarcoma of spleen with unusual clinical and histologic features. Arch Pathol Lab Med 115(10):1042, 1991

230. Ravalli S, Vincent RA, Beaton HL: Acute appendicitis secondary to Kaposi's sarcoma in the acquired immunodeficiency syndrome. NY State J Med 91(9):401, 1991

231. Chetty R, Slavin JL, Miller RA: Kaposi's sarcoma presenting as acute appendicitis in an HIV-1 positive patient. Histopathology 23(6):590, 1993

232. Deziel DJ, Saclarides TJ, Marshall JS, Yaremko LM: Appendiceal Kaposi's sarcoma: A cause of right lower quadrant pain in the acquired immune deficiency syndrome. Am J Gastroenterol 86(7):901, 1991

233. Wien FE, Samanta A, Venkataseshan VS, Kiernan TW: Gastric hemorrhage and Kaposi's sarcoma treated with radiotherapy. NJ Med 88:42, 1991

234. Bossuyt L, Van den Oord JJ, Degreef H: Lymphangioma-like variant of AIDS-associated Kaposi's sarcoma with pronounced edema formation. Dermatology 190:324, 1995

235. Allen PJ, Gillespie DL, Redfield RR, Gomez ER: Lower extremity lymphedema caused by acquired immune deficiency syndrome-related Kaposi's sarcoma: Case report and review of the literature. J Vasc Surg 22:178, 1995

236. Oehler RL, Sinnott JT, Arepally G, Dunn YP: Kaposi's sarcoma mimicking cellulitis. Postgrad Med 94:139, 1993

237. Leal R, Lewin M, Ahmad I, Korula J: Peritoneal Kaposi's sarcoma: A cause of ascites in acquired immunodeficiency syndrome. Dig Dis Sci 39:206, 1994

238. Fife KM, Talbot DC, Mortimer P, et al.: Chylous ascites in Kaposi's sarcoma: A case report. Br J Dermatol 126:378, 1992

239. Priest ER, Weiss R: Chylothorax with Kaposi's sarcoma. South Med J, 84:806, 1991

240. Macasaet MA, Duerr A, Thelmo W, et al.: Kaposi sarcoma presenting as a vulvar mass. Obstet Gynecol 86:695, 1995

241. Sadaghdar H, Eden E: Pulmonary Kaposi's sarcoma presenting as fulminant respiratory failure. Chest 100:858, 1991

242. Suster S: Primary sarcomas of the lung. Semin Diagn Pathol 12:140, 1995

243. Roux FJ, Bancal C, Dombret MC, et al.: Pulmonary Kaposi's sarcoma revealed by a solitary nodule in a patient with acquired immunodeficiency syndrome (review). Am J Respir Crit Care Med 149:1041, 1994

244. Raaf HN, Raaf JH: Sarcomas related to the heart and vasculature. Semin Surg Oncol 10:374, 1994

245. Mollison LC, Mijch A, McBride G, Dwyer B: Hypothyroidism due to destruction of the thyroid by Kaposi's sarcoma. Rev Infect Dis 13:826, 1991

246. Levin M, Hertzberg L: Kaposi's sarcoma of the bone marrow presenting with fever of unknown origin. Med Pediatr Oncol 22:410, 1994

247. Isenbarger DW, Aronson NE: Lytic vertebral lesions: An unusual manifestation of AIDS-associated Kaposi's sarcoma (review). Clin Infect Dis 19:751, 1994

248. Langford A, Pohle HD, Reichart P: Primary intraosseous AIDS-associated Kaposi's sarcoma. Report of two cases with initial jaw involvement. Int J Oral Maxillofac Surg 20:366, 1991

249. Conant MA: Management of human immunodeficiency virus-associated malignancies. Recent Results Cancer Res 139:423, 1995

250. Northfelt DW: Treatment of Kaposi's sarcoma. Current guidelines and future perspectives. Drugs 48:569, 1994

251. Kahn JO, Northfelt DW, Miles SA: AIDS-associated Kaposi's sarcoma. AIDS Clin Rev 261, 1992

252. Mischel PS, Vinters HV: Coccidioidomycosis of the central nervous system: Neuropathological and vasculo-pathic manifestations and clinical correlates. Clin Infect Dis 20:400, 1995

253. Trattner A, Reizis Z, David M, et al.: The therapeutic effect of intralesional interferon in classical Kaposi's sarcoma. Br J Dermatol, 129:590, 1993

254. Boudreaux AA, Smith LL, Cosby CD, et al.: Intralesional vinblastine for cutaneous Kaposi's sarcoma associated with acquired immunodeficiency syndrome. A clinical trial to evaluate efficacy and discomfort associated with infection. J Am Acad Dermatol 28:61, 1993

255. Epstein JB: Treatment of oral Kaposi's sarcoma with intralesional vinblastine. Cancer 71:1722, 1993

256. Hebeda KM, Huizing MT, Brouwer PA, et al.: Photodynamic therapy in AIDS-related cutaneous Kaposi's sarcoma. J Acquir Immune Defic Syndr Hum Retrovirol 10:61, 1995

257. Piedbois P, Frikha H, Martin L, et al.: Radiotherapy in the management of epidemic Kaposi's sarcoma. Int J Radiat Oncol Biol Phys 30:1207, 1994

258. Piccinno R, Caccialanza M, Cusini M: Role of radiotherapy in the treatment of epidemic Kaposi's sarcoma: Experience with sixty-five cases. J Am Acad Dermatol 32:1000, 1995

259. Stelzer KJ, Griffin TW: A randomized prospective trial of radiation therapy for AIDS-associated Kaposi's sarcoma. Int J Radiat Oncol Biol Phys 27:1057, 1993

260. Meyer JL: Whole-lung irradiation for Kaposi's sarcoma. Am J Clin Oncol 16:372, 1993

261. Le Bourgeois JP, Frikha H, Piedbois P, et al.: Radiotherapy in the management of epidemic Kaposi's sarcoma of the oral cavity, the eyelid, and the genitals. Radiother Oncol 30:236, 1994

262. Garbe C: Perspective of cytokine treatment in malignant skin tumors. Recent Results Cancer Res 139:349, 1995

263. Mauss S, Jablonski H: Efficacy, safety, and tolerance of low-dose, long-term interferon-alpha 2b and zidovudine in early-stage AIDS-associated Kaposi's sarcoma. J Acquir Immune Defic Syndr Hum Retrovirol 10:157, 1995

264. Paredes J, Kahn JO, Tong WP, et al.: Weekly oral etoposide in patients with Kaposi's sarcoma associated with human immunodeficiency virus infection: A phase I multicenter trial of the AIDS clinical trial group. J Acquir Immune Defic Syndr Hum Retrovirol 9:138, 1995

265. Saville MW, Lietzau J, Pluda JM, et al.: Treatment of HIV-associated Kaposi's sarcoma with paclitaxel. Lancet 346:26, 1995

266. Morfeldt L, Torssander J: Long-term remission of Kaposi's sarcoma following foscarnet treatment in HIV-infected patients. Scand J Infect Dis 26:749, 1994

267. Bakker PJ, Danner SA, ten Napel CH, et al.: Treatment of poor prognosis epidemic Kaposi's sarcoma with doxorubicin, bleomycin, vindesine, and recombinant human granulocyte-monocyte colony stimulating factor (rh GM-CSF). Eur J Cancer 31A:188, 1995

268. Gill PS, Miles SA, Mitsuyasu RT, et al.: Phase I AIDS Clinical Trials Group (075) study of adriamycin, bleomycin, and vincristine chemotherapy with zidovudine in the treatment of AIDS-related Kaposi's sarcoma. AIDS 8:1695, 1994

269. Harrison M, Tomlinson D, Stewart S: Liposomal-entrapped doxorubicin: An active agent in AIDS-related Kaposi's sarcoma. J Clin Oncol 13:914, 1995

270. Wagner D, Kern WV, Kern P: Liposomal doxorubicin in AIDS-related Kaposi's sarcoma: Long-term experiences. Clin Investig 72:417, 1994

271. James ND, Coker RJ, Tomlinson D, et al.: Liposomal doxorubicin (Doxil): An effective new treatment for Kaposi's sarcoma in AIDS. Clin Oncol (R Coll Radiol) 6:294, 1994

272. Scadden DT, Bering HA, Levine JD, et al.: Granulocyte-macrophage colony-stimulating factor mitigates the neutropenia of combined interferon alfa and zidovudine treatment of acquired immune deficiency syndrome-associated Kaposi's sarcoma. J Clin Oncol 9:802, 1991

273. Alonso K, Pontiggia P, Nardi C, et al.: Systemic hyperthermia in the treatment of HIV-related Kaposi's sarcoma. A phase I study. Biomed Pharmacother 46:21, 1992

274. Logan WD Jr., Alonso K: Total body hyperthermia in the treatment of Kaposi's sarcoma in an HIV positive patient. Med Oncol Tumor Pharmacother 8:45, 1991

275. Bailey J, Pluda JM, Foli A, et al.: Phase I/II study of intermittent all-trans-retinoic acid, alone and in combination with interferon alfa-2a, in patients with epidemic Kaposi's sarcoma. J Clin Oncol 13:1966, 1995

276. Lunardi-Iskandar Y, Bryan JL, Zeman RA, et al.: Tumorigenesis and metastasis of neoplastic Kaposi's sarcoma cell line in immunodeficient mice blocked by a human pregnancy hormone. Nature 375:64, 1995

277. Harris PJ: Treatment of Kaposi's sarcoma and other manifestations of AIDS with human chorionic gonadotropin. Lancet 346:118, 1995

278. Carmeli Y, Mevorach D, Kaminski N, Raz E: Regression of Kaposi's sarcoma after intravenous immunoglobulin treatment for polymyositis. Cancer 73:2859, 1994

279. Lee WA, Hutchins GM: Cluster analysis of the metastatic patterns of human immunodeficiency virus-associated Kaposi's sarcoma. Hum Pathol 23:306, 1992

280. Miles SA, Wang H, Elashoff R, Mitsuyasu RT: Improved survival for patients with AIDS-related Kaposi's sarcoma. J Clin Oncol 12:1910, 1994

281. Orfanos CE, Husak R, Wolfer U, Garbe C: Kaposi's sarcoma: A reevaluation (review). Recent Results Cancer Res 139:275, 1995

282. Tambussi G, Repetto L, Torri V, et al.: Epidemic HIV-related Kaposi's sarcoma: A retrospective analysis and validation of TIS staging. GICAT. Gruppo Italiano Collaborativo AIDS e Tumori. Ann Oncol 6:383, 1995

283. McKenzie R, Travis WD, Dolan SA, et al.: The causes of death in patients with human immunodeficiency virus infection: A clinical and pathologic study with emphasis on the role of pulmonary diseases. Medicine 70:326, 1991

284. Weiss SW, Sobin LH: WHO Classification of Soft Tissue Tumors. Berlin, Springer-Verlag, 1994

285. Murad TM, Von Haam E, Murthy MSN: Ultrastructure of a hemangiopericytoma and a glomus tumor. Cancer 22:1239, 1968

286. Battifora H: Hemangiopericytoma: Ultrastructural study of five cases. Cancer 31:1418, 1973

287. Tocker C: Glomangioma: An ultrastructural study. Cancer 23:487, 1969

288. Venkatachalan MA, Greally JG: Fine structure of glomus tumor: Similarity of glomus cells to smooth muscle. Cancer 23:1176, 1969

289. Tarnowski WM, Hashimoto K: Multiple glomus tumors: An ultrastructural study. J Invest Dermatol 52:474, 1969

290. Shugart RR, Soule EH, Johnson EW: Glomus tumors. Surg Gynecol Obstet 117:334, 1963

291. Brindley GV: Glomus tumor of the mediastinum. J Thorac Surg 18:417, 1949

292. Appelman HD, Helwig EB: Glomus tumors of the stomach. Cancer 23:203, 1969

293. Banner EA, Winkelman RK: Glomus tumor of vagina: Report of a case. Obstet Gynecol 9:326, 1957

294. Albrecht S, Zbieranowski I: Incidental glomus coccygeum: When a normal structure looks like a tumor. Am J Surg Pathol 14:922, 1990

295. Duncan L, Halverson J, DeSchryver-Kecskemeti K: Glomus tumors of the coccyx: A curable cause of coccygodymia. Arch Pathol Lab Med 115:78, 1991

296. Lattes R, Bull DC: A case of glomus tumor with primary involvement of bone. Ann Surg 127:187, 1948

297. Haque S, Modlin IM, West AB: Multiple glomus tumors of the stomach with intravascular spread. Am J Surg Pathol 16:291, 1992

298. Riveros M, Pack GT: The glomus tumors: Report of 20 cases. Ann Surg 133:394, 1951

299. Tsuneyoshi M, Enjoji M: Glomus tumor: A clinicopathologic and electron microscopic study. Cancer 50:1601, 1981

300. Aiba M, Hirayama A, Kuramuochi S: Glomangiosarcoma in a glomus tumor: An immunohistochemical and ultrastructural study. Cancer 61:1467, 1988

301. Gould EW, Manivel JC, Albores-Saavedra J, et al.: Locally infiltrative glomus tumors and glomangiosarcomas: A clinical ultrastructural and immunohistochemical study. Cancer 65:310, 1992

302. Stout AP, Murray MR: Hemangiopericytoma: A vascular tumor featuring Zimmerman's pericytes. Ann Surg 116:26, 1942

303. Stout AP: Hemangiopericytoma: A study of twenty-five new cases. Cancer 2:1027, 1949

304. Maltoni C, Lefemine G: Carcinogenicity bioassays of vinyl chloride: Current results. Ann NY Acad Sci 245:175, 1975

305. Prout MN, Davis HL Jr.: Hemangiopericytoma of the bladder after polyvinyl alcohol exposure. Cancer 39:1328, 1977

306. Enzinger M, Smith BH: Hemangiopericytoma: An analysis of 106 cases. Hum Pathol 7:61, 1976

307. McMaster MJ, Soule EH, Ivins JC: Hemangiopericytoma: A clinicopathologic study and long-term follow-up of 60 patients. Cancer 36:2232, 1975

308. O'Brien B, Brasfield RD: Hemangiopericytoma. Cancer 18:249, 1965

309. Backwinkle KD, Diddams JA: Hemangiopericytoma:

Report of a case and comprehensive review of the literature. Cancer 25:896, 1970

310. Angerval L, Kindblom LG, Nielsen JM, et al.: Hemangiopericytoma: A clinicopathologic, angiographic and microangiographic study. Cancer 42:4212, 1978

311. McCormack LJ, Gallivan WP: Hemangiopericytoma. Cancer 7:595, 1954

312. Ferguson JO, Clagett OT, McDonald JR: Hemangiopericytoma (glomus tumor) of the mediastinum—Review of literature and report of case. Surgery 36:320, 1954

313. Ernst CB, Abell MR, Kahn DR: Malignant hemangiopericytoma of the stomach. Surgery 58:351, 1965

314. Spiro RH, Brockunier A, Brunscwig A: Pelvic hemangiopericytoma. Obstet Gynecol 24:402,1964

315. Wilbanks GD, Szymanska Z, Miller AW: Pelvic hemangiopericytoma: Report of four patients and review of the literature. Am J Obstet Gynecol 123:555, 1975

316. Baglio CM, Growson CN: Hemangiopericytoma of urachus: Report of a case. J Urol 91:660, 1964

317. Lenczyk JM: Nasal hemangiopericytoma. Arch Otolaryngol 87:110, 1968

318. Lal H, Sanyal B, Pant GC, et al.: Hemangiopericytoma: Report of three cases regarding role of radiation therapy. Am J Roentgenol Radiat Ther Nucl Med 126:887, 1976

319. Mira JG, Chu FCH, Fortner JG: The role of radiotherapy in the management of malignant hemangiopericytoma: Report of eleven new cases and review of the literature. Cancer 39:1254, 1977

320. DasGupta TK, Ghosh BC: Principles of Diagnosis and Management of Soft Tissue Sarcomas. In: Nyhus LM (ed) Surg Ann NY: Appleton Century Croft, 1975

# 13

# Tumors of the Lymphatic Tissue

Tumor and tumorlike conditions of the lymphatic tissue can be clinically divided as follows:

A. Benign
   1. Lymphangiomas
      a. Papillary
      b. Cavernous
      c. Cystic hygroma
   2. Lymphangiectasis
      a. Local
      b. Regional
   3. Lymphangiomyoma and lymphangiomyomatosis
B. Malignant
   1. Lymphangiosarcoma
      a. Postmastectomy (Stewart-Treves syndrome)
      b. Not associated with mastectomy (e.g., arising from congenital edema of extremity)

## ■ BENIGN TUMORS

### LYMPHANGIOMA

Lymphangiomas are less common than hemangiomas. Although benign, they possess a remarkable power for continued growth, infiltration, and progressive extension over adjacent skin throughout childhood and adolescence, and occasionally even in adult life. Invariably, they are congenital malformations of the lymphatic system, and most are manifest in infancy. The condition of lymphangiectasis with edema due to lymphatic obstruc-

tion is not to be confused with the aforementioned lymphangiomas, which are hamartomatous growths. Nevertheless, lymphangiectasis or chronic lymphatic obstruction due to any cause should be considered in this relationship because it is sometimes a preneoplastic state, which ultimately results in lymphangiosarcoma.

Lymphangiomas can conceptually be viewed as blockage of lymphatic channels in any given location, with resultant ectasia of the channels and proliferation and infiltration of the surrounding structures. Their anatomic confines frequently determine their size, shape, and clinical characteristics; thus, lymphangiomas can be classified into three types: (1) simple or papillary, (2) cavernous, and (3) cystic hygroma.

### SIMPLE OR PAPILLARY LYMPHANGIOMA

Simple or papillary lymphangioma is composed of agminated, minute lymphatic cysts situated superficially in the skin and subcutaneous tissue and in the mucous membrane of the oral cavity.

### CAVERNOUS LYMPHANGIOMA

Cavernous lymphangioma is usually more discrete, of greater bulk, situated subcutaneously, and compressible but not fluctuant (Fig. 13–1). It is supported by a fibrous tissue lattice, which is interspersed with small multilocular cysts that are lined with smooth endothelial membrane containing lymph. The superadjacent skin may or may not be involved with tiny wartlike blobs that are pathognomonic of lymphangiomas. The cavernous variety is found in deeper locations where the

449

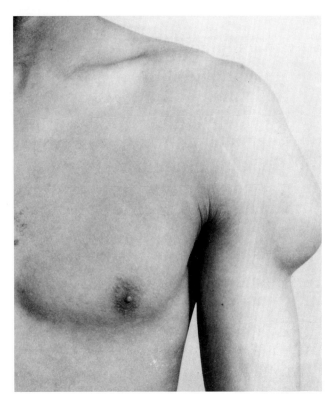

**Figure 13–1.** Simple papillary lymphangioma of the arm in a 29-year-old man. The lesion, 6 × 5 cm, was totally excised.

**TABLE 13–1. ANATOMIC DISTRIBUTION OF CAVERNOUS LYMPHANGIOMAS IN FOUR SERIES***

| Anatomic Site | Harkins and Sabiston[4] (1960) | Bill and Sumner[2] (1965) | Fonkalsrud[1] (1974) | Present Series (1996) |
|---|---|---|---|---|
| Head and neck | 14 | 35 | 9 | 3 |
| Trunk | 2 | 18 | 7 | 1 |
| Lower extremity | 8 | 3 | 9 | 4 |
| Upper extremity | 3 | 21 | 3 | 2 |
| Other locations | — | 6 | — | 3 |
| Total | 27 | 83 | 28 | 13 |

*The areas involved were tabulated rather than the total number of cases. Thus, a single extensive tumor involving the neck, axilla, and upper arm has been recorded three times.

anatomic boundaries prevent the development of large saccules, such as occurs in cystic hygromas. This type of lymphangioma is commonly encountered in the extremities, the trunk, the retroperitoneum, and the viscera.

Table 13–1 shows the incidence of cavernous lymphangiomas in different sites. Unlike cystic hygromas, they are relatively uncommon and sometimes are associated with hemangiomas. Eight (28.5 percent) of 28 patients in Fonkalsrud's[1] group had associated hemangiomas. In our series of 17 cases in the extremities, 9 were associated with hemangiomas. Of the other locations of cavernous lymphangioma (Table 13–1), Bill and Sumner[2] found five in the mediastinum and one in the mesentery. In our present series, two were in the pancreas, two in the retroperitoneum, and two in the pelvis.

This tumor occurs with about equal frequency in both sexes. The most common complaint is the presence of a gradually enlarging mass. Rapid expansion may be produced by hemorrhage or infection. In infancy, respiratory distress sometimes occurs if these lesions are located in the throat and neck, and may require emergency intervention. Although most of these lesions are diagnosed in infancy and childhood,[1–5] they occasionally are encountered in adult life, particularly in the viscera, retroperitoneum, and mediastinum.[2,6–15]

In our present series, two instances of retroperitoneal lymphangioma were encountered. One instance occurred in a 19-year-old boy with a history of a gradually enlarging abdomen over a period of three months. Clinical examination suggested ascites, but paracentesis revealed clear fluid, which yielded no clue regarding cytologic diagnosis. All the radiologic examinations were inconclusive as to the nature of the abdominal disease. He was operated on, and an enormous cyst was found completely filling the abdominal cavity. The cyst was excised in its entirety. The microscopic diagnosis was cystic and cavernous lymphangioma. Seventeen years later, he is still free of any evidence of recurrence.

In general, cavernous lymphangiomas require complete excision in most anatomic sites. For infants, if possible, the operation should be delayed. In symptomatic and enlarging lesions, this luxury of waiting must sometimes be foregone, and early operation becomes mandatory.[4] In some patients, complete excision is not possible, and staged resections are necessary. Staged procedures become essential in large lymphangiomas of the head and neck region: for example, those involving the tongue,[16] the floor of the mouth, and the cheek. The need for staged excision of extensive lymphangiomas of the trunk and the extremities is relatively infrequent (Fig. 13–2A and 13–2B). Amputation of an extremity for extensive lymphangioma has been reported by Harkins and Sabiston,[4] but the need for such an operation is extremely rare, and every effort should be made to avoid it. There is no evidence that a benign lymphangioma can become malignant, and therefore an aggressive surgical approach such as amputation must be tempered with judicious conservatism. Rarely, a lymphangioma infiltrating the surrounding structure makes either a part or all of the extremity totally useless, and, under these circumstances, an amputation might be indicated. Radiation therapy for lymphangioma has been tried,[3,4] but it should be avoided in the management of a benign lesion.

A visceral lymphangioma certainly requires total extirpation. Rarely, lymphangiomas of the pan-

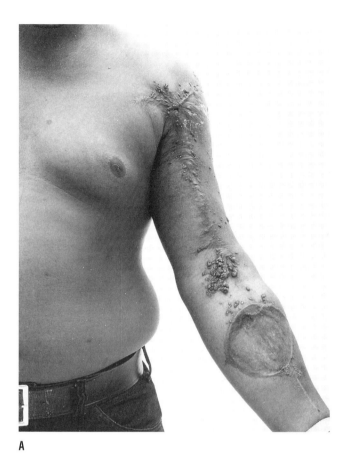

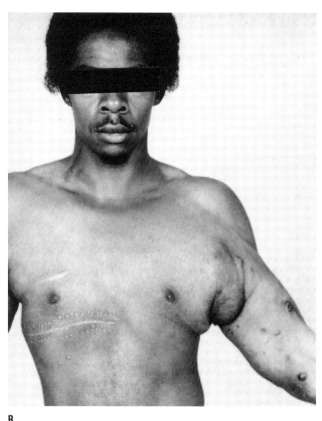

A

B

**Figure 13–2. (A)** A 46-year-old man with extensive cutaneous lymphangioma of the left arm and forearm. The extent of the skin involvement abruptly ends at the left shoulder. He sought medical opinion because of constant rupture of the cystlike spaces and persistent drainage complicated by recurrent episodes of infection. The skin graft area shows the area of first excision, which was performed two years prior to his visit to the University of Illinois Hospital. Since then, he has required four staged excisions, with gratifying results. **(B)** A 26-year-old man with extensive involvement of the left upper extremity with both cavernous and papillary lymphangiomas (anterior view).

creas[10,12,14,17] and duodenum[15] have been described, but the exact incidence is impossible to assess. Usually, only larger lesions in certain unusual sites in the gastrointestinal tract are reported.

We have encountered two instances of cavernous lymphangioma of the pancreas. One patient with involvement of the head of the pancreas was seen in consultation. After a pancreaticoduodenectomy performed elsewhere, the patient is doing well and apparently is back to normal activity. The second patient was an 18-year-old boy who was operated on by one of us (Fig. 13–3). Lymphangioma involved the body and neck of the pancreas. He was treated by subtotal pancreatectomy and is still well 15 years later.

## LYMPHANGIOMAS OF THE BONE

The first case of lymphangioma of the bone was reported by Bickel and Broders[18] in 1947. The patient was a five-year-old girl. Several additional cases in all age groups have since been reported.[19–26] The lesion in some instances progresses to multiple pathologic fractures; in other instances, it remains stationary for a long

period of time. Similar to several other pathologic types, the lesion is seen in x-rays as a lytic defect in the shafts of the long bones. Therefore, the diagnosis is always made after a biopsy. No specific form of therapy is known for this entity.

## CYSTIC HYGROMA

Cystic hygroma is the generally accepted term for a lymphangioma that arises in the posterior cervical triangle or supraclavicular fossa (Fig. 13–4). However, these lymphatic cysts also occur in other parts of the head and neck, axillae, and the groin.[1–5] In general, the larger lesions are found close to the large veins and lymphatic ducts.[1,2] Groups of hyperplastic nodes are frequently present.

The patient presents with a painless mass in the neck (Fig. 13–4). The cyst may become evident only after trauma or an upper respiratory tract infection. The natural history varies from progressive, static, or intermittent growth, to rare regressive spontaneous disappearance. Although congenital, these tumors are not always evident at birth, when perhaps 75 percent are

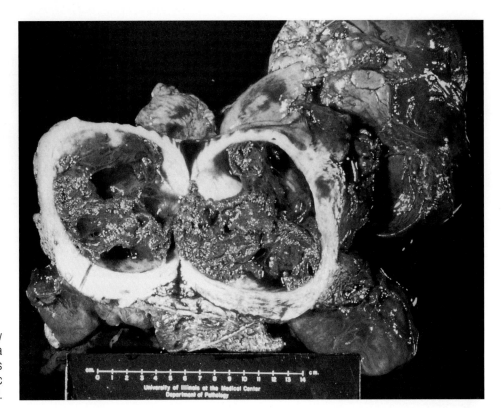

**Figure 13–3.** Subtotal pancreatectomy specimen showing a large lymphangioma of the body and tail of pancreas. Patient's mother first noticed a small epigastric mass when the patient was six years old.

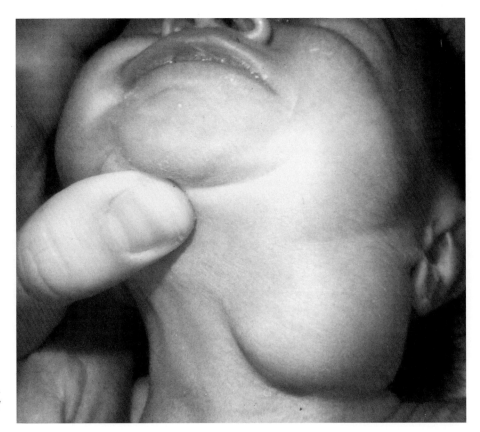

**Figure 13–4.** Cystic hygroma in a newborn. This lesion was excised without any difficulty 16 years ago.

noted.[1,4,5] Approximately 90 percent of these tumors are found by age 2, although the age may vary from birth to the late thirties. The lesion, rarely, arises de novo in adults.

Signs and symptoms may include distortion of the face or neck; respiratory stridor with cyanosis by compression or mediastinal extension; dysphagia secondary to inflammation, infection, or compression; spontaneous infection with concomitant upper respiratory tract infection; sudden increase in size by spontaneous hemorrhage, which may be fatal; and brachial plexus compression with pain or hyperesthesia.

These tumors are diffuse and poorly circumscribed. The overlying skin is usually normal, but if it is thinned by stretching, atrophy of the subcutaneous tissue may occur. Blue venous coloration and light transmission may result. On palpation, the tumors are soft, nontender, noncompressible, poorly delineated, cystic, and often adherent to the skin. Trabeculae or fibrotic areas may be palpable within the bulk of the mass. Usually located beneath the platysma muscle, they may penetrate deeply into the neck and perhaps extend into the mediastinum or axilla.

The treatment of cystic hygromas is excision as soon as it is feasible. However, keen judgment must be exercised to avoid injury to the nerves in the neck during resection of a tumor that in most instances is only cosmetically deforming. We have seen infants whose accessory nerve or hypoglossal nerve, or both, have been injured during operation for a cystic hygroma. Excision of hygromas must not be undertaken when the cyst is inflamed or infected. Recurrence is rare after adequate excision.

## LYMPHANGIECTASIS

Lymphangiectasis is an uncommon malformation of infancy and childhood resulting in chylous ascites or chylothorax. Fonkalsrud[1] described his experience with eight children: five boys and three girls. He found a variety of lymphatic involvement. Four children had small, multiple lymphangiectatic cysts of the mesentery, three had similar cystic involvement of the mediastinum, and one had both mediastinal and intra-abdominal lymphatic cysts. Chylous ascites were noted in two children; chylothorax in one. Treatment of these lesions is indeed problematic. Total excision of all the cysts is sometimes impossible. Frequently, partial resection and unroofing has to be resorted to, but this method results in recurrence of the ascites. Fonkalsrud[1] commented that, since lymphangiectasis without the complications is not a fatal disease, attempts should only be made to keep the expansion and compression of the vital structures in check. He also suggested that, in some instances, after the first year of

life, lymphangiectasis becomes less prominent and may be self-limiting.

### Systemic Lymphangiectasis

Infrequently, lymphangiomas are found to involve the entire extremity, extending from the shoulder to the fingertips or from the groin to the toes (Fig. 13–5A to 13–5C). Systemic lymphangiectasis is a congenital deformity in which all the structures of the entire limb are involved with lymphangiectasis, resulting in a grotesquely swollen and deformed extremity. In certain instances, the situation becomes such that the patient requests a major amputation, such as a hip joint disarticulation or forequarter amputation. In general, these amputations should be avoided, but in some instances they may become necessary.

## LYMPHEDEMA

*Congenital Lymphedema.*  Although the exact pathophysiologic factors of congenital lymphedema are not yet clear, it has been postulated to be due to underdevelopment of the superficial lymphatic system. In instances in which the congenital lymphedema of an extremity is encountered in the absence of a familial predilection, the term *lymphedema praecox* is generally used. In patients in whom a family history of edematous extremities is obtained, the term *Milroy's disease* has been used.

In the normal extremity, subcutaneous lymphatic channels accompany the main superficial veins to the lymph nodes in the groin or axilla. Similarly, deep lymphatic trunks accompany deep blood vessels of the extremities. The communications between these two systems in normal circumstances are found in the ankle, calf, popliteal fossa, and the adductor canal in the lower extremities; and in the epitrochlear area in the upper extremities. In congenital lymphedema, the hypoplastic or absent superficial lymphatic network of the involved extremity is unable to collect lymph, which then pools in subcutaneous fat until the hydrostatic pressure of the tissue exceeds the oncotic pressure of the superficial venous system, and venous decompression occurs. The deep lymphatic system of the extremities in patients with congenital lymphedema usually is normal, in contrast to lymphangiectasis of the extremities, in which both systems are involved.

The clinical manifestations of congenital edema (lymphedema praecox) are often evident only after adolescence, although the malformation is present from birth. Fonkalsrud[1] found that in 13 (33 percent) of 39 patients, the manifestations became apparent during adolescence. In some of the patients reported by Fonkalsrud[1] and Fonkalsrud and Coulson,[27] the edema

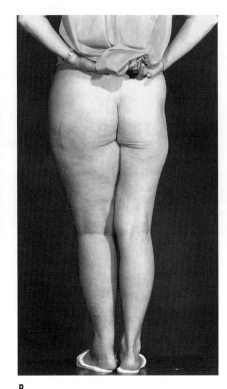

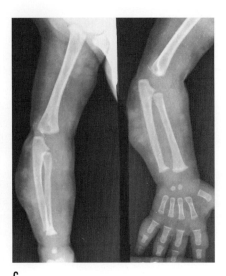

**Figure 13–5.** **(A)** Sixteen-month-old girl with extensive regional lymphangiomatosis of the left lower extremity. Posterior view shows involvement from the toes to the buttock. **(B)** Posterior view of extensive lymphangiomatosis of the left lower extremity in a 45-year-old woman. Note difference of circumference at the midthigh between the two extremities. **(C)** Extensive lymphangioma of the right upper extremity in a male infant. There will be considerable deformity as the child grows older.

was bilateral, and in some, the extremity edema was associated with exudative enteropathy. The clinical features usually are characterized by the enlarged edematous extremity or extremities, resulting in cosmetic deformity, which in extreme cases might be functional as well.

Milroy[28] described familial lymphedema in a family of six generations comprising 97 persons, 23 percent of whom had congenital lymphedema. The basic factors related to the lymphedema, however, were similar to those in the more common nonfamilial congenital type of lymphedema.

Chronic obstructive lymphedema of the extremities in the adult is usually iatrogenically produced by either radical radiation therapy or radical axillary or groin dissections, sometimes with a combination of both these methods. Infrequently, the lymphatic obstruction is secondary to infection. Parasitic infestation resulting in massive extremity edema with massive skin changes is still relatively common in some parts of the world.

The chronically lymphedematous extremity poses a unique challenge in management.[1,2,4,6,27,29] However, the only relevance of this anomaly to the present discussion is the development of lymphangiosarcoma in such an extremity. The details of this aspect are discussed in the section on malignant tumors of the lymphatic system.

## LYMPHANGIOMYOMA

Lymphangiomyoma is a rare benign disorder of the lymphatic system that was first recognized and described in 1966 by Cornog and Enterline.[30] It is characterized by a proliferation of smooth muscles within the lymphatics and lymph nodes of the mediastinum and retroperitoneum and frequently the lung parenchyma. Cornog and Enterline[30] reviewed 20 cases and concluded that the lesion occurred in a striking preponderance in women of childbearing age and is usually multifocal in distribution. The lesion often involves the thoracic duct, has a constant association with chylothorax, and a frequent association with pulmonary disease, consisting of lymphangiectatic honeycombing with the proliferation of smooth muscle and a typical lipid pneumonia, possibly of chylous origin. Following reappraisal of a previously published paper by Enterline and Roberts,[31] Cornog and Enterline[30] concluded that the term *lymphangiopericytoma*, used by Enterline and Roberts[31] should be substituted by the term *lymphangiomyoma*. Based on their observations, Cornog and Enterline[30] suggested that the pulmonary cystic and muscular lesions associated with this entity are an independent expression of a tendency to malformation, as seen in tuberous sclerosis, but in part might be secondary to mediastinal lesions. These authors found no evidence of local infiltration or metastases in their 20 cases. Based on all the available information,[32,33] these lesions can be considered hamartomous and are referred to as *lymphangiomyoma*; when the disease involves large segments of the lymphatic system, the term *lymphangiomyomatosis* has been used.

Following Cornog and Enterline's[30] publication, several other reports have appeared.[30,31,33–41] It is apparent that, although this anomaly or hamartomatous malformation may occur in multiple sites, the pulmonary involvement (being the most dramatic) receives most of the attention.[32,35,39,41–49] In 1975, Corrin and co-workers[35] published a comprehensive review of pulmonary lymphangiomyomatosis. Documented cases of this entity are still rare, and most of these have been in women in the reproductive age group, the major complaint being breathlessness. This is usually progressive, and death from pulmonary insufficiency results within 10 to 15 years. Functional changes in the lungs are obstructive or restrictive, or both. Pneumothorax, chylous effusions, and hemoptysis are major complications. Radiographically, the lesions initially appear as fine, linear or nodular, predominantly basal densities, and progress to a pattern of bullous change or honeycombing. Like eosinophilic granulomas, they involve all portions of the lungs, including the region of the costophrenic sinuses. There may be associated pleural effusion. A progressively increasing lung volume is characteristic. The lesions consist of an irregular nodular or laminar random proliferation of smooth muscle cells within all portions of the lung, with loss of parenchyma leading to honeycombing. Proliferated muscle can obstruct bronchioles (with air-trapping and formation of bullae, often complicated by pneumothorax), venules (with pulmonary hemorrhage and hemosiderosis accompanied clinically by hemoptysis), and lymphatics (with chylothorax or chyloperitoneum). Both thoracic and abdominal lymph nodes and the thoracic duct can also be involved in the myoproliferative process, with formation of subsidiary minute channels and obstruction. Renal or perirenal angiomyolipomas can also occur.[50] Cagnano et al.[32] reported a case which had associated cavernous angioma of the liver, meningioma, and a papillary cancer of the thyroid. Identical pulmonary lesions occasionally occur in tuberous sclerosis. The possibility of a relationship between tuberous sclerosis and lymphangiomyomatosis has been alluded to.[51] One feature of note in pulmonary lesions of tuberous sclerosis is the presence of adenomatoid proliferations of the epithelium. The similarities between these entities are such that it is more likely than not that they are interrelated. As stated earlier, no malignant transformation in these cases has yet been documented.

The treatment of extensive lymphangiomyomatosis is essentially symptomatic; the greatest challenge is control of pleural effusion (chylothorax). Multiple methods have been advocated, including castration,[44] interferon-α,[45] and tamoxifen.[49] However, long-range control of the disease is not yet at hand and, as has already been mentioned, most of these patients die within 10 to 15 years of the onset of this disease. Therefore, whether these suggested therapeutic interventions will actually be beneficial is still undetermined. Infrequently, the localized form of this disease can be excised; however, both the surgeon and patient must be prepared for multiple excisions because this is frequently multicentric in it presentation.

## ■ MALIGNANT TUMORS

### LYMPHANGIOSARCOMA

In 1948, Stewart and Treves[52] described an unusual tumor that developed in an edematous upper extremity following radical mastectomy long after the breast cancer was apparently controlled. After some initial confusion and controversy regarding the true identity of the tumor, it became apparent that a lymphangiosarcoma had developed in an edematous extremity, not to be confused with recurrent or metastatic breast cancer. Since the original description by Stewart and Treves,[52] the occurrence of lymphangiosarcoma associated with chronic lymphedema due to any cause has become well recognized. Woodward and co-workers[53] found that through December, 1970, there were 186 such cases reported in the literature, 162 of which occurred after radical mastectomy and 24 after other causes of edema. For the sake of clarity of presentation, discussion will be divided into lymphangiosarcomas associated with postmastectomy lymphedema and the sarcomas arising in other types of an edematous extremity.

## Postmastectomy Lymphangiosarcoma (Stewart-Treves Syndrome)

The average age of the patient at the time of onset of lymphangiosarcoma is about 63 years, although younger patients (44 years) and older patients (84 years) have been described.[53,54] We have treated four such cases, in which the patients were 59, 65, 71, and 73 years of age. As expected, the overwhelming number of patients are women; however, Woodward and co-authors[53] found two instances in men in their review of the literature. No racial predilection has been noted for this cancer.

Lymphangiosarcoma usually appears in an edematous extremity several years after classical radical mastectomy with or without additional radiation therapy of the axilla or the groin. Although the exact time of appearance of the tumor cannot be accurately pinpointed, it is estimated that at least 10 years elapse between the mastectomy and clinical manifestation of lymphangiosarcoma in the ipsilateral upper extremity. Apparently, the tumor can be identified as early as 1 year after mastectomy and as late as 26 years.[53] In the 151 cases in which the interval was recorded, lymphangiosarcoma first appeared at a median interval of 10 years, 4 months (Fig. 13–6).

In our series, lymphangiosarcoma first became clinically apparent in the upper arm in two patients and in the forearm in the remaining patient (Fig. 13–7A and 13–7B). Woodward et al.,[53] in their review of 90 reported cases, found that in 68 (75.5 percent) the lesion was initially recognized in the arm, in the elbow, and the forearm.

Usually the arm that is the site of tumorigenesis is swollen and hypertrophied, with brawny, atrophic, hyperkeratotic, suffused, purplish skin. Function is limited, with accompanying pain in some instances. Initially, a bluish or purplish macular or nodular lesion is seen; the lesion enlarges, and, with time, a confluence of a number of these lesions makes the diagnosis simple (Fig. 13–7B).

***Treatment.*** Various methods of treatment have been tried for postmastectomy lymphangiosarcoma.[3,52,53] Herrmann and Ariel,[54] in 1967, reviewed the results of

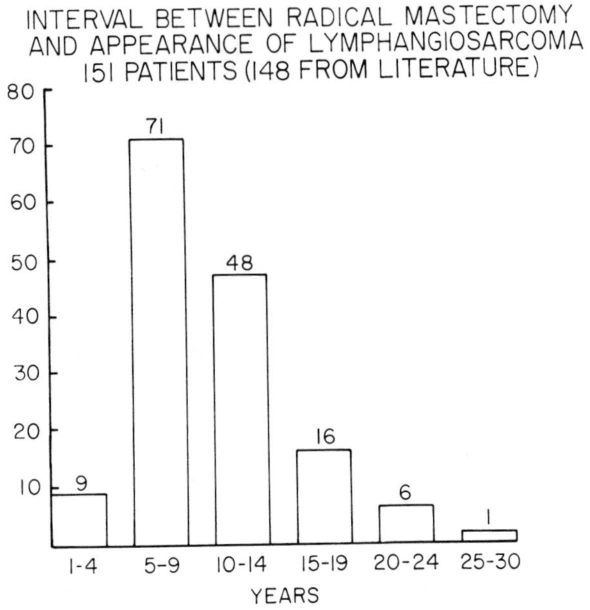

**Figure 13–6.** Histogram showing the interval of appearance of lymphangiosarcoma after radical mastectomy.

treatment in 91 reported cases and concluded that the prognosis was poor in this disease and that neither surgery nor radiation therapy influenced the end result in any appreciable manner. However, after this pessimistic report, several comprehensive reviews were published[53,55–59] showing that the results of treatment were not as depressing as had been thought. Woodward et al.,[53] reviewing the Mayo Clinic experience in 21 patients, found that initial treatment consisted of the following: primary amputation, 10 patients; irradiation, 6 patients; local excision, 2 patients; irradiation and chemotherapy, 1 patient; and chemotherapy, 1 patient. One patient with advanced disease received no treatment. Of the 10 patients treated with amputation, there were 4 five-year survivors (40 percent); 1 of the 4 had metastases after five years. In contrast, none of the six patients treated with radiation therapy alone survived for five years, nor did either of the two patients treated with local excision, both of whom had local recurrence. These authors found no beneficial effect from chemotherapy as a primary form of treatment. In our series of four patients with postmastectomy lymphangiosarcoma, three were treated by forequarter amputation. One is still disease-free at the end of 10 years, and the other two died of metastatic disease within 5 years. The remaining patient, who was treated with combined radiation, systemic chemotherapy, and immunotherapy, lived for 18 months.

In 129 of the 162 cases of lymphangiosarcoma collected by Woodward and co-workers,[53] the median survival rate was 19 months. Woodward and his co-workers[53] compared the published survival rates of 61

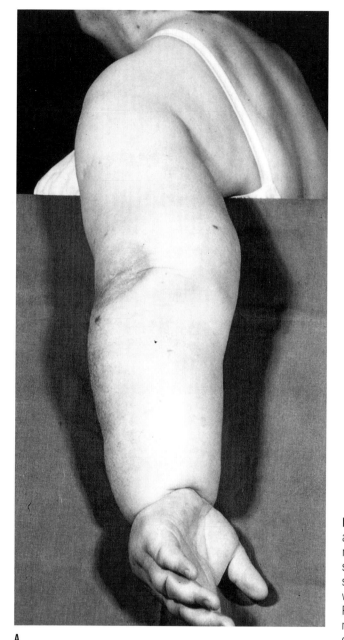

A

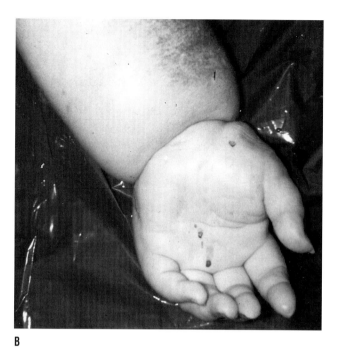

B

**Figure 13–7. (A)** A small pigmented lesion in the posterolateral aspect of the arm was the first sign of a lymphangiosarcoma that developed in a lymphedematous extremity following radical mastectomy eight years earlier. Careful scrutiny shows several minute lesions on the arm and another lesion below the skin graft. An apparent attempt for control of the initial lesions was made by wide local excision when the tumor recurred, before the patient was referred. **(B)** Postmastectomy lymphangiosarcoma showing confluence of multiple cutaneous lesions in the forearm and the wrist, indicating an advanced stage of the disease.

patients treated either by forequarter amputation or by shoulder disarticulation with those of 48 patients treated by radiation therapy alone and found that those subjected to amputation had a slightly better prognosis. The difference was significant at two years ($p = 0.05$), but of borderline significance at one year ($p = 0.06$). There are too few patients treated by either method to allow comparisons of survival rates. Of the 11 patients who survived for more than five years, 7 were treated by amputation (4 by forequarter amputation and 3 by shoulder disarticulation), 2 by wide excision, and 1 by radiation therapy (17-year survival). The remaining patient received intra-arterially administered radioactive yttrium.[54]

The incidence of local recurrence after a major amputation is lower than in patients treated by radiation therapy. The failure of amputation is usually metastatic disease, whereas, in the irradiated group, local failure precedes distant disease. Based on our limited experience and the experience of other authors,[52–54] it appears that radical ablative operation probably offers a better opportunity for cure.

### Lymphangiosarcoma Not Associated with Mastectomy

As pointed out earlier, lymphangiosarcoma can occur in any chronically edematous area (Fig. 13–8). Lymphangiosarcoma of the anterior abdominal wall has been reported in the edematous anterior abdominal

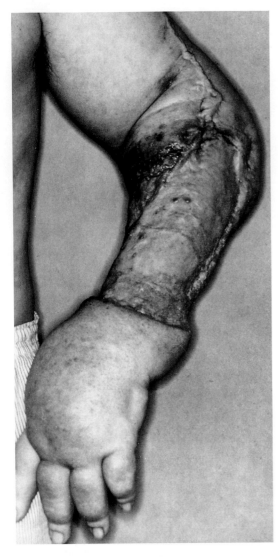

**Figure 13–8.** Lymphangiosarcoma arising in an apparently congenitally lymphedematous left upper extremity of a 46-year-old man. Several attempts at local excision failed, and the patient was then referred. A forequarter amputation was performed, resulting in a five-and-a-half year disease-free survival (Table 13–2).

wall following bilateral lymphadenectomy for carcinoma of the penis.[60] Only a handful of patients have been found with lymphangiosarcoma in a chronically edematous extremity not associated with the aftermath of radical mastectomy (Table 13–2).[61–84] As in the postmastectomy variety, the results of treatment are not encouraging.

### EXTRANODAL LYMPHOMA

A malignant lymphoma occasionally may be encountered in the somatic tissues and may mimic a soft somatic tissue neoplasm (Fig. 13–9). For example, the initial presentation of malignant lymphoma may be an anterior abdominal wall tumor resembling a lipoma. In other instances, the tumors might be encountered in the gastrointestinal tract, conjunctiva, maxillary antrum, breast, and various other locations. The diagnosis is established by means of microscopic examination of the biopsy specimen. An initial attempt in diagnosis with fine-needle aspiration cytology should be considered. Frequently, this would avoid an unnecessary wide excision of a lymphoma arising in extranodal locations. Once the diagnosis of malignant lymphoma is made, the treatment is based on the histologic type and the extent of disease.

### EXTRAMEDULLARY PLASMACYTOMA

Extramedullary plasmacytomas are uncommon tumors that usually originate in the nose, nasal sinuses, oropharynx, bronchi,[85] gastrointestinal tract,[85–92] and even the meninges.[93] They tend to remain localized for long periods before spreading to other sites. Plasma cell tumors may also originate in the intestine. Since the normal plasma cells in the nasopharynx and intestine mainly synthesize immunoglobulin A (IgA), it is not surprising that most of the plasma cell tumors that develop in these sites likewise produce IgA. In rare instances, local manifestation of this entity resembles a soft tissue sarcoma. A palpable tumor or a lesion that can be seen in x-rays of the skeletal system automatically means the disease is of several years' duration. If the treatment reduces the mass, the prognosis is improved, although most patients will eventually die of the disease. The presence of M-protein in a patient with a soft tissue tumor is diagnostic of myeloma.

In general, the treatment is nonsurgical and consists of treatment of symptoms, as well as use of systemic chemotherapy. In an apparently localized plasma cell tumor, if there is no indication of systemic disease, the tumor should be treated primarily by means of radiation therapy (e.g., in solitary lesions of the nose or nasopharynx). In rare instances, the local lesion can be excised with good response. We have had two patients in whom local excision was performed. One was a 51-year-old woman whom we followed up for five years without any evidence of progression of disease, after excision at another medical center of an apparently solitary plasmacytoma located at the medial end of the left clavicle. The second one, whom we treated, was a 66-year-old woman with a large (15 × 12 cm) left scapular mass causing extreme difficulty of motion. A biopsy showed a plasma cell tumor and elevated M-protein. A subtotal scapulectomy was performed. Immediately following the operation, there was a fall of M-protein levels and she improved. She received localized radiation therapy and remained well for five years, after which

**TABLE 13–2.  TWENTY-EIGHT REPORTED CASES OF LYMPHANGIOSARCOMA NOT ASSOCIATED WITH MASTECTOMY**

| Author(s) | Publi- cation Year | Age | Site | Cause of Lymphedema | Duration of Lymphedema (yr) | Treatment | Comments |
|---|---|---|---|---|---|---|---|
| Lowenstein[61] | 1908 | 56 | L arm | Traumatic | 6 | Amputation | Alive, 2 yr |
| Kettle[62] | 1918 | 44 | R leg | Idiopathic | 40 | Hip disarticulation | Alive, 3 yr |
| Nather[63] | 1921 | 59 | R leg | Traumatic | 11/12 | Amputation | Alive, 1 yr |
| Aegerter and Peale[64] | 1942 | 40 | R leg | Idiopathic | 29 | Amputation | Dead, 6 yr |
| Martorell[65] | 1951 | 44 | R leg | Infection | | Radiation therapy and amputation | Dead, 4 yr |
| Raven and Christie[66] | 1954 | 56 | L arm | Extensive nevus | ? | Excision and forequarter amputation | Dead, postop |
| Aird et al.[67] | 1956 | 60 | R leg | Idiopathic | 8 | Amputation | Dead, 3 yr |
| Liszauer and Ross[68] | 1957 | 28 | R leg | Congenital | 28 | Excision | Dead, 8 mo |
| Whittle[69] | 1959 | 31 | R leg | Idiopathic | 11 | Chemotherapy | Dead, 6 mo |
| Francis and Lindquist[70] | 1960 | 52 | L thigh | Fibrosarcoma of the proximal femur | 5 | Hemipelvectomy | Dead, postop |
| Scott et al.[71] | 1960 | 46 | L hand | Congenital | 46 | Amputation | Dead, 4 yr |
| Taswell et al.[72] | 1962 | 18 | L arm | Congenital | 18 | Shoulder disarticulation | Dead, 11 mo |
| Ibid | 1962 | 65 | L leg | Idiopathic | 37 | Amputation | Alive, 15 yr |
| De Jager[73] | 1963 | 43 | R leg | Tibial chondroma | ? | Amputation | Dead, 2 yr |
| Ibid | 1963 | 64 | R forearm | Abscess of second rib | 22 | Radiation therapy | Alive, 3 yr |
| Ibid | 1963 | 44 | R thigh | Tuberculosis | ? | ? | Dead |
| Vandaele et al.[74] | 1963 | 35 | R leg | Idiopathic | 26 | Amputation | Alive, 10 mo |
| Gray et al.[75] | 1966 | 65 | L arm | Axillary node dissection; radiation therapy | 8 | Forequarter amputation | Dead, 9 mo |
| Prudden and Wolarsky[76] | 1967 | 28 | R thigh | Congenital | Intermittently for years | Hemipelvectomy | Alive, 10 mo |
| Danese et al.[77] | 1967 | 26 | L hand | Idiopathic | 17 | None | Dead, 4 mo |
| Huriez et al.[78] | 1968 | 35 | R leg | Idiopathic | 26 | Amputation | Alive, 10 mo |
| McBride et al.[79] | 1969 | — | R thigh | Carcinoma of cervix | — | | — |
| Bunch[80] | 1969 | 13 | L axilla | Congenital | 13 | Forequarter amputation | Dead, 3 mo |
| Finlay-Jones[81] | 1970 | 34 | L thigh | Congenital | 34 | Excision, radiation therapy | Dead, 2½ yr |
| Merrick et al.[82] | 1971 | 52 | L arm | Congenital | 52 | Forequarter amputation | Dead, 2½ yr with metastases |
| Das Gupta | 1981 | 36 | R arm | Congenital | 36 | Forequarter amputation | 2½ yr N.E.D.* |
| Das Gupta | 1984 | 54 | L lower extremity | Congenital | 53 | Mid-thigh amputation and adjuvant chemotherapy | 10 yr N.E.D.* |
| Das Gupta** | 1993 | 59 | L lower extremity | Post-radical Groin dissection | 13 | Hip joint disarticulation | 1½ yr, Died of metastatic lymphangiosarcoma |

*No evidence of disease.
**This patient had a radical groin dissection of malignant melanoma of the left thigh. Immediately after lymphadenectomy, she developed giant lymphedema. This could not be controlled or reduced by any known method(s). Thirteen years later, she developed lymphangiosarcoma of the leg, which continued to progress cephalad and a hip joint disarticulation was performed. She died of metastatic lymphangiosarcoma 1½ years post-disarticulation.

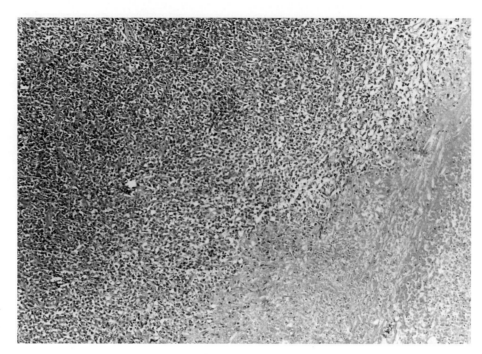

**Figure 13–9.** Extranodal malignant lymphoma of the subcutaneous tissue. (H & E. Original magnification × 65.)

systemic manifestations became evident and she died seven years after her original operation.

## REFERENCES

1. Fonkalsrud EW: Surgical management of congenital malformations of the lymphatic system. Am J Surg 128:152, 1974
2. Bill AH, Sumner DS: A unified concept of lymphangioma and cystic hygroma. Surg Gynecol Obstet 120:79, 1965
3. Pack GT, Ariel IR: Tumors of the Soft Somatic Tissues. New York, Hoeber-Harper, 1958, p 472
4. Harkins GA, Sabiston DC: Lymphangioma in infancy and childhood. Surgery 47:822, 1960
5. Woodring AJ: Cervical cystic hygroma. A review of the literature and report of an unusual case. Ann Otol Rhin Laryngol 77:978, 1968
6. Beahrs OH: Chylous cysts of the abdomen. Surg Clin N Am 30:1081, 1950
7. Eliason EL: Perforated chylous cyst of mesentery. Ann Surg 101:1452, 1935
8. Harrow BR: Retroperitoneal lymphatic cyst (cystic lymphangioma). J Urol 77:82, 1957
9. Handelsman JC, Ravitch MM: Chylous cysts of the mesentery in children. Ann Surg 140:185, 1954
10. Farrel WJ: Intra-abdominal cystic lymphangioma. Am J Surg 108:790, 1964
11. Lynn RB: Cystic lymphangioma of the adrenal associated with arterial hypertension. Canad J Surg 8:92, 1965
12. Sturim HS: Intra-abdominal cystic lymphangiomas. Am J Surg 109:807, 1965
13. Sarrias BA: Two cases of cystic lymphangioma of the mesentery. Bull Soc Int Chir 30 (Sept–Dec):519, 1971
14. Pack GT, Trinidad SS, Lisa JR: Rare primary somatic tumors of the pancreas. Arch Surg 77:1000, 1958
15. Elliot RL, Williams RD, Bayles D, Griffin J: Lymphangioma of the duodenum. One report with light and electron microscopic observations. Ann Surg 163:1, 86, 1966
16. Litzow TJ, Lash H: Lymphangiomas of the tongue. Proc Staff Meet Mayo Clin 36:229, 1961
17. Gonzales LE, Zapatero AH, Fernandez EP: Lymphangioma of the pancreas. Chir Ghastroent 10:225, 1976
18. Bickel WH, Broders AC: Primary lymphangioma of the ilium. Report of a case. J Bone Joint Surg 29A:517, 1947
19. Harris R, Prandoni AG: Generalized primary lymphangiomas of bone: Report of case associated with congenital lymphedema of forearm. Ann Intern Med 33:1302, 1950
20. Cohen J, Graig JM: Multiple lymphangiectases of bone. J Bone Joint Surg 37A:585, 1955
21. Falkmer S, Tilling G: Primary lymphangioma of bone. Acta Orthop Scand 26:99, 1956
22. Hayes JT, Brody GL: Cystic lymphangiectasis of bone. J Bone Joint Surg 45A:107, 1961
23. Shopfner CE, Allen RP: Lymphangioma of bone. Radiology 76:449, 1961
24. Rosenquist CJ, Wolfe FC: Lymphangioma of bone. J Bone Joint Surg 50A:158, 1968
25. Brower AC, Culver JE Jr., Keats TE: Diffuse cystic angiomatosis of bone: Report of two cases. Am J Roentgenol 118:456, 1973
26. Asch MJ, Cohen AH, Moore TC: Hepatic and splenic lymphangiomatosis with skeletal involvement: Report of a case and review of the literature. Surgery 76:334, 1974
27. Fonkalsrud EW, Coulson WF: Management of congenital lymphedema in infants and children. Ann Surg 177:280, 1973

28. Milroy WF: An undescribed variety of hereditary oedema. NY Med J 56:505, 1892

29. Ravitch MM: Radical treatment of massive mixed angiomas (hemolymphangiomas) in infants and children. Ann Surg 134:228, 1951

30. Cornog JL, Enterline HT: Lymphangiomyoma. A benign lesion of chyliferous lymphatics synonymous with lymphangiopericytoma. Cancer 19:1909, 1966

31. Enterline HT, Roberts B: Lymphangiopericytoma. Cancer 8:582, 1955

32. Cagnano M, Benharroch D, Geffen DB: Pulmonary lymphangiomyomatosis: Report of a case with multiple soft tissue tumors. Arch Pathol Lab Med 115:1257, 1991

33. Eliasson AH, Phillips YY, Tenholder MF: Treatment of lymphangioleiomyomatosis: A meta-analysis. Chest 96:1352, 1989

34. Wolff M: Lymphangiomyoma: Clinicopathologic study and ultrastructural confirmation of its histogenesis. Cancer 31:988, 1975

35. Corrin B, Liebow A, Friedman PJ: Pulmonary lymphangiomyomatosis. Am J Pathol 79:347, 1975

36. Edwards WH, Thompson RC, Varsa EW: Lymphangiomatosis and massive osteolysis of the cervical spine: A case report and review of the literature. Clin Orthop 177:222, 1983

37. Ramani P, Shah A: Lymphangiomatosis: Histologic and immunohistochemical analysis of four cases. Am J Surg Pathol 17:329, 1993

38. Bhattacharyya AK, Balogh K: Retroperitoneal lymphangioleiomyomatosis: A 36-year benign course in a postmenopausal woman. Cancer 56:1144, 1985

39. Gray SR, Carrington CB, Cornog JL: Lymphangiomyomatosis: Report of a case with ureteral involvement and chyluria. Cancer 35:490, 1975

40. Taylor JR, Ryu J, Colby TV, et al.: Lymphangioleiomyomatosis: Clinical course in 32 patients. N Engl J Med 323:1254, 1990

41. Vazquez JJ, Fernandez-Cuervo L, Fidalgo B: Lymphangiomyomatosis: Morphogenetic study and ultrastructural confirmation of the histogenesis of the lung lesion. Cancer 37:2321, 1976

42. Kreisman H, Robitailler Y, Dionne P, Palayew N: Lymphangiomyomatosis syndrome with hyperparathyroidism (a case report). Cancer 42:364, 1978

43. Colley MH, Geppert E, Franklin WA: Immunohistochemical detection of steroid receptors in a case of pulmonary lymphangioleiomyomatosis. Am J Surg Pathol 13:803, 1989

44. Kitzsteiner KA, Mallen RG: Pulmonary lymphangiomyomatosis: Treatment with castration. Cancer 46:2248, 1980

45. Klein M, Kreiger O, Ruckser R, et al.: Treatment of lymphangioleiomyomatosis by ovariectomy, interferon, alpha 2b, and tamoxifen: A case report. Arch Gynecol Obstet 252:99, 1992

46. Luna CM, Gene R, Jolly EC, et al.: Pulmonary lymphangiomyomatosis associated with tuberous sclerosis: Treatment with tamoxifen and tetracycline-pleurodesis. Chest 88:473, 1985

47. Rosendal J: A case of diffuse myomatosis and cyst formation in the lung. Acta Radiol 23:138, 1942

48. Sinclair W, Wright JL, Churg A: Lymphangioleiomyomatosis presenting in a postmenopausal woman. Thorax 40:475, 1985

49. Tomasian A, Greenberg MS, Rumerman H: Tamoxifen for lymphangioleiomyomatosis. N Engl J Med 306:745, 1982

50. Montforet WJ, Kohnen PW: Angiolipomas in a case of lymphangiomyomatous syndrome. Relationships to tuberous sclerosis. Cancer 34:317, 1974

51. Kaku T, Toyoshima S, Enjoji M: Tuberous sclerosis with pulmonary and lymph node involvement: Relationship to lymphangiomyomatosis. Acta Pathol Jpn 33:395, 1983

52. Stewart FW, Treves N: Lymphangiosarcoma in postmastectomy lymphedema: A report of six cases in elephantiasis chirurgica. Cancer 1:64, 1948

53. Woodward AH, Ivins JE, Soule EH: Lymphangiosarcoma arising in chronic lymphedematous extremities. Cancer 30:562, 1972

54. Herrmann JP, Ariel IM: Therapy of lymphangiosarcoma of the chronically edematous limb. Am J Roentgenol 99:393, 1967

55. Tragus ET, Wagner DE: Current therapy for postmastectomy lymphangiosarcoma. Arch Surg 97:839, 1968

56. Schreiber H, Barry FM, Russell WC, et al.: Stewart-Treves syndrome: A lethal complication of postmastectomy lymphedema and regional immune deficiency. Arch Surg 114:82, 1979

57. Sordillo EM, Sordillo PP, Hajdu SI, et al.: Lymphangiosarcoma after filarial infection. J Dermatol Surg Oncol 7:235, 1981

58. Sordillo PP, Chapman R, Hajdu SI, et al.: Lymphangiosarcoma. Cancer 48:1674, 1981

59. Yap BS, Yap HY, McBride CM, et al.: Chemotherapy for postmastectomy lymphangiosarcoma. Cancer 47:853, 1981

60. Calnan J, Cowdell RH: Lymphangioendothelioma of the anterior abdominal wall: Report of a case. Br J Surg 46:375, 1959

61. Lowenstein S: Der Atiologische Zusammenhand zwischen akutem einmaligem. Trauma und Sarcoma: ein Beitrag zur Aetiologie der malignen tomoren. Beitr Klin Chir 48:780, 1906

62. Kettle EH: Tumors arising from endothelium. Proc Roy Soc Med 11:19, 1918

63. Nather K: Uber ein malignes Lymphangioendotheliom der Haut des Fusses. Virchows Arch Path Anat 231:540, 1921

64. Aegerter EE, Peale AR: Kaposi's sarcoma: A critical survey. Arch Pathol 34:413, 1942

65. Martorell F: Tumorigenic lymphedema. Angiology 2:386, 1951

66. Raven RW, Christie AC: Hemangiosarcoma: A case with lymphatic and hematogenous metastases. Br J Surg 41:483, 1954

67. Aird I, Weinbren K, Walter L: Angiosarcoma in a limb the

seat of spontaneous lymphoedema. Br J Cancer 10:424, 1956

68. Liszauer S, Ross RC: Lymphangiosarcoma in lymphoedema. Can Med Assoc J 76:475, 1957
69. Whittle RJM: An angiosarcoma associated with an oedematous limb: A case report. J Fac Radiol 10:111, 1959
70. Francis KC, Lindquist HD: Lymphangiosarcoma of the lower extremity involved with chronic lymphedema. Am J Surg 100:617, 1960
71. Scott RB, Nydick I, Conway H: Lymphangiosarcoma arising in lymphedema. Am J Med 28:1008, 1960
72. Taswell HF, Soule HH, Conventry MB: Lymphangiosarcoma arising in chronic lymphedematous extremities. J Bone Joint Surg 44A:277, 1962
73. De Jager H: Oorspronkelijke Stukken: Secundair lymfangiosarcoom. Ned Tijdechr Geneeskd 107:1344, 1963
74. Vandaele R, Van Craeynest W, Haven E, Dupont A: Lymphangiosarcome sur lymphangiosarcome sur lymphoedeme primitif du bras. Bull Soc Fr Dermatol Syphiligr 70:722, 1963
75. Gray GF Jr, Gonzales-Licea A, Hartman WH, Woods AC: Angiosarcoma in lymphedema: An unusual case of Stewart-Treves syndrome. Bull Johns Hopkins Hosp 119:117, 1966
76. Prudden JF, Wolarsky ER: Lymphangiosarcoma of the thigh: Case Report. Arch Surg 94:276, 1967
77. Danese CA, Grishman E, Oh C, Brieling DA: Malignant vascular tumors of the lymphedematous extremity. Ann Surg 166:245, 1967
78. Huriez C, Desmons F, Agache P, et al.: Lymphangiosarcome sur elephantiasis monstreux de la jambe chez une femme agee 35 ans. Bull Soc Fr Dermatol Syphiligr 75:10, 1968
79. McBride CM, Reeder JW, Smith JL: Angiosarcoma in the lymphaedematous limb. South Med J 62:378, 1969
80. Bunch GH: Discussion, Lymphangiosarcoma following post-mastectomy lymphedema (Barnett WO, Hardy JD, Hendrix JH). Ann Surg 169:968, 1969
81. Finlay-Jones LR: Lymphangiosarcoma of the thigh: A case report. Cancer 26:722, 1970
82. Merrick TA, Erlandson RA, Hajdu SI: Lymphangiosarcoma of a congenitally lymphedematous arm. Arch Pathol 91:365, 1971
83. Devi L, Bahuleyan CK: Lymphangiosarcoma of the lower extremity associated with chronic lymphedema of filarial origin. Indian J Cancer 14:176, 1977
84. Muller R, Hajdu SI, Brennan MF: Lymphangiosarcoma associated with chronic filarial lymphedema. Cancer 59:174, 1987
85. Stout AP, Kenney FR: Primary plasma cell tumors of the upper air passages and oral cavity. Cancer 2:261, 1949
86. Ahmed N, Ramos S, Sika J, et al.: Primary esophageal plasmacytoma. Cancer 38:943, 1976
87. Douglass HO Jr, Sika IV, LeVeen HH: Plasmacytoma—A not so rare tumor of the small intestine. Cancer 28:456, 1971
88. Godaro JE, Fox JE, Levinson JJ: Primary gastric plasmacytoma—Case report and review of literature. J Digest Dis 18:508, 1973
89. Hellwig CA: Extramedullary plasma cell tumors as observed in various locations. Arch Pathol 36:95, 1943
90. Line DH, Lewis RH: Gastric plasmacytoma. Gut 10:233, 1969
91. Carson CP, Ackerman LV, Maltby JE: Plasma cell myeloma. A clinical, pathological and roentgenologic review of 90 cases. Am J Clin Pathol 25:849, 1955
92. Hampton JM, Gandy JR: Plasmacytoma of gastrointestinal tract. Ann Surg 145:415, 1957
93. Mancilla-Jemenez R, Tavassoli FA: Solitary meningeal plasmacytoma: Report of a case with electron microscopic and immunohistologic observations. Cancer 38:798, 1976

# 14

# Heterotopic Bone and Cartilage

## ■ BENIGN TUMORS

### LOCALIZED MYOSITIS OSSIFICANS

Solitary myositis ossificans is a rare clinical entity, probably related to chronic minimal trauma. A common example is the bony hard mass that develops in the medial aspect of the thigh of horseback riders, which has been termed *rider's bone*. A localized hard tumor along the long axis of a muscle, which on routine roentgenographic examination shows the presence of osseous tissue, suggests a diagnosis of myositis ossificans. If the patient provides a history of chronic trauma, this diagnosis becomes more likely. In a number of instances, however, there is no such history of chronic trauma (Fig. 14–1). For example, a diagnosis of osseous metaplasia of the breast[1–3] must be established by histologic examination. Local excision is the treatment for symptomatic solitary myositis ossificans.

In rare instances, this tumor can develop into an osteogenic sarcoma. Pack and Ariel[4] described one such case. In 1956, Fine and Stout[5] made an extensive study of the published cases and those in the files of Columbia University's Department of Surgical Pathology and found a total of 46. In 2 of their own cases and in 10 published cases, malignant change in a benign tumor could be suggested. However, in only 1 of these 12 cases was a histologic diagnosis of solitary myositis ossificans made in a preexisting tumor, and this had been left untreated. In all other instances, the diagnosis of a malignant change in a preexisting myositis ossificans was made on the basis of the history of a preexisting tumor of long duration. Using long intervals as the

criterion for accepting the hypothesis that malignant transformation can occur in a preexisting site of ossification, Fine and Stout[5] found that, in 7 (15.2 percent) of their 46 cases, extraskeletal osteogenic sarcoma developed in a preexisting solitary myositis ossificans. More recently, Eckhart et al.[6] essentially came to the same conclusion as was originally proposed by Fine and Stout[5] (i.e., the diagnosis can only be made based on a long interval between appearance of a heterotopic bone and osseous sarcoma).

### PROGRESSIVE MYOSITIS OSSIFICANS

Progressive myositis ossificans is extremely rare and is distinctly different from the localized or solitary form.[7] Rosenstein[8] noted a group of characteristic symptoms that sharply differentiate this condition from the localized form. These symptoms are (1) ossification of a muscle with no apparent cause; (2) manifestation of the disease at birth or in early life; (3) progressive and unrelenting course, unaffected by any treatment; and (4) association with several congenital anomalies, especially of the fingers and toes. Rosenstein[8] collected 119 cases and added one of his own. Pack and Braund[9] described one patient with progressive myositis ossificans in whom osteogenic sarcoma developed in the back muscles.

In general, progressive growth with associated ossification of muscles continues until most of the muscles from the skull to the feet are involved. It occurs most frequently in boys, but the disease is so rare that no sex or race ratio can be established.

## CHONDROMA OF SOFT PARTS

Benign extraskeletal chondroma is rare.[10] Most cases occur in the hands and feet;[10,11] however, its most predominant site is the finger, where over 80 percent of these tumors are encountered. A few cases have been observed in such sites as the tongue[12] or cheek.[13] Extraskeletal chondromas are usually characterized by a slow-growing mass in the fingers or digits, which is seldom painful or tender. These tumors are benign, although Chung and Enzinger[11] reported that, in 10 of 56 (18 percent) patients, the tumor recurred once. Ideally, these tumors should be treated by excision with a satisfactory margin, and any attempt at a radical soft tissue excision or amputation should be avoided.

## ■ MALIGNANT TUMORS

### EXTRASKELETAL OR EXTRAOSSEOUS OSTEOGENIC SARCOMA

Although extraskeletal bone formation is not uncommon under a variety of stimuli, the occurrence of osteogenic sarcoma outside the skeletal system is rare. The first documented case was reported by Boneti[14] in 1700, followed by case reports by Morgagni[15] in 1763, Müller[16] in 1838, and Cooper[17] in 1845. In the early part of this century, Coley,[18] Rhoades and Blumgart,[19] and Mallory[20] further described this entity. After Wilson's[21] report in 1941, Schaffer,[22] in 1952, collected 44 patients from the literature who were presumed to have had extraosseous osteogenic sarcoma. Fine and Stout[5] found only 1 case in a review of 147 cases of osteogenic sarcoma and reports of 864 surgical specimens and 9,065 autopsies. They made a critical study of published cases and were reluctant to accept several as genuine extraosseous osteogenic sarcomas. They did,[5] however, obtain clinical and microscopic data on 12 acceptable cases and added these to the 34 previously established cases. Kauffman and Stout,[23] in 1963, reported two additional cases of this tumor in children.

With the establishment and acceptance of this tumor as a firm clinicopathologic entity, several additional case reports appeared in the literature.[24–27] In 1968, Das Gupta, Hajdu, and Foote[28] described the natural history of nine cases of extraosseous osteogenic sarcoma treated at Memorial Sloan-Kettering Cancer Center. Subsequently, Allan and Soule,[29] Wurlitzen and co-workers,[30] and Rao et al.[31] reported the experience at the Mayo Clinic, M.D. Anderson Tumor Institute, and Roswell Park Memorial Institute, respectively. In 1978, Dahn and associates[32] reported the only instance of extraskeletal osteosarcoma arising in the soft tissues of an organ (larynx).

The etiologic factors in extraosseous osteogenic sarcoma, as in most other sarcomas, are still unknown.

The relationship of localized myositis ossificans to extraosseous osteogenic sarcoma has already been discussed, but, even though a preexisting solitary myositis ossificans may have malignant transformation, the incidence is extremely rare and does not require serious clinical consideration. However, as with fibrosarcomas and osteogenic sarcomas, radiation-induced extraosseous osteogenic sarcomas have been reported, albeit rarely.[23,26,33,34] A review of the case histories of the patients studied shows that, once extraskeletal osteogenic sarcoma develops in an irradiated area, the prognosis is grave. Considering the large number of patients with seminoma, retinoblastoma, and several forms of malignant lymphoma treated solely by radiation therapy, remarkably few cases have been documented.

Extraskeletal osteogenic sarcoma occurs in all age groups. Although, in the review of Fine and Stout,[5] the disease was seen most often in elderly men, in our experience, there has been no age, sex, or race predilection. Our youngest patient was a 31-year-old woman. We have treated 10 cases of extraskeletal osteogenic sarcoma at the University of Illinois Hospital. The ages of the patients ranged from 31 to 82 years (Table 14–1). The location of the tumors corresponded generally with that of osteogenic sarcoma of the extremities, especially the lower. A similar preponderance in the lower extremities has also been reported by other authors.[28–31,35] In our group of 10 patients, six tumors were located in the lower extremity, two in the trunk, one in the right pleura, and one in an upper extremity (Fig. 14–2A to 14–2D).

It is difficult to draw guidelines for diagnostic criteria in the patients studied. In the soft somatic tissues, a tumor showing intrinsic calcifications along with elevated serum alkaline phosphatase levels should arouse clinical suspicion of an extraosseous osteogenic sarcoma. However, this should be distinguished from malignant fibrous histiocytoma with bone and cartilage formation.[36] Bhagavan and Dorfman[36] suggested that malignant fibrous histiocytomas with osteoid and chondroid elements are less aggressive than extraskeletal osteosarcomas or chondrosarcomas. The final diagnosis, of course, depends on the histologic findings. Although general guidelines regarding management cannot be formed on the basis of the small number of cases reported, wide excision, when possible, is most likely the ideal method of management (Fig. 14–3A to 14–3C).[28,31–33]

Of the 10 patients treated by us at the University of Illinois, only four (40 percent) survived five years or longer. The remaining six died at various intervals after initiation of primary treatment (Table 14–1). One patient died of unrelated causes. A review of the cases gleaned from the published case histories[37] shows that

**TABLE 14–1. CLINICAL SUMMARY OF 10 PATIENTS WITH EXTRAOSSEOUS OSTEOGENIC SARCOMA TREATED AT THE UNIVERSITY OF ILLINOIS HOSPITAL**

| Patient No. | Age/Sex | Primary Site | Status of Primary | Treatment at U of I | Local Recurrence | End Results |
|---|---|---|---|---|---|---|
| 1 | 47/M | Posterior thigh | Intact primary 5 × 6 cm (Fig. 14–2A) | Muscle group resection | — | Living and well 15 yrs after treatment |
| 2 | 58/M | Pleura | Exploratory thoracotomy elsewhere and diagnosis established | Radiation therapy and chemotherapy | — | DODD 18 mos. after diagnosis |
| 3 | 69/F | Soft tissue of lateral chest wall | Intact primary, 4 × 5 cm tumor | Chest wall resection | — | 11 yrs, NED |
| 4 | 82/M | Medial aspect of left thigh | Primary treated with 6,000 rads prior to U of I admission with a large 5 × 5 cm persistent ulcer | Wide soft tissue resection; residual tumor (microscopic only) | — | Died 2 mos. later of unrelated cause |
| 5 | 42/M | Lateral aspect of left arm | Intact primary 4 × 5 cm | Wide soft tissue excision | — | 5 yr, NED |
| 6 | 68/M | Thigh | 9-cm oval tumor in infragluteal fold | Wide excision | — | DODD with multiple recurrence within 1 year of diagnosis |
| 7 | 53/F | Lateral wall | Multiple local excisions | Recurrent ulcerating tumor | Chest wall resection | DODD 2 years later |
| 8 | 31/F | Buttock | Multiple local excisions | 6-cm oval tumor in the region of the previous scar | Wide excision | NED 7 yrs |
| 9 | 50/F | Thigh | Multiple local excisions | Recurrent 18 cm | Hemipelvectomy | DODD 3.5 yrs later |
| 10 | 31/F | Thigh | Primary tumor locally excised for biopsy | No obvious primary tumor | Groin dissection and hip disarticulation | Living 4 yrs after treatment without any evidence of metastases |

Abbreviations: DODD, died of diffuse disease; NED, no evidence of disease.

the overall five-year disease-free survival rate is abysmal. Although the incidence of local recurrence reported in the past is high,[28–31] it appears that initial radical resection will reduce the incidence of local recurrence. This was evident in our small series, even though some of these patients were referred to us with recurrent tumors.

Although the role of radiation therapy for these tumors has not been adequately evaluated, it does not seem to have been beneficial in the cases reported thus far. In the few cases in which it has been used, the results have not been satisfactory. Similarly, systemic chemotherapy has not been found to be useful. In our patient with pleural osteogenic sarcoma, various combinations were found to be of no value. The role of chemotherapy has not been ascertained.

## EXTRASKELETAL CHONDROSARCOMA

Extraskeletal chondrosarcoma is a rare tumor originally described in 1953 by Stout and Verner,[38] who collected a series of seven such cases. These authors described the histologic features and tried to correlate the biologic behavior with the morphology of these tumors. Subsequently, additional cases have been recognized and reported.[39–47] Since its original description, it has been recognized that, under the general heading of extraskeletal chondrosarcoma, two subtypes can be identified: (1) extraskeletal myxoid chondrosarcoma and (2) extraskeletal mesenchymal chondrosarcoma. These tumors have different morphologic characteristics and behavior. In 1972, Enzinger and Shiraki[48] reviewed 34 cases of extraskeletal chondrosarcoma

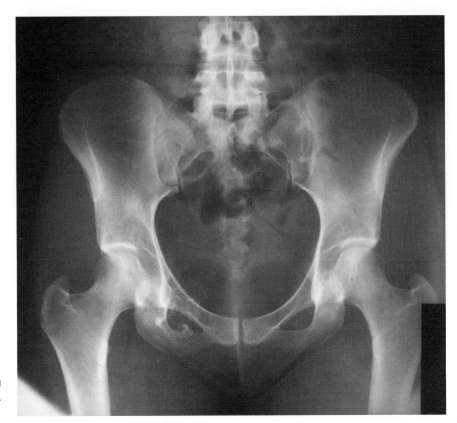

**Figure 14–1.** Heterotopic bone formation within right side of the pelvis in a 22-year-old woman. She was operated on, and the bone was removed.

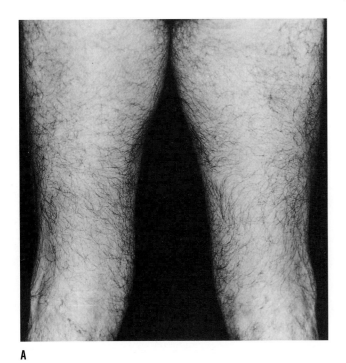

A

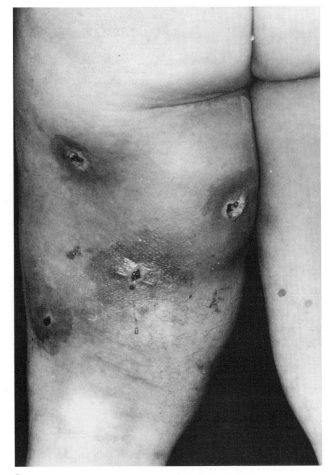

B

**Figure 14–2. (A)** Extraskeletal osteosarcoma in a 47-year-old man. Living disease-free fifteen years later. **(B)** Locally recurrent tumor in a 50-year-old woman. *(Continued.)*

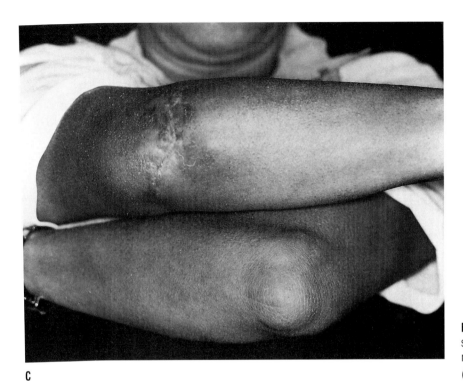

C

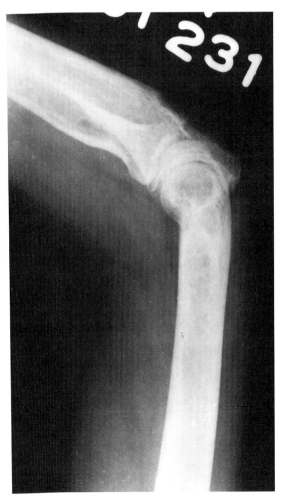

D

**Figure 14–2** *(continued)*. **(C)** Scar induration and swelling in the right elbow. **(D)** Preoperative x-ray of right elbow showing bone destruction in ulna. *(Courtesy of* Annals of Surgery.[28]*)*

from the files of the Armed Forces Institute of Pathology (AFIP) and essentially described the histologic characteristics of this subset of tumors. Since then, Martin et al.[49] and Hajdu et al.[50] have further refined the diagnostic and taxonomic characteristics of this tumor.

### Extraskeletal Myxoid Chondrosarcoma

Extraskeletal myxoid chondrosarcoma usually occurs in older individuals. It is equally prevalent in both sexes and seems to have no racial predilection. The etiologic factors are not known. Of interest is a case of chondrosarcoma of the chest associated with lucite spheres used as a plombage for compression of the tuberculous cavity, reported by Thompson and Entin.[42]

In most instances, the neoplasm occurs as a single, slow-growing, firm, superficial or deep nodule, or else a localized soft tissue swelling. The growth rate is much slower than in the mesenchymal variety. These tumors are usually deep-seated and most frequently encountered in the lower extremities. Enzinger and Shiraki[48] found that, in 29 (85 percent) of 34 patients, the primary tumor was in a lower extremity. Similar observations have recently been made by Meis et al.[51] and Saleh et al.[52] These tumors have also been described in the tongue,[53] thoracic wall,[23,40] and urinary bladder.[23,40] We have encountered chondrosarcomas in 12 patients, seven of which occurred in men and five in women. Six of these tumors were located in the trunk and six in the extremities. The clinical courses of these patients are summarized in Table 14–2,

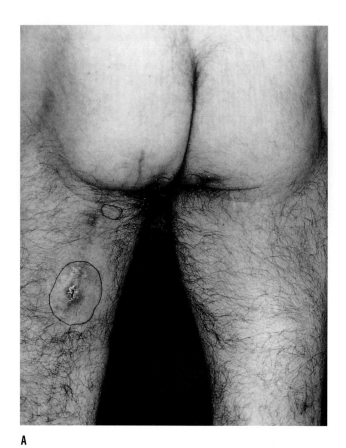

A

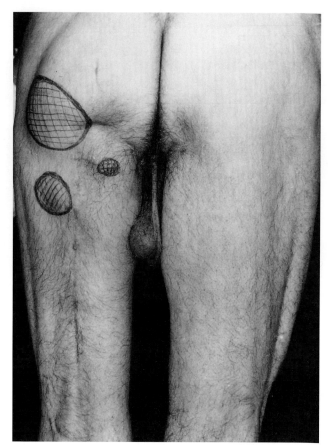

C

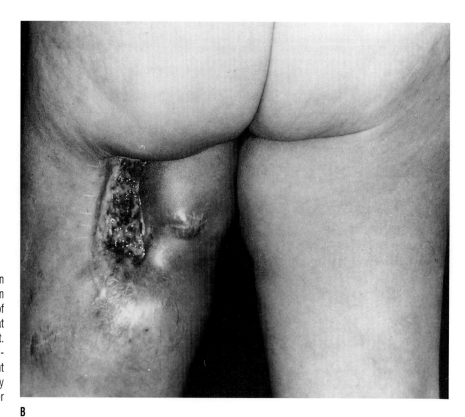

B

**Figure 14–3. (A)** Although the primary excision appeared to be adequate, this 57-year-old man was referred with a recurrence in the middle of the scar. During reoperation it was observed that the original excision was not as wide as thought. **(B)** Ulcerating recurrence after inadequate multiple excisions and radiation therapy. Patient refused hemipelvectomy, and was treated only palliatively. **(C)** Local recurrence in the posterior thigh. *(Courtesy of* Annals of Surgery.[28]*)*

**TABLE 14–2.  CLINICAL COURSE OF TWELVE PATIENTS WITH EXTRASKELETAL CHRONDROSARCOMA TREATED AT THE UNIVERSITY OF ILLINOIS HOSPITAL**

| Patient No. | Initial Treatment | Course | Status |
|---|---|---|---|
| 1 | Surgery + XRT | No Recurrence | AN at 133 mos. |
| 2 | Surgery + XRT + AC | No Recurrence | AN at 112 mos. |
| 3 | Surgery + XRT | No Recurrence | AN at 109 mos. |
| 4 | Surgery | No Recurrence | AN at 99 mos. |
| 5 | Surgery | No Recurrence | AN at 87 mos. |
| 6 | Surgery | No Recurrence | AN at 24 mos. |
| 7 | Surgery | Local recurrence at 19 mos.—resected + XRT; local recurrence at 38 mos.—resected; local recurrence at 96 mos.—resected + AC | AN at 114 mos. |
| 8 | Surgery | Local recurrence at 34 mos.—resected + XRT; local recurrence at 72 mos.—resected; local recurrence at 95 mos.—resected; local recurrence at 121 mos.—resected + AC; lung metastases at 145 mos.—resected; local recurrence at 148 mos.—XRT | DODD at 181 mos. |
| 9 | Surgery | Lung mets at 31 mos.—resected + AC; lung mets at 38 mos.—resected; lung mets at 50 mos.—resected; brain mets at 54 mos.—palliative XRT | DODD at 71 mos. |
| 10 | Surgery | Lung metastases at 5 mos.—resected; Lung metastases 12 mos.—resected + AC; Local recurrence at 18 mos.—palliative resection | DODD at 24 mos. |
| 11 | Surgery | Pelvic recurrence at 17 mos.—no treatment | DODD at 19 mos. |
| 12 | Surgery + XRT | Presented with lung metastases—resected with primary; RN/lung metastases at 7 mos.—resected + AC | DODD at 9 mos. |

Abbreviations: AC, adjuvant chemotherapy; AN, alive, no evidence of disease; DODD, died of diffuse disease; RN, regional lymph nodes; XRT, adjuvant radiation.

and Figure 14–4 shows the disease-free survival in relation to grade and mutant p53 protein expression. Adequate wide excision or muscle group resection appears to be the best form of treatment for extraskeletal myxoid chondrosarcomas. Radiation therapy and chemotherapy probably have little effect.

Enzinger and Shiraki[48] pointed out that, although the clinical behavior of these sarcomas may vary considerably, extraskeletal myxoid chondrosarcomas are certainly far less aggressive than chondrosarcomas of the bone.[39] This observation has been echoed by Smith and his co-workers.[47] One of our patients underwent excision of the gluteal muscles with subsequent good functional quality and satisfactory end results, whereas, in a similar patient reported by Stout and Verner,[38] a hemipelvectomy was performed. If an initial approach of aggressive wide excision is taken, the possibility of local recurrence, which appears to be a frequent complication in most of the published literature, can be avoided; furthermore, with this type of wide excision, little or no functional deformity results.

### Extraskeletal Mesenchymal Chondrosarcoma

Extraskeletal mesenchymal chondrosarcoma was originally described in 1959 by Lichtenstein and Bernstein.[54] Since then, several authors have published a number of case reports.[55–57] This tumor differs from its myxoid counterpart by virtue of the fact that it is more aggressive in nature and tends to metastasize rapidly.[58] We have treated only four patients with extraskeletal mesenchymal chondrosarcoma. All but one died within two years of initial presentation, and one patient is living disease-free four years after primary therapy. We have treated this variety of extraskeletal chondrosarcoma in the same manner as the more indolent myxoid type. It is quite possible that this mesenchymal variety might be a candidate for consideration of adjuvant chemotherapy.

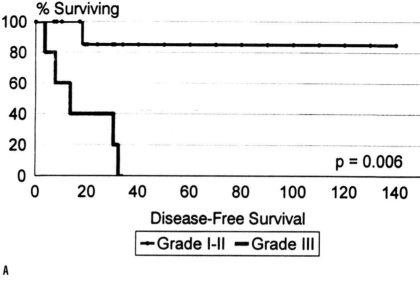

A

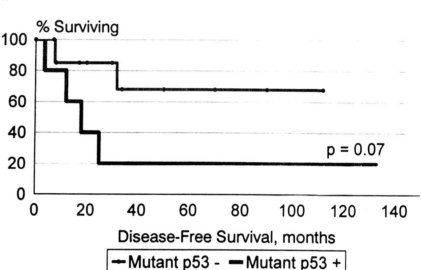

B

**Figure 14–4.** Disease-free survival curve for patients with extraskeletal chondrosarcoma according to **(A)** tumor grade and **(B)** mutant p53 protein expression.

## REFERENCES

1. Willis RA: The Borderland of Embryology and Pathology, chap 14. London, Butterworth, 1958, p 506
2. France CJ, O'Connell JP: Osseous metaplasia in the human mammary gland. Arch Surg 100:238, 1970
3. Ling HW, Stewart IS: A bony tumor of the breast. Br Med J 2:364, 1955
4. Pack GT, Ariel IM: Tumors of the Soft Somatic Tissues: A Clinical Technique. New York, Hoeber-Harper, 1958, p 332
5. Fine G, Stout AP: Osteogenic sarcoma of the extraskeletal soft tissue. Cancer 9:1027, 1956
6. Eckhart JJ, Ivins JC, Perry HO, et al.: Osteosarcoma arising in heterotopic ossification of dermatomyositis: Case report and review of the literature. Cancer 48:1256, 1981
7. Ryan KJ: Myositis ossificans progressive: Review of the literature and report of a case. J Pediatr 27:348, 1945
8. Rosenstein J: A contribution to the study of myositis ossificans progressive. Ann Surg 68:485, 1918
9. Pack GT, Braund RR: The development of sarcoma in myositis ossificans: Report of 3 cases. JAMA 119:776, 1942
10. Dahlin DC, Salvador AH: Cartilaginous tumors of the soft tissues of the hand and feet. Mayo Clin Proc 49:721, 1974
11. Chung EB, Enzinger FM: Chondroma of soft parts. Cancer 41:1414, 1978
12. Bamachandran K, Viswannthan R: Chondroma of the tongue. Report of a case. Oral Surg 25:487, 1968
13. Hankey GT, Waterhouse JP: A calcifying chondroma in the cheek. Br J Oral Surg 5:239, 1968
14. Boneti T: De ventris tumors, in Sepulchretum, sive anatomia practica excadaveribus morbo denatis. Geneva, Cramer et Parachon, Vol 3, Sect 21, Obs 61, 1700, p 522
15. Morgagni G: The Seats and Causes of Diseases. Translated by B. Alexander. London, A. Millar and T. Cadell. Vol 3, letter L, Obs 41, 1769, p 63

16. Müller J: Uber den feinern Bau der Drankhaften Gesehwulste. Berlin, G. Reimer, 1838, p 48

17. Cooper A: The Anatomy and Diseases of the Breast. Philadelphia, Lea & Blanchard, 1845, p 47

18. Coley WB: Myositis ossificans traumatica: A report of three cases illustrating the difficulties of diagnosis from sarcoma. Ann Surg 57:305, 1913

19. Rhoades CP, Blumgart H: Two osteoblastomas not connected with bone, histologically identical with osteogenic sarcoma and clinically benign. Am J Pathol 4:363, 1928

20. Mallory TB: A group of metaplastic and neoplastic bone and cartilage containing tumor of soft parts. Am J Pathol 9:765, 1933

21. Wilson H: Extraskeletal ossifying tumors. Ann Surg 113: 95 1941

22. Schaffer LW Jr.: Extraskeletal osteochondrosarcoma— Review of literature and report of a case. Am Surg 18:739, 1952

23. Kauffman SL, Stout AP: Extraskeletal osteogenic sarcomas and chondrosarcomas in children. Cancer 16:432, 1963

24. Lowry K Jr., Doyle-Hanes C: Osteosarcoma of extraskeletal soft tissue: A case report. Am Surg 30:97, 1964

25. Yannopoulos K, Bom AF, Griffiths CO, Crikelair GF: Osteosarcoma arising in fibrous dysplasia of the facial bones: Case report and review of the literature. Am J Surg 107:556, 1964

26. Boyer CW Jr., Nawin JJ: Extraskeletal osteogenic sarcoma: A late complication of radiation therapy. Cancer 18:628, 1965

27. Lewis RJ, Lotz MJ, Beazley RM: Extraosseous osteosarcoma: Case report and approach to therapy. Ann Surg 40: 597, 1974

28. Das Gupta TK, Hajdu SI, Foote FW Jr.: Extraosseous osteogenic sarcoma. Ann Surg 168:1011, 1968

29. Allan CJ, Soule EII: Osteogenic sarcoma of the somatic soft tissue: A clinicopathologic study of 26 cases and review of the literature. Cancer 27:1121, 1971

30. Wurlitzen F, Ayala A, Ronsdahl M: Extraosseous osteogenic sarcoma. Arch Surg 105:691, 1972

31. Rao U, Cheng A, Didolkar MS: Extraosseous osteogenic sarcoma. Clinicopathological study of eight cases and review of the literature. Cancer 41:1488, 1978

32. Dahn LJ, Schaffer SD, Carder HM, Vellios F: Osteosarcoma of the soft tissue of the larynx: Report of a case with light and electron microscopic studies. Cancer 42:2343, 1978

33. Auerbach O, Friedman M, Weiss L, Amory HI: Extraskeletal osteogenic sarcoma arising in irradiated tissue. Cancer 4:1095, 1951

34. Laskin WB, Silverman TA, Enzinger FM: Postradiation soft tissue sarcomas: An analysis of 53 cases. Cancer 62: 2330, 1988

35. Sordillo PP, Hajdu SI, Magill GB, et al.: Extraosseous osteogenic sarcoma: A review of 48 patients. Cancer 51: 727, 1983

36. Bhagavan BS, Dorfman HD: The significance of bone and cartilage formation in malignant fibrous histiocytoma of soft tissue. Cancer 49:480, 1982

37. Bane BL, Evans HL, Ro JY, et al.: Extraskeletal osteosarcoma: A clinicopathologic review of 26 cases. Cancer 65: 2726, 1990

38. Stout AP, Verner EW: Chondrosarcoma of the extraskeletal soft tissue. Cancer 6:581, 1953

39. Dahlin DC, Henderson ED: Chondrosarcoma—A surgical and pathological problem. Review of 212 cases. J Bone Joint Surg 38A:1025, 1956

40. Goldenberg RR, Cohen P, Steinlauf P: Chondrosarcoma of the extraskeletal soft tissues. J Bone Joint Surg 49A: 1487, 1967

41. Korns ME: Primary chondrosarcoma of extraskeletal soft tissue. Arch Pathol 83:13, 1967

42. Thompson JR, Entin SD: Primary extraskeletal chondrosarcoma: Report of a case arising in conjunction with extrapleural lucite ball plombage. Cancer 23:940, 1969

43. Angervall L, Enerback L, Knutson H: Chondrosarcoma of soft tissue origin. Cancer 32:507, 1973

44. Steiner GC, Mirra JM, Bullough PG: Mesenchymal chondrosarcoma: A study of the ultrastructure. Cancer 32:926, 1973

45. Yao-Shi F, Kay S: A comparative ultrastructural study of mesenchymal chondrosarcoma and myxoid chondrosarcoma. Cancer 33:1531, 1974

46. Pittman MR, Keller EE: Mesenchymal chondrosarcoma: Report of a case. J Oral Surg 32:443, 1974

47. Smith MT, Farinacci CJ, Carpenter HA, Bannayan GA: Extraskeletal myxoid chondrosarcoma: A clinicopathological study. Cancer 37:821, 1976

48. Enzinger FM, Shiraki M: Extraskeletal myxoid chondrosarcoma: An analysis of 34 cases. Hum Pathol 3:421, 1972

49. Martin RF, Melnick PJ, Warner NE, et al.: Chordoid sarcoma. Am J Clin Pathol 59:623, 1973

50. Hajdu SI, Shuh MH, Fortner JG: Tendosynovial sarcoma: A clinicopathologic study of 136 cases. Cancer 39:1201, 1977

51. Meis JM, Martz KL: Extraskeletal myxoid chondrosarcoma: A clinicopathologic study of 120 cases. Lab Invest 66:9A, 1992

52. Saleh G, Evans HL, Ro JY, et al.: Extraskeletal myxoid chondrosarcoma: A clinicopathologic study of ten patients with long-term follow-up. Cancer 70:2827, 1992

53. Vassar PS: Chondrosarcoma of the tongue: A case report. Arch Pathol 65:261, 1958

54. Lichtenstein L, Bernstein D: Unusual benign and malignant chondroid tumors of bone: A survey of some mesenchymal cartilage tumors and malignant chondroblastic tumors including a few multicentric ones and chondromyxoid fibromas. Cancer 12:1142, 1959

55. Dahlin DC, Henderson ED: Mesenchymal chondrosarcoma: Further observations on a new entity. Cancer 15: 40, 1962

56. Salvador AH, Beabont JW, Dahlin DC: Mesenchymal chondrosarcoma: Observations of 30 new cases. Cancer 28:605, 1971

57. Shapiro LG, Vanel D, Conanet D, et al.: Extraskeletal mesenchymal chondrosarcoma. Radiology 186:819, 1993

58. Guccion JG, Font RL, Enzinger FM, et al.: Extraskeletal mesenchymal chondrosarcoma. Arch Pathol 95:336, 1973

# 15

# Undetermined Histogenesis

Although the number of benign and malignant tumors of uncertain histogenesis is decreasing, there are still some in which the correct histogenetic type is difficult or almost impossible to determine. In the absence of such classification, the clinical features of these diverse groups are described in this section. Currently, these entities are classified as follows.

A. Benign Tumors
　1. Myxoma (with all variants)
　2. Benign mesenchymoma
　3. Ossifying fibromyxoid tumor of the soft tissue
　4. Amyloid tumors
　5. Other tumorlike conditions
B. Malignant Tumors
　1. Alveolar soft part sarcoma
　2. Epithelioid sarcoma
　3. Malignant extrarenal rhabdoid tumor
　4. Malignant mesenchymoma
　5. Malignant mesothelioma

## ■ BENIGN TUMORS

### MYXOMA (WITH ALL ITS VARIANTS)

Clinically, the most significant example of myxoma is the intramuscular variety (intramuscular myxoma). The existence of this entity was originally emphasized by Stout[1] and later by Enzinger.[2] Awareness of this particular entity is important inasmuch as these tumors can mimic myxoid liposarcomas or, occasionally, rhabdomyosarcomas. Solitary intramuscular myxomas, in spite of their size and rate of growth, are benign and require only simple excision.

Myxomas can occur at various anatomic locations, most notably in the heart (atrial variety) and occasionally near large weight-bearing joints, mimicking the common variety of soft tissue sarcomas and osteosarcomas. The term *aggressive angiomyosarcoma* was coined by Steepes and Rosai[3] for a slow-growing myxoid neoplasm that occurs chiefly in the genital and pelvic region of adults, especially in women. These tumors have a distinct morphologic appearance and can be easily distinguished from intramuscular myxomas. Although these tumors can grow rapidly and sometimes attain a large size, they are benign and should be treated by conservative resection.

### BENIGN MESENCHYMOMA

In 1938, Tauber and colleagues[4] used the term *mesenchymoma* to describe an unusual tumor of the scalp composed of undifferentiated cells of possible mesenchymal origin. Stout, in 1948,[5] applied this term to designate a group of tumors composed of at least two differentiated mesenchymal elements not ordinarily found together in a given tumor. He reported eight such cases. Since that time, a few additional case reports have appeared in the literature.[6,7] A clinicopathologic diagnosis of benign mesenchymoma must be made with great caution. We have encountered only a few patients whose soft tissue tumors could be so designated. These tumors are treated by local excision.

There are other benign tumors (e.g., ossifying fibromyxoid tumors, parachordoma, and amyloid tumors of the soft tissues). Some of these tumors or tumorlike conditions architecturally resemble malignant tumors; thus, extreme caution must be exercised before instituting any form of therapy, be it excisional and/or radiation therapy. A conservative excision is the central dogma in the management.

# MALIGNANT TUMORS

## ALVEOLAR SOFT PART SARCOMA

The alveolar soft part sarcoma was first described by Christopherson, Foote, and Stewart[6] in 1952. Costero[8] and Udekwu and Pulvertaft[7] later published specific histopathologic evidence which indicated that alveolar soft part sarcoma was an unusual type of malignant mesenchymal tumor. Although rare,[9] clinically these tumors have a distinct history of slow growth, local infiltration, and delayed visceral metastases.

They occur in all age groups from neonates to adults in their seventh decade, but are most commonly encountered in young adults between the ages of 20 and 35 years; they are far more common in women than in men. The average age of discovery in women is 20 years and in men about 10 years later. There seems to be no racial predilection.

The usual history is of a comparatively slow-growing asymptomatic mass located in one of the extremities. Of the original 12 cases reported by Christopherson et al.,[6] 10 were in an extremity. The tumor may also arise from the anterior abdominal wall, the perianal region, the retroperitoneum,[10] or the head and neck region.[6,11–20] It is always associated with skeletal muscles or musculofascial planes, and it is usually well circumscribed.

Lieberman and co-workers[13] analyzed 53 cases of alveolar soft part sarcoma seen at Memorial Sloan-Kettering Cancer Center and presented survival data on 46 patients. We have treated 17 patients with this tumor. Twelve were women, and five were men; ages ranged from 21 to 69 years old. The clinical history in these patients is usually characterized by a slow-growing mass, most commonly located in the lower extremity or less frequently in the upper extremity and trunk. Alveolar soft part sarcomas in the head and neck region are extremely rare. Up to 1979, only 11 cases were recorded.[6,11,15,16–21] In a more recent publication, Enzinger and Weiss[22] reported that, in the files of the Armed Forces Institute of Pathology (AFIP), alveolar soft part sarcomas of the head and neck region constitute 27 percent in a series of 143 patients.

Alveolar soft part sarcoma runs an indolent but inexorable course, with a tendency to metastasize to lungs, liver, skeleton, and, infrequently, to the lymph nodes. In Lieberman and co-workers' series,[13] three patients had lung metastases 15 years after the onset of illness.

Treatment for alveolar soft part sarcoma is wide soft tissue resection. A major amputation is seldom indicated. In our experience to date, no patient with extremity soft part sarcoma required an amputation for local control of the primary tumor. Four (24 percent) of the 17 had their tumors located in the trunk; in only one was the tumor located in the periorbital region. In all five of these instances, radical excision was the primary therapy. Based on a five-year survival analysis, it appears that radical excision alone is adequate. However, in larger lesions or lesions located in the head and neck area, a combination of radiation therapy and systemic chemotherapy probably is in order.

In a more recent publication, Lieberman et al.[23] analyzed the case histories of 91 patients. In patients who presented without metastases, these authors found a 77 percent survival rate at two years, 60 percent at five years, and 38 percent at ten years. Auerbach and Brooks[24] reported an overall survival rate of 67 percent at five years.[24] Of the 17 patients treated by us, 12 (71 percent) are living at the end of five years, and 8 (47 percent) remain disease-free at the end of ten years after treatment of the primary tumor. These neoplasms have a propensity to recur at a late date and also have the potential to metastasize after a long time. However, currently, no data justify the routine use of adjuvant chemotherapy, and it appears that an adequate wide excision is sufficient for local control of these tumors.

## EPITHELIOID SARCOMA

*Epithelioid sarcoma* is a term that was introduced by Enzinger[25] in 1970 to designate a group of unusual sarcomas that are likely to be confused with synovial sarcomas or granulomatous processes and ulcerating squamous cell carcinomas. Since the definitive article by Enzinger, several other authors have described the clinicopathologic characteristics of epithelioid sarcoma.[26–38] Santiago et al.[30] suggested that, in the past, these tumors were probably recognized by other authors,[38–43] but under different names.

Epithelioid sarcoma is usually encountered in adult males.[35,44] Of Enzinger's[25] 62 patients, 49 were male, and 13 were female. In the University of Illinois group, five of the eight patients were men. These tumors are most frequently seen in patients between the ages of 20 and 50 years, although both extremes in age have been reported.[30,32,35,36,44] The oldest patient in our group was 62 years old, and the youngest was 11. No racial predilection has been observed.

## Anatomic Location

Epithelioid sarcomas occur predominantly in the extremities.[25,29,30,32,35–38] Enzinger noted that, with the exception of 2 of his 62 patients (in whom the tumors were in the scalp), the lesions were located in the upper extremities in 38 patients, and were located in the lower extremities in 22 patients. Bryan et al.[37] reported that, of 85 primary soft tissue sarcomas and 16 primary bone tumors involving the hand and forearm in the files of the Mayo Clinic, 13 were epithelioid sarcomas, making this tumor third in frequency, after fibrosarcoma and rhabdomyosarcoma. In our series of eight cases, one was in the posterior trunk, four were in the forearm and hand, one was in the elbow, and two were in the lower extremities. Rarely, epithelioid sarcoma has been reported in the penis[28] and in bone.[31]

Patients with epithelioid sarcoma usually present with a small innocuous-looking lump in an extremity. These tumors are known for their relatively slow rate of growth. Nodules near the skin surface frequently become elevated and, at a later stage of growth, can become ulcerated, giving rise to the appearance of an ulcerating pyogenic granuloma. Deep-seated lesions fixed to the tendons or fascia are generally large and less well defined. Infrequently, these tumors are associated with pain or tenderness. They are relatively less common in the trunk. The incidence of regional node metastases has been variously described by different authors. Enzinger[25] found metastasis in 6 of 62 patients (9.6 percent), and Santiago and co-workers[30] in 3 of 9 (33 percent). Bryan et al.[37] observed metastases in 3 of 13 patients (23 percent). In our present series of eight patients, three (38 percent) had regional node metastases. Frequently, clinicopathologic distinction of tumor from synovial cell sarcoma, malignant giant cell tumor, and malignant melanoma of soft parts is difficult. In Table 15–1, the clinicopathologic characteristics of these diverse groups of tumors are summarized. In two of our three patients with metastases, the tumors were locally recurrent following inadequate excision. This incidence of regional node metastases probably represents the incidence in advanced and locally recurrent tumors. In stage 1 primary tumors, the true incidence is much lower, probably about 10 percent. However, because of this uncertainty, it is recommended that the regional node-bearing area be taken into consideration during initial planning of therapy.

## Treatment

The primary treatment for epithelioid sarcoma should be wide excision and regional node dissection. The major objective is either to eliminate or reduce the possibility of local recurrence. Most authors[27,28,33,34,45] have found that conservative local excision is associated with a high rate of local recurrence, resulting in poor prognosis and end results. In the University of Illinois material, an initial aggressive surgical approach, with adjuvant chemotherapy and, occasionally, radiation therapy, resulted in an excellent salvage rate of these patients. Seven of the eight (87 percent) were disease-free at the end of two years. Of the four eligible for 10-year end-result analysis, three are alive with no evidence of recurrence or metastasis, and the fourth patient died of unrelated causes.

Primary curative radiation therapy alone has not been tried in our patients, and the published data are sparse. However, it appears that postoperative radiation therapy along with adjuvant chemotherapy might be a useful addition to the therapeutic armamentarium. Two of our patients who are living 10 years after original treatment received postoperative radiation therapy.

The role of chemotherapy, either in an adjuvant setting or in metastatic disease, still remains doubtful. However, in locally recurrent tumors and in metastatic disease, adriamycin-based chemotherapy probably should be considered.

## End Results

The end results of treatment of epithelioid sarcoma, and the prognostic factors, are difficult to ascertain. Most of the published reports have been by pathologists,[25,28–30,32,36] and the type of treatment described is based only on reported data in the charts, or from letters by clinicians. We have found that the definition of "wide" radical excision varies among surgeons. Patients have been referred to the University of Illinois with the notation that a wide excision had been performed when in reality the primary tumor was only enucleated. Sometimes, a tumor of the upper anterior leg has been treated with a below-knee amputation with a minimal margin of unaffected tissue, resulting in eventual failure of the primary treatment. Therefore, the statement that epithelioid sarcoma continues to progress relentlessly after adequate excision should be viewed with extreme caution.

In our material, 87 percent of the patients lived disease-free for two years and 75 percent for ten years. Soule and Enriquez[33] suggested that the prognosis is somewhat better for superficially located tumors, and this appears to be a tenable hypothesis.

## MALIGNANT EXTRARENAL RHABDOID TUMOR

Malignant extrarenal rhabdoid tumor is extremely rare and resembles rhabdomyosarcoma. It is probably a variant of Wilms' tumor, but can occur in other parts of the body. Establishment of diagnosis is difficult, and the

**TABLE 15–1. CHARACTERISTICS OF FOUR DIFFERENT MALIGNANT TUMORS OF DIVERSE HISTOGENESIS WITH CONSIDERABLE SIMILARITY OF CLINICAL PRESENTATION**

| Factors | Synovial Sarcoma | Malignant Giant Cell Tumors of Tendon Sheath | Epithelioid Sarcoma | Clear Cell Sarcoma (Malignant Melanoma of Soft Parts) |
|---|---|---|---|---|
| Age | 20–40 yr | 30–50 yr | 10–50 yr | 20–70 yr |
| Sex | M:F 1:1 | M:F 1:2 | M:F 4:1 | F:M |
| Common site | Extremities near major joints | Tendon sheaths over distal part of the extremities | Distal extremities (digits and toes also can be site of primary) | Extremities |
| Common clinical presentation | Painless tumor with relatively rapid increase in size | Small tumor usually attached to a tendon mobile in one axis | Painless tumor, slow-growing, frequently ulcerated, and resembling a pyogenic granuloma | Tumor is frequently associated with discomfort and occasionally with pain |
| Incidence of regional node metastases | 10–25% | 20–25% | 35–40% | 20–25% |
| Roentgenographic findings | Calcific stippling; occasional bone formation | Frequent erosion of the superficial cortex of the adjacent bone | No specific findings | Nothing significant |
| Histologic characteristics | Biphasic appearance (characteristic monophasic appearance not infrequent) | Lack of biphasic pattern and overall rarity of pseudoglandular clefts. Pleomorphic and phagocytic multinucleated giant cells with occasional bone formation | An admixture of granulomatous and pseudocarcinomatous pattern | Uniform pattern of compact nests/fascicles with clear cytoplasm contiguous to adjacent tendons or aponeuroses |
| Treatment | Wide excision with regional node dissection in pleomorphic types and radiation therapy. For low-grade, wide excision alone is adequate. | Same as synovial sarcoma. Because of location, frequently needs amputation. Same as synovial sarcoma. Because of location, frequently needs amputation. | Same as synovial sarcoma. Incidence of regional node involvement, especially in recurrent cases, is high. Additional radiation therapy and chemotherapy are beneficial. | Same as synovial sarcoma. Wide excision and, if indicated, simultaneous regional node dissection. |
| Local recurrence | + | + | ++ | − |

treatment is wide excision. Because of the rarity of the disease, logical decisions regarding management are well nigh impossible.

## MALIGNANT MESENCHYMOMA

Malignant mesenchymoma is rarely encountered today. As described in Chapter 5, if, in an unusual situation, the exact histogenesis of the given tumor cannot be adequately documented, the management of the tumor should depend on the predominant malignant tissue component. For example, a tumor containing different tissue elements with a preponderance of malignant lipoblasts should be treated as an undifferentiated liposarcoma (grade 3 or 4). Caution should be exercised so that this does not become a catch-all diagnosis.

In any event, where this diagnosis is inescapable, the method of management is extremely hard to define. Thus, the most logical approach would entail a wide excision. End-result data cannot properly be described.

## MALIGNANT MESOTHELIOMA

Some malignant mesotheliomas, for example pleural or peritoneal mesotheliomas, are rare malignant neoplasms. Because of the association of pleural mesothelioma with asbestos exposure, this type of malignancy has engendered considerable curiosity; however, the neoplasm is rare, and general guidelines for management are not yet possible. Strictly speaking, pleural mesotheliomas are soft somatic tissue neoplasms, but seldom are they treated as such. In the unusual instance

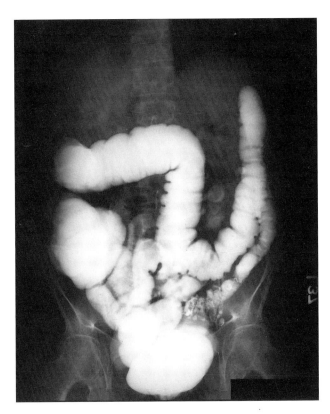

**Figure 15–1.** Peritoneal mesothelioma in a 55-year-old woman. Note the impingement of the sigmoid due to serosal implants and pressure. This patient was first seen because of changing bowel habits. The diagnosis was established by exploratory celiotomy. Treatment consisted of removal of peritoneal implants and segmental resection of the sigmoid colon.

in which the diagnosis can be made early, a pleurectomy might be of some value. However, in most instances, the diagnosis is made after the patient has massive pleural effusion, and the treatment becomes palliative, with judicious thoracentesis, radiation therapy, and chemotherapy. Long-term cures are rare.

A clinical diagnosis of peritoneal or pelvic mesothelioma is based on abdominal or pelvic symptoms. These tumors can be operated on by removing the gross tumor along with the adjacent viscera, but the incidence of local recurrence is extremely high (Fig. 15–1).

## REFERENCES

1. Stout AP: Myxoma, the tumor of primitive mesenchyme. Ann Surg 127:706, 1948
2. Enzinger FM: Intramuscular myxoma. Am J Clin Pathol 43:104, 1965
3. Steepes TA, Rosai J: Aggressive angiomyosarcoma of the female pelvis and perineum: Report of nine cases. A distinctive type of gynecologic soft tissue neoplasm. Am J Surg Pathol 7:463, 1983
4. Tauber EB, Goldman L, Bassett C: Mesenchymoma, a new type of urban tumor. Arch Dermatol Syph 37:444, 1938
5. Stout AP: Mesenchymoma, the mixed tumor of mesenchymal derivatives. Ann Surg 127:278, 1948
6. Christopherson WM, Foote JW Jr., Stewart FW: Alveolar soft part sarcomas: Structurally characteristic tumors of uncertain histogenesis. Cancer 5:100, 1952
7. Udekwu FA, Pulvertaft FJ: Studies of an alveolar soft tissue sarcoma. Br J Cancer 19:744, 1965
8. Costero I: Recent advances in the knowledge concerning chemodectomas. Lab Invest 12:270, 1963
9. Ekfors TO, Kalimo H, Rantakokko V, et al.: Alveolar soft part sarcoma. A report of two cases with some histochemical and ultrastructural observations. Cancer 43:1672, 1979
10. Mathew T: Evidence supporting neural crest origin of an alveolar soft part sarcoma: An ultrastructural study. Cancer 50:507, 1982
11. Buchanan G: Two rare tumors involving the infratemporal fossa: Alveolar soft part sarcoma and haemangiopericytoma. J Laryngol Otol (London): 89:375, 1975
12. Balfour RS: The alveolar soft-part sarcoma: Review of the literature and report of case. J Oral Surg 32:214, 1974
13. Lieberman PH, Foote FW Jr., Stewart FW, et al.: Alveolar soft part sarcoma. JAMA 198:1047, 1966
14. Olson RAJ, Perkins KD: Alveolar soft-part sarcoma in the oral cavity: Report of a case. J Oral Surg 34:73, 1976
15. Smetana HF, Scott WF Jr.: Malignant tumors of nonchromaffin paraganglia. Milit Surg 190:330, 1951
16. Caldwell JB, Hughes KW, Fadell EJ: Alveolar soft-part sarcoma of the tongue: Report of a case. J Oral Surg 14:342, 1956
17. Ushijima H, Tamura Z: A report of two cases of alveolar soft-part sarcoma and their histological variations. Acta Pathol Jpn (Suppl) 7:851, 1957
18. Vakil VV, Sirsat MV: The natural history of alveolar soft-part sarcomas. Indian J Pathol Bacteriol 6:19, 1963
19. Gingrass R, Mladick R, Pickrell L, Punyahotra V: Malignant nonchromaffin paraganglioma or alveolar soft-part sarcoma in the temporal region. Plast Reconstr Surg 40:463, 1967
20. Varghese S, Nair G, Joseph TA: Orbital malignant nonchromaffin paraganglioma: Alveolar soft tissue sarcoma. Br J Ophthalmol 52:713, 1968
21. Spector RA, Travis LW, Smith J: Alveolar soft part sarcoma of the head and neck. Laryngoscope 89:1301, 1979
22. Enzinger FM, Weiss SW: Malignant soft tissue tumors of uncertain type. In Enzinger FM, Weiss SW (eds): Soft Tissue Tumors, 3rd ed. St. Louis, Mosby-Yearbook, 1995, p 1067
23. Lieberman PH, Brennan MF, Kimmel M, et al.: Alveolar soft part sarcoma: A clinicopathologic study of half a century. Cancer 63:1, 1989
24. Auerbach HE, Brooks JJ: Alveolar soft part sarcoma: A clinicopathologic and immunohistochemical study. Cancer 60:66, 1987
25. Enzinger FM: Epithelioid sarcoma: A sarcoma simulating a granuloma or a carcinoma. Cancer 26:1029, 1970
26. Suit HD, Russell WO, Martin RG: Sarcoma of soft tissues:

Clinical and histopathological parameters and response to treatment. Cancer 35:1478, 1975

27. Moore SW, Wheeler JE, Hefter LG: Epithelioid sarcoma masquerading as Peyronie's disease. Cancer 35:1706, 1975

28. Dehner LP, Smith BH: Soft tissue tumors of the penis. Cancer 25:1431, 1970

29. Mackenzie DH: Two types of soft tissue sarcoma of uncertain histogenesis. Br J Cancer 25:458, 1972

30. Santiago H, Feinerman LK, Lattes R: Epithelioid sarcoma: A clinical and pathologic study of nine cases. Human Pathol 3:133, 1972

31. DeLuca FN, Nevasier RJ: Epithelioid sarcoma involving a bone. Clin Orthop 107:168, 1975

32. Fisher ER, Hormvat B: The fibrocytic derivation of the so-called epithelioid sarcoma. Cancer 30:1074, 1972

33. Soule EH, Enriquez P: Atypical fibrous histiocytoma, malignant fibrous histiocytoma, malignant histiocytoma, and epithelioid sarcoma: A comparative study of 65 tumors. Cancer 30:128, 1972

34. Bloustein PA, Silverberg SG, Waddell WR: Epithelioid sarcoma: Case report with an ultrastructural review, histogenetic discussion, and chemotherapeutic treatment. Cancer 38:2390, 1976

35. Males JL, Lain KC: Epithelioid sarcoma in XO/XX Turner's syndrome. Arch Pathol 94:214, 1972

36. Pratt J, Woodruff JM, Marcove RC: Epithelioid sarcoma: An analysis of 22 cases indicating prognostic significance of vascular invasion and regional lymph node metastases. Cancer 41:1472, 1978

37. Bryan RS, Soule EH, Dobyns JH, et al.: Primary epithelioid sarcoma of the hand and forearm. J Bone Joint Surg 56A:458, 1974

38. Tsuneyoshi M, Enjoji M, Shinohara N: Epithelioid sarcoma: A clinicopathologic and electron microscopic study. Acta Pathol Jpn 30(3):411, 1980

39. Berger L: Synovial sarcomas in serous bursae and tendon sheaths. Am J Cancer 34:501, 1938

40. Black WC: Synovioma of the hand. Report of a case. Am J Cancer 28:481, 1936

41. DeSanto DA, Tennant R, Rosahn PD: Synovial sarcomas in joints, bursae, and tendon sheaths. Surg Gynecol Obstet 72:951, 1941

42. Bliss BO, Reed RJ: Large cell sarcomas of tendons sheath: Malignant giant cell tumors of tendon sheath. Am J Clin Pathol 49:776, 1968

43. Eisenstein R: Giant-cell tumor of tendon sheath: Its histogenesis as studied in the electron microscope. J Bone Joint Surg 50A:476, 1968

44. Tsuneyoshi M, Enjoji M, Kubo T: Clear cell sarcoma of tendon and aponeuroses: A comparative study of 13 cases with a provisional subgrouping into the melanotic and synovial types. Cancer 42(1):243, 1978

45. Hoffman GJ, Carter D: Clear-cell sarcoma of tendon and aponeuroses with melanin. Arch Pathol 95:22, 1973

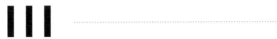

# Principles of Treatment

# 16

# Surgical Treatment

The spectrum of surgical techniques used in treating primary soft somatic tissue tumors ranges from simple excision of a benign lipoma to the most challenging of radical excisions, such as a quarterectomy. In any given sarcoma, the surgeon, before making a decision to operate, must take into consideration such factors as the histologic type and grade, the anatomic location, the fixity to or mobility from the surrounding tissue, the presence of regional or distant metastases, and, finally, his or her own experience and familiarity with sarcomas in general.

The technical aspects of excision of a benign tumor such as a lipoma are simple, and usually the local excision methods described herein cover the principles of management of other benign tumors. However, in some specific instances, modifications in the techniques of local excision are required—for example, excision of a palmar or plantar fibromatosis.

The purpose of surgical treatment is eradication of the primary tumor. Unless an aggressive initial approach is undertaken, the therapy program will ultimately fail in most patients. Thus, on balance, a major operation might be the only opportunity a patient has for living, and the surgeon cannot deny the patient that opportunity. With the use of multimodal therapy, however, the need and indications for major ablative procedures are becoming less and less. No patient should be denied the ideal therapy on the basis of chronological age alone. For example, a total cystectomy, if indicated, should be performed in an infant with rhabdomyosarcoma of the urinary bladder. Similarly, an elderly patient with a sarcoma arising in an extremity should have appropriate resection. Once all the facts

are provided, the patient (or parents) should have the opportunity to make the final decision. Scrutiny of the results of treatment of soft tissue sarcomas shows that, in most instances, the incidence of local recurrence is directly proportional to the inadequacy of treatment of the primary.[1-6] Therefore, unless there is a systemic contraindication that might in itself be life-threatening, the patient should have the opportunity for appropriate resection.

The following general guidelines have been developed in defining contraindications to a major operation, including amputation:

1. Associated unrelated systemic disease of such severity that an operation of any magnitude might endanger life: for example, severe bilateral emphysema or extensive myocardial disease, end-stage renal disease treated by dialysis, or life-threatening asthma.
2. In most instances, the presence of synchronous metastases constitutes a contraindication for a major operation.
3. Inability of the patient to cope psychologically with a major operation, especially an amputation. However, in our experience, when an in-depth discussion is carried on, most patients recognize the need for the operation and accept it. The clinician must not try to "sell" any form of therapy to a patient; rather, it is his or her responsibility to provide the patient with all the pertinent facts and allow the patient to make the decision.
4. Finally, in an unusual instance in which the

rehabilitation of a patient, either psychological, social, or functional, poses an enormous problem, a major operation is preferably avoided. However, this is applicable only when a suitable alternative is available and the patient or the family is aware of that alternative.

After careful assessment of the type of excision or amputation necessary, the surgeon must proceed with the optimum type of operation, without compromise for cosmetic or emotional reasons. It cannot be overemphasized that inadequate initial excision increases the incidence of local recurrence. Most clinicians have observed that a locally recurrent sarcoma is more aggressive than the primary tumor and carries a graver prognosis for the patient. The old adage that the first surgeon has the best opportunity for cure is substantially true.

## ■ INDICATIONS AND TECHNIQUES FOR LOCAL EXCISION

### LIMITED LOCAL EXCISION

This method is used in the management of most benign soft tissue sarcomas. It is also a means of obtaining biopsy material from tumors clinically suggestive of malignancy.

### Technique

***Anesthesia.***   The excision can be performed under local, regional, or general endotracheal anesthesia, depending upon the age of the patient and the location and size of the tumor.

***Steps of Operation.***   After the patient is anesthetized and properly positioned, an elliptical skin incision is made over the prominent part of the tumor (Fig. 16–1A, inset). The skin is elevated on both sides of the tumor, delineating its extent (Fig. 16–1A, right). The tumor is then dissected from the surrounding muscles or other structures (Fig. 16–1B) and delivered out of the wound (Fig. 16–1C). Following removal of the tumor and after adequate hemostasis, the wound is closed in layers (Fig. 16–1D).

Almost all soft tissue sarcomas have a pseudocapsule, and enucleation will leave the peripheral part of the tumor behind. Although lipomas are usually enucleated, as a general principle it is judicious to avoid enucleation of any other soft tissue tumor, even if it appears benign.

If there is any question in the mind of the surgeon as to the benignancy of the tumor, a frozen section diagnosis should be obtained to determine whether the tumor represents a sarcoma. If the tumor is found to be malignant, then it is certainly appropriate to delay the definitive therapy until all relevant data are in hand. However, with a proper index of suspicion and the increasing use of diagnostic aids such as computed axial tomography (CAT) scan and magnetic resonance imaging (MRI), and with increasing proficiency in the use of fine-needle aspiration biopsy (FNAB), instances of unexpected surprises are becoming rare.

Limited local excision of sarcomas is seldom indicated. Therefore, the method of local excision described above should be reserved for benign tumors: for example, lipomas, neurofibromas, and/or benign fibrous tissue tumors. For all practical purposes, this method can also be used as a diagnostic method in a suspected sarcoma of relatively small dimensions. But if the tumor is large, a wedge biopsy is certainly indicated to obtain a correct microscopic diagnosis.

### WIDE LOCAL EXCISION

Wide local excision, if adequate, has a definite place in the management of soft tissue sarcomas. The definition of wide excision is somewhat confusing and frequently is misinterpreted by a clinician not familiar with the management of soft tissue sarcomas.

The term *wide excision* means a three-dimensional excision of the tumor. It is frequently a conceptual problem, and often it is not recognized that a soft tissue tumor grows in all directions (Fig. 16–2). With routine use of preoperative MRI in suspected sarcomas, it is not difficult to estimate the extent of the extension of the tumor, especially its deeper margin. The extent of the lateral excision of the surrounding tissues depends on the type of tumor. Furthermore, for a skin incision to encompass the entire extent of the tumor frequently requires an imaginative approach with due consideration of function and cosmesis, since an unconventional scar frequently results.

In such a complicated and rare neoplastic problem as soft tissue sarcoma, a comprehensive list of indications or contraindications for operations cannot be given. Frequently, the decision for a specific operation in a given patient will be guided by the surgeon's knowledge and experience with the tumor, as well as by the procedure itself. However, there are some guidelines that will help the surgeon in making the decision.

### Indications

1. Most low- or intermediate-grade, superficial malignant tumors (e.g., dermatofibrosarcoma protuberans, cutaneous leiomyosarcoma, superficially located desmoids [abdominal wall], etc.).

2. Low-grade, superficially located (subcutis) sarcomas (e.g., well-differentiated liposarcomas).

3. Certain embryonal types of rhabdomyosarcoma, especially those arising in the head and neck region of children.

4. With the increasing use of adjuvant radiotherapy, some high-grade sarcomas can now be treated by wide local excision or variants thereof.

5. All other benign tumors or malignant tumors of intermediate malignancy, the prime examples of benign tumors being intermuscular or intramuscular lipomas, angiolipomas, and desmoids in certain anatomic sites.

### Contraindications

1. Wide local excision is generally not indicated in the management of high-grade or anaplastic sarcomas of most histologic types, especially those located in the deeper compartments. These tumors should be managed by more extensive resections.

2. Wide local excision is not usually indicated for sarcomas arising in an extremity when a basic defect in the extremity is the cause of development of the sarcoma; for example, lymphangiosarcoma arising in an arm with postmastectomy or congenital edema. Similarly, in patients with neurofibromatosis, a malignant schwannoma arising in an extremity is usually associated with plexiform neuromas of the major nerve bundles. In such instances, an elective major amputation is the treatment of choice.

### Technique

*Anesthesia.*   Wide local excision should be performed under general endotracheal anesthesia. Although seldom needed, an adequate supply of blood or blood substitute should be kept available in case it is needed during the operation. Additionally, in large tumors, provision must be made for appropriate reconstruction of the operated area.

*Steps of Operation.*   The skin incision is made in an elliptical manner over the protruding part of the tumor (Fig. 16–2), excising the redundant skin along with the tumor. The incision is deepened through the subcutaneous tissue, and flaps are raised on all sides to delineate the boundaries of the tumor (Fig. 16–3A). The dissection, with adequate margins on all sides, is then carried deep to the tumor. In a subcutaneous tumor, the deeper excision line extends beneath the deep fascia. Inclusion of the deep fascia is an essential step of the operation. When the tumor is attached to the underlying muscle parenchyma (Fig. 16–3B), this segment of the muscle must be included in the resection. Following such a three-dimensional excision, the tumor and the surrounding normal tissues are removed (Fig. 16–3C). When indicated, the wound margins should be checked for residual tumor by means of frozen sections. The wound is then closed with suction catheters in place to drain serous fluid collection. In patients in whom the overlying skin needs larger excision, the defect is usually covered with a split-thickness skin graft (Fig. 16–3D).

The postoperative course after such an operation is usually smooth, and very little extra care is required. If a skin graft is used, the postoperative management is similar to that for any other wound requiring a split-thickness skin graft.

Wide local excision has several variants, and, although these are termed differently, the basic concepts in the treatment, being the same, will be included in this section on wide local excision. They are as follows:

1. Muscle group excision (wide soft tissue resection)
2. Minor amputation of either the upper or lower extremities
3. Subtotal scapulectomy
4. Tikhoff-Linberg operation
5. Chest wall resection
6. Abdominal wall resection
7. Excision of retroperitoneal tumors
8. Excision of intrathoracic tumors

### MUSCLE GROUP EXCISION (WIDE SOFT TISSUE RESECTION)

Excision of the group of muscles surrounding and underlying a soft tissue tumor is increasingly becoming the method of choice in the treatment of a large number of sarcomas located in the extremities. This operation takes into consideration the fact that all soft tissue sarcomas spread locally along the muscle bundles or the tissue planes. *It may be more appropriate to use the term* major soft tissue resection, *since, in a number of instances, the excised specimen usually consists of segments (bundles) of a number of muscles.*

### Indications

The indications for muscle group excision or major soft tissue resection are as follows:

1. Differentiated liposarcoma, rhabdomyosarcoma, leiomyosarcoma, malignant fibrous tissue, and synovial and angiomatous tissue

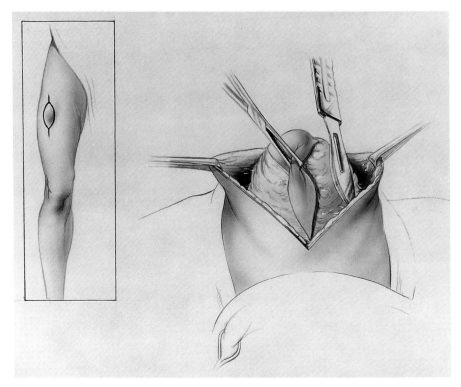

**Figure 16–1. (A)** *Inset:* Elliptical skin incision over a tumor of the thigh. The dimensions of the ellipse and the skin to be removed vary with the size of the tumor. For a tumor less than 3 cm in diameter, skin excision frequently is not required. *Right:* Skin flaps are being raised for a proposed limited excision. **(B)** A benign tumor is being dissected. Underlying muscles are free of any invasion. Occasionally, some of these tumors infiltrate the muscles (intermuscular lipoma), requiring excision of parts of the muscle as well. *(Continued.)*

**A**

tumors arising in a location where the muscle groups can be excised and a cure can be achieved (e.g., in the buttocks, the lateral or medial compartments of the thigh, or the lateral and medial aspects of the arm).

2. Malignant schwannomas either in the lateral compartment of the thigh or the lateral aspect of the arm, when they arise in a cutaneous nerve in these regions. This is because, in these instances, the proximal end of the nerve can be excised.

### Contraindications

The location of the tumor, however well differentiated it might be, may preclude a proper muscle group excision: for example, sarcomas located distal to the elbow or the knee cannot be adequately treated by this procedure, nor can tumors located in the groin or axilla. In essence, if there is any doubt because of the anatomic location of the tumor, the operation should not be attempted. In all high-grade sarcomas, in addition to the muscle group of excision or wide soft tissue resection, adjuvant radiation therapy is invariably indicated.

### Technique

***Anesthesia.*** In our experience, major soft tissue resection is best performed when the patient is under general anesthesia. The operation can be time-consuming

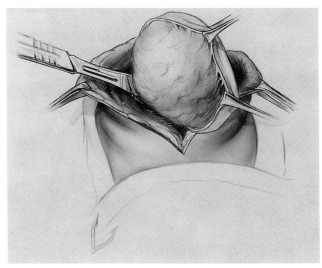

**B**

and might require blood transfusion, so adequate preparation should be made.

***Position of the Patient.*** The patient should be positioned in order to provide best access and exposure of the group of muscles requiring excision. For example, excision of the gluteal muscles requires that the patient be in the prone position; excision of the lateral compartment muscles of the right thigh requires that the patient be positioned on a semi-left lateral decubitus.

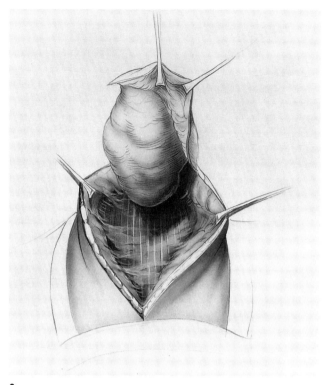

C

***Steps of Operation.***   An elliptical incision is made, encompassing the tumor and extending vertically along the entire course of attachment of the muscles to be excised (Fig. 16–4A). The incision is deepened to include the subcutaneous tissue, and skin flaps are raised on both sides (Fig. 16–4B). The dissection is then started on the proximal aspect of the excision.

The medial attachment of the muscle group is dissected, and the dissection is carried out from the proximal to the distal attachments (Fig. 16–4B). This stage of the operation provides the first opportunity for inspection and evaluation of the undersurface of the tumor. Although, with routine use of preoperative MRI, the deep extension of the tumor can usually be assessed before the operation, the deep margin of the tumor must be examined thoroughly and, if needed, checked by frozen section. When the free margin is assured, the operation proceeds, and the lateral line of attachment of the muscle group is excised (Fig. 16–4C). Ideally, one should be able to remove the entire muscle group containing the tumor without handling the tumor (Fig. 16–4D), but if the tumor is found infiltrating the adjacent bone, segment(s) of the affected bone must be included in this type of operation. In the event that this is not possible (albeit rarely), the procedure should be

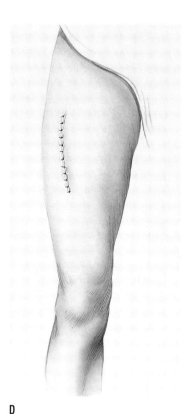

D

**Figure 16–1** *(continued).* **(C)** A benign subcutaneous lipoma is being removed. Note that the tumor is free of any attachment to the underlying muscle bed. **(D)** The wound has been closed in layers.

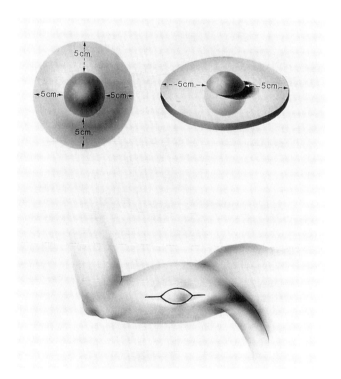

**Figure 16–2.** *Above, left:* Conceptual rendition of the extent of three-dimensional extension of a spheroidal tumor. Although most tumors of the soft tissues are oblate spheroids, for artistic clarity, the tumor is sketched as a perfect spheroid. *Right:* The deeper extension of the tumor is comprehensible. *Below:* An elliptical skin incision is made over a subcutaneous tumor of the arm, with consideration of the extension.

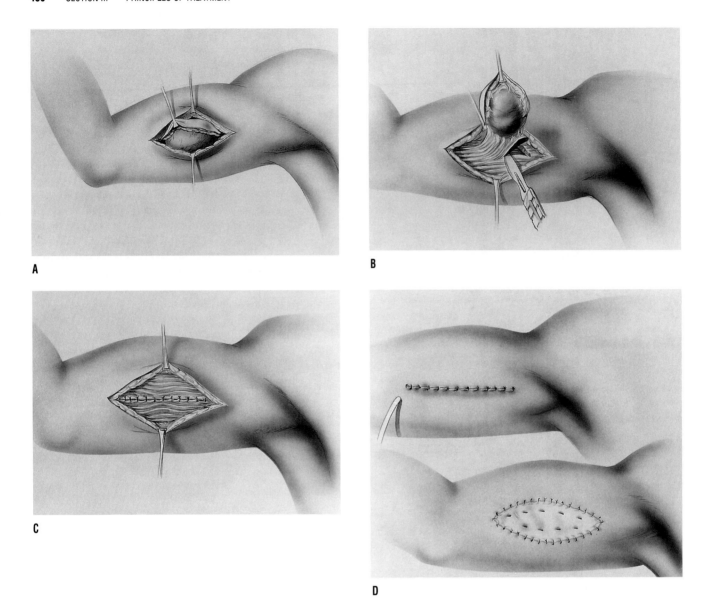

**Figure 16–3.** **(A)** The skin flaps are being raised, delineating the margins of the tumor. **(B)** The deeper extent of the tumor is being dissected. **(C)** The tumor has been excised, and the muscle bed is sutured. **(D)** The skin margins can be closed primarily or can be covered with a split-thickness skin graft.

terminated, and, in an extremity, an appropriate amputation should be resorted to. Notably, in centers where sarcomas are routinely treated, in about 95 percent of the cases, these decisions can be made preoperatively, and the patient can be appropriately apprised of the situation.

Once the specimen is removed, the resected ends of the muscles are attached to the surrounding muscles with intact nerve supply. The wound is then closed in layers. Suction catheters are placed to avoid collection of any serum (Fig. 16–4E). If the ellipse of skin included in the operation is large, the defect can be covered by a split-thickness skin graft.

When the general principles of good surgical technique are applied, the postoperative course is smooth

and the patients may not require any special type of management. Although, initially, it seems they will be unable to either walk or move their arms, within a few weeks most patients, with proper physical therapy, can return to normal activity. The residual deformity, if any, is so minimal that frequently an untrained observer fails to recognize it. The fibrosarcoma shown in Fig. 16–4F was removed from a 61-year-old woman who was able to resume all her preoperative activities within six months. The patient has remained well for more than 11 years. Thus, from a rehabilitation standpoint, this type of operation, whenever feasible, constitutes one of the ideal forms of treatment of soft tissue sarcomas of the extremities.

# RADICAL EXCISION OF THE BUTTOCK (GLUTEAL GROUP EXCISION)

Planning the exact technique to be applied in excising different groups of muscles for a malignant tumor at any given anatomic site requires a thorough familiarity with the regional anatomy and the ability to modify the surgical technique in accordance with the principles of operation discussed above. One such modification is the technique of excision of the gluteal group of muscles for sarcomas of the buttocks.[7] Because of the specific modifications, the operative technique is described here in detail.

## Indications

Radical excision is indicated in all well-differentiated sarcomas of the buttock area that are well circumscribed and can be extirpated by excising the gluteal group of muscles.

It is advisable to discuss the limits of this operation in detail with the patient, since, in some instances, the tumor will be found to be more extensive than originally assessed clinically, requiring a hemipelvectomy or excision of part of the sacrum, coccyx, and iliac crest. Before operating, the surgeon should obtain permission to extend the operation if necessary.

## Contraindications

This operation is not recommended if the tumor extends into the pelvis through the sciatic foramen (dumbbell-shaped tumors), or if there is extensive local recurrence.

## Technique

*Position of the Patient.* Sometimes, because of the vascularity of a tumor, ligation of the internal iliac vessel or some of the gluteal branches may become necessary; thus, if indicated, the patient should be in a supine position, then in the prone position.

*Steps of Operation.* Extensive examination of the abdomen and pelvis (CAT scan and MRI) is essential before performing this operation. It is not uncommon for a tumor in the buttock to have an intrapelvic extension or vice versa; thus, the surgical approach must be tailored to meet the individual patient's needs. Sometimes, due to the extensive vascularity of a given tumor, the ipsolateral internal iliac vessel needs to be ligated, through a separate lower abdominal incision. The ligature should be applied above the superior gluteal branch of the artery; otherwise, the bleeding is not curtailed and this step becomes a technical exercise without any benefit. After this step, the laparotomy wound is closed, and the patient is placed in the prone posi-

tion. The patient is then prepared, and the operative field is so draped that the entire buttock, most of the posterior thigh, and part of the lateral and medial aspects of the body are within the operative field.

A generous elliptical skin incision is made, with the tumor in the central position (Fig. 16–5A). The skin flaps are raised on both sides (Fig. 16–5B). The proximal attachment of the gluteus maximus muscle from the lateral edge of the sacrum and coccyx and from the posterior portion of the iliac crest is exposed medially (Fig. 16–5C), and its distal attachment into the greater trochanter of the femur and into the ileotibial band is exposed laterally (Fig. 16–5D). A vertical incision is then made through the distal attachment of the gluteus maximus muscle, and the muscle is lifted medially (Fig. 16–5E). This exposes the underlying piriformis muscle, and the sciatic nerve is seen emerging from the sciatic foramen underneath the inferior margin of the muscle. The inferior gluteal vessels are identified, ligated, and resected (Fig.16–5E). At this stage of the operation, the extent of the tumor is reassessed, and, if indicated, excision of the gluteus maximus muscle alone might be resorted to. In most instances, however, we have found that, to achieve an adequate margin, the gluteus medius and piriformis muscles must be excised. Therefore, the tendinous distal attachment of the piriformis muscle is then resected, and the incision is carried superiorly to include the distal attachment of the gluteus medius muscle to the trochanter of the femur (Fig. 16–5E and 16–5F). By exploring underneath these muscles, the deeper extension of the tumor is reassessed, and if the deeper margin is free of any tumor extension, then the entire muscle mass is retracted medially and the proximal attachments of these muscles are excised (Fig. 16–5G). Following removal of the muscles along with the tumor, proper hemostasis is obtained.

This operation naturally leaves a large operative defect, which can be closed either by approximating the skin margins, by rotation of a flap, or by a split-thickness skin graft. Although it is preferable to attempt either a primary closure (Fig. 16–5H) or rotation of a flap, split-thickness skin grafts over this area, even immediately over the sciatic nerve, are reasonably well tolerated, and we have used them in several instances.

In some cases, this operation can be extended medially and proximally to incorporate the coccyx, part of the outer table of the sacrum, and the posterior lip of the iliac crest (Fig. 16–6) laterally and distally to include the proximal portions of the muscles of the posterior thigh. The decision to extend the limits of this operation lies largely in the experience of the surgeon and his or her familiarity with sarcomas. To develop general guidelines is neither possible nor desirable. However, if the tumor is found to be infiltrating the sciatic nerve or the bones and, in the opinion of the surgeon, resection will not result in cure, the operation should be abandoned in favor of a hemipelvectomy.

A resection of the buttock is well tolerated by the patient and, in spite of resection of these muscles, he or she is able to walk. The patient may have a waddling gait (Trendelenberg's symptom), which frequently is not noticeable to an inexperienced observer.

## RESECTION OF THE SACRUM

Resection of tumors involving the sacrum may present challenging problems to the surgeon. The most common indication for extensive resection of the sacrum is chordoma of the sacrum. Other malignant tumors of the sacrum—for example, chondrosarcoma, malignant fibrous histiocytoma, or Ewing's sarcoma of the bone—may also necessitate resection of the sacrum. Minor sacral resection (resection of the fifth sacral vertebra and fourth sacral vertebra) is usually accomplished without any technical problem. Resection of the distal sacrum is usually done through a posterior approach. However, further proximal resection of the sacrum (especially at the level of the second sacral vertebra) or removal of a portion of the first sacral vertebra necessitates major planning and meticulous approach. Since first and second sacral nerves are important for function of the anal sphincter and urethral sphincter, before resection of the sacrum at this level, patients should be advised of possible loss of control of these sphincters.

### Technique

Patients for major sacral resection should have meticulous preoperative preparation, including assessment of cardiac and pulmonary function. Patients should have a mechanical and antibiotic bowel prep and be blood typed and crossmatched for possible requirement of transfusion.

***Position of the Patient.***   Sacral resection can be performed using several positions. One approach is a combined abdominal lateral sacral position. In this case, the patient is placed in the right lateral position with the left side of the pelvis elevated to the extent that the whole sacrum is in the field of operation. The left knee is folded at 90 degrees and placed over the right knee and leg with a firm pillow between the knees. This position is usually adequate for resection of the lower part of the sacrum, with a combined anterior approach to the midline and a posterior approach of the sacrum to the posterior midline. However, for a near total sacral resection at the level of the junction of the first and second sacral vertebra, or removal of half of the body of the first sacral vertebra, this position is not ade-

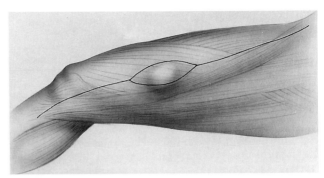

**A**

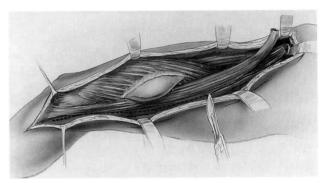

**B**

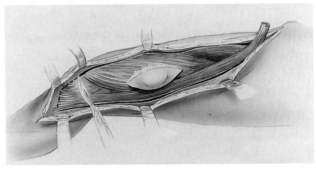

**C**

**Figure 16–4. (A)** Incision line for a proposed muscle group excision of the anteromedial aspect of the thigh. An ellipse is designed at the most prominent part of the tumor. **(B)** The skin flaps on both sides have been raised. The proximal attachment of the sartorius muscle is resected. The dotted line shows the medial margin of the resection. Resection is continued from the proximal to the distal end. **(C)** The lateral margin of resection has been defined, and the muscles are being resected at the distal end. *(Continued.)*

quate. For all major sacral resection, we advise that the patient should be operated on first in the supine position with mobilization of the abdominal viscera from the sacrum and ligation of the blood vessel followed by a posterior approach in the prone position—the same principle as has been described in the operation of extremely vascular sarcomas of the buttock.

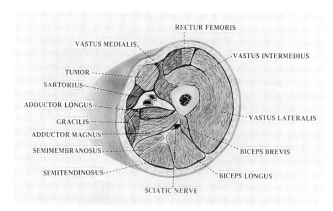

D

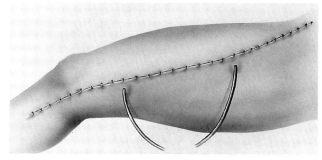

E

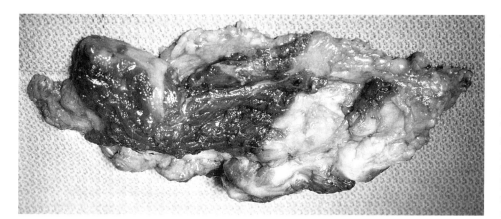

F

**Figure 16–4** *(continued).* **(D)** A transverse section through the middle of the thigh, showing relation of the tumor to the surrounding muscles. The shaded muscles, along with the tumor, are being resected. If such a margin is adhered to, the chances of handling the tumor are minimized. **(E)** The wound is closed with a suction catheter in place. Although a large muscle mass was removed, there is no impairment of activity. All our patients have been able to resume their preoperative activities within four to six months after the operation. **(F)** The resected specimen of a muscle group excision of the thigh. This was a low-grade fibrosarcoma in a 61-year-old woman. The patient resumed all her preoperative activities within six months and has remained disease-free for the last ten years.

***Steps of Operation.*** After appropriate preoperative and anesthetic preparation, the patient is anesthetized (Figs. 16–6 to 16–8). Initially, the patient is placed in a supine position, and the abdomen is prepared and draped in the usual manner. The incision is made curvilinear from the anterior superior iliac spine on one side to the other side, 2 cm above and parallel to the inguinal ligament and symphysis pubis. The skin and subcutaneous tissue are cut along the line of the incision, and the abdominal muscles are exposed. The abdominal muscles are divided on either side from the anterior superior iliac spine to the lateral aspect of the rectus sheath, up to the level of the peritoneum. Thereafter, the parietal peritoneum is pushed medially to expose the common iliac, internal iliac, and external iliac vessels. This retroperitoneal approach provides easy visualization of the vessels. Proper exposure is obtained using a self-retaining retractor (Buchwalter retractor).

The common iliac artery is traced cephalad to its division into internal and external iliac arteries. The internal iliac artery is further dissected, and the anterior and posterior branches are exposed. The posterior branch is then ligated and resected on both sides, and the anterior branches are retracted anteriorly and lat-

erally. Following this, the internal iliac vein is exposed on both sides, dissected free, and ligated close to its junction with the external iliac vein. Thereafter, it is religated distally and divided between suture ligatures.

Afterwards, if there is no involvement of the rectum by the tumor, the rectum is mobilized from the anterior surface of the sacrum. If the rectum is found to be adherent to the tumors, then it can be removed along with the sacrum transperitoneally after ligation of the vessels as described above. In contrast, if the rectum is free, it is mobilized and lifted anteriorly. The obturator vessels and nerves are then identified and preserved. The median sacral artery and middle sacral vein are ligated. The anterior surface of the sacrum and the area of the anterior aspect of the sacroiliac joint are visualized. Any large vein crossing the line of resection is divided between suture ligatures; ligation of these veins will prevent rapid blood loss during the actual resection of the sacrum.

After adequate mobilization of the rectum and ligation of the posterior branches of the internal iliac artery, and after both internal iliac veins and all the branches and tributaries of the pelvic vein crossing over the sacroiliac joint are ligated, two laparotomy pads are

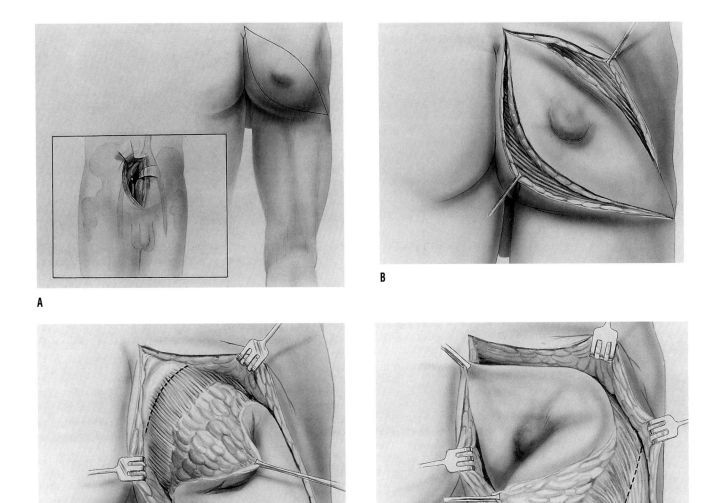

**Figure 16–5.** **(A)** *Inset:* Preliminary exploratory celiotomy with ligation of internal iliac artery is a helpful initial step before excision of a buttock tumor. *Right:* Elliptical skin incision is shown. The width of the skin ellipse to be removed depends on the size of the primary tumor and the histologic diagnosis. **(B)** Skin flaps are raised on both sides in the same manner as for radical mastectomy. **(C)** Medial proximal attachment of gluteus maximus muscle is exposed. Dotted line represents the future line resection of the muscle. **(D)** Distal attachment of gluteus maximus muscle with the proposed line of resection. *(Continued.)*

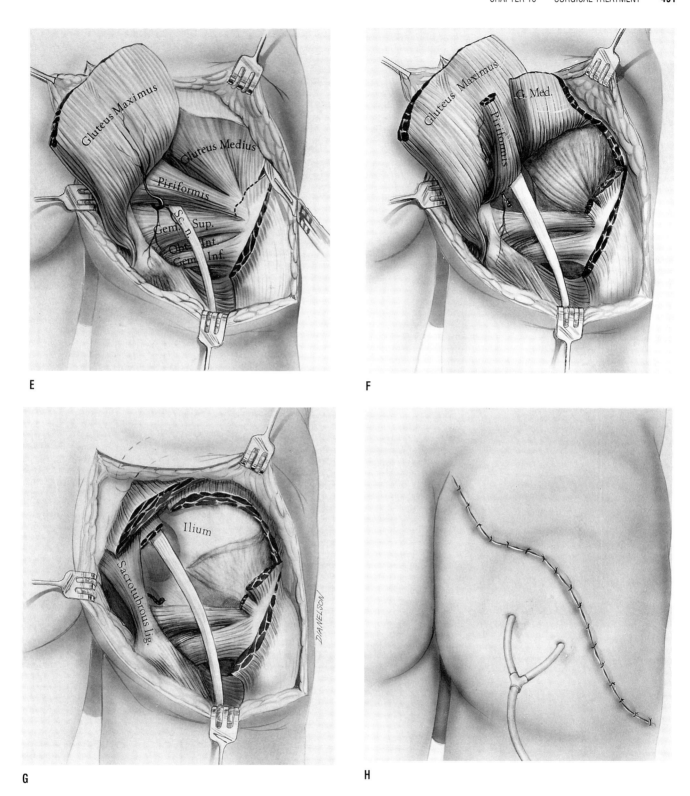

E

F

G

H

**Figure 16–5** *(continued).* **(E)** Distal attachment of the gluteus maximus muscle resected and retracted proximally. The piriformis muscle, sciatic nerve, inferior gluteal vessels, and gluteus medius muscle are seen. The dotted line represents the line of resection of the gluteus medius and piriformis muscles. **(F)** The distal attachments of the piriformis and gluteus medius muscles are resected and retracted proximally. **(G)** The muscles have been resected proximally and the specimen removed. The cut margins of the glutei and the piriformis are easily discernible. **(H)** Appearance of the operative site after a primary closure. Suction catheters are attached to wall suction.

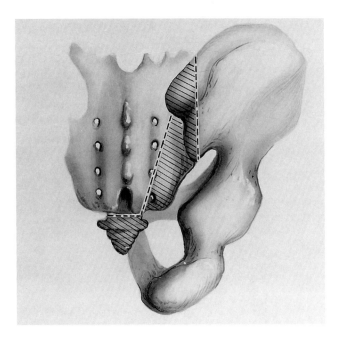

**Figure 16–6.** Diagram of pelvic skeleton from the back. The dotted lines show the extent to which bones can be excised along with this operation without creating any appreciable deformity.

placed between the anterior surface of the sacrum and rectum. The abdominal wound is then closed. We usually close in one layer, using a nonabsorbable suture such as #0 Prolene. The skin and subcutaneous tissues are closed in layers, and the anterior incision is closed completely. The patient is placed in the prone position with a pillow underneath the pelvis so that the gluteal

region is slightly raised upward. Then the patient's back is prepared and draped from the L1–L2 vertebral region down to the tip of the coccyx and on either side up to the greater trochanter. A midline starting incision is made from the L4–L5 region and extending down to the tip of the coccyx. The cephalic part of the incision is further extended in a T-shaped manner. Skin flaps are raised on either side, and the origin of the gluteus maximus muscle is identified on either side of the sacrum and the coccyx. The gluteus maximus muscle is then detached from the sacral and coccygeal origins and is retracted laterally. Care should be taken at this time for proper hemostasis and to avoid injuring the sciatic nerve. If the resection is below the level of the second sacral vertebra, it is also important to identify and preserve the pudendal nerve, which would lie just posterior to the ischial spine. At this time, the endococcygeal raphe should be divided, and the presacral space should be entered from the posterior aspect. The ligamentous attachments between the sacrum and the ischium are identified posteriorly. The dorsal sacrococcygeal ligament is initially divided, and, higher up, the long dorsal sacroiliac ligaments are also divided. After division of the posterior ligaments, the exposed anterior ligament, which is the sacrotuberous ligament, is divided. Further superiorly, after identification of the pudendal nerve, the sacrospinous ligament is divided.

Following this, the greater sciatic foramen is entered, the ventral sacroiliac ligaments are identified, and the sciatic nerve is identified and retracted out of harm's way. The piriformis muscles are detached on both sides. The skin flaps along with subcutaneous tis-

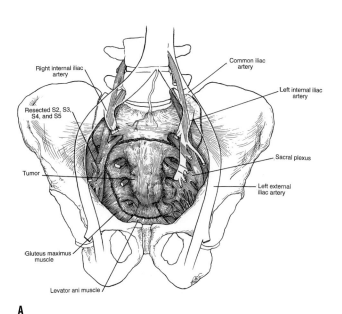

A

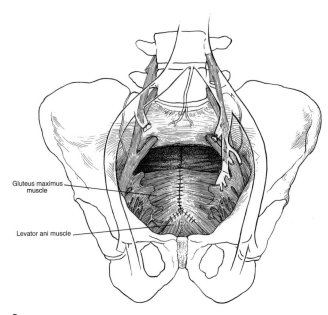

B

**Figure 16–7. (A)** Schematic rendition of the pelvis when all the structures are removed, exposing the sacrum anteriorly. **(B)** The repair of the posterior part of the pelvis and the pelvic floor after resection of the sacrum *(anterior view).*

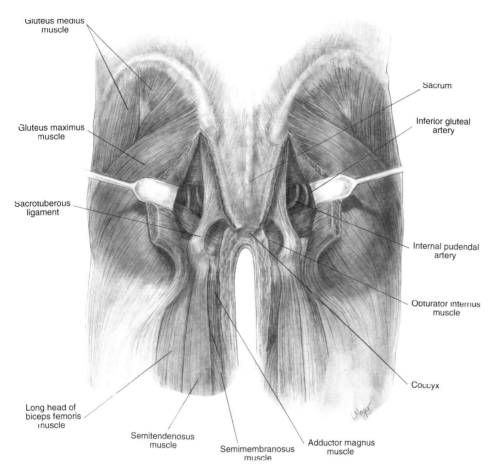

Gluteus medius
muscle

Gluteus maximus
muscle

Sacrotuberous
ligament

Long head of
biceps femoris
muscle

Semitendenosus
muscle

Semimembranosus
muscle

Adductor magnus
muscle

Sacrum

Inferior gluteal
artery

Internal pudendal
artery

Obturator internus
muscle

Coccyx

**Figure 16–8.** Posterior view of the sacrum prior to resection.

sue are raised so that the lower aspect of the sacroiliac joint is identified. Resection of a portion of the first sacral vertebra will require entering the sacroiliac joint, which is a synovial joint. The articular surface of the sacroiliac joint is uneven, with irregular elevations and depressions. These uneven areas keep the joint stable, with restricted movement. To remove a portion of the first sacral vertebra, the lower portion of the sacroiliac joint is identified, and a portion of the joint capsule is opened. After this, the body of the sacrum is divided in a transverse manner, encompassing the entire posterior surface of the sacrum at that level. The first and second sacral nerve roots are then identified and preserved. At this time, the dural sac is identified, which extends to the junction of the second and third sacral body. The dural sac is ligated at the level of resection and divided between the ligatures. Then the rest of the body of the first sacral vertebra is divided, and the specimen is removed. Proper hemostasis is obtained. Usually, with appropriate ligation of the posterior branches of the internal iliac arteries and of the internal iliac veins and division of the tributaries of the internal iliac vein crossing the space between the sacrum and iliac bone, the bleeding is minimal. After appropriate hemostasis, the gluteal muscles, especially in the lower portions, are

approximated together. Suction catheters are placed on either side, and the subcutaneous tissue is closed with interrupted suture. The skin is closed with interrupted suture.

## CONSERVATIVE AMPUTATION

The minor and conservative amputations to be discussed herein must be considered as variants of the wide local excision already described. A minor amputation is resorted to only when the sarcoma is well differentiated and is located in an area in the extremity where a conservative amputation is feasible.

### MINOR OR CONSERVATIVE AMPUTATIONS OF THE UPPER EXTREMITIES

In conservative amputations of the hand, it is essential to bear in mind that retention of any of the fingers will be most rewarding to the patient. Even if the thumb and only one other finger are preserved, the patient will have a functioning hand.

Amputations at the level of the wrist, midforearm, or below the elbow are seldom indicated in the management of soft tissue sarcomas. With the increasing use of radiation therapy, the indications for minor amputations, especially of the upper extremities, have become rarer still. The technical considerations for these operations are standard and will not be discussed.

There are, however, two types of conservative amputations in the upper extremities that are sometimes used in the management of soft tissue sarcomas—subtotal scapulectomy and en bloc resection of the shoulder girdle (Tikhoff-Linberg operation). Although the indications for such operations are few, it is appropriate to discuss the indications and techniques of these two unusual operations.

## Subtotal Scapulectomy

A procedure for removal of tumors in the scapular region was originally described by Syme[8] in 1864. In his monograph, he described three patients in whom he had performed this operation, showing it to be feasible and practical. However, de Nancrede,[9] in his presidential address to the American Surgical Association in 1909, categorically stated that scapulectomy was an inferior operation. Thereafter, it fell into disrepute, and only occasional reports of results with this operation were published. Pack and Ariel[10] mentioned this procedure in 1958 but did not elaborate either for or against it. It is thus apparent that the indications for scapulectomy have never been clearly defined; consequently, the end results sometimes have been unsatisfactory. Scapulectomy has a limited role in surgery for neoplastic disease, and strict criteria must be set up for its performance; otherwise, a perfectly suitable operative procedure will not be properly used.[11]

***Indications.*** Scapulectomy is indicated in the following types of tumors:

Soft tissue sarcomas

Low-grade fibrosarcoma invading the scapular muscles

Aggressive fibromatoses (desmoids) infiltrating the scapular muscles

Liposarcoma arising from the adipose tissue in the scapular region, with local infiltration

Bone tumors

Primary malignant bone tumors arising in the scapula (this is rare); however, scapulectomy may be useful in unusual cases of a low-grade skeletal or extraskeletal chondrosarcoma or giant cell tumor of the scapula

***Contraindications.*** Scapulectomy is definitely contraindicated if the sarcoma is located in the superior pole of the scapula, or if the tumor extends beyond the scapula and the muscles immediately attached to the scapula.

### Technique

*Position of the Patient.* The patient is placed in the prone position with the arm resting in a 90-degree abduction on an arm board. The arm should be draped so that an assistant can move the arm as required during the operation (Fig. 16–9A).

*Steps of Operation.* An elliptical skin incision is then made, encompassing the tumor and extending from the tip of the acromion superolaterally to the paravertebral region inferomedially. The lower end of the incision can be extended to cross the midline if the tumor is so large as to make this necessary (Fig. 16–9A).

The medial and lateral skin flaps are raised, and the superficial dorsal muscular attachment of the scapula is identified. The attachment of the trapezius muscle to the scapula is identified and resected. Reflection of the trapezius muscle exposes the supraspinatous muscle superiorly and rhomboid major inferiorly (Fig. 16–9B). The attachment of the deltoid muscle to the lateral tip of the scapular spine is similarly resected and retracted superomedially, exposing the remainder of the supraspinatus muscle. At this stage, the rhomboid major muscle at the vertebral border, the latissimus dorsi muscle inferiorly, the teres major and minor muscles laterally, and the infraspinous muscle can be easily identified.

The insertion of the latissimus dorsi muscle at the tip of the scapula is then excised, and the muscle is retracted downward, exposing the tip of the scapula (Fig. 16–9C). The tip is then held by an assistant with a straight clamp and pulled inferolaterally. This provides traction to the muscles at the vertebral border and excision of their scapular attachment is made simple (Fig. 16–9C).

The muscular attachments in the superior angle of the scapula are then resected along the vertebral border of the scapula. The levator scapulae and the rhomboids, easily delineated, are then cut. This maneuver can be quite simple if the assistant maintains constant traction at the tip of the scapula. The inferior tip of the scapula is then rotated, and a medial pull is applied while the arm is abducted (Fig. 16–9D). The lateral muscles, teres major and minor, and the long head of the triceps (Fig. 16–9B) are then resected, protecting the axillary neurovascular bundle. Next, the supraspinatus tendons and the attachment of serratus anterior muscles are cut (Fig. 16–9D). The shoulder joint is then exposed and identified, and the scapular spine is cut near the acromion process by use of an osteotome. Thus, the acromioclavicular joint is kept intact. The only muscle remaining attached to the scapula, humerus, and shoulder joint is the subscapularis, which is resected under the guidance of the operator's finger (Fig.16–9E, Part 1).

A Gigli's saw is then passed around the neck of the scapula, avoiding the glenohumeral joint. The scapula is resected and the specimen removed, care being taken to avoid injury to the glenohumeral joint (Fig. 16–9E, Parts 2 and 3). This part of the resection can also be accomplished by means of a Stryker saw. The sole objective is to resect the neck of the scapula without injuring the glenohumeral joint and the axillary vessels and nerves.

After proper hemostasis is achieved, the cut edge of the trapezius muscle is sutured to the deltoid muscle at the line of the previous position of the spine of the scapula (Fig. 16–9F). The lateral margins of these muscular stitches incorporate the remnant of the acromion process. The teres major and minor muscles are sutured to the chest wall (Fig. 16–9F).

The suction catheter beneath each skin flap is then brought out through normal skin, the wound is closed by interrupted subcutaneous chromic catgut sutures, and the skin margins are apposed by interrupted 3-0 nylon stitches. A firm pressure dressing is applied, and the arm is placed in a sling in adduction. The long-term result of this operation is quite satisfactory (Fig. 16–9G).

## En Bloc Resection of the Shoulder Girdle (Tikhoff-Linberg Operation)

Tikhoff-Linberg operation encompasses total scapulectomy, partial or complete excision of the clavicle, and resection of the head and neck of the humerus with preservation of the arm, brachial plexus, and subclavian vessels.

The operation was first planned by Tikhoff[12] in 1900 under the name "resectointerscapulothoracica" as an alternative to forequarter amputation. However, Linberg[13] first described the technique of the operation, while discussing the management of malignant tumors of the shoulder girdle. Pack and Baldwin[14] discussed indications for the operation and described one patient on whom they operated.

### Indications

1. Low-grade fibrosarcoma or well-differentiated liposarcoma located in the superior pole of the scapula or in the region of the lateral third of the clavicle.
2. Localized chondrosarcoma of the scapula or clavicle, not infiltrating the surrounding muscles.

### Contraindications

1. This operation is not indicated in any high-grade sarcoma of this region.

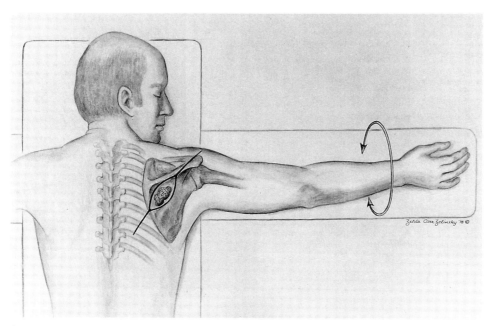

**Figure 16–9. (A)** The position of the patient and the incision for a tumor located in the center of the scapular region are shown. The arm should be draped in such a way that an assistant can freely move the arm to facilitate excision of muscular attachments. *(Continued.)*

A

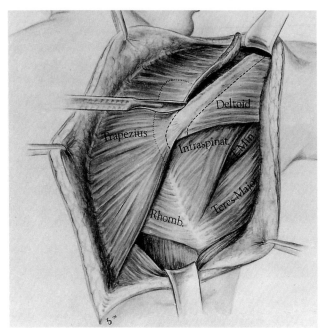

B

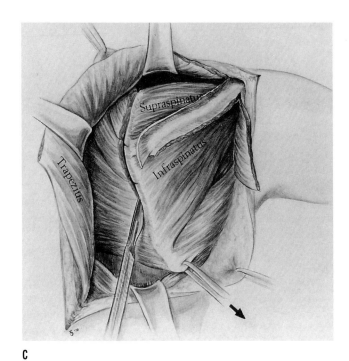

C

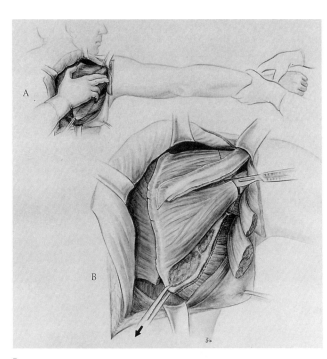

D

**Figure 16–9** *(continued).* **(B)** The scapular muscles are exposed after raising the skin flaps. The trapezius muscle is then resected at the scapular spine. The dotted line shows the site of excision of the deltoid attachment. Reflection of the trapezius exposes the supraspinatus muscle. **(C)** Trapezius and deltoid muscles are reflected, and the latissimus dorsi are retracted downward. An assistant is pulling the lip laterally *(arrow).* This maneuver makes resection of the muscle attached to the vertebral border quite simple. **(D)** *Part 1:* Palpation of the axillary contents. *Part 2:* The tip of the scapula is now pulled inferomedially, and the lateral muscles are cut. The dotted line shows the line of resection of the supraspinatus, infraspinatus, and serratus anterior muscles. *(Continued.)*

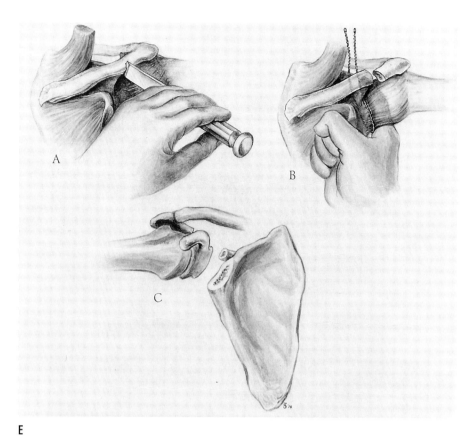

E

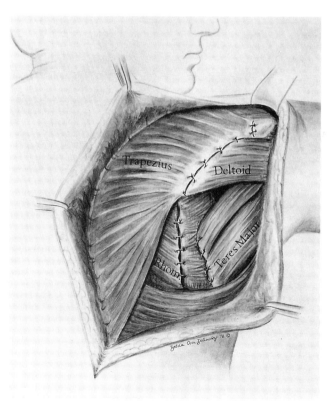

F

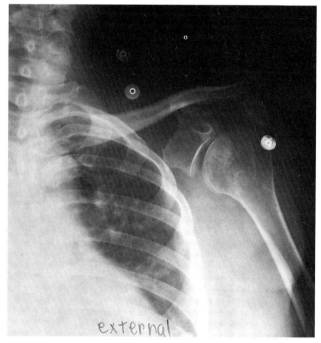

G

**Figure 16–9** *(continued).* **(E)** *Part 1:* The scapular spine is cut with an osteotome. The subscapularis muscle is cut under the guidance of the operator's finger. *Part 2:* A Gigli's saw is then passed around the neck of the scapula (any other saw can also be used). *Part 3:* The specimen is removed. **(F)** Suture line between deltoid and trapezius muscles. The acromion process is shown at the top. The teres major and minor muscles are attached to the rib cage. **(G)** Roentgenogram showing the shoulder joint *(left)* in patient who underwent subtotal scapulectomy nine years ago. Patient has good use of her arm.

2. Any patient with sarcoma of the scapula that infiltrates the subscapularis muscle is not a candidate for this operation.

One of the most important accomplishments of this operation is the preservation of a relatively useful forearm and hand.

### Technique

*Position of the Patient.* The patient lies on the unaffected side in a modified lateral position. The arm is prepared and draped so as to be included in the operative field and is positioned so that the assistant can manipulate it during the operation.

*Steps of Operation.* A racquet incision is made along the anterior surface of the clavicle and is extended laterally over the deltoid about 5 cm below the acromion process (Fig. 16–10A). The second part of the incision is usually begun at the midclavicular line anteriorly and is extended posteriorly over the neck, near the medial border, and around the inferior tip of the scapula, to be connected with the distal arm of the racquet (Fig. 16–10D, inset).

Following this outlining of the skin incision, the dissection is started anteriorly along the anterior border of the clavicle and extended laterally, exposing the deltoid muscle (Fig. 16–10A). The clavicle is then resected at the junction of the medial third and lateral two-thirds by means of a Gigli's saw. The pectoralis major muscle, including the clavicular head anteriorly and the deltoid laterally, is resected, exposing the coracoid process. The resected medial and lateral parts of the clavicle are retracted from the operative field. The pectoralis minor muscle attached to the coracoid process is exposed and resected (Fig. 16–10B). With the resection of the pectoralis minor muscle near the tip of the coracoid process, access is gained to the axillary contents (Fig. 16–10C). The anterior circumflex humeral artery and subscapular vessels are defined, ligated, and resected. The resected lateral part of the clavicle is retracted laterally, further exposing the brachial plexus (Fig. 16–10C). The incision is then carried along the vertebral border of the scapula, and the muscles are resected in a manner identical to that shown for the technique of scapulectomy (Figs. 16–10D and 16–10E). The posterior incision is then connected with the lateral arm of the racquet, and the remaining portion of the deltoid, the long head of the triceps, and the teres major muscle are divided (Fig. 16–10F). The surgical neck of the humerus is then exposed and, after ensuring the safety of the radial nerve, is resected and the specimen removed (Fig. 16–10F, inset).

The humerus is then suspended by ligatures to the remaining trapezius muscle or to a rib (Fig. 16–10G).

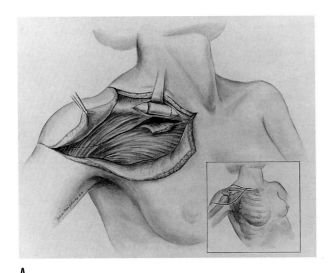

**A**

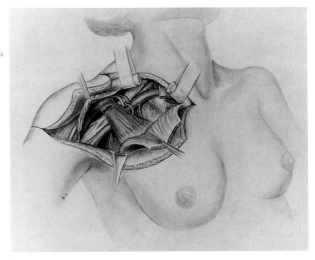

**B**

**Figure 16–10. (A)** With the patient in a modified lateral position, the incision is started on the anterior surface of the clavicle. The lateral handle of the racquet is extended along the clavicle laterally over the deltoid 5 cm below the acromion process, the medial handle over the neck to the back *(inset)*, and then along the medial border to the tip of the scapula, and there laterally to meet the lateral handle of the racquet over the lateral aspect of the arm (see *inset*, Fig. 16–10D). Anterior incision is deepened. The clavicle is resected at the junction of the lateral two-thirds and medial third. Dotted line is the line of resection of the muscles. **(B)** Pectoralis major muscle anteriorly and the deltoid laterally are resected, exposing the coracoid process and the pectoralis minor muscle. The pectoralis minor muscle at its attachment to the coracoid process is then excised. *(Continued.)*

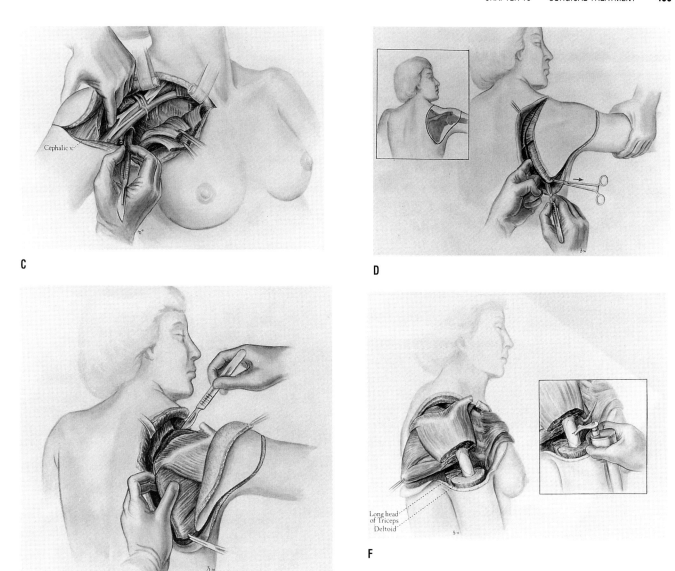

**Figure 16–10** *(continued).* **(C)** Resection of anterior muscle attachments is completed, exposing the axillary contents and the brachial plexus. **(D)** The posterior incision is deepened, and vertebral attachments of the scapula are severed. The inset shows the posterolateral part of the incision. **(E)** All the posterior muscles have been resected, including the trapezius muscle; the tip of the scapula is pulled inferolaterally. **(F)** The distal part of the deltoid and long head of the triceps are cut, and the surgical neck of the humerus is exposed. The inset shows the line of resection of the humerus, following which the specimen is removed. *(Continued.)*

The trapezius and deltoid muscles are then sutured together, covering the defect (Fig. 16–10H). The skin is closed with suction catheters in place (Fig. 16–10I).

At the completion of the operation, the arm, forearm, and hand are intact. The functions of the forearm and hand are retained, but the shoulder and upper arm movements are no longer possible. With appropriate physiotherapy and training, the patient will have reasonable use of the forearm and the hand (Figs. 16–11A and 16–11B).

## MINOR OR CONSERVATIVE AMPUTATIONS OF THE LOWER EXTREMITIES

In considering limited amputations of the foot, one must bear in mind that a retention arch will permit use of the foot. If possible, a transmetatarsal amputation is satisfactory insofar as a functional foot is concerned. Of the variety of other conservative amputations practiced and described, few, if any, apply to the management of soft tissue sarcomas. A below-the-knee amputation occa-

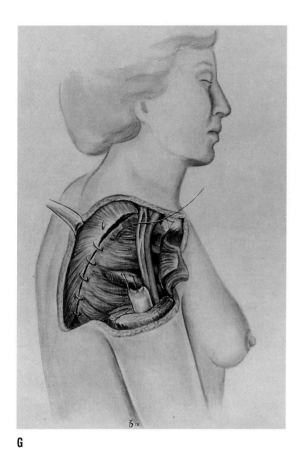

G

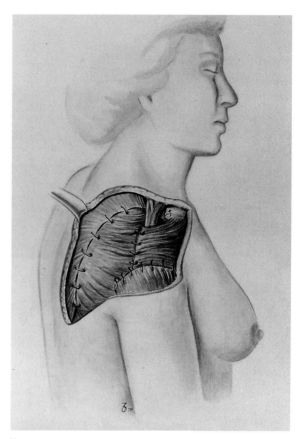

H

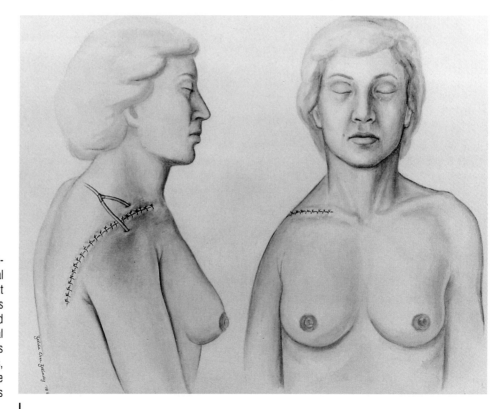

**Figure 16–10** *(continued).* **(G)** The distal humerus is anchored to the lateral chest wall with several monofilament sutures. **(H)** The ends of the muscles are approximated with interrupted absorbable sutures covering the brachial plexus and the vessels. **(I)** The wound is closed with interrupted nylon sutures, and suction catheters are placed. The appearance of the shoulder after this resection is cosmetically tolerable.

I

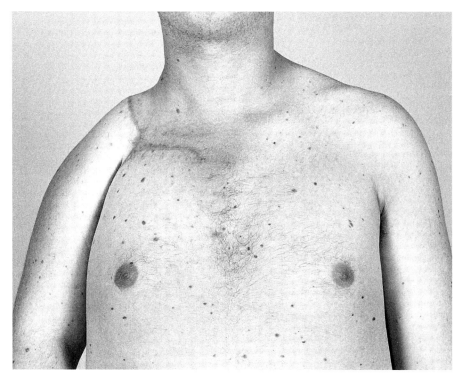

**A**

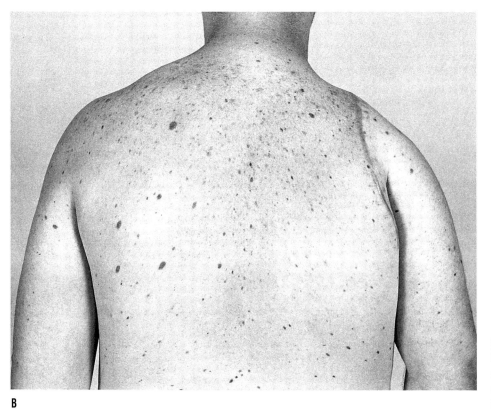

**B**

**Figure 16–11. (A)** Anterior and **(B)** posterior views of a patient who underwent an en bloc resection of the shoulder girdle. The functions of hand and forearm are intact.

sionally applies. The technique is standard and can be found in any textbook of orthopedic surgery.

## CHEST WALL RESECTION

Resection of a part of the anterior, lateral, or posterior part of the thoracic cage is occasionally required for tumors arising in these sites. The basic surgical concept is the same as that for an adequate wide excision, the only modification being that necessitated by the location of the tumor.

### Indications

1. All soft tissue sarcomas, osteosarcomas, and chondrosarcomas arising from the tissues of the chest wall.
2. Locally recurrent skin cancers invading the ribs or the perichondrium.

### Contraindications

There are relatively few contraindications for a chest wall resection in the management of soft tissue sarcomas of the thoracic cage. In some highly malignant tumors to which judicious radiotherapy can be applied without injuring the underlying lung and pleura, a massive resection of the thoracic cage should be avoided; for example, rhabdomyosarcoma located in the chest wall.

### Technique

***Steps of Operation.***   The technical aspects of chest wall resection are simple. After assessing the resectability of a given tumor, the extent of the resection is outlined, and the appropriate number of ribs on either side of the tumor is resected (Figs. 16–12A to 16–12C). The resected segment of the ribs must be adequate in length; otherwise, extension of the tumor along the marrow of the ribs will be overlooked, resulting in an inadequate operation. We perform intrapleural chest wall resections rather than extrapleural, since on several occasions we have found the undersurface of the tumors in intimate contact with the pleura.

The reconstruction following chest wall resection, however, is laden with diverse ideas and techniques. The major area of discord has been in the type of material to be used for replacing the lost chest wall. We used to employ bovine fascia lata (Fig. 16–12D) for reconstruction and found it to be satisfactory. However, due to its lack of availability, we currently use Gore-Tex mesh as our synthetic material of choice. The end result after these repairs is excellent and our patients have been able to resume normal activity (Figs. 16–13A and 16–13B). In selected instances, various types of myocutaneous flaps are being used for improved cosmetic and functional results.

## ABDOMINAL WALL RESECTION

The anterior abdomen is often the site of several types of tumors, most notably abdominal wall desmoids (aggressive fibromatosis). Frequently, it is stated that the incidence of local recurrence in this anatomic location following excision is very high. A fatalistic attitude of acceptance of local recurrence by most authors reporting on this subject is commonly found in the literature.[15] The recurrence rate can be reduced to a minimum, however, if the proper concept of wide excision is applied. To accomplish this, the anterior abdominal wall must be excised totally, including the underlying peritoneum. A 3- to 5-cm margin on all sides of the primary tumor should be mapped out, and a block of tissue containing skin, fascia, anterior abdominal wall musculature, and the underlying peritoneum must be resected (Figs. 16–14A and 16–14B). The defect is closed by using synthetic material (Fig. 16–14C). The skin is closed with interrupted sutures. In our hands, application of this principle has lowered the incidence of recurrence to a minimum, and there is no functional handicap after this operation (Fig. 16–15). Similarly, in some patients, abdominal wall defects can be effectively closed by myocutaneous flaps.

## EXCISION OF RETROPERITONEAL TUMORS

Retroperitoneal sarcomas are indeed difficult to operate on. The boundaries of the retroperitoneum are varied, and the surgeon may be confronted with a sarcoma of immense size. Therefore, it is not possible to describe the steps of the operation. The surgeon should plan the extent of the operation after a preliminary exploration of the abdominal cavity and assessment of the situation. We try to ascertain the extent of the tumor and its relation to the aorta and inferior vena cava by extensive use of preoperative investigative techniques (Chapter 4). Adequate exposure is always the key to the excision of these retroperitoneal tumors. Figure 16–16 shows the incisions that have been found useful in our hands. Multiple variations of these basic incisions can be adopted as the situation dictates. During the operation, adherence to surrounding organs is ascertained, and a plan for resection is outlined. Frequently, all or part of several viscera must be excised.

The recurrence rate of these tumors is high, and some patients need multiple operations. One of our patients with a retroperitoneal liposarcoma required 11

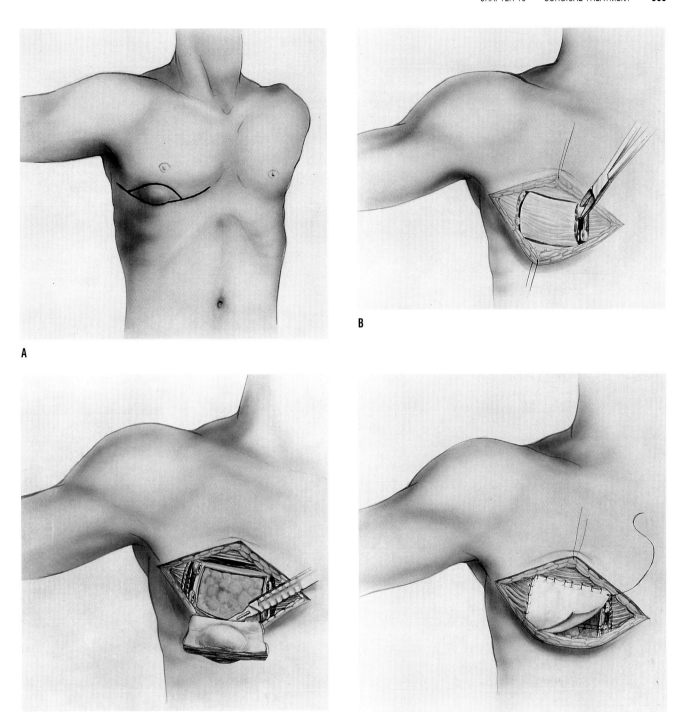

**Figure 16–12.** **(A)** A tumor of the anterior chest wall. The proposed incision is shown. **(B)** The skin flaps have been raised, the resectability assessed, and the ribs are being resected. **(C)** Segment of the chest wall being moved. Unaffected lung can be seen underneath. **(D)** Chest wall being repaired by synthetic material.

procedures. Currently, intraoperative radiation therapy is being investigated as a means of reducing the incidence of local recurrence. Reliable data have not yet been generated to ascertain whether this would reduce the rate of local recurrence after excision of retroperitoneal tumors.

## EXCISION OF INTRATHORACIC TUMORS

Mediastinal soft tissue tumors are less common, and, unlike in their retroperitoneal counterpart, surgical management is relatively simple. Once a mediastinal tumor is diagnosed and the patient properly assessed,

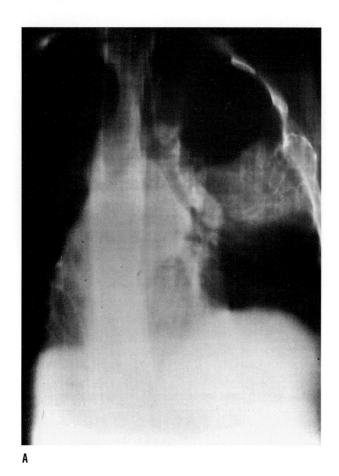

A

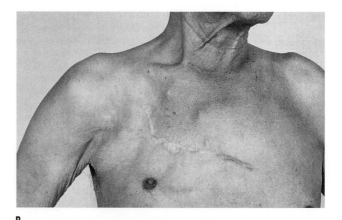

B

**Figure 16–13. (A)** Roentgenogram of chest showing a fibrosarcoma tumor of the chest wall in a 9-year-old girl. Following chest wall resection, she has remained well for 22 years. **(B)** Another patient, a 56-year-old man, two years after chest wall resection and repair with bovine fascia lata for a myxoid liposarcoma of the pectoral region.

an exploratory thoracotomy is performed, and the tumor is approached. If it is truly a soft tissue tumor, it is excised. With today's advances in anesthesia and postoperative management techniques, the results of the operation are usually excellent.

### WIDE EXCISION AND IN-CONTINUITY NODE DISSECTION

The well-known concept of excision of the primary tumor and simultaneous dissection of the regional node-bearing area, as proposed by Halstead[16] for cancer of the breast, is seldom required for the management of soft tissue sarcomas. Rarely do these tumors metastasize to the regional nodes of the neck, axillae, or groin. However, in some instances of high-grade synovial sarcoma, rhabdomyosarcoma (all types), and other sundry sarcomas, regional node metastases may occur (details are described under each type elsewhere in this book). Therefore, the concept of wide excision with in-continuity regional node dissection should be kept in mind.

The procedure to be applied must be tailored to a given patient, and it must be planned with the concept of wide excision of the primary sarcoma, as described earlier, with extension of the excision in-continuity to include the regional node-bearing area. Because of the location of the primary tumor, bizarre types of incision lines often will result, but this should not deter the surgeon from undertaking these operations.

### ■ INDICATIONS AND TECHNIQUES FOR RADICAL AMPUTATION

The principles governing the choice of a radical amputation of an extremity are varied. Probably, the single most important factor is the clinical experience of the surgeon treating the patient. However, when all the available information is considered, it is possible to develop certain guidelines to apply when planning amputations for sarcomas. These are as follows:

1. Many sarcomas extend imperceptibly proximally along the muscular or fascial planes, sometimes making it difficult to assess the extent of the disease.
2. Fibrosarcomas extend along the fascial plane, and along all the fascial attachments proximally, distally, and deep to the tumor.
3. Malignant schwannomas extend along the nerve sheath, and with the coexistent beading of the nerves commonly seen in plexiform neuroma, it is often difficult to be certain of the level of excision, even with appropriate use of rapid histologic techniques for examination of the margins of the resected specimens.
4. Invasion of a soft tissue sarcoma to the underlying bone or blood vessels and nerves usually requires an amputation.

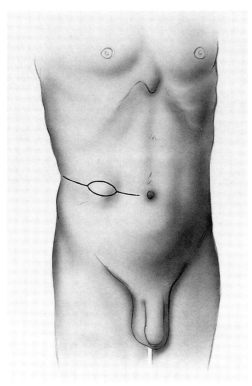

**A**

5. Sarcomas of any histologic type that persistently recur after primary therapy: The need for a major amputation becomes more acute after a number of local recurrences.

Based on the five points above, the general principles to be applied in making a decision for or against an amputation can be used. However, before making the decision, all other options for therapy must be evaluated.

The surgeon performing amputations for soft tissue sarcomas does not have wide latitude in selecting the site of amputation, as in the management of trauma or peripheral vascular disorders. This does not imply that a thorough consideration of a good functional prosthesis is not advocated, but rather that prosthetic considerations should not interfere with the potential cure. We have seen a number of patients in whom, for the sake of a better prosthesis, inadequate amputations have been performed with resultant local recurrences in the stump. Local recurrence after a major amputation is indeed a failure of treatment, and every attempt should be made to avoid it.

**Figure 16–14. (A)** Proposed skin incision for an anterior abdominal wall tumor. **(B)** Skin flaps have been raised, the line of resection is outlined, and the resection is begun in the medial end. Extent of resection is shown by the dotted line. **(C)** Specimen has been removed, including the parietal peritoneum. Small intestine can easily be seen. Defect is being closed with a synthetic material. Following this repair, we have not come across any abdominal wall hernia in an otherwise healthy person.

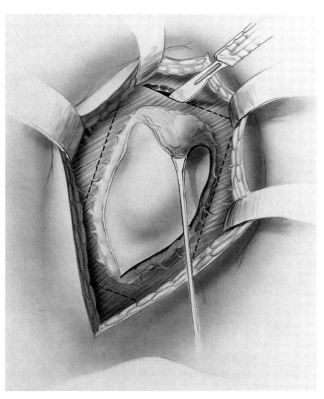

**B**

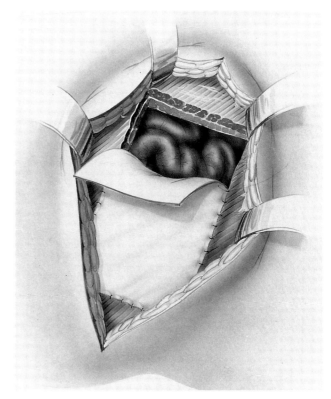

**C**

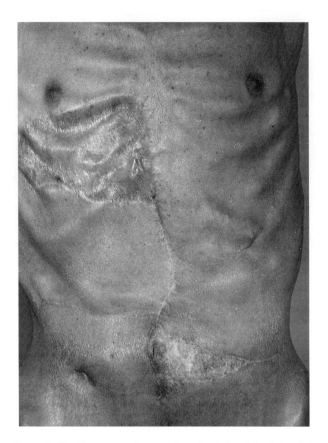

**Figure 16–15.** Three years after resection of anterior abdominal wall for hemangiopericytoma. Patient had no disability.

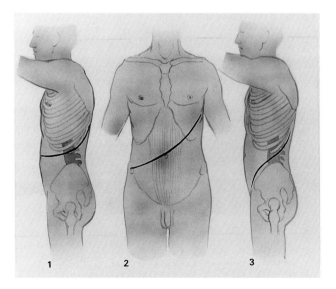

**Figure 16–16.** Three types of incision are shown. The transverse incision usually is best for most retroperitoneal structures. However, the lateral might be of value in tumors of the renal region with a need for entry into the thoracic cavity in situations in which the tumors are located in association with the adrenal, or behind the liver bed.

With the combination of radiation therapy and chemotherapy, the need for radical amputation has decreased in most sarcomas (see Chapter 19), and the patients can be well treated with multimodal therapy. The types of tumors and the kinds of patients in whom such multimodality therapy is possible have been described in Chapter 19 and the chapters dealing with specific tumor types.

## PREOPERATIVE CARE FOR PATIENTS UNDERGOING RADICAL AMPUTATIONS

Preoperative preparation of patients who will undergo radical amputation is essentially the same as that for any other major operation. There are excellent monographs dealing with this subject alone, and the reader is urged to consult them. However, it is important to note here that all major limb ablative procedures are operations of major magnitude, and the patient must be adequately evaluated regarding cardiopulmonary and renal status, underlying infection, and any other concomitant feature that might produce postoperative complications.

We advocate an in-depth discussion with the patient and loved ones of the indications for and against the proposed amputation. We have found that a well-informed patient always adjusts better to the deformity and has fewer associated symptoms: for example, phantom limb syndrome or similar complaints. As a result of the discussion, the patient will feel less hostility and that he or she is still a useful member of society. We strongly recommend that a major amputation not be "sold" to a patient, and if he or she has any doubt, such an operation should be abandoned. The objective of the surgical oncologist is to provide all the necessary information, then let the patient make the final decision.

A preliminary exploratory laparotomy used to be an essential first step for most patients undergoing a major amputation; however, with increasing use of abdominal and pelvic CAT scan and/or MRI, the need for this step is by and large eliminated. In any event, for patients requiring either a hip joint disarticulation or a hemipelvectomy, we routinely use preoperative cleansing of the colon and evaluation of the urinary bladder, and in male patients, the prostate as well.

## RADICAL AMPUTATIONS OF THE UPPER EXTREMITY

### Mid-Arm Amputation

There are few indications for mid-arm amputation. This operation is indicated when the tumor is located in the forearm and amputation must be above the common flexor or extensor attachments in the lower end of the humerus. Occasionally, in cases of tumors of the hand and forearm in which there are palpable nodes in the axilla, a mid-arm amputation with axillary dissection can be resorted to instead of a forequarter amputation (Fig. 16–17). The technique is standard, and will not be repeated here.

## Shoulder Joint Disarticulation

Shoulder joint disarticulation has little value in the management of soft tissue sarcomas. We have seldom used this operation for the management of any of our patients. Although there can be an occasional application of this technique, we think that, in most of these patients, the better operation would be a forequarter amputation. The technical aspects of shoulder disarticulation are standard and can be found in any textbook of operative orthopedics; thus, we will not discuss it in this chapter.

## Interscapulothoracic Amputation (Forequarter Amputation or Berger's Amputation)

In an interscapulothoracic amputation, the entire upper extremity and the shoulder girdle and its muscular attachments are removed. The first interscapu-

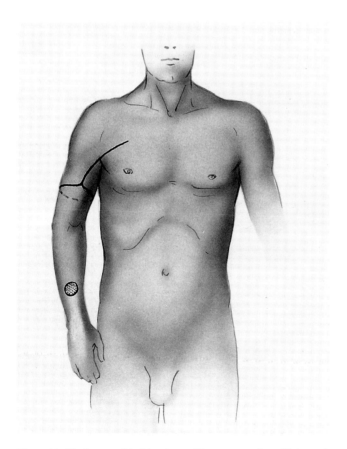

**Figure 16–17.** Suggested incision for a mid-arm amputation with in-continuity axillary node dissection for a tumor of the forearm.

lothoracic amputation for cancer was performed by Crosby[17] in 1836 for removal of an osteosarcoma. The technique of the operation, however, was standardized by Berger[18] in 1887. This classic operation still bears his name. Since the turn of the century, it has been increasingly used for the management of sarcomas of the upper extremities. Pack and associates[19] published an elegant review of the operation in 1942 and reported on their series of 31 patients so treated at Memorial Sloan-Kettering Cancer Center. Subsequently, Moseley[20] published a review on forequarter amputations. Interested readers should review these classic works. With the development of better anesthesia and blood transfusion methods, this operation has become less of a technical feat than it used to be.[21–23]

### Indications

1. All malignant tumors of the upper arm, axilla, and shoulder region that are not amenable to local control by means of multimodal therapy.
2. Bone sarcomas proximal to the elbow, particularly those involving the upper end of the humerus or those extending into the medullary cavity of the humerus, where a bone graft is contraindicated, or those osteosarcomas that extensively involve the surrounding soft tissues.
3. All malignant tumors infiltrating the capsule of the shoulder joint, the deltoid, subscapularis, and pectoral muscles.
4. Tumors of the shoulder girdle for which an attempted Tikhoff-Linberg operation or a scapulectomy procedure has been deemed unsuitable.
5. Aggressive fibromatoses of the upper arm that are symptomatic, especially those infiltrating the brachial plexus or the periosteum of the humerus.

**Contraindications.** The usual contraindications to any major surgical procedure because of systemic disease apply. Additionally, sarcomas that are deemed sensitive to chemotherapy and radiation therapy should not be treated by this operation. Patients with such tumors in an upper extremity should be treated with regional chemotherapy, wide soft tissue resection, and adjuvant radiation therapy and chemotherapy, or both. We think that adoption of this policy will further reduce the need for forequarter amputation in the management of soft tissue sarcomas of the upper extremities.

### Technique

*Anesthesia.* Standard endotracheal anesthesia is generally used.

*Position of the Patient.*   The patient is placed on his or her back with the affected shoulder elevated so that the skin of the upper arm, axilla, and the skin of both the anterior and posterior chest wall up to the midline can be prepared and draped to be included in the operative site.

*Steps of Operation.*   A linear incision is first made over the medial third of the clavicle (Fig. 16–18A). This incision is deepened to the periosteum, and the periosteum is elevated by means of a periosteal elevator. The clavicle is resected with a Gigli's saw (Fig. 16–18B). Through this window, the subclavian vessels are exposed, with the artery lying deeper than the vein (Fig. 16–18C). The subclavian vessels are then individually ligated and resected. It is our practice to double-ligate the proximal end of these structures using 2-0 silk and do the suture ligature with 3-0 silk (Fig. 16–18D). Ligation of the superficial cervical and descending scapular arteries along with the transverse cervical vessels will prevent excessive blood loss during the rest of the operation. After ligating the vessels, the skin incision is extended laterally to the tip of the acromion process, then downwards anteriorly toward the axilla (Fig. 16–18D). The arm is then drawn across the body, and

the posterior flap is outlined by an incision of the skin along the vertebral border of the scapula, which unites with the inferior tip of the anterior incision at the lateral margin of the axillary fold (Fig. 16–18E).

The arm is then brought back to its original position, and the anterior incision is deepened up to the pectoral muscles. Resection of the pectoralis major and minor muscles provides excellent exposure of the brachial plexus (Fig. 16–18F). The brachial plexus is then resected as proximally as possible. The arm is brought forward again, and the patient is rotated anterolaterally. The posterior incision is then deepened, exposing the trapezius muscle, and the muscles attached to the vertebral border of the scapula are sequentially resected (Figs. 16–18G and 16–18H). This step of the operation is similar to that described for subtotal scapulectomy. With detachment of the scapula, the amputation is complete, and the extremity is removed (Fig. 16–18I). After proper hemostasis, the wound is closed, using absorbable sutures for muscle and subcutaneous tissue and interrupted 3-0 nylon sutures for skin. Suction catheters are left behind (Fig. 16–18J).

The exposure of the subclavian vessels through the window described above sometimes becomes difficult.

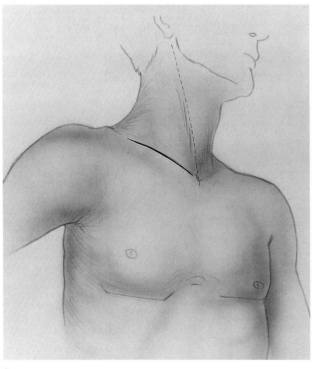

**A**

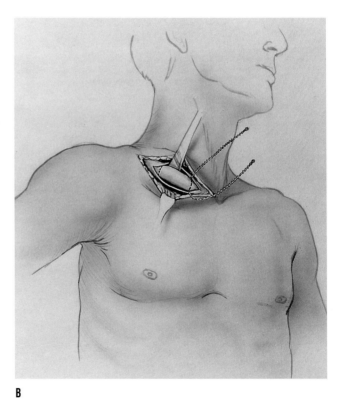

**B**

**Figure 16–18.** **(A)** The deep line represents the first step of the incision in forequarter amputation. The dotted line in the neck shows the incision that can be used for a concomitant neck dissection when indicated. **(B)** Incision has been deepened. The clavicle is exposed, clavicular periosteum is incised, and the clavicle resected with a Gigli's saw. *(Continued.)*

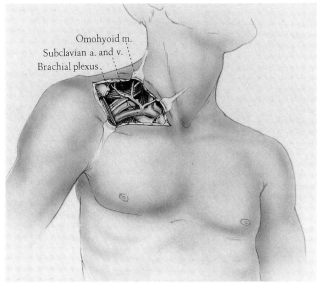

C

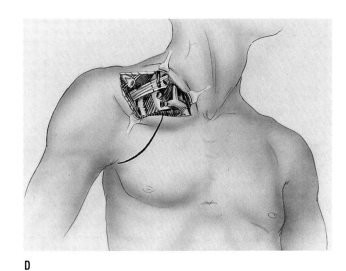

D

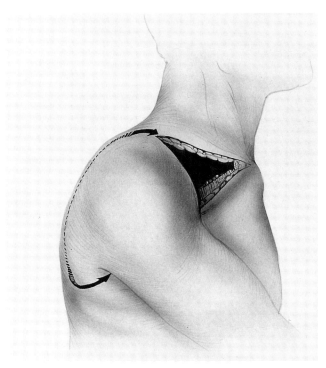

E

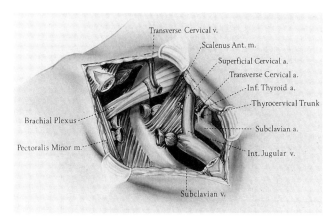

F

**Figure 16–18** *(continued).* **(C)** The middle segment of the clavicle has been removed. The subclavian vessels (artery and vein) and the brachial plexus can be seen. **(D)** The vessels are ligated and resected. Dotted line shows the proposed line of resection of the brachial plexus, and the dark line shows the skin incision to the axilla. The anterior skin incision is sometimes extended to the axilla before ligation of the vascular bundle. **(E)** Artistic rendition of the incision in the back along the vertebral border of the scapula. This incision, bound by arrows, is extended from the acromion process, and, encircling the tip of the scapula, reaches the anterior axillary incision, as seen in Fig. 16–18D. **(Γ)** Anterior view of the completed axillary resection. Vessels are resected; brachial plexus is being cut. All the anterior structures are resected, completing the anterior separation of the extremity. *(Continued.)*

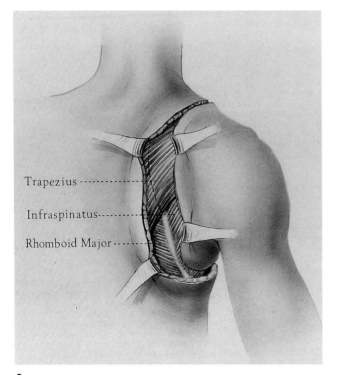

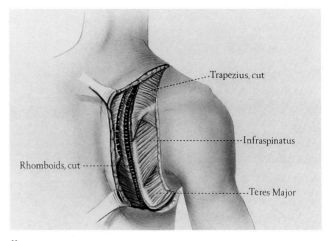

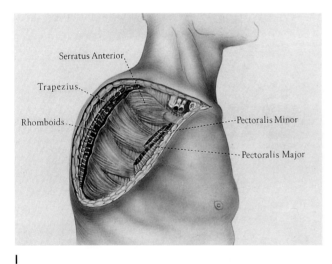

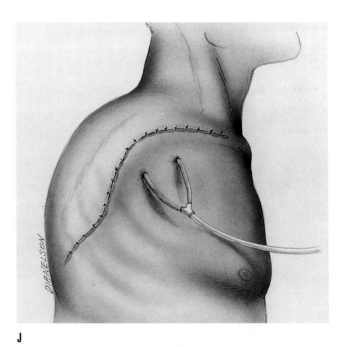

**Figure 16–18** *(continued).* **(G)** Posterior excision is begun. First layers of the muscles are exposed and resected. **(H)** The deeper muscles attached to the verte-bral border of the scapula are sequentially resected. **(I)** Appearance of the wound after the extremity has been separated. **(J)** Wound closed, with suction drainage.

In such cases, following resection of the clavicle, the ligation of the vessels is postponed until the anterior incision is carried through the pectoral muscles into the axilla. With this dissection, the axillary vein and artery come into view, and ligation of the vessels becomes relatively simple. The rest of the operative steps are the same as above.

Occasionally, an unusual location of the primary tumor (for example, over the superior aspect of the shoulder) will prevent adequate exposure of the sub-clavian vessels by the method described above. For such cases, Nadler and Phelan[21] have described a posterior method for approaching the subclavian vessels as well as for assessing the resectability of the tumor. In these patients, the posterior skin incision is first deepened, and the pleural cavity is entered through the bed of the second rib. If the lesion is resectable, the subclavian vessels are identified and ligated within the chest cavity. Care should be taken to avoid injury to the innominate vessels on the right side, and the vagus and phrenic nerves on both sides. The chest wall defect is closed with a synthetic material, as described in chest wall resection.

Bowden[22] described a method of extending forequarter amputation to include an ipsilateral neck dissection (Fig. 16–18A). This extension of the operation is useful in tumors of the axilla or shoulder that could metastasize to neck nodes: for example, some cases of rhabdomyosarcoma or synovial cell sarcoma.

In a number of patients, the operation can be extended to include resection of the chest wall, radical mastectomy, excision of part of the intrathoracic viscus, and so forth. All these modifications are applied whenever indicated, and in our hands these extended operations have been useful in a few selected patients.

Although the operation is dramatic and mutilating, in properly selected patients, operative complications or problems are minimal. Blood loss is usually less than one liter. The incidence of traumatic neuroma is high following an interscapulothoracic amputation.[24] In our hands, the only satisfactory method for reduction of the incidence has been sharp excision of the plexi at the most proximal point. This allows the individual roots to retract without getting encased in the fibrous scar of the incision. Sometimes reexcision of these painful neuromas becomes necessary.

The postoperative course is usually smooth. The patient is ambulatory the day after the amputation and, in uncomplicated cases, can be discharged within a few days. Most patients adjust to this operation well and continue to function adequately as useful members of society (Fig. 16–19).

A forequarter operation becomes complicated, however, in patients with recurrent tumors who have been previously irradiated to the maximum tolerable dose. In such instances, the major problem is postoperative wound healing, since, in a number of patients, the skin flaps necrose, leaving a large defect. Frequently, the closure of these defects taxes the imagination of the best of plastic surgeons.

## RADICAL AMPUTATIONS OF THE LOWER EXTREMITIES

### Above-the-Knee or Midthigh Amputations

Amputations above the knee joint for soft tissue sarcomas arising in the foot or in the leg have a definite place in the armamentarium of surgical treatment. The usual indications for such an operation are fibrosarcomas, synovial sarcomas, rhabdomyosarcomas, and liposarcomas arising in the leg. The technical aspects of a midthigh amputation are well known and will not be repeated. In certain instances (e.g., in rhabdomyosarcomas and synovial sarcomas), above-the-knee amputation is combined with a radical groin dissection (Fig. 16–20).[25] The technique of groin dissection is described in detail in combination with hip joint disarticulation (see below).

### Hip Joint Disarticulation

Amputation of a lower extremity through the hip joint is a formidable procedure and should be undertaken only when the indications for this operation are unassailable.

Hip joint disarticulation apparently was first performed by Walter Bonchear of Bardstown, Kentucky, in August of 1806, but an account was never published. Frank[26] described Bonchear's performance of this operation, without anesthesia, in a 17-year-old boy with a comminuted multiple fracture of the femur. The earliest recorded instance of an anatomically well-conceived hip joint disarticulation was that of Sir Astley Cooper.[27] The operation was performed at Guy's Hospital on January 16, 1824, on a 40-year-old man, again without anesthesia. The patient did well and was free of disease one year after the operation. The courage, imagination, and perseverance of the patients, as well as of the surgeons, in those earlier days of extended surgery is indeed unimaginable in today's technologically advanced environment. Today, with the advances in anesthesia and transfusion, the operation of hip joint disarticulation has become a relatively routine procedure. Most of the credit for application of this operation to the management of soft tissue sarcomas should go to the late George T. Pack and his colleagues at Memorial Sloan-Kettering Cancer Center.[1,4,10]

*Indications.*   Patients with malignant tumors of the soft somatic tissues of the thigh and upper leg that cannot be locally controlled by multimodal limb-sparing surgery are candidates for hip joint disarticulation. However, this operation should only be undertaken when all methods of sparing the affected limb have failed.

*Technique*

*Steps of Operation.*   An anterior racquet incision is most suitable (Fig. 16–21A, inset [left hip]). The vertical part of the incision is carried downward and outward across the anterior aspect of the thigh, coursing just above the greater trochanter. The medial incision is similarly carried across the thigh about 4 cm below the genitofemoral fold. The two incisions join posteriorly at the infragluteal fold. Although an attempt is always made to adhere to this classic racquet incision, deciding the

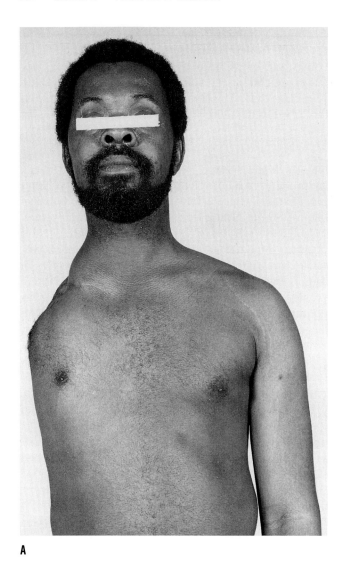

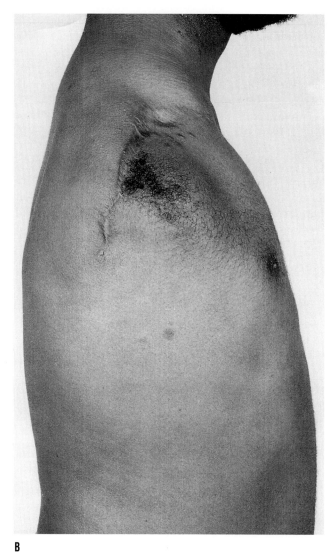

**Figure 16–19. (A)** Anterior and **(B)** lateral views of a 31-year-old man who underwent a forequarter amputation for a low-grade fibrosarcoma nine years ago. He has remained well and active.

amount of skin to be sacrificed depends on the location of the tumor. Frequently, this decision results in several modifications of the standard skin incision.

A detailed description of the subsequent steps of the operation will be found in the following section dealing with hip joint disarticulation and radical groin dissection. The minor differences in steps between these two operations will be pointed out as they occur.

### Hip Joint Disarticulation and Radical Groin Dissection

***Indications.***   Rhabdomyosarcomas, synovial cell sarcomas, malignant fibrous histiocytomas, and certain other highly anaplastic sarcomas that have proven (clinically and histologically) regional node metastasis should be treated by combined hip joint disarticulation and radical groin dissection.

*Steps of Operation.*   The vertical incision extends from the subcostal region inferiorly on a straight line crossing the midpoint of the inguinal ligament and is continued about 4 cm below, on the skin of the thigh. The lateral arm of the incision is carried laterally, just above the greater trochanter. The medial incision is similarly carried across the medial aspect of the thigh about 4 cm below the inguinal fold (Fig. 16–21A, inset [right hip]). As before, the skin incision in the thigh might require modification, depending on the amount of skin to be excised in a given patient.

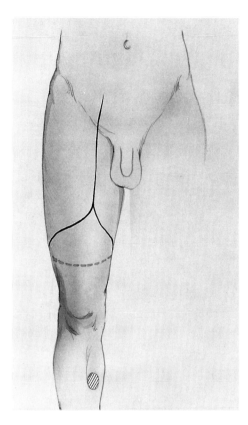

**Figure 16–20.** Incision for midthigh amputation and radical groin dissection. For indications of this type of composite operation, see text.

The vertical incision on the anterior abdominal wall is deepened up to the midinguinal point. The anterior abdominal wall muscles and the peritoneum are incised along the same line as the skin incision (Fig. 16–21A). When indicated, the peritoneal cavity is explored (Fig. 16–21B), and if necessary, questionable areas in the liver or other viscera and the para-aortic nodes are examined by means of frozen section. If there is any evidence of intra-abdominal metastases, the proposed hip joint disarticulation is not carried out. Upon completion of the exploration, the peritoneum is closed (Fig. 16–21B). Next, the retroperitoneal area is exposed by pushing the peritoneal contents medially with a sponge stick, which can be accomplished with relative ease and without any blood loss (Fig. 16–21C). This method will expose the bifurcation of the aorta and the formation of the inferior vena cava proximally to the iliac vessels distally. The ureter will be seen reflected along with the posterior peritoneum medially.

The deep part of the groin dissection is then begun about 2 cm above the bifurcation of the aorta and carried distally to include the iliac and obturator group of nodes. The most proximal part is marked with metal clips, and the areolar tissue containing the nodes

is dissected distally (Fig. 16–21D). The dissection includes the adventitial layer of both the external iliac artery and vein distally from the bifurcation of the common iliac vessels. These vessels are ligated and resected about two centimeters from the bifurcation. The resected blood vessels and their areolar envelope, along with the nodes, are dissected distally. The obturator contents are dissected out from the obturator fossa and the perivesical fat (Fig. 16–21E). In contrast to the conventional radical groin dissection described earlier,[25] the dissection is not carried to the femoral triangle, since that part is included when the limb is removed at the level of the hip joint.

Following the deep node dissection, the hip joint disarticulation is begun. Both the external iliac artery and vein have been previously ligated and resected. The inguinal ligament and the femoral nerves are then resected. The medial and lateral incisions of the thigh are deepened, and thick flaps are developed both medially up to the pubis and laterally to the greater trochanter. The anterior compartment muscles are then resected. The limb is abducted by an assistant, and the medial compartment muscles are then resected at their point of proximal attachment (Fig. 16–21F). The limb is then adducted and the tensor fascia lata resected. This completes the dissection of the anterior aspects of the hip joint. The limb is then adducted and internally rotated. As a result, the greater trochanter comes into view, and the lateral muscles attached to the greater trochanter are resected.

After this, the limb is rotated, and the gluteal group of muscles is resected. The capsule of the hip joint is exposed and incised. The ligamentum teres is then exposed and resected, and the head of the femur is delivered out of the acetabulum (Fig. 16–21G). The limb is now attached only posteriorly by the sciatic nerve and the hamstring muscles. These are resected and the limb removed.

Following removal of the specimen, the bleeding points are caught and ligated. Any extra muscle or fat is trimmed. The acetabular cavity is curetted to remove as much of the synovial surface as possible; otherwise, the membrane secretes synovial fluid for a prolonged period. The wound is then closed, with adequate drains (Fig. 16–21H), and a firm pressure dressing is applied.

If node dissection is not indicated, the superior limit of the incision is initially deepened to expose the inguinal ligament, which is resected. Following this, femoral vessels are dissected, isolated, and individually ligated and resected. The femoral nerve is then divided. The technique of severing the limb is the same as described above.

Sometimes it is possible to cut the anterior muscles lower than the contemplated line of resection. In such instances, these muscles can be used to plug the acetab-

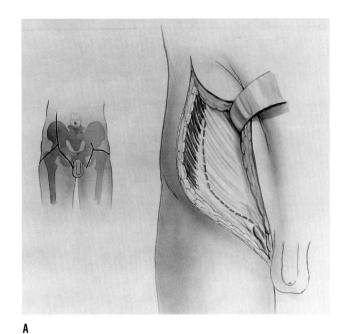

**A**

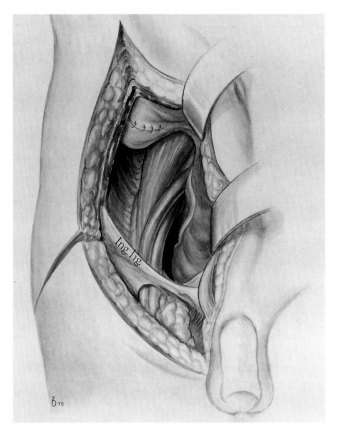

**C**

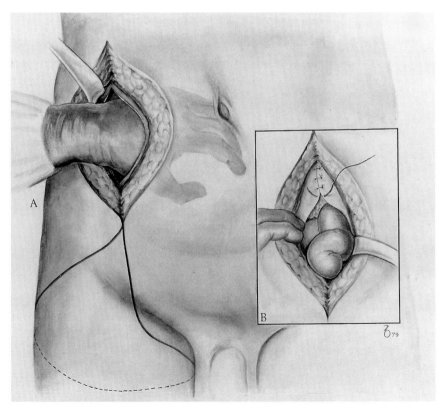

**B**

**Figure 16–21. (A)** *Inset:* Outline of incision for a hip joint disarticulation and ipsilateral radical groin dissection. Incision for a standard hip joint disarticulation is shown on left. *Right:* Upper abdominal incision used for exploratory celiotomy. **(B)** *Left:* The peritoneal cavity is entered through the upper part of the incision. Exploratory laparotomy constitutes examination of the intra-abdominal viscera and para-aortic nodes. The entire incision, including the posterior extent in the back of the thigh, is outlined. The inset *(right)* shows the peritoneum being closed. **(C)** The peritoneum, with its contents, has been pushed medially. On the upper part of the diagram, the recently sutured peritoneum is seen. The ureter can be observed to be adherent to the posterior peritoneum retracted medially. The external iliac vessels, psoas major, and iliacus muscles are apparent. The femoral vessels distal to the inguinal ligament can be seen at the lower part of the diagram. *(Continued.)*

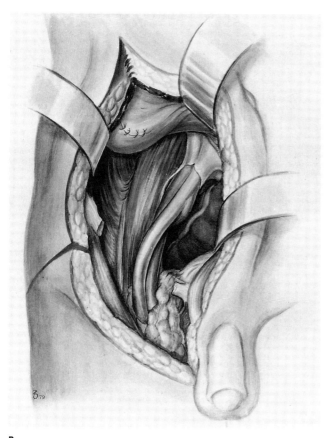

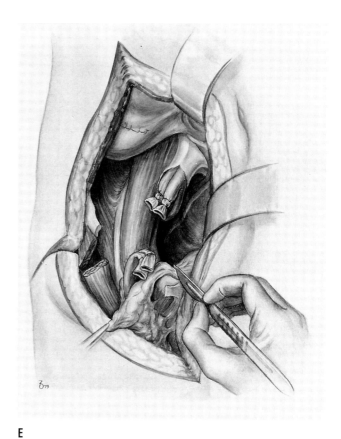

E

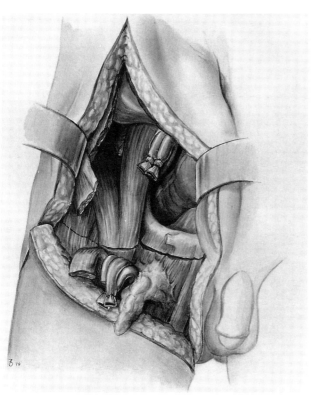

F

**Figure 16–21** *(continued).* **(D)** Dissection is initiated at the bifurcation of the aorta or the formation of the inferior vena cava. The dissection includes the adventitial layer of the external iliac vessels, along with the nodes. In this diagram, the inguinal ligament is resected medially, exposing the obturator fat pad at the lower end. The spermatic cord and the urinary bladder are retracted medially. The internal iliac artery is seen curving into the pelvic cavity. **(E)** The external iliac vessels are ligated and resected. The areolar tissue and the nodes, along with the vessels, are pushed distally towards the inguinal ligament. The obturator contents are identified and dissected free from the adherent perivesical fat. The femoral nerve is seen emerging lateral to the psoas major muscle. It is resected at this level. The sartorius muscle is already resected. The outline of the ureter attached to the posterior wall of the peritoneum should always be visible during the dissection. **(F)** The obturator dissection is completed. The anterior and lateral muscles are resected, with patient in supine position. The extremity is then abducted, and the medial compartment muscles are resected. The cut ends of the vessels and femoral nerve are seen in the lower end of the diagram. *(Continued.)*

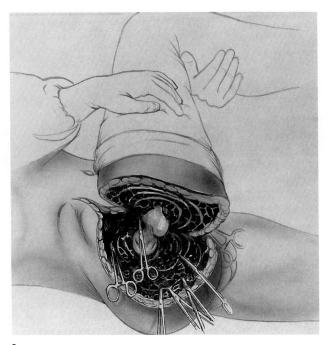

G

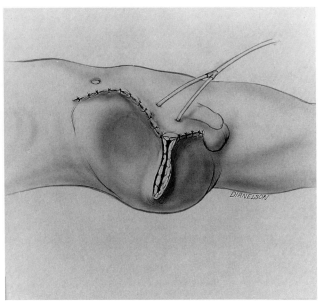

H

**Figure 16–21** *(continued).* **(G)** The extremity is adducted and internally rotated. All the lateral muscles to the greater trochanter are being cut, then the gluteal muscles are resected. The femoral head is delivered out of the acetabular cavity. Ligamentum teres, clearly seen in this diagram, is cut. The limb is now attached posteriorly by the sciatic nerve and hamstring muscles; these are cut and the extremity removed. **(H)** The Y-shaped wound closure. Once the wound heals, a prosthesis can easily be fitted.

ular cavity. This step, although desirable, is not essential and should not be performed at the risk of jeopardizing a good cancer operation. The operative blood loss seldom is more than one liter.

The postoperative course of these patients is relatively smooth. Usually, they are up and about by the second day. With physiotherapy, the patients shortly can be taught to use a crutch, and can be discharged within three or four days. Wound healing is not a problem in nonirradiated patients. The problem of phantom pain is similar to that in other major amputations and is infrequently a physiologic or rehabilitative problem (see pages 522–523).

### Hemipelvectomy (Sacroiliac Disarticulation or Hindquarter Amputation)

***Historical Background.*** The operation was first performed by Girard[28,29] in 1895. The principles of the surgical procedure were laid down by J. Hogarth Pringle[30] in 1916. Pringle reviewed the literature and described his own two cases. Subsequently, the literature was reviewed by Judin[31] in 1926, by Gordon-Taylor and Wiles[32] in 1935, by Sugarbaker and Ackerman[33] in 1945, and again by Gordon-Taylor and Paley[34] in 1946.

In 1952, Gordon-Taylor and Monroe[35] described the technique used in their 64 cases. Pack and Ehrlich,[36] in 1946, and Pack,[37] in 1956, reviewed both the technical and the end result experience at Memorial Sloan-Kettering Cancer Center. These reports provide an insight into the development of this operation.

In the last few decades, the operative mortality has been reduced from approximately 45 percent to an acceptable level of less than 5 percent in most of the centers engaged in this type of radical amputation.

A radical procedure such as hemipelvectomy should be used only when the indications are clearly defined and standardized. In its evolutionary phase, the operation was either performed with bravado by some surgeons, or abandoned out of fear by others. As a result, the proper place for this operation in the therapeutic armamentarium of the cancer surgeon was never defined. In recent years, however, hemipelvectomy as an operative technique has become reasonably standardized and is being performed in several centers in the United States and elsewhere with decreasing morbidity and mortality. The novelty of a "big operation" has now worn off, and the extent of the operation and the indications and contraindications can be adequately defined. In properly selected cases, this operation provides a good end result.

**Definition.**   The term *hemipelvectomy* means removal of one side of the pelvis along with the buttock and the entire lower extremity. The operative limit in the pelvis usually is through the sacroiliac synchondrosis and pubic symphysis. However, this operation can be extended and can be performed by cutting through the sacrum and lumbar vertebrae, or can be modified by resecting through the innominate bone.

Other names that have been used to describe this operation are sacroilial disarticulation, and interinnominoabdominal, hindquarter, and interpelvicabdominal amputation.

**Indications.**   Hemipelvectomy as a curative operation is indicated in the following clinical settings:

1. Any recurrent sarcoma that has failed multimodal therapy and is located in the upper part of the thigh, buttock, inguinal, and/or pubic region.
2. A well-differentiated soft tissue sarcoma located in the upper part of the thigh, extending to the inguinal ligament or to the pubic symphysis, a situation in which a clear proximal margin of the resection cannot be accomplished without resorting to this operation: for example, a low-grade fibrosarcoma that has infiltrated the areas mentioned above, or the adjacent femur or the major blood vessels and nerves. Hemangiopericytoma, malignant schwannoma, and similar tumors in this region might also require a hemipelvectomy.
3. Primary or recurrent malignant osseous and periosteal tumors of the upper femur, if the tumor has extended to or through the hip joint; and similar neoplasms of the innominate bones.
4. Primary soft tissue sarcomas of the iliac fossa or upper thigh, extending through the obturator foramen.
5. Soft tissue sarcomas of the buttock, extending to the pelvis through the sciatic notch, which cannot be extirpated by excision of the buttocks.

**Contraindications**

1. Any soft tissue sarcoma that can be treated by either muscle group excision or hip joint disarticulation, alone or in conjunction with node dissection.
2. Soft tissue sarcomas that can be well treated by multimodal therapy must receive this combined modality limb-sparing operation before embarking on a hemipelvectomy.
3. In some instances of highly anaplastic soft tissue sarcomas in which there is minimal life expec-

tancy: for example, in highly anaplastic fibrosarcoma. In these patients, the operation neither cures nor serves as an effective measure of palliation.
4. Hemipelvectomy is not an optimum operation for patients with psychological disorders, even though the tumor can be eradicated.

**Preoperative Preparation.**   The general principles of preoperative preparation have been described earlier. We recommend preparation of the colon as though the patient were undergoing a colon resection. An intravenous pyelogram and cystoscopic evaluation of the urinary bladder are also indicated. In female patients, antibiotic vaginal suppositories are used for three to five days before the operation.

### Technique

*Anesthesia.*   General endotracheal anesthesia is usually employed in our hospitals. Use of adjuvant epidural anesthesia for the first 48 hours after the operation is excellent for postoperative pain control.

*Positioning of the Patient.*   The patient is placed on the table, lying on the side opposite to the lesion, and is turned slightly onto the back (45-degree angle). The position is maintained by a support against the lower ribs and dorsal spine, well clear of the iliac crest. The limb is kept free and is prepared and draped within the operative field. The ipsilateral arm is supported at the ether screen. Care should be taken to avoid sustained pressure on the brachial plexus on the contralateral side. The table is then rotated toward the surgeon's side to about 20 degrees, allowing easier access to the anterior abdominal wall. An in-dwelling urinary catheter is attached to a urinal. In male patients, the scrotum is either sutured or taped to the opposite thigh. Meticulous preparation and draping of the entire side are essential; otherwise, movement of the limb during the operation can contaminate the operative field.

*Steps Of Operation.*   The preliminary incision is lateral and vertical, extending from the subcostal margin down about 4 to 5 cm laterally to the level of the umbilicus. The medial arm of the incision is then carried medially 3 cm higher and parallel to the inguinal ligament up to the pubic tubercle. The posterolateral limb of the incision extends to the greater trochanter and along the infragluteal groove to the perineum. It is then joined with the medial end of the anterior incision at the superior border of the symphysis pubis (Fig. 16–22A). The incision described above is the standard one we use whenever feasible. In some instances, however, the skin incision must be modified because of the

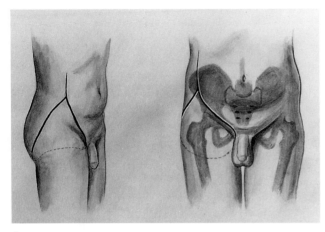

**A**

**Figure 16–22.** **(A)** Anterolateral and anterior views of incision for a conventional hemipelvectomy. **(B)** The anterior abdominal wall muscles are cut along the line of the skin incision. In male patients, the spermatic cord is identified and protected. The rectus muscle is detached from the pubis. The spermatic cord is retracted laterally to show the line of resection of the rectus abdominis muscle. In this diagram, the inguinal ligament is still in place. **(C)** Exploratory celiotomy has been completed, and the anterior abdominal wall muscles are cut laterally and at the pubic symphysis. In male patients, the spermatic cord is moved out of harm's way. The retroperitoneal space is seen. Ureter is seen adherent to the posterior peritoneum. Silk sutures are placed around the iliac vessels. If the operation becomes feasible, these sutures will be tied and the vessel resected. In this diagram, the inguinal ligament has been resected. **(D)** Anterior view of the pelvic contents for orientation. *(Continued.)*

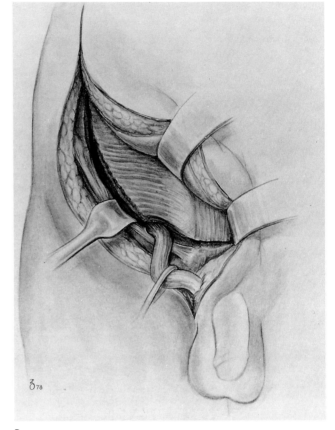

**B**

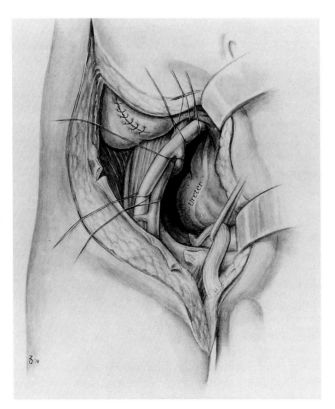

**C**

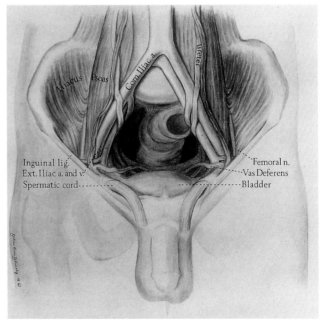

**D**

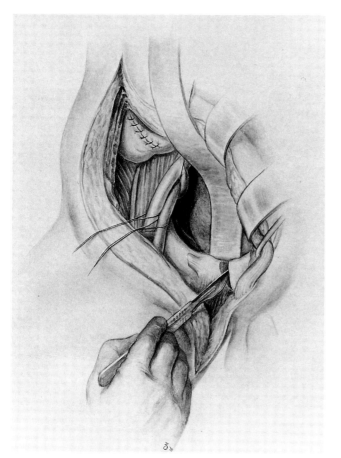

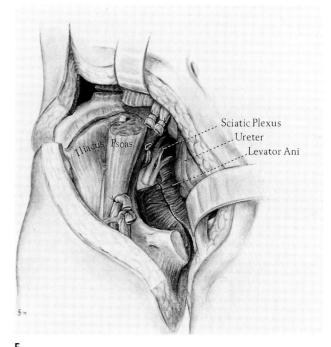

F

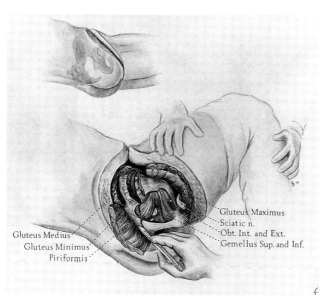

G

**Figure 16–22** *(continued).* **(E)** Pubic symphysis has been exposed and skeletonized. In most instances, the symphysis can be cut with a scalpel. Care should be taken to avoid injury to the urethra. A small malleable metallic retractor can be used for this purpose. The muscles of the inner aspect of the thigh can be resected at this stage by moderate abduction of the extremity. **(F)** With separation of the pubic symphysis, the extremity is abducted and pressed downward, and if no contraindication to hemipelvectomy is found, the iliac vessels are ligated and resected. The perineal muscles are cut along the line shown. Injury to the rectum is avoided by reflecting it away from the operative field. The iliac crest is also skeletonized at this juncture. **(G)** The posterior flap, as shown in the inset, is then raised. The posterior attachments of the gluteal muscles are resected with the leg held in extreme adduction. The remaining posterior muscles and sciatic nerve are cut. Following completion of the entire posterior dissection, the extremity is held in extreme abduction, and all the remaining attachments of the medial muscles of the thigh are severed. *(Continued.)*

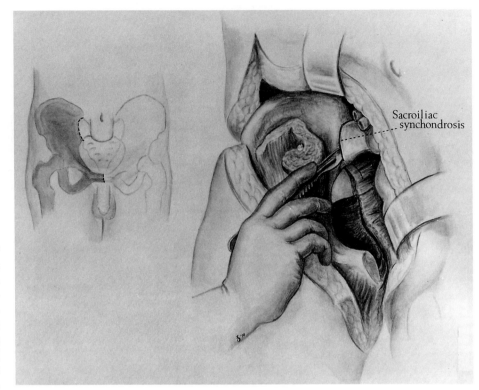

**Figure 16–22** *(continued).* **(H)** The only major attachment is the sacroiliac synchondrosis. The space is being entered at the superior end by the means of a scalpel. If the scalpel is now maneuvered at an angle of 45 degrees, the synchrondiosis can be cut. We seldom use any bone-cutting instruments. The inset shows the line of sacroiliac joint; pubic symphysis and shaded part of the pelvic skeleton constitute the upper part of the specimen. **(I)** The wound after removal of the extremity. The sacrum and the peritoneal contents can be seen. **(J)** Appearance after wound closure.

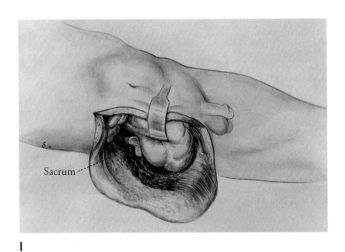

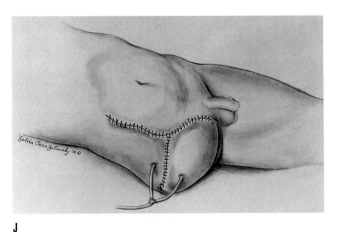

size, location, and concomitant fungation of the tumor, or because of the effects of previous irradiation of the area. These modifications might include a large anterior flap or a large gluteal flap. The decision as to the type of modification best suited for a given patient depends mostly on the experience of the operating surgeon.

The upper part of the vertical incision in the lateral abdominal wall is deepened, and the peritoneal cavity is entered. Following adequate exploration of the abdomen, if no contraindication to hemipelvectomy is

found, the operation proceeds. The peritoneum is closed with 2-0 chromic catgut suture. The lower part of the skin incision is then deepened, and the anterior abdominal wall muscles are cut along the line of the incision. The rectus abdominis muscle is resected at its attachment to the pubis and the inguinal ligament at the iliac crest and pubic tubercle (Fig. 16–22B). This results in detaching the anterior abdominal wall from the bony pelvis, forming the anterior flap. The peritoneal cavity is then pushed medially by means of sponge sticks. In male patients, the spermatic cord is preserved carefully. By placing packs and using refractors, the entire lateral wall of the pelvis from the sacroiliac synchondrosis to the pubic symphysis is brought into view. The intestines are held medially and upward, and the urinary bladder is held medially and downward, care being taken not to injure the ureter. The common iliac vessels are dissected out, and 1-0 silk ties are placed around all these vessels (Fig. 16–22C). For purposes of orientation, an anatomic diagram is included (Fig. 16–22D). This shows the bifurcation of the aorta, formation of the inferior vena cava proximally, and the contents of the lateral wall of the pelvis up to the symphysis pubis distally. It is better not to ligate the vessels at this stage, since once they are ligated, the surgeon is committed to performing the operation. We advocate a thorough reassessment of the resectability of the tumor at this stage of the operation, and if no contraindications for a hemipelvectomy are found, then proceed to the next stage of the operation.

In this stage, the pubic symphysis is exposed, skeletonized, and divided (Fig. 16–22E). This is easily accomplished by using the scalpel; seldom is there a need for a Gigli's saw or a chisel. Care must be taken to protect the urethra below, and it is advisable to put a narrow malleable retractor immediately below the symphysis. Following separation of the pubic symphysis, the incision is deepened inferiorly along the previously outlined skin incision at the inner aspect of the thigh (Fig. 16–22E). At this stage, some bleeding might be incurred, especially in male patients, due to cutting of the vascular erectile tissue. We advocate that the resectability of the tumor be reassessed for the second time. If the tumor is found to be unresectable for cure, it is possible to close the wound by wiring the pubic symphysis, and the patient can be rehabilitated insofar as the use of the limb is concerned. However, if there are no contraindications for a curative hemipelvectomy, the surgeon should proceed with the third stage of the operation.

The iliac vessels are then ligated. The common iliac, external iliac, and internal iliac vessels are doubly ligated and resected in the same locations where the original ties were placed (Fig. 16–22F). The femoral nerve trunk located laterally to the vessels is also resected at this stage.

The anterior dissection is then continued. The crest of the ileum is skeletonized, including resection of the attachment of the quadratus lumborum muscle. The iliopsoas muscles are transected high. The assistant then flexes the knee and pushes it down to the surface of the table, exposing the piriformis and levator ani muscles. These are resected as high as possible (Fig. 16–22F), care being taken to avoid injury to the rectum or bladder. This completes the anterior dissection, and the sacroiliac synchondrosis is then exposed. All the major bleeding points are caught and ligated. A packing is placed in the pelvic space.

The posterior flap is then raised, first by extending the skin incision as far back as the sacrum (Fig. 16–22G). The table is then tilted to the opposite direction, making the patient lie on the lateral decubitus. With the extremity held in extreme adduction, the posterior attachments of the gluteal muscles are then divided, and the remainder of the posterior dissection is completed (Fig. 16–22G). The limb is then flexed and abducted sharply, and all the remaining medial muscle attachments are cut.

At this stage, the limb is attached only at the sacroiliac synchondrosis. We consider severance of this synchondrosis as the penultimate phase of the operation. The limb, as before, is flexed and moved by the assistant so that the surgeon can find the uppermost part of the synchondrosis. Once the scalpel is in this space, the assistant sharply abducts the limb. The surgeon, by placing the blade of the scalpel at an angle of 45 degrees, can easily cut through the synchondrosis (Fig. 16–22H). We have seldom found the need for use of chisels, saws, or any other bone-cutting instruments.

The limb is now attached to the patient by the ligaments of the sacrum. These are resected, the gluteal arteries are caught, ligated, and resected, and the specimen is removed (Fig. 16–22I). Dry packs are placed on the exposed surface.

After removal of the limb, meticulous care is taken to obtain perfect hemostasis. It is essential that all the nerve trunks are cut sharply and allowed to retract. This reduces the incidence of traumatic neuromas. We have found that use of local anesthetic in the proximal end of the nerve trunk invariably reduces the incidence of postoperative pain and occasionally reduces the intensity of the phantom limb syndrome as well.

The anterior abdominal wall is closed with a Penrose drain in the retroperitoneal space, and the skin incision is closed, using suction catheters (Fig. 16–22J). An Ace bandage pressure dressing is kept in place for about five to six days postoperatively.

*Postoperative Management.*   It is expected that the blood volume loss will be corrected either during the operation or within two to three hours thereafter. Following this immediate management, care is taken to record blood pressure, urinary output, wound drainage, and hematocrit. Based on these, the intravenous administration of fluids and blood is monitored. Patients should have nasogastric suction until the bowel sounds appear. Frequently, the urinary bladder develops some paresis. The Foley catheter should be kept in place until the patient regains bladder control. Excluding these usual problems, seldom in well-selected cases are there any major complications. Phantom limb pain and development of neuromas are accepted problems associated with any radical amputation, and we think there is no higher incidence with hemipelvectomy. Proper physiotherapy often reduces these problems.

Wound healing can sometimes be complicated by skin flap necrosis. This is more common in patients with a large tumor or in those who have had prior irradiation. It has been our experience that the problem of skin flap necrosis, although annoying, has never been unmanageable. As soon as possible, patients should be encouraged to use crutches and move about. Usually, a well-motivated patient can maneuver on a plane surface by the end of two weeks. A cooperative and competent physiotherapist with a good program can make a patient self-reliant within four weeks (Figs. 16–23A and 16–23B). Although the use of a prosthesis after hemipelvectomy is not always as satisfactory as in cases of amputations performed at lower levels, some excellent prosthetic results are still possible.

The operation of hemipelvectomy can be extended by including part of the sacrum or parts of the vertebrae. These types of extension are seldom required but, when indicated, can be accomplished without any associated increase in morbidity. However, care must be taken to avoid injury to the dura, thereby incurring spinal fluid leak.

A modified and limited type of hemipelvectomy was first described by Sherman and Duthie[38] in 1960. This essentially consists of excising the innominate bone and not separating the extremity at the sacroiliac synchondrosis. The level of excision of the innominate bone depends on the type and location of the tumors. If feasible, the presence of the iliac crest and a relatively stable sacroiliac joint provides a better prosthesis and better rehabilitation.

## ■ REHABILITATION OF PATIENTS WHO HAVE UNDERGONE AMPUTATION

The principles of rehabilitation of patients with soft tissue sarcomas are similar to those for cancer patients in general. However, since most of these tumors are located in the extremities, the rehabilitation plan for patients who have undergone one of the types of amputation described above would include consideration of the following two major points: first, the association of phantom limb pain and second, the acquisition of an appropriately fitting prosthesis.

The phantom limb is a phenomenon that has long aroused curiosity. How is it that one feels a limb that is not there? Yet, once one thinks about the anatomy and physiology of the situation, the phantom limb phenomenon is to be expected. All the nerves coming from the limb are still there; they still make connections at

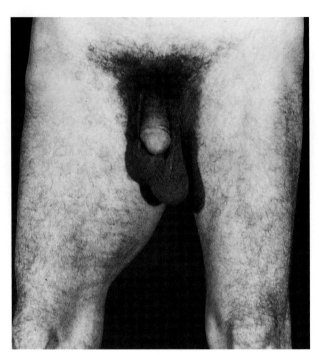

A

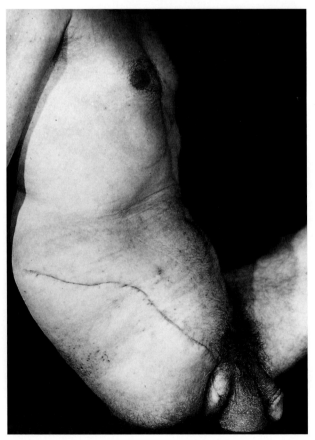

B

**Figure 16–23. (A)** Fifty-year-old man with extensive liposarcoma of the thigh. **(B)** Appearance six months later. Note the excellent wound-healing process.

various levels of the central nervous system, and, finally, these connections link to the part of the brain where afferent nerve impulses evoke sensation. The phantom limb sensation occurs in 95 percent or more of all people who have had a limb or part of a limb amputated. In that other 5 percent or less, the limb may still be conjured up by concentrating on it or by trying to move it.

In most limb amputations, the cut nerves end up in neuromas.[39] One assumes that these nerve fibers can work and that they frequently fire impulses to the central nervous system. Not only is this likely, but it is reinforced by the effect of blocking the cut nerves of the neuroma with a local anesthetic. When these nerve fibers are blocked this way, there is a great reduction or even total loss of the sensation of the phantom limb.

A few people who have had parts of their bodies amputated experience constant pain in the stump or in the phantom, or both. In such patients, blocking the neuromas with local anesthetics almost always temporarily stops the pain. Many suggestions have been proffered as to why some patients have pain and others do not.

Wall and Gutnick[40] induced neuromas in the cut sciatic nerve of rats and recorded a compound potential from the posterior rootlets entering the spinal cord. As expected, they found that the nerve fibers of these neuromas were continually active. Their discharge of impulses could be increased by pressure or tapping on the neuromas, and it could be stopped by anesthetizing the neuromas with local anesthetic solution—all similar to the situation in man.

A more interesting finding was the effect of electrical stimulation of the chronically divided nerve. The nerve in which the neuroma had been induced was divided so that it no longer reached the spinal cord. Electrodes were then placed on the nerve, and it was stimulated rapidly for a few seconds. The electrical excitation caused a marked reduction in the nerve's spontaneous activity for as long as an hour. This finding may suggest that, if the nerve fibers can be induced to fire off maximally, they may stop firing spontaneously for a prolonged period.

During the past few years, the transcutaneous electrical stimulation of nerves has been introduced for many painful conditions, including painful amputation stumps and painful phantom limbs. This treatment is based on Melzack and Wall's gate control theory of pain.[11] The theory states that whether an input to the spinal cord finally causes pain depends on the amount of input in large myelinated efferent fibers on the one hand and small myelinated and nonmyelinated fibers on the other. Both groups of fibers are said to affect the small neurons of the *substantia gelatinosa* of the posterior horn. The large fibers excite these neurons, and the small fibers inhibit them. These substantia gelati-

nosa neurons are inhibitory. Thus, when these neurons are inhibited, their inhibitory action on the efferent fibers is not excited, and a massive afferent input enters the spinal cord, resulting in pain. In contrast, when these neurons are excited, they exert presynaptic inhibition on afferent fibers, and the input to the spinal cord is moderate and pain does not occur. Excitation of the large afferent fibers thus reduces the input to the spinal cord and closes the gate.

Wall and Gutnick[40] suggested an alternative way in which electrical stimulation might act. It could do so by preventing nerve impulses from being fired spontaneously, and since it is this firing that causes both the pain and the phantom sensation, both could be stopped by electrical stimulation. The mechanism by which antidromic stimulation stops impulse generation after stimulation has stopped is unknown.[40,42–45] Wall and Gutnick[40] suggested that the excitability of small nerve fibers within the neuron is altered by electrical stimulation because these endings are abnormal and do not behave in the same way as normal nerve fibers.

This appears to be the first logical explanation for the phantom limb pain syndrome, as well as a practical therapeutic recommendation for control of this syndrome. We routinely infiltrate the cut end of the nerve trunks with anesthesia. Although this is not a panacea, it appears to lower the incidence and intensity of the phantom limb syndrome. In patients with intractable pain, its use might help considerably.[46,47]

Patients should be fitted with a prosthesis as soon after amputation as feasible. Most amputations are performed in the lower extremities, and, excluding hemipelvectomy or hip joint disarticulation, the prosthesis can be fitted within eight weeks. Early physical therapy after a temporary prosthesis is exceptionally valuable in rehabilitating the patient. In the upper extremities, the problem is the lack of available functionally useful prostheses. Be that as it may, if and when an upper extremity amputation is performed, a rigid cast and some form of prosthesis must be used as early as possible after the operation.

## REFERENCES

1. Pack GT: The definition of inoperability of cancer. Ann Surg 127:1105, 1948
2. Pack GT, Anglem TJ: Tumors of the soft somatic tissues in infancy and childhood. J Pediatr 15:372, 1939
3. Stout AP: Sarcomas of the soft parts. J Missouri State Med Assoc 44:329, 1947
4. Pack GT: Argument for radicalism in cancer surgery. Am Surg 17:271, 1951
5. Barber JR, Coventry MD, McDonald JR: The spread of soft tissue sarcomata of the extremities along peripheral nerve trunks. J Bone Joint Surg 39A:534, 1957

6. Bowden L, Booher RF: The principles and technique of resection of soft part sarcoma. Surgery 44:963, 1958

7. Bowden L, Booher R: Surgical consideration in the treatment of sarcomas of the buttock. Cancer 6:89, 1953

8. Syme J: Excision of the Scapula (monograph). Edinburgh, Edmonstom & Douglas, 1864

9. de Nancrede CBG: The end results after total excision of the scapula for sarcoma. Ann Surg 50:1, 1909

10. Pack GT, Ariel IR: Tumors of the Soft Somatic Tissues. New York, Hoeber-Harper, 1958

11. Das Gupta TK: Scapulectomy: Indications and technique. Surgery 67:601, 1970

12. Tikhoff P: On tumors. Med Obozr Mosk 53:81, 1900

13. Linberg BE: Interscapulothoracic resection for malignant tumors of the shoulder joint region. J Bone Joint Surg 10A:344, 1928

14. Pack GT, Baldwin JC: The Tikhoff-Linberg resection of shoulder girdle—Case report. Surgery 38:753, 1955

15. Brasfield RD, Das Gupta TK: Desmoids of the anterior abdominal wall. Surgery 65:241, 1969

16. Halstead WS: The results of radical operation for the cure of cancer of the breast. Ann Surg 46:80, 1907

17. Crosby AB: The first operation on record for removal of the entire arm, scapula, and three fourths of the clavicle by Dixie Crosby. Med Rec 10:753, 1875

18. Berger P: L'amputation du membre superieur dans la contiguite du tronc (amputation interscapulothoracique). Paris, G. Masson, 1887

19. Pack GT, McNeer G, Coley BL: Interscapulothoracic amputation for malignant tumors of the upper extremity: A report of 31 consecutive cases. Surg Gynecol Obstet 74:171, 1942

20. Moseley HF: The Forequarter Amputation. Edinburgh, Churchill Livingstone, 1957

21. Nadler SJ, Phelan JT: A technique of interscapulothoracic amputation. Surg Gynecol Obstet 122:359, 1966

22. Bowden L: A more thorough in-continuity neck and axillary dissection. Ann Surg 141:481, 1956

23. Fanus N, Didolkar MS, Hoyoke ED, Elias EG: Evaluation of forequarter amputation in malignant diseases. Surg Gynecol Obstet 142:381, 1976

24. Das Gupta TK, Brasfield RD: Amputation neuromas in cancer patients. NY State J Med 69:2129, 1969

25. Das Gupta TK: Radical groin dissection. Surg Gynecol Obstet 129:1275, 1969

26. Frank L: Lest we forget. Am J Surg 20:160, 1933

27. Eckoff N: An account of Sir Astley Cooper's first case of amputation at the hip joint, January 16, 1824. Guy's Hosp Rep 89:9, 1939

28. Girard C: Sur la desarticulation interilioabdominale. Congres Francais Chir, 9:823, 1895

29. Girard C: Sur la desarticulation interilioabdominal. Rev Chir (Paris) 18:1141, 1898

30. Pringle JH: The interpelvic-abdominal amputation with notes on two cases. Br J Surg 4:283, 1916

31. Judin SS: Ilioabdominal amputation in a case of sarcoma; recovery, pregnancy, and birth of a living child. Surg Gynecol Obstet 43:668, 1926

32. Gordon-Taylor GI, Wiles P: Interinnominoabdominal (hindquarter) amputation. Br J Surg 22:671, 1935

33. Sugarbaker ED, Ackerman L: Disarticulation of the innominate bone for malignant tumor of the pelvic parietes and upper thigh. Surg Gynecol Obstet 81:36, 1943

34. Gordon-Taylor G, Paley D: A further review of the interinnominoabdominal operation based on 21 personal cases. Br J Surg 34:61, 1946

35. Gordon-Taylor G, Monroe R: The technique and management of hindquarter amputation. Br J Surg 39:536, 1952

36. Pack GT, Ehrlich HE: Exarticulation of the lower extremities for malignant tumor: Hip joint disarticulation (with or without deep iliac dissection) and sacroiliac disarticulation (hemipelvectomy). Ann Surg 124:1, 1946

37. Pack GT: Major exarticulations for malignant neoplasms of the extremities; interscapulothoracic amputation, hip joint disarticulation, and interilioabdominal amputation: A report of end results in 228 cases. J Bone Joint Surg 38A:249, 1956

38. Sherman CD Jr., Duthie RB: Modified hemipelvectomy. Cancer 13:51, 1960

39. Ramon y Cajal S: Degeneration and Regeneration in the Nervous System. London, Oxford University Press, 1928

40. Wall PD, Gutnick M: Properties of afferent nerve impulses originating from a neuroma. Nature 248:740, 1974

41. Melzack R, Wall PD: Pain mechanisms: A new theory. Science 150:971, 1965

42. Diamond J: The effects of injecting acetylcholine into normal and regenerating nerves. J Physiol (London) 145:611, 1959

43. Basbaum AI: Effects of central lesions on disorders produced by multiple dorsal rhizotomy in rats. Exp Neurol 42:490, 1970

44. Catton WT: Some properties of frog skin mechanoreceptors. J Physiol (London) 141:305, 1958

45. Wall PD, Johnson AJ: Changes associated with posttetanic potentiation of a monosynaptic reflex. J Neurophysiol 21:148, 1958

46. Wall PD, Wickelgren B: Afferent hyperpolarization and post-tetanic potentiation of a monosynaptic reflex. J Physiol (London) 196:135, 1968

47. Wall PD, Sweet WH: Temporary ablation of pain in man. Science 155:108, 1967

# 17

# Radiation Therapy
# of Soft Tissue Tumors

Radiation therapy (RT) occupies an important role in the management of patients with soft tissue tumors. A wide variety of benign and malignant soft tissue neoplasms, including desmoid tumors, uterine sarcoma, and sarcomas of the extremity and retroperitoneum, are currently treated with RT. Radiation therapy is also an important component in the multidisciplinary treatment of childhood rhabdomyosarcoma.

In the recent past, however, RT played virtually no role in managing patients with soft tissue tumors. Although proposed soon after the discovery of x-rays,[1] its use quickly dropped out of favor. The disappointing outcomes seen in large, inoperable tumors treated with low doses during the orthovoltage era resulted in the widely held belief that soft tissue neoplasms were radioresistant. It was not until the 1960s, with the pioneering work of Cade,[2] and later Perry and Chu[3] and McNeer et al.,[4] that radioresistance was finally brought into question. More recently, a number of clinical reviews[5–9] and radiobiological studies[10,11] have dismissed this belief and firmly established the present role of RT in the management of these tumors.

Soft tissue neoplasms represent a diverse spectrum of diseases, ranging from benign (but locally aggressive) fibromatoses to high-grade sarcomas of the retroperitoneum and extremity. Moreover, soft tissue tumors, notably rhabdomyosarcoma, often arise in children. Thus, the radiation oncologist involved in the care of patients with soft tissue neoplasms must possess a thorough knowledge of not only the behavior, patterns of spread, and treatment of these varied tumors, but also of the potential sequelae of therapy in both adults and children. This chapter provides an overview of the radiotherapeutic management, treatment techniques, outcomes, and sequelae in adult and pediatric patients undergoing RT for benign and malignant tumors of the soft tissues.

## ■ RADIOBIOLOGY

Soft tissue tumors are often labeled *radioresistant*, due to their slow rate of regression even after high doses of radiation. However, radiosensitivity is confused here with radioresponsiveness. *Radiosensitivity* refers to the inherent cellular response of tumors to radiation, specifically the percentage of cells surviving a given radiation dose. In contrast, *radioresponsiveness* refers to how rapidly a tumor disappears after the initiation of treatment. Radioresponsiveness depends on a variety of tumor kinetic factors (growth fraction, cell loss, etc.) and the inherent radiosensitivity of the tumor. Although a radioresponsive tumor is radiosensitive, a poorly responsive tumor, as in the case of soft tissue neoplasms, is not necessarily radioresistant.[12]

In vitro analysis provides important insight into the inherent cellular response of human tumors to radiation.[12] Established cell lines in the laboratory are exposed to various doses of radiation, and the proportion of surviving cells is calculated. The relationship between radiation dose and the proportion of surviving cells is graphically represented as a survival curve. A semilogarithmic plot is used, with dose on the x-axis and survival fraction on the y-axis. Since the initial description of the first clonogenic in vitro radiation survival curve in a cervical carcinoma cell line by Puck and

Marcus in 1956,[13] many cell lines of various types of human tumors,[14–17] including adult and pediatric soft tissue tumors,[10,18] have been analyzed.

Several models have been proposed for analyzing radiation survival data.[19] The linear-quadratic (LQ) model assumes two components to cell kill: (1) alpha, the linear component, which is proportional to the dose (D), and (2) beta, the quadratic component, which is proportional to the dose squared ($D^2$). The multi-hit (MH) model describes three parameters: (1) $D_o$, which refers to the terminal slope, and (2) n (extrapolation number) and (3) $D_q$ (quasi-threshold dose), both of which refer to the shoulder region of the survival curve. Several other model-free parameters have been proposed, including $\overline{D}$ (mean inactivation dose),[20] which represents the area under the survival curve, and the survival fraction (SF-2) after a dose of 2 Gy.[21] These various parameters provide a means of quantitatively describing the radiosensitivity of established tumor cell lines. Mathematically, $D_o$ represents the dose of radiation needed to reduce the survival fraction by one natural log; thus, it is a direct measure of inherent radiosensitivity.[12] Cells with a more linear initial portion of the survival curve (larger alpha) are also considered more radiosensitive. $\overline{D}$ and SF-2 are both inversely proportional to the degree of cellular radiosensitivity.[20,21]

In vitro survival curve analysis has consistently demonstrated that both adult and pediatric soft tissue tumor cell lines are radiosensitive. Weichselbaum et al.[12] compared the radiation survival data of cell lines established from untreated soft tissue sarcomas and epithelial tumors of the head and neck. Overall, the 13 soft tissue sarcoma cell lines were *more* radiosensitive than the 20 epithelial head and neck cell lines. The sarcoma cell lines exhibited a higher alpha ($p < 0.005$), lower $\overline{D}$ ($p < 0.001$), and lower SF-2 ($p < 0.0005$).[10] In an analysis of rhabdomyosarcoma cell lines, Kelland and co-workers[18] reported mean values for $D_o$, n, alpha, and beta of $1.27 \pm 0.03$, $1.49 \pm 0.14$, $0.64 \pm 0.002$, and $0.014 \pm 0.001$, respectively. In addition, a SF-2 of only 0.26 was noted. These results clearly demonstrate the fallacy of the long-held belief that soft tissue tumors are radioresistant.

# ■ RADIOTHERAPEUTIC MANAGEMENT

## BENIGN TUMORS

Benign soft tissue tumors and tumorlike conditions are often asymptomatic and thus require no treatment. When necessary, the treatment of choice is typically surgery. However, RT is occasionally used, notably after incomplete resection and in patients with unresectable disease. Importantly, RT is the primary treatment in a select group of benign soft tissue tumors, including temporal bone chemodectomas and juvenile angiofibromas with intracranial extension. The radiotherapeutic management of the most commonly encountered benign soft tissue tumors and tumorlike conditions is discussed below.

## Desmoids

The traditional method of treatment in patients with desmoid tumors (aggressive fibromatosis) is surgery.[22–26] However, RT is often used following incomplete surgery and in patients with unresectable or recurrent disease.[27–36] Doses and techniques are similar to those used in low-grade soft tissue sarcomas. Although high rates of local control are possible with RT alone, regression rates are often protracted. A full response may not be seen for several months to years after treatment.[27,32]

## Keloids

Radiation therapy is an important mode in managing keloids.[37–44] Radiation therapy effectively reduces the high rate of recurrence seen in many patients after surgical excision.[45–48] Low total doses of RT (10–12 Gy) are associated with high rates of control without untoward sequelae. Controversy exists regarding the importance of treatment timing in patients with keloids.[37,38,43] Many radiation oncologists believe that RT is most effective in the immediate postoperative period and thus insist on commencing treatment on the day of surgery or soon thereafter. However, this opinion is not shared by all.

## Dermatofibrosarcoma Protuberans

Although a low-grade soft tissue sarcoma, dermatofibrosarcoma protuberans is commonly considered along with the benign neoplasms. Treatment approaches are similar to those used in patients with desmoids, with surgery occupying a primary role.[49–51] Radiation therapy is indicated following incomplete surgery and in patients with unresectable or recurrent disease.[52–54] Doses and techniques are similar to those employed in low-grade soft tissue sarcomas.

## Penile Fibromatosis (Peyronie's Disease)

Various treatment approaches, including local and systemic medication, ultrasound, and surgery, have been used in patients with Peyronie's disease (induratio penis plastica). Although less used, RT offers an alternative and effective means of therapy. Treatment is administered with low-energy (orthovoltage) techniques. Radiation therapy by itself achieves high response rates, with less pain, less penile curvature, and less induration.[55–59]

## Chemodectoma (Glomus Body Tumor)

The appropriate therapy in patients with glomus body tumors depends upon a number of factors, including tumor size and location. Patients with small (less than 5 cm) carotid body tumors are typically treated with surgery alone.[60] However, patients with large carotid body[61,62] or with temporal bone chemodectomas should undergo definitive RT. Although comparable control rates are possible either with surgery[63–69] or RT[66,67,70–74] in patients with temporal bone chemodectomas, RT is associated with less morbidity.[75] As in many other benign soft tissue tumors, regression rates are often quite protracted following RT alone.

## Juvenile Angiofibroma

Juvenile angiofibromas are benign, vascular tumors that are managed either with surgery or RT. The selection of therapy depends upon the tumor size and its extent. Patients with small resectable tumors (without evidence of intracranial extension) are best treated with surgery.[76,77] However, larger tumors and all tumors with evidence of intracranial extension should instead undergo RT.[78–84] Moderate doses of radiation (30–36 Gy) are associated with high rates of local control with low risk of untoward sequelae.

## Hemangioma

Most patients with hemangiomas require no treatment. However, when treatment is indicated, RT is often the treatment of choice. Treatment indications in adults and children include symptomatic visceral and bone lesions as well as unsightly cutaneous lesions of infancy. Hemangiomas are very responsive to RT. Even large tumors are controlled with moderate doses of radiation.[85–88]

## MALIGNANT TUMORS

Malignant soft tissue tumors (sarcomas), like their benign counterparts, represent a wide spectrum of diseases in both adults and children. The indications for and treatment of various soft tissue sarcomas depend upon a number of factors, including disease site, histology, extent of resection, and the age of the patient. The general management of the more common soft tissue sarcomas is described below. The discussion is limited to sarcomas of the trunk, extremities, head and neck, retroperitoneum, and uterus. In addition, Kaposi's sarcoma and childhood rhabdomyosarcoma are discussed separately due to their unique behavior and therapy. Although soft tissue sarcomas arise in a number of other sites, including the central nervous system,[89] lungs,[90] heart,[91] breast,[92] and gastrointestinal[93] and genitourinary[94] tracts, experience with RT in many of these sites is limited and often anecdotal.[95–97] Interested readers are directed to the referenced texts and journals.

## Extremity/Truncal Sarcomas

The primary treatment of soft tissue sarcomas of the extremities and trunk was formerly radical surgery (amputation or compartmental resection).[98,99] However, numerous retrospective trials[6–9,11,100,101] and a prospective randomized trial[102] demonstrated that RT showed local control and survival equivalent to that of conservative (limb-sparing) approaches with radical surgery. Radical surgery is now reserved for patients in whom excision and RT are not feasible. Similar approaches have been applied successfully in children with nonrhabdomyosarcomatous tumors.[103] An alternative limb-sparing approach is the use of concomitant chemoradiotherapy before conservative surgery.[104–107] Although technically demanding, multimodal approaches have been extended to patients with distal extremity (hand, wrist, foot) tumors.[108–110]

Limb-sparing approaches consist of wide excision with either preoperative or postoperative RT. These approaches combine limited surgery (removal of the clinically apparent disease) and moderate dose wide-field irradiation (sterilization of the residual microscopic disease in normal surrounding tissue). The goal is to avoid the necessity and resultant cosmetic and functional sequelae of either extensive surgical resection or high-dose irradiation. Controversy exists regarding the optimal sequencing of RT and surgery,[111] the optimal treatment volume[8,11] and radiation dose,[9,11] the roles of brachytherapy[112–119] and combined chemoradiotherapy,[104–107] and the use of conservative surgery alone in select patients.[120–122]

Unresectable extremity or truncal sarcomas are managed with radiation alone[5,123–127] or in combination with radiosensitizers.[128] Several groups have explored the use of particle beam (neutron) therapy either alone or in combination with photons.[125–127] Neutron beams, unlike traditional photon therapy, consist of densely ionizing radiation. Densely ionizing beams depend less on the presence of oxygen and thus theoretically offer an advantage, particularly in large tumors. Although a nihilistic attitude is frequently adopted, RT can control a subset of unresectable soft tissue tumors.

## Head/Neck Sarcomas

The behavior and treatment of soft tissue sarcomas of the head and neck are analogous to tumors in the extremity and trunk. Radiation therapy is frequently given in conjunction with conservative surgery.[129–133] However, an important exception is the treatment of angiosarcoma (hemangiosarcoma). These aggressive tumors are notoriously infiltrative and are associated with high rates of recurrence even after extensive surgery. Wide-field RT offers the best chance of control in patients with angiosarcoma of the face or scalp.[133–135]

## Sarcomas of the Retroperitoneum

Soft tissue sarcomas arising in the retroperitoneum often present in an advanced state with involvement of surrounding structures and are associated with high rates of local recurrence following surgery alone.[136] Radiation therapy is thus commonly used either before or after surgery. Techniques include external beam radiation therapy (EBRT) and/or intraoperative radiation therapy (IORT).[137–142] These tumors have been the subject of a number of prospective[137,140] and randomized trials[138,142] at the National Cancer Institute (NCI).

## Uterine Sarcomas

Soft tissue sarcomas of the uterus, like their epithelial counterparts, are primarily managed by surgery (total abdominal hysterectomy and bilateral salpingo-oophorectomy) (TAHBSO). Radiation therapy has been used in patients with uterine sarcomas after surgery, in an attempt to decrease the risk of pelvic and vaginal recurrences, and in patients with unresectable or recurrent disease.[143–150] Treatment techniques involve a combination of pelvic EBRT and afterloading intracavitary brachytherapy. In patients with intact uteri, intrauterine sources are placed with the aid of a tandem and Heyman-Simon capsules. The vaginal vault is irradiated with the aid of colpostats placed in the lateral fornices. Doses are similar to those used in patients with epithelial tumors.

## Kaposi's Sarcoma

Radiation therapy occupies an important role in the treatment of both AIDS-associated (epidemic) and non-AIDS-associated (classic) Kaposi's sarcoma. However, due to the very different natural histories of classic and epidemic Kaposi's sarcoma, the specific indications for and treatment of the two types differ considerably. Nonetheless, RT is associated with high local control rates in both types, with minimal risk of late sequelae.[151–159]

## Rhabdomyosarcoma

The optimal approach to patients with childhood rhabdomyosarcoma is multimodal therapy consisting of chemotherapy, radiation therapy, and surgery. Important insights into the behavior and treatment of rhabdomyosarcoma have resulted from careful and systematic study by the Intergroup Rhabdomyosarcoma Study (IRS).[160–162] The role of RT in rhabdomyosarcoma has

evolved through the various IRS studies. At present, RT is used primarily in patients with incomplete surgery (microscopic positive margins), involved regional lymph nodes, locally advanced (unresectable) disease, and metastatic disease (groups II–IV). However, RT is also indicated after a complete resection in patients with unfavorable disease histology (group I, unfavorable histology).[163] A current area of particular interest is the use of altered fractionation regimens in patients with locally advanced (group III) disease.[164]

## ■ RADIATION THERAPY TECHNIQUES

The technical approach to patients with soft tissue neoplasms depends on factors including the disease site, tumor histology, tumor grade, extent of resection, and patient age. A full description of the technical approach to each of the various benign and malignant soft tissue tumors in both adults and children is beyond the scope of this chapter. Interested readers are directed to the referenced texts and journals. The following section outlines the approach to patients with sarcomas of the extremities. In addition, the technical details of brachytherapy and IORT are described.

### TREATMENT VOLUME

Delineation of the treatment volume in patients with extremity soft tissue sarcomas requires a thorough knowledge of limb anatomy, including the major vessels, nerves, and origin and insertion of the different muscle groups. The muscle groups of the proximal upper and lower extremities are divided into separate compartments by tough, fibrous septa. The arm consists of two compartments (flexor, extensor), whereas the thigh consists of three compartments (extensor, flexor, adductor). The compartmental nature of the extremities results in the unique pattern of spread seen in extremity soft tissue sarcomas. *Tumors arising within a compartment spread longitudinally through (along muscle and fascial planes), not transversely between, compartments.* Generous margins are thus necessary proximally and distally to the tumor or tumor bed. Conversely, the low risk of transverse spread allows the sparing of neighboring uninvolved tissue lateral to the tumor or tumor bed.

Controversy exists regarding the optimal volume of treatment in sarcomas of the extremities and trunk. Most investigators advocate generous coverage proximally and distally (5–10 cm), depending on the grade of the tumor.[6,7,11,101] Others feel that the entire compartment from origin to insertion of the involved muscle groups should be irradiated.[104,165] Clearly, small (less than 5 cm) margins are inadequate due to a higher rate of local failure (predominantly marginal or geographic misses).[11] However, no added benefit is seen, even in high-grade tumors, in terms of local control between field margins of 5 to 9.9 cm around the tumor bed and scar versus margins of greater than 10 cm or inclusion of the entire compartment.[8,11] Moreover, the risk of severe late sequelae has been correlated with field length.[166,167] Currently, we recommend a margin of 5 cm for low-grade tumors and 5 to 7 cm for high-grade tumors. A transverse margin of 2 to 3 cm is probably sufficient, provided that the entire transverse diameter of the involved compartment is included. Failure to include the entire transverse diameter of the compartment is associated with a higher rate of local failure.[8]

Several important caveats exist in the design of the treatment volume in patients with extremity soft tissue sarcomas. First and foremost, the entire circumference of the limb should never be included. Irradiation of the entire limb circumference is associated with significant late sequelae including chronic edema and fibrosis.[6,167] A minimum of a 1-cm strip of soft tissue should be spared throughout the entire treatment. Other caveats include avoiding treatment of the entire circumference of adjacent bone and joint space. The initial treatment volume includes all potential areas at risk for subclinical disease, including drain sites, areas of present (and previous) ecchymosis, and the surgical scar. At the time of simulation, these areas should be outlined with wire. Generous use of surgical clips and the use and placement of a longitudinal incision are essential. Examples of initial treatment volumes are shown in Figures 17–1 and 17–2.

Shrinking field techniques are used in patients with extremity soft tissue sarcomas. Most radiation oncologists use 1 or 2 field reductions; the final (high-dose) volume encompasses the tumor or tumor bed with a small (2 cm) margin. Patients treated with preoperative RT do not require field reductions unless doses in excess of 50 Gy are used. It is essential to review contours at several levels (central axis as well as 2 cm from the inferior and superior field edges), due to often marked variations in the external contour over the length of the field. All available imaging studies, including computed tomography (CT) and magnetic resonance (MR), should be used in the treatment planning process. Simple opposed anteroposterior fields are rarely sufficient or appropriate. Instead, opposed oblique or wedged pair fields are usually required. Computer-assisted treatment planning is beneficial in difficult situations.[110] Bolus, wedges, and tissue compensation are used as necessary. Example treatment plans are shown in Figures 17–3 and 17–4.

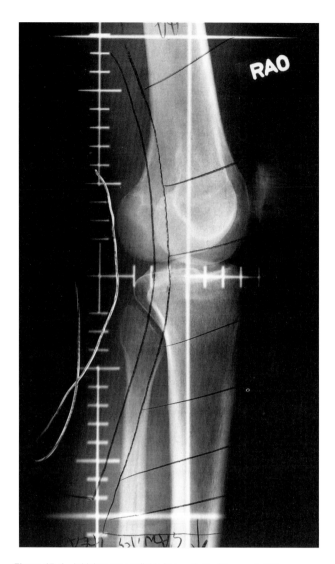

**Figure 17–1.** Initial treatment fields in a patient with a grade 3 liposarcoma of the lower extremity following wide excision. Care is taken to include the entire scar and tumor bed with a generous margin.

## PATIENT IMMOBILIZATION

Successful treatment of a patient with an extremity sarcoma requires proper immobilization. Immobilization aids in the day-to-day reproducibility by properly positioning the limb and minimizing rotation. At the time of simulation, a variety of positions should be evaluated. Selection of the optimal position combines experience and ingenuity. Two different positions are shown in Figures 17–5 and 17–6. Occasionally, the opposite limb may require immobilization to remove it from the treatment field. Thermoplastic or foam cradles are commonly used in most radiation oncology departments to immobilize patients. Attention is given to the placement of the surgical scar within the treatment field. If the scar is treated tangentially, no bolus is necessary.

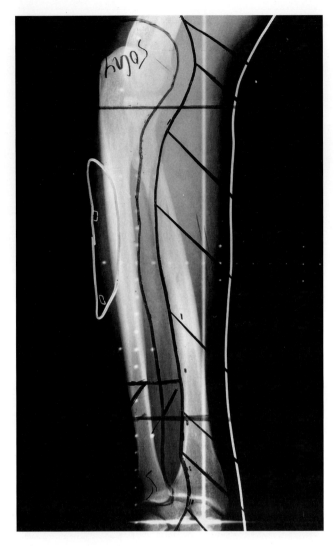

**Figure 17–2.** Initial treatment fields in a patient with a grade 2 malignant fibrous histiocytoma of the upper extremity.

Otherwise, bolus is indicated to prevent underdosage and a possible scar recurrence. Doses to all areas of concern should be verified by the use of thermoluminescence dosimetry (TLD).

## RADIATION DOSE

Extremity soft tissue sarcomas are treated with high doses, even in the postoperative setting. Initially, doses of 70–75 Gy were used.[7] Presently, patients undergoing preoperative RT receive 45–50 Gy (often supplemented with a 10–14 Gy boost either intraoperatively or postoperatively). Patients treated postoperatively receive total doses in the range of 63–66 Gy via a shrinking field technique, depending upon the tumor grade and margin status. Treatment should be administered with 4–6 mV photons to avoid potential underdosage of superficial tissues. Patients with unresectable disease require doses in the range of 70–75 Gy.

The optimal radiation dose in patients treated with postoperative RT is controversial. Most investigators use 63–66 Gy after a wide excision.[6,7,9] However, lower doses may be equally efficacious. In a review of the University of Chicago experience, Mundt et al.[11] noted no difference in terms of the local control between patients receiving doses of 60–63.0 Gy versus 64–66 Gy. Investigators at the Mallinckrodt Institute also noted no difference in local control between doses of 60–64.9 Gy and 65 Gy.[8] Moreover, late sequelae have been correlated with higher total doses.[11,167] We currently recommend a total dose of 60 Gy in patients with negative margins who have been treated with wide local excision. Patients with close or positive margins require higher doses (65–70 Gy) or preferably reexcision, due to the significant risk of local recurrence.[9]

## BRACHYTHERAPY

Brachytherapy involves the use of implanted radioactive sources to deliver high doses of radiation to a localized volume. In patients with soft tissue sarcomas, the most commonly used source is [192]Ir. Brachytherapy is appealing because, compared to EBRT, it allows the delivery of higher doses in a shorter period of time. However, brachytherapy requires considerable expertise and close cooperation between the radiation and surgical oncologists. In addition, brachytherapy has minimal penetration outside the implanted volume and also necessitates exposure of the medical and nursing staff.

Treatment planning in patients treated with brachytherapy begins with the delineation of the treatment volume. The tumor (or tumor bed) and surrounding areas at risk are marked by clips in the operating room (OR) by the surgical and radiation oncologists. Stainless steel needles are placed percutaneously, through which nylon afterloading catheters are inserted. Catheters are placed 1 cm apart and parallel. The treatment volume should include a margin (1.5–2 cm) of uninvolved tissue.[114] Catheters are loaded on postoperative day 3 with [192]Ir seeds. Immediate loading is discouraged due to a higher rate of wound complications.[114] A set of orthogonal films are obtained before loading, and, with the aid of treatment planning, software plans are generated. Most radiation oncologists prescribe 20–25 Gy as a boost (in conjunction with EBRT) or 40–45 Gy with brachytherapy alone.[114,116,118] Typically, dose rates of 40–60 Gy/hr are used. After completion of treatment, the catheters and sources are removed, and the patient is discharged.

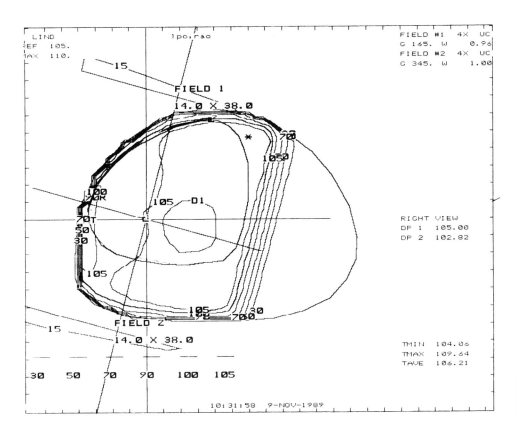

**Figure 17–3.** Isodose curves in a patient with a grade 3 liposarcoma of the thigh.

## INTRAOPERATIVE RADIOTHERAPY

Intraoperative radiotherapy is an alternative means of delivering high doses of radiation to a limited volume while minimizing the treatment of surrounding tissues. As with brachytherapy, close cooperation between the radiation and surgical oncologists and considerable expertise are required. However, unlike brachytherapy, treatment is completed on the day of surgery, and there is no additional hospital stay nor exposure of medical and nursing personnel. Treatment is administered with high-energy electrons directed at the tumor or tumor bed in the operating room. A major problem with IORT is equipment. IORT requires either a dedicated linear accelerator in the OR or transport of the patient to and from the RT department. Few centers in the United States possess a dedicated accelerator. Transport to and treatment in a busy department are not easy. Concerns range from infection control to allotting time on a busy therapy machine.[168]

Treatment is often given in conjunction with EBRT. Four to six weeks after the completion of EBRT, the patient is taken to the OR, and resection of the residual tumor is attempted. The surgical bed and/or tumor is clipped, and the proper cone size is selected, which encompasses the designated treatment volume. Cones are available in a variety of diameters (4–9 cm)

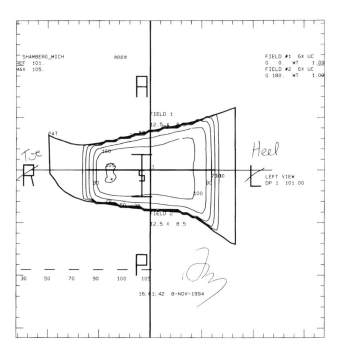

**Figure 17–4.** Isodose curves in a patient with a grade 2 malignant fibrous histiocytoma of the foot.

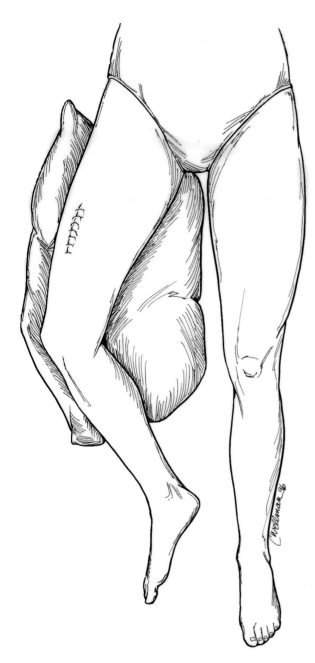

**Figure 17–5.** "Frogleg" position for the treatment of anterior thigh lesions.

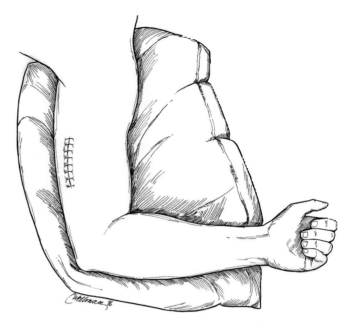

**Figure 17–6.** "Throwing" position for the treatment of upper extremity tumors.

and have either flat or beveled ends.[140,168] The cone is positioned and secured at the proper angle to ensure coverage of the tumor volume while minimizing the treatment of neighboring uninvolved structures. If a dedicated machine is not available, the patient is draped and transported to the RT department. The treatment cone is attached ("docked") to the machine head. The treatment field must be visualized before treatment in order to ensure proper cone position and the absence of all critical structures (notably small bowel) from the treatment field. High-energy electrons (10–18 Mev) are preferred due to the ability to limit dosage to underlying normal structures.[168] If lower energy electrons are used, bolus may be necessary. It is useful to place TLDs on the tumor or tumor bed. Doses used range from 15–25 Gy in a single fraction.[138,139] After completion of therapy, the patient is returned to OR, closed, and taken to the recovery room.

## ■ TREATMENT RESULTS

### BENIGN TUMORS

#### Desmoid Tumors

The outcome of patients with desmoid tumors treated with surgery, RT, or a combination of surgery and RT is shown in Table 17–1. Local control rates in patients treated with surgery alone range from 41.6 to 85.7 percent and average about 63 percent.[22–26] RT alone or in conjunction with surgery resection is associated with local control rates ranging from 68.4 to 100 percent.[27–36]

Local recurrence is frequent in patients treated with surgery alone, particularly if wide local excision is not performed. Masson and Soule[24] reported the outcome of 22 patients with desmoid tumors treated with surgery alone. The type of surgery ranged from simple excision to radical resection. Thirteen patients (59.1 percent) recurred locally. Reitamo[23] noted a recurrence rate of 24 percent in 68 patients with desmoid tumors following complete removal. Das Gupta et al.[26] reported recurrence in 18 of 45 patients (40 percent) undergoing wide excision and one of seven patients (14.3 percent) treated with radical surgery (amputation or compartmental resection).

**TABLE 17–1. OUTCOME OF PATIENTS WITH DESMOID TUMORS TREATED WITH SURGERY, RADIATION THERAPY, OR RADIATION THERAPY AND SURGERY**

| Surgery | | | Radiotherapy | | | |
|---|---|---|---|---|---|---|
| Author | Type of Surgery | Control | Author | Dose (Gy) | Control (RT) | Control (RT + S) |
| Musgrove et al.[22] | Various | 17/30 (56.6%) | Wara et al.[29] | 50–55 | 13/16 (81.2%) | |
| Reitamo[23] | CE | 52/68 (76.4%) | Greenberg et al.[28] | 30–68.6 | 8/9 (88.8%) | |
| Masson and Soule[24] | Various | 9/22 (40.9%) | Leibel et al.[27] | 40.8–61.2 | 13/19 (68.4%)* | |
| Khorsand and Karakousis[25] | Various | 5/12 (41.6%) | Kiel and Suit[30] | 22–70.9 | 8/10 (80%) | 5/7 (71.4%) |
| Das Gupta et al.[26] | WE | 27/45 (60%) | Benninghoff and Robbins[31] | 20–40 | 1/1 (100%) | 2/3 (66.6%) |
| | Radical | 6/7 (85.7%) | Hill et al.[33] | 51–61 | 4/4 (100%) | |
| Spears et al.[35] | Various | 58%† | Sherman et al.[32] | 50–76.2 | 10/14 (71.4%) | 24/31 (77.4%) |
| | | | Spears et al.[35] | 10–72 | 93%† | 71%† |
| | | | Kamath et al.[36] | 35–70 | | 44/53 (83%) |
| Total | | 116/184 (63.0%) | | | 57/73 (78.1%) | 75/94 (79.8%) |

Abbreviations: CE, complete excision; RT, radiation therapy; S, surgery; WE, wide excision.
*Contains several RT + S patients.
†5-year actuarial rates, crude numbers not available.

Adjuvant RT can reduce the rate of failure in patients undergoing surgery alone. Sherman et al.[32] treated 31 patients with postoperative RT. Total doses ranged from 50–76.2 Gy. Twenty-four patients (77.4 percent) were controlled. Of note, a poorer local control rate was seen in patients with a history of two or more previous surgeries (66 percent versus 88 percent) ($p = 0.17$). Late sequelae were infrequent. In a review of the Massachusetts General Hospital (MGH) experience, Kiel and Suit[30] reported the outcome of seven patients treated with RT and surgery (3 postoperative, 4 preoperative). Doses ranged from 22–70.9 Gy in 1.8–2.0 Gy daily fractions. While all three patients treated postoperatively due to microscopic positive margins were controlled, only two of the four patients treated preoperatively remained without evidence of disease. In a recent update of the MGH experience, Spears et al.[35] reported a five-year actuarial control rate of 71 percent in 40 patients treated with RT and surgery versus 58 percent in 37 patients treated with surgery alone. A statistically significant improvement in local control was seen in patients with gross positive and microscopic positive margins. Complication rates continued to remain low. Kamath et al.[36] reported the outcome of 53 patients with desmoid tumors treated with incomplete resection and postoperative RT (35–70 Gy).[36] Local control was achieved in 83 percent of patients. Local control rates were similar in patients with microscopic positive and gross positive margins (79 percent versus 88 percent). Of the nine local recurrences, four were on the field margin, and four were just outside the treatment volume.

Several investigators have reported high rates of control in patients treated with RT alone. Liebel et al.[27]

treated 19 patients with desmoid tumors with total doses ranging from 40.8 to 61.2 Gy. Thirteen patients (68.4 percent) were controlled at a median follow-up of 18 years. The ultimate local control (with salvage therapy) was 89 percent. Regression rates were often protracted, with complete responses requiring from 8 to 24 months. Complication rates were low (one patient with moderate fibrosis and decreased range of motion, one patient with mild lower extremity edema). Overall, cosmesis was judged excellent in most patients. Other investigators using RT alone have also reported high rates of control (despite slow regression rates) with minimal risk of late sequelae.[28–31]

The optimal radiation dose in patients with desmoid tumors is unclear. None of the above reports demonstrates a clear dose response. Of note, Sherman et al.[32] reported in-field recurrences over the entire range of doses used (57–66 Gy). Since all grade 3 complications occurred in patients treated above 60 Gy, the authors recommended a total dose of 50–55 Gy. In contrast, Suit[34] feels that higher doses (55–60 Gy in 1.8–2.0 Gy daily fractions) are necessary. Moreover, he recommends 60–65 Gy in patients with recurrent disease and/or disease in anatomical sites not feasible to salvage surgery.[34] Nonetheless, generous field margins are indicated in all patients, due to the risk of marginal recurrence.[27,30,36]

## Keloids

Table 17–2 lists the outcome of patients with keloids treated with excision alone, RT alone, or combined therapy. Excision alone (with or without adjuvant steroid injections) is associated with a local recurrence rate of approximately 50 percent.[45–48] Local control

**TABLE 17–2. OUTCOME OF PATIENTS WITH KELOIDS TREATED WITH SURGERY (EXCISION), RADIATION THERAPY, OR COMBINED SURGERY (EXCISION) AND RADIATION THERAPY**

| Surgery | | Radiotherapy | | | |
|---|---|---|---|---|---|
| Author | Control | Author | Dose (Gy) | Control (RT) | Control (RT+S) |
| Conway et al.[45]* | 15/28 (53.5%) | Borok et al.[44] | 10–18 | | 366/375 (97.6%) |
| Cosman et al.[46] | 116/248 (46.7%) | Kovalic and Perez[37] | 10–20 | | 82/112 (73.2%) |
| Singleton and Gross[47] | 10/54 (18.5%) | Lo et al.[43] | 2–20 | 41/85 (48.2%) | 146/168 (86.9%) |
| Ramakrishnan et al.[39] | 86/108 (79.6%) | King and Salzman[38] | 10–30 | 15/57 (26.3%) | 23/32 (71.8%) |
| | | Ramakrishnan et al.[39] | 16 | | 35/36 (97.2%) |
| | | Hintz[40] | 15–18 | | 186/259 (71.8%) |
| | | Malaker et al.[41] | 20 | | 24/30 (80%) |
| | | Levy et al.[42] | 15–18 | | 31/35 (88.5%) |
| Total | 227/438 (51.8%) | | | 56/142 (39.4%) | 893/1047 (85.3%) |

Abbreviations: RT, radiation therapy; S, surgery (excision).
*Includes treatment with postoperative steroid injections.

rates in patients treated for keloids with RT with or without surgery range from 26.3 to 97.6 percent. Series treating patients with excision and postoperative RT report control rates of approximately 90 percent.[37–44]

Excision alone is clearly not an effective means of controlling most patients with keloids. Cosman et al.[46] noted a recurrence rate of approximately 47 percent in 248 patients following excision. In a review of the literature, Garb and co-workers[48] noted a recurrence rate of 75 percent in patients treated with surgery alone. Others have noted similarly high rates of recurrence following excision alone.[39,45,47]

Excision and postoperative RT can control most patients with keloids. Borok and colleagues[44] analyzed the outcome of 375 keloids in 250 patients treated with RT following surgical excision. Nine (2.4 percent) failed locally. However, seven of the nine failures underwent post RT ear piercing. Excluding these patients, the local failure rate was only 0.53 percent. Cosmesis was judged as excellent in most (92 percent). One patient developed a progressive pigment disturbance within the treated field. Of note, no patients developed a second skin malignancy. Others have reported equally low rates of recurrence in patients treated with excision and postoperative RT.[37–40,42,43]

In contrast, the local control of keloids treated with RT alone is poor. Lo et al.[43] treated 253 patients with keloids at the Lahey Clinic with either RT alone

(85) or excision and postoperative RT (168). Total doses ranged from 2–20 Gy. Local control was achieved in approximately 87 percent of the patients treated with surgery and RT versus 48 percent in patients treated with RT alone. No significant complications were noted in either group. King and Salzman[38] noted a control rate of only 26.3 percent in 57 patients treated with 10–30 Gy without excision. Radiation therapy alone is thus not indicated unless surgical excision cannot be performed.

An area of controversy in the management of patients with keloids is the importance of treatment timing. Lo and co-workers[43] reported poorer local control in patients treated after three days (65.7 percent) compared to those receiving treatment within three days (85.7 percent). In contrast, Kovalic and Perez[37] noted no difference in control rates in patients treated within 24 hours compared to those treated after 24 hours. Similarly, King and Salzman[38] noted no difference in control between patients treated immediately postoperatively and those treated within 10 days of surgery. Our current recommendation in patients with keloids is surgical excision and postoperative RT (12 Gy in 3–4 fractions). Although it is prudent to commence therapy in a timely fashion (2–3 days), it is not imperative to treat immediately following surgery. Treatment should be given with small, localized fields encompassing the tumor bed and incision with a small margin. Low-

**TABLE 17–3. OUTCOME OF PATIENTS WITH DERMATOFIBROSARCOMA PROTUBERANS TREATED WITH SURGERY, RADIATION THERAPY, OR RADIATION THERAPY AND SURGERY**

| Surgery | | | Radiotherapy | | | |
|---|---|---|---|---|---|---|
| Author | Type of Surgery | Control | Author | Dose (Gy) | Control (RT) | Control R+S[†] |
| O'Sullivan et al.[54] | WE | 16/16 (100%) | O'Sullivan et al.[54] | 50–60 | | 17/19 |
| | < WE* | 8/11 (72.7%) | Marks et al.[52] | 66.7–75 | 3/3 (100%) | |
| Roses et al.[49] | Various | 32/48 (66.6%) | | 60–67 | | 6/7 |
| Barnes et al.[50] | Various | 8/17 (47%) | Pack and Tabah[53] | Not known | | 5/7 |
| Buckhardt et al.[51] | Various | 37/52 (71.1%) | | | | |
| Total | | 101/144 (70.1%) | | | 3/3 (100%) | 28/33 (84.8%) |

Abbreviations: RT, radiation therapy; S, surgery; WE, wide excision.
*Close/microscopic positive margins.
†Majority incomplete excisions.

energy electrons (4–6 Mev) with bolus or orthovoltage techniques are ideal.

## Dermatofibrosarcoma Protuberans

The outcome of patients with dermatofibrosarcoma protuberans treated with surgery alone, RT alone, or combined modality therapy is shown in Table 17–3. Local control rates after surgery alone range from 47 to 100 percent, depending on the type of resection performed.[49–51] Local control in patients undergoing incomplete surgery and postoperative RT is approximately 85 percent.[52–54]

The outcome of patients with dermatofibrosarcoma protuberans treated with wide excision alone is excellent. O'Sullivan et al.[54] at MGH reported a local control rate of 100 percent in 16 patients treated with wide excision. However, patients with close or microscopic positive margins had a local recurrence rate of 27.3 percent. Roses and co-workers[49] evaluated the impact of surgical margin status on the local control of 48 patients with dermatofibrosarcoma protuberans. Overall, the local recurrence rate was 33.3 percent. However, patients treated with a margin of smaller than 2 cm had a higher rate of local recurrence than patients treated with margins of larger than 2 cm (40.7 percent versus 23.8 percent). Others have noted local recurrence rates ranging from 30 to 50 percent following surgery alone.[50,51]

Several series have examined the outcome of patients with dermatofibrosarcoma protuberans treated with postoperative RT following incomplete resection. Marks and others[52] reported the outcome of ten patients treated with either RT alone (3) or RT following incomplete resection (7). Two of the patients undergoing RT alone achieved a complete response. The third patient continued to regress at 33 months of follow-up. Six patients treated postoperatively with RT (60–67 Gy) were locally controlled.[52] A large series was recently reported by O'Sullivan and co-workers.[54] Nineteen patients received postoperative RT (50–60 Gy) for either microscopic positive (18) or close (1) margins. Local control was 89.5 percent. Patients treated with wide excision and who have negative margins do not require adjuvant RT. However, patients undergoing less than complete excision should receive postoperative RT. Recommended doses and techniques are similar to those used in other low-grade soft tissue sarcomas.

## Peyronie's Disease

Table 17–4 summarizes the outcome of patients with Peyronie's disease treated with RT alone. Radiation therapy can reduce the distressing symptoms and resultant sexual dysfunction in most patients with Peyronie's disease. Overall, decreased pain, curvature, and induration are seen in 81.1 percent, 33.5 percent, and 50.4 percent of patients, respectively.[55–59]

Several investigators have reported favorable results with RT alone in Peyronie's disease. Rodrigues et al.[55] treated 38 patients with Peyronie's disease with a total dose of 9 Gy in three fractions over five days with 200–250 kVp photons. Sixteen patients required a second course of therapy due to minimal improvement. Overall, 76 percent of patients reported improvement in pain, 48 percent in curvature, and 47 percent in sexual function. No radiation-induced morbidity was seen in patients receiving either one or two courses of therapy. Mira and co-workers[58] reviewed the outcome of 56 patients treated with RT alone. Most patients received 18 Gy in 6 Gy fractions on alternating days with low-energy (orthovoltage) techniques. Response rates varied by the presenting symptom. While pain symptoms decreased in 79.5 percent of patients, curvature and induration decreased in 38 percent and 43.7 percent of patients, respectively. The most rapid response rate was seen in patients presenting with pain (2.8 months).

**TABLE 17–4. OUTCOME OF PATIENTS WITH PEYRONIE'S DISEASE TREATED WITH RADIATION THERAPY**

| Author | No. Patients | Dose (Gy) | Results | | | |
|---|---|---|---|---|---|---|
| | | | Improved Sex life | Decreased Curvature | Decreased Pain | Decreased Induration |
| Rodrigues et al.[55] | 38 | 9–18 | 18/38 (47.4%) | 17/35 (48.5%) | 20/26 (76.9%) | |
| Carson and Coughlin[56] | 40 | 6–16 | | 2/32 (6.25%) | 11/14 (78.5%) | 4/30 (13.3%) |
| Griff[57] | 17 | 6–18 | | | 8/9 (88.8%) | |
| Mira et al.[58] | 56 | 2–19.9 | | 16/42 (38%) | 31/39 (79.4%) | 21/48 (43.7%) |
| Ariathurai et al.[59] | 40 | 10 | | 15/40 (37.5%) | 33/39 (84.6%) | 34/39 (87.1%) |
| Total | | | 18/38 (47.4%) | 50/149 (33.5%) | 103/127 (81.1%) | 59/117 (50.4%) |

Maximum responses in curvature and induration were seen at 6.5 and 9.1 months, respectively. Others have reported similarly favorable results with RT alone.[57,59]

A less favorable experience with RT alone was reported by Carson and co-workers.[56] A total of 40 patients were treated with total doses ranging from 6 to 16 Gy. Although 78.5 percent of patients presenting with pain responded, induration and curvature improved in only 13.3 percent and 6.25 percent, respectively. Responses were more common in younger patients with a shorter history of disease. However, these poor results are most likely due to the excessive protraction of therapy in this study. Reported treatment intervals ranged from 10 to 90 days.

The optimal radiation dose and fractionation scheme in patients with Peyronie's disease are unclear. Rodrigues et al.[55] administered 9 Gy in three fractions. However, 42.1 percent of patients required a second course of therapy due to minimal improvement. In the study by Mira and co-workers,[58] most patients received 18 Gy in six fractions. Regimens of 15–18 Gy in five to six fractions delivered over two to three weeks are reasonable. Treatment fields should include the entire penile shaft, because the efficacy of smaller treatment volumes is unknown. Low-energy electrons with bolus or orthovoltage techniques are recommended.

## Chemodectoma (Glomus Body Tumor)

The outcome of patients with temporal bone chemodectomas treated with either surgery or RT is shown in Table 17–5. Local control rates in patients treated with surgery and with RT are approximately 87 percent and 93 percent, respectively.[63–74] Springate and Weichselbaum[75] performed a comprehensive review of the modern surgery and radiation series of patients with temporal bone chemodectomas published between 1932 and 1983. Although comparable control rates were noted in patients treated with RT or surgery, patients undergoing surgery had a higher rate of complications. Reported complication rates in surgery alone series range from 4 to 100 percent (cranial nerve palsies, spinal fluid leaks, and perioperative death). In contrast, severe acute and late sequelae are uncommon following RT.[75] Radiation therapy should thus be considered the treatment of choice in patients with temporal bone chemodectomas.

Patients with small (less than 5 cm) resectable carotid chemodectomas are controlled with surgery,[60] but RT can control patients with large, unresectable tumors and patients unsuited for surgery.[61,62] As in temporal bone chemodectomas, moderate-dose RT (45–50 Gy in 1.8–2.0 Gy fractions) is recommended. Treatment should include the tumor and a small mar-

**TABLE 17–5. OUTCOME OF PATIENTS WITH TEMPORAL BONE CHEMODECTOMAS TREATED WITH SURGERY OR RADIATION THERAPY**

| Surgery | | Radiotherapy | | |
|---|---|---|---|---|
| Author | Control | Author | Dose (Gy) | Control |
| Kim et al.[66] | 10/17 (58.8%) | Kim et al.[66] | 13–62 | 15/17 (88.2%) |
| Cece et al.[64] | 16/17 (94.1%) | Cole et al.[73] | 20.9–57 | 18/20 (90%) |
| Brown[63] | 158/174 (90.8%) | Cummings et al.[70] | 35/3 wks | 34/36 (94.4%) |
| Jackson et al.[65] | 87/89 (97.7%) | Dickens et al.[74] | NS | 15/15 (100%) |
| Newman et al.[68] | 3/14 (21.4%) | Hatfield et al.[71] | 15–45 | 4/4 (100%) |
| Thomsen et al.[67] | 4/6 (66.6%) | Thomsen et al.[67] | 50–60 | 8/10 (80%) |
| Spector et al.[69] | 57/68 (83.8%) | Reddy et al.[72] | 22–56 | 9/9 (100%) |
| Total | 335/385 (87.0%) | | | 103/111 (92.8%) |

**TABLE 17–6. OUTCOME OF PATIENTS WITH JUVENILE ANGIOFIBROMA TREATED WITH SURGERY OR RADIATION THERAPY**

| Surgery | | | Radiation Therapy | | |
|---|---|---|---|---|---|
| Author | Stage | Control | Author | Dose (Gy) | Control |
| Witt et al.[77] | Various | 18/24 (75%) | Cummings et al.[78,79] | 30–35 | 54/55 (98.1%) |
| Jones et al.[76] | I–IIA | 17/17 (100%) | Sinha and Aziz[80] | 30–36 | 6/7 (85.7%) |
| | IIB–IIC | 9/11 (81.8%) | Cherlow et al.[81] | 30–50 | 8/10 (80%) |
| | III | 6/12 (50%) | Briant et al.[82] | 30 | 17/22 (77.2%) |
| Cherlow et al.[81] | Various | 15/22 (68.1%) | Jereb et al.[83] | 30–40 | 47/69 (68.1%) |
| Total | | 65/86 (75.6%) | | | 132/163 (80.1%) |

gin. Wedged pair treatment techniques limiting dosage to the surrounding tissues are ideal.

## Juvenile Angiofibroma

Table 17–6 summarizes the outcome of patients with juvenile nasopharyngeal angiofibroma treated by surgery or RT. Local control rates in patients treated with surgery range from 50 to 100 percent, depending on the extent of disease.[76,77,81] Local control in the RT series is approximately 81 percent.[78–84] In patients with limited disease, surgical excision is associated with high rates of control. However, when disease spreads beyond the confines of the nasopharynx, particularly with intracranial extension, surgical resection is less successful. Jones et al.[76] reported a 100 percent control rate in 17 patients with disease either confined to the nasopharynx (stage I) or with minimal extension to the pterygopalatine fossa (stage IIA). In contrast, patients with evidence of disease filling the pterygopalatine fossa and/or extending into the orbit (stage IIB) or into the cheek or infratemporal fossa (stage IIC) had a local control rate of 81.8 percent with surgery alone. Moreover, only 50 percent of patients with evidence of intracranial extension (stage III) were controlled with resection alone. Other investigators have reported local recurrence rates of 25 to 32 percent with surgery alone.[77,81]

Radiation therapy is associated with high rates of control in patients with juvenile angiofibroma, even when there is evidence of intracranial extension. Cummings and co-workers[78,79] treated 55 patients with juvenile angiofibroma of the nasopharynx with moderate doses of radiation (30–35 Gy). Forty-five (82 percent) were controlled with a follow-up of 3 to 26 years. However, a repeat course of 30 Gy successfully salvaged 8 of the 10 treatment failures. The ultimate local control was thus 96 percent. No untoward sequelae were observed in either the single-course or repeat-course patients. Two second malignancies (basal cell carcinoma and thyroid carcinoma) were noted respectively 13 and 14 years after treatment. Eleven of 13 patients

with nasopharyngeal angiofibroma were controlled with RT alone (36–52 Gy) at Washington University. However, sequelae were frequent, including xerostomia and dental problems later in life.[84] Cherlow et al.[81] reported a control rate of 80 percent in 10 patients treated with RT alone. All but one had evidence of intracranial extension. Radiation doses ranged from 30–50 Gy in 1.8–2.0 Gy daily fractions. Eight of the RT patients (72.7 percent) were controlled. Other investigators have reported similarly favorable outcomes with RT alone, even in patients with significant extension outside the confines of the nasopharynx.[80,82,83]

The optimal treatment of patients with juvenile angiofibroma should thus be based on the extent of disease. Radiation therapy is indicated in cases with locally advanced disease, particularly with evidence of intracranial extension. In patients with localized, resectable disease, surgery is preferable, in light of possible late sequelae.[78,79,84] Moderate doses of radiation (30–36 Gy in 15–18 fractions) are recommended. These tumors are notoriously infiltrative and thus treatment fields should be comprehensive in order to decrease the risk of a marginal recurrence. In the event of a local recurrence, consideration of a repeat course of RT is advisable in lieu of surgical salvage.[78–80]

## Hemangioma

The outcome of patients with hemangiomas treated with RT alone is summarized in Table 17–7. Radiation therapy is associated with high response rates and control in both visceral and cutaneous hemangiomas in adults and children.[85–88]

Several series have reported favorable results in patients with visceral and bone hemangiomas undergoing RT. Faria et al.[85] treated nine adult patients with symptomatic vertebral body hemangiomas. Total doses ranged from 30–40 Gy in 2–3 Gy daily fractions. Seven patients (77.8 percent) experienced a complete or near complete response, with a follow-up of 6 to 62 months. No significant sequelae were reported. Park and

**TABLE 17-7. OUTCOME OF PATIENTS WITH HEMANGIOMAS TREATED WITH RADIATION THERAPY**

| Author | No. Patients | Site | Dose (Gy) | Results |
|---|---|---|---|---|
| Faria et al.[85] | 9 | Vertebrae | 30–40 | 77.8 CR or near CR |
| Schild et al.[86] | 13 | Various | 6.25–40 | 81.8% response (36.4% CR) |
| Park and Phillips[87] | 5 | Liver | 13–20 | 80% controlled |
| Donaldson et al.[88] | 99 | Cutaneous | 15* | 69% CR |

Abbreviations: CR, complete response.
*Interstitial brachytherapy ([90]Y).

Phillips[87] controlled four of five unresectable liver hemangiomas with RT (13–20 Gy). No early or late hepatic sequelae were noted. Schild et al.[86] treated 13 patients with unresectable hemangiomas arising in various sites (extremity, 5; vertebral body, 3; face, 2; pituitary, 1; pelvis, 1; liver, 1) with 6.25–40 Gy in 1.6–2.5 Gy daily fractions. In 11 evaluable patients, 9 (81.8 percent) responded, 4 (36.4 percent) completely. None of the responders relapsed. The authors noted more success with doses greater than 30 Gy. Two of four patients (50 percent) responded with doses greater than 30 Gy versus only two of seven (29 percent) with doses less than 30 Gy. These results demonstrate the use of moderate-dose (30–40 Gy) RT in patients with symptomatic visceral and bone lesions.

Cutaneous hemangiomas of infancy have also been successfully treated with RT. Donaldson et al.[88] reviewed the outcome of 99 infants (median age, 10.7 months) treated at the Institute Gustave Roussey with interstitial [90]Y brachytherapy. A total of 123 implants were performed, with total doses ranging from 9–25 Gy. Most received 15 Gy over 2.5 hr prescribed to 2 mm depth. Sixty-eight (69 percent) achieved a complete response. Regression rates were often slow, with only 60 percent of complete responders achieving a complete response by six months. Cosmesis was judged to be good/average in most (92 percent) patients. Treatment decisions in infants with cutaneous hemangiomas need to be weighed against the high reported spontaneous regression rate.[169] Interstitial techniques in infants clearly require considerable experience and expertise.

## MALIGNANT TUMORS

### Extremity/Trunk Sarcomas

***Conservative Surgery and Adjuvant Radiation Therapy.*** The outcome of patients with extremity and trunk soft tissue sarcomas treated with conservative surgery and adjuvant RT is summarized in Table 17-8. Local recurrence rates range approximately from 8 to 22 percent depending on the type of surgery and sequencing of treatment. Ultimate limb preservation rates range approximately from 84 to 97 percent.[6–9,11,100–102,111,166,170–172]

**TABLE 17-8. OUTCOME OF PATIENTS WITH SOFT TISSUE SARCOMAS OF THE EXTREMITIES AND TRUNK TREATED WITH CONSERVATIVE SURGERY AND ADJUVANT RADIATION THERAPY**

| Author | Institution | No. Patients | Dose (Gy) | Local Failure | Complications | Limb Preservation |
|---|---|---|---|---|---|---|
| **Preoperative RT** | | | | | | |
| Brant et al.[100] | University of Florida | 58 | 50–60[a] | 10.4% | 16% | 87% |
| Barkley et al.[101] | MDAH | 110 | 50–60 | 10% | 14% | 97.3% |
| Suit et al.[6,111] | MGH | 60 | 50–56 | 14% | 26.7% | NS |
| Zlotecki et al.[166] | University of Florida | 142 | 50.4[a] | 8% | 21–54%[b] | 85% |
| **Postoperative RT** | | | | | | |
| Pao and Pilepich[8] | Mallinckrodt | 50 | 45–69 | 13% | 16% | 90% |
| Fein et al.[9] | Fox Chase | 67 | 39.6–71 | 22% | 7.5% | NS |
| Lindberg et al.[7] | MDAH | 300 | 60–75 | 22.3% | 6.5% | 84.5% |
| Mundt et al.[11] | University of Chicago | 50 | 60–68 | 17.5% | 14.5% | 84.4% |
| Leibel et al.[170] | UCSF | 29 | 50–75 | 10% | 27.6% | 96% |
| Suit et al.[6,111] | MGH | 110 | 66–68 | 16% | 5%[c] | NS |
| Rosenberg et al.[102] | NCI | 27 | 50–70 | 14.8% | NS | 96.3% |
| Robinson et al.[171] | Royal Marsden | 79[d] | 40–60 | 8% | 12.7% | NS |

Abbreviations: NS, not stated; RT, radiation therapy.
[a]1.2–1.25 Gy bid.
[b]Depending upon field length.
[c]Reference 172.
[d]Also includes a subset of patients treated with preoperative RT (two groups not analyzed separately).

Early experience with conservative surgery and adjuvant RT in patients with extremity and truncal soft tissue sarcomas was presented by Leibel et al.[170] at the University of California at San Francisco (UCSF). In a total of 81 patients, 47 patients were treated with either surgery alone, 29 patients with conservative surgery and RT, and 5 patients with RT alone. Total doses of 50–75 Gy were prescribed with shrinking field techniques. Patients with negative margins received 60–65 Gy, whereas patients with gross disease received 70 Gy. Local control was achieved in 89.6 percent of the limb-sparing group and 87.5 percent of the patients undergoing amputation. Two recurrences were noted just outside the field edge, emphasizing the necessity of generous field margins. Despite no prophylactic treatment of the draining lymph nodes (with either surgery or RT), only 5 percent of patients failed regionally. Complications included soft tissue necrosis requiring skin grafting (2), severe fibrosis (3) and chronic edema (2).

Several centers have reported the use of preoperative RT in patients with soft tissue sarcomas of the extremities. Barkeley et al.[101] at the M.D. Anderson Hospital (MDAH) and Tumor Institute treated 110 patients with preoperative RT and conservative surgery. Seventy-eight tumors (70.9 percent) were larger than 10 cm, and 57 (51.8 percent) were high grade. Most patients received 50 Gy; 15 received 60 Gy. No intraoperative or postoperative boosts were given. The local recurrence rate was 10 percent. Complications (edema, soft tissue necrosis, fracture, and fibrosis) occurred in 14 percent. In a recent review of the University of Florida experience, Zlotecki et al.[166] studied 142 patients treated with preoperative RT. Most patients received 50.4 Gy in 1.2 Gy twice daily fractions. The 5- and 10-year actuarial local control rates were respectively 92 percent and 88 percent. Limb preservation was achieved in 85 percent. Other centers have reported similarly favorable outcomes with preoperative RT and conservative surgery.[100,111]

Favorable results have also been reported in patients treated with conservative surgery and postoperative RT. Lindberg and co-workers[7] treated 300 extremity and trunk sarcomas with conservative surgery followed in three to four weeks by postoperative RT. Doses were initially 70–75 Gy (before 1971). Subsequently, low-grade tumors received 60 Gy and grade 2–3 tumors received 65 Gy. The overall local recurrence rate was 22.3 percent. However, the high recurrence rate is explained, in part, by the fact that many patients underwent a simple "shelling out" procedure, not wide excision. Of note, no difference in local control was seen with the use of lower total doses. Significant complications were seen in 6.5 percent of patients. Limb preservation was achieved in 84.5 percent of

patients. Mundt et al.[11] recently reviewed the outcome of 50 patients treated with postoperative RT at the University of Chicago. The local control of patients treated with adequate field margins (greater than 5 cm surrounding the tumor bed/scar) was 87.6 percent. The ultimate limb preservation rate was 84.4 percent. Comparable results with postoperative RT have been reported by Pao and Pilepich,[8] Fein et al.,[9] Suit et al.,[6] and Robinson et al.[171]

The optimal sequencing of surgery and RT in patients with extremity and truncal soft tissue sarcomas is unclear. The selection of preoperative or postoperative RT depends upon a number of factors, including the institution, preferences of the treating surgeon and radiation oncologists, and characteristics of the lesion (size, grade, location, involvement of neurovascular structures). In general, comparable results in terms of local control and limb preservation have been reported with both preoperative and postoperative RT. The relative merits of each approach have been described in detail.[6] While preoperative fields include only the tumor and surrounding tissues known and suspected of harboring subclinical disease, postoperative fields must include all tissues handled surgically, drain sites, areas of ecchymosis, and the surgical scar. Preoperative RT increases the resectability rate in patients with large tumors and also results in the inactivation of most tumor cells, which in turn may lower the risk of tumor dissemination at the time of surgery. However, postoperative RT allows a better delineation of tumor extent and does not increase surgical morbidity or delay surgery. In addition, postoperative RT allows the pathological analysis of the complete, untreated tumor specimen.

In a review of the MGH experience, Suit et al.[111] reported five-year actuarial local control rates of 80 percent and 92 percent in patients treated with postoperative and preoperative RT, respectively. While no difference was seen in tumors smaller than 10 cm, local control rates were superior in larger tumors treated with preoperative RT. At the University of Chicago, our preference is for postoperative RT in most patients. However, in patients with tumors involving neighboring critical structures (bone, neurovascular bundle) or in whom amputation would be required, preoperative RT is recommended. Size per se is not an indication for preoperative RT.

Conservative surgery with adjuvant RT was compared against radical surgery in a prospective, randomized trial conducted at the NCI. Forty-three adult patients with high-grade extremity soft tissue sarcomas were randomized to receive either conservative surgery and postoperative RT (n = 27) or amputation (n = 16). A 2:1 randomization scheme was used favoring the conservative surgery group. Limb-sparing treatment consisted of wide local excision followed by 60–70 Gy postoperative EBRT delivered with shrinking field techniques. Both groups received adjuvant combination chemotherapy. The five-year actuarial disease-free survival (71 percent versus 78 percent) ($p = 0.75$) and overall survival (83 percent versus 88 percent) ($p = 0.99$) rates were similar in the two groups. A slight benefit in terms of local control was seen favoring the radical surgery group (85.2 percent versus 100 percent) ($p = 0.06$). However, the sole significant factor on multivariate analysis in terms of local control was final surgical margin status.[102]

The importance of surgical margin status in patients treated with postoperative RT has also been described by several other investigators.[8,9,166] Fein et al.[9] reported the outcome of 67 patients treated with postoperative RT at the Fox Chase Cancer Center. Of these, ten patients had close margins, 17 patients had microscopic positive margins, and 1 patient had grossly positive margins. Doses ranged from 39.6–71 Gy. Thirteen patients received brachytherapy. The five-year actuarial local control was 87 percent. Patients with positive margins had significantly poorer local control than patients with close or negative margins (56 percent versus 100 percent) ($p = 0.002$). Margin status was an independent negative prognostic factor for local control on multivariate analysis. Other factors (overall treatment time and surgery–RT interval) did not reach statistical significance. It is thus prudent to achieve, whenever possible, negative pathological margins in patients treated with postoperative RT.

An alternative to adjuvant RT alone is the use of preoperative chemoradiotherapy. In a series of reports, Eilber and co-workers[104,105] at the University of California at Los Angeles (UCLA) reported their experience with intra-arterial doxorubicin and rapid fractionation preoperative RT followed by surgery. Treatment consisted of intra-arterial doxorubicin (90 mg over three days) and 35 Gy in 10 fractions administered with wide margins (often whole compartment). In the initial 77 patients, the five-year local control and survival were 95 percent and 65 percent, respectively. However, more than 25 percent of patients required surgery due to wound complications. The RT dose was subsequently decreased to 17.5 Gy in five fractions. Although the significant sequelae rate dropped to 15 percent, the local control also decreased to 86 percent. In addition, the incidence of tumor necrosis decreased from 80 percent to 20 percent. In the present protocol, a total dose of 28 Gy in seven fractions is given. Other centers have reported favorable results with preoperative chemoradiotherapy.[106,107] Although promising, preoperative chemotherapy with rapid fractionation RT remains an experimental approach and cannot be recommended in patients outside of a clinical trial.

It is unclear whether all patients with sarcomas of the extremity and trunk require adjuvant RT after conservative surgery. In a review of the NCI experience, Marcus et al.[120] reported a significantly lower rate of local recurrence in patients treated with adjuvant RT (4.5 percent versus 30.7 percent) ($p = 0.0008$). However, the benefit was almost exclusively seen in patients with positive margins. Small (less than 5 cm) tumors had a very low rate of recurrence following conservative surgery alone. The NCI is currently conducting a prospective, randomized trial comparing the outcome of completely resected small, low-grade tumors with and without adjuvant RT. Until the results of this important study are available, it remains unclear whether RT is necessary in low-grade patients after wide excision.

A second group of patients who may not require adjuvant RT following conservative surgery are patients with subcutaneous sarcomas. In a review of 40 subcutaneous sarcomas treated with wide excision alone, Rydholm et al.[121] noted no failures in 32 patients. Mundt et al.[122] recently analyzed the outcomes of 62 patients with subcutaneous soft tissue sarcomas of the extremity treated at the University of Chicago. Forty-five tumors (72.5 percent) were 5 cm in size and 30 (48.4 percent) were grade 3. A total of 57 patients underwent conservative surgery (51 patients, wide local excision; 6 patients, marginal excision). Thirty (58.8 percent) of the patients treated with wide excision did not receive adjuvant RT. The local control of patients treated with wide excision was similar with and without adjuvant RT (92.3 percent versus 100 percent) ($p = 0.23$). Of note, none of 22 tumors smaller than 5 cm or 8 tumors larger than 5 cm recurred locally following wide excision alone. Our current policy is to omit adjuvant RT in all patients with subcutaneous extremity soft tissue sarcomas treated with wide excision in whom negative margins are achieved.

**Brachytherapy.**  The outcome of patients with extremity and truncal soft tissue sarcomas treated with interstitial brachytherapy is shown in Table 17–9. Local failure rates range from 5 to 33 percent.[112–119]

Several investigators have used interstitial brachytherapy without EBRT in patients undergoing conservative surgery.[114,115,118] Shiu and co-workers[114] at the Memorial Sloan-Kettering Cancer Center (MSKCC) treated 33 patients with locally advanced extremity soft tissue sarcomas with brachytherapy and conservative surgery. Treatment consisted of a total dose of 40 Gy given over four to five days to the tumor bed with an interstitial $^{192}$Ir implant. Supplemental EBRT was administered to only seven patients. At a median follow-up of 36 months, the local recurrence rate was 18 percent. Wound complications occurred in 11 patients (33

**TABLE 17–9. OUTCOMES OF PATIENTS WITH EXTREMITY AND TRUNCAL SOFT TISSUE SARCOMAS TREATED WITH BRACHYTHERAPY**

| Author | No. Patients | EBRT | BT Dose (Gy) | Local Control | Complications | Functional Limb |
|---|---|---|---|---|---|---|
| Shiu et al.[116] | 33 | 21.2% | 40 | 82% | Wound, 33% Neuritis, 6.1% | 79% |
| Shray et al.[117] | 65 | 93.8% | 10–20 | 92.1% | Wound, 9.8% | 96% |
| Mills and Hering[119] | 17 | 100% | 125–135 TDF | 94.1% | Wound, 17.6% | NS |
| Habrand et al.[118] | 48 | 8.3% | 60 | 66.7% | NS | NS |
| Zelefsky et al.[115] | 45 | 28.9% | 44 | 79% | Neuritis, 9% | 84% |
| Brennan et al.[112] | 52 | 0% | 40–45 | 95% | NS | NS |

Abbreviations: BT, brachytherapy; EBRT, external beam radiotherapy; NS, not stated; TDF, time-dose fractionation.

percent). As noted earlier, the authors reported a higher rate of complications when the catheters were loaded within 72 hours of surgery.

In a subsequent report, investigators at MSKCC reported the outcome of a prospective randomized trial of brachytherapy in conjunction with conservative surgery. A total of 117 patients were randomized to either adjuvant brachytherapy (n = 52) or no further local therapy following wide excision (n = 65). Treatment consisted of 40–45 Gy over four to five days. The four-year actuarial local control was superior in the patients treated with brachytherapy (95 percent versus 54 percent) ($p = 0.06$). The local control benefit was most pronounced in patients with high-grade tumors (100 percent versus 82 percent) ($p = 0.03$).[112]

An important limitation of brachytherapy is highlighted in a trial by Habrand et al.[118] Forty-eight patients underwent conservative surgery and adjuvant brachytherapy (median dose, 60 Gy). Only four patients (8.3 percent) received supplemental EBRT. While two patients (4.2 percent) recurred locally (within the implant volume), 14 (29 percent) relapsed on the edge of the brachytherapy volume. These results clearly demonstrate that, although high doses are delivered to the tumor bed with brachytherapy, supplemental EBRT is beneficial due to the presence of subclinical disease in the surrounding tissues.

Series that combine brachytherapy and EBRT report consistently low rates of marginal and local recurrences. Shray et al.[117] treated 65 patients with conservative surgery, EBRT, and brachytherapy. A dose of 50 Gy was delivered preoperatively, and, at the time of surgery, catheters were positioned in order to deliver an additional 10–20 Gy. The recurrence rates within the implant volume and at the edge of the implant volume were 1.5 percent and 6.2 percent, respectively. Good/excellent limb function was achieved in 96 percent of patients. These results support the use of wide-field moderate-dose EBRT in conjunction with a brachytherapy boost. In select cases (e.g., patients with

recurrent disease following full-course EBRT), brachytherapy alone combined with conservative surgery remains appropriate.

A possible role for brachytherapy lies in patients with positive surgical margins due to anatomic constraints limiting wide resection. Zelefsky and co-workers[115] reported the outcome of 45 patients with positive margins due to involvement of the neurovascular bundle. Despite attempted surgery, 11 patients had gross positive, and 34 had microscopic positive disease. Catheters were placed directly on the neurovascular bundle. The median dose was 44 Gy. The five-year disease-free survival and local control were 69 percent and 79 percent, respectively. Only four (9 percent) developed radiation neuritis at 6–20 months. All four patients received doses greater than 90 Gy to the neurovascular bundle. Compared to reports using EBRT in patients with positive margins, the high rate of local control with brachytherapy (79 percent) is impressive. Similar favorable results have been reported in tumors in anatomically difficult locations (popliteal and antecubital fossae), which preclude the ability to obtain wide margins.[116]

***Unresectable Disease.*** The outcome of patients with unresectable sarcomas of the extremities and trunk treated with RT alone or in combination with radiosensitizers is shown in Table 17–10. Local control rates in patients treated with photons alone or neutrons (with and without photons) range approximately from 28 to 63.6 percent and 32 to 69 percent, respectively.[5,123–128]

Radiation therapy alone can control a subset of patients with unresectable disease. Early experience with photons alone was reported by Windeyer and colleagues.[124] Twenty-two patients received RT alone (60–85 Gy) over five to nine weeks. Responses were seen in 19 out of 22 (86.3 percent) patients, with 14 (63.6 percent) achieving a complete response. McNeer et al.[4] treated 25 patients with doses ranging from 20–75 Gy. Local control and survival were both 56 per-

**TABLE 17–10. OUTCOME OF PATIENTS WITH UNRESECTABLE SOFT TISSUE SARCOMAS OF THE EXTREMITIES AND TRUNK TREATED WITH RADIATION THERAPY**

| Author | No. Patients | Dose (Gy) | Local Control |
|---|---|---|---|
| **Photons Alone** | | | |
| Slater et al.[123] | 57 | 44–88 | 28% |
| Tepper and Suit[5] | 51 | 64–66 | 33% |
| Windeyer et al.[124] | 22 | 60–85 | 63.6% |
| McNeer et al.[4] | 25 | 20–75 | 56% |
| **Neutrons with and without Photons** | | | |
| Slater et al.[123] | 15 | 7.44–22.6[a] | 32% |
| Pelton et al.[125] | 11 | 13.6–20[a] | 54% |
| Cohen et al.[126] | 26 | 18–26[a] | 50% |
| Salinas et al.[127] | 29 | 45–80[b] | 69% |
| **RT + Radiosensitizers** | | | |
| Kinsella and Glatstein[128] | 10 | 40–50[c] (misonidazole) | 100% |
| | 5 | 50–60 (BUdR) | 60% |
| | 14 | 46–60.5[d] (IUdR) | 85.7% |

Abbreviations: BUdR, bromodeoxyuridine; IUdR, iododeoxyuridine.
[a] Doses in neutron Gy.
[b] In photon Gy equivalents.
[c] 4–4.5 Gy daily fractions.
[d] 1.5 Gy twice daily fractions.

cent. More recently, Tepper and Suit,[5] demonstrated that local control in patients treated with RT alone depends on tumor size. In a series of 51 patients treated with photons alone (64–66 Gy), the five-year local control was 33 percent. However, small tumors (less than 5 cm) had a local control of 87.5 percent versus 53 percent in 5 to 10 cm tumors and only 30 percent in tumors larger than 10 cm.

Several investigators have explored the use of neutrons either alone or in combination with photons. Pelton et al.[125] treated 11 inoperable patients with neutrons with and without photons. Total doses in patients treated with neutrons alone ranged from 13.6 to 20 neutron Gy. Local control was achieved in 54 percent of patients. Of note, 36 percent of patients experienced severe late sequelae, most notably severe fibrosis. Others have reported high rates of severe late sequelae in patients treated with neutrons.[123] A review of 12 of 287 neutron studies in the United States and Europe revealed overall local control and severe late sequelae rates of 50 percent and 30 percent, respectively.[125] Although theoretically appealing, the role of neutrons in the management of unresectable soft tissue sarcomas remains unclear. Comparable local control rates with a lower risk of late sequelae are achieved with photons alone. The routine use of neutrons in these patients is not recommended.

A promising approach in the treatment of patients with unresectable soft tissue sarcomas is the use of radiosensitizers. Kinsella and Glatstein[128] at NCI treated 29 patients with large (5–33 cm), unresectable tumors with RT in conjunction with three different radiosensitizers. The initial 10 patients received 40–50 Gy in 4–4.5 Gy daily fractions given twice weekly and preceded by the hypoxic cell sensitizer, misonidazole (2 g/m$^2$). Although no complete responses were noted, all 10 patients remained free of local progression. Due to a high rate of late sequelae (20 percent), the next 19 patients received a total dose of 46–60 Gy. Five of these patients received the dosage in conventional fractionation (1.8–2 Gy/day). Five of these patients received the dosage in conjunction with bromodeoxyuridine (BUdR), and 14 received the dosage in accelerated fractionation (1.5 Gy twice daily) in conjunction with iododeoxyuridine (IUdR). Three of the five patients achieved local control with BUdR, versus 12 of 14 with IUdR. Of note, two patients with "persistent disease" were found to have no evidence of viable tumor at autopsy. Moreover, six patients achieved a complete response.

### Head and Neck Sarcoma

The outcome of patients with soft tissue sarcomas of the head and neck is shown in Table 17–11. The local control in patients with nonangiosarcoma histologies ranges from 69 to 78.3 percent.[129–133] The local control and survival are less favorable in patients with angiosarcomas of the face and scalp.[133–135]

Only a few centers have published their experience with conservative surgery and adjuvant RT in patients with soft tissue (nonangiosarcoma) sarcomas of the head and neck. Goepfert and co-workers[129] treated 23 patients with conservative surgery and adjuvant RT (median dose = 60 Gy). Only three patients (13 percent) received elective nodal RT. Local control was achieved in 78.3 percent of patients. In a recent review of 46 patients at MGH, Willers and co-workers[133] reported five-year actuarial local-regional control, survival, and freedom-from-distant metastases of 69 percent, 74 percent, and 83 percent, respectively. Comparable results have been reported earlier by McKenna et al.[131] Although extensive experience is lacking, conservative surgery and adjuvant RT is a reasonable approach in patients with head and neck soft tissue sarcomas. Dose recommendations are similar to those in patients with extremity sarcomas.

Angiosarcomas of the head and neck have a poor outcome. Holden et al.[134] treated 45 patients with scalp and face angiosarcomas with 25–66 Gy (93.8 percent with RT alone). Only 13 patients survived two years, of whom eight (61.5 percent) were controlled. Despite the use of generous margins, marginal recurrences were common. Morales et al.[135] treated six patients and reported local and marginal recurrences in four.

**TABLE 17–11. OUTCOME OF PATIENTS WITH SOFT TISSUE SARCOMAS OF THE HEAD AND NECK TREATED WITH RADIATION THERAPY AND CONSERVATIVE SURGERY**

| Author | No. Patients | Dose (Gy) | Local Control |
|---|---|---|---|
| **Nonangiosarcomas** | | | |
| McKenna et al.[131] | 16 | 60–63 | 75% |
| Goepfert et al.[129] | 23 | 60 (median) | 78.3% |
| Willers et al.[133] | 46 | 36–79.2 | 69% |
| **Angiosarcomas** | | | |
| Holden et al.[134] | 45* | 25–66 | — |
| Morales et al.[135] | 6 | 50–70 | 33% |
| Willers et al.[133] | 11 | 36–79.2 | 24% |

*Only 13 patients survived two years; 8 were controlled (61.5 percent).

Willers and colleagues[133] treated 11 face and scalp angiosarcomas with either RT or surgery and RT. The five-year actuarial local-regional control, survival, and freedom-from-distant metastases were 24 percent, 31 percent, and 42 percent, respectively. High-dose RT with generous margins is recommended in patients with angiosarcomas of the face and scalp, particularly when surgery cannot be performed.

## Sarcomas of the Retroperitoneum

The outcome of patients with retroperitoneal soft tissue sarcomas treated with surgery and adjuvant RT is shown in Table 17–12. Local control rates range from 20 to 41.2 percent without adjuvant IORT[139,141,142] and 57 to 75 percent with IORT.[137–139,140,142]

Several investigators have reported the outcomes of patients with retroperitoneal soft tissue sarcomas

**TABLE 17–12. OUTCOME OF PATIENTS WITH RETROPERITONEAL SARCOMAS TREATED WITH SURGERY AND ADJUVANT RADIATION THERAPY**

| Author | No. Patients | EBRT Dose (Gy) | IORT Dose (Gy) | Local Control |
|---|---|---|---|---|
| **EBRT** | | | | |
| Tepper et al.[139] | 17 | 24.5–69.0 | NA | 41.2% |
| Fein et al.[141] | 21 | 36–90 | NA | 33.3% |
| Sindelar et al.[142] | 20 | 50–55 | NA | 20.0% |
| **EBRT + IORT** | | | | |
| Kinsella et al.[140] | 11 | 45 | 20 | 63.6% |
| Tepper et al.[130] | 12 | 40–50 | 10–20 | 66.7% |
| Willett et al.[137] | 12 | 40–50 | 10–20 | 75.0% |
| Sindelar et al.[142] | 15 | 35–40 | 20 | 60.0% |
| Glenn et al.[138]* | 37 | 50.4 | 20 | 56.8 |

Abbreviations: EBRT, external beam radiation therapy; IORT, intraoperative radiation therapy.
*Includes a subset of patients not treated with IORT.

treated with surgery and EBRT alone. Tepper et al.[139] treated 23 patients (17, definitive; 6, palliative) with surgery and postoperative EBRT (24.5–69 Gy). The five-year local control and survival rates in the definitive group were both 54 percent. Local control rates were higher in patients treated with complete resection versus less than complete resection or biopsy alone (71 percent versus 50 percent). Local control rates were also higher in patients treated with doses of greater than 60 than ones less than 60 Gy (83 percent versus 18.2 percent). Fein et al.[141] reported two-year actuarial local control and survival rates of 72 percent and 69 percent, respectively, in 21 patients treated with surgery and adjuvant EBRT (median dose = 54 Gy). Improved local control was seen in patients treated with doses greater than 55.2 Gy.

The use of adjuvant IORT in patients with retroperitoneal sarcomas has been the subject of several reports. Tepper et al.[139] treated 20 patients with retroperitoneal soft tissue sarcoma with IORT in addition to surgery and EBRT (40–50 Gy). Nineteen (95 percent) received EBRT dose before surgery, in an attempt to increase the resectability rate. The IORT dose depended on the extent of residual disease (15 Gy, microscopic disease; 20 Gy, gross disease). Of 17 evaluable patients, 12 (70.6 percent) received IORT. Local control was achieved in 9 out of 10 patients (90 percent) treated for microscopic disease and in 1 out of 2 patients (50 percent) treated for gross disease. Complication rates were low except for the development of a radiation-induced neuropathy in 2 out of 12 patients (17 percent). Willett et al.[137] reported four-year actuarial local control and disease-free survival rates of 81 percent and 64 percent, respectively, in 20 patients with retroperitoneal sarcomas, of whom 12 received adjuvant IORT. Local control was achieved in 9 out of 10 patients (90 percent) treated with microscopic disease only following surgery.

The role of adjuvant IORT was evaluated in a prospective randomized trial conducted at NCI. Thirty-five patients were randomized to receive either 20 Gy IORT and 35–40 Gy postoperative EBRT or 50–55 Gy EBRT alone. Both groups underwent maximal surgical resection. No difference was seen in median survival rates (45 versus 52 months) or median disease-free survival (19 versus 38 months) between patients treated with IORT versus without IORT. However, a lower local-regional recurrence rate was seen in the IORT group (40 percent versus 80 percent). Although patients treated with IORT had a higher rate of radiation-induced enteritis (13.3 percent versus 50 percent), a higher rate of peripheral neuropathy was seen (60 percent versus 5 percent).[142] Further study is clearly necessary to define the role of IORT in patients with retroperitoneal soft tissue sarcomas.

**TABLE 17–13. OUTCOME OF PATIENTS WITH UTERINE SARCOMAS TREATED WITH SURGERY OR SURGERY AND ADJUVANT POSTOPERATIVE PELVIC RADIATION THERAPY**

| | | Pelvic Recurrence | | Survival | |
| --- | --- | --- | --- | --- | --- |
| Author | Stage | Surgery | S + RT | Surgery | S + RT |
| Perez et al.[143] | I | 3/6 (50%) | 1/3 (33%) | 50%[a] | 64.7%[a] |
| | II | 1/1 (100%) | 6/8 (75%) | 0%[a] | 37.5%[a] |
| Vongtama et al.[148] | I–II | 35/61 (57.3%) | 8/31 (25.8%) | 40% | 53–54% |
| Disaia et al.[149] | I | 3/5 (60%) | 5/24 (20.8%) | 40%[b] | 58.3%[b] |
| | II | 5/5 (100%) | 1/11 (9%) | 0%[b] | 27.3%[b] |
| Badid et al.[150] | I | 23/46 (50%) | 5/27 (18.5%) | 56.5%[c] | 74.1%[c] |
| Salazar et al.[147] | I–II | 12/19 (63.1%) | 7/20 (35%) | 88%[d] | 42%[d] |
| Omura et al.[144] | I–II | 19/97 (19.5%) | 5/59 (8.4%) | NS | NS |
| Total | I | 29/57 (50.9%) | 11/54 (20.4%) | | |
| | II | 6/6 (100%) | 7/19 (36.8%) | | |
| | I–II | 66/177 (37.3%) | 20/110 (18.2%) | | |

Abbreviations: NS, not stated; RT, radiation therapy; S, surgery.
[a]3-year crude survivals.
[b]Stage I only.
[c]5-year crude survivals.
[d]2-year crude survivals.

## Uterine Sarcomas

The outcome of patients with early stage uterine sarcomas treated with and without adjuvant postoperative RT is shown in Table 17–13. Pelvic control is achieved in approximately 60 percent of stage I–II patients with surgery alone and in 80 percent of patients treated with surgery and RT.[143–150]

Numerous investigators have retrospectively compared the outcome of patients with early stage uterine sarcoma treated with surgery alone or with surgery and adjuvant pelvic RT. Perez et al.[143] treated 54 stage I–II patients with either RT alone, surgery alone, or surgery and RT. Radiation therapy consisted of whole pelvic RT (10–20 Gy) followed by an intracavitary insertion (Heyman-Simon capsules, tandem, and ovoids) and parametrial boosting (total parametrial dose of 45–50 Gy). The intrauterine dose for the resectable and unresectable patients were 5,000 and 7,500–8,000 mg/hr, respectively. Although no difference was noted in terms of survival in resectable patients treated with or without RT, pelvic recurrence rates were significantly lower in stage I–II patients treated with RT in addition to surgery (36 percent versus 57.1 percent). Other investigators have reported consistently better pelvic control rates in stage I–II uterine sarcoma patients with the use of adjuvant RT.[144–150] The impact of RT on survival, however, remains unclear. While several reports noted better survival with RT,[143,149,150] others did not.[146]

Uterine sarcomas have been the subject of two prospective, randomized trials conducted by the Gynecology Oncology Group (GOG). In the initial study, 156 stage I–II patients were randomized to receive either adjuvant adriamycin or no chemotherapy. The use of pelvic RT was left to the discretion of the treating physician. While no difference was seen in recurrence rates between the chemotherapy and control groups, the 59 patients treated with pelvic RT had significantly lower rates of pelvic (23 percent versus 54 percent) and vaginal (3.4 percent versus 15.5 percent) recurrence than the 97 patients treated with surgery alone.[144] A second trial was initiated, randomizing patients with completely resected disease to receive either 50 Gy pelvic RT or observation. Unfortunately, the trial was discontinued due to poor accrual. The above results suggest that adjuvant RT is beneficial in patients with resectable uterine sarcoma undergoing TAHBSO. Although no clear difference in survival has been demonstrated in the retrospective series, treatment provides improved pelvic control. Doses and techniques similar to those used in patients with epithelial uterine carcinoma are recommended.

Although fewer data are available, promising results have also been reported using RT alone in patients with medically inoperable or unresectable disease.[143,146] A number of important issues, however, remain to be defined. First, unlike their epithelial counterparts, uterine sarcomas have a propensity to fail in the upper abdomen.[147] This raises the question of whether whole-abdominal RT might prove beneficial. To answer this question, GOG is currently randomizing optimally debulked uterine sarcoma patients to receive either whole-abdominal RT or combination chemotherapy. Until the results of this ongoing study are available, the role of whole-abdominal RT in these patients remains unclear and is not recommended off-protocol. A second important issue is the optimal timing of RT and surgery. The available data suggest that preoperative and postoperative RT are equally efficacious.[143,146,149]

## Kaposi's Sarcoma

The outcome of patients with either epidemic or classic Kaposi's sarcoma treated with RT is shown in Table 17–14. Local control rates range from 30 to 85 percent in patients with classic and 62 to 91 percent in patients with epidemic Kaposi's sarcoma treated with RT.[151–159]

Radiation therapy is an effective means of controlling disease in patients with classic Kaposi's sarcoma. Cooper et al.[152] reviewed the outcome of 82 patients with classic Kaposi's sarcoma treated at New York University Hospital (NYU). Most patients were elderly (median age = 74) with lesions on the lower extremity (90.2 percent). Radiation therapy doses and fractionation schemes varied from 6.5 to 35 Gy in 1–10 fractions. All patients received local field RT only. Local control was best in patients treated with doses of 2,750 in 10 fractions or higher (1,200 ret). Of note, patients treated with large single-fraction regimens achieved the same rate of local control. Hamilton et al.[153] and Nisce et al.[154] also noted high response and control rates with RT alone in patients with classic Kaposi's sarcoma.

The optimal dose and treatment volume in patients with classic Kaposi's sarcoma are unclear. In his classic study, Cohen et al.[151] noted greater than 85 percent local control with doses of 8.4 Gy in one fraction. Cooper[152] noted local control of 85 percent in patients treated with doses of 27.5 Gy in 10 fractions versus 30 percent with lower doses ($p = 0.0007$). Others recommend doses from 8–30 Gy in 1–10 fractions. Our current recommendation in most patients is 8 Gy in one fraction. However, in patients with distal extremity lesions, particularly with involvement of the sole of the foot, more protracted regimens are recommended. Small treatment volumes are used, encompassing the lesion(s) with a small margin. Low-energy electron (with bolus) or orthovoltage techniques are ideal. No benefit was seen with the use of more extended fields in patients with localized disease.[152] In patients with diffuse cutaneous involvement, high response rates have been reported with total or subtotal skin EBRT.[154]

Several investigators have reported favorable results in patients with epidemic Kaposi's sarcoma treated with RT. In a series of reports, Cooper and co-workers[155] at NYU reviewed the outcome of 129 patients with 226 lesions, all treated with local RT alone. Small lesions received 3,000 in 10 fractions; larger lesions received 800 in one fraction. A total of 154 sites (68 percent) achieved a complete response. Of note, 45 additional patients had only a small area of residual dis-

**TABLE 17–14. OUTCOME OF PATIENTS WITH KAPOSI'S SARCOMA TREATED WITH RADIATION THERAPY**

| Author | No. of Patients | Dose/ Technique | Control |
|---|---|---|---|
| **Classic (Non-AIDS associated) KS** | | | |
| Cohen[151] | 38 | Various TD and fx | 65.8% |
| Cooper[152] | 82 | <1,200 ret | 30% |
| | | 1,200 ret | 85% |
| Hamilton et al.[153] | 91 | NS | 66.3% CR |
| Nisce et al.[154] | 20 | 4 Gy (TSEB or STSEB) | 85% CR |
| **Epidemic (AIDS-associated) KS** | | | |
| Cooper et al.[155] | 226* | 8–30 Gy/1–10 fx | 91% |
| Berson et al.[158] | 375* | 1.5–25 Gy/1–15 fx | 62%† |
| Chak et al.[159] | 72* | 20 Gy | 86.8% |

Abbreviations: AIDS, acquired immunodeficiency syndrome; CR, complete response; fx, fraction; KS, Kaposi's sarcoma; STSEB, subtotal skin electron beam; TD, total dose; TSEB, total skin electron beam.
*Number of total sites.
†At 12 months.

coloration. The overall local control rate was 91 percent. The response rates were a function of the presenting symptom. Complete response rates were highest in patients presenting with bleeding lesions (75 percent), lowest in patients presenting with impaired function (30 percent) and edema (30 percent). No significant complications were noted.[155–157] Favorable results were also reported by Berson and others[158] at the UCSF. A total of 375 sites in 187 patients were treated with RT. The fields used depended on the extent of disease. Four major fractionation schemes were used: 6–8 Gy in one fraction, 3–4 Gy in 10 fractions, 18–25 Gy in 10–15 fractions, and 15–16 in 10 fractions. Response rate was 93 percent. No difference in control or response was noted among the various schemes. Freedom-from-relapse was 62 percent at 12 months and 46 percent at 24 months. No untoward sequelae were noted.

As in classic Kaposi's sarcoma, the optimal dose and fractionation scheme in epidemic Kaposi's sarcoma is unclear. Given the high response rates, minimal risk of sequelae, and short life expectancy of these patients, a total dose of 8 Gy in one fraction administered to a local field is recommended. More protracted regimens should be used in patients with oropharyngeal (mucosal) lesions. Treatment should be restricted to lesions which are painful, result in functional impairment, or are disfiguring.[155]

## Rhabdomyosarcoma

The outcome of patients with childhood rhabdomyosarcoma depends on a number of factors, including the disease site, histology, and disease group. In the most recent IRS protocol (IRS-III), the five-year actuarial progression-free and overall survivals in 1,062 children were 71 percent and 63 percent, respectively.[162]

Group I patients have a favorable outcome following surgery and combination chemotherapy.[162] Radiation therapy is not necessary in most patients. In IRS-1, group I patients were randomized to receive either postoperative RT (with age-adjusted total doses of 40–60 Gy) or no further local therapy. All patients received combination chemotherapy, consisting of vincristine, actinomycin-D, and cyclophosphamide. Patients treated with RT had similar local control (91.5 percent versus 92.3 percent) and survival (81 percent versus 93 percent) as patients not receiving RT.[160] Adjuvant RT was not administered to group I patients in the second IRS protocol. However, a later analysis demonstrated a higher local failure rate in patients with unfavorable histology (alveolar or unclassified).[163] Adjuvant RT was thus reinstated in IRS-III in group I patients with unfavorable histology.[162] Local control in group II patients (microscopic positive margins and/or positive lymph nodes) is approximately 90 percent in patients treated with combination chemotherapy and postoperative RT (41.4 Gy).[173,174]

Local recurrence is a problem in most group III and IV patients. Local-regional recurrence occurred in 22 percent of group III and 30 percent of group IV patients treated on IRS-II with total doses of 40–55 Gy.[164,174] Although higher doses (55–65 Gy) are associated with lower local recurrence rates,[175] such doses are not desirable in young patients, due to the increased risk of late sequelae. To address this problem, IRS-IV currently randomizes patients with group III disease to receive either conventional dose RT (50.4 Gy) or hyperfractionated RT consisting of 59.4 Gy in 1.1 Gy twice daily fractions. In a recently published pilot study (IRS IV-P) of 204 group III and 80 group IV patients, hyperfractionated RT was felt to be feasible and tolerable. Although 75 percent of group III and 65 percent group IV patients experienced severe or life-threatening toxicity, most were hematopoietic and explained by the chemotherapy.[164] Until the results of IRS-IV are available, hyperfractionated RT in patients with group III–IV disease remains an experimental approach and is not recommended outside a controlled clinical trial.

Rhabdomyosarcoma arising in parameningeal head and neck sites has a poor outcome despite aggressive combined modality therapy. In IRS-1, 57 patients with parameningeal disease were treated (40, group III; 17, group IV). Twenty (35 percent) had evidence of direct meningeal extension either at diagnosis or within 12 months of treatment. Meningeal extension was found to be a grave prognostic sign, with 90 percent of patients dying of their disease.[176] In subsequent IRS protocols, patients received more aggressive therapy,

consisting of craniospinal RT in addition to treatment of the primary site. More aggressive therapy was associated with an improved three-year survival and decreased failure in the meninges.[161] More recently, the routine use of craniospinal and whole-brain RT has been questioned.[177] Currently, most patients with parameningeal rhabdomyosarcoma should receive localized RT to the primary and adjacent meninges.[178] Cranial RT is added in patients with parenchymal metastases. Spinal RT is the recommended RT in patients with evidence of involvement of the cerebral spinal fluid.[162]

Radiation therapy may not be necessary in all group III patients. Currently, children with group III bladder and prostate primaries receive RT instead of surgery only when total cystectomy is required. In children who respond to chemotherapy and can be managed with less than total cystectomy, surgery is the recommended local modality. Similarly, in children with chemosensitive disease of the vulva, vagina, or uterus in whom resection can be accomplished with negative margins, RT can be omitted. RT should be given postoperatively to all patients with positive gross or microscopic margins.[162]

Radiation therapy remains a fundamental component in the management of children with orbital rhabdomyosarcoma. Wharam et al.[179] reviewed the outcome of 127 children with orbital rhabdomyosarcoma treated on IRS protocols. Total RT doses ranged from 30–64 Gy (50 percent received from 45–55 Gy). Wedged pair beam portals were used in most patients. The local control was 94 percent in group III disease (98 percent after surgical salvage).[179] However, toxicity was significant, including cataracts, facial asymmetry, and orbital hypoplasia.[180]

Radiation therapy also occupies an important role in the management of children with paratesticular and extremity rhabdomyosarcoma. In paratesticular disease, RT is indicated in patients with involved para-aortic lymph nodes. Treatment fields in these patients resemble those used in patients with testicular seminoma.[181] Patients with resectable extremity primaries are managed with limb-sparing approaches. No advantage has been shown with the use of radical surgery over conservative approaches.[182] Group I favorable histology patients receive conservative surgery and combination chemotherapy. Patients with unfavorable histology group I disease and group II–IV disease are treated with RT. Treatment volumes are smaller than those used in adult soft tissue sarcomas. The treatment volume includes the pretreatment volume plus a 2-cm margin. Elective nodal RT is not indicated. As in all patients with extremity tumors, care must be given to avoid irradiation of the entire limb circumference. Moreover, joints and adjacent growth plates should be excluded from the treatment field whenever possible.

## ■ FUTURE DIRECTIONS

New treatment strategies are clearly needed in many types of soft tissue sarcomas. Effective adjuvant chemotherapeutic regimens addressing both micrometastatic and local disease would be a welcome development. New agents that are both cytotoxic and radiosensitizing may evolve. A new method of gene-targeted radiotherapy in which cytokines/toxins are activated locally may improve the local control of larger tumors and perhaps treat some subclasses of distant metastases. Finally, radiolabelled monoclonal antibodies to sarcomas may prove effective in treating local and distant disease.

## REFERENCES

1. Pusey WA: Cases of sarcoma and of Hodgkin's disease treated by exposure to X-rays: A preliminary report. JAMA 38:166, 1902
2. Cade S: Soft tissue tumors: Their natural history and treatment. Proc R Soc Med 44:19, 1951
3. Perry H, Chu F: Radiation therapy in the palliative management of soft tissue sarcomas. Cancer 15:179, 1962
4. McNeer GP, Cantin J, Chu F, Nickson J: Effectiveness of radiation therapy in the management of sarcomas of the soft tissue. Cancer 22:391, 1968
5. Tepper JE, Suit H: Radiation therapy alone for sarcomas of the soft tissues. Cancer 56:475, 1985
6. Suit HD, Mankin HJ, Wood WC, et al.: Treatment of the patient with stage M$_o$ soft tissue sarcoma. J Clin Oncol 6:854, 1988
7. Lindberg RD, Martin RG, Romsdahl MM, Barkley HT: Conservative surgery and postoperative radiotherapy in 300 adults with soft-tissue sarcomas. Cancer 47:2391, 1981
8. Pao WJ, Pilepich MV: Postoperative radiotherapy in the treatment of extremity soft tissue sarcomas. Int J Radiat Oncol Biol Phys 19:907, 1990
9. Fein DA, Lee WR, Lanciano RM, et al.: Management of extremity soft tissue sarcomas with limb-sparing surgery and postoperative irradiation: Do total dose, overall treatment time and surgery-radiotherapy interval impact on local control? Int J Radiat Oncol Biol Phys 32:969, 1995
10. Weichselbaum RR, Beckett M, Vijayakumar S, et al.: Radiobiological characterization of head and neck and sarcoma cell lines derived from patients prior to radiotherapy. Int J Radiat Oncol Biol Phys 19:313, 1990
11. Mundt A, Awan A, Sibley G, et al.: Conservative surgery and adjuvant radiation therapy in the management of adult soft tissue sarcomas of the extremities: Clinical and radiobiological results. Int J Radiat Oncol Biol Phys 32:977, 1995
12. Weichselbaum R, Hallahan D, Chen G: Biological and physical basis to radiation oncology. In Holland J, Frei E, Bast R, et al. (eds): Cancer Medicine. Malvern, Lea & Febriger, 1993
13. Puck TT, Marcus PI: Action of x-rays on mammalian cells. J Exper Med 103:653, 1956
14. Gerwick L, Kornblith P, Burlett P, et al.: Radiosensitivity of cultured glioblastoma cells. Radiology 125:231, 1977
15. Nilsson S, Carlson J, Larson E, Ponten J: Survival of irradiated glia and glioma cells studied with a new cloning technique. Int J Radiat Oncol Biol Phys 7:267, 1980
16. Barranco S, Romsdahl M, Humphrey R: The radiation response of human melanoma cells grown in vitro. Cancer Res 31:830, 1971
17. Drewinko B, Yang L, Romsdahl M: Radiation response of cultured CEA producing colon adenocarcinoma cells. Int J Radiat Oncol Biol Phys 2:1109, 1977
18. Kelland LR, Bingle L, Edwards S, Steel G: High intrinsic radiosensitivity of a newly established and characterised human embryonal rhabdomyosarcoma cell line. Br J Cancer 59:160, 1989
19. Hall E: Cell survival curves. In Hall EJ (ed): Radiobiology for the Radiologist. Philadelphia, J.B. Lippincott, 1994
20. Fertil B, Dertingen H, Courdi A, Malaise EP: Mean inactivation dose: A useful concept for intercomparison of human cell survival curves. Radiat Res 99:75, 1984
21. Tucker B: Is the mean inactivation dose a good measure of cell radiosensitivity. Radiat Res 105:18, 1986
22. Musgrove J, McDonald J: Extra-abdominal desmoid tumors: Their differential diagnosis and treatment. Arch Pathol 45:513, 1948
23. Reitamo J: Desmoids: Choice of treatment, results, and complications. Arch Surg 129:1318, 1983
24. Masson J, Soule E: Desmoid tumors of the head and neck. Am J Surg 112:615, 1966
25. Khorsand J, Karakousis C: Desmoid tumors and their management. Am J Surg 149:215, 1985
26. Das Gupta T, Brasfield R, O'Hara J: Extra-abdominal desmoids: A clinicopathological study. Ann Surg 170:109, 1969
27. Leibel A, Wara W, Hill D, et al.: Desmoid tumors: Local control and patterns of relapse following radiation therapy. Int J Radiat Oncol Biol Phys 9:1167, 1983
28. Greenberg HM, Goebel R, Weichselbaum R, et al.: Radiation therapy in the treatment of aggressive fibromatoses. Int J Radiat Oncol Biol Phys 7:305, 1981
29. Wara W, Phillips T, Hill D, et al.: Desmoid tumors: Treatment and prognosis. Radiology 124:225, 1977
30. Kiel K, Suit H: Radiation therapy in the treatment of aggressive fibromatoses (desmoid tumors). Cancer 54:2051, 1984
31. Benninghoff D, Robbins R: The nature and treatment of desmoid tumors. Am J Roentgenol 91:132, 1964
32. Sherman N, Romsdahl M, Evans H, et al.: Desmoid tumors: A 20-year radiotherapy experience. Int J Radiat Oncol Biol Phys 19:37, 1990
33. Hill D, Newman H, Phillips T: Radiation therapy of desmoid tumors. Am J Roentgenol 117:84, 1973
34. Suit H: Radiation dose and response of desmoid tumors (editorial). Int J Radiat Oncol Biol Phys 19:225, 1990
35. Spears M, Jennings L, Efird J, et al.: Indications for radiation therapy and surgery in the treatment of fibromatosis. Int J Radiat Oncol Biol Phys 32(suppl 1):288, 1995

36. Kamath S, Parson J, Marcus R, et al.: Radiotherapy for aggressive fibromatosis. Int J Radiat Oncol Biol Phys 32 (suppl 1):289, 1995

37. Kovalic J, Perez C: Radiation therapy following keloidectomy: A 20-year experience. Int J Radiat Oncol Biol Phys 17:77, 1989

38. King G, Salzman F: Keloid scars: An analysis of 89 patients. Surg Clin North Am 50:595, 1970

39. Ramakrishnan K, Thomas K, Sundararajan C: Study of 1,000 patients with keloids in South India. Plast Reconstr Surg 53:276, 1974

40. Hintz B: Radiotherapy for keloid treatment. J Natl Med Assoc 65:71, 1973

41. Malaker K, Ellis F, Paine C: Keloid scars: A new method of treatment combining surgery with interstitial radiotherapy. Clin Radiol 27:179, 1976

42. Levy D, Salter M, Roth R: Postoperative irradiation in the prevention of keloids. Am J Roentgenol 127:509, 1976

43. Lo TC, Seckel B, Salzman F, Wright K: Single-dose electron beam irradiation in the treatment and prevention of keloids and hypertrophic scars. Radiother Oncol 19:267, 1990

44. Borok T, Bray M, Sinclair I, et al.: Role of ionizing irradiation in 393 keloids. Int J Radiat Oncol Biol Phys 15:865, 1988

45. Conway H, Gillette R, Smith J, Findley A: Differential diagnosis of keloids and hypertrophic scars by tissue cultures techniques with notes on therapy of keloids by surgery and decadron. Plast Reconstr Surg 25:117, 1960

46. Cosman B, Crikelair G, Ju D, et al.: The surgical treatment of keloids. Plast Reconstr Surg 27:335, 1961

47. Singleton M, Gross C: Management of keloids by surgical excision and local injection of a steroid. South Med J 64:1377, 1971

48. Garb J, Stone M: Keloids: Review of the literature and a report of 80 cases. Am J Surg 58:315, 1942

49. Roses D, Valensi Q, LaTrenta G, Harris M: Surgical treatment of dermatofibrosarcoma protuberans. Surg Gynecol Obstet 162:449, 1986

50. Barnes L, Coleman J, Johnson J: Dermatofibrosarcoma protuberans of the head and neck. Arch Otolaryngol 10:398, 1984

51. Buckhardt B, Soule E, Winkelman R, Ivins J: Dermatofibrosarcoma protuberans—A study of 56 cases. Am J Surg 111:638, 1966

52. Marks L, Suit H, Rosenberg A, Wood W: Dermatofibrosarcoma protuberans treated with radiation therapy. Int J Radiat Oncol Biol Phys 17:379, 1989

53. Pack G, Tabah E: Dermatofibrosarcoma protuberans: A report of 39 cases. Arch Surg 62:391, 1951

54. O'Sullivan B, Catton C, Bell R, et al.: Treatment outcome in dermatofibrosarcoma protuberans referred to a radiation oncology practice. Int J Radiat Oncol Biol Phys 32 (suppl 1):289, 1995

55. Rodrigues CI, Njo KH, Karim AB: Results of radiotherapy and vitamin E in the treatment of Peyronies disease. Int J Radiat Oncol Biol Phys 31:571, 1995

56. Carson C, Coughlin P: Radiation therapy for Peyronies disease: Is there a place? J Urol 134:684, 1985

57. Griff L: Peyronie's disease. Am J Roentgenol 100:916, 1967

58. Mira J, Chahbazian C, del Regato J: The value of radiotherapy for Peyronie's disease: Presentation of 56 new case studies and a review of the literature. Int J Radiat Oncol Biol Phys 6:161, 1980

59. Ariathurai SV, Kimball W, Wilson A, et al.: Radiation therapy in the treatment of Peyronie's disease (abstr). Int J Radiat Oncol Biol Phys 9(suppl 1):105, 1983

60. Warren K: Symposium on surgical lesions of the neck and upper mediastinum: Tumors of the carotid body: Recognition and treatment. Surg Clin North Am 53:677, 1953

61. Guedea W, Medenhall W, Parsons J, Million R: Radiotherapy of chemodectoma of the carotid body and ganglion nodosum. Head Neck 13:509, 1991

62. Valdagni R, Amichetti M: Radiation therapy of carotid body tumors. Am J Clin Oncol 13:45, 1990

63. Brown J: Glomus jugulare tumors revisited: A ten-year statistical follow-up of 231 cases. Laryngoscope 95:284, 1985

64. Cece J, Lawson W, Biller H, et al.: Complications in the management of large glomus jugulare tumors. Laryngoscope 97:152, 1987

65. Jackson C, Glassock M, Nissen A, Schwaber M: Glomus tumor surgery: The approach, results, and problems. Otolaryngol Clin North Am 15:897, 1982

66. Kim J, Elkon D, Lim M, Constable W: Optimum dose of radiotherapy for chemodectomas of the middle ear. Int J Radiat Oncol Biol Phys 6:815, 1980

67. Thomsen K, Elbrønd O, Anderson A: Glomus jugulare tumours: A series of 21 cases. J Laryngol 89:1113, 1975

68. Newman H, Rowe J, Phillips T: Radiation therapy of glomus jugulare tumors. Am J Roentgenol Radiat Ther Nucl Med 118:663, 1973

69. Spector G, Gado M, Ciralsky R, et al.: Neurologic implications of glomus jugulare tumors in the head and neck. Laryngoscope 85:1387, 1875

70. Cummings B, Beale F, Garrett P, et al.: The treatment of glomus tumors in the temporal bone by megavoltage radiation. Cancer 53:2635, 1984

71. Hatfield P, James A, Schultz D: Chemodectomas of the glomus jugulare. Cancer 30:1164, 1972

72. Reddy E, Mansfield C, Hatman G: Chemodectomas of the glomus jugulare. Cancer 52:337, 1983

73. Cole J: Glomus jugulare tumor. Laryngoscope 87:1244, 1977

74. Dickens W, Million R, Cassisi N, Singleton G: Chemodectomas arising in temporal bone structures. Laryngoscope 92:188, 1982

75. Springate C, Weichselbaum R: Radiation or surgery for chemodectoma of the temporal bone: A review of local control and complications. Head Neck 12:303, 1990

76. Jones G, Desanto L, Bremer J, Neel H: Juvenile angiofibroma. Arch Otolaryngol Head Neck Surg 112:1191, 1986

77. Witt T, Shoh J, Sternberg S: Juvenile angiofibroma: A 30-year clinical review. Am J Surg 146:521, 1983

78. Cummings B, Stone E, Blend R: The results of treatment and late toxicity of megavoltage radiation for juvenile

angiofibroma (abstr). Int J Radiat Oncol Biol Phys 9 (suppl 1):81, 1983

79. Cummings B, Blend R, Fitzpatrick P, et al.: Primary radiation therapy for juvenile nasopharyngeal angiofibroma. Laryngoscope 94:1599, 1984

80. Sinha P, Aziz H: Juvenile nasopharyngeal angiofibroma. A report of 7 cases. Radiology 127:501, 1978

81. Cherlow J, Clacaterra J, Juillard G, Parker R: Radiation therapy or surgery in 33 cases of juvenile angiofibroma of the nasopharynx (abstr). Int J Radiat Oncol Biol Phys 9 (suppl 1):81, 1983

82. Briant T, Fitzpatrick P, Berman J: Nasopharyngeal angiofibroma: A twenty year study. Laryngoscope 88: 1247, 1978

83. Jereb B, Anggard A, Baryd I: Juvenile nasopharyngeal angiofibroma: A clinical study of 69 cases. Acta Radiol Ther Phys Biol 9:302, 1970

84. Perez C, Amendola B, Lindberg R, Marcial-Vega V: Unusual nonepithelial tumors of the head and neck. In Perez C, Brady L (eds): Principles and Practice of Radiation Oncology. Philadelphia, J.B. Lippincott, p 762, 1992

85. Faria S, Schlupp W, Chiminazzo H: Radiotherapy in the treatment of vertebral hemangiomas. Int J Radiat Oncol Biol Phys 11:387, 1985

86. Schild S, Buskirk S, Frick L, Cupps R: Radiotherapy for large symptomatic hemangiomas. Int J Radiat Oncol Biol Phys 21:729, 1991

87. Park W, Phillips R: The role of radiation therapy in the management of hemangiomas of the liver. JAMA 212: 1496, 1970

88. Donaldson S, Chassagne D, Sancho-Garnier H, Beyer H: Hemangiomas of infancy: Results of $^{90}$Y interstitial therapy: A retrospective study. Int J Radiat Oncol Biol Phys 5:1, 1979

89. Thomas H, Dolman C, Berry K: Malignant meningioma: Clinical and pathological features. J Neurosurg 55:929, 1981

90. Nascimento A, Unni K, Bernatz P: Sarcomas of the lung. Mayo Clin Proc 57:355, 1982

91. Harris H: Angiosarcoma of the heart. J Clin Pathol 13: 205, 1960

92. Barnes L, Pietruszka M: Sarcomas of the breast: A clinicopathologic analysis of ten cases. Cancer 40:1577, 1977

93. Goodner J, Miller T, Watson W: Sarcoma of the esophagus. Am J Roentgenol Radiat Ther Nucl Med 89:134, 1963

94. Sen S, Malek R, Farrow G, Lieber M: Sarcoma and carcinosarcoma of the bladder in adults. J Urol 133:29, 1985

95. Luk K, Caderao J, Leavens M: Radiotherapy for treatment of meningioma and meningiosarcoma. Cancer Bull 31:220, 1979

96. Antman K, Corson J, Greenberger J, Wilson R: Multimodality therapy in the management of angiosarcoma of the breast. Int Surg 61:463, 1982

97. Celik C, Lopez C, Douglas H: Advanced leiomyosarcoma of the stomach. J Surg Oncol 26:83, 1984

98. Simon M, Enneking W: The management of soft-tissue sarcomas of the extremities. J Bone Joint Surg 58A:317, 1976

99. Lawrence W, Donegan W, Natarajan N, et al.: Adult soft tissue sarcomas. A pattern of care survey of the American college of surgeons. Ann Surg 205:349, 1987

100. Brant T, Parsons J, Marcus R, et al.: Preoperative irradiation for soft tissue sarcomas of the trunk and extremities in adults. Int J Radiat Oncol Biol Phys 19:899, 1990

101. Barkley H, Martin R, Romsdahl M, et al.: Treatment of soft tissue sarcomas by preoperative irradiation and conservative surgical resection. Int J Radiat Oncol Biol Phys 14:693, 1988

102. Rosenberg S, Tepper J, Glatstein E, et al.: The treatment of soft tissue sarcomas of the extremities: Prospective randomized evaluations of (1) limb-sparing surgery plus radiation compared with amputation and (2) the role of adjuvant chemotherapy. Ann Surg 196:305, 1982

103. Brizel D, Weinstein H, Hunt M: Failure patterns and survival in pediatric soft tissue sarcoma. Int J Radiat Oncol Biol Phys 15:37, 1988

104. Eilber F, Eckhardt J, Morton D: Advances in the treatment of sarcomas of the extremity: Current status of limb salvage. Cancer 54:2695, 1984

105. Rosen G: Chemotherapy of sarcomas. In Eilber F, Morton D, Sondak V, Economou J (eds): The Soft Tissue Sarcomas. Orlando, Grune & Stratton, 1987; p 83

106. Goodnight J, Bargar W, Voegell T, Blaisdell F: Limb-sparing surgery for extremity sarcomas after preoperative intra-arterial doxorubicin and radiation therapy. Am J Surg 150:109, 1985

107. Denton J, Dunham W, Salter M, et al.: Preoperative regional chemotherapy and rapid-fraction irradiation for sarcomas of the soft tissue and bone. Surg Gynecol Obstet 158:545, 1984

108. Kinsella TJ, Loeffler JS, Fraas BA, Tepper J: Extremity preservation by combined modality therapy in sarcomas of the hand and foot: An analysis of local control, disease free survival and functional result. Int J Radiat Oncol Biol Phys 9:1115, 1983

109. Okunieff P, Suit H, Proppe K: Extremity preservation by combined modality treatment of sarcomas of the hand and wrist. Int J Radiat Oncol Biol Phys 12:1923, 1987

110. Chun L, Crawford S, Mundt A, Vijayakumar S: Computer aided treatment design in the treatment of a soft tissue sarcoma of the distal extremity: A case report. Med Dosim 9:56, 1993

111. Suit H, Mankin H, Wood W, Proppe K: Preoperative, intraoperative and postoperative radiation in the treatment of primary soft tissue sarcoma. Cancer 55:2659, 1985

112. Brennan M, Hilaris B, Shiu M, et al.: Local recurrence in adult soft tissue sarcoma: A randomized trial of brachytherapy. Arch Surg 122:1289, 1987

113. Arbeit J, Hilaris B, Brennan M: Wound complications in the multimodality treatment of extremity and superficial truncal sarcomas. J Clin Oncol 5:480, 1987

114. Shiu M, Turnbull A, Nori D, et al.: Control of locally advanced extremity soft tissue sarcomas by function saving resection and brachytherapy. Cancer 53:1385, 1984

115. Zelefsky M, Nori D, Shiu M, Brennan M: Limb salvage in soft tissue sarcomas involving neurovascular structures

using combined surgical resection and brachytherapy. Int J Radiat Oncol Biol Phys 19:913, 1990

116. Shiu M, Collin C, Hilaris B, et al.: Limb preservation and tumor control in the treatment of popliteal and antecubital soft tissue sarcomas. Cancer 57:1632, 1986

117. Schray M, Gunderson L, Sim F, et al.: Soft tissue sarcoma. Integration of brachytherapy, resection, and external irradiation. Cancer 66:451, 1990

118. Habrand J, Gerbaulet A, Pejovic M, et al.: Twenty years experience of interstitial iridium brachytherapy in the management of soft tissue sarcoma. Int J Radiat Oncol Biol Phys 20:405, 1991

119. Mills E, Hering E: Management of soft tissue tumours by limited surgery combined with tumor bed irradiation using brachytherapy and supplemental teletherapy. Br J Radiol 54:312, 1981

120. Marcus S, Merino M, Glatstein E, et al.: Long-term outcome in 87 patients with low-grade soft-tissue sarcoma. Arch Surg 128:1336, 1993

121. Rydholm A, Gustafson P, Rööser B, et al.: Limb-sparing surgery without radiotherapy based on anatomic location of soft tissue sarcoma. J Clin Oncol 9:1757, 1991

122. Mundt A, Gibbs P, Peabody T, et al.: Localized subcutaneous soft tissue sarcoma: Implications for the use of adjuvant radiation therapy. Int J Radiat Oncol Biol Phys (abstr) 32:166, 1995

123. Slater J, McNeese M, Peters L: Radiation therapy for unresectable soft tissue sarcomas. Int J Radiat Oncol Biol Phys 12:1729, 1986

124. Windeyer B, Dische S, Mansfield C: The place of radiotherapy in the management of fibrosarcomas of the soft tissues. Clin Radiol 17:32, 1966

125. Pelton J, Del Rowe J, Bolen J, et al.: Fast neutron radiotherapy for soft tissue sarcomas. University of Washington experience and review of the worlds literature. Am J Clin Oncol 9:397, 1986

126. Cohen L, Hendrickson F, Mansell J, et al.: Response of sarcomas of bone and of soft tissue to neutron beam therapy. Int J Radiat Oncol Biol Phys 10:821, 1984

127. Salinas R, Hussey D, Fletcher G, et al.: Experience with fast neutron therapy for locally advanced sarcomas. Int J Radiat Oncol Biol Phys 6:267, 1980

128. Kinsella T, Glatstein E: Clinical experience with intravenous radiosensitizers in unresectable sarcoma. Cancer 59:908, 1987

129. Goepfert H, Lindberg R, Sinkovics J, Ayala A: Soft tissue sarcoma of the head and neck after puberty: Treatment by surgery and postoperative radiation therapy. Arch Otolaryngol 103:365, 1977

130. Abbatucci J, Boulier N, De Ranieri J, et al.: Local control and survival in soft tissue sarcomas of the limbs, trunk walls, and head and neck: A study of 113 cases. Int J Radiat Oncol Biol Phys 12:579, 1986

131. McKenna W, Barnes M, Kinsella T, et al.: Combined modality treatment of adult soft tissue sarcomas of the head and neck. Int J Radiat Oncol Biol Phys 13:1127, 1987

132. Marcus R, Brant T, Mancuso A: Adult mesenchymal tumors presenting in the head and neck. In Million R, Cassisi N (eds): Management of Head and Neck Cancer:

A Multidisciplinary Approach. Philadelphia, J.B. Lippincott, 1994

133. Willers H, Hug E, Spiro I, et al.: Adult soft tissue sarcoma of the head and neck treated by radiation and surgery or radiation alone: Patterns of failure and prognostic factors. Int J Radiat Oncol Biol Phys 32 (suppl 1):290, 1995

134. Holden CA, Spittle MF, Jones EW: Angiosarcoma of the face and scalp, prognosis and treatment. Cancer 59: 1046, 1987

135. Morales P, Lindberg R, Barkley H: Soft tissue angiosarcomas. Int J Radiat Oncol Biol Phys 7:1655, 1981

136. Cody H, Turnbull A, Fortner J, Hajdu S: The continuing challenge of retroperitoneal sarcomas. Cancer 47:2147, 1981

137. Willett C, Suit H, Tepper J, et al.: Intraoperative electron beam radiation therapy for retroperitoneal soft tissue sarcomas. Cancer 68:278, 1991

138. Glenn J, Sindelar W, Kinsella T, et al.: Results of multimodality therapy of resectable soft tissue sarcomas of the retroperitoneum. Surgery 97:316, 1985

139. Tepper J, Suit H, Wood W, et al.: Radiation therapy of retroperitoneal soft tissue sarcoma. Int J Radiat Oncol Biol Phys 10:825, 1984

140. Kinsella T, Sindelar W, Rosenberg S, Glatstein E: Wide excision combined with intraoperative radiation therapy and external beam radiotherapy in retroperitoneal soft tissue tumors. Int J Radiat Oncol Biol Phys 9 (suppl 1):92, 1983

141. Fein D, Corn B, Lanciano R, et al.: Management of retroperitoneal sarcomas: Does dose escalation impact on locoregional control? Int J Radiat Oncol Biol Phys 31:129, 1995

142. Sindelar W, Kinsella T, Chen P, et al.: Intraoperative radiotherapy in retroperitoneal sarcomas: Final results of a prospective, randomized, clinical trial. Arch Surg 128:402, 1993

143. Perez C, Askin F, Baglan R, et al.: Effects of irradiation on mixed mullerian tumors of the uterus. Cancer 43: 1274, 1979

144. Omura G, Blessing J, Major F, et al.: A randomized clinical trial of adjuvant adriamycin in uterine sarcomas: A gynecologic oncology group study. J Clin Oncol 3:1240, 1985

145. Hornback N, Omura G, Major F: Observations on the use of adjuvant radiation therapy in patients with stage I and II uterine sarcoma. Int J Radiat Oncol Biol Phys 12:2127, 1986

146. Salazar O, Bonfiglio T, Patten S, et al.: Uterine sarcomas: Analysis of failure patterns with special emphasis on the use of adjuvant radiation therapy. Cancer 42:1161, 1978

147. Salazar O, Bonfiglio T, Patten S, et al.: Uterine sarcomas: Natural history, treatment, and prognosis. Cancer 42: 1152, 1978

148. Vongtama V, Karlen J, Piver S, et al.: Treatment results and prognostic factors in stage I and II sarcomas of the corpus uteri. Am J Roentgenol 126:139, 1976

149. Disaia P, Castro J, Rutledge F: Mixed mesodermal sarcoma of the uterus. Am J Roentgenol 117:632, 1973

150. Badid A, Vongtama V, Kurohara S, Webster J: Radio-

therapy in the treatment of sarcomas of the corpus uteri. Cancer 24:724, 1969

151. Cohen L: Dose, time, and volume parameters in radiotherapy of Kaposi's sarcoma. Br J Radiol 35:485, 1962

152. Cooper J: The influence of dose on long-term control of classic (non-AIDS associated) Kaposi's sarcoma by radiotherapy. Int J Radiat Oncol Biol Phys 15:1141, 1988

153. Hamilton C, Cummings B, Harwood A: Radiotherapy of Kaposi's sarcoma. Int J Radiat Oncol Biol Phys 12:1931, 1986

154. Nisce L, Safai B, Poussin-Rosillo H: Once weekly total and subtotal skin electron beam therapy for Kaposi's sarcoma. Cancer 47:640, 1981

155. Cooper J, Steinfeld A, Lerch I: Intentions and outcomes in the radiotherapeutic management of epidemic Kaposi's sarcoma. Int J Radiat Oncol Biol Phys 20:419, 1991

156. Cooper J, Fried P: Defining the role of radiation therapy for epidemic Kaposi's sarcoma. Int J Radiat Oncol Biol Phys 13:35, 1987

157. Cooper J, Fried P, Laubenstein L: Initial observations on the effect of radiotherapy on epidemic Kaposi's sarcoma. JAMA 252:934, 1984

158. Berson A, Quivey J, Harris J, Wara W: Radiation therapy for AIDS-related Kaposi's sarcoma. Int J Radiat Oncol Biol Phys 19:569, 1988

159. Chak L, Gill P, Lawrence A, et al.: Radiation therapy for AIDS-related Kaposi's sarcoma. J Clin Oncol 6:863, 1988

160. Maurer H, Beltangady M, Gehan E: The Intergroup Rhabdomyosarcoma Study-I. A final report. Cancer 61:209, 1988

161. Maurer H, Gehan E, Beltganady M: The Intergroup Rhabdomyosarcoma Study-II. Cancer 71:1904, 1993

162. Crist W, Gehan E, Ragab A: The third Intergroup Rhabdomyosarcoma Study. J Clin Oncol 13:610, 1995

163. Tefft M, Wharam M, Ruyman F, et al.: Radiotherapy for rhabdomyosarcoma in children: A report from the Intergroup Rhabdomyosarcoma Study #2 (IRS-2). Proc Am Soc Clin Oncol 4:234, 1985

164. Donaldson S, Asmar L, Breneman J, et al.: Hyperfractionated radiation therapy in children with rhabdomyosarcoma—Results of an intergroup rhabdomyosarcoma pilot study. Int J Radiat Oncol Biol Phys 32:903, 1995

165. Tepper J, Rosenberg S, Glatstein E: Radiation therapy technique in soft tissue sarcomas of the extremity: Policies of treatment at the National Cancer Institute. Int J Radiat Oncol Biol Phys 8:263, 1982

166. Zlotecki R, Parsons J, Marcus R, et al.: Preoperative radiotherapy for adult soft tissue sarcomas. Int J Radiat Oncol Biol Phys 32 (suppl 1):288, 1995

167. Stinson S, Delaney T, Greenberg J, et al.: Acute and long-term effects of limb-function of combined modality

168. Tepper J, Calvo I: Intraoperative radiation therapy. In Perez C, Brady L (eds): Principles and Practice of Radiation Oncology. Philadelphia, J.B. Lippincott, 1992, p 388

169. Modlin J: Capillary hemangioma of the skin. Surgery 38:169, 1955

170. Leibel S, Tranbaugh R, Wara W, et al.: Soft tissue sarcomas of the extremities: Survival and patterns of failure with conservative surgery and postoperative irradiation compared with surgery alone. Cancer 50:1076, 1982

171. Robinson M, Barr L, Fisher C, et al.: Treatment of extremity soft tissue sarcomas with surgery and radiation therapy. Radiother Oncol 18:221, 1990

172. Wood W, Suit H, Mankin H, et al.: Radiation and conservative surgery in the treatment of soft tissue sarcomas. Am J Surg 147:537, 1984

173. Tefft M, Lindberg R, Gehan E: Radiation therapy combined with systemic chemotherapy of rhabdomyosarcoma in children: Local control of patients enrolled in the Intergroup Rhabdomyosarcoma Study. NCI Monogr 56:75, 1981

174. Tefft M, Wharam M, Gehan E: Local and regional control by radiation of rhabdomyosarcoma in IRS-II. Int J Radiat Oncol Biol Phys 15 (suppl 1):159, 1988

175. Jereb B, Cham W, Lattin P, et al.: Local control of embryonal rhabdomyosarcoma in children by radiation therapy when combined with concomitant chemotherapy. Int J Radiat Oncol Biol Phys 1:217, 1976

176. Tefft M, Fernandez C, Donaldson M, et al.: Incidence of meningeal involvement by rhabdomyosarcoma of the head and neck in children: A report of the Intergroup Rhabdomyosarcoma Study (IRS). Cancer 42:253, 1978

177. Gasparini M, Lombardi F, Gianni M, et al.: Questionable role of central nervous system radioprophylaxis in the therapeutic management of childhood rhabdomyosarcoma with meningeal extension. J Clin Oncol 8:1854, 1990

178. Tarbell N, Schwenn N, Delorey M: Extent of bone erosion predicts survival in non-orbital rhabdomyosarcoma of the head and neck in children. Proc Am Soc Clin Oncol 6:41, 1987

179. Wharam M, Bettangady M, Hays D, et al.: Localized orbital rhabdomyosarcoma. Ophthalmology 94:251, 1987

180. Heyn R, Ragab A, Raney B: Late effects of treatment in orbital rhabdomyosarcoma in children: A report from the Intergroup Rhabdomyosarcoma Study. Cancer 57:1738, 1986

181. Raney R, Hayes D, Lawrence W, et al.: Paratesticular rhabdomyosarcoma in childhood. Cancer 42:729, 1978

182. Malogolowkin M, Ortega J: Rhabdomyosarcoma in childhood. Pediatr Ann 17:251, 1988

# 18

# Chemotherapy in the Treatment of Soft Tissue Sarcomas

Soft tissue sarcomas represent a family of at least 20 tumor types arising in connective tissue. The American Cancer Society estimates that approximately 6,000 new cases arise each year.[1] Histologically, they are heterogeneous; however, biologically, they fall in distinct groups with a similar natural history. The most important prognostic factors are the grade and size of the primary tumor. Other prognostic factors that influence the ultimate outcome include extent of disease, depth, and site of the primary tumor. The most common site of metastases for most of these tumors is the pulmonary parenchymal tissue. Resection of pulmonary metastases is clearly an integral part of the management of a patient with metastatic sarcoma. Complete resection of all gross metastatic disease reportedly results in five-year disease-free survival of 10–30 percent. A small fraction of these patients may be cured with this procedure alone; however, for most patients, systemic chemotherapy is the most sound therapeutic approach.[2–5]

## ■ CHEMOTHERAPY STUDIES IN PATIENTS WITH ADVANCED DISEASE

The history of sarcoma chemotherapy dates back to the early 1970s, when doxorubicin (Adriamycin [A]) was introduced as a new experimental chemotherapy agent. Responses to doxorubicin in patients with sarcomas were noted in a number of phase I and broad phase II studies. The Southwest Oncology Group (SWOG) performed a phase II study, including 55 patients with sarcomas, 49 of whom were evaluable. Overall response rate was 31 percent, and complete remission rate was 4 percent.[6] Subsequently, while conducting a dose-response study of single-agent doxorubicin, SWOG duplicated its results in 51 patients, 48 of whom were evaluable. The overall response rate was 31 percent, and the complete remission rate was 2 percent.[7] "Good-risk" patients included in the dose-response study showed a significantly higher response rate in patients treated with 75 mg/m$^2$ (37 percent) than those treated with 45 mg/m$^2$ (18 percent) ($p = 0.05$).

In a broad phase II study of dacarbazine (DTIC), the overall response rate in 53 evaluable patients with sarcomas was 17 percent.[8] Despite this low response rate and the unpleasant nausea and vomiting associated with DTIC administration, Gottlieb added dacarbazine to doxorubicin (ADIC = doxorubicin [Adriamycin] + dacarbazine [DTIC]) and obtained a 42 percent overall response rate and an 11 percent complete remission rate in 218 evaluable patients with sarcomas.[9] Two hundred fifty four patients were entered in this study, and their overall response rate was 36 percent. This represented an improvement over the results achieved with single-agent doxorubicin.

One reason for the success of the regimen was that, because of the predominantly nonmyelosuppressive toxicities of DTIC, doxorubicin could be given at 60 mg/m$^2$ and DTIC at 250 mg/m$^2$ daily for five days in the combination regimen. While histologic diagnoses were not subject to a subsequent pathology review and were certainly incorrect to some extent, an important finding from that study was the relative lack of responsiveness of chondrosarcoma compared with other histologic types. There were no responses in

12 evaluable patients with chondrosarcoma, while the response rate in other histologic types ranged from 33 to 55 percent.

Another critical finding in that study was that patients with primary tumors of the gastrointestinal tract had the lowest response rate of any primary site. Leiomyosarcoma is the predominant histology in the gastrointestinal tract, just as in the uterus and genitourinary tract. Nonetheless, patients with primary gastrointestinal tumors had only a 21 percent response rate, compared with 53 percent for patients with uterine or genitourinary primary tumors. Subsequently, addition of vincristine (VADIC = vincristine + doxorubicin [Adriamycin] + dacarbazine [DTIC]) in the chemotherapy of 107 evaluable patients provided no further improvement in the overall response rate, which was 42 percent, with a complete remission rate of 9 percent.[10]

In a later study involving fewer institutions, cyclophosphamide was added to the regimen to form the familiar CyVADIC regimen.[11] The 136 evaluable patients displayed a 14 percent complete remission rate and a 55 percent overall response rate. Based on these results, SWOG undertook a large randomized study comparing CyVADIC and CyVADACT, the latter of which substituted Actinomycin-D (an agent known to be effective in treating embryonal rhabdomyosarcoma in children) for dacarbazine.[11] The cyclophosphamide, vincristine, and doxorubicin doses were identical in both regimens.

Of 270 patients entered into the CyVADIC regimen, 221 were evaluable; of 261 entered into the CyVADACT regimen, 225 were evaluable. The overall response rates for evaluable patients were 50 percent for CyVADIC, compared with 30 percent for CyVADACT ($p = 0.02$). For all eligible patients, the CyVADIC regimen was also superior, but the response rates were lower: 42 percent for CyVADIC, compared with 34 percent for CyVADACT ($p = 0.07$). Complete response rates did not differ, ranging from 10 to 14 percent.

Because doxorubicin is central to the treatment of patients with sarcomas, a major concern in maximizing doxorubicin administration is its cardiac toxicity. Having demonstrated that cardiac toxicity could be substantially reduced by 96-hour continuous intravenous infusion,[12] we incorporated a continuous infusion schedule into our sarcoma chemotherapy program. The final analysis of the VADIC and ADIC regimens showed no advantage for the addition of vincristine, so we eliminated vincristine except for patients with small cell sarcomas. The resulting regimen, CyADIC, gave cyclophosphamide on day 1 and doxorubicin and DTIC as a four-day infusion. The doxorubicin and DTIC doses were divided and mixed together in a Travenol infusor and given daily for four consecutive days.

Results of that regimen in a pilot study of 51 patients showed a 53 percent overall response rate and a 14 percent complete response rate, equivalent to those seen with rapid infusion of the same drugs.[13]

In a subsequent study conducted by SWOG (which varied only in the schedule of doxorubicin administration), it was confirmed that either continuous or rapid infusion of doxorubicin produced similar results.[14] Response rates in that study were substantially lower than in previous studies, possibly because, after the introduction of computed tomography, many patients previously assessed as having partial response were reclassified into a lesser response category.

Quite some time lapsed before the next active agent for treating soft tissue sarcomas (ifosfamide) was introduced. A number of investigators have studied ifosfamide as a single agent. Antman and colleagues[15] evaluated 124 patients with previously treated sarcomas and obtained a 24 percent response rate, using a dose of 2 g/m$^2$ for four days. In that study, the authors noted a superior response rate when the drug was given for four hours each day, compared to a continuous 24-hour infusion. Patients with soft tissue sarcomas receiving a four-hour infusion had a response rate of 26 percent, compared with 9 percent for continuous infusion ($p = 0.03$).

In a series of four studies involving 232 evaluable patients with sarcomas, we obtained a 15 percent response rate and a 3 percent complete remission rate.[16] Those studies confirmed Antman's observation of a decreased response rate with continuous infusion administration of ifosfamide. When the drug was given by one- or two-hour infusion at a total dose of 8 g/m$^2$, we observed a 14 percent response rate in 44 patients. In contrast, when the drug was given by continuous infusion, only one response (6 percent) in 17 patients was obtained. In addition, our studies demonstrated a dose-response relationship. When administered by one- or two-hour infusion at a total dose of 6 g/m$^2$, the overall response rate was 10 percent; at 8 g/m$^2$, the response rate was 14 percent; and at 10 g/m$^2$, the response rate was 21 percent.

We have also evaluated high-dose ifosfamide (total dose = 14 g/m$^2$) plus granulocyte colony-stimulating factor (G-CSF) as a single-agent salvage therapy in patients whose disease did not respond to previous doxorubicin-based chemotherapy. In a 37-patient phase II study in which high-dose ifosfamide was administered as a continuous infusion after a loading dose, the objective response rate was 17 percent. In a more recent pilot study evaluating the same total dose of ifosfamide, a similar patient population in whom ifosfamide was administered as a 2 g/m$^2$ infusion for two hours every 12 hours for seven doses displayed a response rate of 45 percent.[17] The sample size in this pilot study is only

12, and we plan to expand this to a formal phase II study to test the true activity of high-dose ifosfamide when administered by short infusion.

Bramwell and colleagues compared ifosfamide at 5 g/m$^2$ with cyclophosphamide at 1.5 g/m$^2$, both by 24-hour continuous infusion.[18] In the 68 evaluable patients treated with ifosfamide, the response rate was 18 percent. In the 67 treated with cyclophosphamide, the response rate was 7 percent. Approximately 40 percent of the patients had had previous chemotherapy, and 60 percent were untreated. In the previously untreated patients, the response rate to ifosfamide was 25 percent, compared with 13 percent for patients treated with cyclophosphamide. For previously treated patients, the response to ifosfamide was 7 percent, compared with zero for patients treated with cyclophosphamide. Although the differences were not statistically significant, the investigators concluded correctly that ifosfamide was the superior agent.

The next logical step was the substitution of ifosfamide for cyclophosphamide in the CyADIC regimen to form the so-called MAID regimen (M refers to the uroprotective agent, MESNA, which is used routinely with ifosfamide). In a phase II study reported by Elias and colleagues,[19] the overall response rate in 105 eligible patients was 47 percent, using 7.5 g/m$^2$ of ifosfamide, 60 mg/m$^2$ of doxorubicin, and 900 mg/m$^2$ of DTIC, all given by continuous infusion. Despite the relatively low doses of both doxorubicin and ifosfamide (especially considering their dose-response relationships), this regimen produced substantial myelosuppression, requiring dose reductions in 43 percent of patients after the first cycle. Bramwell and colleagues[20] used ifosfamide at 5 g/m$^2$ as a 24-hour infusion together with 50 mg/m$^2$ of doxorubicin and 850 mg/m$^2$ of DTIC as bolus injections.[20] In 40 patients, they obtained an overall response rate of 25 percent, with a complete remission rate of 5 percent.

A comparison of the two studies indicates the inherent problem with MAID. As with the single agents doxorubicin and ifosfamide, there appears to be a dose-response relationship for the combination. Unfortunately, even the relatively low doses of doxorubicin and ifosfamide used in the Bramwell regimen caused substantial toxicity, requiring dose reductions. A simultaneously conducted intergroup trial compared doxorubicin (60 mg/m$^2$) plus dacarbazine (1,000 mg/m$^2$) to the same drugs and doses plus ifosfamide (7.5 g/m$^2$ at the initiation of the study, later reduced to 6 g/m$^2$) in 340 eligible patients with advanced soft tissue sarcomas. Patients receiving the three-drug regimen achieved a significantly higher response rate (32 percent versus 17 percent; $p < 0.002$) and a longer time to progression (six months versus four months; $p < 0.02$), with significantly more myelosuppression. The survival advantage

for patients receiving doxorubicin + DTIC (12 months versus 13 months; $p = 0.04$) was not significant by multivariate analysis.[21]

The Eastern Cooperative Oncology Group (ECOG) conducted a prospective randomized three-arm trial comparing doxorubicin alone at 80 mg/m$^2$, versus a combination of doxorubicin (60 mg/m$^2$) plus ifosfamide (7.5 g/m$^2$), versus a three-drug regimen (MAP = mitomycin 8 mg/m$^2$ + doxorubicin 40 mg/m$^2$ + cisplatin 60 mg/m$^2$), in 262 assessable patients with advanced soft tissue sarcomas. The objective response rates were 20 percent, 34 percent, and 32 percent, respectively, and the complete response rates were 2 percent, 3 percent, and 7 percent, respectively. The doxorubicin and ifosfamide combination, therefore, resulted in a statistically significant improvement in objective response rate, at the expense of significantly more hematopoietic toxicity and no difference in survival.[22]

The EORTC (European Organisation for Research and Treatment of Cancer) recently reported the results of their randomized phase III study conducted by 35 centers using 663 eligible patients, comparing adriamycin alone at 75 mg/m$^2$ to CyVADIC and doxorubicin (50 mg/m$^2$) plus ifosfamide (5 g/m$^2$). The response rates in the three arms were respectively 23 percent, 28 percent, and 28 percent; the median durations of responses were respectively 46 weeks, 48 weeks, and 44 weeks; and the median survivals were respectively 52 weeks, 51 weeks, and 55 weeks (Table 18–1).[23] Apparently, combining the two most effective drugs in treating soft tissue sarcomas (i.e., adriamycin and ifosfamide) with or without dacarbazine may improve partial response rates without significantly affecting complete response rates and survival. One probable explanation is that, given the overlapping myelosuppressive toxicity, one is forced to compromise the dose-intensity of each of the two most active drugs, thereby defeating the underlying purpose.

Interestingly, an older ECOG study in 200 patients with advanced soft tissue sarcomas randomized to single-agent adriamycin (70 mg/m$^2$) versus adriamycin (50 mg/m$^2$) + vincristine (1.4 mg/m$^2$) versus vincristine (1.4 mg/m$^2$) + actinomycin D (0.4 mg/m$^2$) + cyclophosphamide (750 mg/m$^2$) reported similar results, with response rates of 27 percent with adriamycin alone at 70 mg/m$^2$ dropping off to 19 percent for adriamycin + vincristine, most likely due to the lower dose of adriamycin. The response rate in the third arm including no adriamycin was the lowest, at 11 percent.[24]

In an attempt to increase the dose intensity of the chemotherapy programs, we and others have employed hematopoietic growth factors. Our first study used granulocyte-macrophage colony-stimulating factor (GM-CSF) in combination with the CyADIC regimen.[25] We

**TABLE 18–1. PHASE III STUDIES OF ADRIAMYCIN + IFOSFAMIDE-BASED REGIMENS**

| Group | Regimen* | No. of Patients | CR (percent) | PR (percent) | TTP (Mos.) | MS (Mos.) |
|-------|----------|-----------------|--------------|--------------|------------|-----------|
| SWOG/CALGB | AD | 170 | 2 | 15 | 4 | 12 |
| | AD | 170 | 2 | 30[†] | 6[†] | 13[†] |
| ECOG | AD | 90 | 2 | 18 | — | 9 |
| | AD | 88 | 3 | 31[†] | — | 12 |
| | AD | 84 | 7 | 25 | — | 10 |
| EORTC | AD | 263 | 4 | 17 | 11.5 | 13 |
| | AD | 258 | 5 | 20 | 12 | 12.8 |
| | AD | 142 | 9 | 18 | 11 | 12.8 |

Abbreviations: A, adriamycin; CR, complete response; Cy, cyclophosphamide; D, dacarbazine; I, ifosfamide; M, mitomycin; P, cisplatin; PR, partial remission.
*Total dose of adriamycin = 60 mg/m$^2$; dacarbazine = 1,000 mg/m$^2$.
[†]$p < 0.05$.

were unwilling to go directly to a MAID regimen until we could demonstrate adequate protection from myelo-suppression with CyADIC. This strategy allowed us to maximize the dose of doxorubicin in the CyADIC regimen and subsequently to maximize the dose of ifos-famide as a single-agent salvage regimen.

Initially, our CyADIC regimen, at escalated dox-orubicin and cyclophosphamide doses of 75 mg/m$^2$ and 750 mg/m$^2$, respectively, was administered until patients demonstrated significant myelosuppression (less than 500 granulocytes/mL). Patients then received a 14-day cycle of GM-CSF delivered by continuous intra-venous infusion. After a one-week rest, chemotherapy was resumed on days 1 to 5, and GM-CSF was added on day 8. Although the duration of severe neutropenia was shortened, all patients experienced neutrophil counts below 500/mL, so we compressed the chemotherapy cycle so that doxorubicin and DTIC were infused on days 1 to 2 and cyclophosphamide was given on day 3, with GM-CSF started on day 4. Using that schedule, we were able to eliminate severe neutropenia in some patients and even escalate doxorubicin doses from 75 to 90 mg/m$^2$.

Laboratory studies in conjunction with our clin-ical trial indicated that administration of GM-CSF increased bone marrow cellularity, granulocyte-macro-phage colony-forming units (GM-CFU), and erythro-cyte burst-forming units (BFU-E). Cellularity remained increased for up to one week after cessation of GM-CSF administration; however, within 24 hours of stopping GM-CSF and up to one week later, both GM-CFU and BFU-E decreased below baseline levels. Thus, GM-CSF was able to provide protection by a combination of factors: (1) stimulating existing myeloid elements after chemotherapy; (2) increasing bone marrow re-serve before the next course of chemotherapy; and (3) putting bone marrow precursors into a relative rest-ing state before the next cycle of chemotherapy. Unfor-tunately, we also discovered that, although we could

protect against granulocyte toxicity from chemotherapy with GM-CSF, thrombocytopenia quickly became dose-limiting.

Our next study employed the same chemotherapy regimen but used PIXY 321, a fusion protein incorp-orating the active sites of GM-CSF and interleukin-3 (IL-3), as a growth factor.[26] When administered at therapeutic doses of 500 to 1000 mg/m$^2$/d following CyADIC chemotherapy, PIXY 321 significantly reduced the degree and duration of neutropenia. Additionally, in comparison with our historical control data of CyADIC alone or with GM-CSF, the mean platelet nadir count in cycle 2 was 1.7-fold higher with PIXY 321, sug-gesting attenuation of cumulative multilineage hemato-poietic toxicity of chemotherapy.

Our subsequent study then added PIXY 321 to the MAID regimen to determine whether the addition of this growth factor allowed us to take full advantage of the combination of the three most effective sarcoma-treating drugs in relatively high doses. A formal analysis of this study is pending; however, nonspecific sympto-matic toxicity makes the regimen difficult for patients to tolerate for more than a few courses. We are cur-rently evaluating the combination of adriamycin and ifosfamide at full therapeutic doses of 75 to 90 mg/m$^2$ and 10 g/m$^2$ respectively, without dacarbazine. If in-deed this regimen is more active (as expected), deliver-ing multiple cycles will require growth factor support for all cell lineages, and the availability of thrombopoi-etin in addition to the currently commercially available growth factors will most likely be helpful. While the strategy of dose intensification with growth factor sup-port seems very promising, its ultimate effect on sur-vival is not yet demonstrated.

The enthusiasm seems to have waned for marrow ablative doses of chemotherapy with or without total body radiation followed by autologous bone marrow rescue. The results of the earlier studies performed in the mid-to-late 1980s have been uniformly disappointing, with very short durations of response, extremely high cost, substantial treatment-related morbidity and mortality, and an obvious lack of improvement in survival.[27,28] Among the most apparent reasons seems to be the absence of an effective, cytoreductive regimen with minimal extramedullary toxicities. With the advent of peripheral blood stem cell support, this approach is being revisited. In solid tumors with a relatively low growth fraction, the concept of higher than usual but not quite myeloablative chemotherapy, given on multiple occasions with aliquots of peripheral blood stem cells along with growth factors, is currently being studied. Stem cells may be a safe and effective addition to growth factors in the studies discussed above.

## ADJUVANT CHEMOTHERAPY

The average five-year disease-free survival in patients with localized disease who have undergone surgical excision of the primary tumor is approximately 50 percent, ranging from 28 to 83 percent as reported in several randomized trials (Table 18–2). This number decreases to less than 20 percent for specific histologic types like rhabdomyosarcoma and extraskeletal Ewing's sarcoma because these tumors have a much higher propensity for systemic micrometastases. Rhabdomyo-

sarcoma and Ewing's sarcoma are responsive to chemotherapy, with a resultant survival advantage; therefore, adjuvant chemotherapy is considered standard therapy for these two soft tissue sarcomas.[29,30]

The issue of adjuvant chemotherapy in all other soft tissue sarcomas remains controversial and generates a significant amount of debate and discussion. Over the last 10 to 15 years, several prospective randomized trials have been conducted to evaluate the role of adjuvant chemotherapy in localized soft tissue sarcomas.[31–42] Five of these randomized trials used single-agent adriamycin. One of these five studies, conducted by the investigators at the Rizzoli Institute in Bologna, Italy, reveals a significant improvement in disease-free survival ($p = 0.015$) as of the last report in 1993, at a median follow-up of 106 months; however, the improvement in overall survival reported in earlier reports lost its statistical significance ($p = 0.06$). The other four single-agent adriamycin studies, conducted by the Boston/ECOG, Intergroup, Scandinavian, and UCLA investigators, did not show any statistically significant benefit to the use of adjuvant adriamycin.

Five other randomized adjuvant trials have used adriamycin-based multi-agent chemotherapy. One of these trials, conducted by the group at Fondation Bergonie in a small group of 59 patients, revealed a sig-

## TABLE 18–2. RANDOMIZED ADJUVANT STUDIES OF SOFT TISSUE SARCOMA

| | | SINGLE-AGENT STUDIES | | | | | |
|---|---|---|---|---|---|---|---|
| | | **Median** | | **DFS (percent)** | | **S (percent)** | |
| Group | Regimen | FU (Mos.) | No. of Patients | OBS | CTx | OBS | CTx |
| Scandinavian | A | 40 | 155 | 60 | 62 | 72 | 72 |
| UCLA | A | 28 | 119 | 54 | 58 | 80 | 85 |
| ISTSS[†] | A | 47 | 86 | 54 | 71 | 55 | 65 |
| Rizzoli Institute | A | 106 | 77 | 32 | 56* | $p = 0.06$ | — |
| DFCI/MGH** | A | 75 | 49 | 62 | 74 | 68 | 68 |
| ECOG | A | 105 | 36 | 55 | 68 | 53 | 65 |
| | | MULTI-AGENT STUDIES | | | | | |
| | | **Median** | | **DFS (percent)** | | **S (percent)** | |
| Group | Regimen | FU (Mos.) | No. of Patients | OBS | CTx | OBS | CTx |
| EORTC | CVAD | 80 | 317 | 65 | 81* | 62 | 67 |
| MDA*** | CVAAd | >120 | 43 | 35 | 54* | 35 | 65 |
| NCI-Extremity | ACM | 85 | 67 | 54 | 75* | 60 | 82 |
| Bergonie | CVAD | 52 | 36 | 32 | 81* | 54 | 87* |
| Mayo Clinic | AVDAd | 64 | 52 | 68 | 88 | 82 | 82 |

Abbreviations: A, adriamycin; AD, actinomycin D; C, cyclophosphamide; CTx, chemotherapy; D, DTIC; DFS, disease-free survival; FU, fluorouracil infusion; M, methotrexate, OBS, observation; S, overall survival; V, vincristine.
*$p < 0.05$.
[†]Intergroup Soft Tissue Sarcoma Study
**Dana Farber Cancer Institute/Massachusetts General Hospital
***M.D. Anderson

nificant improvement in overall survival ($p = 0.002$) in favor of the CyVADIC arm. Three of the other four trials, including the ones conducted by the M.D. Anderson Cancer Center, National Cancer Institute (NCI), and EORTC, revealed a statistically significantly better relapse-free survival and numerically superior overall survival in favor of chemotherapy, but these findings fail to attain statistical significance.

The apparent conclusion derived by a casual reader of the above data may well be that adjuvant chemotherapy is not beneficial in soft tissue sarcomas since randomized studies have failed to show a significant survival advantage. Criticisms of the above-mentioned studies include the following: inadequate sample size, inappropriate patient selection due to inclusion of low-risk patients ($T_1$ tumors, low- or intermediate-grade tumors), suboptimal chemotherapy by current standards, and other confounding factors like uncertainties in the timing and actual dose of chemotherapy received, dose-reductions that may not be considered necessary by current standards, and so forth. These criticisms challenge the validity of the apparent conclusion and make the data difficult to interpret. However, a recent report of pooled data from published prospective randomized adjuvant studies reveals a disease-free (68 percent versus 53 percent, $p < 0.00001$) and overall survival advantage (81 percent versus 71 percent, $p = 0.0005$) for adjuvant chemotherapy in soft tissue sarcomas of the extremities.[43]

Given this controversy, the question, Is adjuvant chemotherapy justifiable? is often posed. The question that should be asked is, How can we improve the prognosis and outcome of the high-risk subset? Major deterrents in the use of adjuvant chemotherapy have been the lack of proven benefit and, more important, the toxicity of chemotherapy and the unjustifiable risk to the nonresponding patient population. In the best of circumstances, 50 percent of the patients with soft tissue sarcomas will not respond to standard chemotherapy.

A better approach to this problem would be to use neoadjuvant or primary chemotherapy, which would enable clinicians to identify patients whose disease is responsive so that they could be treated aggressively with some hope of improving the ultimate outcome. Conversely, the nonresponding group of patients could be spared the toxicities of prolonged, ineffective chemotherapy. Also, with continually improving supportive care, the availability of growth factors, and improved antiemetics and antibiotics, the morbidity of chemotherapy is being significantly diminished, making it reasonable and justifiable to treat the high-risk population in a controlled clinical research setting.

Newer data further support the use of chemotherapy in the management of high-risk patients with sarcomas of the extremities. A meta-analysis of individual patient data from all the adjuvant chemotherapy trials noted above indicated significant improvement in metastasis-free survival ($p = 0.003$), and a trend toward improved survival ($p = 0.087$) for all patients randomized to receive chemotherapy.[44] The study differs from that of Zalupski in that patients were included regardless of primary site, leading one to wonder about the results for patients with extremity sarcomas. However, this study has the advantage of updated analysis of individual patient data.

Recently, Frustaci presented preliminary results from the Italian cooperative study that randomized patients with large (>5 cm), high-grade spindle-cell or pleomorphic sarcomas of the extremities to receive or not receive adjuvant chemotherapy with epirubicin, 120 mg/m$^2$ (equivalent to doxorubicin at 80 mg/m$^2$), plus ifosfamide, 9 mg/m$^2$.[45] The study was stopped because of the major benefit in relapse-free survival ($p = 0.001$) and overall survival ($p = 0.007$). The study is important because it is the first to use "modern" dose-intensive chemotherapy for soft tissue sarcomas in the adjuvant setting and because it is so strongly positive.

## CHEMOTHERAPY FOR LOW- AND INTERMEDIATE-GRADE TUMORS

Desmoid tumors are locally aggressive neoplasms with no metastatic potential and no tendency to dedifferentiate. The vast majority of them are cured with local therapy consisting of surgery with or without radiation therapy. In select situations, they present as huge primaries requiring surgical procedures that may impose significant functional limitations, or they present as part of Gardner's syndrome, with mesenteric fibromatosis encasing the mesenteric vasculature. In these cases, chemotherapy has been shown to be effective in cytoreduction, enabling less radical surgical procedures.[46–47]

Our experience at the M.D. Anderson Cancer Center has been with doxorubicin- and dacarbazine-based chemotherapy. Durable objective remissions were observed in six of nine evaluable patients. Two other patients, who were evaluated only by physical examination, also achieved tumor reduction, enabling resection of previously deemed unresectable tumors in the axilla and pelvis, respectively. Hormonal therapy with tamoxifen, toremifene (a triphenylethylene derivative chemically related to tamoxifen), or progesterone has been reported to be effective in desmoid tumors.[48–50] The precise response rates are unclear due to small numbers and varying definitions of response used by the reporting investigators; however, the true objective response rates seem to be in the neighborhood of 20 to 25 percent, with a similar proportion of patients experiencing subjective improvement in symptoms and performance status without an objective response on radiographic studies. Data from a multi-institutional trial of toremifene in desmoid tumors conducted in the United States is pending formal analysis.

Unlike desmoid tumors, intermediate-grade tumors, like myxoid liposarcoma, myxoid malignant fibrous histiocytoma, and extraskeletal myxoid chondrosarcoma, have definite metastatic potential. Fortunately, they tend to be indolent, with a long natural history. Myxoid liposarcoma and malignant fibrous histiocytoma respond to standard doxorubicin-based chemotherapy similar to other soft tissue sarcomas. In reviewing our experience with doxorubicin- and dacarbazine-based chemotherapy in myxoid liposarcoma in a cohort of 21 patients seen over a five-year period, we found the response rate to be 44 percent.[51] A similar review of our experience with doxorubicin- and dacarbazine-based chemotherapy in myxoid malignant fibrous histiocytoma revealed a response rate of 27 percent.[52] Extraskeletal myxoid chondrosarcoma, on the other hand, like skeletal chondrosarcoma, seems to be refractory to standard soft tissue sarcoma chemotherapy.[53]

## ■ BIOLOGIC THERAPY

Limited information is available on the role of biologic therapy in soft tissue sarcomas. The M.D. Anderson Cancer Center conducted a phase II study of alpha-interferon 2-β in 30 patients with chemotherapy-refractory soft tissue sarcomas.[54] α-interferon 2-β was administered subcutaneously at a dose of 10 mU/m$^2$ three times a week. Two patients achieved a partial response. Given the anti-angiogenesis effects of interferon, we tried this regimen in 24 patients with leiomyosarcomas, resulting in only one partial response. Our ongoing study of interferon and cis-retinoic acid in indolent angiosarcomas has shown a definite effect of the regimen. We also studied the combination of 5-fluorouracil infusion (750 mg/m$^2$ over 24 hours × 5 days) and interferon (5 mU/m$^2$ subcutaneously days 1 to 6) repeated every 2 to 3 weeks in 28 evaluable chemotherapy-refractory sarcomas; we observed no objective responses.[55]

The more recent use of biologic agents in soft tissue sarcomas has been in the form of hyperthermic isolation limb perfusion. Eggermont et al.[56] treated 16 patients with unresectable or recurrent extremity soft tissue sarcomas with tumor necrosis factor, gamma interferon, and melphalan. Six patients achieved a complete remission, and five patients achieved a partial response, enabling limb-sparing surgery in most patients. This is clearly an effective treatment for local

extirpation of the tumor with minimal functional compromise but no systemic effect. (See pages 569–570, Chapter 19 for a detailed description.)

In summary, researchers continue to try to improve the quality and quantity of responses of soft tissue sarcomas to chemotherapy. These efforts have become more feasible with the availability of various growth factors, such as G-CSF, GM-CSF, and erythropoietin. The availability of thrombopoietin for clinical trials (anticipated in the near future) should help significantly with the dose-limiting thrombocytopenia and improve the ability to maintain dose-intensity. In a tumor where the two most effective drugs (i.e., adriamycin and ifosfamide) have a steep dose-response curve, full therapeutic doses of both these drugs given concomitantly should improve the frequency and quality of responses. If indeed this is accomplished, adjuvant therapy issues will have to be reinvestigated with the use of modern chemotherapy in a multi-institutional study with a large enough number of appropriately selected patients to resolve the long-lived controversy of chemotherapy's role and effectiveness in management of soft tissue sarcomas. While current areas of research support, including dose intensification with growth factor, seem quite promising, identification of newer, more effective drugs offers the best hope for future benefit. Patients should be encouraged to participate in research protocols designed to help answer relevant questions in order to deter an otherwise lethal problem.

## REFERENCES

1. Wingo PA, Tong T, Bolden S: Cancer statistics. CA J Clin 45:12, 1995
2. Putnam JG Jr., Roth JA, Wesley MN, et al.: Analysis of prognostic factors in patients undergoing resection of pulmonary metastasis from soft tissues sarcomas. J Thorac Cardiovasc Surg 87:260, 1984
3. Joseph WL, Morton DL, Adkins PC: Prognostic significance of tumor doubling time and evaluating operability in pulmonary metastatic disease. J Thorac Cardiovasc Surg 61:23, 1971
4. Roth JA, Putnam JB, Wesley MN: Deferring determinants of prognosis following resection of pulmonary metastasis from osteogenetic and soft tissue sarcoma patients. Cancer 55:1361, 1985
5. Creagan ET, Fleming TR, Edmonson JH, et al.: Pulmonary resection for metastatic non-osteogenic sarcoma. Cancer 44:1908, 1979
6. O'Bryan RM, Luce JK, Talley RW, et al.: Phase II evaluation of adriamycin in human neoplasia. Cancer 32:1, 1973
7. O'Bryan R, Baker L, Gottlieb J, et al.: Dose-response evaluation of adriamycin in human neoplasia. Cancer 39:1940, 1977
8. Gottlieb J, Benjamin R, Baker L, et al.: Role of DTIC

(NSC 45388) in the chemotherapy of sarcomas. Cancer Treat Rep 60:199, 1976

9. Gottlieb J, Baker L, Quagliana J, et al.: Chemotherapy of sarcomas with a combination of adriamycin and dimethyl triazeno imidazole carboxamide. Cancer 30:1632, 1972

10. Gottlieb JA, Baker LH, O'Bryan RM, et al.: Adriamycin (NSC-123127) used alone and in combination for soft tissue and bony sarcomas. Cancer Chemother Rep 6:271, 1975

11. Benjamin R, Baker L, Rodriquez V, et al.: The chemotherapy of soft tissue sarcomas in adults. In Martin RG, Ayala AG (eds): Management of Primary Bone and Soft Tissue Tumors. Chicago, Year Book Medical Publishers, p 309, 1977

12. Legha S, Benjamin R, Mackay B, et al.: Reduction of doxorubicin cardiotoxicity by prolonged continuous intravenous infusion. Ann Intern Med 96:133, 1982

13. Benjamin R, Yap B: Infusion chemotherapy for soft tissue sarcomas. In Baker L (ed): Soft Tissue Sarcoma. The Hague, Martinus Nijhoff, p 109, 1983

14. Zalupski M, Metch B, Balcerzak S, et al.: Phase III comparison of doxorubicin and dacarbazine given by bolus versus infusion in patients with soft-tissue sarcomas: A Southwest Oncology Group Study. J Natl Cancer Inst 83: 926, 1991

15. Antman KH, Ryan L, Elias A, et al.: Response to ifosfamide and mesna: 124 previously treated patients with metastatic or unresectable sarcoma. J Clin Oncol 7:126, 1989

16. Benjamin RS, Legha SS, Patel SR, Nicaise C: Single-agent ifosfamide studies in sarcomas of soft tissue and bone: The M. D. Anderson Experience. Cancer Chemother Pharmacol 31(2):S174, 1993

17. Patel SR, Hays C, Papadopoulos NE, et al.: Pilot study of high-dose ifosfamide + G-CSF in patients with bone and soft-tissue sarcomas. Proc Am Soc Clin Oncol (abstr) 14:516, 1995

18. Bramwell V, Mouridsen H, Santoro A, et al.: Cyclophosphamide versus ifosfamide: Final report of a randomized phase II trial in adult soft tissue sarcomas. Eur J Cancer Clin Oncol 23:311, 1987

19. Elias A, Ryan L, Sulkes A, et al.: Response to mesna, doxorubicin, ifosfamide, and dacarbazine in 108 patients with metastatic or unresectable sarcoma and no prior chemotherapy. J Clin Oncol 7:1208, 1989

20. Bramwell V, Quirt I, Warr D, et al.: Combination chemotherapy with doxorubicin, dacarbazine, and ifosfamide in advanced adult soft tissue sarcoma. J Natl Cancer Inst 81:1496, 1989

21. Antman KH, Crowley J, Balcerzak SP, et al.: An intergroup phase III randomized study of doxorubicin and dacarbazine with or without ifosfamide and mesna in advanced soft tissue and bone sarcomas. J Clin Oncol 11: 1276, 1993

22. Edmonson JH, Ryan LM, Blum RH, et al.: Randomized comparison of doxorubicin alone versus ifosfamide plus doxorubicin or mitomycin, doxorubicin and cisplatin against soft tissue sarcomas. J Clin Oncol 11:1269, 1993

23. Santoro A, Tursz T, Mouridsen H, et al.: Doxorubicin vs. CyVADIC vs. doxorubicin plus ifosfamide in first-line treatment of advanced soft-tissue sarcomas: A randomized study of the EORTC soft-tissue and bone sarcoma group. J Clin Oncol 13:1537, 1995

24. Schoenfeld DA, Rosenbaum C, Horton J, et al.: A comparison of adriamycin versus vincristine and adriamycin, versus vincristine, actinomycin-D and cyclophosphamide for advanced sarcoma. Cancer 50:2757, 1982

25. Vadhan-Raj S, Broxmeyer H, Hittelman W, et al.: Abrogating chemotherapy-induced myelosuppression by recombinant granulocyte-macrophage colony-stimulating factor in patients with sarcoma: Protection at the progenitor cell level. J Clin Oncol 10:1266, 1992

26. Vadhan-Raj S, Papadopoulos NE, Burgess M, et al.: Effects of PIXY 321, a granulocyte-macrophage colony-stimulating factor/Interleukin-3 fusion protein, on chemotherapy-induced multilineage myelosuppression in patients with sarcoma. J Clin Oncol 12:715, 1994

27. Cheson BD, Lacerna L, Leyland-Jones B, et al.: Autologous bone marrow transplantation current status in future directions. Ann Intern Med 110:51, 1989

28. Antman K, Paul Eder J, Frei E: High-dose chemotherapy with bone marrow support for solid tumors. Important Adv Oncol 221, 1987

29. Razek A, Perez C, Tefft M, et al.: Local control related to radiation dose, volume and site of primary lesion in Ewing's sarcoma. Cancer 46:516, 1980

30. Maurer HM, Beltangady M, Gehan EA, et al.: The Intergroup Rhabdomyosarcoma Study I. A final report. Cancer 61:209, 1988

31. Bramwell V, Rouesse J, Steward W, et al.: European experience of adjuvant chemotherapy for soft-tissue sarcoma: Interim report of a randomized trial of CyVADIC versus control. In Ryan JR, Baker LH (eds): Recent Concepts in Sarcoma Treatment. Dordrecht, Netherlands: Kluwer Academic, 1988, p 157

32. Ravaud A, Nguyen BB, Coindre JM, et al.: Adjuvant chemotherapy with CyVADIC in high-risk soft tissue sarcoma: a randomized prospective trial. In Salmon SE (ed): Adjuvant Therapy of Cancer, vol. VI. Philadelphia, WB Saunders, 1990, p 556

33. Benjamin RS, Terjanian TO, Fenoglio CJ, et al.: The importance of combination chemotherapy for adjuvant treatment of high-risk patients with soft-tissue sarcomas of the extremities. In Salmon SE (ed): Adjuvant Therapy of Cancer, vol. V. Orlando, Grune & Stratton, 1987, p 735

34. Chang A, Kinsella T, Glatstein E, et al.: Adjuvant chemotherapy for patients with high-grade soft-tissue sarcomas of the extremity. J Clin Oncol 6:1491, 1988

35. Edmonson JH, Flemming TR, Ivins JC Jr., et al.: Randomized study of systemic chemotherapy following complete excision of non-osseous sarcomas. J Clin Oncol 2: 1390, 1984

36. Omura GA, Major FJ, Blessing JA, et al.: A randomized clinical trial of adjuvant Adriamycin in uterine sarcomas: A GOG study. J Clin Oncol 3:1240, 1985

37. Alvegard TA, Sigurdsson H, Mouridsen H, et al.: Adjuvant chemotherapy with doxorubicin in high-grade soft-tissue sarcoma: A randomized trial of the Scandinavian Sarcoma Group. J Clin Oncol 7:1504, 1989

38. Eilber FR, Giuliano AE, Huth JF, et al.: Adjuvant adria-

mycin in high-grade extremity soft-tissue sarcomas—A randomized prospective trial. Proc Am Soc Clin Oncol 5:488, 1986

39. Picci P, Bacci G, Gherlinzoni F, et al.: Results of a randomized trial for the treatment of localized soft-tissue tumors of the extremities in adult patients. In Ryan JR, Baker LH (eds): Recent Concepts in Sarcoma Treatment. Dordrecht, Netherlands: Kluwer Academic, 1988, p 144

40. Gherlinzoni F, Bacci G, Picci P, et al.: A randomized trial for the treatment of high-grade soft-tissue sarcomas of the extremities: preliminary observations. J Clin Oncol 4:552, 1986

41. Antman K, Ryan L, Borden E, et al.: Pooled results from three randomized adjuvant studies of doxorubicin versus observation in soft-tissue sarcomas: 10-year results and review of the literature. In Salmon SE (ed): Adjuvant Therapy of Cancer, vol. VI. Philadelphia, WB Saunders, 1990, p 529

42. Antman KH, Amato D, Lerner H, et al.: ECOG and Dana Farber Cancer Institute/MGH Study. In Salmon SE (ed): Adjuvant Therapy of Cancer, vol. V. Orlando, Grune & Stratton, 1984, p 611

43. Zalupski M, Ryan J, Hussein M, et al.: Defining the role of adjuvant chemotherapy for patients with soft-tissue sarcoma of the extremities. In Salmon SE (ed): Adjuvant therapy of Cancer, vol. VII. Philadelphia, JB Lippincott, 1993, p 385

44. Tierney J: A meta-analysis using individual patient data from randomised clinical trial (RCTS) of adjuvant chemotherapy for soft tissue sarcomas (STS). J Clin Oncol 14:1751, 1997

45. Frustaci S, Gherlinzoni F, DePaoli A, et al.: Preliminary results of an adjuvant randomized trial in high risk extremity soft tissue sarcomas (STS): The interim analysis. Proc Am Soc Clin Oncol 1997, p 469a

46. Patel SR, Evans HL, Benjamin RS: Combination chemotherapy in adult desmoid tumors. Cancer 72:3244, 1993

47. Weiss AJ, Lackman RD: Low-dose chemotherapy of desmoid tumors. Cancer 64:1192, 1989

48. Brooks MD, Ebbs SR, Colletta AA, Baum M: Desmoid tumors treated with Triphenylethylenes. Eur J Cancer 28A:1014, 1992

49. Kinzbrunner B, Ritter S, Domingo J, Rosenthal CJ: Remission of rapidly growing Desmoid tumors after tamoxifen therapy. Cancer 52:2201, 1983

50. Lanari A: Effect of progesterone in Desmoid tumors (aggressive fibromatosis). N Engl J Med 309:1523, 1983

51. Patel SR, Burgess MA, Plager C, et al.: Myxoid Liposarcoma—Experience with chemotherapy. Cancer 74:1265, 1994

52. Patel SR, Plager C, Papadopoulos N, et al.: Myxoid malignant fibrous histiocytoma—Experience with chemotherapy. Am J Clin Oncol 18:528, 1995

53. Patel SR, Burgess MA, Papadopoulos N, et al.: Extraskeletal myxoid chondrosarcoma—Long-term experience with chemotherapy. Am J Clin Oncol 18(2):161, 1995

54. Salem P, Benjamin RS, Howard J, et al.: Phase II trial of recombinant interferon alpha-2-b in the treatment of advanced metastatic and refractory sarcomas. Proc Am Assoc Cancer Res 33:200, 1991

55. Plager C, Howard J, Papadopoulos NEJ, et al.: A phase II study of 5-fluorouracil infusion, and interferon alpha in metastatic sarcomas. Proc Am Assoc Cancer Res (abstr) 33:229, 1992

56. Eggermont AMM, Lienard D, Schraffordt K, et al.: Limb salvage by high-dose TNF-alpha, interferon-gamma and melphalan isolated limb perfusion in patients with irresectable soft-tissue sarcomas. Proc Am Soc Clin Oncol (abstr) 11:412, 1992

# 19

# Combined Modality Treatment

The management of malignant mesenchymal tumors has undergone considerable change in recent years. The hitherto accepted dictum of radical operation or radical radiation therapy is no longer considered the prima facie mode of treatment; rather, the guiding principle has become judicious conservatism, with the appropriate combination of surgery and radiation therapy for managing the primary tumors and chemotherapy for eradication of micrometastases.[1–11] Because most sarcomas arise in the extremities (especially the lower extremity), multimodal treatment with sparing of the affected limb has become the goal in the management of extremity soft tissue sarcomas. Although this multimodal treatment program is highly desirable, its proper role must be established, and our enthusiasm, which is sometimes unwarranted, should not cloud good clinical judgment.

To gain a proper perspective on the evolution of combined modality treatment therapy, let us trace the history of the development of each individual form of treatment used to manage soft tissue sarcomas. In this evolutionary scale, surgical treatment was the first form used.

## ■ SURGERY

The established practice of radical surgery was based on the poor results of limited local excision of primary tumors.[12–17] Analysis of the data generated by various authors[12–14,16,18,19] showed that the more radical the excision of the primary tumor, the lower the incidence of local recurrence.[12,15,18,19] Abbas et al.[12] found that

the incidence of local recurrence was 65 percent after limited local excision, 36 percent after wide resection, and 8 percent after amputation. Based on these and other historic observations, the concept of major amputation for control of primary soft tissue sarcomas of the extremities was derived.[12–15,17–19] Because the lower extremity is the most common site for adult soft tissue sarcomas, the proper treatment of these tumors has generated the highest amount of controversy. In 1975, Shiu et al.[17] stated that major amputation or disarticulation offers the surest means of eradication of a soft tissue sarcoma in terms of obtaining the widest margin of resection. In their retrospective series from Memorial Sloan-Kettering Cancer Center, they found the incidence of local recurrence after resection to be 28 percent, but after amputation only 7 percent.[17]

Our results at the University of Illinois were also similar (i.e., 8 percent after a major amputation).[20] However, in recent years, we have observed that better control of local recurrence frequently does not translate into prolonged life or increased disease-free survival. In fact, in a more recent publication from Memorial Sloan-Kettering Cancer Center, Willard and his associates[21] also made a similar observation.

It appears, therefore, that judiciously applied regional surgical treatment in itself can bring the incidence of local recurrence down to an acceptable minimum (for details, see Chapter 16 on surgical techniques). However, the factors that influence distant dissemination include the size, histologic type, grade, and several other biologic factors. Furthermore, local control of the primary tumor in itself is not synonymous with control of metastases.[22] It has become clear, at least in sarcomas of the extremities, that, although amputation is a useful mode of treatment, it cannot be equated with cure; hence, an alternative form of management, with preservation of a functional limb, is the goal of modern treatment strategies for extremity sarcomas.

# ■ RADIOTHERAPY

Clinical trials of radiation therapy as a primary treatment of soft tissue sarcomas have in the past been disappointing, with local tumor control achieved in fewer than 5 percent of patients.[23,24] However, with advances in technology, sufficient numbers of soft tissue sarcoma patients have been treated, and results have been encouraging enough to warrant optimism (for details, see Chapter 17 on Radiation Therapy). There is now adequate clinical experience to state that radiation therapy controls certain forms of primary soft tissue sarcomas.[4,23,24] Preoperative irradiation appears to sterilize well-oxygenated tumor cells located on the periphery of the neoplasm, thereby rendering the tumor more amenable to wide excision alone. It is now generally accepted that this type of conservative operation combined with radiation therapy at radical dose levels can control most primary sarcomas and avoid a deformity or loss of limb.

The concept has evolved that microscopic tumors can be controlled with doses of radiation that allow good cosmetic and functional results, thereby avoiding disabling operations. This is founded on the biological principle that effective "log kill" of well-oxygenated microscopic tumor can be achieved using radiation dose, such as 4,500 to 5,000 cGy. *The problem of radiation resistance by hypoxic tumor cells at the center of the mass is circumvented by subsequent resection.*

Based on this operational hypothesis, Suit et al.[25] described the Massachusetts General Hospital experience with 36 soft tissue sarcoma patients who were treated by *preoperative* radiation therapy followed by conservative surgery. In 33 of these patients, the tumors were greater than 5 cm. The radiation dose was 5,000 to 6,000 cGy (200 cGy, five times per week), followed in approximately three weeks by conservative excision; a booster dose to the tumor bed was given intraoperatively or postoperatively. Local control was achieved in 31 of 33 patients (follow-up periods ranged from three months to eight years). Although this was an uncontrolled and inconclusive study, it pointed out the need for further investigation of the role of preoperative radiation therapy.

Simultaneously with Suit et al.,[25] Lindberg et al.[26] described the beneficial role of *postoperative* radiation therapy for 300 patients treated at the M.D. Anderson

Cancer Center. These authors reported absolute two- and five-year survival rates of 74 percent and 61 percent, respectively, and an overall local recurrence rate of 22 percent. Lindberg et al.[26] emphasized that radical-dose radiation therapy after conservative local excision was as effective as radical surgery (i.e., major amputation). However, positive margins (both gross and microscopic involvement), which are usually encountered with limited excision, are generally recognized to be associated with increased local recurrence in spite of all the advances made in the technique(s) of radiation therapy.[27,28] Therefore, the acceptable minimum indicated in managing these malignant mesenchymal tumors must be a radical soft tissue resection along with currently available radical radiation therapy methods.

# ■ CHEMOTHERAPY

Despite reasonable control of local disease, distant metastases are common in most high-grade soft tissue sarcomas. The most commonly used chemotherapeutic agents in soft tissues sarcomas before 1970 were cyclophosphamide, actinomycin D, and vincristine, given alone or in combination. In 1970, Jacobs[29] reviewed several individual series and found that 56 of 238 patients (23.5 percent) showed an objective response to these drugs. However, when the childhood cases of rhabdomyosarcoma were eliminated, the response rate was found to be only 18 percent (32 of 179 cases), and only a small number of long-term remissions was reported.

In 1969, DiMarco et al.[30] reported encouraging results in initial trials treating soft tissue sarcomas with Adriamycin (doxorubicin). These data were later confirmed by Benjamin et al.[31] in 1973. Definite activity was also noted during the initial investigations with 5-(3,3-dimethyl-1-triazeno)imidazole-4-carboxamide (DTIC), a synthetic congener of the naturally occurring purine precursors 5- (or 4-)-aminoimidazole 4-(or 5)-carboxamide.[32] During initial single-agent trials with either Adriamycin or DTIC, most centers achieved response rates of 29 percent and 15 percent, respectively.[33] Gottlieb et al.[33,34] later found that DTIC lengthened duration of remission. In 1974, they reported that a combination of Adriamycin and DTIC in 200 evaluable patients with all types of soft tissue and bone sarcomas resulted in 22 complete responses and 63 partial responses (overall rate = 42.5 percent).

A review of currently published data shows that doxorubicin is central to the treatment of adults with metastatic soft tissues sarcomas. However, the limiting factor in using doxorubicin is its cardiac toxicity. The extent of cardiac toxicity was reduced by using 96-hour continuous intravenous infusions,[35] and this became more or less a standard form of administration of doxorubicin.[35] Based on data generated from a number of studies, vincristine was excluded from the multi-agent chemotherapy regimen(s) (see Chapter 18 for details). Thus, until recently, the most effective regimen was CyADIC (cyclophosphamide, Adriamycin, and DTIC). Quite some time passed before the next active agent, ifosfamide, was introduced. This agent singly was extensively studied by Antman and colleagues[1] and Legha and his colleagues.[35] Once the efficacy was established, the next step was to compare the relative efficacy of ifosfamide and cyclophosphamide.[35] Having established a response rate for ifosfamide of 25 percent compared to 13 percent for cyclophosphamide, it was only a matter of time until ifosfamide replaced cyclophosphamide in the CyADIC regimen. Thus, the MAID (M referring to the uroprotective agent MESNA) regimen has come into current popularity. For a detailed discussion of this and other regimens, see Chapter 18.

## ■ COMBINED MODALITIES

As has already been mentioned, in adults, the lower extremity is the most frequent site of development of soft tissue sarcomas, followed by the upper extremity; therefore, an important consideration in managing soft tissue sarcomas is the attempt to salvage a limb by using all three methods of treatment described above. In these anatomical sites, combining all three treatment modes has become the major objective. Several authors have obtained data suggesting that combined modality treatment can indeed salvage a tumor-bearing limb without jeopardizing the disease-free interval. In 1976, Morton et al.[16] reported that multimodal management of extremity skeletal and soft tissue sarcomas with preoperative Adriamycin and radiation therapy, radical resection, and postoperative chemotherapy or chemo-immunotherapy, resulted in preservation of a functional extremity in 13 of 14 patients. The disease-free interval varied between 4 and 34 months. These authors concluded that the results of the combined modality approach were significantly better than those obtained by one method alone.

Rosenberg et al.[36] reported the results of their prospective randomized study of 43 adults with extremity soft tissues sarcomas. The study was conducted as follows. Between May 1975 and April 1983, 43 adult patients with high-grade soft tissue sarcomas of the extremities were assigned randomly to receive either amputation at or above the joint proximal to the tumor, including all involved muscle groups, or to receive a limb-sparing resection plus adjuvant radiation therapy. The limb-sparing resection group received wide local excision followed by 5,000 cGy to the entire anatomical area at risk of local spread and 6,000 to 7,000 cGy to the tumor bed. Both randomization groups received postoperative chemotherapy with doxorubicin (maximum cumulative dose 550 mg/m$^2$), cyclophosphamide, and high-dose methotrexate. Twenty-seven patients were assigned randomly to receive limb-sparing resection and radiotherapy, whereas 16 had amputation only (randomization was 2:1). There were four local recurrences in the limb-sparing group and none in the amputation group ($p = 0.06$, generalized Wilcoxon test). However, there were no differences between the limb-sparing group and the amputation treatment groups in either the disease-free survival rate (71 percent and 75 percent at 5 years; $p = 0.75$) or overall survival rate (83 percent and 88 percent at 5 years; $p = 0.99$). Multivariate analysis indicated that the only correlate of local recurrence was the final margin of resection. Patients with positive margins of resection were more likely to recur locally than those with negative margins ($p < 0.0001$), even when postoperative radiotherapy was used.

The simultaneous prospective randomized study by these investigators[36] of postoperative chemotherapy in 65 patients with high-grade soft tissue sarcoma of the extremities revealed better results in those receiving chemotherapy than in those who did not, in both three-year continuous disease-free rates (92 percent versus 60 percent; $p = 0.0008$) and in overall survival (95 percent versus 74 percent; $p = 0.04$). The authors concluded that the combination of limb-sparing surgery, radiation therapy, and adjuvant chemotherapy was successful as treatment in most adult patients with soft tissue sarcomas of the extremity.

We conducted a similar study at the University of Illinois.[37,38] A total of 55 patients with extremity soft tissue sarcoma were entered into the protocol. All patients were evaluated in the Department of Surgical Oncology at the University of Illinois. The number of patients in the protocol represented approximately 10 percent of the extremity soft tissue sarcoma seen by the Department from 1978–1991. The gender distribution of the 55 adult patients with soft tissue sarcoma who were enrolled in the protocol was 26 men and 29 women. The average age was 47 years (range, 17 to 79 years). The soft tissue sarcomas were located as follows: upper extremity, 11 patients; lower extremity, 40 patients; and buttock, 4 patients. The histologic diagnosis and grades of the soft tissue sarcomas are shown in Table 19–1.

The patients received identical preoperative regimens of intra-arterial doxorubicin with concomitant radiation.[37] An arterial catheter was inserted using the Seldinger technique, and its position was confirmed with arteriography. An infusion of doxoru-

**TABLE 19–1. HISTOLOGIC DIAGNOSES AND GRADES***

| Cell Type | Grade 1 | Grade 2 | Grade 3 | Total |
|---|---|---|---|---|
| Malignant fibrous histiocytoma | 1 | 2 | 12 | 17[†] |
| Synovial cell sarcoma | 1 | 6 | 1 | 9[†] |
| Rhabdomyosarcoma | — | — | 8 | 8 |
| Liposarcoma | 3 | 1 | 1 | 5 |
| Hemangiopericytoma | 2 | 2 | 1 | 5 |
| Leiomyosarcoma | — | 1 | 2 | 3 |
| Extraskeletal sarcoma | — | 1 | 2 | 3 |
| Other | — | — | 5 | 5 |
| Total | 7 | 13 | 32 | 55[†] |

*Histologic diagnosis by stage and grade. The cell types listed in the category "other" consisted of one each of lymphangiosarcoma, malignant schwannoma, epithelioid sarcoma, and clear cell sarcoma.
[†]Three patients' original slides were unavailable for grading: two had malignant fibrous histiocytomas, and one had a synovial cell sarcoma.

bicin ($10/m^2/d$) in heparinized saline was administered for 10 days. Within 24 hours of the infusion, radiation therapy was begun, with either a cobalt-60 teletherapy unit or a 6-MeV linear accelerator. The treated volume encompassed the entire muscle compartment from its origin to its insertion, sparing at least a 2-cm strip of normal tissue. Parallel opposed anterior-posterior or lateral fields were used. A total preoperative dose of 25 cGy was given in 10 daily fractions over two weeks.

One to six weeks after the concomitant chemoradiation therapy, all patients underwent resection. Wide en bloc resections of the tumor masses were performed in each case.[38,39]

After operation, the patients whose margins were considered close received additional radiation therapy, which was begun three weeks postoperatively and was administered in 1.8-Gy daily fractions five days per week. The additional postoperative radiation dose was determined by the time-dose fractionation tables described previously,[40] to compensate for the interruption of radiation therapy necessitated by surgery.

After patients completed radiation therapy, adjuvant chemotherapy was administered. Those receiving chemotherapy before 1984 were treated with cycles of doxorubicin ($60$ mg/$m^2$) and dacarbazine ($1.0$ g/$m^2$), the details of which have been reported previously.[18] Patients treated after 1984 received doxorubicin ($50$ mg/$m^2$) and dacarbazine ($1.25$ mg/$m^2$), with or without the addition of vincristine ($3$ mg/$m^2$) and/or cyclophosphamide ($500$ mg/$m^2$). Hematopoietic toxicity was mild and was found in five patients (9 percent), with stomatitis in two (4 percent) and severe skin reactions in three (5 percent).

All patients were followed monthly for the first year after treatment. Thereafter, the follow-up was less frequent, with a minimum of biannual consultations after five years of disease-free survival. The overall and disease-free survival rates were computed according to the method of Kaplan and Meier.[41] Staging was completed as set forth in the manual prepared by the American Joint Committee on Cancer.[42] No patient with a stage 1 lesion required an amputation; 13 patients (27 percent) with stage II tumors eventually underwent amputation. The stages of the tumors and the distribution of the amputations are shown in Table 19–2. A total of 14 patients (25 percent) experienced some treatment-related toxicity. The median follow-up among survivors was 97 months.

The overall and disease-free survival curves are shown in Figure 19–1. The overall and disease-free survival rates at five years were 69 percent and 51 percent, respectively. Those at 10 years were 65 percent and 42 percent, respectively. Of the deaths from disease, 66 percent occurred within the first two years of follow-up and 90 percent within the first five years. The longest disease-free interval was 8.5 years. The grade of the tumor significantly affected survival; patients with grade 1 lesions had no disease-related mortality. The five-year survival rates of patients with grades 2 and 3 soft tissue sarcomas were statistically similar: 69 percent and 61 percent, respectively. Twenty-nine patients are currently free of disease.

The ultimate limb-salvage rate was 81 percent. Furthermore, the overall survival rates between patients undergoing amputation and those not requiring amputation did not differ significantly (64 percent versus 68 percent). However, the disease-free survival rate at five years was significantly shorter in patients requiring amputation (24 percent versus 58 percent; $p = 0.0113$).[38]

The local in-field failure rate was 15 percent (eight patients). One patient had an isolated, out-of-field nodal failure and is currently free of disease three years

**TABLE 19–2. STAGE AND LIMB LOSS***

| Stage | No. of Patients | Amputation |
|---|---|---|
| IA | 1 | 0 |
| IB | 6 | 2 |
| IIA | 5 | 0 |
| IIB | 8 | 2 |
| IIIA | 5 | 0 |
| IIIB | 24 | 6 |
| IVA | 1 | 0 |
| IVB | 2 | 0 |

*Distribution by stage[42] and the number requiring amputation.

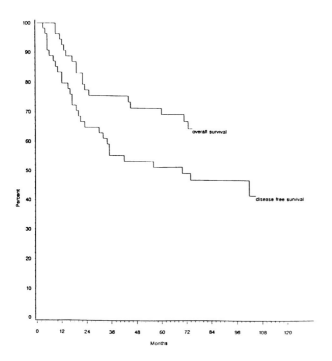

**Figure 19–1.** Preoperative multimodality treatment for soft tissue sarcoma.

after a radical groin dissection. Distant metastases were found in a total of 20 patients. Of these patients, 19 were pulmonary, and 1 was cerebral. Of the 19 patients with pulmonary metastases, 3 had synchronous metastases at other sites. Two patients had both local recurrences and pulmonary metastases; one is now free of disease after a hemipelvectomy and pulmonary resection.

Postoperative radiation therapy was administered to 27 patients whose tumors were judged to have close margins. Among these patients, an average of 32 Gy (range, 18 to 54 Gy) of additional radiation was given.[40] The dose of postoperative radiation depended on the time between preoperative and postoperative treatment.[40] Only one (3.7 percent) patient receiving postoperative radiation had a local recurrence. This is in sharp contrast with the 28 patients who did not receive postoperative radiation, 7 of whom (25 percent) experienced local failure. Thus, the difference in local recurrence between the group that received postoperative radiation and the one that did not was statistically significant ($p = 0.026$, by Fisher's exact test).

Limb-salvage protocols have taken several forms: chemotherapy alone,[43–45] radiation therapy alone,[25] or a combination of the two. Preoperative chemotherapy has been used, with some success, to improve limb salvage.[44,45] However, the use of doxorubicin-based preoperative chemotherapy has been shown to have only a 40 percent response rate.[43,45] Furthermore, when this

regimen was combined with limb-sparing resections, local recurrence rates up to 34 percent have been reported.[43] Preoperative chemotherapy alone offers the unique advantage of determination of in vivo sensitivity to chemotherapy. Patients responding to preoperative chemotherapy have longer survival times than do those who do not respond. However, the limb-salvage rates are lower than those reported in other multimodality protocols; therefore, the advantage of chemosensitivity determination must be weighed against the advantages of other neoadjuvant regimens when the risk of limb loss is high.

Preoperative radiation therapy alone as a limb-sparing regimen in soft tissue sarcoma has also been used successfully.[25] This regimen generally involves 50 to 60 Gy delivered over five to six weeks, which has resulted in a five-year local control rate of 86 percent,[45] with 75 percent initial limb salvage among those cases initially judged unresectable. However, 15 percent of patients had wound-healing delays, necessitating remedial surgical procedures in 12 percent.[46] Furthermore, the local control rate was much lower in very large lesions.[46,47]

Because of the obvious gravity of amputation, it seemed prudent to combine chemotherapy with radiation therapy in a preoperative limb-salvage protocol. This approach was pioneered by the group at the University of California at Los Angeles.[48] In two consecutive trials, they combined intra-arterial doxorubicin (30 mg/d for three days) with 35 Gy or 17.5 Gy in 250 cGy fractions.[49] Using these protocols, the authors found results similar to those found in the initial report of our data.[48] Similar reports, with minor variations in dosing and radiation schedules, have also been published, with relatively short follow-ups.[2,49–54] These studies revealed limb-salvage rates of 80 to 97 percent, with local recurrence rates of 0 to 11 percent. Our study confirms these earlier findings. Furthermore, 81 percent ultimate limb-salvage rate and 15 percent local recurrence rate in our study suggest that the early results of those studies should be durable on long-term follow-up.

The complications of this protocol are significant, with 26 percent experiencing an adverse treatment-related morbidity. The most serious complications of the protocol were related to intra-arterial infusion. The 7 percent incidence of treatment-related morbidity requiring surgery is notable. However, with the increased use of systemic chemotherapy, intra-arterial catheter-related complications have been obviated. For all practical purposes, currently, intra-arterial infusion chemotherapy for soft tissue sarcoma is not indicated.[55–57]

The long-term results of this preoperative protocol for adults with limb-threatening soft tissue sarcoma clearly justify the use of a multimodal approach.

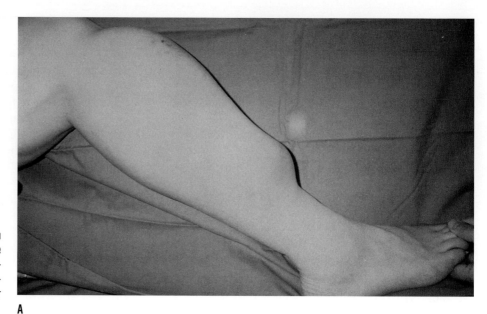

**Figure 19–2. (A)** Large liposarcoma in anterior lateral aspect of the right leg. The tumor was attached to the fibula and essentially completely replaced the anterior compartment and extended to the posterior compartment. *(Continued.)*

**A**

Adding routine postoperative radiation to such a regimen improves the local control rate still further. Implicit in this approach is the participation of a team experienced in the complex care of patients with limb-threatening soft tissue sarcoma.

Multimodal therapy using resection and radiation remains the method of choice for limb salvage in high-grade soft tissue sarcomas of the extremities. However, several treatment-related short- and long-term complications are encountered with these limb-salvage procedures when radiation is one of its components. These treatment-related complications include delayed wound healing, long bone fracture, limb contracture, loss of limb function, and occasional need for amputation as a result of complication of therapy.[49,58–61] Radiation therapy plays a major role in tumor control, but is also believed to be related to or contributing to most of these complications. Decreasing the dose of radiation decreases the incidence of complication but simultaneously increases the incidence of local recurrence.[61] Preservation of good functional capacity of the extremity is achieved in approximately 70 percent of the cases following multimodal therapy using radiation, especially after treatment of lower limb sarcoma. Isolated limb perfusion using different chemotherapeutic agents has been suggested as a treatment modality for extremity soft tissue sarcomas. Isolated limb perfusion for soft tissue sarcoma was initially proposed and performed by Krementz et al.[62] In a series of 113 patients with soft tissue sarcoma of the extremities treated between 1957 and 1975, these authors reported an early response rate in 83 percent of the cases. However, complete response was rare. In our series, among 22 patients with primary sarcomas of the extremities, 2 patients had complete response, 3 patients had par-

tial response with reduction of the tumor by more than 50 percent of the size, and 14 patients had minor responses. Among 21 patients treated with isolated limb perfusion for recurrent soft tissue sarcoma, 2 patients had complete responses, 8 had partial responses, and 8 had minor responses of less than 50 percent reduction in tumor size. Most of the patients in this series were treated either by melphalan or a combination of melphalan, nitrogen mustard, and actinomycin D. As reported by Krementz et al.,[62] the incidence of local recurrence was 24 percent in patients with isolated limb perfusion performed for primary tumor. Other investigators also found similar response using melphalan for isolated limb perfusion for extremity soft tissue sarcomas.[63–65] Using perfusion and more conservative excision for sarcoma of the limbs, McBride[63] reported a 9 percent local recurrence rate, and Stehlin et al.[64] reported a 16 percent local recurrence rate after isolated limb perfusion and excision. Several other investigators, including Ghussen et al.,[65] Lethi et al.,[66] and Hoekstra et al.,[67] reported local recurrence rates varying from 7 to 10 percent.

Doxorubicin remains the most effective agent against soft tissue sarcomas and a logical choice for use in isolated limb perfusion for soft tissue sarcomas. Several investigators have used doxorubicin for isolated limb perfusion in soft tissue sarcoma with mixed results.[68–71] Klaase et al.[70] reported a 0 percent response rate in 22 patients with high-grade soft tissue sarcomas. Three of the patients required amputation due to toxicity secondary to the use of Adriamycin for isolated limb perfusion. It is our opinion that the high toxicity reported by these authors is partly due to lack of strict adherence to the principle of doxorubicin kinetics during isolated limb perfusion and inadequate

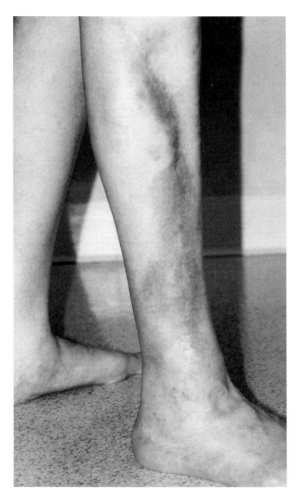

**Figure 19–2** *(continued).* **(B)** Same patient one year postoperatively following isolated limb perfusion with Adriamycin and resection of the tumor mass. Currently, patient is free of disease eighteen months after the procedure.

information on ideal dose for doxorubicin during isolated limb perfusion. Technical factors in isolated limb perfusion may also have contributed to this increased toxicity. In contrast, Braat et al.[68] reported only one incident of local recurrence among 14 patients treated with perfusion alone or perfusion and resection following the use of Adriamycin as a chemotherapeutic agent for isolated limb perfusion.

We have treated 11 patients with high-grade soft tissue sarcoma of the extremity by isolated normothermic limb perfusion using doxorubicin. These lesions were located below midthigh, and most were near the joints or distal extremities. All were resected either immediatcly after perfusion or shortly thereafter (Fig. 19–2 A & B). Only one of the 11 patients showed recurrence in extremity, and this patient also simultaneously demonstrated evidence of systemic metastasis. Morbidity in this group included delayed wound healing in one patient and pulmonary embolism in another. All

patients had excellent limb function, and there was no evidence of any limb contracture or joint problem. In our opinion, doxorubicin is an excellent agent for isolated limb perfusion for the treatment of soft tissue sarcoma at a dose between 0.3 mg and 0.4 mg/kg of body weight. One concern about the use of doxorubicin for isolated limb perfusion is that heparin use results in precipitation of doxorubicin from solution. However, we demonstrated that the concentration of doxorubicin is minimally affected in perfusate-containing plasma after adding heparin. Isolated perfusion can be performed safely without precipitation of doxorubicin by heparin up to a concentration of 5 U/mL of heparin and 60 µg/mL of doxorubicin in plasma-containing perfusate.[72] In a canine model, we have also demonstrated Adriamycin in the cell nucleus following isolated limb perfusion with doxorubicin.[73] However, it is noteworthy that Adriamycin binds to the surface of the tubing and the surface of the oxygenator. Thus, with use of a standard oxygenator and three meters of 6.4 mm-diameter pump tubing, the loss of Adriamycin from the perfusate is approximately 30 percent of the total concentration.[72] *This loss of Adriamycin in the perfusate apparatus and tubing must be accounted for, for proper dosage of doxorubicin during isolated limb perfusion.*

Recently, Lienard et al.[74] reported on the efficacy of high-dose recombinant tumor necrosis factor-alpha (TNF-$\alpha$) in combination with interferon-$\gamma$ (IFN-$\gamma$), and of melphalan in isolated limb perfusion of sarcoma. Since then, a number of other authors have reported on the efficacy of TNF-$\alpha$ and melphalan in the treatment of high-grade soft tissue sarcoma of the extremity isolated limb perfusion.[75–77] Recently, Eggermont and colleagues[77] have reported on isolated limb perfusion for nonresectable extremity soft tissue sarcomas using high-dose TFN-$\alpha$ in combination with IFN-$\gamma$ and melphalan. These authors used TFN-$\alpha$ at a dose of 4 mg for lower extremity and 3 mg for upper extremity. Using this high dose for advanced soft tissue sarcoma, they reported a complete response in 36 percent of the patients and a partial response in 51 percent. Among patients with a single lesion of high-grade soft tissue sarcoma treated with a high dose of TNF-$\alpha$ and melphalan with IFN-$\gamma$ followed by resection, the local recurrence rate was 6 percent. However, when a subsequent resection was not performed, the local recurrence rate was 18 percent. Among patients perfused for multiple tumors in the extremity, the local recurrence rate was 30 percent. The incidence of cardiovascular, pulmonary, renal, or significant hepatic toxicity secondary to perfusion with high-dose TNF-$\alpha$ was reasonably low. Excellent limb function was achieved in 80 percent of the patients. Although the exact mechanisms of tumor necrosis after TNF-$\alpha$ and melphalan perfusion remains uncertain, one proposed mechanism is destruction of endothelial cells of tumor blood vessels. Recently, Hill et al.[75] reported the results of isolated limb perfusion with low-dose TNF-$\alpha$ and melphalan, with the TNF concentration in the perfusate varying from 0.5 to 0.75 $\mu$g/mL, which is approximately five- to six-fold lower than reported by Eggermont et al.[77]

With this low-dose TNF-$\alpha$ and melphalan perfusion, Hill et al.[75] reported a 100 percent complete response rate without use of any interferon. However, adding melphalan to TNF-$\alpha$ perfusion appears to be critical, since all available data suggest that response to TNF-$\alpha$ without melphalan appears to be low and short-lived.[77,78]

Isolated limb perfusion is an excellent method for limb sparing in soft tissue sarcomas of the extremities, with adequate local control. A number of chemotherapeutic agents have shown efficacy in isolated perfusion systems. Among these, adriamycin and a combination of TNF-$\alpha$ and melphalan appear to be the most promising. Early reports in the literature suggest that TNF-$\alpha$ with melphalan, even in a low dose, is effective in control of soft tissue sarcoma of the extremity. These preliminary encouraging data await a well-designed multi-institutional randomized clinical trial.

## REFERENCES

1. Antman KH, Corson J, Greenberger J, et al.: Multimodality therapy in the management of angiosarcoma of the breast. Cancer 50:2000, 1982
2. Sordillo PP, Magill GB, Schauer PK, et al.: Preliminary trial of combination therapy with Adriamycin and radiation in sarcomas and other malignant tumors. J Surg Oncol 21:23, 1982
3. Rosen G, Juergens H, Caparros B, et al.: Combination chemotherapy (T-6) in the multidisciplinary treatment of Ewing's sarcoma. Natl Cancer Inst Monogr 56:289, 1981
4. Perez CA, Tefft M, Nesbit ME Jr., et al.: Radiation therapy in the multimodal management of Ewing's sarcoma of bone: Report of the intergroup of Ewing's sarcoma study. Natl Cancer Inst Monogr 56:263, 1981
5. Kaufman JJ, Gelbard M: Leiomyosarcoma of renal vein and inferior vena cava. Urology 18:173, 1981
6. Middleton AW Jr., Elman AJ, Stewart JR, et al.: Combined modality therapy with conservation of organ function in childhood genitourinary rhabdomyosarcoma. Urology 18:42, 1981
7. Ransom JJ, Pratt CB, Hustu HO, et al.: Retroperitoneal rhabdomyosarcoma in children: Results in multimodality therapy. Cancer 45:845, 1980
8. King DR, Clatworthy HW Jr.: The pediatric patient with sarcoma. Semin Oncol 8:215, 1981
9. Mandard AM, Chasle J, Manard JC, et al.: The pathologist's role in a multidisciplinary approach for soft part tissues sarcoma: A reappraisal (39 cases). J Surg Oncol 17:69, 1981
10. DeVita VT Jr., Henney JE, Weiss RB: Advances in the multimodal primary management of cancer. Adv Intern Med 26:115, 1980
11. Cruz AB Jr., Thames EA Jr., Aust JB et al.: Combination chemotherapy for soft-tissue sarcomas: A phase III study. J Surg Oncol 11:313, 1979
12. Abbas JS, Holyoke ED, Moore R, et al.: The surgical treatment and outcome of soft-tissue sarcoma. Arch Surg 116:765, 1981
13. Cantin J, McNeer GP, Chu FC, et al.: The problem of local recurrence after treatment of soft tissue sarcoma. Ann Surg 168:47, 1968
14. Castro GG, Hajdu S II, Fortner JG: Surgical therapy of fibrosarcoma of the extremities: A reappraisal. Arch Surg 107:284, 1973
15. Eilber FR, Mirra JJ, Grant TT, et al.: Is amputation necessary for sarcomas? Ann Surg 192:431, 1980
16. Morton DL, Eilber FR, Townsend CM Jr., et al.: Limb salvage from a multidisciplinary treatment approach for skeletal and soft tissue sarcomas of the extremity. Ann Surg 184:268, 1976
17. Shiu MH, Castro EB, Hajdu S, et al.: Surgical treatment of 297 soft-tissue sarcomas of the lower extremities. Ann Surg 182:597, 1975
18. Das Gupta TK, Patel M, Chaudhuri PK, et al.: The role of chemotherapy as an adjuvant to surgery in the initial treatment of primary soft tissue sarcomas in adults. J Surg Oncol 19:139, 1982
19. Pritchard DJ, Soule EH, Taylor WF, et al.: Fibrosarcoma: A clinicopathological and statistical study of 199 tumors of the soft tissues of the extremities and trunk. Cancer 33:888, 1974
20. Das Gupta TK: Tumors of the Soft Tissues. East Norwalk, CT, Appleton-Century-Crofts, 1983
21. Willard WC, Hajdu SI, Casper ES, Brennan MF: Comparison of amputation with limb-sparing operations for adult soft tissue sarcoma of the extremity. Ann Surg 215:269, 1992
22. Gaynor JJ, Tan CC, Casper ES, et al.: Refinement of clinicopathologic staging for localized soft tissue sarcoma of the extremity: A study of 423 adults. J Clin Oncol 10:1317, 1992
23. Suit HD: Soft tissue sarcomas (excluding rhabdomyosarcoma): Radiotherapy applications. Natl Cancer Inst Monogr 56:245, 1981
24. Liebner EJ: Radiation therapy. In Das Gupta TK (ed): Tumors of the Soft Tissues. East Norwalk, CT, Appleton-Century-Crofts, 1983, p 271
25. Suit HD, Proppe KH, Mankin HJ, et al.: Preoperative radiation therapy for sarcoma soft tissue. Cancer 47:2269, 1981
26. Lindberg RD, Martin RG, Romsdahl MM, et al.: Conservative surgery and postoperative radiotherapy in 300 adults with soft-tissue sarcomas. Cancer 47:2391, 1981
27. O'Connor MI, Pritchard DJ, Gunderson LL: Integration of limb-sparing surgery, brachytherapy, and external-beam irradiation in the treatment of soft-tissue sarcomas. Clin Orthop Rel Res 289:73, 1993
28. Markhede G, Angervall L, Stener B: A multivariate analysis of the prognosis after surgical treatment of malignant soft-tissue tumors. Cancer 49:1721, 1982
29. Jacobs EM: Combination chemotherapy of metastatic testicular germinal cell tumors and soft part sarcomas. Cancer 25:324, 1970

30. DiMarco A, Gaetani NM, Scarpinato B: Adriamycin (NSC-123-127): A new antibiotic with antitumor activity. Cancer Chemother Rep 53:33, 1969

31. Benjamin RS, Riggs CE Jr., Bachur NR: Pharmacokinetics and metabolism of Adriamycin in man. Clin Pharmacol Ther 14:592, 1973

32. Gottlieb JA: Combination chemotherapy for metastatic sarcoma. Cancer Chem Rep 58:265, 1974

33. Gottlieb JA, Benjamin RS, Baker LH, et al.: Role of DTIC (NSC-45388) in chemotherapy of sarcomas. Cancer Treat Rep 60:199, 1976

34. Gottlieb JA, Baker LH, Quagliana JM, et al.: Chemotherapy of sarcomas with a combination of Adriamycin and dimethyltriazenoimidazole carboxamide. Cancer 30:1632, 1972

35. Legha S, Benjamin R, Mackay B, et al.: Reduction of doxorubicin cardiotoxicity by prolonged continuous intravenous infusion. Ann Intern Med 96:133, 1982

36. Rosenberg SA, Tepper J, Glatstein E, et al.: The treatment of soft-tissue sarcomas of the extremities. Ann Surg 196:305, 1982

37. Mantravadi RVP, Trippon MJ, Patel MK, et al.: Limb salvage in extremity soft tissue sarcoma: Combined modality therapy. Radiology 152:523, 1984

38. Levine EA, Trippon MJ, Das Gupta TK: Preoperative multimodality treatment for soft tissue sarcomas. Cancer 71:3685, 1993

39. Das Gupta TK: Tumors of the soft tissues. East Norwalk, CT, Appleton-Century-Crofts, 1983, p 209

40. Orton CG, Ellis F: A simplification in the use of NSD concept in practical radiotherapy. J Radiol 46:529, 1973

41. Kaplan EL, Meier P: Nonparametric estimation from incomplete observations. J Am Stat Assoc 53:457, 1958

42. Beahrs OH, Henson DE, Hutter RVP, Myers M: Manual for staging of cancer. 4th ed. Philadelphia, JB Lippincott, 1992, p 131

43. Pezzi CM, Pollock RE, Evans HL, et al.: Preoperative chemotherapy for soft-tissue sarcomas of the extremities. Ann Surg 211:476, 1990

44. Lokich JJ: Preoperative chemotherapy for soft tissue sarcomas. Surg Gynecol Obstet 148:512, 1979

45. Rouesse JG, Friedman S, Sevin DM, et al.: Preoperative induction chemotherapy in the treatment of locally advanced soft tissue sarcomas. Cancer 60:296, 1987

46. Suit DH, Mankin HJ, Wood WC, Proppe KH: Preoperative, intraoperative, and postoperative radiation in the treatment of primary soft tissue sarcoma. Cancer 55:2659, 1985

47. Tepper JE, Suit HD: Radiation therapy of soft tissue sarcomas. Cancer 55:2273, 1985

48. Eilber FR, Morton DL, Eckardt J, et al.: Limb salvage for skeletal and soft tissue sarcoma. Cancer 53:2579, 1984

49. Eilber FR, Giuliano AE, Huth J, et al.: Limb salvage for high-grade soft tissue sarcomas of the extremity: Experience at University of California, Los Angeles. Cancer Treatment Symp 3:49, 1985

50. Hoekstra HJ, Koops HS, Molenaar WM, et al.: A combination of intra-arterial chemotherapy, preoperative and postoperative radiotherapy, and surgery as limb-saving treatment of primarily unresectable high-grade soft tissue sarcomas. Cancer 63:59, 1989

51. Goodnight JE, Bargar WL, Voegell T, Blaisdell FW: Limb-sparing surgery for extremity sarcomas after preoperative intraarterial doxorubicin and radiation therapy. Am J Surg 150:109, 1985

52. Temple WJ, Russell JA, Arthur K, et al.: Neoadjuvant treatment in conservative surgery of peripheral sarcomas. Can J Surg 32:361, 1984

53. Denton JW, Dunham WK, Salter M, et al.: Preoperative regional chemotherapy and rapid-function irradiation for sarcomas of the soft tissue and bone. Surg Gynecol Obstet 158:545, 1984

54. Wanebo H, Temple WJ, Popp MB, et al.: Combination regional therapy for extremity sarcoma. Arch Surg 125:355, 1990

55. Bramwell VHC: Intra-arterial chemotherapy of soft tissue sarcomas. Semin Surg Oncol 4:66, 1988

56. Eilber FR, Giuliano JF, Huth JF, et al.: Intravenous (IV) vs. intraarterial (IA) Adriamycin, 2800r radiation and surgical excision for extremity soft tissue sarcomas: A randomized prospective trial. Proc Am Soc Clin Oncol 9:309, 1990

57. Winkler K, Bielack S, Delling G, et al.: Effect of intraarterial versus intravenous cisplatin, in addition to systemic doxorubicin, high-dose methotrexate, and ifosfamide, on histologic tumor response in osteosarcoma (study COSS-86). Cancer 66:1703, 1990

58. Blum RH: An overview of studies with Adriamycin (NSC 123 127). United States Cancer Chemother 6:247, 1975

59. Delaney TF, Stinson SF, Greenburg J, et al.: Effect on limb function of combined modality, limb sparing therapy for extremity, soft tissue sarcomas. Proc Am Soc Clin Oncol (abstr) 10:1243, 1991

60. Lindberg R: Treatment of localized soft tissue sarcomas in adults at M.D. Anderson Hospital and Tumor Institute. Cancer Treat Symp 3:59, 1985

61. Huth JF, Eilber FR: Pre-operative intra-arterial chemotherapy. Cancer Treat Res 44:103, 1989

62. Krementz ET, Carter RD, Sutherland CM, Hutton I: Chemotherapy of sarcomas of the limbs by regional perfusion. Ann Surg 185:555, 1977

63. McBride CM: Sarcomas of the limbs: Results of adjuvant chemotherapy using isolation perfusion. Arch Surg 109:304, 1974

64. Stehlin JS, de Ipolyi PD, Giovanella BC: Soft tissue sarcomas of the extremity: Multidisciplinary therapy employing hyperthermic perfusion. Am J Surg 130:643, 1975

65. Ghussen F, Nagel K: Die regionale hypertherme cytostatica-perfusion als alternative bei der behandlung van malignen weichgeweburumoren der extremitaten. Chirurg Berlin 55:505, 1954

66. Lethi PM, Stephens MH, Janoff K: Improved survival for soft tissue sarcoma of the extremities by regional hyperthermic perfusion, local excision, and radiation therapy. Surg Gynecol Obstet 162:149, 1986

67. Hoekstra HJ, Schaffordt Koops H, et al.: Results of isolated regional perfusion in the treatment of malignant soft tissue tumors of the extremities. Cancer 60:1703, 1987

68. Braat RP, Wieberdink I, van Slooten EN, Olthuis G:

Regional perfusion with Adriamycin in soft tissue sarcomas. Recent Results Cancer Res 86:260, 1983

69. Chaudhuri PK, Mucci SJ, Crist KA: Isolated-limb perfusion for high-grade soft-tissue sarcomas. Reg Cancer Treat 4:213, 1982

70. Klaase JM, Kroon BBR, Benckhuijsen C, et al.: Results of regional isolation perfusion with cytostatics in patients with soft tissue tumors of the extremities. Cancer 64:616, 1989

71. Rossi CR, Vecchiato A, Foletto M, et al.: Phase II study on neoadjuvant hyperthermic-antiblastic perfusion with Doxorubicin in patients with intermediate or high grade limb sarcomas. Cancer 73:2140, 1994

72. Mucci SJ, Crist KA, Chaudhuri B, Chaudhuri PK: Pharmacokinetics of doxorubicin during isolated perfusion. I. The effect of heparin on doxorubicin concentration. Reg Cancer Treat 4:110, 1991

73. Briele HA, Djuric M, Walker MJ, et al.: Kinetics and toxicity of Doxorubicin (Adriamycin A) in isolation perfusion of canine hind limb. Surg Forum 11:429, 1980

74. Lienard D, Delmotte JJ, Renard N: High doses of rTNF-α in combination with TFN-gamma and melphalan in isolation perfusion of the limbs for melanoma and sarcoma. Clin Oncol 10:52, 1992

75. Hill S, Fawcett WJ, Sheldon J: Low-dose tumour necrosis factor α and melphalan in hyperthermic isolated limb perfusion. Br J Surg 80:995, 1993

76. Vaglini M, Belli F, Ammatuna M, et al.: Treatment of primary or relapsing limb cancer by isolation perfusion with high-dose alpha-tumor necrosis factor, gamma-interferon, and melphalan. Cancer 73:483, 1994

77. Eggermont AMM, Schaffordt Koops H, et al.: Isolated limb perfusion with high-dose necrosis factor-α in combination with Interferon-γ and melphalan for nonresectable extremity soft tissue sarcoma: A multicenter trial. J Clin Oncol 14:2653, 1996

78. Manusama E, Nooijen PTGA, Stavast J, et al.: Synergistic antitumour effect of recombinant tumour necrosis factor α with melphalan in isolated limb perfusion in the rat. Br J Surg 83:551, 1996

# 20

# Immunology and Immunotherapy

Recent advances in the field of immunology have focused attention on potential immunologically mediated therapeutic modalities in the treatment of metastatic sarcomas. Investigation in the areas of monoclonal antibodies (MoAbs), ctyokines, and cell-mediated cytotoxicity have resulted in new diagnostic and therapeutic reagents. Although considerable advances have been made since the first edition of this book was published, much still remains to be accomplished before the true role of immunotherapy in the management of metastatic soft tissue sarcomas is established.

Because bone and soft tissue sarcomas in general are rare, the individual subtypes are even less common. Although this has hampered the development of tumor-specific MoAbs, some progress has been made, and a number of antibodies have been generated that seem to recognize antigens shared by several subsets of malignant mesenchymal tumors. Several investigators have reported murine MoAbs that react to a broad range of human sarcomas. Bartal, Lavie, and colleagues[1,2] have raised an antibody originally directed against antigens in human malignant fibrous histiocytoma (MFH) cell lines. This antibody has since been shown to bind to most sarcomas, including Kaposi's.[3] Unfortunately, it also binds to several carcinomas, making it less useful in differentiating sarcoma from carcinoma.

Miettinen reported on the use of murine MoAb HHF-035, which has been raised against muscle.[4] Muscle actins are present in normal skeletal and smooth muscle, pericytes of small vessels, and in myoepithelial cells. Well-differentiated rhabdomyosarcomas and leio-

myosarcomas stain positive with this antibody. Further, Schmidt et al.[5] confirmed the observations of Miettinen and proposed that this antibody is highly sensitive and specific for tumors with myogenic differentiation. The major problem of MoAb HHF-035 is that it helps to identify the myogenic origin in only 25 percent of the pleomorphic (undifferentiated) sarcomas, thus somewhat limiting the practicality of this MoAb.

In 1983, Brown,[6] working in our laboratory, developed hybridoma cells derived from a mouse that was immunized with plasma membranes prepared from the fresh tumor tissues of a patient with MFH. Supernatants from the resultant hybridoma clones were screened for positive antibody binding to tumor cell membranes and negative binding to cell membrane preparations of normal tissues using a solid-phase radioimmunoassay. Two distinct monoclonal immunoglobulin G1 (IgG1) ($\kappa$) antibodies, 19–14 and 19–24, were identified that showed identical patterns of reactivity with a large panel of tissues. Both antibodies displayed high levels of binding to membranes prepared from most MFHs and osteogenic sarcoma tumors tested. Moderate levels of binding were obtained with melanoma, colorectal carcinoma, and first-trimester fetal membranes. Weak or no significant binding was observed with membranes from a variety of autologous and allogeneic normal adult tissues. Antibody reactivities could be specifically removed by absorption with MFH and osteosarcoma membranes but not with adult muscle membranes. An electrophoretic analysis of immunoprecipitated membrane antigens indicated that antibodies 19–14 and 19–24 reacted with the same protein, a monomer with an approximate molecular weight of 102,000 D (termed *p102*). The antigen was detected in membrane preparations of MFH, osteosarcoma, and first-trimester fetus, but was not present in normal adult spleen. However, a small amount of antigen of molecular weight 107,000 D was precipitated from a normal adult liver preparation, which suggests that related antigens may be present in low levels in some normal tissues. High levels of p102 antigen were also found in all sarcoma and carcinoma cell lines and neonatal skin fibroblasts tested.

The results of the immunoprecipitation and SDS/PAGE analysis indicated that both antibodies 19–14 and 19–24 were binding to a monomeric protein antigen of approximately 102,000 D. This membrane protein (p102) was detected in 51 of 53 human sarcomas. Antigen expression in various histologic subtypes apparently depends on the amount of fibrous tissue matrix present in the actual sarcoma specimen. Lectin affinity absorption indicated that p102 was a mannose-containing glycoprotein, with an isoelectric point (pI) 4.7, and $5.9 \times 10^5$ binding sites per cultured human HT-1080 fibrosarcoma cell.

Based on these and other in vitro studies, an in vivo study using soft tissue sarcoma xenograft was designed.[7] $^{125}$I-labeled monoclonal antibody 19–24 (mouse isotype IgG1) was evaluated for its potential use in the clinical radioimmunodetection of sarcoma. Chromatographic and electrophoretic analyses indicated that the labeled preparation was relatively pure. Binding studies in vitro demonstrated that specificity for the antigen was retained after iodination and indicated that the labeled antibody possessed an immunoreactivity in excess of 90 percent and a binding constant of $8.1 \times 10^9$ M$^{-1}$.

When administered to athymic NCr-nu/nu mice bearing 1-cm diameter human fibrosarcoma HT-1080 xenografts, the labeled antibody preferentially localized in tumor deposits. Maximum tumor-to-blood radioactivity ratios (2.2–3.4) were obtained seven days after antibody injection. Specificity of the localization was confirmed with a control mouse IgG1 antibody and by using a nonreactive xenograft. Distinct tumor images (Fig. 20–1) were obtained by computed tomography (CT), demonstrating the possible clinical use of the labeled antibody.

In a similar vein, indium-111 ($^{111}$In)-labeled monoclonal antibodies have been used in human sarcoma xenografts.[8] In order to study localization of metastatic tumors with a radiolabeled monoclonal antibody, a pulmonary metastases model was devised in athymic mice. Metastatic pulmonary sarcoma colonies were verified by histologic examination. The murine monoclonal antibody (MoAb 19–24) directed against a human sarcoma antigen was labeled with $^{111}$In by use of the linker 1-(p-isothiocyanatobenzyl)-diethylenetriaminepentaacetic acid (SCN-Bz-DTPA). An unrelated mouse IgG MoAb P3 was similarly labeled as a negative control. In the

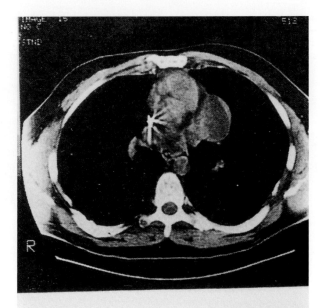

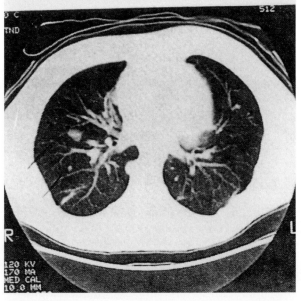

**Figure 20–1. (A & B)** Noncontrast CT of the chest (top) demonstrates a 5.5 cm × 4.0 cm left hilar mass, and at the level of the aortopulmonary window (bottom) two parenchymal soft tissue nodules in the right lower lobe measuring 2.0 cm × 1.5 cm and 1.0 cm × 1.0 cm, 2 cm below the level of the aortopulmonary window (lung windows).

group given MoAb 19–24, the percent injected dose uptake per gram of lung tissue bearing tumor colonies (30.1 percent, 29.6 percent, and 27.7 percent on days 1, 2, and 3, respectively) was significantly ($p < 0.05$) higher than in those receiving labeled MoAb P3. Hepatic activities of both $^{111}$In-MoAb 19–24 and $^{111}$In-MoAb P3 were low. The tumor colonies in the lungs demonstrated the clearest images on day 3. The specific binding of $^{111}$In-SCN-Bz-DTPA-labeled MoAb 19–24 to pulmonary xenografts without appreciable liver uptake indicated that it might be a useful tool in the clinical

**TABLE 20–1. DETAILS OF PATIENTS RECEIVING RADIOLABELED MoABs\***

| Patient | Age/Sex | $^{125}$I dose (µCi) | Presumed Diagnosis | Comments |
|---------|---------|---------------------|--------------------|----------|
| 1 | 54/M | 250 | Recurrent leiomyosarcoma of groin | Adjacent superficial inguinal nodes positive |
| 2 | 53/F | 250 | Pulmonic MFH metastasis | Presumed diagnosis confirmed by autopsy |
| 3 | 17/M | 250 | Recurrent aggressive fibromatosis of arm | NED |
| 4 | 66/F | 250 | Recurrent fibrosarcoma of thorax | Tumor was cystic |
| 5 | 60/F | 250 | Residual MFH of arm | Tumor < 1.0 mm; sequential MoAb study done[a] |
| 6 | 13/F | 250 | Pulmonic osteogenic sarcoma metastases | 11 tumors present |
| 7 | 54/M | 250 | Residual MFH of foot | Tumor < 1.0 mm; sequential MoAb study done |
| 8 | 64/F | 250 | Recurrent MFH of thigh | NED |
| 9 | 40/F | 250 | Hepatic leiomyosarcoma metastases | Sequential MoAb study done |
| 10 | 36/F | 250 | Recurrent leiomyosarcoma of pelvis | 2 tumors present |
| 11 | 56/F | 500 | Recurrent MFH of sacrum | |
| 12 | 61/M | 500 | Pulmonic MFH metastases | Sequential MoAb study done |
| 13 | 28/M | 500 | Recurrent aggressive fibromatosis of chest wall | 2 tumors present |
| 14 | 37/F | 500 | Recurrent aggressive fibromatosis of shoulder | NED |
| 15 | 29/M | 500 | Recurrent Ewing's sarcoma of abdomen | |
| 16 | 56/M | 500 | Recurrent fibrosarcoma of thorax | |

Abbreviations: MFH, malignant fibrous histiocytoma; NED, no evidence of disease.
[a]Sequential MoAb studies consisted of injection of nonspecific $^{125}$I-labeled MoAb P3 followed by specific $^{125}$I-labeled MoAb 19–24 with an isotope clearance interval between dosages.
\**From* Cancer Immunol Immunother *33:341, 1991.*

localization of occult or radiologically detectable pulmonary metastatic sarcomas.

These types of xenograft studies led us to initiate a phase I trial using $^{125}$I-MoAb 19–24.[9] A group of 16 sarcoma patients with suspected advanced disease were studied with a radiolabeled antisarcoma monoclonal antibody (MoAb 19–24) in an attempt to localize tumor deposits. All 16 patients received $^{125}$I-MoAb 19–24 and then had external probe analysis and imaging performed. Confirmation of tumor deposits was performed at surgery or by autopsy. From patients who were operated on, both tumor and normal tissues as well as blood were studied and analyzed for radioactivity. Tumor-to-blood ratios ranged from 0.6 to 36.8. The details of patient characteristics and the localization results are summarized in Tables 20–1 and 20–2. Analysis of the operative specimens after injection of radiolabeled MoAb 19–24 is shown in Table 20–3. In this context, it is interesting to note that all 16 of these patients, and subsequently a number of other metastatic sarcoma patients, were initially analyzed with an external probe and then imaged. It was observed that external probe examination had an overall sensitivity of 83.3 percent and specificity of 100 percent. The scintigraphic results showed an overall sensitivity of 78.9 percent and specificity of 100 percent.

In order to use these sarcoma-specific MoAbs in the immunotherapy of sarcoma-bearing athymic mice, we attempted to conjugate daunomycin (DAU) or adriamycin (ADR) with them.[10] When ADR was linked via a biotin-avidin-biotin bridge, the molar ratios of ADR:total protein ranged from 2 to 7.5. No significant differences were observed between the binding ability of the ADR-MoAb conjugate and that of the unconjugated MoAb 19–24 to fresh sarcoma tissue membranes. The ADR-MoAb conjugate also retained the ability to compete with MoAb 19–24 for binding to sarcoma-associated antigen pl02. In vitro cytotoxicity studies using human fibrosarcoma cells showed that the ADR-MoAb conjugate maintained 40 percent of the efficacy of free ADR. Thus, it was evident that another method of coupling ADR or DAU to MoAb 19–24 was needed if a therapeutically acceptable linkage was to be produced. We therefore developed a method of coupling these anthracycline drugs via a dextran bridge and found this to be more effective.[10]

**TABLE 20–2. LOCALIZATION RESULTS IN PATIENTS RECEIVING RADIOLABELED MoABs\***

| Patient | Probe | Image | Gamma-Counting Ratio[a] |
|---------|-------|-------|-------------------------|
| 1 | Positive | Positive | 34.3 |
| 2 | Positive | Positive | [b] |
| 3 | Negative | Negative | No tumor |
| 4 | Negative | Negative | 1.1 |
| 5 | Negative | Negative | Tumor <1 mm[c] |
| 6 | Positive | Positive | 1.9–28.3 |
| 7 | Negative | Negative | Tumor <1 mm[c] |
| 8 | Negative | Negative | No tumor |
| 9 | Negative | Negative | 0.6–9.1 |
| 10 | Positive | Positive | 6.3–36.8 |
| 11 | Positive | Positive | [b] |
| 12 | Positive | Positive | [b] |
| 13 | Positive | Positive | 5.4–6.3 |
| 14 | Negative | Negative | No tumor |
| 15 | Positive | Positive | [b] |
| 16 | Positive | Positive | [c] |

[a]Tissue activity divided by blood activity.
[b]Tumor localization confirmed by autopsy.
[c]Tumor confirmed at time of surgery but insufficient specimen obtained, radioactivity of the tissue could not be measured.
*From Cancer Immunol Immunother 33:341, 1991.*

In different preparations, the DAU:total protein molar ratio ranged from 1.9 to 6.1. In vitro cytotoxicity studies using human fibrosarcoma cells showed that, at 10 μg/mL concentration, this immunoconjugate was 79.4 percent as efficient as free DAU and, at 1 μg/mL concentration, 36.8 percent as efficient. Control non-specific murine MoAb P3 immunoconjugates were relatively ineffective.

The biodistribution of $^{14}$C-ADR, $^{125}$I-labeled MoAb 19–24, and $^{125}$I-labeled 19–24 immunoconjugate was also evaluated over a 24-hour period in tumor and normal tissues of athymic mice bearing a human fibrosarcoma xenograft. Poor uptake of radiolabeled ADR by the tumor tissue was observed. The level of $^{14}$C radioactivity in the tumor tissue never exceeded 1 percent of the total injected dose and was 24.8-fold lower than the radioactivity found in the spleen. Tumor tissue uptake of radiolabeled monoclonal antibody 19–24 was characterized by the high tumor tissue-to-blood ratio of 1.62 ± 0.28 (SD). However, for monoclonal antibody 19–24 immunoconjugates, this ratio decreased to 0.66 ± 0.05, which was still higher than normal (liver, 0.48 ± 0.02; lung, 0.48 ± 0.07; spleen, 0.28 ± 0.01) or nonspecific MoAb P3 immunoconjugates (0.22 ± 0.03). These data suggest that ADR or DAU linked to MoAb should be less cytotoxic to normal tissues. Further in vivo experiments showed that the maximal tolerated dose (MTD) of free DAU by athymic mice was 4 μg DAU/g, but, for DAU linked to MoAb, it was more than 25 μg DAU/g. The therapeutic efficacy of DAU-DEX-MoAb 19–24 immunoconjugate in the human fibrosarcoma xenograft model is shown in Table 20–4. Thus, it appears that, compared to free DAU, monoclonal antibody 19–24 immunoconjugates may be more efficient and less cytotoxic to normal tissues.[10]

## ■ CHIMERIC (HUMANIZED) MoAb

Limits to using murine MoAbs as carriers of cytotoxic substances for cancer treatment include cytotoxicity, allergic reaction, and patient's immune response to foreign (xenogeneic) immunoglobulin G (IgG). One approach to overcoming the human response to murine MoAbs is to construct, through recombinant DNA technology, murine/human chimeric MoAb in which the mouse variable (V) region of heavy (H) and light (L) chains is linked to the constant region of human IgG.[11,12] A number of methods have been developed to produce chimeric (humanized) MoAbs. In the most frequently used strategy, the rodent constant (C) regions of heavy (H) and light (L) chains are replaced by the constant regions of human IgG. The chimeric MoAb will be expressed in myeloma cells.[13–15] In another strategy, the antigen-binding site of mouse MoAb, which consists of three hypervariable regions (complementary-determining regions [CDRs]), is transplanted to human IgG.[16,17] Finally, the best solution would be to use human MoAb(s) as carriers of cytotoxic substances. However, generation of human sarcoma-specific MoAb(s) with a high-binding affinity is still unpredictable. Although, theoretically, human MoAbs should be less immunogeneic, it has not been proven; in contrast, recent studies demonstrated that human MoAb LiCO 16.88 had a short half-life of 24.0 ± 1.2 hours and was immunogenic in humans.[18] We assume that the presence of the hypervariable regions in human MoAb is responsible for the production of human anti-idiotypic antibodies. It is germane also to recognize that repeated use of murine monoclonals, however specific they might be, is neither feasible nor prudent. Thus, there is a lot of activity in constructing either a chimera or a single-chain specific monoclonal antibody.

In our laboratory, we are pursuing both these lines of investigation. Extensive work is in progress on the preparation of humanized (chimeric) MoAb 19–24. Total cytoplasmic RNA, including mRNA, has been isolated from hybridoma cells producing antisarcoma MoAb 19–24. The isolated RNA was transcribed into the cDNA of mouse MoAb light (L) and heavy (H) chain variable (V) regions. Four primers described previously,[19] modified by adding Eco RI restriction site,[20] were used to synthesize VL and VH 19–24 DNA regions by polymerase chain reaction (PCR). The amplified

**TABLE 20–3. ANALYSIS OF OPERATIVE SPECIMENS AFTER INJECTION OF RADIOLABELED MoAB 19–24***

| Patient[a] | Tissue | Activity[b] | Tissue/blood Ratio[c] |
|---|---|---|---|
| 1 | Groin tumor | 8.93 | 34.3 |
|  | Normal tissue | 0.06–0.26 | 0.2–1.0 |
| 2 | [d] | | |
| 3 | NED | | |
| 4 | Thorax tumor | 0.19 | 1.1 |
|  | Normal tissue | 0.04–0.18 | 0.2–1.0 |
| 5 | [e] | | |
| 6 | Pulmonic metastasis 1 | 9.43 | 28.3 |
|  | Pulmonic metastasis 2 | 7.00 | 21.0 |
|  | Pulmonic metastasis 3 | 6.74 | 20.2 |
|  | Pulmonic metastasis 4 | 5.72 | 17.2 |
|  | Pulmonic metastasis 5 | 5.27 | 15.8 |
|  | Pulmonic metastasis 6 | 4.16 | 12.5 |
|  | Pulmonic metastasis 7 | 3.96 | 11.9 |
|  | Pulmonic metastasis 8 | 3.32 | 10.0 |
|  | Pulmonic metastasis 9 | 3.12 | 9.4 |
|  | Pulmonic metastasis 10 | 0.93 | 2.8 |
|  | Pulmonic metastasis 11 | 0.63 | 1.9 |
|  | Normal lung | 2.21 | 6.6 |
|  | Blood | 0.33 | 1.0 |
| 7 | [f] | | |
| 8 | NED | | |
| 9 | Hepatic metastasis 1 | 4.99 | 9.1 |
|  | Hepatic metastasis 2 | 1.00 | 1.8 |
|  | Hepatic metastasis 3 | 0.69 | 1.3 |
|  | Hepatic metastasis 4 | 0.48 | 0.9 |
|  | Hepatic metastasis 5 | 0.39 | 0.7 |
|  | Hepatic metastasis 6 | 0.35 | 0.6 |
|  | Normal tissue | 0.30–0.55 | 0.5–1.0 |
| 10 | Pelvic tumor | 13.22 | 36.0 |
|  | Pelvic tumor | 13.49 | 36.8 |
|  | Left ovarian tumor | 10.17 | 27.7 |
|  | Right ovarian tumor | 2.30 | 6.3 |
|  | Normal tissue | 0.05–0.64 | 0.1–1.7 |
| 11 | [d] | | |
| 12 | [d] | | |
| 13 | Chest wall tumor 1 | 1.70 | 6.3 |
|  | Chest wall tumor 2 | 1.46 | 5.4 |
|  | Normal tissue | 0.07–0.27 | 0 3–1.0 |
| 14 | NED | | |
| 15 | [d] | | |
| 16 | [e] | | |

Abbreviations: NED, no evidence of disease.
[a]Patients were injected with 300 μg MoAb 19–24 labeled with 250–500 μCi $^{125}$I; tissues were obtained 2–3 days later.
[b]Calculated as percentage injected dose per gram of tissue × 1000.
[c]Tissue activity divided by blood activity.
[d]No biopsies performed, tumor confirmed by autopsy at later date.
[e]Tumor confirmed at time of surgery but insufficient specimen obtained; radioactivity of the tissue could not be measured.
*From Cancer Immunol Immunother *33:341, 1991.*

cDNA for VL and VH 19–24 genes has been cloned into the plasmid pGEM-4Z. Competent *Escherichia coli* cells have been transformed with ligated pGEM-4Z/INSERT (VL or VH), and recombinants have been isolated and further tested for the insert. In the construct that contains the human variable light lysosome gene and the gene for the human constant (kappa) chain, the vari-able light gene has been replaced by the mouse VL gene of MoAb 19–24 and is ready for transfection of nonsecreting myeloma cells. Similarly, in the construct that contains the human variable heavy lysosome gene and human IgG1 gene, the variable heavy gene will be replaced by the mouse VH gene of MoAb 19–24. The process is labor-intensive, and progress is slow, but it

**TABLE 20–4. EFFECT OF DAU-DEX-MOAB (19–24) IMMUNOCONJUGATES ON THE SURVIVAL OF ATHYMIC MICE[a]**

| | Total Dose (μg DAU/g)[b] | Route | Tumor size before treatment X±SD (cm³) | Tumor size at the end point X±SD (cm³) | Survival time X±SD (days)[c] |
|---|---|---|---|---|---|
| Daunomycin (DAU) | | | | | |
| | 4 | i.p. | 0.27±0.06 | 3.55±0.72 | 27.3±1.3 |
| | 10 | i.p. | 0.33±0.13 | 1.14±0.47 | 25.6±0.9 |
| DAU-DEX-MoAb (19–24) | | | | | |
| | 5 | i.v. | palpable[d] | 3.62±0.43 | 26.6±2.2 |
| | 5 | i.p. | p.27±0.19 | 3.88±0.88[e] | 31.0±3.0[e] |
| | 25 | i.p. | palpable | 3.94±0.25[f] | 53.3±4.7[f] |
| | 35 | i.p. | 0.00 or palpable | 1.32±1.70 | 45.2±7.3 |
| DAU-DEX-P3 | | | | | |
| | 25 | i.p. | 0.27±0.10 | 3.67±0.67 | 26.3±2.9 |
| | 35 | i.p. | 0.00 or palpable | 1.95±1.28 | 33.6±2.5 |
| Intact MoAb 19–24 (1 mg/g) | | | | | |
| | 0 | i.p. | 0.17±0.11 | 3.69±0.49 | 25.7±0.4 |
| Control | | | | | |
| | 0 | — | — | 4.44±0.73 | 24.4±1.7 |

Abbreviations: i.p., intraperitoneally; i.v., intravenously; SD, standard deviation.
[a]Given subcutaneous injection of $2 \times 10^6$ HT-1080 fibrosarcoma cells. Mean values (X) were calculated from a group of five mice.
[b]Schedule: every 3 days; four injections on days 0, 3, 6, and 9.
[c]Palpable: less than 0.5 cm³.
[d]Time from the initial injection of tumor cells.
[e]Mean value calculated from four mice; one mouse sacrificed because of ulcer.
[f]Mean value calculated from four mice; one mouse completely cured (no tumor after 75 days).

appears that, in the near future, a workable chimeric sarcoma-specific monoclonal antibody will be available for human xenograft experiments.

## ■ SINGLE-CHAIN ANTIBODY AGAINST HUMAN SARCOMA-ASSOCIATED ANTIGEN

Limitations in the use of murine monoclonal antibodies for human tumor diagnosis and therapy led to development of single-chain antibodies (FVs). The single-chain FVs, each consisting of VH—linker—VL, have shown a number of advantages over the intact mouse IgG MoAbs.[21–24] These antibodies comprise about 25 kD, as compared to the 150 kD for an intact IgG molecule. The small size of these antibodies favors their rapid penetration into tumor tissues and fast blood clearance, resulting in increased tumor-to-blood ratio.[25] In addition, the single-chain FVs showed similar affinity to antigens and decreased immunogenicity (which caused severe immune response in human bodies) compared to the mouse parent IgG MoAbs.[25] Furthermore, they can be produced economically in bacteria[26] or yeast,[27] and manipulated by genetic engineering to form antitumor fusion proteins with additional effector functions.[28,29]

Some single-chain FVs that recognize tumor-associated antigens have been generated and characterized for their potential in tumor immunother-apy.[25,26,29–32] Recombinant single-chain immunotoxins were reported to kill tumor cells in vitro and to regress human tumor xenografts in athymic mice.[33–39] T-cell surface-expressed chimeric single-chain FV/receptors, each composed of an extracellular single-chain FV and a cytoplasmic domain of T-cell receptor(TCR) gamma (γ) or CD3 zeta (ζ) chain, were also engineered to activate T cells, leading to retargeting of the activated T cells to tumor cells.[28,40] In addition, bispecific single-chain antibodies were used to target T cells to tumor cells.[41]

Over the years, MoAbs against human sarcoma-associated antigens have been generated in our laboratory.[6,7,8,10,42–46] Among them, MoAb 29–13 was well characterized, showing affinity and specificity to the human sarcoma-associated antigen p200. Engineering and primary characterization of the recombinant gene encoding the single-chain FV2913 has been accomplished. In this study, the renatured single-chain FV2913 was used in immunohistochemical staining of 99 frozen sections of human sarcomas and other tissues. Results from this study revealed the comparable affinity and specificity to the sarcoma-associated antigen p200 between the single-chain FV2913 and the intact parent MoAb 29–13.

The single-chain FV2913 recombinant gene, consisting of VH—linker—VL, was constructed with reverse transcription polymerase chain reaction (RT-PCR). This gene was cloned and expressed in E. coli.

The renatured single-chain FV2913 was used in the immunostaining study. Engineering of the recombinant single chain FV2913 gene essentially consisted of the following steps. Total RNA prepared from hybridoma cells was used to synthesize the first-strand cDNA. After 30 cycles of PCR, the VH and VL DNA fragments were isolated, purified, and cloned into the cloning vector pGEM-4Z. At least 10 JM109 transformants were analyzed for VH and VL inserts, respectively, by restriction digestion and DNA agarose gel electrophoresis. DNA sequences of three clones for either VH or VL were compared, showing 377 bps of VH and 337 bps of VL DNA. The PCR product of the single-chain FV2913 gene, synthesized through the second run of RT-PCR, was cloned into the expression vector pQE-60. The insert of the recombinant plasmid was confirmed by restriction digestion and DNA sequencing. The DNA sequence of the 741 bp length of the single-chain FV2913 gene consists of VH and VL regions connected by a linker DNA coding for (GGGGS)$_3$ (Fig. 20–2). The single-chain FV2913 gene contained the translation

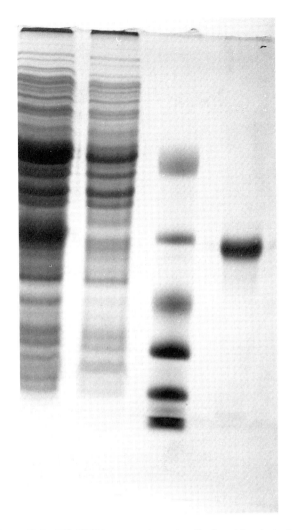

**Figure 20–3.** SDS-PAGE for expression and purification of the single-chain FV2913. *Lane 1:* expression induced by isopropylthiogalactoside (IPTG); an extra protein band was observed at the position of about 28 kD; *Lane 2:* non-induced sample; *Lane 3:* prestained molecular weight of proteins: ovalbumin 43,050, carbonic anhydrase 29,150, β-lactoglobulin 18,800, lysozyme 16,525, bovine trypsin inhibitor 6,420, and insulin 3,066; and *Lane 4:* the purified single-chain FV2913 with the size of about 28 kD.

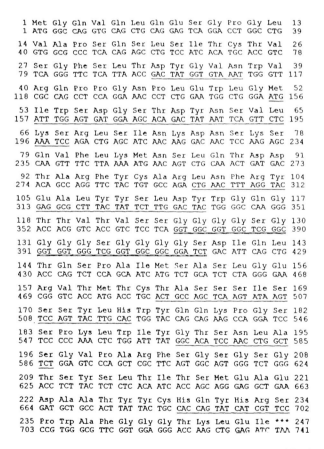

```
  1 Met Gly Gln Val Gln Leu Gln Glu Ser Gly Pro Gly Leu  13
  1 ATG GGC CAG GTG CAG CTG CAG GAG TCA GGA CCT GGC CTG  39

 14 Val Ala Pro Ser Gln Ser Leu Ser Ile Thr Cys Thr Val  26
 40 GTG GCG CCC TCA CAG AGC CTG TCC ATC ACA TGC ACC GTC  78

 27 Ser Gly Phe Ser Leu Thr Asp Tyr Gly Val Asn Trp Val  39
 79 TCA GGG TTC TCA TTA ACC GAC TAT GGT GTA AAT TGG GTT 117

 40 Arg Gln Pro Pro Gly Asn Pro Leu Glu Trp Leu Gly Met  52
118 CGC CAG CCT CCA GGA AAC CCT CTG GAA TGG CTG GGA ATG 156

 53 Ile Trp Ser Asp Gly Ser Thr Asp Tyr Asn Ser Val Leu  65
157 ATT TGG AGT GAT GGA AGC ACA GAC TAT AAT TCA GTT CTC 195

 66 Lys Ser Arg Leu Ser Ile Asn Lys Asp Asn Ser Lys Ser  78
196 AAA TCC AGA CTG AGC ATC AAC AAG GAC AAC TCC AAG AGC 234

 79 Gln Val Phe Leu Lys Met Asn Ser Leu Gln Thr Asp Asp  91
235 CAA GTT TTC TTA AAA ATG AAC AGT CTG CAA ACT GAT GAC 273

 92 Thr Ala Arg Phe Tyr Cys Ala Arg Leu Asn Phe Arg Tyr 104
274 ACA GCC AGG TTC TAC TGT GCC AGA CTG AAC TTT AGG TAC 312

105 Glu Ala Leu Tyr Tyr Ser Leu Asp Tyr Trp Gly Gln Gly 117
313 GAG GCG CTT TAC TAT TCT TTG GAC TAC TGG GGC CAA GGG 351

118 Thr Thr Val Thr Val Ser Ser Gly Gly Gly Gly Ser Gly 130
352 ACC ACG GTC ACC GTC TCC TCA GGT GGC GGT GGC TCG GGC 390

131 Gly Gly Gly Ser Gly Gly Gly Gly Ser Asp Ile Gln Leu 143
391 GGT GGT GGG TCG GGT GGC GGC GGA TCT GAC ATT CAG CTG 429

144 Thr Gln Ser Pro Ala Ile Met Ser Ala Ser Leu Gly Glu 156
430 ACC CAG TCT CCA GCA ATC ATG TCT GCA TCT CTA GGG GAA 468

157 Arg Val Thr Met Thr Cys Thr Ala Ser Ser Ser Ile Ser 169
469 CGG GTC ACC ATG ACC TGC ACT GCC AGC TCA AGT ATA AGT 507

170 Ser Ser Tyr Leu His Trp Tyr Gln Gln Lys Pro Gly Ser 182
508 TCC AGT TAC TTG CAC TGG TAC CAG CAG AAG CCA GGA TCC 546

183 Ser Pro Lys Leu Trp Ile Tyr Gly Thr Ser Asn Leu Ala 195
547 TCC CCC AAA CTC TGG ATT TAT GGC ACA TCC AAC CTG GCT 585

196 Ser Gly Val Pro Ala Arg Phe Ser Gly Ser Gly Ser Gly 208
586 TCT GGA GTC CCA GCT CGC TTC AGT GGC AGT GGG TCT GGG 624

209 Thr Ser Tyr Ser Leu Thr Ile Thr Ser Met Glu Ala Glu 221
625 ACC TCT TAC TCT CTC ACA ATC ACC AGC AGG GAG GCT GAA 663

222 Asp Ala Ala Thr Tyr Tyr Cys His Gln Tyr His Arg Ser 234
664 GAT GCT GCC ACT TAT TAC TGC CAC CAG TAT CAT CGT TCC 702

235 Pro Trp Ala Phe Gly Gly Gly Thr Lys Leu Glu Ile *** 247
703 CCG TGG GCG TTC GGT GGA GGG ACC AAG CTG GAG ATC TAA 741
```

**Figure 20–2.** DNA sequence and translated amino-acid sequence of the single-chain FV2913. The single-chain FV2913 gene is composed of VH and VL variable domains connected by the linker coding for a short peptide (GGGGS)$_3$. The single-chain FV2913 is 741 bp in length. The linker region is double-underlined, and the complementary-determining regions (CDR) for both VH and VL are single-underlined.

start codon ATG in the Nco I site at the 5′ end and the Bgl II site at the 3′ end of the gene. The stop codon TAA in the Hind III site is contained in the expression vector pQE-60. The 6-Histidine "tag" between Bgl II and Hind III is available for affinity purification.

After induction by adding isopropylthiogalactoside (IPTG) to the culture medium, the single-chain FV2913 protein was expressed. The induced and noninduced samples were electrophoresed on a 15 percent polyacrylamide running gel and stained with Coomassie Blue. An extra band of protein was observed in the induced sample (Fig. 20–3). The purified single-chain FV2913 was also electrophoresed on the same gel, showing the size of about 28 kD (Fig. 20–3). The purified and renatured single-chain FV2913 was used to test

**TABLE 20–5. IMMUNOREACTIVITY OF MONOCLONAL ANTIBODY 29–13 AND SINGLE-CHAIN ANTIBODY FV2913 WITH SARCOMA-ASSOCIATED ANTIGEN P200 IN HUMAN FROZEN TISSUES (IMMUNOALKALINE-PHOSPHOTASE STAINING[a])**

| Sarcomas | Staining Ratio[b] | Other Tissues | Staining Ratio |
|---|---|---|---|
| Osteosarcoma | 2:2 | Merkel cell carcinoma | 0:1 |
| Liposarcoma | 11:13 | Basal cell carcinoma | 0:1 |
| Rhabdomyosarcoma | 5:6 | Colon cancer | 0:1 |
| Malignant fibrous histiocytoma | 7:8 | Esophadenocarcinoma | 1:1 |
| Leiomyosarcoma | 9:13 | Melanoma | 0:6 |
| Ewing's sarcoma | 3:5 | Skin | 0:2 |
| Fibrosarcoma | 6:9 | Lymph node | 0:1 |
| Synovial cell sarcoma | 5:5 | Muscle | 0:2 |
| Schwannoma | 4:6 | Lung | 0:3 |
| Hemangiopericytoma | 1:1 | Spleen | 0:2 |
| Cystosarcoma | 1:1 | Liver | 0:3 |
| Dermatofibrosarcoma protuberans | 3:3 | Kidney | 0:2 |
| Epithelioid cell sarcoma | 1:1 | Fat | 0:1 |
| Chondrosarcoma | 2:3 | | |
| Desmoid | 2:2 | | |

[a]The intact MoAb 29–13 (1:200 dilution of the culture medium) and the renatured single-chain FV2913 were used as primary antibodies respectively. Goat anti-mouse IgG heavy chain conjugated to alkaline phosphatase (1:50 dilution) was used as the secondary antibody.
[b]Staining ratio = positive staining:total specimens tested.

its binding function to the sarcoma-associated antigen p200 contained in the sarcoma tissues.

Ninety-nine specimens of different human sarcomas, other tumors, and normal tissues were used in the study of immunohistochemical staining. Table 20–5 summarizes the results of immunostaining data. The results from the renatured single-chain FV2913 were consistent with those from the parent intact MoAb 29–13. The ratios of positive staining:total number of tested specimens for each class of human tissues were as follows: osteosarcoma (2:2), liposarcoma (11:13), rhabdomyosarcoma (5:6), malignant fibrous histiocytoma (7:8), leiomyosarcoma (9:13), Ewing's sarcoma (3:5), synovial cell sarcoma (5:5), fibrosarcoma (6:9), schwannoma (4:6), dermatofibrosarcoma protuberans (3:3), chondrosarcoma (2:3), desmoid (2:2), hemangiopericytoma (1:1), cystosarcoma (1:1), and epithelioid cell sarcoma (1:1). No positive staining was observed in any epithelial cancer nor in specimens of normal tissues (e.g., skin, lymph node, muscle, lung, spleen, liver and kidney). Figure 20–4 shows the immunostaining of liposarcoma frozen tissue sections. The single-chain FV2913 gave rise to positive staining (Fig. 20–4A), comparable to the parent intact MoAb 29–13 (Fig. 20–4B), when they were used as the respective primary antibody. However, the other primary antibody—MoAb P3, an unrelated mouse IgG—led to a negative staining (Fig. 20–4C).

DNA sequence of the single-chain FV2913 gene (Fig. 20–2) consists of the conservative framework and three complementary-determining regions (CDRs) for either VH or VL. As expected, the CDRs for both VH and VL of the single-chain FV2913 gene showed great diversity in comparison with the CDRs of VHs and VLs of other MoAb genes.[36] The diversity of CDR sequences determined the affinity and specificity of antibody/antigen binding.

The single-chain FV2913 gene was expressed under IPTG induction (Fig. 20–3). Yield of the single-chain FV2913 was about 0.5–1 mg from 1 L of culture. The renatured single-chain FV2913 was confirmed to carry specificity and affinity to the sarcoma-associated antigen p200 by the immunohistochemical staining studies (Fig. 20–4 and Table 20–5). According to the immunostaining data of 99 specimens, 62 of 78 (80 percent) sarcoma specimens were positively stained when either the single-chain FV2913 or the parent intact MoAb 29–13 was used as the primary antibody. None of the normal tissues, and only 1 out of 10 other tumors, were observed as positive staining. This indicated that the sarcoma-associated antigen p200 expressed in sarcomas was recognized by the renatured single-chain FV2913. Some sarcomas (20 percent) showing negative staining might be due to heterogeneous expression of the sarcoma-associated antigen p200.

The consistency of affinity and specificity to the sarcoma-associated antigen p200 of the single-chain FV2913 and the parent intact MoAb 29–13 indicated the potential of the single-chain FV2913 for sarcoma immunodiagnosis and immunotherapy. These results correspond with the radioimmunoassay data of the parent intact MoAb 29–13 reported previously,[42] suggesting that immunostaining with the single-chain FV2913 as the primary antibody is useful in diagnostic analysis

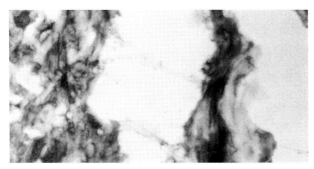

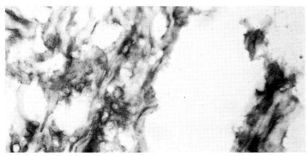

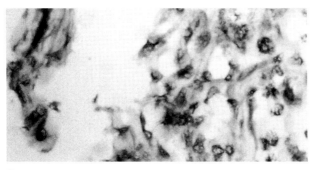

**Figure 20–4.** Immunohistochemical staining of human liposarcoma specimens. **(A)** Positive staining using single-chain FV2913 as the primary antibody. **(B)** Positive staining using the MoAb 29–13 as the primary antibody. **(C)** Negative staining using the MoAb P3 as the primary antibody.

of human sarcomas, especially in sarcomas of fibrous tissue origin (i.e., fibrosarcoma, malignant fibrous histiocytoma, desmoid, and dermatofibrosarcoma protuberans). Heterogeneous expression of the sarcoma-associated antigen p200 was observed (Table 20–5) in 75 specimens of 15 subsets of sarcomas. Antigen expression not only varies between histologically similar sarcomas from different individuals, but also between different locations within a large tumor. Therefore, it appears that the logical way to effectively detect expression of sarcoma-associated antigens with the immunostaining method is to use a combination of different single-chain FVs against various sarcoma-associated antigens.

# ■ INTERFERONS

Interferons are cellular proteins that have a broad range of immunomodulatory and antiproliferative effects. Hoffman et al.[47] evaluated the effect of recombinant human leukocyte interferon (rIFN-2) on the in vitro growth of human bone sarcomas. They were able to demonstrate a dose-dependent inhibition of $^{3}$H thymidine incorporation by sarcoma cells. Despite high doses ($10^{4}$ U/mL), they were not able to completely block the uptake. They then went on to evaluate the effect of rIFN-α2 on human sarcoma growth in a nude mouse model. Three of four human sarcoma cell lines tested in this fashion demonstrated sensitivity to rIFN-α2. Unfortunately, this sensitivity was evidenced by growth retardation only and required high daily doses (20,000 μ) to achieve it. Additionally, this was seen only when the rIFN-α2 was administered either before or shortly after tumor administration. No effect was seen on established metastasis.

Harris et al.[48] evaluated the effect of fibroblast interferon (beta-interferon) in 20 patients with metastatic soft tissue sarcomas. Only one patient exhibited a brief (10 weeks) partial response with intravenous therapy. Toxicity was rated as moderate, with only one patient suffering severe granulocytopenia. Similarly, Edmonson et al.[49] evaluated the effect of rIFN-α2 in 20 patients with metastatic bone sarcomas. Using the intramuscular route, three patients exhibited brief (1, 2, and 3 months) partial responses. Toxicity was modest, with no significant problems reported. The efficacy of interferons, therefore, remains to be established. Whether IFN in combination with currently available chemotherapy will be beneficial or not will require further scrutiny.

# ■ CELL-MEDIATED THERAPY

Adoptive immunotherapy is a therapeutic approach in which tumor immune cells are administered to the tumor-bearing host in an effort to mediate tumor regression. The identification of interleukin 2 (IL-2) as an agent able to cause proliferation and activation of human T-lymphocytes provided the impetus for the rapid application of this form of therapy.[50] Subsequent work by North and other researchers[51–54] demonstrated that the administration of activated lymphocytes in conjunction with IL-2 could effect the regression of metastasis and subsequent cure of mice with various forms of malignancies.

In late 1985, Rosenberg et al.[55] reported for the first time the use of lymphokine-activated killer (LAK) cells in humans.[55] LAK cells are peripheral blood lymphocytes that have been removed from the patient by leukophereses, incubated in vitro with IL-2, and then returned to the patient along with systemic IL-2 infusions. In this first report of 25 patients, they demonstrated 11 objective regressions. Although 4 of the 25 patients had sarcomas of various histologic subtypes, no responses were seen in this subgroup. When this report was updated, an additional two patients with sarcomas had been treated again without response.[56] West et al.[57] reported a similar treatment approach using constant infusion rather than bolus IL-2. In this trial of 40 patients, none had metastatic sarcomas. Because the experience with this form of therapy in patients with sarcomas is limited, the National Cancer Institute IL-2/LAK Extramural Working Group is currently evaluating it (along with various other forms of malignancies) in a national study.

LAK cells have been found to have a broad range of specificity. They will kill a large variety of tumors without regard to major histocompatibility antigens. In an attempt to generate a more specifically cytotoxic cell, Rosenberg et al.[58,59] have investigated ways of expanding tumor-infiltrating lymphocytes (TIL). In several recent reports, they have demonstrated the ability to effectively expand the population of lymphocytes that are found in tumor nodules. It is hoped that this population of lymphocytes has naturally developed immunity to the tumor and that, when expanded to adequate numbers, they will be effective in mediating tumor regression. In fact, in animal studies, the TILs have been found to be 50 to 100 times more effective than LAK cells at killing tumor cells. Successful generation of TIL from tumors removed from sarcoma patients has been reported.[59] Clinical trials using TIL have been initiated by the National Cancer Institute. However, preliminary results do not appear encouraging.

In an attempt to overcome the problems encountered in the recovery and expansion of TIL, Slovin et al.[60,61] have developed the concept of the "educated" lymphocyte. Educated lymphocytes are T-lymphocytes derived from the peripheral blood that have been sensitized or "educated" in vitro with the patient's autologous irradiated tumor cells and IL-2. T-cell clones isolated in this manner have been found to be specifically cytotoxic for the patient's autologous tumor cells, as well as other histologic types of sarcomas, providing they share at least one major histocompatibility complex determinant.[60] No cross-reactivity was seen with various carcinomas or normal cells. Recently, clinical trials using educated lymphocytes in conjunction with cyclophosphamide and IL-2 have also been initiated. It is too premature to try to draw any conclusions regarding the overall efficacy of the method in general and sarcomas in particular.

During the past five years, many investigators have demonstrated the effectiveness of granulocyte-macrophage colony-stimulating factor (GM-CSF) and other cytokines in the immune destruction of rodent tumors when the cytokine gene is transduced into irradiated tumor cells[62,63] or when controlled-release cytokine depots are implanted with the tumor cells.[64] Under these conditions, not only are the tumor cells destroyed, but also this treatment causes the host mice to destroy any further injected cells of this same lineage. Thus, the principle has been established that GM-CSF (and perhaps other cytokines) may enhance antitumor immunity, and such GM-CSF-based autologous tumor vaccines are currently being prepared and used in human studies.[65] If current efforts against human renal adenocarcinoma, prostate cancer, lung cancer, and melanoma are at all successful in enhancing antitumor immunity, cytokine gene transduction undoubtedly will be studied in sarcomas as well, both alone and with chemotherapy. In general, systemic infusion of GM-CSF in mice has been found insufficient to generate effective autologous tumor vaccines; however, at least one early phase I human study of molgramostim (recombinant human [rh]GM-CSF, nonglycosylated *Escherichia coli*-derived; Schering-Plough/Sandoz, Kenilworth, NJ) suggested possible antisarcoma activity from this GM-CSF preparation infused alone into heavily pretreated patients.[66] Conceivably, a small but tumor-selective enhancement of immune recognition and host rejection might provide the additional tumor-cell control required to permit total tumor destruction in some metastatic sarcomas already partially responsive to chemotherapy. Although such speculative views must be based currently more on hope than on hard data, the concept that cytokines or other agents of cytoimmune enhancement soon might become therapeutically relevant against sarcomas is no longer difficult to imagine.[67]

# ■ TUMOR NECROSIS FACTOR

Although tumor necrosis factor (TNF) in purified form is currently available, its overall usefulness in the management of soft tissue sarcomas remains to be investigated. Administration of TNF-α has a marked effect on a variety of murine tumors.[68] The initial response in vivo is a hemorrhagic infarction/necrosis of the tumor, evident as early as 30 minutes to six hours after bolus TNF administration.[69] TNF acts primarily on host endothelial cells in the tumor microenvironment, to increase procoagulant activity with thrombosis and platelet aggregation in the tumor microenvironment. This effect, which is specific for the tumor vasculature, is apparently induced by factors produced by the tumor cells priming the local endothelial cell response to TNF.[70]

Currently, TNF-α has only been tried in isolated limb perfusion in unresectable sarcoma, with supposedly good results (see Chapter 19 for further details).

## REFERENCES

1. Bartal AH, Lavie E, Boazi M, et al.: Human sarcoma-associated murine monoclonal antibody labeled with Indium-111, Gallium-67, and Iodine-125. NCI Monogr 3:153, 1987

2. Lavie E, Boazi M, Weininger J, et al.: Labeling of sarcoma associated monoclonal antibody with $^{111}$In $^{67}$Ga and $^{125}$I. Radiother Oncol 8:129, 1987

3. Bartal AH, Luchtiz C, Friedman-Birnbaum R, et al.: The interaction of Kaposi's sarcoma with monoclonal antibodies to human sarcoma and connective tissue differentiation antigens. Cancer 56:1071, 1985

4. Miettinen M: Antibody specific to muscle actins in the diagnosis and classification of soft tissue tumors. Am J Pathol 130:205, 1988

5. Schmidt RA, Cone R, Haas JE, et al.: Diagnosis of rhabdomyosarcomas with HHF-35, a monoclonal antibody directed against muscle actins. Am J Pathol 131:19, 1988

6. Brown JM: Detection of a human sarcoma-associated antigen with monoclonal antibodies. Cancer Res 43:2113, 1983

7. Brown JM, Greager JA, Pavel DG, Das Gupta TK: Localization of radiolabeled monoclonal antibody in a human soft tissue sarcoma xenograft. J Natl Cancer Inst 75:637, 1985

8. Greager JA, Chao T-C, Blend MJ, et al.: Localization of pulmonary human sarcoma xenografts in athymic nude mice with indium-111-labeled monoclonal antibodies. J Nucl Med 31:1378, 1990

9. Greager JA, Chao T-C, Brown JM, et al.: Localization of human sarcoma with radiolabeled monoclonal antibody—A follow-up report. Cancer Immunol Immunother 33:341, 1991

10. Stastny JJ, Das Gupta TK: The use of daunomycin-antibody immunoconjugates in managing soft tissue sarcomas: Nude mouse xenograft model. Cancer Res 53:5740, 1993

11. Morrison SL, Schlom J: Recombinant chimeric monoclonal antibodies. In DeVita VT, Hellman S, Rosenberg SA (eds.) Important Advances in Oncology, Philadelphia, J.B. Lippincott, 1990, p 3

12. Winter G, Milstein C: Man-made antibodies Nature (Lond) 349:293, 1991

13. Morrison SL, Johnson MJ, Herzenberg LA, Oi VT: Chimeric human antibody molecules: Mouse antigen-binding domains with human constant region domains. Proc Natl Acad Sci U S A 81:6851, 1984

14. Steplewski Z, Sun LK, Shearman CW, et al.: Biological activity of human-mouse IgG1, IgG2, IgG3, and IgG4 chimeric monoclonal antibodies with antitumor specificity. Proc Natl Acad Sci U S A 85:4852, 1988

15. Hutzell P, Kashmiri S, Colcher D, et al.: Generation and characterization of recombinant/chimeric B72.3 (human gamma 1). Cancer Res 51:181, 1991

16. Jones PT, Dear PH, Foote J, et al.: Replacing the complementarity-determining regions in a human antibody with those from a mouse. Nature (Lond) 321:522, 1986

17. Caron PC, Co MS, Bull MK, et al.: Biological and immunological features of humanized M195 (anti-CD33) monoclonal antibodies. Cancer Res 52:6761, 1992

18. Rosenblum MG, Levin B, Roh M, et al.: Clinical pharmacology and tissue disposition studies of $^{131}$I-labeled anti-colorectal carcinoma human monoclonal antibody LiCO 16.88. Cancer Immunol Immunother 39:397, 1994

19. Orlandi R, Gussow DF, Jones PT, Winter G: Cloning immunoglobulin variable domains for expression by the polymerase chain reaction. Proc Natl Acad Sci U S A 86:3833, 1989

20. Chen H, Stastny JJ, Das Gupta TK: Molecular cloning and sequence analysis of a single-chain antibody 29–13 against human sarcoma-associated antigen p200. Proc Amer Assoc Cancer Res 35:525, 1994

21. Jain RK: Delivery of novel therapeutic agents in tumors: Physiological barriers and strategies. J Natl Cancer Inst 81:570, 1989

22. Bolhuis RLH, Sturm E, Braakman E: T-cell targeting in cancer therapy. Cancer Immunol Immunother 34:1, 1991

23. Schroff RW, Foon KA, Beatty SA, et al.: Human anti-murine immunoglobulin responses in patients receiving monoclonal antibody therapy. Cancer Res 45:879, 1983

24. Shaaler DL, Bartholomew RM, Smith LM, Dillman RO: Human immune response to multiple injections of murine monoclonal IgG. J Immunol 135:1530, 1985

25. Colcher D, Bird R, Roselli M, et al.: In vitro tumor targeting of a recombinant single-chain antigen-binding protein. J Natl Cancer Inst 82:1191, 1990

26. Milenic DE, Yokota T, Filpula DR, et al.: Construction, binding properties, metabolism, and tumor targeting of a single-chain FV derived from the pancarcinoma monoclonal antibody CC49. Cancer Res 51:6363, 1991

27. Ridder R, Schmitz R, Legay F, Gram H: Generation of rabbit monoclonal antibody fragments from a combinatorial phage display library and their production in the yeast pichia pastoris. Biotechnology 13:255, 1995

28. Eshhar Z, Waks T, Gross G, Schindler DG: Specific activation and targeting of cytotoxic lymphocytes through chimeric single chains consisting of antibody-binding domains and the or subunits of the immunoglobulin and T-cell receptors. Proc Natl Acad Sci U S A 90:720, 1993

29. Wels W, Harwerth IM, Mueller M, et al.: Selective inhibition of tumor cell growth by a recombinant single-chain antibody-toxin specific for the erbB-2 receptor. Cancer Res 52:6310, 1993

30. Hwu P, Shafer GE, Treisman J, et al.: Lysis of ovarian cancer cells by human lymphocytes redirected with a chimeric gene composed of an antibody variable region and the Fc receptor chain. J Exp Med 178:361, 1993

31. Wels W, Harwerth IM, Hynes NE, Groner B: Diminution of antibodies directed against tumor cell surface epi-

topes: A single-chain Fv fusion molecule specifically recognizes the extracellular domain of the c-erbB-2 receptor. J Steroid Biochem Mol Biol 43:1, 1992

32. Goshorn SC, Svensson HP, Kerr DE, et al.: Genetic construction, expression, and characterization of a single-chain anti-carcinoma antibody fused to B-lactamase. Cancer Res 53:2123, 1993

33. Chaudhary VK, Batra JK, Gallo MG, et al.: A rapid method of cloning functional variable-region antibody genes in Escherichia coli as single-chain immunotoxins. Proc Natl Acad Sci U S A 87:1066, 1990

34. Chaudhary VK, Gallo MG, FitzGerald DJ, Pastan I: A recombinant single-chain immunotoxin composed of anti-Tac variable regions and a truncated diphtheria toxin. Proc Natl Acad Sci U S A 87:9491, 1990

35. Brinkmann U, Pai LH, Fitzgerald DJ, et al.: B3(Fv)-PE38KDEL, a single-chain immunotoxin that causes complete regression of a human carcinoma in mice. Proc Natl Acad Sci U S A 88:8616, 1991

36. Kreitman RJ, Schneider WP, Queen C, et al.: Mik-B1(Fv)-PE40, a recombinant immunotoxin cytotoxic toward cells bearing the B-chain of the IL-2 receptor. J Immunol 149:2810, 1991

37. Batra JK, Fitzgerald DJ, Chaudhary VK, Pastan I: Single-chain immunotoxins directed at the human transferrin receptor containing Pseudomonas Exotoxin A or diphtheria toxin: Anti-TFR(Fv)-PE40 and DT388-anti-TFR(Fv). Mol Cell Biol 11:2200, 1991

38. Brinkmann U, Buchner J, Pastan I: Independent domain folding of Pseudomonas exotoxin and single-chain immunotoxins: Influence of interdomain connections. Proc Natl Acad Sci U S A 89:3075, 1992

39. Huston JS, Levinson D, Mudgett-Hunter M, et al.: Protein engineering of antibody binding sites: Recovery of specific activity in an anti-digoxin single-chain Fv analogue produced in Escherichia coli. Proc Natl Acad Sci U S A 85:5879, 1988

40. Brocker T, Peter A, Traunecker A, Karjalainen K: New simplified molecular design for functional T-cell receptor. Eur J Immunol 23:1435, 1993

41. Zhu Z, Zapata G, Shalaby R, et al.: High level secretion of a humanized bispecific diabody from Escherichia coli. Biotechnology 14:192, 1996

42. Stastny JJ, Brown JM, Beattie CW, Das Gupta TK: Monoclonal antibody identification and characterization of two human sarcoma-associated antigens. Cancer Res 51:3768, 1991

43. Brown JM, Stastny JJ, Beattie CW, Das Gupta TK: Monoclonal antibody characterization of sarcoma-associated antigen p102. Anticancer Res 11:1565, 1991

44. Blend MJ, Greager JA, Atcher RW, et al.: Improved sarcoma imaging and reduced hepatic activity with IN-111-SCN-Bz-DTPA linked to MOAB 19–24. J Nucl Med 29(11):1810, 1988

45. Greager JA, Brown JM, Pavel DG, et al.: Localization of human sarcoma with radiolabeled monoclonal antibody. Cancer Immunol Immunother 23:148, 1986

46. Mohamed G, Kuzmanoff KM, Stastny JJ, Das Gupta TK: In vitro cytotoxicity of the conjugate Adriamycin with anti-sarcoma monoclonal antibody 19–24. Anticancer Res 12:529, 1992

47. Hoffman V, Groscurth P, Morant R, et al.: Effects of leukocyte interferon (E. Coli) on human bone sarcoma growth in vitro and in the nude mouse. Eur J Cancer Clin Oncol 21:859, 1985

48. Harris J, Das Gupta T, Vogelzang N, et al.: Treatment of soft tissue sarcoma with fibroblast interferon (B-Interferon): An American Cancer Society/Illinois Cancer Council Study. Cancer Treat Rep 70:293, 1986

49. Edmonson JH, Long HJ, Frytak S, et al.: Phase II study of recombinant alfa-2a interferon in patients with advanced bone sarcomas. Cancer Treat Rep 71:747, 1987

50. Morgan DA, Ruscetti FU, Gallo RC: Selective in vitro growth of T-lymphocytes from normal bone marrows. Science 193:1007, 1976

51. North RJ: Cyclophosphamide-facilitated adoptive immunotherapy of an established tumor depends on elimination of tumor-induced suppressor T cells. J Exp Med 55:1063, 1982

52. Cheever MA, Greenberg DD, Gillisd S, et al.: Specific, adoptive immunotherapy of murine leukemia with cells secondarily sensitized in vitro and expanded by culture with interleukin 2. Prog Cancer Res Ther 22:127, 1982

53. Mazumder A, Rosenberg SA: Successful immunotherapy of natural killer resistant established pulmonary metastases by the intravenous adoptive transfer of syngeneic lymphocytes activated in vitro by interleukin-2. J Exp Med 159:495, 1984

54. Mule JJ, Shu S, Schwartz SL, et al.: Adoptive immunotherapy of established pulmonary metastases with LAK cells and recombinant interleukin-2. Science 225:1487, 1984

55. Rosenberg SA, Lotte MT, Muul LM, et al.: Observations on the systemic administration of autologous lymphokine activated killer cells and recombinant interleukin-2 to patients with metastatic cancer. N Engl J Med 313:1485, 1985

56. Rosenberg SA, Lotze MT, Muul LM, et al.: A progress report on the treatment of 157 patients with advanced cancer using lymphokine-activated killer cells and interleukin-2 or high dose interleukin-2 alone. N Engl J Med 315:889, 1987

57. West WH, Tauer KW, Jannelli JR: Constant-infusion recombinant interleukin-2 in adoptive immunotherapy of advanced cancer. N Engl J Med 316:898, 1987

58. Rosenberg SA, Spiess D, Lafreniere R: A new approach to the adoptive immunotherapy of cancer using tumor infiltrating lymphocytes. Science 233:1318, 1986

59. Topalian SL, Muul LM, Solomon D, et al.: Expansion of human tumor infiltrating lymphocytes for use in immunotherapy trials. Immunol Methods 102:127, 1987

60. Slovin SF, Lackman RD, Ferrone S, et al.: Analysis of cellular immune response to sarcomas as using cytotoxic T-cell clones. Proc Am Assoc Cancer Res 27:360, 1986

61. Slovin SF, Lackman RD, Ferrone S, et al.: Cellular immune response to human sarcomas: Cytotoxic T-cell clones reactive with autologous sarcomas. I. Development Phenotype and Specificity. J Immunol 137:3042, 1986

62. Pardoll DM, Golumbek P, Levitsky H, et al.: Molecular engineering of the antitumor response. Bone Marrow Transplant 9(1):S182, 1992

63. Dranoff G, Jaffee E, Lozenby A, et al.: Vaccination with irradiated tumor cells engineered to secrete murine gran-

ulocyte-macrophage colony stimulating factor stimulates potent, specific and long-lasting antitumor immunity. Proc Natl Acad Sci U S A 90:3539, 1993

64. Golumbek PT, Axhari R, Jaffee EM, et al.: Controlled release, biodegradable cytokine depots: A new approach in cancer vaccine design. Cancer Res 53:5841, 1993

65. Rankin EM, Spits H, Orsini D, et al.: A phase I study of vaccination with autologous GM-CSF-transduced and irradiated tumor cells in patients with advanced melanoma. Proc Am Soc Clin Oncol (abstr) 14:226, 1995

66. Steward WP, Scarffe JH, Austin R, et al.: Recombinant human granulocyte-macrophage colony-stimulating factor given as daily short infusions: A phase I dose-toxicity study. Br J Cancer 59:142, 1989

67. Zitvogel L, Tahara H, Robbins PD, et al.: Cancer gene therapy using a cytokine, IL-12 and a constimulatory sig-

nal molecule B7.1. Proc Am Soc Clin Oncol (abstr) 14:226, 1995

68. Sugarman BJ, Aggarwal BB, Hass PE, et al.: Recombinant human tumor necrosis factor: Effects on proliferation of normal and transformed cells in vitro. Science 230:943, 1985

69. Asher A, Mulø JJ, Reichert CM, et al.: Studies on the antitumor efficacy of systemically administered recombinant tumor necrosis factor against several murine tumors in vivo. J Immunol 138:963, 1987

70. Clauss M, Murray JC, Vianna M, et al.: A polypeptide factor produced by fibrosarcoma cells that induces endothelial tissue factor and enhances the procoagulant response to tumor necrosis factor/cachectin. J Biol Chem 265:7078, 1990

# IV

## Mesenchymal Tumors in Children

# 21

# Soft Tissue Sarcomas in Children

Soft tissue sarcomas are malignant neoplasms derived from primitive mesenchyme. The latter is composed of mesenchymal cells, which principally give rise to fibrous tissue, muscle, cartilage, and bone. Consequently, soft tissue sarcomas may occasionally contain elements or structures derived from the multipotential derivatives of the mesenchymal cell (see Chapters 2 and 5 for details).

## ■ EPIDEMIOLOGY

Soft tissue sarcomas are the sixth most common form of childhood cancer.[1] They occur at a rate of 8.4 cases per million in Caucasian children per year and 3.9 cases per million in African-American children per year.[1] (See Chapter 1 for details). The incidence and cure rates for rhabdomyosarcoma by primary site are presented in Tables 21–1 and 21–2. Rhabdomyosarcoma in children may be considered the prototype soft tissue sarcoma. We present and consider it as the paradigm of this group of cancers. More specific details of other soft tissue sarcomas will be provided in their respective sections.

## ■ ETIOLOGY

Rhabdomyosarcoma arises from tissue that imitates normal striated muscle (Fig. 21–1). It is the most common soft tissue sarcoma in patients under the age of 15 years and accounts for 5 to 8 percent of childhood cancer cases.[1] Approximately 250 new cases are diag-

nosed annually in the United States.[2] Males are more likely to be affected than females. The etiology is unknown. An association with neurofibromatosis has been suggested with the report of rhabdomyosarcomatous differentiation within the neurogenic component.[3] Such peripheral nerve tumors with rhabdomyosarcomatous differentiation have been designated *malignant triton tumors.* An increased incidence of congenital anomalies has also been noted in children with rhabdomyosarcoma.[4] Li and Fraumeni[5] reported an association between maternal breast cancer and soft tissue sarcoma in the offspring. This has been designated *Li-Fraumeni syndrome.* The syndrome is categorized by germline mutations in the p53 tumor suppressor gene located on chromosome 17. The syndrome has also been described as autosomal dominant in five families.[6]

## ■ PATHOLOGY

Rhabdomyosarcoma has conventionally been classified into the following pathologic entities: embryonal rhabdomyosarcoma sarcoma, alveolar rhabdomyosarcoma, pleomorphic rhabdomyosarcoma, and extraosseous Ewing's sarcoma.

Current thinking, however, considers extraosseous Ewing's sarcoma a derivative of primitive neuroectodermal tissue. From an ontogenic standpoint, these tumors are grouped together with neuroblastomas or malignant ganglioneuromas. However, from a clinical standpoint, at least in children, it appears to behave similarly to rhabdomyosarcomas (see Chapter 5 for further details).

**TABLE 21–1. RHABDOMYOSARCOMA DISTRIBUTION BY PRIMARY SITE***

| Primary Site | Percentage |
| --- | --- |
| Head and Neck | 34 |
| Genitourinary Tract | 25 |
| Extremities | 17 |
| Trunk | 10 |
| Retroperitoneum | 11 |
| Miscellaneous | 3 |

*Average from collected series; percentages may not add up.

## EMBRYONAL RHABDOMYOSARCOMA SARCOMA

Embryonal sarcoma is the most common variety and accounts for approximately 50 percent of rhabdomyosarcomas. It is composed primarily of spindle-shaped rhabdomyoblasts and small round cells in which longitudinal striations may be found (Fig. 21–2). Solid embryonal rhabdomyosarcoma occurs within deep or superficial structures not covered by mucosa. Botryoid rhabdomyosarcoma is a histologic variation of the embryonal type and is almost exclusively a tumor of young children (Fig. 21–3). It arises in structures covered by mucosa and apposite to a body cavity (e.g., bladder or nasopharynx).[7]

## ALVEOLAR RHABDOMYOSARCOMA

Alveolar rhabdomyosarcoma was described by Riopelle and Theriault[8] and formally characterized by Enzinger and Shiraki.[9] The tumor tends to grow in cords that have cleftlike spaces resembling "alveoli" (Fig. 21–4).[8] It is the second most common type and accounts for

**TABLE 21–2. RHABDOMYOSARCOMA CURE RATE (PRINCIPALLY LOCO-REGIONAL DISEASE)***

| Primary Site | Percentage |
| --- | --- |
| Head and neck | 80 |
| Parameningeal | 55 |
| Extremities | 75 |
| Genitourinary tract | 80 |
| Paratesticular | 90 |
| Trunk | 50 |
| Retroperitoneum | 40 |
| Perineal | 48 |
| Intrathoracic | 24 |
| Miscellaneous | 25–50 |

*Average from collected series; percentages may not add up.

approximately 20 percent of rhabdomyosarcomas. The rhabdomyoblasts are often mixed with large cells that exhibit a prominent eosinophilic cytoplasm.

## PLEOMORPHIC (ADULT-TYPE) RHABDOMYOSARCOMA

Pleomorphic rhabdomyosarcoma is more common in adults but has also been observed in children. It is composed of large pleomorphic cells (Fig. 21–5). These tumors have been described as straplike, with multiple nuclei in tandem; racket-shaped, with cytoplasmic tails; and large round cells, with giant nuclei and multinucleated giant cells.

## EXTRAOSSEOUS EWING'S SARCOMA

Extraosseous Ewing's sarcoma is a relatively new entity that is now clinically included in the category of rhab-

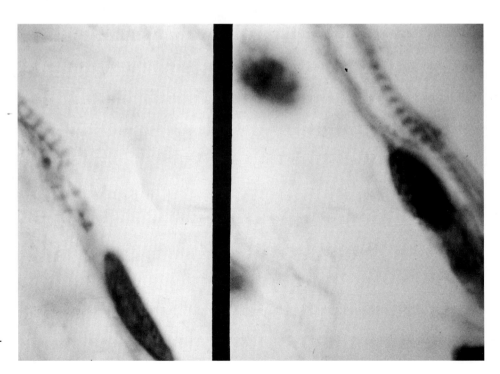

**Figure 21–1.** Cross-striations in a skeletal muscle cell.

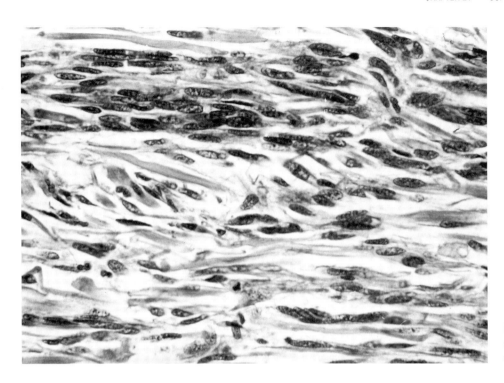

**Figure 21–2.** Embryonal rhabdomyosarcoma. The tumor has a dominant spindle cell component.

domyosarcoma.[10,11] This tumor is composed of small, round or oval anaplastic cells of uniform size with giant cytoplasm (Fig. 21–6). PAS-positive diastase material, which may be arranged in pseudorosette formation, is usually evident within the cells. In general, the tumor is located in soft tissue and has morphologic characteristics similar to that of Ewing's sarcoma of bone (Also see page 386, Chapter 10).

## ■ PROGNOSIS

Embryonal and botryoid rhabdomyosarcomas are generally characterized by a favorable prognosis. The alveolar type has a poor prognosis, and the pleomorphic type has the worst prognosis. Newton[12] recently published a classification system that appears reproducible and highly predictive of outcome (Table 21–3).

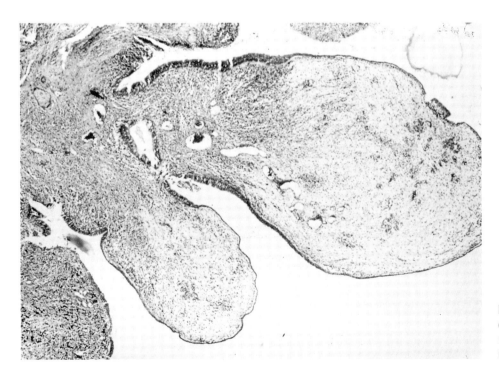

**Figure 21–3.** Botryoid rhabdomyosarcoma. The tumor is similar to embryonal rhabdomyosarcoma and covered by a lining of mucosal cells.

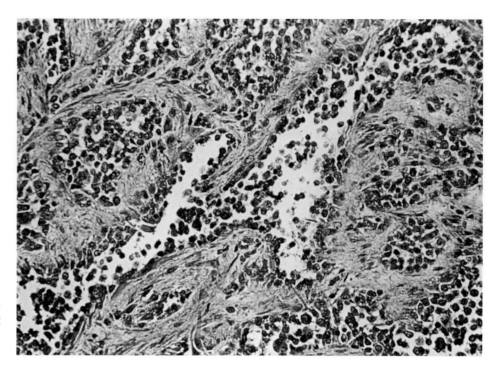

**Figure 21–4.** Alveolar rhabdomyosarcoma. The alveolar pattern is reminiscent of the alveoli of the lung but is composed of high-grade tumor cells.

## ■ PATHOLOGIC DIAGNOSIS

The pathologic diagnosis of rhabdomyosarcoma is initially attempted with light microscopy. Cross-striation mimicking striated muscle is used to identify tumor. Unfortunately, cross-striations are often inapparent on routine hematoxylin and eosin sections. Immunocytochemical examination with antibodies directed against skeletal muscle and other myogenous proteins are usually more reliable. These include skeletal muscle myosin, myoglobin, creatine kinase-MM, skeletal muscle actin, desmin, vimentin, neuron-specific enolase, and Z-band protein.[13–18] Desmin and muscle-specific actin are probably the most sensitive markers used to identify rhabdomyosarcoma, although they are not specific for skeletal muscle. A relationship between marker predominance and prognosis has been suggested.[19,20]

Electron microscopy may be extremely useful in supporting a diagnosis of rhabdomyosarcoma, particularly if the tumors are primitive. However, the investi-

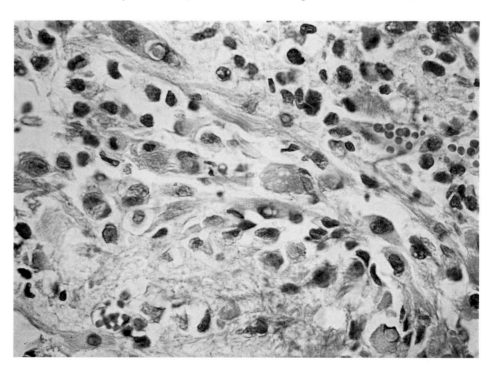

**Figure 21–5.** Pleomorphic rhabdomyosarcoma. High-grade tumor cells are present.

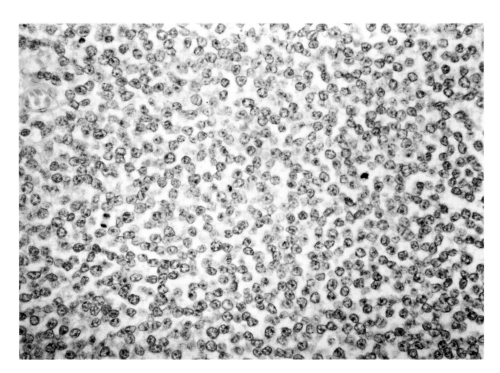

**Figure 21–6.** Extraosseous Ewing's sarcoma. This tumor is characterized by a monotonous appearance of small, round blue cells.

gation may not be completely reliable, and, in many instances, immunocytochemistry with light microscopy may also be necessary.

## DIFFERENTIAL DIAGNOSIS

Rhabdomyosarcoma must be differentiated from other soft tissue sarcomas. Most prominent are the following: fibroblastic, neurogenic, and primitive neuroectodermal tumor (PNET). Well-differentiated soft tissue entities such as synovial sarcoma, fibrosarcoma, alveolar soft part sarcoma, and hemangiopericytoma may occasionally be confused with rhabdomyosarcoma. Non-Hodgkin's lymphoma and neuroblastoma may also (rarely) mimic rhabdomyosarcoma.

**TABLE 21–3. CLASSIFICATION OF CHILDHOOD RHABDOMYOSARCOMA**

| |
|---|
| **Superior prognosis** |
| Botryoid RMS |
| Spindle cell RMS |
| **Intermediate prognosis** |
| Embryonal RMS |
| **Poor prognosis** |
| Alveolar RMS |
| Undifferentiated sarcoma |
| **Subtypes whose prognosis is not presently evaluable** |
| RMS with rhabdoid features |

Abbreviations: RMS, rhabdomyosarcoma.
Adapted from Newton et al.,[12] with permission.

## ■ CHROMOSOMAL AND MOLECULAR CHARACTERISTICS

Various chromosomal abnormalities in soft tissue sarcomas have been reported. Whether these are expressions or alterations of oncogene abnormality is unknown. Translocation in alveolar rhabdomyosarcoma, t(2;13), and extra Chromosome 2 material in embryonal rhabdomyosarcoma patients are well documented.[21] This observation is also supported by investigators who noted a t(2;13) (q35; q14) translocation in the alveolar and other varieties of rhabdomyosarcoma.[22,23] The characteristic abnormality in alveolar rhabdomyosarcoma involving chromosomes 2 and 13, t(2;13) (q35;q14),[22,24] also affects the PAX3 gene in band 2q35 and the FKHR gene in band 13q14.[25,26] Further, although t(2;13) has been found in most cases of alveolar rhabdomyosarcoma, several cases have a variant, t(1;13) (p36;q14), which juxtaposes the PAX7 gene on Chromosome 1p36 with the FKHR gene on Chromosome 13q14.[27] This fusion produces a chimeric transcript in which the PAX7 DNA-binding domains are similar to those of PAX3.[28] Alterations in the p53 gene and in the retinoblastoma gene have also been documented[29,30] (See Chapters 5 and 6 for further details).

Identification of genes disrupted by tumor-specific translocations has permitted the development of sensitive and specific molecular diagnostic assays. These may be performed by reverse transcriptase/polymerase chain reaction (RT-PCR), which has been used to detect chimeric messenger RNA molecules in tumors with t(2;13) rearrangements.[25,28,31] Further, fluorescence in situ hybridization (FISH) may also identify tumor-specific derivative chromosomes with this translocation.[32]

Embryonal and alveolar tumors also possess other genetic abnormalities. Over 50 percent may have diverse p53 mutations.[33] Embryonal tumors have also been reported to possess more point mutations of the N-ras and K-ras proto-oncogenes than the alveolar cases. Finally, N-myc gene amplification may be an exclusive feature of approximately 10 percent of alveolar tumors.[34,35] The discovery of these abnormalities, in particular the PAX-FKHR gene, could provide specific molecular targets for future intervention. This may also stimulate investigation of the efficacy of gene-based therapy.

## THERAPEUTIC AND DIAGNOSTIC IMPLICATIONS OF CHROMOSOMAL AND MOLECULAR ABERRATIONS

Embryonal rhabdomyosarcoma with hyperdiploid characteristics may be more sensitive to chemotherapy and radiation therapy than similar cases without these cytogenetic features.[36–40] In contrast, near tetraploidy (which is usually of the alveolar variety) generally does poorly.[36] Hyperdiploidy also reportedly conferred the best prognosis and diploidy the worst.[36]

## ■ TUMOR LOCATION

Embryonal rhabdomyosarcoma generally occurs in the head and neck region or genitourinary tract. The botryoid type is usually found in the bladder, vagina, or nasopharynx. The alveolar variety is more frequently encountered in the extremities and trunk. The remaining types of rhabdomyosarcoma, which include pleomorphic, undifferentiated, extraosseous Ewing's sarcoma, and other rare entities, are usually found in the extremities and trunk.

## ■ AGE DISTRIBUTION

Embryonal and botryoid rhabdomyosarcomas usually occur in infants and young children (0 to 12 years), whereas the alveolar and other varieties arise in the older population (6 to 20 years).

## ■ BIOPSY

Microscopic diagnosis before initiating any therapy program is usually obtained either by resecting a wedge of the tumor (incisional biopsy) or excising the entire tumor, especially smaller ones (excisional biopsy).

More recently, cytologic examination of specimens obtained by fine-needle aspiration or core biopsies is being employed. Although fine-needle aspiration biopsy is an extremely useful method, it should not be relied upon unless the pathologist is adept in interpreting the cytologic details and in using immunocytochemical methods. Needle biopsy may also be used to document recurrent or residual disease or to plan excisional strategies. Bone marrow examination (needle aspiration and biopsy) is usually performed to confirm suspected or established cases of dissemination.

## ■ BIOLOGICAL BEHAVIOR

### PRIMARY TUMOR

Rhabdomyosarcoma may occur at any site where striated muscle is located. The tumor spreads locally by contiguity and continuity, and infiltrates into surrounding tissues. It metastasizes to draining lymph nodes and eventually to the lungs. It may also spread by hematologic dissemination to the lungs and to other parts of the body. This includes invasion into the bone marrow, which may be microscopic. In the parameningeal region, it may infiltrate the bone and meninges and contaminate the cerebrospinal fluid.

### INVASION OF REGIONAL LYMPH NODES

Invasion of regional lymph nodes generally varies with the site and pathologic variety of the tumor. Most tumors must be considered able to infiltrate into the regional lymph nodes. However, nodal infiltration is not common in head and neck tumors, except in advanced stages. It is extremely rare in orbital rhabdomyosarcoma. Invasion into regional lymph nodes may complicate tumors arising in paratesticular structures; however, it is more likely to occur with tumors in the extremities. Any regional lymph node suspected of harboring metastases at any site should be removed and submitted for pathologic examination.

## ■ STAGING

Various staging systems have been developed. Many are surgical-pathologic in nature and are dictated by the degree to which the tumor has been extirpated. The system developed by the Intergroup Rhabdomyosarcoma Study group (IRS) has been widely publicized.[41] It has been used in studies I–III and is outlined in Table 21–4. The system has been found to be particularly useful for its prognostic value.[42] Tumors may also be categorized without regard to the extent of resection—

**TABLE 21–4. INTERGROUP RHABDOMYOSARCOMA STUDY CLINICAL GROUPING SYSTEM**

| | |
|---|---|
| Group I | Localized tumor, completely removed; no tumor cells at margins or in regional lymph nodes. |
| Group II | Localized tumor, grossly removed but with tumor cells at margins, in regional lymph nodes, or both. |
| Group III | Localized tumor sampled by biopsy only or incompletely removed, with visible residual tumor, with or without tumor cells in regional lymph nodes. |
| Group IV | Distant metastases at any site, including tumor cells or implants in the pleural or peritoneal cavity or in the cerebrospinal fluid. |

**TABLE 21–5. TNM STAGING SYSTEM FOR RHABDOMYOSARCOMA**

| Stage | Sites | T[a] | Size | N[b] | M[c] |
|---|---|---|---|---|---|
| 1 | Orbit<br>Head and neck (excluding parameningeal)[d]<br><br>Genitourinary (non-bladder/nonprostate) | $T_1$ or $T_2$ | a or b | $N_0$ or $N_1$ or $N_x$ | $M_0$ |
| 2 | Bladder/prostate<br>Extremity<br>Cranial parameningeal<br>Other (includes trunk, retroperitoneum, etc.) | $T_1$ or $T_2$ | a | $N_0$ or $N_x$ | $M_0$ |
| 3 | Bladder/prostate<br>Extremity<br>Cranial parameningeal<br>Other (includes trunk retroperitoneum, etc.) | $T_1$ or $T_2$ | a<br>b | $N_1$<br>$N_0$ or $N_1$ or $N_x$ | $M_0$<br>$M_0$ |
| 4 | All | $T_1$ or $T_2$ | a or b | $N_0$ or $N_1$ | $M_1$ |

[a]Tumor (T):
| | | |
|---|---|---|
| | $T(site)_1$ | Confined to anatomic site of origin |
| | a | < 5 cm diameter |
| | b | ≥ 5 cm diameter |
| | $T(site)_2$ | Extension and/or fixation to surrounding tissue |
| | a | < 5 cm diameter |
| | b | ≥ 5 cm diameter |

[b]Regional nodes (N):
| | | |
|---|---|---|
| | $N_0$ | Regional nodes not clinically involved |
| | $N_1$ | Regional nodes clinically involved by neoplasm |
| | $N_x$ | Clinical status of regional nodes unknown (especially sites that preclude lymph node evaluation) |

[c]Metastasis (M):
| | | |
|---|---|---|
| | $M_0$ | No distant metastasis |
| | $M_1$ | Metastasis present |

[d]Arising in nasopharynx/nasal cavity, paranasal sinuses, middle ear/mastoid, or parapharyngeal area/pterygopalatine/infratemporal fossae.

the TNM system (i.e., tumor, node, metastasis). This classification system, based upon pretreatment assessment of the extent and location of the tumor, is outlined in Table 21–5. The system recently has also been adopted by the IRS.[43]

## ◼ CLINICAL PRESENTATION

Clinical manifestations depend on the size and location of the tumor. Signs and symptoms also manifest as a consequence of dissemination to other organs and structures.

### HEAD AND NECK REGION

The head and neck, including the orbit, is the most common site for the occurrence of rhabdomyosarcoma. Overall, 34 percent of rhabdomyosarcomas appear in the head and neck: 16 percent cranial or parameningeal, 8 percent orbital, and 10 percent in other sites. Most of these tumors are unresectable for cosmetic reasons or because of their location. Most are embryonal cell tumors and can be classified in clinical group III. Tumors of the orbit are usually diagnosed early, possibly because the face is continually exposed to observation. They occasionally manifest with proptosis and occasionally ophthalmoplegia.[44,45] These tumors rarely metastasize to the draining cervical lymph nodes except in the advanced stages. Notwithstanding, any suspicious lymph node should be excised or included in the radiation port.

The parameningeal region incorporates the nasal cavity, parameningeal sinuses, middle ear, mastoid, and pterygoid and infratemporal fossae. These tumors usually produce obstruction with or without mucopurulent or sanguineous discharge. Invasion into the meninges may result in cranial nerve palsies.[46] Involvement of the middle ear and mastoid sometimes affects the facial nerve. The tumor may also metastasize to the lungs and bones.

### GENITOURINARY TRACT

Rhabdomyosarcomas of the bladder, prostate, vagina, and uterus account for approximately 25 percent of the cases. The embryonal type, with or without botryoid configuration, is the most common. Rhabdomyosarcomas of the spermatic cord and paratesticular area account for approximately 8 percent of cases. In most patients, the disease is localized (group I or II).

Paratesticular tumors produce painless unilateral scrotal or inguinal enlargement. The regional retroperitoneal lymph nodes may be involved.[47] Bladder tumors usually grow intraluminally and appear polypoid on gross or endoscopic examination. Hematuria, urinary obstruction, and occasionally extrusion of mucosanguineous tissue may occur. Prostate tumors usually produce large pelvic masses and urinary obstruction.

Vaginal tumors are generally botryoid in type and occasionally present with a mucosanguineous discharge or extrusion of mucosanguineous tissue. Cervical and uterine sarcomas may appear as a mass or glistening grapelike vesicles on the infant's diaper. Vaginal tumors usually appear at an age younger than the uterine forms (mean age 2 years versus over 14 years). They generally respond more favorably to treatment.[48,49]

## EXTREMITY

Primary tumors of the extremity account for approximately 17 percent of all cases. They are associated with the highest incidence of relapse and the lowest survival rate.[50–52] The alveolar subtype carries a worse prognosis. They are generally characterized by widespread dissemination[53] and regional lymph node involvement.[50–52,54,55] The affected part of the limb usually presents with swelling. It is frequently painless but later becomes tender. Surgical or needle biopsy of the lymph nodes should be performed if any involvement is suspected. Metastases to the lungs are frequently found, even in the early stages. However, the lungs may occasionally be bypassed, with dissemination detected in the skeleton, bone marrow, and other organs.

## TRUNK AND THORAX

Rhabdomyosarcoma of the trunk comprises approximately 10 percent of all cases.[56] This includes tumors of the chest wall, paraspinal region, and abdominal wall. The histologic subtype is generally of the alveolar variety, although extraosseous Ewing's sarcoma and undifferentiated sarcoma are not unusual. Extraosseous Ewing's sarcoma of the thoracic wall is frequently referred to as Askin's tumor. Approximately 30 percent of these cases are associated with distant metastases and pleural effusion. Tumors of the trunk tend to recur locally. Distant spread is not uncommon, despite wide local excision.[56,57]

## LESS FREQUENT SITES OF INVOLVEMENT

Tumors of the retroperitoneum, excluding genitourinary tract, account for approximately 11 percent of cases. They are usually of the embryonal type.[58] Hepatobiliary tract rhabdomyosarcoma may arise in the bile ducts or ampulla of Vater.[59] These tumors account for approximately 2 percent of the cases. Most are of the embryonal type.[60] Most children present with fever, jaundice, abdominal pain, and increasing abdominal girth. Extension of tumor into the liver and regional lymph nodes is not uncommon. Failure is usually the result of local recurrence with invasion into the liver.

Tumors in the intrathoracic, thoracic, and retroperitoneal-pelvic regions are often silent and usually become large before presentation.[61–63] These lesions are rare. Tumor histology of intrathoracic lesions may be of the embryonal, alveolar, undifferentiated, or extraosseous Ewing's sarcoma type.

Perineal and perianal tumors often have regional lymph node involvement.[64,65] Perineal lesions are usually characterized by the alveolar histologic subtype.

Other unusual primary sites include liver, brain, trachea, heart, and ovary.[66–72]

## ■ DIAGNOSTIC STUDIES

Plain radiographs of the affected region are invariably obtained. This may be followed by examination by ultrasound, computerized axial tomography (CT), and/or nuclear magnetic resonance (MRI). The latter two investigations may be particularly useful in determining involvement of the base of the skull (see also Chapter 4). Radionuclide studies using $^{99m}$TC-diphosphonate may reveal skeletal infiltration. Radiographic examination of the chest is used to demonstrate metastases to the lungs. A CT examination, particularly if the chest radiograph is negative, may also be requested for this purpose. The nature of the imaging study to be performed is dictated by the site and size of the tumor and its attendant complications. These investigations include CT, MRI, ultrasonography, angiography, and contrast studies.

## ■ TREATMENT

The evolution of treatment for childhood cancer has expanded areas of overlapping skill into multidisciplinary programs. At present, five major disciplines are used in clinical practice: surgery, radiation therapy, chemotherapy, biological response modifiers, and, to a limited extent, immunotherapy. Before initiating treatment, a strategy for overall care is formulated by interdisciplinary consultation. The potential contribution of each discipline is exploited to maximum advantage. The tactics and strategies are then carefully integrated and individualized for each patient.

### SURGERY

#### Primary Tumor

Primary surgery to extirpate the presenting tumor with adequate margins is a time-honored and fundamental principle. This treatment should receive serious initial consideration, provided that the disease can be extirpated with no (or minimal) mutilation and functional debilitation. If microscopic disease still appears to be present after the initial surgical procedure, it may be appropriate to consider reoperation, provided the earlier prerequisites can be honored.

Second-look surgical procedures may also be performed after initial treatment with chemotherapy and/or radiation therapy. This strategy may be adopted to prevent mutilating procedures of the bladder, prostate, vagina, and uterus. In these circumstances, surgery is generally implemented two to three months after the administration of chemotherapy (see below). The intent is to identify response, reduce the size of the tumor, and extirpate resistant or residual disease.

## Lymph Nodes

Surgical exploration of suspected lymph node involvement should be considered in patients with primary tumors of the extremity, genitourinary sites, or paratesticular sites.[54] If paratesticular lymph node involvement is suspected, the initial procedure should be limited to random sampling, since the question of routine lymph node dissection for stage I disease is debatable (see below). The orbit, head and neck, and trunk rarely have lymph node involvement unless the disease is fairly advanced.[54]

## RADIATION THERAPY

### Primary Tumor

Radiation therapy is administered to achieve primary tumor control when the latter is not feasible by surgical extirpation. It is also occasionally administered after initial treatment with surgery and/or chemotherapy if there is any question of residual (viable) microscopic tumor. CT and/or MRI may assist in planning the radiation ports. Generally, 4,000 to 6,000 cGy are administered over four to six weeks. In patients under six years of age, 4,500 cGy may be used for tumors larger than 5 cm in diameter. For children over six years, the dose may be escalated to 5,040 cGy. If the tumor is smaller than 5 cm in diameter, a reduction to 4,140 cGy in children under six years of age, and 4,500 cGy for those over six years, may be considered. The standard daily dose fraction is 180 cGy (see Chapter 17 for further details).

### Lymph Nodes and Metastatic Sites

Radiation therapy may be administered initially as definitive treatment or following primary treatment to regional lymph node metastases with chemotherapy and/or surgery. It may also be administered to sites of metastatic disease. Generally, the dose is 1,440 cGy to the whole lung and 3,060 cGy to the abdomen. Limited areas in the abdomen may receive a boost to a total dose of 4,500 cGy. Bone lesions generally receive 5,040 cGy and soft tissue metastases 4,140 cGy.

Careful consideration and appropriate adjustments in dosage should be made when radiation therapy is juxtaposed with radiopotentiating agents (e.g., actinomycin-D and/or adriamycin). Treatment with chemotherapy may be continued during radiation therapy, provided radiopotentiating agents are withheld and that the other components do not induce an inordinate amount of myelosuppression (e.g., vincristine).

Hyperfractionation programs are currently being investigated. These programs involve treatment with a large number of small fractions in the same overall period as conventional radiation therapy. The rationale is to enhance tumor control and concurrently retain or possibly reduce the same degree of delayed radiation injury. Brachytherapy is also being investigated in selected institutions. This practice appears particularly suited for patients with small residual lesions or for those with tumors in the retroperitoneum and pelvis. The intent is to ensure minimum injury to the surrounding sites.

## CHEMOTHERAPY

Chemotherapy has been found to be potentially beneficial when administered in accordance with the following tactics and strategies.

1. Preoperative treatment with or without radiation therapy to facilitate surgical removal of large tumors by reduction in tumor volume. In these circumstances, the large tumor initially may be considered inoperable.
2. Concurrent treatment with or before radiation therapy for lesions in surgically inaccessible sites (e.g., nasopharynx).
3. Concurrent treatment with or before radiation therapy to avoid mutilating operative procedures in specific sites (e.g., rhabdomyosarcoma of the eye, genitourinary tract, and extremities). Surgery may subsequently be used if the response is sufficient and if its application will avoid mutilation and retain function.
4. Concurrent treatment with or before radiation therapy to eradicate metastases (e.g., pulmonary metastases). Residual metastases after treatment with chemotherapy and radiation therapy may also possibly be rendered resectable by surgery.
5. Palliative administration for disseminated disease. In these circumstances, radiation therapy may be administered before, concurrent with, or after treatment with chemotherapy.
6. "Adjuvant" therapy for micrometastases. This is the most frequent category in which chemotherapy is employed.

A large number of communications attest to the efficacy of chemotherapy administered as "adjuvant" treatment. The rationale underlying its administration in this category is based upon the recognition that surgery and radiation therapy do not always control the primary tumor. In most malignant conditions, disseminated microscopic foci of tumor (micrometastases) are present at diagnosis, and eradication of the latter requires a systemic approach. This is generally accomplished through chemotherapy. Experimentally, such therapy was shown to be most effective if applied when the tumor burden was at its nadir. It produced longer disease-free intervals, increases in survival, and a high percentage of cures.[73-76] The tactic is extrapolated into clinical strategies after the primary tumor is extirpated by radiation therapy and/or surgery.

## Chemotherapy Regimens

Various chemotherapeutic agents have been found to be effective in treating rhabdomyosarcoma. These agents are recorded in Table 21–6. To improve the efficacy of treatment, agents with different mechanisms of action and minimal or nonoverlapping toxicity were used. The two most common combinations investigated in sequential studies were vincristine and actinomycin-D (VA) versus vincristine, actinomycin-D, and cyclophosphamide (CTX). The latter combination was designated VAC and administered in a variety of doses and schedules.

With the discovery in the 1960s that antineoplastic agents were effective in sarcomas, particularly rhabdomyosarcoma, a number of therapeutic trials were initiated. Studies by Wilbur[77] in the early 1970s demonstrated that the combination of VAC with radiation therapy could increase the complete response rate in newly diagnosed patients. Similar studies at the Dana Farber Cancer Institute (formerly the Children's Cancer Research Foundation), also demonstrated that actinomycin-D, VA, and VAC sequentially increased survival when used as postoperative treatment (Fig. 21–7).[78-80]

After the efficacy of VAC had been established, adriamycin was added (A-VAC or VACA) (Table 21–7). More recently, ifosfamide (IFX) and etoposide (VP-16,

occasionally administered also with carboplatin [ICE]), were incorporated into the chemotherapeutic regimens. In general, less intense combinations are used for patients with favorable histology and localized disease, and more aggressive treatment is used for patients with extensive or advanced disease.

## ■ INTERGROUP RHABDOMYOSARCOMA STUDIES

Because of the relative rarity of rhabdomyosarcoma and its biologic heterogeneity, in 1972, three pediatric cooperative cancer groups combined to form the conglomerate IRS. The objective was to combine their resources and attain a more rapid answer to investigative studies. To date, three consecutive trials have been

**TABLE 21–6. RESPONSE OF RHABDOMYOSARCOMA TO SINGLE AGENTS**

| Agent | Complete and Partial Response (%) |
|---|---|
| Vincristine | 59 |
| Cyclophosphamide | 54 |
| Ifosfamide | 40 |
| Mitomycin-C | 36 |
| Etoposide | 33 |
| Adriamycin | 31 |
| Actinomycin-D | 24 |
| Cisplatin | 21 |
| Imidazole carboxamide | 1 |
| 5-Fluorouracil | 0 |

Adapted from Green and Jaffe,[78] and augmented to include ifosfamide, cisplatin, and etoposide from the recent literature.

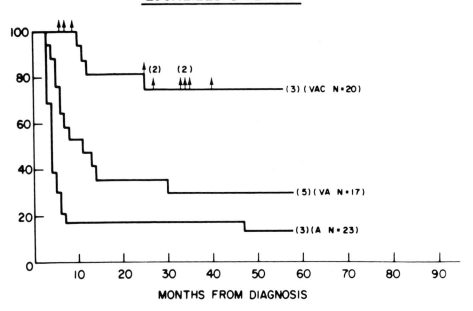

**RHABDOMYOSARCOMA LOCALIZED DISEASE**

**Figure 21–7.** Sequential escalation of tumor-free survival in patients receiving chemotherapeutic agents in combination (*V* = vincristine; *A* = adriamycin-D; *C* = cyclophosphamide).

**TABLE 21–7. SELECTED EXAMPLES OF CHEMOTHERAPY REGIMENS\***

| Drug | Dose | Schedule |
|---|---|---|
| | ***A-VAC (Similar to VADRC and VACA)*** | |
| | ***Initial Phase (Adriamycin)*** | |
| Vincristine | 1.5 mg/m$^2$ (max. 2 mg) | Weekly × 12 if tolerated. Subsequently with each Adriamycin and cyclophosphamide dose. |
| Adriamycin | 60 mg/m$^2$ by continuous 24-hr infusion (usually diluted in 480 cc of 5% dextrose water) | Every 3 wk provided ejection fraction above 60. Six courses. |
| Cyclophosphamide | 600 mg/m$^2$ | Every 3 wk. Six courses |
| | ***VAC Phase (Actinomycin-D)*** | |
| Vincristine | 1.5 mg/m$^2$ (max. 2 mg) | Every 3–4 wk |
| Actinomycin D | 0.25 mg/m$^2$ (max. dose 0.5 mg) | Daily × 3 every 3–4 wk |
| Cyclophosphamide | 300 mg/m$^2$ | Daily × 3 every 3–4 wk |
| | ***"Regular" VAC therapy*** | |
| Vincristine | 2 mg/m$^2$ (max. 2 mg) | Weekly × 12 |
| Actinomycin D | 0.015 mg/kg (max. dose 0.5 mg) | Daily × 5 every 4 wk |
| Cyclophosphamide | 10 mg/kg | Daily × 3 every 4 wk |
| | ***"ICE" Regimen*** | |
| Ifosfamide | 1.5 gm/mg$^2$ with MESNA uroprotectant | Every 3–4 wk |
| Carboplatin | 150 mg/m$^2$ | Single dose, every 3–4 wk |
| Etoposide | 100 mg/m$^2$ | Every 3–4 wk |

\*Total duration of treatment is generally one to two years. Therapy is usually not administered unless the following parameters are met: (1) leukocyte count over 2,000 (total phagocyte count over 500) and (2) platelet count over 75,000. Consult individual protocols for full details.

conducted and analyzed: IRS-I, 1972 to 1978; IRS-II, 1978 to 1984; and IRS-III, 1984 to 1991.[81–84] The results of these consecutive studies have been published.[82–84] A brief summary of the overall published results follows. Selected reports from other institutions and groups are also presented.

### IRS-I AND IRS-II

#### Group I Disease

IRS-I reported no significant difference in survival in patients with group I (note that the term *group* is used as opposed to *stage*) disease when treated with VAC or VAC plus radiation therapy.[82] This observation was important because it permitted cure without the potential adverse effects of radiation therapy in this category of patients. IRS-II demonstrated that CTX should not be withdrawn from standard VAC therapy if radiation therapy was withheld in patients with group I disease.[82,83] At five years, more patients treated with VAC were alive and disease-free than those treated with VA, although overall survival was comparable (85 percent).

#### Group II Disease

IRS-I demonstrated that patients derived equal benefit from VAC plus radiation or intensified VA plus radiation. Disease-free survival at five years was approximately 70 percent.

IRS-II reported that repetitive pulse VAC courses and a more intensive schedule (compared to that used in group II patients in IRS-I) did not boost survival above the results obtained with intensified VA. Treatment included postoperative radiation therapy. Further, patients in group I and group II with alveolar rhabdomyosarcoma fared more poorly than those with other histologic varieties.

#### Group III and Group IV Disease

In IRS-I, patients with advanced disease were treated with a single course of VAC followed by intensive VAC maintenance. Several patients were also treated with adriamycin and radiation therapy to the tumor bed and metastatic sites. These additional tactics did not improve the outcome. Overall survival at five years was 52 percent in group III patients and 20 percent in group IV.

In group III patients, IRS-II, in comparison to IRS-I, also introduced a more intense pulse VAC regimen with or without Adriamycin. The results were superior to those achieved with less intense treatment. At five years, disease-free survival was approximately 69 percent in IRS-II, compared to 59 percent in IRS-I ($p = 0.01$).

### IRS-III

IRS-III attempted to improve the treatment outcome by means of a risk-based protocol. Surgery or multi-agent chemotherapy with or without radiation therapy was employed. The overall outcome was significantly better than IRS-II (five-year disease-free survival 65 percent ± 2 percent versus 55 percent ± 2 percent $p = <0.001$).

Patients with group I favorable histology tumor fared just as well on a one-year regimen of VA as a comparable group treated with VA plus CTX. Patients with group III tumors, excluding those in special pelvic, orbit, or other selected nonparameningeal sites, attained a better outcome with a more intense regimen than pulse VAC or VAC-Vadr C (the latter had been used in IRS-II). The five-year disease-free survival was 62 percent versus 52 percent ($p < 0.01$).

## IRS-IV AND IRS-V

IRS-IV has recently been closed and will be analyzed. IRS-V has been initiated. Physicians interested in participating should obtain details from members of the IRS organization.

## NATIONAL CANCER INSTITUTE

The National Cancer Institute (NCI) used an intensive regimen of vincristine, adriamycin, and CTX (Vadr C) in combination with radiation therapy for group III and group IV patients. The group III patients had tumors in the chest wall, retroperitoneum, perineum, and extremity. Treatment was followed by total body radiation and autologous bone marrow transplant in patients who achieved complete remission.[85] Actuarial disease-free and overall survival at 24 months were 68 percent and 48 percent, respectively. More recently, NCI reported that, with the administration of IFX and VP-16, three complete and six partial responses were obtained in 13 previously treated patients.[86] It also appeared that IFX was superior to CTX, particularly for some CTX-resistant tumors.

## INTERNATIONAL SOCIETY FOR PEDIATRIC ONCOLOGY

Promising results were achieved with IVA (IFX, vincristine, and actinomycin-D) in a study conducted by the International Society for Pediatric Oncology (SIOP).[87,88] This was used as front-line chemotherapy for patients with node metastases based on the TNM study (stages I–III). The response was 89 percent; however, the relapse rate was high. Patients who did not receive local radiation generally developed local recurrences. (See below for treatment of recurrent or residual disease).

## ■ TREATMENT OF TUMORS IN SPECIAL ANATOMIC SITES

## HEAD AND NECK REGION

If cosmetically permissible, tumors should be surgically resected. However, most are inoperable, and chemotherapy and radiation therapy generally constitute the essential components of treatment. Chemotherapy is administered initially for several weeks. A response is invariably obtained (Fig. 21–8A to 21–8B). This is followed by radiation therapy (Fig. 21–9A and 21–9B). The latter is usually effective, and most patients may be expected to survive. Unfortunately, late complications frequently occur. These include cataract and hypoplasia of the orbit, lacrimal duct stenosis, and changes in the cornea and retina.[89] In an effort to avoid radiation therapy, SIOP advocated exclusive treatment with chemotherapy. Investigators reported that the procedure, with curative intent, was feasible in many of the patients.[90]

Survival for tumors of the head and neck using a multidisciplinary approach is in excess of 80 percent.[91] Results were not influenced by primary site, histologic findings, or the presence of adenopathy. Patients with group III tumors and those younger than 5 years of age at diagnosis had a somewhat lower survival.

## PARAMENINGEAL RHABDOMYOSARCOMAS

Parameningeal disease may be diagnosed or suspected in patients with meningeal symptoms, cranial nerve palsies, and/or bone erosion at the base of the skull. Patients may also (rarely) exhibit tumor cells in the cerebrospinal fluid. Those without evidence of neurologic involvement or radiologic signs of invasion of the base of the skull are considered to be at low risk for this complication.

In IRS-I, patients with parameningeal disease had a 45 percent survival rate. This escalated to 65 percent in IRS-II ($p < 0.001$).[92] The improved survival followed extension of the radiation therapy portal to encompass all known sites of primary disease with a 2-cm margin of meninges. Treatment also commenced as soon as possible after diagnosis (in IRS-I, there was a six-week delay). Intrathecal chemotherapy was also administered. This comprised arabinosylcytosine, hydrocortisone, and methotrexate with leucovorin rescue. The drugs were injected into the cerebrospinal fluid for two to three days, until the tumor cells were cleared. Maintenance therapy was then administered every two to eight weeks for two years. Alternatively, the combination was given less frequently for 18 months if tumor cells were absent from the cerebrospinal fluid initially and if chemical and/or radiologic parameters of high-risk were still present.

It is difficult to justify or understand the rationale for intrathecal chemotherapy, because the recommended agents are minimally, if at all, active in rhabdomyosarcoma (see Table 21–4). The radiation therapy administered concurrently with chemotherapy was more likely responsible for eradication of disease. This premise has been adopted in the more recent IRS studies. Intrathecal chemotherapy for meningeal disease is

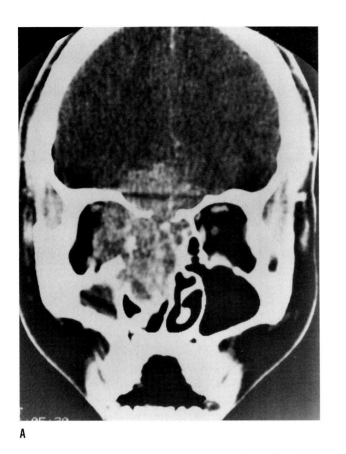 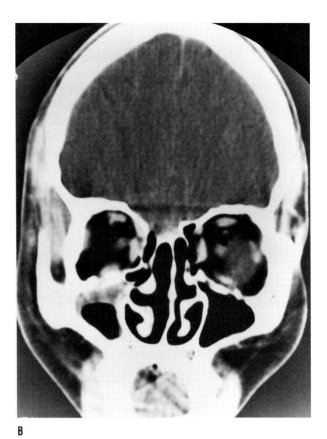

A

B

**Figure 21–8.** **(A)** Rhabdomyosarcoma of the right orbital maxillary facial area. **(B)** After four courses of VAC chemotherapy, the tumor has almost completely disappeared.

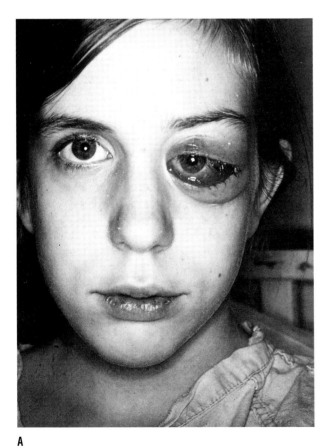 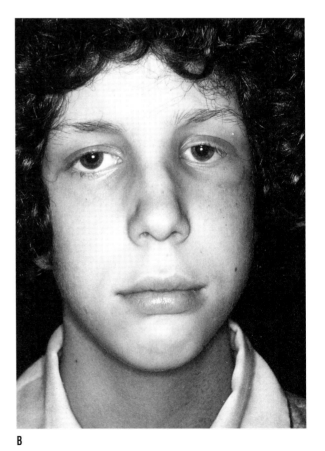

A

B

**Figure 21–9.** **(A)** Rhabdomyosarcoma of the left orbit. **(B)** After three courses of VAC chemotherapy, the tumor has been markedly reduced.

not prescribed; radiation therapy is considered the fulcrum of treatment. It is delivered as follows:

1. If the base of the skull is not involved, and if there is no neurologic abnormality, and if the cerebrospinal fluid cytology is normal, the portal of radiation incorporates a margin of the meninges extending 2 cm above the base of the skull.
2. The dose of radiation to the primary parameningeal tumor is 4,500 to 5,040 cGy, depending upon the patient's age, tumor size, and group.
3. The affected area is included in 90 percent of the isodose line. Radiation therapy of the whole brain and spinal meninges is not required.

In IRS-II, treatment for parameningeal rhabdomyosarcoma began as soon as possible after diagnosis; in the absence of intracranial extension, more recent approaches permit initiation of treatment with chemotherapy and introduction of radiation therapy after 9 to 15 weeks. Patients with intracranial extension of tumor, erosion of the base of the skull, or cranial nerve palsy are treated with radiation therapy as soon as possible after diagnosis. Systemic chemotherapy is also administered.

Radiation therapy to the cerebrospinal axis should be administered if malignant cells are detected in the cerebrospinal fluid. The dose varies from 2,400 to 3,600 cGy depending on age (above or below six years). However, detection of malignant cells in the cerebrospinal fluid is extremely rare. (IRS-IV, at the time of this review, still advocated the administration of arabinosyl cytosine, hydrocortisone, and methotrexate with leucovorin rescue for the treatment of malignant cells in the cerebrospinal fluid. However, as indicated earlier, it has not been prescribed in IRS-V.)

## EXTREMITY

Every attempt is made to achieve limb salvage with surgical extirpation of the primary tumor in the extremities. If this is impossible, radiation therapy may be administered. However, growth retardation of the limb is to be anticipated. This complication sometimes renders radiation therapy impractical for patients under 7 years of age. If local control with radiation therapy is unlikely, amputation becomes the treatment of choice. Additionally, regional lymph node biopsy is recommended in all cases, and a complete lymphadenectomy should only be performed if there is microscopic evidence of regional lymph node metastases. Sometimes, postoperative radiation therapy to the regional node-bearing area is also indicated. The role of lymphadenectomy alone or in combination with postoperative radiation therapy is sometimes difficult to establish.

The five-year survival rate for extremity tumors is about 75 percent.

## GENITOURINARY TRACT

IRS-I used primary surgery for tumors of the bladder, prostate, vagina, and uterus. In contrast, IRS-II introduced repetitive pulse VAC therapy in addition to surgery and/or radiation therapy. Survival was similar (IRS-I, 78 percent and IRS-II, 68 percent; $p = 0.45$).[93] Based on these experiences, current strategies are designed to attain preservation of the bladder and other organs: chemotherapy is used as primary treatment followed by radiation therapy and/or surgery. An example of a response attained with chemotherapy is presented in Figure 21–10A to 21–10D.

Chemotherapy is usually administered for two to three months. This generally permits some form of surgical excision. If residual microscopic disease is present after surgery, radiation therapy (approximately 4,000 cGy over four weeks) is administered. This is followed by additional postoperative adjuvant chemotherapy. Limited surgery comprises partial cystectomy, "tumorectomy," or partial vaginovulvectomy.[80,94–96] If surgery cannot be performed after initial treatment with chemotherapy, radiation therapy should be administered. In contrast, organ extirpation or pelvic exenteration may be requested if radiation therapy is not feasible. Suspicious bilateral pelvic or para-aortic lymph nodes should be evaluated.

In IRS-III, patients with group III special pelvic primary tumors (bladder, prostate, vagina, and uterus) also benefited from more complex therapy. Adding adriamycin and cisplatin or actinomycin-D plus etoposide to VAC, with or without second-look surgery, improved the outcome. This was evident by comparing the results obtained in IRS-II, where VAC was employed with or without second-look surgery. Survival improved significantly: 83 percent in IRS-III versus 72 percent in IRS-II. The bladder salvage rate also doubled. This was attributed to more intensive therapy.[84]

Preservation of major pelvic organs, particularly in patients with localized sarcoma of the bladder, prostate, vagina, uterus, and cervix, appears possible. However, unfortunately, only about 25 percent of patients usually avoid severe mutilating procedures. Five-year survival rates of about 80 percent have been reported for genitourinary tumors. Tumors of the dome of the bladder have a better prognosis than those of the trigone.[80,93,94,97]

## PARATESTICULAR RHABDOMYOSARCOMA

About 26 percent of paratesticular rhabdomyosarcomas have retroperitoneal lymph node involvement at diagnosis.[47] Mechanisms to determine retroperitoneal

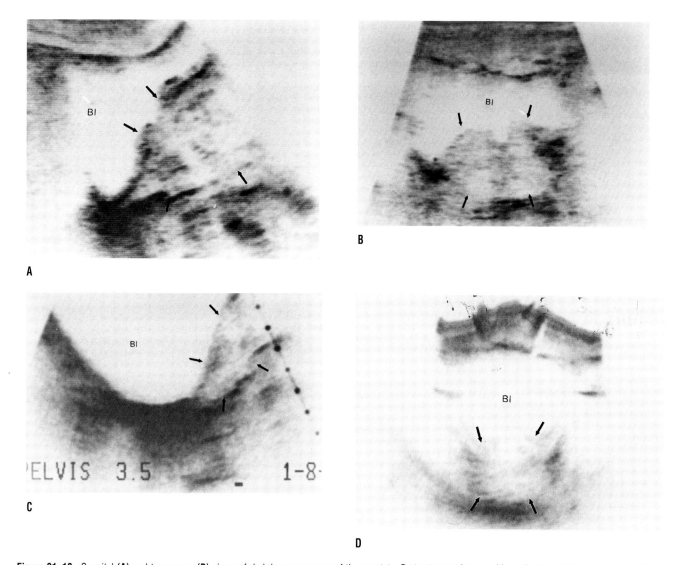

**Figure 21–10.** Saggital **(A)** and transverse **(B)** views of rhabdomyosarcoma of the prostate. Pretreatment ultrasound investigation of the pelvis demonstrating a solid mass *(arrows)* measuring 8.5 × 8 × 5.5 cm, rising from the prostate and indenting the base of the urinary bladder *(Bl)*. Saggital **(C)** and transverse **(D)** views of rhabdomyosarcoma of the prostate posttreatment ultrasound investigation. After two courses of VAC chemotherapy, the mass shown in Figure 21–10A and 21–10B has markedly regressed. The tumor now measures 6 × 6 × 2.5 cm.

lymph node involvement are controversial. Retroperitoneal lymphadenectomy is the most reliable; however, the procedure is associated with retrograde ejaculation. In an effort to avoid the complication, examination of retroperitoneal nodes by other methods has been advocated. These include bipedal lymphangiography and/or evaluation of the lymph nodes by means of a CT scan or MRI.[98,99] However, these investigations may not be completely reliable. Wiener[99] noted that at least 14 percent of patients with negative imaging studies may have positive retroperitoneal nodes by biopsy. Thus, despite the presence of normal imaging studies, it may still be prudent to perform a laparotomy and to sample suspicious nodes. The contralateral retroperitoneal lymph nodes are rarely involved but should also be inspected. Positive lymph nodes are associated with decreased survival.[99] Treatment of positive nodes usu-

ally involves lymphadenectomy, regional radiation therapy, and chemotherapy.

If radical orchiectomy is required, hemiscrotectomy should also be performed. Scrotal radiation should be delivered to patients in whom there is a suggestion of residual microscopic disease. During the period of radiation therapy, the contralateral testis should be transposed to the thigh and reimplanted into the scrotum upon completion of treatment. The five-year survival rate is in the vicinity of 90 percent.

## LESS COMMONLY INVOLVED SITES

For tumors in less commonly involved sites, general principles for their treatment should be applied. These principles comprise surgical excision of the primary tumor with generous margins, followed by radiation therapy for suspected or established (residual) localized disease, and aggressive multi-agent chemotherapy.

### Rhabdomyosarcoma of the Trunk

Spinal axis radiation does not appear to be indicated in most patients with rhabdomyosarcoma of the trunk, because the lesions rarely extend into the meninges. Overall survival at five years is approximately 50 percent.[83] Paraspinal lesions have the best prognosis.

### Retroperitoneum

Regional lymph nodes are frequently involved in retroperitoneal tumors. The five-year-survival rate is approximately 40 percent.[83]

### Perineal Lesions

Relapse-free survival at three years is approximately 48 percent in patients with perineal lesions.[100]

### Intrathoracic Lesions

Intrathoracic tumors are generally unresectable, but surgery should be considered, particularly if reduction in size can be achieved with radiation therapy and chemotherapy. The two-year relapse-free survival is 24 percent.[61]

### Bile Duct Lesions

A number of survivors with bile duct lesions have been reported.[60]

## ■ TREATING RHABDOMYOSARCOMA EXCLUSIVELY WITH CHEMOTHERAPY

Several investigators have claimed that treatment exclusively with intensive chemotherapy could achieve cure in patients with rhabdomyosarcoma of the head and neck[90] and bladder.[95,101] This experience could not be duplicated by investigators at the M.D. Anderson Cancer Center.[102] Most patients relapsed at or before seven months while undergoing primary treatment with chemotherapy. This interval appeared to be the maximum delay permissible before introducing definitive treatment with radiation therapy and/or surgery to achieve optimum results.[102] Since overt manifestations of disease were detected at seven months,[102] it appeared that a more accurate estimate for intervention could be obtained by considering the doubling time for sarcomas: 11 to 125 days with a median of 25. Extrapolating from these data, it appears prudent to intervene 25 to 50 days (i.e., double 25 days) prior to the seven-month appearance of overt disease (i.e., at approximately five months). This extrapolation was confirmed by deter-

mining the optimum disease-free survival in 52 patients subjected to definitive treatment (surgery and radiation therapy) at different time intervals. The best survival (70 percent) was attained in patients treated with definitive therapy at or before five months. This was compared to a 15 percent survival in patients in whom definitive therapy was implemented after five months (see Fig. 21–11).

### METASTATIC DISEASE

Metastases spread by contiguity and continuity and via the lymphatic and hematologic systems. The most common sites are the lung (60 percent), regional lymph nodes (30 percent), bone (30 percent), liver (20 percent), and brain (20 percent). Bone marrow may also be involved.[53,103] Patients with primary tumors of the extremity frequently present with metastases to the lungs and regional lymph nodes. Genitourinary lesions also metastasize to regional lymph nodes and the lungs. Pratt[104] noted an association between antemortem bone marrow involvement and heart metastasis.

### SURVIVAL FOLLOWING RECURRENCE

Survival after recurrence is possible, provided aggressive multidisciplinary treatment is implemented. Overall survival rate at five years was reported at approximately 17 percent, with figures varying from 5 to 30 percent.[82,83] Patients who develop recurrence should be evaluated for persistent local disease at the primary site and distant metastases. Surgery and/or radiation therapy in such patients usually has a limited role because the disease is generally disseminated. Under these circumstances, provided aggressive "conventional" therapy has previously been used, strategies incorporating investigational or experimental tactics may be explored. These include phase I-II agents and autologous bone marrow transplantation. At the present time, however, the latter has not shown any advantage over conventional chemotherapy and radiation therapy regimens.[85,105] The role of bone marrow transplantation in patients with recurrent, extensive, or persistent disease remains to be defined.

### COMPLICATIONS OF CHEMOTHERAPY AND SUPPORTIVE CARE

Chemotherapeutic agents may induce a variety of side effects and complications. The most important are severe myelosuppression, superimposed infection, ulceration of the buccal mucosa, and gastroenteritis. The last may be further complicated by poor nutrition, culminating in cachexia. In an effort to prevent neutropenia and superimposed infection, granulocyte colony-stimulating factor (G-CSF) may be prescribed immediately after completion of a course of chemotherapy. It

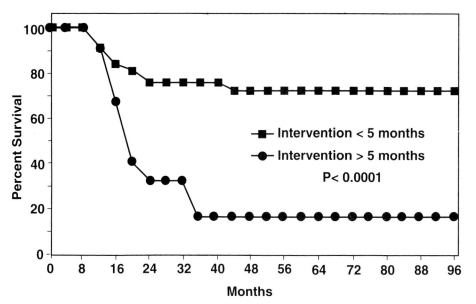

**Figure 21–11.** Optimum disease-free survival (Kaplan-Meier plot) attained with five-month delay before beginning definitive therapy (surgery and/or radiation therapy). Survival with a five-month delay was 70 percent; patients treated after five months had a 15 percent survival ($p < 0.0001$). Less significant curves attained with definitive intervention at other times are omitted. *(Reproduced with permission from Int J Oncol 7:855, 1995).*

has little benefit, if any, if administered during the period of severe myelosuppression. The drug is particularly indicated if efforts are being made to escalate dose intensity. Blood and platelet transfusions may also be required.

Patients who develop severe neutropenia and superimposed infection will require antibiotic therapy pending restoration of the blood count. In some centers, trimethoprim and sulfamethoxazole (Bactrim/Sulfa) are prescribed as a prophylaxis against infection. If severe mucositis develops, nasogastric tube feedings or hyperalimentation may be indicated. Gastrostomy feedings have also been found to be particularly useful. Most chemotherapeutic agents are currently administered with the use of a double lumen central line. In these circumstances, an external catheter or portacath may be used. Treatment should be administered in centers where facilities to combat infections and complications are readily available.

### FOLLOW-UP EVALUATION

Patients should be examined at three- to four-week intervals during chemotherapy. Evaluation of the status of the primary tumor should be performed at each visit. Radiographic examination of the chest (the most common site for the development of pulmonary metastases) should be obtained initially and at three- to six-week intervals during the first two years. The interval may subsequently be extended so that, by the end of the fifth year, radiographic examination of the chest is obtained annually. Radiographic studies of sites previously exposed to radiation therapy should be obtained at annual intervals. The intent is to identify delayed

radiation injury to the bones and soft tissue and to detect the possible development of a second malignant neoplasm. Other investigations should be obtained as dictated by the patient's status and an understanding of the delayed consequences of chemotherapy.

### ■ NONRHABDOMYOSARCOMA SOFT TISSUE SARCOMAS

These tumors are less common than rhabdomyosarcoma and demonstrate considerably more heterogeneity in tissue type and evolution. Many of the principles outlined for the treatment of rhabdomyosarcoma may be extrapolated to the management of nonrhabdomyosarcoma soft tissue sarcomas. Ascendancy rests in the multidisciplinary approach with surgical extirpation as the major component. In general, the role of chemotherapy is debatable, because regression in nonrhabdomyosarcoma soft tissue tumors has rarely been reported. However, periodically, the possibility that microscopic disease may be responsive to chemotherapy receives serious consideration.

### SYNOVIAL CELL SARCOMA

Synovial cell sarcomas should be surgically resected. Chemotherapy was considered beneficial by the German Cooperative Group, which reported an increased five-year survival of 74 percent in 31 patients.[106] Survival rate was somewhat better for patients with completely resected tumors (84 percent) than for those with residual tumors (58 percent). Chemotherapy consisted of vincristine, actinomycin-D and IFX, and adriamycin. Most children also received local radiation therapy.

Similar experiences were reported by the St. Jude Children's Research Hospital.[107]

Survival apparently depends on size of tumor (tumors larger than 5 cm have a poorer outlook), location (proximal tumors have a worse prognosis), and the possibility of achieving adequate surgical margins. In one series, localized radiation therapy appeared beneficial in patients with marginal resections, while the role of chemotherapy was uncertain.[108]

## ALVEOLAR SOFT PART SARCOMA

Alveolar soft part sarcomas occur in adolescence and young adults and have been detected in a variety of structures, including deep soft tissues of the extremities. It usually presents as a painless palpable nodule that has been present for a prolonged period before diagnosis. Metastases have been reported in the lungs, bone, liver, and brain.[109–111]

Surgical resection should be attempted in all cases. Unfortunately, local recurrence is common. Metastases may occur in as many as 30 percent of cases.[112] Radiation therapy may be effective in achieving control of the primary lesion and/or pulmonary metastases.[113]

The five-year survival rate varies from 27 to 59 percent.[114] Metastases may appear late, even after a disease-free interval of 15 to 20 years. Younger patients probably have a better prognosis.[109]

## FIBROSARCOMA

Complete surgical removal is the treatment of choice for fibrosarcomas. The likelihood of metastases is small but increases after five years and approaches that of adults in children over 10 years (50 percent).[115] In older patients, it may be reasonable to administer postoperative adjuvant chemotherapy. In young children, particularly in the toddler, because of the rather indolent nature of the disease, the question of postoperative adjuvant treatment is undefined.

## DERMATOFIBROSARCOMA PROTUBERANS

Dermatofibrosarcoma protuberans is a rare low-grade sarcoma of the skin. It may occur at any age and may even be present at birth. Ten to 16 percent are found in the first decade of life, with a slight male preponderance.[116] Lesions occur most frequently in the trunk or proximal part of the limbs. Initially, they grow slowly and later enter a period of rapid growth. The tumors are frequently fixed to the skin and do not invade deeply. They rarely metastasize. The treatment of choice is wide surgical excision. Radiation therapy does not appear to be effective and the role of chemotherapy is unknown. With adequate surgical excision, prognosis is excellent. There are occasional reports of malignant regression and fibrosarcomatous change.[117]

## MALIGNANT FIBROUS HISTIOCYTOMA

Malignant fibrous histiocytomas are composed predominantly of pleomorphic sarcoma cells and are characterized by a whirled growth pattern.[118] Many sarcomas previously classified as pleomorphic rhabdomyosarcoma or neurofibrosarcoma have been reclassified as malignant fibrous histiocytoma. These tumors appear to be one of the most common soft tissue sarcomas in adults. They frequently occur as a painless mass deeply situated in the lower extremity. Also affected may be the head and neck, the retroperitoneal region, and bone.

The treatment of choice is local excision. Postoperative radiation therapy is recommended if the margins are inadequate. Responses to chemotherapy have also been noted.[119] Malignant fibrous histiocytomas appear to have a better prognosis in children than in adults.[120] The five-year survival rate has varied from 27 to 53 percent.[121–123]

## NEUROGENIC SARCOMA

Tumors of the peripheral nerve sheath (MPNST) have also been termed *malignant schwannoma, neurofibrosarcoma*, or *neurogenic sarcoma*.[124,125] Approximately 20 to 69 percent of the reported cases occur in association with neurofibromatosis, and 4.6 percent of patients with this disease have developed neurofibrosarcoma.[124,126,127] The usual presentation is a painful, enlarging mass that may cause neurologic problems. A long history of symptoms may be noted in patients with neurofibromatosis. Pain or sudden enlargement of any existing neurofibroma should suggest the possibility of malignancy. The tumors are usually close to major nerves.

The treatment is wide local excision or even amputation. In the absence of adequate excision, local recurrence and distant metastases are highly probable. The degree of surgical excision correlates with prognosis.[128] Postoperative radiation therapy in patients with an incomplete excision may reduce the rate of local recurrence. Some reports suggest that chemotherapy, particularly vincristine, adriamycin, cyclophosphamide, and actinomycin-D, may have activity against the tumor.[125,128]

## ANGIOSARCOMA

Angiosarcoma is an uncommon malignant tumor of the vascular endothelium. It has also been designated hemangioblastoma, hemangioendothelioma, lymphangiosarcoma, hemangiosarcoma, and angiosarcoma. The term *angiosarcoma* is generally used to encompass both hemangiosarcoma and lymphangiosarcoma.[129]

In children, angiosarcomas of the liver may arise from a preexisting infantile hemangioendothelioma.[130] The most common presenting manifestation is abdominal enlargement.[131] Multiple cutaneous hemangiomas in patients with hepatic angiosarcoma may also be present.[132] Cases have been reported of angiosarcoma developing after radiation therapy.[133] Factor VIII-associated antigen produced by endothelial tumor cells may be detected in angiosarcoma.[134,135] Angiosarcoma of the bone affects all age groups and usually manifests with pain. Radiologically, the lesions are often multifocal.[136]

Wide surgical excision is the treatment of choice. In bone, surgical removal should also be attempted. Postoperative radiotherapy may be needed to eradicate microscopic foci of tumor. Experience with chemotherapy is limited.[137] The prognosis is improved in patients with tumors smaller than 5 cm. Angiosarcoma of the liver in children carries an extremely grave prognosis.[131]

## HEMANGIOPERICYTOMA

Hemangiopericytoma is a rare vascular tumor characterized by proliferation of cells that surround and compress capillaries.[138] It may arise wherever capillaries are found. The most common site is the lower extremity. The tumors are usually deep-seated and attached to muscle, deep fascia, or periosteum. Wide surgical excision is the treatment of choice. Amputation may be necessary if the tumor is located in an extremity. Radiation therapy may possibly decrease local recurrence. Chemotherapy has occasionally been used, and regression has been observed with vincristine and actinomycin-D[139] or adriamycin in combination with other agents.[140]

Overall survival rate varies from 59 to 75 percent.[141,142] Metastases have been known to develop as long as 14 years after treatment of the primary tumor.[143]

## EPITHELIOID SARCOMA

Epithelioid sarcoma is a rare soft tissue sarcoma that occurs most frequently in adolescence in young adults. The tumor is usually found in the extremities, the hand and forearm being the most common locations. Pain and limitation of function are minimal, which may explain the typical delay before the tumor is brought to medical attention. The tumors generally present as superficial nodules and grow proximally along tendons and facial planes, giving rise to local recurrence.

Optimum treatment comprises wide surgical excision. This should be en bloc or amputation. Radiation may be partially effective in reducing the tumor size. There does not appear to be any evidence that chemotherapy is effective.

In the absence of adequate local control, the prognosis is poor. Metastases have been known to occur many years after excision of the primary tumor.

## LEIOMYOSARCOMA

Leiomyosarcoma is a malignant tumor of the smooth muscle. Recent studies have demonstrated an association between leiomyosarcoma in young people with acquired immunodeficiency syndrome (AIDS) and Epstein-Barr virus.[144] Childhood leiomyosarcomas have been reported in a variety of anatomic sites, including the gastrointestinal tract, particularly the stomach.[145] Gastric pain and gastrointestinal bleeding appear to be the main presenting symptoms.

Complete excision is the treatment of choice. Radiotherapy as primary treatment did not appear to be effective.[146] A variety of chemotherapeutic agents, including a combination of mitomycin-C, adriamycin, and cisplatin, yielded a 28 percent objective response.[119] Lack[145] reported that 3 of 10 children were disease-free one to five years after diagnosis.[145] In another series, among 9 of 15 children in whom adequate follow-up data were available, 8 were well three months to five years after diagnosis.[147]

## FIBROMATOSIS

Fibromatosis includes a range of dysplastic lesions of connective tissue that may occur anywhere in the body. Fibromatosis in a child may be classified as congenital, infantile, or juvenile, and is different from that found in adults.

Treatment of congenital generalized fibromatosis is wide local excision. Spontaneous regression has also been described, and, therefore, conservative treatment following biopsy may be considered. Radiation therapy in high doses has also been used to control proliferation of the fibrous tissue. Treatment with vincristine, actinomycin, and cyclophosphamide for 3 weeks to 13 months has also been shown to cause good short-term responses.[148] The outlook is better for patients with involvement of the skin, subcutaneous tissue, muscle, and bone, and less favorable for those with vessel involvement.

## AGGRESSIVE FIBROMATOSIS

Aggressive fibromatosis is a group of nonmetastasizing, local invasive fibrous lesions. They present as firm diffuse masses that may have been present for months before rapidly increasing in size. Typically, the lesions are painless, firm, and manifest as an enlarging mass. The treatment of choice is surgical excision.[149]

## DESMOID TUMORS

Desmoid tumors are locally aggressive, nonmetastasizing tumors of fibroblastic origin. They have also been reported in association with cerebrospinal fluid, shunt tubing, and other foreign body implants.[150] The terms *desmoid* and *aggressive fibromatosis* have also been used to describe tumors of musculoaponeurotic tissue.

Clinically, intra-abdominal or extra-abdominal desmoids present as firm, fixed tumors and are often painful masses in the skeletal muscle or fascia. The desmoid tumor must be differentiated from fibrosarcoma or reactive fibrosis. Histologically, it may be distinguished from low-grade fibrosarcoma by normal mitosis and lack of a pseudocapsule; clinically, by failure to metastasize.

The treatment of choice is surgical excision. Amputation may be necessary for local recurrence in the extremities. Radiation therapy has been used for repeated local recurrent tumors with variable conflicting results. Antiestrogenic agents such as tamoxifen and testolactone have been investigated, in an effort to alter the estrogen effect implicated in accelerating tumor growth.[151–153] The role of chemotherapy is not established. However, vincristine, actinomycin-D, adriamycin, dacarbazine, and cyclophosphamide have been used in various combinations with variable success.[151,154] The prognosis for long-term survival is generally good, but there is a high rate of local recurrence. Death may occur when the tumor involves vital structures.

## ■ SUMMARY

The tactics and strategies used to treat rhabdomyosarcoma can generally be used to treat other soft tissue sarcomas. Resectability and size of primary lesion, histopathologic grade, and occasionally tumor location are important determinants of prognosis. Patients with high-grade tumors have a lower likelihood of survival. It is not uncommon for postoperative adjuvant chemotherapy to be advocated in an effort to prevent the development of pulmonary metastases. The role of chemotherapy, however, remains to be defined. Similarly, the efficacy of radiation therapy needs further investigation.

## REFERENCES

1. Young JL, Miller RW: Incidence of malignant tumors in U.S. children. J Pediatr 86:254, 1975

2. Miller RW: Deaths from childhood cancer sibs. N Engl J Med 279:122, 1968

3. Woodruff JM, Chernik NL, Smith MC, et al.: Peripheral nerve tumors with rhabdomyosarcomatous differentiation (malignant "Triton" tumors). Cancer 32:426, 1973

4. Ruymann FB, Maddux HR, Ragab A, et al.: Congenital anomalies associated with rhabdomyosarcoma: An autopsy study of 115 cases. A report from the Intergroup Rhabdomyosarcoma Study. Med Pediatr Oncol 16:33, 1987

5. Li FP, Fraumeni JF Jr.: Prospective study of a family cancer syndrome. JAMA 267:2692, 1982

6. Malkin D, Li RFP, Strong L, et al.: Germline p53 mutations in a familial syndrome of breast cancer, sarcomas, and other neoplasms. Science 250:1233, 1990

7. Stobbe CD, Dargeon HW: Embryonal rhabdomyosarcoma of the head and neck in children in adolescence. Cancer 3:816, 1950

8. Riopelle JL, Theriault JP: Sur une meconnue de sarcoma des partes molles: Rhabdomyosarcoma alevulaire. Ann Anat Pathol 1:88, 1956

9. Enzinger FM, Sheraki M: Alveolar rhabdomyosarcoma: Analysis of 110 cases. Cancer 24:18, 1969

10. Angervall L, Enzinger FM: Extraskeletal neoplasm resembling Ewing's sarcoma. Cancer 36:240, 1975

11. Dickman PS, Triche TJ: Extraosseous Ewing's sarcoma versus primitive rhabdomyosarcoma: Diagnostic criteria and clinical correlation. Hum Pathol 17:881, 1986

12. Newton WA, Gehan EA, Weber BL, et al.: Classification of rhabdomyosarcomas and related sarcomas. Pathologic aspects and proposal for a new classification—an Intergroup Rhabdomyosarcoma Study. Cancer 76:1073, 1995

13. Corson JM, Pinkus GS: Intracellular myoglobin—A specific marker for skeletal muscle differentiation in soft tissue sarcomas: An immunoperoxidase study. Am J Pathol 103:384, 1981

14. Brooks JJ: Immunohistochemistry of soft tissue tumors: Myoglobin as a tumor marker for rhabdomyosarcoma. Cancer 50:1757, 1982

15. Tsokos M, Howard R, Costa J: Immunohistochemical study of alveolar and embryonal rhabdomyosarcoma. Lab Invest 48:148, 1983

16. De Jong ASH, van Kessel-van Vark M, Albus-Lutter CE, et al.: Skeletal muscle actin as tumor marker in the diagnosis of rhabdomyosarcoma in childhood. Am J Surg Pathol 9:467, 1985

17. Molenaar WM, Oosterhuis JW, Oosterhuis AM, Ramaekers FCS: Mesenchymal and muscle-specific intermediate filaments (vimentin and desmin) in relation to differentiation in childhood rhabdomyosarcomas. Hum Pathol 16:838, 1985

18. Altmannsberger M, Weber K, Droste R, Osborn M: Desmin is a specific marker for rhabdomyosarcomas of human and rat origin. Am J Pathol 118:85, 1985

19. Dias P, Kumar P, Marsen HB, et al.: Evaluation of desmin as a diagnostic and prognostic marker of childhood rhabdomyosarcomas and embryonal sarcomas. Br J Cancer 56:361, 1987

20. Schmidt D, Reimann O, Treuner J, Harms D: Cellular

differentiation and prognosis in embryonal rhabdomyo-sarcoma: A report from the Cooperative Soft Tissue Sarcoma Study 1981 (CWS 81). Virchows Arch [A] 409:183, 1986

21. Wang-Wuu S, Soukup S, Ballard E, et al.: Chromosomal analysis of sixteen human rhabdomyosarcomas. Cancer Res 48:983, 1988

22. Douglass EC, Valentine M, Etcubanas E, et al.: A specific chromosomal abnormality in rhabdomyosarcoma. Cytogenet Cell Genet 45:148, 1977

23. Valentine M, Douglass BC, Look AT: Closely linked loci on the long arm of chromosome 13 flank a specific 2:13 translocation breakpoint in childhood rhabdomyosarcoma. Cytogenet Cell Genet 52:128, 1989

24. Turc-Garel C, Lizand-Noule S, Justrabo S, et al.: Consistent chromosomal translocations in alveolar rhabdomyosarcomas. Cancer Genet Cytogenet 19:361, 1986

25. Shapiro DN, Sublett JE, Li B, et al.: Fusion of PAX3 to a member of the forkhead family of transcription factors in human alveolar rhabdomyosarcoma. Cancer Res 53:5108, 1993

26. Barr FG, Galili N, Holick J, et al.: Rearrangement of the PAX3 paired box gene in the paediatric solid tumour alveolar rhabdomyosarcoma. Nat Genet 3:113, 1993

27. Douglass EC, Rowe ST, Valentine M, et al.: Variant translocations of chromosome B in alveolar rhabdomyosarcoma. Genes Chromosom Cancer 3:480, 1991

28. Davis RJ, D'Cruz CM, Lovell MA, et al.: Fusion of PAX7 to FKHR by the variant t(1;13)(p36;q14) translocation in alveolar rhabdomyosarcoma. Cancer Res 54:2869, 1994

29. Levine AJ: Tumor suppressor genes. Bioessays 12:60, 1990

30. Reismann PT, Simon MA, Lee W, Slamon DJ: Studies of the retinoblastoma gene in human sarcomas. Oncogene 4:839, 1989

31. Galili N, Davis RJ, Fredericks WJ, et al.: PAX3 in the solid tumor alveolar rhabdomyosarcoma. Nat Genet 5:230, 1993

32. Biegel JN, Nycum LM, Valentine V, et al.: Detention of the t(2:13) (q35;q14). Chromosomal translocation of PAX3-FKHR tumor in alveolar rhabdomyosarcoma by fluorescence in situ hybridization genes. Chromosom Cancer 12:186, 1995

33. Felix CA, Kappel CC, Mitsudomi T, et al.: Frequency and diversity of p53 mutations in childhood rhabdomyosarcoma. Cancer Res 52:2243, 1992

34. Dias P, Kumar P, Marsden HB, et al.: N-myc gene is amplified in alveolar rhabdomyosarcomas (RMS) but not in embryonal RMS. Int J Cancer 45:593, 1990

35. Stratton MR, Fisher C, Gusterson BA, et al.: Detection of point mutations in N-ras and K-ras genes of human embryonal rhabdomyosarcomas using oligonucleotide probes and the polymerase chain reaction. Cancer Res 49:6324, 1989

36. Shapiro DN, Parham DM, Douglass EC, et al.: Relationship of tumor cell ploidy to histologic subtype and treatment outcome in children and adolescents with unresectable rhabdomyosarcoma. J Clin Oncol 9:159, 1991

37. Wijnaedts LLD, van der Linder JC, van Dreats PJ, et al.: Prognostic importance of DNA flow cytometric variables in rhabdomyosarcomas. J Clin Pathol 40:948, 1993

38. Niggli FK, Powell JE, Parkes SE, et al.: DNA ploidy and proliferative activity (S-phase) in childhood soft-tissue sarcomas: Their value as prognostic indicators. Br J Cancer 69:1106, 1994

39. Mathieu MC, Niggli F, Vielh P, et al.: Prognostic value of flow cytometric DNA ploidy in childhood rhabdomyosarcomas enrolled in SIOP-MMT 89 Study. Med Pediatr Oncol (abstr) 23:223, 1994

40. Kilpatrick SE, Teot LA, Geisinger KR, et al.: Relationship of DNA ploidy to histology and prognosis in rhabdomyosarcoma: Comparison of flow cytometry and image analysis. Cancer 74:3227, 1994

41. Maurer HM: The Intergroup Rhabdomyosarcoma Study (IRS): Objectives and clinical staging classification. J Pediatr Surg 10:977, 1975

42. Gehan EA, Glover FN, Maurer HM, et al.: Prognostic factors in children with rhabdomyosarcoma. NCI Monogr 56:83, 1981

43. Lawrence W Jr., Gehan EA, Hays DM, et al.: Prognostic significance of staging factors of the UICC staging system in childhood rhabdomyosarcoma: A report from the Intergroup Rhabdomyosarcoma Study (IRS-II). J Clin Oncol 5:46, 1987

44. Sagerman RH, Tretter P, Ellsworth RM: The treatment of orbital rhabdomyosarcoma of children with primary radiation therapy. Am J Roentgenol Radiat Ther Nucl Med 114:31, 1972

45. Wharam M, Beltangady M, Heyn R, et al.: Localized orbital rhabdomyosarcoma: An interim report of the Intergroup Rhabdomyosarcoma Study Committee. Ophthalmology 94:251, 1987

46. Tefft M, Fernandez C, Donaldson M, et al.: Incidence of meningeal involvement by rhabdomyosarcoma of the head and neck in children. Cancer 42:253, 1978

47. Raney RB Jr., Tefft M, Lawrence W Jr., et al.: Paratesticular sarcoma in childhood and adolescence: A report from the Intergroup Rhabdomyosarcoma Studies I and II, 1973–1983. Cancer 60:2337, 1987

48. Hays DM, Shimada H, Raney RB Jr., et al.: Clinical staging and treatment results in rhabdomyosarcoma of the female genital tract among children and adolescents. Cancer 61:1893, 1988

49. Hays DM, Shimada H, Raney RB Jr., et al.: Sarcomas of the vagina and uterus: The Intergroup Rhabdomyosarcoma Study (IRS). J Pediatr Surg 20:718, 1985

50. Hays DM, Soule EH, Lawrence W Jr., et al.: Extremity lesions in the Intergroup Rhabdomyosarcoma Study (IRS-I): A preliminary report. Cancer 49:1, 1982

51. Heyn R, Beltangady M, Hays D, et al.: Results of intensive therapy in children with localized alveolar extremity rhabdomyosarcoma: A report from the Intergroup Rhabdomyosarcoma Study. J Clin Oncol 7:200, 1989

52. Lawrence W Jr., Hays DM, Heyn R, et al.: Surgical lessons from the Intergroup Rhabdomyosarcoma Study pertaining to extremity tumors. World J Surg 12:676, 1988

53. Shimada H, Newton WA, Soule EH, et al.: Pathology of fatal rhabdomyosarcoma: Report from the Intergroup

Rhabdomyosarcoma Study (IRS-I and II). Cancer 59: 459, 1987

54. Lawrence W Jr., Hays DM, Heyn R, et al.: Lymphatic metastases in childhood rhabdomyosarcoma: A report from the Intergroup Rhabdomyosarcoma Study. Cancer 60:910, 1987

55. Hays DM, Newton WJ, Soule EH, et al.: Mortality among children with rhabdomyosarcoma of the alveolar histologic subtype. J Pediatr Surg 18:412, 1983

56. Raney RB Jr., Ragab AH, Ruymann FB, et al.: Soft-tissue sarcoma of the trunk in childhood: Results of the Intergroup Rhabdomyosarcoma Study. Cancer 49:2612, 1982

57. Ortega JA, Wharam M, Gehan EA, et al.: Clinical features and results of therapy for children with paraspinal soft tissue sarcoma: A report of the Intergroup Rhabdomyosarcoma Study. J Clin Oncol 9:796, 1991

58. Crist WM, Raney RB, Tefft M, et al.: Soft tissue sarcomas arising in the retroperitoneal space in children: A report from the Intergroup Rhabdomyosarcoma Study (IRS) Committee. Cancer 56:2125, 1985

59. Hays DM, Sayder WH: Botryoid sarcoma (rhabdomyosarcoma of the bile ducts). Am J Dis Child 110:595, 1965

60. Ruymann FB, Raney RB Jr., Crist WM, et al.: Rhabdomyosarcoma of the biliary tract in childhood: A report from the Intergroup Rhabdomyosarcoma Study. Cancer 56:575, 1985

61. Crist WM, Raney RB Jr., Newton W, et al.: Intrathoracic soft tissue sarcomas in children. Cancer 50:598, 1982

62. Crist WM, Raney RB, Tefft M, et al.: Soft tissue sarcomas arising in the retroperitoneal space in children: A report from the Intergroup Rhabdomyosarcoma Study Committee. Cancer 56:2125, 1985

63. Ransom JL, Pratt CB, Hustu HO, et al.: Retroperitoneal rhabdomyosarcoma in children: Results of multimodality therapy. Cancer 45:845, 1980

64. Srouji MN, Donaldson MH, Chatter J, Koblinger CS: Perianal rhabdomyosarcoma in childhood. Cancer 38:1008, 1976

65. Raney RB, Crist WM, Hays DM, et al.: Soft tissue sarcoma of the perineal anal region in childhood. A report from the Intergroup Rhabdomyosarcoma Study (IRS). Cancer 65:2787, 1990

66. Harris MB, Shen S, Weiner MA, et al.: Treatment of primary undifferentiated sarcoma of the liver with surgery and chemotherapy. Cancer 54:2859, 1984

67. Stocker JT, Ishak KG: Undifferentiated (embryonal) sarcoma of the liver: A report of 31 cases. Cancer 42:336, 1978

68. Horowitz ME, Etcubanas E, Webber BL, et al.: Hepatic undifferentiated (embryonal) sarcoma and rhabdomyosarcoma in children. Cancer 59:396, 1987

69. Dropcho EJ, Allen JC: Primary intracranial rhabdomyosarcoma: Case report and review of the literature. J Neurooncol 5:139, 1987

70. Kedar A, Cantrel G, Rosen G: Rhabdomyosarcoma of the trachea. J Laryngol Otol 102:735, 1988

71. Schmaltz AA, Apitz J: Primary rhabdomyosarcoma of the heart. Pediatr Cardiol 2:73, 1982

72. Nunez C, Abboud SC, Lemon NC, Kemp JA: Ovarian rhabdomyosarcoma presenting as leukemia. Cancer 52:297, 1983

73. Schabel FM Jr.: The use of tumor growth kinetics in planning "curative" chemotherapy of advanced solid tumors. Cancer Res 29:2384, 1969

74. Skipper HE, Schabel FM Jr., Wilcox WS: Experimental evaluation of potential anti-cancer agents: XIII. On the criteria and kinetics associated with "curability" of experimental leukemia. Cancer Chemother Rep 35:1, 1964

75. Laster WR Jr., Mays JG, Simpson-Herron L, et al.: Success and failure in the treatment of solid tumors: II. Kinetic parameters and "cell cure" of moderately advanced carcinoma 755. Cancer Chemother Rep 53:169, 1969

76. Wilcox WS: The last surviving cancer cell: The chances of killing it. Cancer Chemother Rep 50:541, 1966

77. Wilbur JR: Combination chemotherapy of embryonal rhabdomyosarcoma. Cancer Chemother Rep 58:281, 1974

78. Green DM, Jaffe N: Progress and controversy in the treatment of childhood rhabdomyosarcoma. Cancer Treat Rev 5:7, 1978

79. Jaffe N, Filler RM, Farber S, et al.: Rhabdomyosarcoma in children. Am J Surg 125:482, 1973

80. Jaffe N, Murray J, Traggis D, et al.: Multidisciplinary treatment for childhood sarcoma Ann J Surg 133:405, 1977

81. Maurer HM, Moon T, Donaldson M, et al.: The Intergroup Rhabdomyosarcoma Study: A preliminary report. Cancer 40:2015, 1977

82. Maurer HM, Beltangady M, Gehan EA, et al.: The Intergroup Rhabdomyosarcoma Study-I: A final report. Cancer 61:209, 1988

83. Maurer H, Gehan EA, Beltangady M, et al.: The Intergroup Rhabdomyosarcoma Study (IRS)-II. Cancer 71:1904, 1993

84. Crist W, Gehan EA, Rajaba AH, et al.: The Third Intergroup Rhabdomyosarcoma Study. J Clin Oncol 13:610, 1995

85. Kinsella TJ, Miser JS, Triche TJ, et al.: Treatment of high-risk sarcomas in children and young adults: Analysis of local control using intensive combined-modality therapy. N C I Monogr 6:291, 1988

86. Miser JS, Kinsella JJ, Triche TJ, et al.: Ifosfamide with mesna uroprotection and etoposide: An effective regimen in the treatment of recurrent sarcomas and other tumors in children and young adults. J Clin Oncol 5:1191, 1987

87. Otter J, Flamant F, Rodary M, et al.: Treatment of malignant mesenchymal tumors (MMT) of childhood with Ifosfamide + Vincristine + Dactinomycin (IVA) as front-line therapy: A preliminary report on a study by the International Society of Pediatric Oncology (SIOP) Proc Annu Symp Comput Appl Med Care (abstr #878) 6:723, 1987

88. Rodary C, Rey A, Olive D, et al.: Prognostic factors in 281 children with non-metastatic rhabdomyosarcoma at diagnosis. Med Pediatr Oncol 16:71, 1988

89. Heyn R, Ragab A, Raney RB Jr., et al.: Late effects of

therapy in orbital rhabdomyosarcoma in children. Cancer 57:1738, 1986

90. Rousseau P, Flamant F, Quintana E, et al.: Primary chemotherapy in rhabdomyosarcomas and other malignant mesenchymal tumor of the orbit: Results of the International Society of Pediatric Oncology MMT 84 Study. J Clin Oncol 12:516, 1994

91. Sutow WW, Lindberg RD, Gehan EA, et al.: Three-year relapse-free survival rates in childhood rhabdomyosarcoma of the head and neck: Report from the Intergroup Rhabdomyosarcoma Study. Cancer 49:2217, 1982

92. Raney RB Jr., Tefft M, Newton WA, et al.: Improved prognosis with intensive treatment of children with cranial soft tissue sarcomas arising in nonorbital parameningeal sites: A report from the Intergroup Rhabdomyosarcoma Study. Cancer 59:147, 1987

93. Raney RB, Gehan EA, Hays DM, et al.: Primary chemotherapy with or without radiation therapy and/or surgery for children with localized sarcoma of the bladder/prostate, vagina, uterus and cervix: A comparison of the results in Intergroup Rhabdomyosarcoma studies I and II. Cancer 66:2077, 1990

94. Hays DM, Raney RB Jr., Lawrence WJ, et al.: Bladder and prostate tumors in the Intergroup Rhabdomyosarcoma Study (IRS-I): Results of therapy. Cancer 50:1472, 1982

95. Ortega JA: A therapeutic approach to childhood pelvic rhabdomyosarcoma without pelvic exenteration. J Pediatr Surg 94:205, 1979

96. Voute PA, Vos A, de Kraker L, Behrendt H: Rhabdomyosarcomas: Chemotherapy and limited supplementary treatment program to avoid mutilation. N C I Monogr 56:121, 1981

97. Hays DM: Pelvic rhabdomyosarcomas in childhood: Diagnosis and concepts of management reviewed. Cancer 45:1810, 1980

98. Olive D, Flamant F, Zucker JM, et al.: Para-aortic lymphadenectomy is not necessary in the treatment of localized paratesticular rhabdomyosarcoma. Cancer 54:1283, 1984

99. Wiener ES, Lawrence W, Hays D, et al.: Retroperitoneal node biopsy in paratesticular rhabdomyosarcoma. J Pediatr Surg 29:171, 1994

100. Raney RB, Crist W, Hays D, et al.: Soft tissue sarcoma of the perineal-anal region in childhood: A report from the Intergroup Rhabdomyosarcoma Studies I and II, 1972–1984. Med Pediatr Oncol (abstr) 16:415, 1988

101. Rivard G, Ortega J, Kettle R, et al.: Intensive chemotherapy as primary treatment for rhabdomyosarcoma of the pelvis. Cancer 30:1593, 1975

102. Jaffe N, Roth II EJ, Woo SY, et al.: Is there a safe therapeutic window for delivery of chemotherapy prior to initiation of surgery and/or radiation therapy for treatment of the primary tumor in children with rhabdomyosarcoma? Int J Oncol 7:855, 1995

103. Raney RB Jr., Tefft M, Maurer HM, et al.: Disease patterns and survival rate in children with metastatic soft-tissue sarcoma: A report from the Intergroup Rhabdomyosarcoma Study (IRS-I). Cancer 62:1257, 1988

104. Pratt CB, Drigger DL, Johnson WW, et al.: Metastatic

105. Ruymann FB: Multiagent chemotherapy with adjuvant whole body radiation in half increments in children with clinical Group IV rhabdomyosarcoma and extraosseous Ewing's sarcoma. Proc Int Soc Ped Oncol, 1984

106. Ladenstein R, Treuner J, Koscielniak E, et al.: Synovial sarcoma of childhood and adolescence: Report of the German CWS-81 Study. Cancer 71:3647, 1993

107. Pappo AS, Fontanesi J, Luo X, et al.: Synovial sarcoma in children and adolescents: The St. Jude Children's Research Hospital experience. J Clin Oncol 12:2360, 1994

108. Choong PLM, Portchard DJ, Sim FH: Long-term survival in high grade soft tissue sarcoma: Prognostic factors in synovial sarcoma. Int J Oncol 7:161, 1995

109. Cordier JF, Barly C, Tabone E: Alveolar soft part sarcoma presenting asymptomatic pulmonary nodules: Report of a case with ultrastructural diagnosis. Thorax 40:203, 1985

110. Evans HL: Alveolar soft part sarcoma: A study of 13 typical examples and one with a histologically atypical component. Cancer 55:912, 1985

111. Lewis AJ: Sarcoma metastatic to the brain. Cancer 61:593, 1988

112. Shen JT, D'Ablaing G, Morow CP: Alveolar soft part sarcoma of the vulva: Report of first case and review of the literature. Gynecol Oncol 13:120, 1982

113. Sherman N, Vavilala M, Pollack R, et al.: Radiation therapy for alveolar soft-part sarcoma. Med Pediatr Oncol 22:380, 1994

114. Komori A, Takeda Y, Kaklichi T: Alveolar soft part sarcoma of the tongue: Report of a case with electron microscopic study. Oral Surg 57:532, 1984

115. Soule EH, Pritchard DJ: Fibrosarcoma in infants and children: A review of 110 cases. Cancer 40:1711, 1977

116. Enzinger FM, Weiss SW: Fibrohistiocytic tumors of intermediate malignancy. In: Soft Tissue Tumors, 2nd ed. St. Louis, CV Mosby, 1988

117. O'Dowd J, Laidler PM: Progression of dermatofibrosarcoma protuberans to malignant fibrous histiocytoma: Report of a case with implications for tumor histogenesis. Hum Pathol 19:368, 1988

118. Weiss SW, Enzinger FM: Malignant fibrous histiocytoma: An analysis of 200 cases. Cancer 41:2250, 1978

119. Edmonson JH, Long NJ, Richardson RL, et al.: Phase II study of a combination of mitomycin, doxorubicin, and cisplatin in advanced sarcomas. Cancer Chemother Pharmacol 15:181, 1985

120. Tracy T Jr., Neifeld SP, De May RM, et al.: Malignant fibrous histiocytomas in children. J Pediatr Surg 19:81, 1984

121. Kearney MM, Soule EH, Ivins JC: Malignant fibrous histiocytoma: A retrospective study of 167 cases. Cancer 45:167, 1980

122. Capanna R, Bertoni F, Bacchinc P, et al.: Malignant fibrous histiocytoma of bone. The experience at the Rizzoli Institute: Report of 90 cases. Cancer 54:177, 1984

123. Bertoni F, Capanna R, Biagini R, et al.: Malignant fi-

brous histiocytoma of soft tissue: An analysis of 78 cases located and deeply seated in the extremities. Cancer 56:356, 1985

124. Enzinger FM, Weiss SW: Neurogenic sarcomas. In: Soft Tissue Tumors, 2nd ed. St. Louis, CV Mosby, 1988

125. Sordillo P, Helson L, Hajdu SI, et al.: Malignant schwannoma—Clinical characteristics survival and response to therapy. Cancer 47:2503, 1981

126. Ducatman BS, Scheithauer BW: Malignant peripheral nerve sheath tumors with divergent differentiation. Cancer 54:1049, 1984

127. Guccion JG, Enzinger FM: Malignant schwannoma associated with von Recklinghausen's neurofibromatosis. Virchows Arch [A] 383:43, 1979

128. Raney RB Jr., Littman P, Jarrett P, et al.: Results of multimodal therapy for children with neurogenic sarcoma. Med Pediatr Oncol 7:229, 1979

129. Enzinger FM, Weiss SW: Malignant vascular tumors. In: Soft Tissue Tumors, 2nd ed. St. Louis, CV Mosby, 1988

130. Alt B, Haber GR, Trigg M, et al.: Angiosarcoma of the liver and spleen in an infant. Pediatr Pathol 4:331, 1985

131. Noronha R, Gonzalez-Crussi F: Hepatic angiosarcoma in childhood. A case report and review of the literature. Am J Surg Pathol 8:863, 1984

132. Falk H, Herbert J, Crowly S, et al.: Epidemiology of hepatic angiosarcoma in the United States: 1964-1974. Environmental Health Perspectives 41:107, 1981

133. Chen KT, Hoffman KD, Hendrics EJ: Angiosarcoma following therapeutic irradiation. Cancer 44:2044, 1979

134. Charman HP, Lowenstein DN, Cho KG, et al.: Primary cerebral angiosarcoma: Case report. J Neurosurg 68:806, 1988

135. Taxy JB, Battiora H: Angiosarcoma of the gastrointestinal tract: A report of three cases. Cancer 2:210, 1988

136. Unni KK, Ivins JC, Beabout JW, et al.: Hemangioma, hemangiopericytoma, and hemangioendothelioma (angiosarcoma) of bone. Cancer 27:1403, 1971

137. Dannaber CL, Tamburro CH, Yam LT: Chemotherapy of vinyl chloride-associated hepatic angiosarcoma. Cancer 47:466, 1981

138. Stout AP, Murray MR: Hemangiopericytoma: Vascular tumor featuring Zimmerman's pericytes. Ann Surg 166:26, 1992

139. Bredt AB, Serpick AA: Metastatic hemangiopericytoma treated with vincristine and actinomycin-D. Cancer 24:266, 1969

140. Beadle GF, Hillcoat BL: Treatment of advanced malignant hemangiopericytoma with combination adriamycin and DTIC: A report of four cases. J Surg Oncol 22:167, 1983

141. Auguste LJ, Razack MS, Sako L: Hemangiopericytoma. J Surg Oncol 20:260, 1982

142. Tang JSH, Gold RH, Bassett LW, et al.: Hemangiopericytoma of bone. Cancer 62:848, 1988

143. Enzinger FM, Smith BH: Hemangiopericytoma. An analysis of 106 cases. Hum Pathol 7:61, 1976

144. McClain KL, Leach CT, Jenson HB, et al.: Association of Epstein-Barr virus with leiomyosarcoma in young people with AIDS. N Engl J Med 332:12, 1995

145. Lack EE: Leiomyosarcomas in childhood: A clinical and pathologic study of 10 cases. Pediatr Pathol 6:181, 1986

146. Lindsay PCC, Ordonez N, Raaf JH: Gastric leiomyosarcoma: Clinical and pathological review of fifty patients. J Surg Oncol 18:399, 1981

147. Angerpointner TA, Weitz H, Haas RJ, et al.: Intestinal leiomyosarcoma I in childhood—Case report and review of the literature. J Pediatr Surg 16:491, 1981

148. Raney B, Evans A, Granowetter L, et al.: Nonsurgical management of children with recurrent or unresectable fibromatosis. Pediatrics 79:394, 1987

149. Rao VN, Horowitz ME, Parham DM, et al.: Challenges in the treatment of childhood fibromatosis. Arch Surg 122:1296, 1987

150. Gonzalez-Darder J, Alacreu JB, Garcia-Vazquez F: Desmoid tumor arising around the distal tubing of a cerebrospinal fluid shunt. Surg Neurol 26:365, 1986

151. Khorsand J, Karakousis CP: Desmoid tumors and their management. Am J Surg 149:215, 1985

152. Kinzbrunner B, Ritter S, Domingo J, et al.: Remission of rapidly growing desmoid tumors after tamoxifen therapy. Cancer 52:2201, 1983

153. Waddell WR, Gerner RE, Reich MP: Nonsteroid antiinflammatory drugs and tamoxifen for desmoid tumors and carcinoma of the stomach. J Surg Oncol 22:197, 1983

154. Goepfert H, Cangir A, Ayala AG, et al.: Chemotherapy of locally aggressive head and neck tumors in the pediatric age group—Desmoid fibromatosis and nasopharyngeal angiofibroma. Am J Surg 144:437, 1982

# Index

Liver (*cont.*)
   hemangiomas of, 414–415, *415*
Localized myositis ossificans, 463
Lumbar region, ganglioneuromas of, 150
Lung(s)
   angiosarcomas of, 423–424
   chemodectomas of, 387(t)
   Kaposi's sarcomas of, 434
   malignant fibrous histiocytomas of, 301–302
   as primary metastatic site, 29, 30
   synovial sarcomas of, 400
Lymph node(s)
   Kaposi's sarcomas of, 428–429
   palisade myofibroblastomas of, 114
Lymphangiectasis, 453
   lymphangioma vs., 449
   systemic, 453, *454*
Lymphangioma(s), 175, 177, *179*
   of bone, 451
   cavernous, 449–451, 450(t), *450–452*
   cystic hygroma as, 451, *452*, 453
   papillary, 449
   simple, 449
Lymphangiomyoma, 177, 179, 455
Lymphangiomyomatosis, 177, 179, 455
Lymphangiosarcoma(s), 179, *180*, 455–458
   angiosarcoma vs., 168
   not associated with mastectomy, 457–458, *458*, 459(t)
   postmastectomy, 9, 179, *180*, 456–457, *456–457*
Lymphatic system
   prenatal development of, 14, 165
   tumors of
      benign, 175, 177, 179, 449–455
      classification of, 18(t), 175
      extramedullary plasmacytomas as, 458, 460
      extranodal lymphomas as, 458, *460*
      lymphangiomas as. *See* Lymphangioma(s)
      lymphangiomyomas as, 177, 179, 455
      lymphangiosarcomas as. *See* Lymphangiosarcoma(s)
      lymphedemas as, 453–454
      malignant, 179, 455–460
Lymphedema(s)
   acquired, 454
   congenital, 453–454
   of extremities, 454, 457–458
   Kaposi's sarcoma and, 434
Lymphocytes
   educated, 582
   natural killer cells and, 581–582
   tumor-infiltrating, 582
Lymphokine-activated killer cells, 581–582
Lymphoma(s)
   extranodal, 458, *460*

   and Kaposi's sarcoma, 431
Lymphosarcoma, anaplastic, 153

Madelung's disease, 71, 246
Maffucci's syndrome
   hemangioma and, 416
   lipomatosis and, 246
Magnetic resonance imaging
   of aggressive fibromatosis, 44, *44–46*
   of angiofibromas, 43, *43*
   of benign schwannomas, 52, *52–55*
   of chondrosarcomas, 56, *57*
   as diagnostic aid, 26
   disadvantages of, 39
   dynamic, 39
   indications for, 39
   of lipomas, 39–40, *40*
   of malignant fibrous histiocytomas, 46, *48*
   of malignant schwannomas, 52–53
   of myositis ossificans, 56–57, *58*
   of paragangliomas, 53, *56*
   of rhabdomyosarcomas, 49, 51, *51*, 327
   tissue characterization in, 39
MAID regimen, 319
   dose-response relationship for, 555
   and PIXY321, 556
Malignant fibrous histiocytoma. *See* Fibrous histiocytoma(s), malignant
Malignant peripheral nerve sheath tumors, *23*, 139–145, 366–379
   in child, 606
   classification of, 139
   clear cell sarcomas as, 144–145, *147*, 378–379
   cytogenetic findings in, 143
   epithelioid, 143
   with glandular differentiation, 143, 377
   granular cell tumors and, 145–146, *148*
   with neurofibromatosis, 139, 142–143, *146*, 374–379
   radiologic evaluation of, 52–53, *54*
   with rhabdomyoblastic differentiation, 143, 377, 589
   secondary, 145–148, *149*
   solitary, 139, 140–142, 367–374
      anatomic distribution of, 368(t), 368–369
      demographic factors in, 367
      electron microscopy of, *135, 141–142, 145*
      end results in, 371, 371(t), 373–374, 374(t)
      of head and neck, 368, *372*
      of lower extremities, 368–369, *374*
      macroscopic findings in, 139, *142–143*
      metastatic, to liver, *377*
      microscopic findings in, 139, 141–142, *144–145*
      with neurofibromatosis, 374–379
      prognosis in, 374, 374(t)
      treatment of, 369, 370